Clinical Nutrition

ENTERAL and TUBE FEEDING

Clinical Nutrition

ENTERAL and TUBE FEEDING

Third Edition

John L. Rombeau, M.D.
Professor of Surgery
University of Pennsylvania School of Medicine
Director, Nutrition Support Service
Department of Veterans Affairs Medical Center
Philadelphia, Pennsylvania

Rolando H. Rolandelli, M.D.
Associate Professor of Surgery
Director, Nutrition Support Service
Allegheny University Hospitals, Center City
Philadelphia, Pennsylvania

W.B. SAUNDERS COMPANY
A Division of Harcourt Brace & Company
Philadelphia   London   Toronto   Montreal   Sydney   Tokyo

W.B. SAUNDERS COMPANY
A Division of Harcourt Brace & Company

The Curtis Center
Independence Square West
Philadelphia, Pennsylvania 19106

Library of Congress Cataloging-in-Publication Data

Clinical nutrition : enteral and tube feeding / [edited by] John L.
   Rombeau, Rolando H. Rolandelli. — 3rd ed.
      p.   cm.
   Includes bibliographical references.
   ISBN 0-7216-2155-4
   1. Enteral feeding. 2. Tube feeding. I. Rombeau, John L.
II. Rolandelli, Rolando.
   [DNLM: 1. Enteral Nutrition. 2. Nutrition. 3. Food, Formulated.
4. Intubation, Gastrointestinal.   WB 410 06415 1997]
RM225.C565   1997
615.8'54—dc20
DNLM/DLC   96-16727

Clinical Nutrition: Enteral and Tube Feeding   ISBN 0–7216–2155–4

Printed in the United States of America

Last digit is the print number: 9 8 7 6 5 4 3 2 1

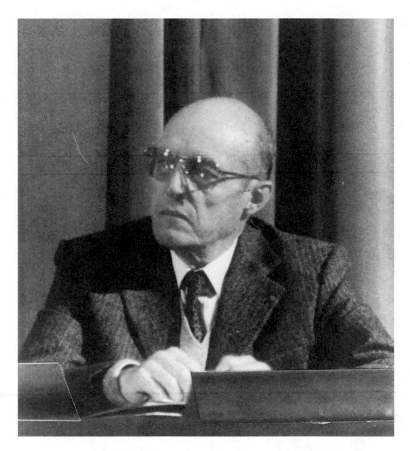

Dr. Etienne Paul Louis Levy 1922–1996

This book is dedicated to Dr. Etienne Paul Louis Levy, Head of the Intensive Care Unit of the Department of Digestive Surgery, Höpital Saint-Antoine, Paris. Dr. Levy's clinical and research contributions have led to major improvements in the care of critically ill patients in need of enteral feeding throughout the world.

DOSAGE NOTICE

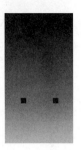

Contributors

Susan S. Baker, M.D., Ph.D.
Associate Professor of Pediatrics, Medical University of South Carolina; Codirector of Pediatric Gastroenterology and Nutrition, Children's Hospital, Charleston, South Carolina
Enteral Nutrition in Pediatrics

Gustavo Bounous, M.D.
Professor of Surgery, McGill University; Senior Scientist, Immunotec Research Corporation, Ltd., Montreal, Quebec, Canada
History of Enteral Feeding: Past and Present Perspectives

Timothy E. Bowling, M.D., M.B.B.S., M.R.C.P.
Consultant Physician in Gastroenterology, North Staffordshire Hospital NHS Trust, Stoke on Trent, England
Diarrhea and Enteral Nutrition

Michael A. Buckmire, M.D.
General Surgery Resident Physician and Nutrition and Metabolism Fellow, Allegheny University of the Health Sciences, Philadelphia, Pennsylvania
Enteral Nutrition in the Surgical Patient

Eduard Cabré, M.D.
Senior Research Fellow, Department of Gastroenterology, Hospital Universitari Germans Trias i Pujol, Badalona, Catalonia, Spain
Enteral Nutrition in Inflammatory Bowel Disease

Mary F. Chan, M.D.
Assistant Professor of Medicine, Washington University School of Medicine; Director of Endoscopy, Barnes Hospital, St. Louis, Missouri
Short-Bowel Syndrome

Jesse C. Chow, Ph.D.
Postdoctoral Fellow, Harvard Medical School and Joslin Diabetes Center, Boston, Massachusetts
The Molecular Biology of Enteral Nutrition and the Gut

Charlene Compher, R.D., M.S.
Nutrition Support Dietitian Clinical Specialist, University of Pennsylvania Medical Center, Philadelphia, Pennsylvania
Dietary Fiber and Its Clinical Applications to Enteral Nutrition

Mark H. DeLegge, M.D.
Gastroenterologist, Charlotte Clinic for Gastrointestinal and Liver Disease, Charlotte, North Carolina
Enteral Nutrition and the Neurologic Diseases

Achilles A. Demetriou, M.D., Ph.D.
Professor of Surgery, University of California Los Angeles School of Medicine; Chairman, Department of Surgery, Cedars-Sinai Medical Center, Los Angeles, California
Enteral Nutrition and Liver Failure

Wilfred Druml, M.D.
Professor of Medicine, Medical Department III, Division of Nephrology, University of Vienna and Vienna General Hospital, Vienna, Austria
Enteral Nutrition in Renal Disease

Marinos Elia, M.D., B.Sc.Hon., F.R.C.P.
Head, Clinical Nutrition Group, Medical Research Council, Dunn Clinical Nutrition Centre; Honorary Consultant Physician, Addenbrooke Hospital, Cambridge, England
Assessment of Nutritional Status and Body Composition

Martha Ericson, R.D., M.S., C.N.S.D.
Nutrition Support Dietitian, The Graduate Hospital, Philadelphia, Pennsylvania
Delivery Systems and Administration of Enteral Nutrition

Maria Esteve-Comas, M.D.
Senior Research Fellow, Department of Gastroenterology, Hospital Universitari Germans Trias i Pujol, Badalona, Catalonia, Spain
Enteral Nutrition in Inflammatory Bowel Disease

Douglas G. Farmer, M.D.
Fellow, Transplantation Surgery, Dumont-University of California Los Angeles Transplant Center, Division of Liver and Pancreas Transplantation, University of California Los Angeles Medical Center, Los Angeles, California
The Role of Enteral Nutrition in Organ and Cellular Transplantation

Fernando Fernández-Bañares, M.D.

Senior Research Fellow, Department of Gastroenterology, Hospital Universitari Germans Trias i Pujol, Badalona, Catalonia, Spain

Enteral Nutrition in Inflammatory Bowel Disease

C. Richard Fleming, M.D.

Professor of Medicine and David Murdock Professor of Nutrition Science, Mayo Medical School, Rochester, Minnesota; Chair, Division of Gastroenterology, Mayo Clinic Jacksonville, Jacksonville, Florida

Physiology of the Gastrointestinal Tract: As Applied to Patients Receiving Tube Enteral Nutrition

Yuman Fong, M.D.

Assistant Professor of Surgery and Cell Biology and Anatomy, Cornell University Medical College; Assistant Attending Physician, Memorial Sloan-Kettering Cancer Center, New York, New York

Enteral Nutrition in the Cancer Patient

Miquel A. Gassull, M.D.

Associate Professor of Medicine, Universidad Autonoma de Barcelona; Head, Department of Gastroenterology, Hospital Universitari Germans Trias i Pujol, Badalona, Catalonia, Spain

Enteral Nutrition in Inflammatory Bowel Disease

Phillip George, M.D.

Emeritus Professor of Pediatrics, University of Tennessee; Associate Medical Officer, UT Medical Group, Inc., Memphis, Tennessee

Managed Care

Maureen E. Geraghty, R.D., L.D., M.S.

Senior Clinical Research Associate, Medical Nutrition Research and Development, Ross Products Division, Abbott Laboratories, Columbus, Ohio

History of Enteral Feeding: Past and Present Perspectives

Scott Craig Goodwin, M.D.

Assistant Professor and Chief, Vascular and Interventional Radiology, University of California Los Angeles, Los Angeles, California

Radiologic Techniques for Enteral Access

Robert C. Gorman, M.D.

Instructor of Surgery, University of Pennsylvania School of Medicine; Chief Surgical Resident, Hospital of the University of Pennsylvania, Philadelphia, Pennsylvania

Minimally Invasive Access to the Gastrointestinal Tract

Michele M. Gottschlich, Ph.D., R.D., C.N.S.D.
Associate Professor, Department of Health and Nutrition Sciences, University of Cincinnati; Director, Nutrition Services, Shriners Burn Institute, Cincinnati, Ohio
Defined Formula Diets

Peggi Guenter, Ph.D., R.N., C.N.S.N.
Clinical Assistant Professor, University of Pennsylvania School of Nursing; Coordinator, Nutrition Support Service, The Graduate Hospital, Philadelphia, Pennsylvania
Delivery Systems and Administration of Enteral Nutrition

Elie Hamaoui, M.D.
Clinical Associate Professor of Medicine, State University of New York Health Sciences Center at Brooklyn; Medical Director, Metabolic Support Service, Maimonides Medical Center, Brooklyn, New York
Complications of Enteral Feeding and Their Prevention

Lawrence E. Harrison, M.D.
Surgical Oncology Fellow, Memorial Sloan-Kettering Cancer Center, New York, New York
Enteral Nutrition in the Cancer Patient

Per-Olof Hasselgren, M.D., Ph.D.
Professor of Surgery, University of Cincinnati, Cincinnati, Ohio
Enteral Nutrition and Protein Metabolism

Lyn Howard, M.B., F.R.C.P.
Professor of Medicine and Associate Professor of Pediatrics, Albany Medical College; Attending Physician, Albany Medical Center, Albany, New York; Consultant DMERC Region C, Blue Cross Blue Shield, Columbia, South Carolina
Home Enteral Nutrition in Adults

Daniel L. Hurley, M.D.
Instructor, Mayo Medical School; Consultant, Division of Endocrinology, Diabetes, and Nutrition and Director, Clinical Endocrine Training Program, Mayo Clinic, Rochester, Minnesota
Enteral Nutrition and Diabetes Mellitus

Andrea M. Hutchins, R.D., M.S., C.N.S.D.
Assistant Clinical Specialist, Department of Food Science and Nutrition, University of Minnesota, St. Paul, Minnesota
Defined Formula Diets

Susan Jones, R.D., C.N.S.D.
Nutrition Support Dietitian, The Graduate Hospital, Philadelphia, Pennsylvania
Delivery Systems and Administration of Enteral Nutrition

Elaine A. Kahaku, B.S.N., C.C.R.N.
Member, American Association of Critical Care Nurses, Los Angeles, California and North American Transplant Coordinators Organization, Pittsburgh, Pennsylvania
Enteral Nutrition and Liver Failure

Donna Reber Katona, R.D.
Dietitian, Pediatric Pulmonology, Children's Hospital of Los Angeles, Los Angeles, California
Nutritional Support in Pancreatic Disease

Darlene G. Kelly, M.D., Ph.D.
Assistant Professor, Mayo Medical School; Consultant, Gastroenterology and Internal Medicine, Mayo Foundation, Rochester, Minnesota
Physiology of the Gastrointestinal Tract: As Applied to Patients Receiving Tube Enteral Nutrition

Donald F. Kirby, M.D.
Professor of Medicine and Chief, Section of Nutrition, Division of Gastroenterology, Medical College of Virginia; Director, Nutrition Support Services, McGuire Veterans Affairs Medical Center, Richmond, Virginia
Enteral Nutrition and the Neurologic Diseases

Samuel Klein, M.D.
Associate Professor of Medicine and Director, Center for Human Nutrition, Washington University School of Medicine, St. Louis, Missouri
Short-Bowel Syndrome

Robert Kodsi, M.D.
Fellow, Gastroenterology, Maimonides Medical Center, Brooklyn, New York
Complications of Enteral Feeding and Their Prevention

Mark J. Koruda, M.D.
Associate Professor, Department of Surgery and Nutrition and Chief, Gastrointestinal Surgery, University of North Carolina, Chapel Hill, North Carolina
Nutrition and Trauma

Donald P. Kotler, M.D.
Associate Professor of Medicine, Columbia University College of Physicians and Surgeons; Associate Chief, Gastrointestinal Division and Director, Gastrointestinal Immunology, St. Luke's-Roosevelt Hospital Center, New York, New York
Enteral Nutrition in HIV Infection

Amy M. Kusske, M.D.

Resident, General Surgery, University of California Los Angeles School of Medicine, Los Angeles, California

Nutritional Support in Pancreatic Disease

John I. Lew, M.D.

Medical Student, University of Pennsylvania School of Medicine; Research Fellow, Hospital of the University of Pennsylvania, Philadelphia, Pennsylvania

Dietary Fiber and Its Clinical Applications to Enteral Nutrition

Timothy O. Lipman, M.D.

Assistant Chief, Gastroenterology, Hepatology, and Nutrition Section, Department of Veterans Affairs Medical Center; Associate Professor of Medicine, Georgetown University School of Medicine, Washington, DC

Enteral Nutrition and Dying: Ethical Issues in the Termination of Enteral Nutrition in Adults

Stan Liu, M.D.

Clinical Instructor, University of California Los Angeles, Los Angeles, California

Radiologic Techniques for Enteral Access

Margaret Malone, Ph.D., B.C.N.S.P.

Professor of Pharmacy, Albany College of Pharmacy; Adjunct Associate Professor of Medicine, Albany Medical College, Albany, New York

Home Enteral Nutrition in Adults

Joel B. Mason, M.D.

Assistant Professor of Medicine and Nutrition, Tufts University and the USDA Jean Mayer Human Nutrition Research Center on Aging at Tufts University; Gastroenterologist and Director, Adult Nutrition Support Service, New England Medical Center, Boston, Massachusetts

Enteral Nutrition in the Elderly

Mark A. McCamish, M.D., Ph.D.

Clinical Associate Professor, Division of Endocrinology, Department of Internal Medicine, Ohio State University; Medical Director, Medical Nutrition Research and Development, Ross Products Division, Abbott Laboratories, Columbus, Ohio

History of Enteral Feeding: Past and Present Perspectives

Barbara T. McKinnon, Pharm.D., B.C.N.S.P.

Assistant Professor of Clinical Pharmacy, University of Tennessee; Director, Business Development, Nova Factor, Memphis, Tennessee

Managed Care

M. Molly McMahon, M.D.

Associate Professor of Medicine, Mayo Medical School; Consultant, Division of Endocrinology, Metabolism, and Internal Medicine, Mayo Clinic and Mayo Foundation, Rochester, Minnesota

Enteral Nutrition and Diabetes Mellitus

Tory A. Meyer, M.D.

Surgical Resident, Department of Surgery, University of Cincinnati, Cincinnati, Ohio

Enteral Nutrition and Protein Metabolism

William E. Mitch, M.D.

Garland Herndon Professor of Medicine and Director, Renal Division, Emory University, Atlanta, Georgia

Enteral Nutrition in Renal Disease

Lyle L. Moldawer, Ph.D.

Professor of Surgery, University of Florida College of Medicine, Gainesville, Florida

Glucose Metabolism

Jon B. Morris, M.D.

Director of Student Education, University of Pennsylvania School of Medicine; Attending Surgeon, Division of Gastrointestinal Surgery and Nutrition Support Services, Hospital of the University of Pennsylvania, Philadelphia, Pennsylvania

Minimally Invasive Access to the Gastrointestinal Tract

Lee M. Oberman, M.D.

Attending Physician, St. Joseph's Hospital and North Side Hospital, Atlanta, Georgia

Enteral Nutrition in HIV Infection

Susan K. Pingleton, M.D.

Professor of Medicine and Director, Division of Pulmonary and Critical Care Medicine, University of Kansas Medical Center, Kansas City, Kansas

Enteral Nutrition and Respiratory Diseases

Basil A. Pruitt, Jr., M.D.

Professor of Surgery, University of Texas Health Science Center, San Antonio, Texas; Commander and Director, United States Army Institute of Surgical Research, Fort Sam Houston, Texas

Enteral Nutrition in Burns

Howard A. Reber, M.D.

Professor of Surgery, University of California Los Angeles School of Medicine; Chief of Surgery, Sepulveda Veterans Administration Medical Center, Los Angeles, California

Nutritional Support in Pancreatic Disease

Rolando H. Rolandelli, M.D.

Associate Professor of Surgery and Director, Nutrition Support Service, Allegheny University Hospitals, Center City, Philadelphia, Pennsylvania

Enteral Nutrition in the Surgical Patient; The Role of Enteral Nutrition in Organ and Cellular Transplantation

Carol J. Rollins, Pharm.D., R.D., M.S.

Clinical Assistant Professor in Pharmacy Practice, University of Arizona College of Pharmacy; Coordinator, Nutrition Support Service and Clinical Pharmacist, Home Infusion Therapy, University Medical Center, Tucson, Arizona

Nutrient-Drug Interactions

John L. Rombeau, M.D.

Professor of Surgery, University of Pennsylvania School of Medicine; Director, Nutrition Support Service, Department of Veterans Affairs Medical Center, Philadelphia, Pennsylvania

Dietary Fiber and Its Clinical Applications to Enteral Nutrition

Edward Saltzman, M.D.

Instructor of Medicine, Tufts University School of Medicine; Scientist III, Jean Mayer USDA Human Nutrition Research Center on Aging at Tufts University; Fellow, Division of Clinical Nutrition, New England Medical Center, Boston, Massachusetts

Enteral Nutrition in the Elderly

Thomas A. Santora, M.D.

Program Director, Surgical Critical Care Fellowship, Director, Surgical Intensive Care Unit, and Associate Director, Trauma/Critical Care Services, Allegheny University of the Health Sciences, Philadelphia, Pennsylvania

Nutrition and Trauma

Renée W. Seto, B.A.

Research Laboratory Technician, Harrison Department of Surgical Research, University of Pennsylvania Medical Center, Philadelphia, Pennsylvania

Dietary Fiber and Its Clinical Applications to Enteral Nutrition

Alan Shenkin, Ph.D., B.Sc., F.R.C.P., F.R.C.Path.

Professor of Clinical Chemistry, University of Liverpool; Honorary Consultant Chemical Pathologist, Royal Liverpool University Hospital, Liverpool, England

Micronutrients

Eva Politzer Shronts, R.D., M.M.Sc., C.N.S.D.

Assistant Clinical Professor, Department of Pharmacy Practice, University of Minnesota College of Pharmacy; Associate Director, Nutrition Support Service, Department of Surgery, University of Minnesota Hospital, Minneapolis, Minnesota
Defined Formula Diets

David B. A. Silk, M.D., M.B.B.S., F.R.C.P.

Consultant Gastroenterologist and Codirector, Department of Gastroenterology and Nutrition, Central Middlesex Hospital NHS Trust, London, England
Diarrhea and Enteral Nutrition

Elissa L. Smith, R.D., M.S.

Clinical Nutritionist, Allegheny University of the Health Sciences, Philadelphia, Pennsylvania
The Role of Enteral Nutrition in Organ and Cellular Transplantation

Robert J. Smith, M.D.

Associate Professor of Medicine, Harvard Medical School; Assistant Director of Research and Head, Metabolism Section, Joslin Diabetes Center; Staff Physician, Brigham and Women's Hospital and New England Deaconess Hospital, Boston, Massachusetts
The Molecular Biology of Enteral Nutrition and the Gut

Margot Roberts Sweed, R.N., M.S.N., C.N.S.N.

Surgical Oncology Clinical Nurse Specialist, Fox Chase Cancer Center, Philadelphia, Pennsylvania
Delivery Systems and Administration of Enteral Nutrition

Cynthia A. Thomson, R.D., M.S., C.N.S.D.

Program Coordinator, Nutrition Curriculum in Medical Education, University of Arizona College of Medicine; Clinical Nutrition Research Specialist, Arizona Prevention Center, University of Arizona, Tucson, Arizona
Nutrient-Drug Interactions

Joan R. Ullrich, R.D.

Nutrition Coordinator, Home Enteral Program, University of California Los Angeles Medical Center, Los Angeles, California
Lipids and Enteral Nutrition

Frederick D. Watanabe, M.D.

Clinical Instructor, University of California Los Angeles; Research Fellow, Departments of Pediatrics and Surgery, Cedars-Sinai Medical Center, Los Angeles, California
Enteral Nutrition and Liver Failure

M. Burress Welborn III, M.D.
Surgical Resident-in-Training, University of Florida College of Medicine, Gainesville, Florida
Glucose Metabolism

Bruce M. Wolf, M.S.
Research Administrator, Oley Foundation, Albany, New York
Home Enteral Nutrition in Adults

Mary Kathryn Wolfson, R.N.
Director, Contract Management, Western Region, Value Rx/HPI, a Value Health Company, Albuquerque, New Mexico
Managed Care

Lorraine S. Young, R.D., M.S.
Senior Research Associate, Home Health Care Research, Department of Surgery, Brigham and Women's Hospital and Laboratories of Surgical Metabolism and Nutrition, Boston, Massachusetts
Therapeutic Effects of Specific Nutrients

Charles J. Yowler, M.D.
Assistant Professor of Surgery, Uniformed Services University of Health Sciences, Bethesda, Maryland; Chief, Burn Study Branch, United States Army Institute of Surgical Research, Fort Sam Houson, Texas
Enteral Nutrition in Burns

Thomas R. Ziegler, M.D., M.S.
Assistant Professor of Medicine, Division of Endocrinology and Metabolism, Department of Medicine, and Instructor in Surgery, Department of Surgery, Emory University School of Medicine; Associate Director, Nutrition and Metabolic Support Service, Emory University Hospital, Atlanta, Georgia
Therapeutic Effects of Specific Nutrients

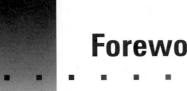

Foreword

Scientific advancements in providing enteral nutrition have stretched the imagination to previously unforeseen vistas. Reflected in *Clinical Nutrition: Enteral and Tube Feeding* are 36 completely revised or entirely new chapters to the third edition of this comprehensive text. Authors of each chapter are recognized authorities in specific aspects of enteral nutrition. It is clear that the entire volume has been designed to approach the multitude of diverse areas relating to enteral nutrition in a unique and systematic way.

This volume is a shining star of the intense, comprehensive, wholehearted authorship of the editor, John L. Rombeau, M.D. His attention and unique, quiet, winning way of managing this tremendous effort are noteworthy. He has brought together a superb group of authors, and his editorship is a major factor in the fruitful completion of the text. Rolando Rolandelli, M.D., Associate Professor of Surgery at Allegheny University of the Health Sciences, is a clinical scientist with a broad range of experience in enteral nutrition. He serves as coeditor, and contributes extensive clinical and scientific knowledge of enteral nutrition that has been invaluable to the reorganization and preparation of this edition.

The opening chapter on the history of enteral nutrition support reminds the reader of the early efforts to nourish patients via the gastrointestinal tract through the oral or anal routes of nutrient delivery. Over the past 5 decades, gigantic strides have been taken to progress to a multitude of approaches to enteral feeding that are creative, unique, and sophisticated, and that have in recent years been life-sustaining methodologies designed and proven to sustain adequate essential nutrients for many patients.

Chapter 2 highlights unique features of the gastrointestinal system that have been effectively used to support enteral nutrition. This has been the key delivery system for the administration of formula diets uniquely designed to provide selected nutrients or total nutrient requirements through a multitude of gut feeding systems. This chapter sets the stage for this volume on enteral feeding.

Macronutrients (proteins, carbohydrates, lipids) are featured in separate chapters to highlight the unique features of these essential nutrients and how they are most effective in gut delivery systems. For example, the liver is the primary organ system involved in regulating glucose availability for metabolism at all times. Likewise, life-essential micronutrients (vitamins and minerals) are also highlighted. A new chapter of special interest discusses the therapeutic effects of selected specific nutrients including omega-3 fatty acids, taurine, arginine, branched-chain amino acids, glutamine, ornithine, and (-ketoglutarate. References to published studies using these specific nutrients provide vistas of future nutritional support.

No text on enteral nutrition would be complete without providing a deeper understanding of the molecular basis of gut utilization of nutrients and the techniques of providing those nutrients through endoscopic, laparoscopic, and radiologic access systems. Over the past few years defined formula diets have been refined, redesigned, and retested to provide all essential nutrients for patients. With unique advances in access to the gut, delivery systems and administration of enteral feeding have become increasingly more sophisticated. Guenter's elegant chapter, Delivery Systems and Administration of Enteral Nutrition, is a superb example of the increased sophistication of modern enteral feeding. These delivery systems have demonstrated effectiveness in the care and management of enteral feeding for a variety of medical circumstances: neurologic disease, surgery, cancer, trauma, critical illness, burns, acquired immunodeficiency syndrome (AIDS), gastrointestinal diseases, diabetes, renal disease, respiratory diseases, organ and cellular transplantation, and short-bowel syndrome. The role of enteral nutrition in organ and cellular transplantation is a unique example of advances that have been made in this clinically oriented situation. Several studies have shown enteral nutrition to be efficacious in certain patients undergoing transplantation; however, larger prospective, randomized studies are needed to confirm the advantages of enteral nutrition.

The circumstances surrounding the medical need for enteral feeding require serious consideration of specific ethical issues. This consideration is an appropriate ending chapter to this text because ethical aspects of enteral feeding permeate all other aspects of the care of patients maintained on enteral nutrition support. One such ethical consideration is the effect of dietary nutrient content on gene expression in multiple body tissues. Information transfer from genes to proteins, protein translation, DNA cloning, recombinant protein products, and genetic modifications and protein expression in intact organisms are examples of molecular biology of enteral nutrition that are likely to expand in the future. While many significant advances in the technology of enteral feeding have taken place in recent years, patient consent and concerns and care of nutrition support must be considered first.

Ethical issues regarding enteral nutrition support may become even more important when we consider the challenges and opportunities of managed care, as well as the rising costs of and access to health care and the security of health care systems. Managed care systems may offer lower-cost health care but perhaps with less freedom to choose the type of care. Today we stand to improve the quality of nutrition care based on appropriate clinical guidelines so we can obtain the best clinical outcome possible. Appropriate application of modern enteral nutrition will be one of the health care systems that will be an effective life-giving support for many patients into the future. This application is a reflection of the intensive research and numerous advances that have occurred in recent years in the scientific development of enteral feeding to effect a holistic nutrition-support system.

ELEANOR A. YOUNG, PH.D., R.D., L.D.

Preface

Enteral nutrition is being prescribed for patients in hospitals and in the home at an unprecedented rate. This increase in use is due in part to results of controlled clinical trials identifying the types of patients who receive the greatest benefits from this feeding method. Improved dietary formulations, technologic advances in enteral access and dietary delivery, reduced costs, and fewer complications when compared to parenteral nutrition have led to the current clinical dictum that the enteral route is the optimal method for feeding most malnourished patients with functioning gastrointestinal tracts and the inability to ingest sufficient nutrients by mouth.

The rationale for publishing the third edition of this book on enteral nutrition is the same as the previous two editions—to provide the highest quality of scientific information combined with the state of the art of clinical techniques and delivery. This book is not intended to be a basic nutrition text. It has been developed to specifically address the scientific rationale and clinical techniques of enteral feeding. The editors strongly believe that understanding the scientific basis of feeding into the gut is a mandatory prerequisite to appropriate clinical utilization and improved patient outcome.

Significant advances in enteral nutrition have occurred since this book was last published in 1990. These advances have provided the rationale for the extensive changes in content in this edition. More than one third of the chapters in this edition (12 chapters) are presented for the first time. For each of these chapters, the selection of authors was based upon proven track records of both scientific and clinical experience in their respective fields.

A new chapter on micronutrients is included. This reflects new information concerning vitamin and trace element requirements of critically ill patients in need of enteral feeding. This information is included in Chapter 7.

Nutritional pharmacotherapy is an exciting new component of enteral feeding. Nutritional pharmacotherapy is defined as the use of nutrients that have major pharmacologic effects as well as confirmed nutritional benefits per se and/or the use of drugs to enhance nutrient utilization or modify the nutritional-metabolic environment of the patient. Examples of these nutrient-drugs include arginine, glutamine, and the omega-3 fatty acids. This information is included in Chapter 8.

As in other areas of medical science, there has been an "explosion" of information concerning the effects of enteral nutrients on the molecular mediation of gastrointestinal structure and function. Moreover, it is now known that nutrients can selectively influence gene expression. This new component of the science of enteral nutrition has great therapeutic promise as discussed in Chapter 9.

The endoscopic placement of feeding tubes for long-term enteral nutrition is now the gold standard for access to the stomach. This technique is safer and less expensive than the traditional method of surgical gastrostomy. Additionally, tubes are now being inserted via laparoscopic techniques. These innovative approaches to enteral access are described in a new chapter (Chapter 11) exclusively dedicated to this topic.

There are now at least five prospective, randomized, controlled clinical trials demonstrating improved clinical outcome in postoperative patients receiving enteral nutrition when compared with the outcomes in individuals receiving the same amounts of nutrients by the parenteral route. The scientific bases for these results and clinical techniques for feeding these patients is presented in Chapter 15.

Transplantation of most major organs is being performed with increasing frequency and success. These operations are often associated with prolonged recoveries and require special diets and techniques of postoperative feeding. This topic is presented for the first time in this book in Chapter 29.

Enteral nutrients are now being prescribed more frequently to malnourished patients with AIDS. The types of diets, rationale for their delivery, and technical expertise required to feed these challenging patients are provided in Chapter 21.

In contrast to traditional teachings, increasing amounts of enteral nutrients are now being given to patients with pancreatitis and respiratory disease. The specifics of feeding these patients are included in Chapters 25 and 28.

There is new evidence that the presence of nutrients within the gut provides a pharmacologic stimulus to intestinal growth and function. These findings have significant implications for feeding patients with short bowel syndrome. This topic is presented in Chapter 34.

Diarrhea remains the single most common and important complication of enteral feeding. New information concerning the pathogenesis of diarrhea and its treatment in enterally fed patients has evolved during the past 5 years. This topic is now exclusively presented in a new Chapter 32.

Clinicians and ethicists continue to debate the appropriateness of enteral nutrition in the terminally ill patient. A chapter on this topic was included in the last edition of this book; however, considerable new information has emerged on this topic. The author and respective content of this chapter (Chapter 35) are new to this edition.

Similar to other aspects of clinical medicine, enteral nutrition is entering the arena of managed care. This very new topic is presented from both the economic and the scientific perspective in Chapter 36.

Each of the contributors has been chosen because of his or her proven clinical expertise and objective documentation of this expertise. Additionally, contributors have been selected because of concurrent experience at the bedside and in the laboratory. Of necessity, one will find areas of conflict among the authors because of differences in interpretation of data, varying clinical experiences and training, and the complexities of enteral feeding of certain types of patients. The editors believe that including different diagnostic and therapeutic approaches to clinical problems enhances the utility of this book.

An important editorial function is to minimize the duplication of content. Every effort has been made to minimize redundancy. Of necessity, content has been repeated, in part, in several chapters. The editors have decided to retain this information in selected chapters to avoid disrupting continuity of the chapter.

We wish to thank Ms. Suzanne Pierson and Ms. Deborah Muto for their editorial and secretarial assistance. The work of Mr. Raymond Kersey and W.B. Saunders is also acknowledged.

The most important goal of this book is to help patients. It is our strong hope that the information contained within this edition will contribute to improved care of the patient in need of enteral feeding both in the hospital and at home. Moreover, it is hoped that the information contained herein will provide a stimulus to basic scientists and clinical researchers to continue scientific investigations to perpetuate the many ongoing advances in enteral nutrition.

JOHN L. ROMBEAU, M.D.
ROLANDO H. ROLANDELLI, M.D.

Contents

1

History of Enteral Feeding: Past and Present Perspectives

Mark A. McCamish
Gustavo Bounous
Maureen E. Geraghty

This chapter will review the history of enteral nutrition, which has depended on the convergence of two major fields of investigation: enteral access devices and enteral nutrition solutions. Obviously the perfect product would not be useful without the ability to deliver it, and vice versa. As enteral access devices evolved over the centuries, so did the nutritional components administered through the tubes.

RECTAL FEEDING

The history of enteral nutrition therapy dates back to the documentation of nutrient enemas first described in ancient papyri from 3500 years ago (Fig. 1–1). Until the 17th century, such publications were largely limited to a description of the syringes and other appliances used to administer these enemas.[1,2] It was less problematic to establish rectal access with these crude devices than to bypass the nasopharnyx or oropharynx with inflexible conduits. With the advent of rubber and the vulcanization process, improvements were made in the properties of the materials used to make enema appliances. A common simplistic form of rectal feeding device was one where rubber tubing, 1/8 inch in diameter, was attached to a small funnel and to a short segment of glass tubing for observation of nutrient flow.[3]

Undoubtedly, the most noted medical case wherein rectal feeding was successfully administered was that of U.S. President James Garfield in 1881. For virtually 79 days following the bullet-induced wound of the assassin, Charles Guiteau, Garfield was maintained by a mixture of peptonized beef broth, beef peptonoids, and whiskey administered rectally every 4 hours.[2]

The documentation of development of rectal devices for nutrient provision was accompanied by a listing of common foods administered through these tubes.[4] The use of milk, grain, broths, and whey was first reported by Egyptian and Greek physicians,[2] and foods added to this repertoire included raw eggs and brandy.[2] A letter in *The Lancet* in 1878 described a physician's use of finely ground hog and beef pancreas administered rectally.[5]

UPPER GASTROINTESTINAL FEEDING

The provision of orogastric or pharyngeal alimentation through a conduit somewhat paralleled that of rectal administration in that it was described as early as the 12th century,[1] yet general acceptance of this practice was not

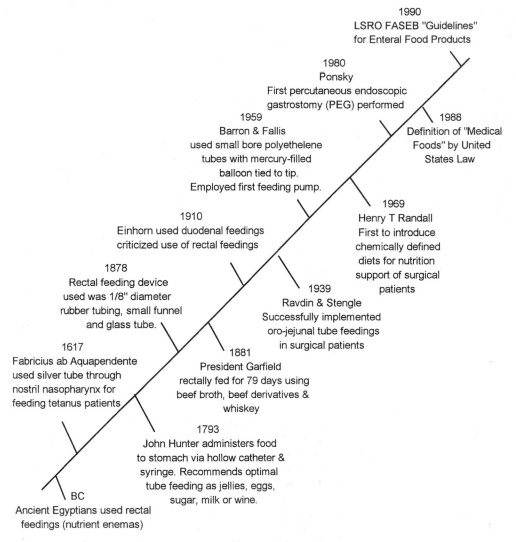

FIGURE 1–1   History of enteral feeding.

demonstrated until the 16th century. The introduction of a nutritional mixture into the esophagus through a hollow tube with a bladder attached to the end was reported in 1598.[6] Soon after, Fabricius ab Aquapendente devised a silver tube that he threaded through the nostril into the nasopharynx for nutrient delivery to tetanus patients.[7] By the mid-17th century, Von Helmont designed flexible leather catheters that Boerhaave suggested be placed nasogastrically.[7,8]

The era of "modern" enteral nutrition support commenced at the end of the 18th century, when John Hunter administered blended food to the stomach through a hollow catheter and syringe.[9] Hunter's initial attempt was made by stimulating the stomach with food de-

livered through the catheter in efforts to resuscitate a patient from near drowning. In 1790, Hunter passed an eel-skin-covered whale bone probe orogastrically for nutrient provision. Hunter noted in his recommendations that optimal tube feeding foods were jellies, eggs beaten with water, sugar, and milk or wine.[9]

Before this time, nutrient mixtures were delivered through the force of gravity, which did not provide consistent or dependable flow rates. With the invention of the first stomach pump toward the end of the 18th century, it became possible not only to provide consistent enteral nutrition, but also to irrigate and empty stomach contents in the event of poisoning.[1,7] Oral hypopharyngeal and nasopharyngeal routes accommodated stomach pump feedings throughout the 19th century and were often employed in mentally ill patients who refused to eat. Tube materials remained rather primitive and uncomfortable throughout the 19th century. In 1872, Clouston described two types of nasoesophageal tubes: one fabricated from elastic rubber and one from gum elastic with a spiral wire. It was noted, however, that for one patient, four strong men were needed to insert the equipment.[10]

DELIVERY OF ENTERAL NUTRITION TO THE DUODENUM AND JEJUNUM

The year 1910 marked a significant breakthrough in enteral nutrition. Max Einhorn proposed that duodenal feeding be implemented in place of rectal feeding whenever gastric feeding was impossible. Einhorn asserted that if oral and gastric feeding were not possible in a patient, rectal feeding was no longer an acceptable feeding route. He pointed out that alternative foods placed in the rectum were inadequately used and that the procedure was associated with complaints of rectal irritation.[11] His device consisted of a rubber tube with a metal weight of 10 to 12 g attached to the distal end.

Einhorn was one of the first to suggest slow administration of liquified food and to provide these at room temperature. His "recipe" generally consisted of 240 ml of milk, one raw egg, and 15 g of lactose. Positive accounts describing the clinical course and outcome of three patients receiving this type of tube feeding were well-received by the medical community. This European tube was immediately adopted and adapted in the United States.[4]

Following the general use of oroduodenal feeding tubes, orojejunal tube feeding in surgical patients was successfully implemented by Ravdin and Stengel in 1939.[12] This practice also highlighted the importance of protein and caloric nutriture in the postoperative period.[4]

ENTERAL FEEDING ACCESS DEVICES

Enteral tube feeding equipment remained rather awkward until 1959 when Barron described a technique where he tied a mercury-filled balloon to the tip of a feeding tube as an insertion aid.[13] Barron and his group also reported on 150 patients in whom gastric or jejunal alimentation was employed using polyethylene tubes with outside diameters of only 1.9 mm (about 6 F). The gastrostomy tubes were 27 inches long, and the jejunal tubes were 6 feet long. A mixture of 500 ml of homogenized milk, 175 g of liver protein hydrolysate, 300 g of a partially hydrolyzed cereal starch, 75 g of powdered milk, and four eggs was successfully administered to these patients either through a 27-inch gastrostomy tube or a 6-foot jejunal tube. Water and electrolyte status was monitored and replaced as necessary.[14]

Barron was also one of the pioneers in the use of a tube feeding pump; feedings were started at 30 ml every 1 or 2 hours and gradually increased to as much as 200 ml/hour.[14] Tincture of opium was used by Barron for patients who developed diarrhea.[4]

The year 1959 also marked the first publication of a textbook addressing enteral tube feeding, which was written by Morton Pareira,[7] a Director of Surgery at Jewish Hospital in St. Louis. This book was based, in part, on the positive experience he and his colleague, Ellman, had with 240 sole source tube feeding patients. Many of Pareira's recommendations in his book (use of a small-bore [< 2.5 mm or 8 F] soft tube; initial feedings delivered by continuous drip or pump; formula dilution to promote adaptation the first few days; provision of free water) are all generally accepted principles now.[4,7] Pareira was also astute in that he recommended home enteral nutrition for select patients.[4]

Over the last 10 years, nasogastric suction tubes have been used occasionally to deliver enteral feedings, but they are not recommended for this purpose. The rubber or polyvinyl chloride (PVC) material of older nasogastric tubes is irritating to patients. In addition, PVC stiffens when exposed to digestive juices, requiring frequent tube replacement. The availability of specifically designed feeding tubes of soft, biocompatible materials has contributed in large measure to enhanced patient tolerance of nasally placed tubes. Most feeding tubes today are made of polyurethane or silicone. Because these materials do not rapidly disintegrate or embrittle in situ, they do not need frequent replacement. Silicone is softer and more flexible than other tube materials, with a greater tendency to stretch and collapse. Polyurethane is stronger than silicone, allowing for a tube of this material to have thinner walls and thus a larger internal diameter (Fig. 1–2).[15] The French (F) unit measures the outer lumen diameter of a tube (each French unit is equal to 0.33 mm). A silicone tube of the same French size as a polyurethane tube has a smaller internal diameter,

ID/OD Ratio

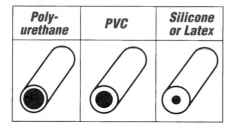

FIGURE 1–2   Comparison of tube diameters.

since the wall thickness must be greater to confer similar strength as the polyurethane tube. The silicone tube provides more flexibility, which may add comfort. The flexibility and decreased internal diameter, however, may lead to kinking or clogging.[16,17]

Although the search for a more perfect material has included the use of polyurethane blends, polyvinyl chloride (PVC), polyurethane, silicone, and other copolymers, flaws still exist. Polymers may become stiffer after prolonged use, and silicone degrades over time due to fungal/microbial colonization.[18] Use of small-bore tubes specially designed for nasoenteric feeding significantly enhances patient comfort and safety, although the risk of clogging and requirement for replacement may be higher.[19] Some physicians still request large-diameter tubes (> 16 F), which tend to cause pressure necrosis in the nasolabial area, esophagitis, pharyngitis, and otitis. They may further compromise lower esophageal sphincter competency, increasing the potential for gastric reflux and pulmonary aspiration. These large tubes generally interfere with swallowing and are more uncomfortable for the patient. Most adults tolerate nasoenteral tubes ranging between 8 and 12 F. Nasogastric tubes are usually 30 to 36 inches long, and tubes placed transpylorically are approximately 43 to 60 inches long.

It has long been thought the transpyloric intubations are facilitated by weighted tubes. Initially, mercury tips were used, but disposal proved to be a problem. Now inert tungsten weights (3 g, 5 g, or 7 g) are found in the weighted tubes, generally in the form of pellets, segments, or powder. There is no significant difference in transpyloric passage between the three weight categories.[20] It is, however, controversial whether weighted tubes are necessary to aid transpyloric passage and to maintain tube placement.[17,21,22] Most tube manufac-turers presently offer both weighted and un-weighted nasoenteral tubes.

Clogging problems were resolved when the small-bore feeding tube was introduced. Tube tips were redesigned to facilitate formula flow. Many tubes now have multiple feeding ports or eyelets to maximize outflow in the distal portion of the tube. The staggered positioning of these eyelets on the sides of the tube a few centimeters from the end, as well as a feeding port at the terminal end of the tube, minimizes the potential for backflow and clogging problems. The portion of the tube on which the eyelets or feeding ports are positioned may be made of a more rigid material than the rest of the tube, which also helps to prevent folding or kinking.

Nasoenteral feeding tubes have become quite advanced and include such features as stylets to aid placement, Y-ports to accommodate irrigation/medication administration, and radiopaque materials for radiographic confirmation of placement. Placement techniques have included blind, endoscopic, fluoroscopic, and surgical techniques. Confirmation of placement has included radiography, pH testing,[23] monitoring electromyographic activity,[24] and sensing tiny electromagnetic coils in the tips of enteral tubes.[25]

By 1980 gastrostomy tube placement experienced a revolutionary improvement. Jeffrey Ponsky, a pediatric surgeon at the Children's Hospital in Cleveland, and his colleague, Michael Gauderer, combined endoscopic techniques and enteral tube placement to develop the nonsurgical gastrostomy known as the percutaneous endoscopic gastrostomy (PEG).[26] Clinicians currently regard this as a preferred access method for long-term enteral nutrition. Newer surgical techniques include laparoscopic gastrostomies[27] and laparoscopic jejunostomies.[28] An excellent review of state-of-the-art enteral access was recently compiled by Minard.[29]

Enteral delivery systems have vastly evolved since the use of a stomach pump in the 18th century. Common systems comprise a pump, feeding set, and administration container. Enteral product can be decanted into containers for delivery or obtained in "Ready to Hang" containers. Pumps deliver product through various mechanisms such as peristaltic or volumetric pumping action. Pumps can provide various alarms for clogging, free flow, or being out of product. The most recent advances provide dual channel pumps for automatic flushing, hydration, and reduced tube clogging,[30,31] which illustrates the technologic advances from the 18th century.

DEVELOPMENT AND REGULATORY CLIMATE OF SPECIALTY ENTERAL FORMULAS

Since John Hunter recommended jellies, eggs, milk, or wine as a nutrient mixture, there have been continual efforts to improve and refine enteral nutrition products. This effort has led to the use of various descriptive terms without national or international consensus on nomenclature. Terminology has included the following descriptors: polymeric, all-purpose, oligomeric, peptide based, predigested, elemental, nutritionally complete, modular, special products for inborn errors of metabolism, foods for special dietary uses, disease specific products, foods for special medical purposes, orphan medical foods, and medical foods. There are legal definitions and clinical use definitions. This section will address the history of the development as well as the regulatory climate of these "medical foods."

As far back as ancient history, foods have been used to maintain the structure, function, and growth of the human organism. One could monitor various nutritional parameters, whether simple or complex, to document that foods/nutrition could maintain "structure/function" or nutritional status. Nitrogen balance is a prime example, and Benjamin[32] was one of the first to document this in long-term studies in 1914 using infants. It would be relatively simple to concentrate on nutrition and its role in maintaining nutritional status. However, as technology has advanced, there has also been an emphasis on "nutritional therapy" of illnesses. This is generally considered an adjunctive therapy, but nevertheless nutritional therapy or treatment is generally accepted by clinicians. This acceptance dates back to at least 1893 when Cutter wrote "One reason why I am now an advocate of food treatment of disease is that I found I could not cure throat cases satisfactorily unless I paid attention to the diet."[33] Unfortunately, the regulatory systems of the world have not kept pace with advancing nutritional science; therefore, nutritional *treatment* of illness or disease is not recognized. This is easily demonstrated by comparing the definitions of drugs vs foods in U.S. law.

The term "drug" is defined in the Federal Food, Drug and Cosmetic Act (Chapter 1, Subsection 201[a] [2]) as "articles recognized in the official *U.S. Pharmacopeia*...and articles intended for use in the diagnoses, cure, mitigation, treatment, or prevention of disease in man or other animals and articles *other than food* [emphasis author's] intended to affect the structure or any function of the body of man." From this definition one can see that foods can affect body structure or function, but any food or nutrition "intended" to treat, cure, mitigate, or prevent disease would be classified as a drug under this definition! The term "medical food" (p. 7) means a food that is formulated to be administered under a physician's supervision and intended for the *specific dietary management* of a disease or condition for which distinctive nutritional requirements are established by medical evaluation (Orphan Drug Law, P.L. 100-290, Apr. 18, 1988).

Two important aspects of the definition of a medical food in the United States are the term "specific dietary management" and the absence of any therapeutic definition. The regulation does not allow a medical food to be used as therapy. Any such "intended use" would only be allowed in the drug definition. Even though clinicians worldwide endorse nutritional "therapy" or treatment, most regulatory agencies do not allow for therapeutic claims—rather, simply for the use of "specific dietary management." A brief discussion of the history of "elemental diets" and their use in the treatment of various disease states will serve to illustrate the *fact* that nutritional therapy is a reality despite the lack of regulatory endorsement.

Chemically Defined Diets: A Historical Overview

The history of "chemically defined" or "elemental diets" dates back to the turn of the century when no one had yet shown that higher animals could satisfy their protein needs by substitution with amino acids or protein hydrolysates. In 1949 and shortly thereafter, a highly purified diet containing amino acid mixtures, sucrose, corn oil, starch, vitamin, and minerals was fed to young men for the first time in the classic studies of Rose on human amino acid requirements.[34] The late 1950s through 1970s marked the "space age" and the time when space diet research was conducted by Greenstein et al[35] and Winitz et al.[36,37] These chemically defined diets were investigated in both rats and healthy human volunteers to provide a "low-residue" diet that would decrease fecal output during space travel. These chemically defined formulas or "elemental" diets consisted of known quantities of crystalline amino acids, simple sugars, essential fatty acids, and vitamins and minerals.[35] Dr. Henry

T. Randall, Professor and Chairman of the De-partment of Surgery at Brown University, was the first to introduce chemically defined diets through fine-bore (5 or 8 F) polyethylene infant feeding tubes for partial or complete nutritional support of seriously ill surgical patients.[38] Positive nitrogen balance and weight gain were reported in some patients with pancreatitis and inflammatory bowel disease. A tracheoesoph-ageal pleural cutaneous fistula closed sponta-neously in a gastrostomy-fed patient receiving a chemically defined formula diet.

Recent advances in infusion delivery sys-tems for continuous enteral feeding have made possible the use of this form of nutrition in sev-eral disease states. Following is a historical overview of the use of elemental diets in vari-ous disease entities that illustrates the benefit of nutritional *therapy*.

Necrosis of the intestinal mucosa without ap-parent vascular occlusion has been reported in patients after cardiac failure, burn, hemorrhage, postoperative hypotension, and sepsis.[39] The concept of using these types of diets in the pro-phylaxis of the intestinal lesions was first pro-posed in 1967[40] following the discovery that pancreatic proteases play an important role in the pathogenesis of acute ischemic enteropa-thy.[41] The use of an elemental diet was then conceived with the object of reducing the con-centration of pancreatic proteases in the intes-tine. The use of protein hydrolysate or synthetic amino acids in place of intact protein decreases the concentration of pancreatic proteases in the intestine, hence reducing the potential for mu-cosal autodigestion.[42]

The prototype diet used in 1967 contained fibrin hydrolysate, sucrose, and small amounts of triglycerides. When dogs ingested this diet exclusively for 3 days before controlled hemor-rhagic hypotension or intestinal ischemia, the resulting intestinal pathology was minimized and survival improved compared with dogs fed standard laboratory chow. The term "elemental diet" was then introduced[43] and has since gained general acceptance even though the term was not "chemically correct." The term "elemental diet" was used partly because an al-ternative, more accurate description would be too lengthy. Similar clinical results were ob-tained with either this prototype diet[44,45] or a commercial elemental diet containing casein hydrolysate[46,47] in dogs,[44,45] rats,[46] and pigs[47] subjected to controlled hemorrhagic hypoten-sion[44,45,47] or severe burns.[46] Because the same types of injury may lead to a defect in the ter-minal digestion of nutrients,[48] elemental diets

are also effectively used as a therapeutic tool following multiple trauma, major surgery, and burns. This was demonstrated in the intensive care unit (ICU) after abdominal surgery, where enteral support with formula containing enzy-matic protein hydrolysate was found to be more effective than an equivalent diet contain-ing whole proteins in restoring plasma amino acid and protein levels.[49]

Pancreatic proteases have also been found to affect adversely the intestine and the sur-vival or irradiated dogs.[50] This similarity be-tween radiation and ischemic enteropathies prompted the use of an elemental diet in the prophylaxis of radiation enteropathy. Thus, mice fed a casein hydrolysate elemental diet in powder form before and after irradiation were found to have better survival and less weight loss than animals eating regular rodent chow. Systematic protection has been associated with accelerated healing of the injured intestinal mucosa in mice and rats.[51,52] Patients fed ex-clusively a casein hydrolysate–based elemental diet during intensive abdominal radiotherapy experienced no severe diarrhea and main-tained body weight and serum protein levels, whereas patients receiving an isocaloric hospi-tal diet lost weight and serum protein and had a 30 percent incidence of severe diarrhea, ne-cessitating interruption of treatment.[53] An ele-mental diet regimen (free amino acid) replac-ing standard hospital food in children receiving whole or hemiabdominal radiotherapy resulted in no cases of severe, acute, or delayed radia-tion enteropathy, whereas the prior incidence was 70 percent for radiation enteritis and 36 percent for delayed enteritis.[54] Patients with bladder cancer, fed exclusively an elemental diet (protein hydrolysate) during preoperative radiotherapy, had normal ileal mucosa and no diarrhea, unlike control patients receiving a hospital diet.[55] Thus "elemental diets" have not only been used to *treat* disease states, they have also been used to *prevent* disease (i.e., ra-diation enteritis). Such intended uses would certainly classify them as drugs and not as medical foods.

Potential injury by pancreatic secretions and dietary protein antigenicity in Crohn's disease also suggested that elemental diets might be needed to treat patients with this syndrome. Stephens and Randall first reported the bene-fits of an elemental diet in one patient with Crohn's disease.[38] In a series of nine patients with Crohn's disease successfully treated with elemental diet, symptoms and nutritional sta-tus improved.[56] The effectiveness of elemental diet as *primary therapy* of this syndrome has been confirmed by several investigators who have frequently reported the superiority of elemental diet to conventional food and standard drug therapy. Chronic intermittent treatment of Crohn's disease with elemental diet has been shown to reverse growth arrest while decreasing prednisone requirements and disease activity index in pediatric patients.[57] Protein hydrolysate was also found to offer an advantage over intact protein as an anti-inflammatory agent in acute Crohn's disease.[58] Clinical remission was found to occur more frequently in patients fed an amino acid-based elemental diet during active Crohn's disease than in corresponding patients fed an equivalent formula diet with intact proteins.[59]

In a recent comparative study an amino acid–based elemental diet was found to be as effective as a protein hydrolysate-based elemental diet as a primary treatment for active Crohn's disease.[60] The reported remissions of symptoms, improved radiologic features, and weight gain in patients receiving an elemental diet strongly suggest reduction of disease activity. Although controversy exists whether to feed a polymeric or an elemental formula, findings suggest that acute attacks of Crohn's disease can be treated by enteral nutritional support. If enteral nutrition is used to correct nutritional insufficiencies, elemental or peptide preparations may be better than polymeric formulas, especially if short bowel syndrome is present.[61]

In conclusion, the use of elemental diet in the management of intestinal disorders constitutes a multifactorial approach to the treatment of patients with these disorders. Such diets reduce intestinal pancreatic protease activity, have low antigenicity, and deliver absorbable nutrients to the intestinal mucosa at a time when mucosal terminal digestion may be impaired. Low-flow enteral infusion of these diets provides continuous nutritional support to the intestinal mucosa, which largely depends on the enteral route for its own nutrition and trophism.[62]

Elemental diets have also been recommended, especially during acute disease events. "Elemental" is a frequently used term to describe a "semisynthetic fiber-free liquid diet containing a full range of basic nutrients for the maintenance of normal physiological functions."[63] In the clinical setting, "elemental" is used to describe a range of formulas that provide protein as free amino acids to formulas that provide protein as peptides. A truly elemental diet would consist of glucose, amino acids, fatty acids, vitamins, and minerals.[63] Therefore, the commonly used term "elemental diet" is a misnomer, since no commercially available enteral diet formula fits all these criteria.[63] However, health care professionals commonly associate elemental diets with the following qualities: hydrolyzed protein, reduced pancreatic secretions, low residue, and rapid absorption.

Unfortunately, there is no consensus on what classifies a product for the descriptive term "elemental." Companies may go to great lengths to classify their products as elemental, including developing an entirely new and thoroughly confusing methodology for quantifying peptide lengths.[64, Table 1] In this novel approach the percentage of peptides present in the product is listed by "number" instead of by weight, which is the classic method. For example, if there are essentially two different length peptides in a mixture, one being a tripeptide (molecular weight 400) and the other a polypeptide of 300 amino acids (molecular weight 40,000), the classic approach would quantitate their contribution to the peptide mix by weight. Thus, if the mixture were half tripeptide and half polypeptide by weight, then 50 percent of the mixture would be three amino acids long and 50 percent would be long polypeptides. However, since the tripeptide is $1/100$ the size of the polypeptide, there are approximately 100 times more molecules of the tripeptide than the polypeptide. Thus, if one expresses this simple equivalent mixture of peptides (by weight) in the "peptide by number method," the mixture would be 99 percent tripeptides and 1 percent polypeptides! Using this approach, any hydrolyzed protein appears to have a higher content of smaller peptides, and this can be used in marketing "elemental" products.[64]

The previous discussion serves to demonstrate the complexity of the history and evolution of enteral nutrition. Products can be classified using multiple terminology, but in reality there are polymeric and oligomeric mixtures, although the term "elemental" is so entrenched that change is not anticipated.

MEDICAL FOODS

Despite the lack of regulatory latitude for developing nutritional *treatments,* several "disease-specific products" have been developed.[65] Some have suggested that "disease-specific" products have limited efficacy;[66] however, it may not generally be understood that disease-specific products are not all designed necessarily to modify or mitigate the disease. Some are designed simply to make it more practical to provide adequate nutrition support to distinct patient categories (i.e., renal disease).[67] These types of products are more classically aligned to the regulatory definition of "medical food," that is, they are designed to provide "specific dietary management."

As one approaches a true disease-specific *therapeutic* nutritional product, there is no consensus on how to demonstrate therapeutic efficacy. The critical factor is regulatory or legal, since there is no regulatory mechanism to obtain nutritional therapy "claims" regardless of what research is performed. Forbes[68] has reviewed the regulatory history and documented that medical foods have been exempted from all key regulations (except their definition in the Orphan Drug Act as previously mentioned). There have been attempts to define how medical foods' efficacy should be demonstrated (contracted by the U.S. Food and Drug Administration [FDA]), yet nothing has been adopted by the regulatory agencies.[65] This review, under FDA contract, stated the following:

> The consultant for this LSRO [Life Sciences Research Organization] review suggested the following as appropriate types of end points for designing clinical trials: nutritional, metabolic, functional, and morbidity and mortality. Despite the difficulties of accurately relating the effects of nutritional support to morbidity and mortality...these end points should be part of the protocol whenever the investigator considers them feasible. An example of a functional endpoint is the ability of a patient with COPD to be weaned from mechanical ventilation.[69]

Such research has been performed,[70] yet since these guidelines suggested by the LSRO have not been enacted as a regulation, it is not possible to make such a product "claim" for *treatment* of patients on ventilators.

Several enteral nutrition products may in fact modify or mitigate disease to some degree. The development of disease-specific products is often based initially on medical nutritional concepts reported in the literature, followed by testing the product for efficacy in the intended patient population. The formulation of enteral nutrition for pulmonary patients demonstrates this point. In 1980 and 1981, it was reported that when glucose provision to nutritionally depleted patients exceeded energy requirements, the respiratory quotient (RQ) increased to 1.0 or greater, reflecting a significant increase in Vco_2.[71] CO_2 retention resulted from this increase in Vco_2 in patients with limited respiratory reserve,[72] which ultimately led to respiratory failure.[73] With this and related research serving as the medical rationale, researchers developed a pulmonary product with modified carbohydrate, fat, and protein distributions. The product was successfully tested in pulmonary patients,[70,74,75] and physicians began to use this disease specific product in similar pulmonary patients.

An enteral formula was also developed for diabetic patients and intended to enhance glycemic control and maintain nutritional status. Products with a low-carbohydrate, high-fiber, high-fat profile have been tested with favorable clinical results in both type I[76] and type II diabetic patients.[77,78] Surrogate markers of diabetes have been used (i.e., glucose level and control) because it was impractical to demonstrate benefits to long-term morbidity such as microvascular or macrovascular complications as in the Diabetes Control and Complications Trial [DCCT].[79]

Copius clinical research has been performed in the area of hepatic encephalopathy, and, although it seems prudent to use a specialized enteral nutrition product in hepatic patients with hepatitis, cirrhosis, or encephalopathy, clinical experts agree that for most patients, "standard nutritionally adequate commercial enteral products alone or with the addition of modular nutrient sources are suitable."[65] At this time there is also no clinical consensus on the efficacy of branched-chain amino acids to improve nitrogen balance and to manage hepatic encephalopathy.[65,80,81] Prominent hepatologists recommend the use of standard formulas (not enriched with branched chains) for most liver patients.[82]

Over the last decade, there has been a plethora of research concerning nutritional status in acquired immunodeficiency syndrome (AIDS) patients. Opportunistic infections, weight loss, diarrhea, anorexia, nausea, and vomiting all impede adequate oral intake. An enteral nutrition formula designed for human immunodeficiency virus (HIV)-positive or AIDS patients has been clinically tested with promising results in terms of body weight and triceps skinfold maintenance and decreased numbers of hospitalizations.[83]

More recently the Dietary Supplement and Health Education Act (DSHEA) was enacted (October 1994). This was driven by the dietary supplement industry after repetitive actions by the FDA to classify individual dietary supplements either as drugs or food additives which are subject to significant regulatory scrutiny as well as premarket approval. This legislation exempts dietary supplements from food additive status and allows certain claims and the use of supportive literature. The actual label requirements are currently being created by an appointed committee. This legislation was a grassroots and industry effort to force limitations onto the FDA and allow for some limited claims for these products.

The current philosophy at the Center for Food Safety and Nutrition at the FDA has been presented at many meetings by Dr. Yetley (*Food Labeling and Nutrition News,* Nov. 2, 1995; 4(5):23–24). Following is a quote from this newsletter abstracting meeting contents: "Any supplement which is deemed to diagnose, cure, mitigate, treat or prevent disease is defined by FDA as a drug, and any claim that involves any of the above verbs, then is a drug claim." Despite many efforts on behalf of industry, academia and several independent groups, therapeutic nutrition is not an option under the existing laws.

Thus, as the history of enteral nutrition unfolded, complex issues arose in terminology, application, and regulation. Resolution of these issues will require herculean efforts by scientists, clinicians, regulators, and, unfortunately, politicians. Efficacy of complex nutritional therapy has already been demonstrated, and further "outcome" studies are needed.[84] As history always points the way to the future, the future for enteral nutrition is bright, but it must depend on valid science, adequate documentation of "efficacy," and a regulatory strategy for approving such documented medical nutritional therapies.

Acknowledgment

We would like to acknowledge the assistance of Tina Zians in the diligent preparation of this manuscript.

REFERENCES

1. Bonsmann M, Hardt W, Lorber CG: The historical development of artificial enteral alimentation. Part 1. Anasthesiol Intensivmed 1993;34:207.
2. Bliss DW: Feeding per rectum: as illustrated in the case of the late President Garfield and others. Med Red 1882;22:64.
3. Jones-Humphreys YM: An easy method of feeding per rectum. Lancet 1878;1:144.
4. Randall HT: The history of enteral nutrition. In Rombeau JL, Caldwell MD (eds): Clinical Nutrition: Enteral and Tube Feeding, Philadelphia: WB Saunders 1984:1–9.
5. Brown-Séquard CE: Feeding per rectum in nervous affections. Lancet 1878;1:144.
6. His W: Zur Geschichte der magenpumpe. Med Klin 1925;21:391.
7. Pareira MD: Therapeutic Nutrition with Tube Feeding. Springfield, IL: Charles C Thomas, 1959.
8. Alcock T: On the immediate treatment of persons poisoned. Lancet 1823;1:372.
9. Hunter J: A case of paralysis of the muscles of deglutition cured by an artifical mode of conveying food and medicines into the stomach. Trans Soc Improve Med Chir Know 1793;1:182.
10. Clouston TS: Forcible feeding. Lancet 1872;2: 797.
11. Einhorn M: Duodenal alimentation. Med Rec 1910;78:92.
12. Stengel A Jr, Ravdin IS: The maintenance of nutrition in surgical patients with a description of the orojejunal method of feeding. Surgery 1939;6:511.
13. Barron J: Tube feeding of post-operative patients. Surg Clin North Am 1959;39:1481.
14. Fallis LS, Barron J: Gastric and jejunal alimentation with fine polyethylene tubes. Arch Surg 1952;65:373.
15. Geraghty ME: Tube feeding equipment update. Dietians in Nutrition (support newsletter), 1989; July/Aug, p.1.
16. Fagerman KE, Lysen LK: Enteral feeding tubes: a comparison and history. Nutr Supp Serv 1987;7:10.
17. Metheny N, Eisenberg P, McSweeney M: Effect of feeding tube properties and three irrigants on clogging rates. Nurs Res 1988;37;165.
18. Gottlieb K, Leya J, Kruss D et al: Intraluminal fungal colonization of gastrostomy tubes. Gastrointest Endosc 1993;39:413.
19. Bohnker GK: Narrow bore nasogastric feeding tube complications. Nutr Clin Prac 1987;2:203.
20. Whatley K, Turner WW, Dey M: Transpyloric passage of feeding tubes. Nutr Supp Serv 1983;3:18.
21. Levenson R, Turner WW, Dyson WW et al: Do weighted nasoenteric feeding tubes facilitate duodenal intubation? J Parenter Enter Nutr 1988;12:135.
22. Payne-James JJ, Rees RG, King C et al: Enteral tube design and its effect on spontaneous transpyloric passage and duration of tube usage. Abstract. J Parenter Enter Nutr 1988;12:215.
23. Metheny NA, Crouse RE, Clark JM et al: pH testing of feeding-tube aspirates to determine placement. Nutr Clin Prac 1994;9:185.
24 Levy H: Pulmonary complications of enteral feeding. In Enteral Nutrition Support for the 1990s: Innovations in Nutrition, Technology, and Techniques. Report of the Twelfth Ross Roundtable on Medical Issues; Ross Products Division, 1992:24–27.
25a. Hirschi R, Karbowski J, Tiefenthal J et al: Tube Placement Verifier. U.S. Patent #5316024. Issued 05/31/94.
25b. Hirschi R: Tube Placement Verifier. U.S. Patent #5325873. Issued 07/05/94.
26. Ponsky JL (ed): Techniques of Percutaneous Gastrostomy. New York: Igaku-Shoin 1988.
27. Duh Q-Y, Way LW: Laparoscopic gastrostomy using T-fasteners as retractors and anchors. Surg Endosc 1993;7:60.
28. Duh Q-Y, Way LW: Prospective evaluation of safety and efficacy of laparoscopic jejunostomy. Surgical Edg 1993;7(3);222.
29. Minard G: Enteral access. Nutr Clin Prac 1994;9:172.
30. Clinical Protocol BC94-2: The effect of automatic flushing on gastrostomy tube clogging rates. FASEB J 1993;7(3):A377.

31. Clinical Protocol BC94-2: The effect of automatic flushing on nasogastric tube clogging rates. J Am Coll Nutr 1993;12(5):598.
32. Benjamin, as reported by Wallace Wm: Nitrogen content of the body and its relation to retention and loss of nitrogen. Fed Proc 1959;18:1125–1129.
33. Cutter E: Medical food ethics now and to come. JAMA 1893;20:239–244.
34. Rose WC: Amino acid requirements of man. Fed Proc 1949;8:546.
35. Greenstein JP, Birnbaum SM, Winitz M et al: Quantitative nutritional studies with water-soluble chemically defined diets. I. Growth, reproduction and lactation in rats. Arch Biochem Biophys 1957;72:396.
36. Winitz M, Graff J, Gallagher N et al: Evaluation of chemical diets as nutrition for man-in-space. Nature 1965;205:741.
37. Winitz M, Seedman DA, Graff J: Studies in metabolic nutrition employing chemically defined diets. I. Extended feeding of normal human adult men. Am J Clin Nutr 1970;23:525.
38. Stephens RV, Randall HT: Use of a concentrated, balanced, liquid elemental diet for nutritional management of catabolic states. Ann Surg 1969;170:642–667.
39. Bounous G: Acute necrosis of the intestinal mucosa. Gastroenterology 1982;82:1457.
40. Bounous G, Sutherland NG, McArdle AH et al: The prophylactic use of an "elemental" diet in experimental shock and intestinal ischemia. Ann Surg 1967;166:312.
41. Bounous G, Hampson LJ, Gurd FN: Cellular nucleotides in hemorrhagic shock: relationship of intestinal metabolic change, to hemorrhagic enteritis and the barrier function of intestinal mucosa. Ann Surg 1964;160:650.
42. Guan D, Ohta H, Green GM: Rat pancreatic secretory response to intraduodenal infusion of elemental vs polymeric defined formula diet. J Parenter Enter Nutr 1994;18:335.
43. Worthen OB, Lorimer JP: Enteral Hyperalimentation with Chemically Defined Elemental Diets: A Source Book. Norwich, NY: Norwich-Eaton Pharmaceuticals, 1979.
44. Cross FS, Akao M, Jones RD: The evaluation of experimental mitral valve prostheses in the dog. Surgery 1969;65:89.
45. McArdle CS, Fisher WD: Cardiac sequelae of hemorrhagic shock. Br J Surg 1973;60:803.
46. Langlois P, Williams HB, Gurd FN: Effect of an elemental diet on mortality rates and gastrointestinal lesions in experimental burns. J Trauma 1972;12:771.
47. Voitk AJ, Chiu C, Gurd FN: Prevention of porcine stress ulcer following hemorrhagic shock with elemental diet. Arch Surg 1972;105:473.
48. Bounous G, Konok G: Intestinal brush border enzymes after short-term mesenteric ischemia. Am J Surg 1977; 133:304.
49. Ziegler F, Ollivier GM, Cynober L et al: Efficiency of enteral nitrogen support in surgical patient: small peptides vs non-degraded proteins. Gut 1990;31:1277.
50. Morgenstern L, Patin CS, Krohn HL: Prolongation of survival in lethally irradiated dogs. Arch Surg 1970;101:586.
51. Hugon J, Bounous G: Elemental diet in the management of the intestinal lesions produced by radiation in the mouse. Can J Surg 1972;15:18.
52. Pageau R, Lallier R, Bounous G: Systemic protection against radiation. I. Effect of an elemental diet on hematopoietic and immunologic systems in rat. Radiat Res 1975;62:357.
53. Bounous G, Lebel E, Shuster J et al: Dietary protection during radiation therapy. Strahlenterapie 1975;149:476.
54. Donaldson SS: Nutritional consequences of radiotherapy. Cancer Res 1977;37:2407.
55. McArdle AH, Reid EC, Laplante MP et al: Prophylaxis against radiation injury: the use of elemental diet prior to and during radiotherapy for invasive bladder cancer and in early postoperative feeding following radical cystectomy and ileal conduit. Arch Surg 1986;121:879.
56. Bounous G, Devroede G, Haddad H et al: Use of elemental diet for intestinal disorders and for the critically ill. Dis Colon Rectum 1974;17:157.
57. Belli DC, Seidman EG, Bouthillier L: Chronic intermittent elemental diet improves growth failure in children with Crohn's disease. Gastroenterology 1988;94:603.
58. Steinhardt HJ, Payer E, Henn K: Enteral nutrition in acute Crohn's disease: effect of whole vs hydrolysed protein on nitrogen economy and intestinal protein loss. Gastroenterology 1988;94:443.
59. Giaffer MH, North G, Holdsworth CD: Controlled trial of polymeric vs elemental diet in treatment of active Crohn's disease. Lancet 1990;335:816.
60. Royal D, Jeejeebhoy KN, Baker JP et al: Comparison of aminoacid vs peptide based enteral diets in active Crohn's disease; clinical and nutritional outcome. Gut 1994;35:783.
61. Russell RI: Review article: dietary and nutritional management of Crohn's disease. Aliment Pharmacol Therap 1991;5:211.
62. Levine GM, Deren JJ, Steiger E et al: Role of oral intake in maintenance of gut mass and disaccharidase activity. Gastroenterology 1974;67:975.
63. Russell RI (ed): Elemental Diets. Boca Raton, FL: CRC Press, 1981:53, 56, 236–241.
64. Donald P, Miller E, Schirmer B et al: Repletion of nutritional parameters in surgical patients receiving peptide *versus* amino acid elemental feedings. Nutr Res 1994;14:3.
65. Talbot JM: Guidelines for the scientific review of enteral food products for special medical purposes. J Parenter Enter Nutr 1991;15 (May–June suppl):99S–174S.
66. Matarese LE: Rationale and efficacy of specialized enteral nutrition. Nutr Clin Prac 1994;9:58.
67. Cockram DB, Moore LW, Acchiardo SR: Response to an oral nutritional supplement for chronic renal failure patients. J Ren Nutr 1994;4:78.
68. Forbes AL: An historical overview of medical foods. In Development of Medical Foods for Rare Diseases. Proceedings of a Workshop, June 9–11, 1991. Bethesda, MD: Life Sciences Research Office, FASEB, 1991.
69. Talbot JM: Guidelines for the scientific review of enteral food products for special medical purposes. J Parenter Enter Nutr 1991;15 (May–June suppl):1475.
70. Al-Saady NM, Blackmore CM, Bennett ED: High fat, low carbohydrate, enteral feeding lowers PaCO$_2$ and reduces the period of ventilation in artificially ventilated patients. Intensive Care Med 1989;15:290.
71. Askanazi J, Carpentier YA, Elwyn DH et al: Influence of total parenteral nutrition on fuel utilization in injury and sepsis. Ann Surt 1980;191:40.
72. Askanazi J, Rosenbaum SH, Hyman AI et al: Respiratory changes induced by the large glucose loads of total parenteral nutrition. JAMA 1980;234:1444.
73. Covelli HD, Black JW, Olsen MS et al: Respiratory failure precipitated by high carbohydrate loads. Ann Intern Med 1981;95:579.
74. Goldstein SA, Askanazi J, Elwyn DH et al: Submaximal exercise in emphysema and malnutrition at two levels

of carbohydrate and fat intake. J Appl Physiol 1989; 67(3):1048.

75. Angelillo VA, Bedi S, Durfee D et al: Effects of low and high carbohydrate feedings in ambulatory patients with chronic obstructive pulmonary disease and chronic hypercapnia. Ann Intern Med 1985;103:883.

76. Peters AL, Davidson MB, Isaac RM: Lack of glucose elevation after simulated tube feeding with a low-carbohydrate, high-fat enteral formula in patients with type I diabetes. Am J Med 1989;87:178.

77. Harley JR, Pohl SL, Isaac RM: Low carbohydrate with fiber enteral formulas: effect on blood glucose excursion in patients with type II diabetes. Abstract. Clin Res 1989;37:141A.

78. Galkowski J, Silverstone FA, Brod M et al: Use of low carbohydrate with fiber enteral formula as a snack for elderly patients with type II diabetes. Abstract. Clin Res 1989;37:89A.

79. DCCT Research Group: The effect of intensive treatment of diabetes on the development and progression of long-term complications in insulin-dependent diabetes mellitus. N Engl J Med 1993;329:977.

80. Eriksson LS, Conn HO: Branched-chain amino acids in the management of hepatic encephalopathy: an analysis of variants. Hepatology 1989;10:228.

81. Marchesini G, Fabbri A, Bianchi GP et al: Nutritional effects of branched-chain amino acid therapy in chronic liver disease. In Branched Chain Amino Acids: Biochemistry, Physiopathology, and Clinical Science. New York: Raven Press, 1992:157–171.

82. Nompleggi DJ, Bonkovsky HL: Nutritional supplementation in chronic liver disease: an analytical review. Hepatology 1994;19:518.

83. Chlebowski RT, Beall G, Grosvenor M: Long-term effects of early nutritional support with new enterotropic peptide-based formula vs. standard enteral formula in HIV-infected patients. Randomized prospective trial. Nutrition 1993;9:507.

84. McCamish MA: Malnutrition and nutrition support interventions: cost benefits outcomes. Nutrition 1993;9:556.

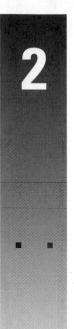

2

Physiology of the Gastrointestinal Tract: As Applied to Patients Receiving Tube Enteral Nutrition

Darlene G. Kelly
C. Richard Fleming

The nutrition practitioner who provides enteral nutrition support will benefit from knowledge of some aspects of gastrointestinal physiology. This chapter will address various topics of gut structure and function including (1) anatomy of the gastrointestinal (GI) tract; (2) GI motility, particularly the function of the lower esophageal sphincter, gastric motor mechanisms that affect acceptance of a meal volume and subsequent emptying into the duodenum, small bowel mixing of chyme with enteric secretions, and colonic transit; (3) gastric and pancreaticobiliary secretion; (4) digestion; and (5) absorption and region of these functions.

ANATOMY OF THE GASTROINTESTINAL TRACT

The mouth masticates food and mixes the bolus with saliva, which is produced by salivary glands lining the mouth, as well as by the parotid, submandibular, and sublingual glands. In addition to lubricating the food bolus, saliva contains the digestive enzyme salivary α–amylase.

The GI tract, extending from the pharynx to the anus, is a mucosa-lined hollow muscular tube. The upper esophagus consists of skeletal muscle, which is in part under voluntary control, while the remainder of the tract, to the level of the anal sphincter, is made up of smooth muscle. The esophagus is approximately 30 to 35 cm long and is lined with squamous epithelium. At its proximal and distal ends are the upper esophageal sphincter and the lower esophageal sphincter, both of which are tonically contracted at rest and relax with swallowing. The esophagus functions primarily as a conduit to transport food from mouth to stomach; it helps to propel the food bolus as a result of peristaltic waves of contraction, which are induced by swallowing.

The stomach provides a receptacle for ingested food and fluid, as well as a grinding function (trituration) that prepares food for controlled entry into the small intestine. Structurally it consists of a complex series of muscular layers that generate the strong contractions needed for trituration. The stomach is lined by a simple columnar epithelium characterized by abundant apical mucus and intercellular tight junctions that provide marked resistance to the effects of the hydrochloric acid the stomach produces.[1] Specialized cells found within the glands of the gastric corpus and antrum include parietal cells, which secrete acid and intrinsic factor, chief cells, which produce the proteolytic enzyme pepsin, and G cells, which synthesize the acid-stimulating hormone gastrin.

The adult small intestine, which functions primarily to absorb nutrients, fluids, and electrolytes, is estimated to be 325 to 785 cm long, depending on the circumstances under which it is measured.[2] The absorptive surface area is magnified from approximately 1 m^2, the surface of a hollow tube of equal length, to more than 200 m^2 (larger than a doubles tennis court) as a result of mucosal folds, fingerlike projections or villi (Fig. 2–1), which are covered by the columnar surface epithelial cells known as enterocytes, and a superimposed fuzzy coat of microvilli (Fig. 2–2) that covers the enterocytes.[3] The villi have a remarkable ability to adapt by changing their height and absorptive capacity as a result of various physiologic conditions. Notably, the villi shorten when deprived of enteral nutrients and become taller and more efficient absorbers during pregnancy or lactation and following resection of the small bowel or colon.[4] This characteristic of intestinal adaptation is an important factor in long-term nutritional support of patients with surgical short-bowel syndrome.

The colon, which is about 150 cm long, acts as an efficient absorber of fluid, a site for salvaging unabsorbed carbohydrate, and a reservoir for fecal material.[5] Proximally, the colon is bounded by the ileocecal valve, a structure formed by reduplication of the mucosa and of circular muscle. This valve functions to prevent reflux of colonic bacteria into the small bowel. The distal extent of the colon is the anus, which is controlled by sphincters composed of smooth muscle and skeletal muscle, the latter of which is under voluntary control. The mucosa of the colon consists of a flat layer of simple columnar epithelium containing large numbers of goblet cells. The colonocytes are active in absorption of water and sodium.

GASTROINTESTINAL MOTILITY

Lower Esophageal Sphincter

The lower esophageal sphincter (LES) is the primary anatomic structure that prevents gastroesophageal reflux. In consists of a 3- to 4-cm-long band of circular smooth muscle fibers that is contracted at rest with a pressure of 10 to 30 mm Hg relative to intragastric pressure. The sphincter, which is under vagal and adrenergic control, relaxes within about 2 seconds of initiation of a swallow and remains open for 6 to 8 seconds until a peristaltic wave traverses the tubular esophagus and the food bolus passes into the stomach. Sphincteric tone is altered by various hormones, medications, foods, and social habits (Table 2–1). Recogni-

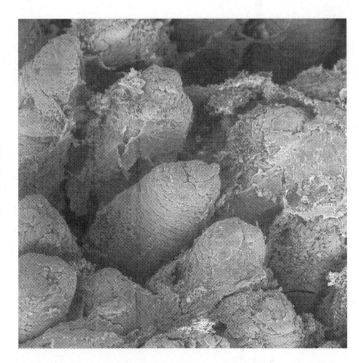

FIGURE 2–1 Scanning electron micrograph of normal intestinal epithelium. The fingerlike villi present throughout the small intestine increase the absorptive surface area by 10-fold. Epithelial cells secrete mucus, which covers the surface of some villi in this micrograph.

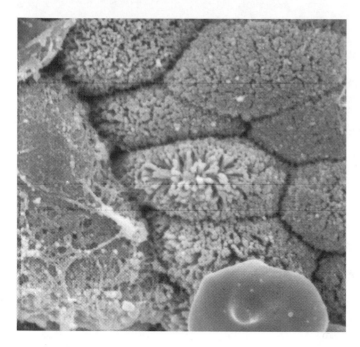

FIGURE 2–2 Scanning electron micrograph of intestinal surface epithelial cells. The cells are studded with microvilli, which are projections that contain digestive enzymes and specialized protein carrier molecules. The microvilli further amplify the surface area by a factor of 100.

tion of these factors may help identify reasons for aspiration in patients who have normal gastroesophageal anatomy and neurologic function.

Intragastric volume also affects gastroesophageal reflux. It has been shown that intragastric volumes of greater than 140 ml can cause reflux in patients with slightly decreased LES

TABLE 2–1 Factors Altering LES Resting Pressure

Increase Sphincter Pressure	Decrease Sphincter Pressure
Gastrin	Secretin
Somatostatin	Cholecystokinin
	Progesterone
β-blocking drugs	Anticholinergic agents
Antacids	Calcium channel blockers
Metoclopramide	Theophylline
Omeprazole	Barbiturates
	Morphine
	Meperidine
Protein meals	Fat
	Chocolate
	Peppermint
	Caffeine
	Alcohol
	Smoking

Modified from Kahrilas PJ: Functional anatomy and physiology of the esophagus. In Castell DO (ed): The Esophagus. Boston: Little Brown & Company, 1992:1–27. Copyright 1992.

resting pressures, while volumes greater than 300 ml are required before reflux occurs in those with normal sphincteric pressures.[6] This has implications for the use of bolus feedings and for safe monitoring of residual intragastric volumes in gastrostomy feedings.

Gastroesophageal Reflux and Aspiration

Often a postpyloric site for nutrient delivery is chosen to attempt to minimize gastroesophageal reflux of tube feeding formula and aspiration pneumonia. Whether postpyloric tube placement achieves this is debatable. In a recent analysis of outpatients in whom enteral feedings were administered through percutaneous endoscopically placed gastrostomy (PEG) or PEGs with jejunal extensions (PEG/J), Taylor and colleagues found that aspiration pneumonia was more frequent in those with PEG/J tubes.[7] An investigation of patients with radiologically placed percutaneous feeding tubes showed that gastrostomy tubes did not induce reflux when studied scintigraphically.[8] Additionally 39 percent of those patients with gastrojejunal extensions of gastrostomy tubes developed pneumonia compared with 25 percent of those with gastrostomies. However, surgical jejunostomies may decrease the incidence of aspiration pneumonia, probably as a result of the more distal site of infusion.[9]

There are no well-designed prospective studies of gastroesophageal reflux of tube feeding formula comparing delivery by nasogastric, nasoenteric, PEG, PEG/J, and surgically placed gastric or jejunal tubes. Whether a feeding tube traversing the LES or the pylorus predisposes to reflux remains to be carefully examined. Furthermore, the precise infusion site of a postpyloric tube is another frequently discussed point: many feel that the ligament of Treitz is the most appropriate level, but until recently attempts at percutaneous endoscopic jejunostomies were rare.[10] This, too, awaits investigation before the proximal versus distal duodenum/jejunum issue can be settled. Clearly, much aspiration pneumonia results from failure to handle secretions rather than regurgitation of tube feedings, and the site used for enteral nutrition will not alter this problem.

Gastric Motor Function

When meals enter the stomach, the fundus accommodates to accept the volume load through a mechanism known as "receptive relaxation," which is a reflex mediated in part by the vagus.[11] This allows filling of the stomach without its developing high intragastric pressures.

As a result of slow sustained tonic contraction, the proximal stomach is also important in controlling gastric emptying of liquids.[12] By regulating transfer of solids toward the pylorus, this portion of the stomach also participates in emptying of solid foods. Peristaltic contractions of the gastric antrum sweep particles toward the pylorus, which allows tiny particles to pass into the duodenum. Larger particles are retropulsed through the orifice of a powerful muscular contraction and in traversing this region undergo shearing and liquefaction.

Factors that control the rates of gastric emptying include the physical form of food (liquids vs solids) as well as chemical constituents (Fig. 2–3). Water is emptied most quickly from the stomach, while liquids containing nutrients empty more slowly.[13] Solids and liquids high in fat are the slowest to be emptied from the stomach. Fluids with high osmolality or high caloric density are emptied more slowly than their more dilute counterparts due to feedback regulation of gastric emptying. Theoretically this controlled emptying process allows optimal matching of nutrient loads and digestive enzymes within the small bowel.

When enteral formulas are delivered to the stomach either by continuous or intermittent feedings, the controlled emptying process for liquids should be intact. By contrast, postpy-

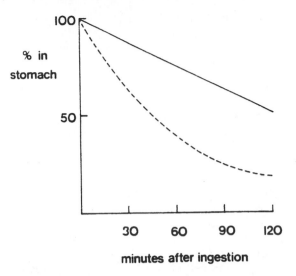

FIGURE 2–3 Emptying patterns of the stomach. The solid line represents emptying of solids from the stomach while more rapid liquid emptying is shown with the dashed line. (From Heading RC: Gastric motility and emptying. In Sircus W, Smith AN [eds]: The Scientific Foundations of Gastroenterology. Philadelphia: WB Saunders, 1980.)

loric infusions bypass this mechanism. Continuous duodenal or jejunal infusions may mimic super-controlled gastric emptying, but intermittent postpyloric feedings, unless presented very slowly, may not be well tolerated. The result may be bowel distention and suboptimal digestion and absorption with resulting diarrhea. In some patients the result may be similar to dumping syndrome that often occurs after a gastrectomy removes the normal pyloric regulation of gastric emptying.

However, in cases of severe gastroparesis, such as may be seen with long-term diabetes, postpyloric feedings may be necessary to prevent weight loss and malnutrition. In these situations a venting gastrostomy may also be required to provide comfort for the patient. Many diabetics with severe gastroparesis have had resolution of symptoms after pancreatic transplantation.

The presence of gastric and transpyloric tubes[14] does not appear to alter gastric emptying rates.[14] Furthermore, duodenogastric reflux is not increased by a thin pliable transpyloric tube. This is important with both temporary nasoenteric tubes and jejunal extensions of gastrostomy tubes.

Small Bowel Motility

Small bowel motor activity can be separated into fasting and fed patterns. Fasting motor activity includes a phase of relative quiescence followed by a period of increasing activity; then comes a short phase of intense activity that is associated with prograde propulsion of any residual materials within the lumen; and finally there is a period of decreasing activity. The cycle recurs every 90 to 100 minutes as long as no food is consumed.[15] This pattern is somewhat analogous to a program of muscle training and may play a part in maintaining smooth muscle health. On feeding, the pattern changes to one of irregular contractions that are effective in mixing chyme within the lumen with digestive juices secreted into the gut. This fed pattern is slowly propulsive and appears to have a role in optimizing contact with the absorptive mucosal surface.

Infusion of an elemental formula into the jejunum, as well as oral intake of the formula or of a test meal consisting of solid foods, interrupts the fasting pattern of motor activity in dogs.[16] However, jejunal infusion results in less stimulation of jejunal-fed pattern motor activity, and with increasing rates of infusion (from 0.5 to 2.5 kcal min^{-1}) or increasing osmolality of the infusate progressive inhibition of jejunal motility occurs, making motor activity less propulsive.[17] Small intestinal motility increases after a meal and causes chyme to enter the proximal colon.[18] However, if unabsorbed nutrients are presented to the ileum, gastric emptying and small bowel transit both slow.[19] This mechanism, termed the "ileal brake," appears to be under hormonal control and presumably occurs in an attempt to maximize contact time of chyme with the absorptive surface.

Colonic Motility

Colonic motility functions to enhance water absorption, to maintain the normal colonic bacterial flora that salvage unabsorbed carbohydrate by fermenting them to produce short chain fatty acids,[5] preferred fuels for colonocytes,[20] and to control timing of defecation. Three separate motor patterns occur in the colon.[18] The pattern of motility in the right colon is retrograde, and this tends to retain the fecal mass in the cecum and ascending colon for storage and fluid absorption. In the midcolon the motor pattern is slowly retrograde. The strong contractile activity of the distal colon moves the fecal mass forward at defecation.

The ingestion of food prompts mass movement of fecal material within the colon and has been termed the "gastrocolic reflex."[18] This re-

sponse begins slowly after a meal and persists for 1 hour or more. The response occurs promptly if food is placed directly into the duodenum,[21] as well as when essential amino acids or sodium oleate are infused into the duodenum.[22]

GASTROINTESTINAL SECRETION

Gastric Secretion

In health, gastric secretion is stimulated by the thought of food and the act of eating (cephalic phase), by the presence of food in the stomach resulting in distention and bathing of the lumen by protein and other food components (gastric phase), and by the presence of amino acids within the small bowel (intestinal phase). Of these three, the gastric phase is quantitatively most important. Gastrin, which is released from the G cells in the gastric antrum, stimulates the parietal cells in the body of the stomach to secrete hydrochloric acid. Vagal stimulation also results in acid secretion. Inhibition of acid secretion results from the presence of hydrochloric acid within the gastric lumen as well as by fat, acid, and hypertonic glucose within the proximal duodenum. Several hormones and gut peptides, such as somatostatin, secretin, cholecystokinin, gastric-inhibitory polypeptide (GIP), and neurotensin, are also inhibitory.

In comparisons of gastric and duodenal nutrient infusion in healthy volunteers, gastric acid secretion was significantly increased above baseline values when an isotonic solution of nutrients was delivered to the stomach.[23] This secretion persisted during the hour following infusion. By contrast, infusion of the solution into the duodenum decreased gastric acid output below basal levels. Gastric emptying was slowed during duodenal infusion compared with gastric infusion; thus residual volume resulting from salivary and gastric secretions remained in the stomach longer when postpyloric feedings were given. Valentine and colleagues measured serial pHs of gastric aspirates from critically ill patients receiving either continuous intragastric or intraduodenal polymeric formulas.[24] Fewer patients receiving duodenal feedings had pH values of ≥5 than did those on intragastric infusions. These authors felt that continuous tube feedings did not provide adequate prophylaxis against gastric stress ulceration.

Continuous intragastric infusions of a polymeric formula into patients requiring mechanical ventilation stimulated gastric acid secretion in a dose-related manner in studies by Rigaud and colleagues.[25] The protein and hemoglobin concentrations in the juice were significantly higher than in normal gastric juice, although there was no clinically significant bleeding during the study.

Layon and coworkers found that gastric pH was < 4.0 for less time during intraduodenal infusion of an enteral polymeric formula than when saline was infused.[26] The antacid dose required to maintain the pH above 4.0 was also significantly less with the nutrient formula. These investigators found that the gastrin levels did not increase from baseline with either infusion nor were they different under the two circumstances, but the GIP level was significantly increased in response to enteral feeding. They hypothesized that elevation of plasma GIP may decrease intragastric volume and acidity independent of change in serum gastrin concentration.

The possible inhibition of gastric acid secretion by duodenal nutrient infusions may be beneficial in the critical care setting where stress ulceration is of concern. However, the observed delay in gastric emptying seen with duodenal infusion may actually predispose to gastroesophageal reflux and potentially to aspiration, possibly offsetting the "acid advantage."

Pancreatic Secretion

Pancreatic secretion, like that of the stomach, has a cephalic phase associated with anticipation of eating and mastication of food. The most potent stimulation of pancreatic secretion, however, results from nutrients within the duodenal lumen.[27] Glucose maximally stimulates secretion, but its effect is not sustained. Essential amino acids cause submaximal but sustained enzyme secretion, and fats cause maximal, sustained secretion. Cholecystokinin (CCK), which is produced and released by the intestinal cells when nutrients are present, stimulates pancreatic enzyme production and release, as well as gallbladder contraction. There is a gradient of CCK production in the small bowel, with most being present in the duodenum.

In healthy subjects, continuous intragastric and intraduodenal polymeric nutrient infusions both stimulated pancreatic enzyme release, but the observed stimulation by intragastric feedings was delayed.[23] The rate of enzyme secretion was directly related to the rate of entry of nutrients into the duodenum and to rises in the plasma concentrations of CCK and pancreatic polypeptide.[28]

Stabile and colleagues made similar observations in dogs, showing that both intraduodenal elemental and full liquid diets caused dose-related increases in pancreatic protein (thus enzyme) outputs over basal rates.[29] They contrasted this with intravenous nutrients, which did not stimulate pancreatic secretion. Contrasting data in dogs showed similar pancreatic protease outputs in controls compared with intravenous nutrients and with elemental diets infused into the stomach or jejunum.[30]

Studies of more distal infusion of nutrient solutions in animals and humans have yielded variable and confusing results. Ileal and colonic infusion fairly consistently inhibit pancreatic secretion, but the nutritional benefit of these is, of course, minimal. Ragins and colleagues used a dog model to show that an elemental diet infused into the jejunum did not increase pancreatic water or bicarbonate output, whereas instilling the diet into the stomach was stimulatory.[31] In dogs, Klein and associates demonstrated decreased pancreatic amylase output in response to jejunal glucose perfusion, no change from baseline with amino acids, and stimulation with fat.[32] Yet when Grant and coworkers infused various diets into the jejunum of a patient receiving total parental nutrition (TPN) following a complicated cholecystectomy, they found that all nutrient-containing solutions stimulated lipase production, even though they decreased amylase and bicarbonate output.[33] The elemental formulas were somewhat less stimulatory than the polymeric formula.

Vidon and coworkers, studying healthy volunteers, found that jejunal infusion of two polymeric formulas suppressed previously stimulated pancreatic secretion.[34] Furthermore, this suppression was more marked with higher calorie infusions. Subsequently the same authors found that high calorie infusions consisting of carbohydrate or lipids decreased pancreatic secretion, and they coined the term "jejunal brake" to describe this phenomenon.[35]

In acute pancreatitis, stimulation of pancreatic enzyme synthesis and subsequent secretion is of concern. Indeed, usual therapy is directed toward reducing enzyme secretion. Traditionally this has taken the form of keeping patients nil per os (NPO). Subsequently, TPN was added to the treatment plans. However, most recently the use of enteral nutrition, often delivered by a nasojejunal tube, has been successful in treating some patients with acute pancreatitis.

DIGESTION

Digestion begins in the mouth where salivary α-amylase can interact with starch. The enzyme has a pH optimum within the neutral range, and when the bolus reaches the acidic environment of the stomach, enzymatic activity stops. How much digestion occurs depends on chewing time and the physical-chemical nature of the food bolus.

Within the stomach acid denatures protein, a process that involves breakdown of the noncovalent protein structure with unfolding of the molecule to expose peptide bonds to proteolytic enzymes. Pepsin is secreted into the stomach in its proenzyme form pepsinogen, and after activation by gastric acid, it begins proteolysis of dietary protein. Pepsin secretion has been shown to be normal in infants given constant-rate intragastric enteral nutrition.[36] Gastric lipase is also secreted by the stomach where it cleaves the 1-α bond of triglyceride, particularly in milk fat.[37] This function may be particularly important in neonates when pancreatic lipolytic function is not completely developed.

The pancreas synthesizes enzymes that provide luminal digestion. Pancreatic α-amylase is secreted in its active form into the lumen where it cleaves the α-1,4 glycosidic bonds of starch to yield maltose and maltotriose and limit dextrins. These products along with the disaccharides undergo further digestion as a result of interaction with brush border disaccharidases and trisaccharidases. Sucrase and lactase are found in highest concentrations in the jejunum, whereas maltase is most abundant in the ileum.[38]

Protein digestion requires several different peptidases, including trypsin, chymotrypsin, elastase, and carboxypeptidase A and B. These enzymes are produced by the pancreas and secreted in their inactive proenzyme forms for subsequent activation within the intestinal lumen. Each of these enzymes is specific for hydrolysis of bonds adjacent to individual amino acids. The peptide products resulting from luminal digestion are about 40 percent amino acids and 60 percent oligopeptides.[39] In addition to luminal digestion, peptides undergo proteolysis at the brush border and intracellularly through interaction with aminopeptidase and specific dipeptidases.

Lipid digestion is somewhat more complicated, in large part because of the hydrophobic nature of long-chain fat. To provide a physical form that can interact with luminal enzymes, lipids first undergo emulsification as a result of the shearing activity in the gastric antrum. Within the duodenum the major pancreatic lipolytic products, lipase and colipase, bind to the surface of the emulsified lipid particles where they hydrolyze ester bonds of the triglycerides. This process requires the detergent action of conjugated bile acids that are released from the liver. Fatty acids released from the lipid droplet (Fig. 2–4) are then incorporated into micelles and can move through the chyme to the mucosal surface for absorption.

Medium-chain triglyceride (MCT) is less hydrophobic than long-chain triglyceride. Because it presents a larger surface area for intra-

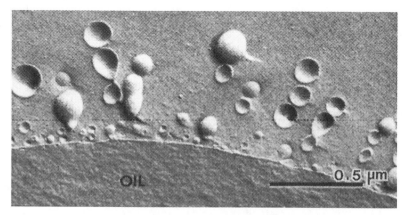

FIGURE 2–4   Freeze fracture electron micrograph demonstrating surface digestion of a lipid droplet. The pancreatic enzyme lipase is anchored to the lipid droplet by colipase. Fatty acids hydrolyzed from triglyceride by enzymatic action are then released from the droplet into the surrounding milieu where they are solubilized by bile acids. (Reprinted from Biochem Biophys Acta, vol. 751, WW Rigler and JS Patton, The production of liquid crystalline product phases by pancreatic lipase in the absence of bile salts. A freeze fracture study, 444-454, 1983 with kind permission of Elsevier Science-NL, Sara Burgerhartstraat 25, 1055 KV Amsterdam, The Netherlands.)

luminal hydrolysis, MCT is more rapidly hydrolyzed and more completely absorbed.[40] The 6 to 10 carbon fatty acids that are released have greater solubility in water than do their longer chain counterparts, so bile is not needed for solubilization. In addition, about 30 percent of MCT is absorbed intact, so pancreatic enzyme activity is less essential. These features of MCT are used clinically in enteral formulas that contain a high percentage of lipids as MCT.

Caliari and associates reported that pancreatic enzyme replacement was essential in severe pancreatic insufficiency resulting from pancreatectomy when either polymeric or elemental enteral diets were used.[41] Both fecal fat and nitrogen losses were responsive to pancreatic supplementation.

ABSORPTION

The general function of the duodenum is to neutralize the acid contained in the chyme that enters it, regulate gastric emptying and secretion, and alter its luminal contents to be iso-osmotic with blood. Osmotic pressures are driving forces for transport of fluid throughout the small bowel and the colon down to the level of the sigmoid colon, where an increasing osmotic gradient can be maintained within the lumen. Digestion occurs primarily in the jejunum, and nutrients are absorbed throughout the small intestine (Fig. 2–5). The colon is instrumental in transporting water and electrolytes.

Carbohydrates are absorbed as monosaccharides at sites adjacent to the brush border enzymes; thus they cannot diffuse away. Galactose and glucose are absorbed by active transport, and fructose is absorbed through facilitated diffusion in an energy-independent process. Glucose is transported by a membrane carrier protein against a concentration gradient as a result of cotransport with sodium, which moves down its concentration gradient.[42] This principle of glucose absorption is the basis for oral rehydration solutions,[43] which are gaining popularity in the enteral rehabilitation of patients with short-bowel syndrome.[44] Although sucrose is almost completely absorbed in the small intestine, Levitt found that up to 20 percent of starch escapes absorption in the small bowel and enters the colon.[45] Within the colon bacteria salvage this starch through fermentation and production of short-chain fatty acids.[5] These act as a primary fuel for the colonocytes.[20]

Although intact proteins can be absorbed early in life, providing antibodies derived from colostrum, this ability is lost during normal de-

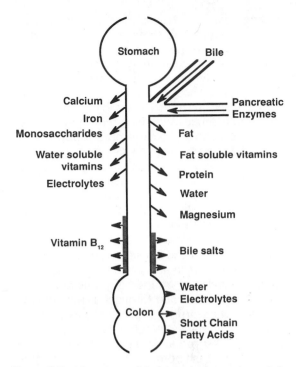

FIGURE 2–5 The sites of intestinal absorption. Calcium, magnesium, and iron are preferentially absorbed from proximal small intestine. The hatched segment indicates that vitamin B_{12} and bile salts are actively absorbed by specialized transport mechanisms that are found in the distal ileum. (Modified from Booth CC: Effect of location along the small intestine on absorption of nutrients. In Code CF, Heidel W [eds]: Handbook of Physiology, sec. 6, vol. III, Baltimore: Williams & Wilkins, 1968.)

velopment. Instead, amino acids and small peptides are the main forms in which proteins are absorbed. Dipeptides and tripeptides compete for transport, but this process is more efficient than transport of individual amino acids.[46] Once small peptides have been transported into the enterocytes, they are hydrolyzed to free amino acids. As for glucose, active cotransport of amino acids with sodium ions occurs from the small intestine. In addition, carrier mechanisms exist for groups of amino acids that share chemical characteristics. Small peptides are absorbed in the jejunum and ileum, but amino acids are primarily absorbed from the jejunum.

Fat is absorbed predominantly in the duodenum and proximal jejunum through efficient passive diffusion. However, if the jejunum is resected, the ileum can transport unabsorbed fatty acids. Fatty acid–binding protein found in the villi helps to direct fatty acids toward the endoplasmic reticulum of the enterocyte for reesterification.[47] Transport of long chain lipids occurs through the lymphatics, while that of MCT is through the portal vein. This characteristic of MCT circulation is important in situations where lymph flow is compromised.

Some minerals and vitamins are absorbed through specialized processes that may have important implications in enteral nutrition. Active absorption of calcium occurs primarily in the duodenum through a vitamin D–dependent transcellular route.[48] However, a passive paracellular route may also be used for calcium transport, and this is present in all parts of the small intestine. Iron is also absorbed most efficiently in the duodenum. At the brush border, ferrous iron is oxidized to the ferric form before interacting with the brush border carrier. This pathway for iron absorption is closely controlled, depending on the body's need for iron. Zinc can be absorbed throughout the small intestine, but absorptive capacity is greatest in the jejunum.[49] Because intraluminal glucose stimulates zinc absorption, it appears that they share a common brush border carrier. Zinc undergoes enterohepatic circulation with secretion in the bile and subsequent reabsorption in the distal small intestine, so in cases of enterocutaneous or biliary fistula, losses can be great. Based on studies of isolated segments of intestine, it appears that magnesium is absorbed primarily in the distal small intestine[50] and the colon[51] by passive diffusion. However, there is also evidence for an active transport mechanism in isolated rat small intestine and descending colon, which is important when magnesium intake is low.[52] Vitamin D given in pharmacologic doses enhances magnesium absorption but also increases urinary excretion. Magnesium loss is prominent in patients with short-bowel syndrome and inflammatory bowel disease.

The absorption of vitamins also involves specialized transport mechanisms, some of which are restricted to regions of the bowel. The fat-soluble vitamins A, D, E, and K require bile for absorption and can become deficient in patients with impaired bile production and release. Vitamin B_{12} is protected from the gastric acid milieu by binding with R protein, which is produced within the stomach.[53] On reaching the small bowel, the vitamin is cleaved from this protein and then combines with intrinsic factor, also a gastric product, for transit through the small intestine. Vitamin B_{12} intrinsic factor complex is actively absorbed by the brush border of the terminal ileum. Although receptors for the vitamin B_{12} intrinsic factor complex were found to be present in this distal three

fifths of human small intestine,[54] resection of more than 80 cm of ileum has been shown to reduce absorption of the vitamin.[55] However, clinical evidence of deficiency usually does not appear for several years due to hepatic storage of vitamin B_{12}. Gastrectomy also causes vitamin B_{12} deficiency over time, but this occurs because of lack of intrinsic factor. In pernicious anemia parietal cell antibodies are produced, causing production of intrinsic factor to cease and subsequent malabsorption of vitamin B_{12}. Furthermore, drugs that inhibit acid secretion by the parietal cells, including H2 blockers,[56] also decrease absorption of this vitamin. Patients frequently use these antiulcer medications for years, and their vitamin B_{12} status should be monitored. All these forms of malabsorption require parenteral administration of the vitamin.

Bile acids are transported to the distal ileum where more than 90 percent of the luminal load is absorbed. Absorbed bile acids enter the portal vein and are cleared by the liver to undergo enterohepatic circulation. When < 100 cm of distal ileum is resected, bile acids are lost into the colon where they are metabolized by bacteria and cause bile acid diarrhea, but hepatic bile acid synthesis can be accelerated sufficiently to expand the bile acid pool for normal fat absorption to occur.[57] In this case dietary fat does not need to be decreased, and the bile-acid-binding resin cholestyramine may be used to treat diarrhea. However, when > 100 cm of distal ileum is resected, the liver can no longer adequately synthesize bile acids, and fat malabsorption occurs. In this situation, fat intake should be decreased, since malabsorbed fat entering the colon causes fatty acid diarrhea, and treatment with cholestyramine only results in further diminished fat absorption and worsening of diarrhea.

Absorption of nutrients from oral solid food was compared with polymeric and elemental tube feedings infused distal to the ligament of Treitz in a study of hospitalized patients reported by Heymsfield and colleagues.[58] All three forms of nutrition resulted in equal absorption of macronutrients as well as potassium, phosphorus, calcium, magnesium, sodium, and chloride. These data suggest that digestion and absorption of nutrient presented to the jejunum is equivalent to that occurring with oral intake. Furthermore, absorption of carbohydrates and protein from polymeric formula infused into the jejunum was equal and efficient whether patients were malnourished or well nourished.[59]

REGIONAL FLUID AND ELECTROLYTE ABSORPTION

Although fluid and electrolyte transport occurs throughout the small intestine and colon, certain regional characteristics of absorption are particularly important in considerations of enteral nutrition support. Approximately 2 L of fluid enter the GI tract daily in the form of food and water, while nearly 7 L are secreted into the gut in the form of salivary, gastric, pancreaticobiliary, and intestinal secretions.[60] Of this fluid load, about 85 percent (7.5 L) is absorbed in the jejunum and ileum, and 1.4 L are absorbed from the colon. The normal colon can increase absorption of water by an additional 4 L/day.[61] The potential importance of the colon in compensating for major small intestinal resection is apparent, and in cases of borderline short-bowel syndrome an intact colon can prevent the need for parenteral fluid support. Intestinal water absorption occurs as a result of flow-down osmotic gradients. Oral rehydration solutions, based on cotransport of sodium and glucose and resulting osmotic shifts of water, can be used to compensate for inadequate water absorption in short-bowel syndrome.[44]

Sodium is absorbed throughout the intestine, although mechanisms involved differ regionally. Permeability of the small intestine to sodium (and water) decreases in a proximal to distal manner. Potassium, by contrast, is absorbed from the proximal small bowel and distal colon but is secreted from the distal small intestine and proximal colon. Chloride is absorbed in exchange for bicarbonate in the ileum and colon. Knowledge of regionality of fluid and electrolyte transport can be helpful in predicting the result of resection of various segments of the intestine and in planning therapeutic programs for affected patients.

Spiller and coworkers reported the effect of very low sodium enteral formulas on transport of sodium and water in jejunal segments of healthy subjects.[62] Sodium absorption was directly proportional to sodium concentration of the perfusate, and with extremely low sodium formulas net secretion occurred. Water absorption, as expected, paralleled sodium transport. This implies that in patients with short-bowel syndrome and end jejunostomies, use of low-sodium formulas may actually result in net loss of sodium and water. Because the ileum and colon have decreased permeability to sodium, patients who have undergone proximal resection with preservation of the distal intestine should not experience this effect.

REFERENCES

1. Kelly DG, Code CF, Lechago J et al: Physiological and morphological characteristics of progressive disruption of the canine gastric mucosal barrier. Dig Dis Sci 1979;24:424–441.
2. Underhill BML: Intestinal length in man. Br Med J 1955;2:1243–1246.
3. Caspary WF: Physiology and pathophysiology of intestinal absorption. Am J Clin Nutr 1992;55:299S–308S.
4. Lo CW, Walker WA: Changes in the gastrointestinal tract during enteral or parenteral feeding. Nutr Rev 1989;47:193–198.
5. Bond JH, Currier BE, Buchwald H et al: Colonic conservation of malabsorbed carbohydrate. Gastroenterology 1980;78:444–447.
6. Ahtaridis G, Snape WS Jr, Cohen S: Lower esophageal sphincter pressure as an index of gastroesophageal acid reflux. Dig Dis Sci 1981;26:993–998.
7. Taylor CA, Larson DE, Ballard DJ et al: Predictors of outcome after percutaneous endoscopic gastrostomy: a community-based study. Mayo Clin Proc 1992;67:1042–1049.
8. Olson DL, Krubsack AJ, Stewart ET: Percutaneous enteral alimentation: gastrostomy versus gastrojejunostomy. Radiology 1993;187:105–108.
9. Burtch GD, Shatney CH: Feeding gastrostomy: assistant or assassin? Am Surg 1985;51:204–207.
10. Shike M, Wallach C, Likier H: Direct percutaneous endoscopic jejunostomies. Gastrointest Endosc 1991;37:62–65.
11. Azpiros F, Malagelada J-R: Vagally mediated gastric relaxation induced by intestinal nutrients in the dog. Am J Physiol 1986;251:G727–G735.
12. Collins PJ, Houghton LA, Read NW et al: Role of the proximal and distal stomach in mixed solid and liquid meal emptying. Gut 1991;32:615–619.
13. Malagelada J-R, Azpiroz F: Determinants of gastric emptying and transit in the small intestine. In Wood JD (ed): Handbook of Physiology, sec. 6, vol. I, Part 2, Chap. 23, Bethesda: American Physiological Society, 1989:909–937.
14. Müller-Lissner SA, Fimmel CJ, Will N et al: Effect of gastric and transpyloric tubes on gastric emptying and duodenogastric reflux. Gastroenterology 1982;83:1276–1279.
15. Szurszewski JH: A migrating electric complex of the canine small intestine. Am J Physiol 1969;217:1757–1763.
16. Schmid HR, Ehrlein HJ, Feinle C: Effects of enteral infusion of nutrients on canine intestinal motor-patterns. J Gastrointest Mot 1992;4:279–292.
17. Schmid H-R, Ehrlein H-J: Effects of enteral infusion of hypertonic saline and nutrients on canine jejunal motor patterns. Dig Dis Sci 93;38:1062–1072.
18. Christensen J: Colonic motility In Wood JD (ed): Handbook of Physiology, sec. 6, vol. I, Part 2, Chap. 24. Bethesda: American Physiological Society, 1989:939–973.
19. Read N, McFarlane A, Kinsman R et al: The effect of infusion of nutrient solutions into the ileum on gastrointestinal transit and plasma levels of neurotensin and enteroglucagon. Gastroenterology 1984;86:274–280.
20. Roediger WEW: Role of anaerobic bacteria in the metabolic welfare of the colonic mucosa in man. Gut 1980;21:793–798.
21. Connell AM, Logan CJH: The role of gastrin in gastroileocolic responses. Am J Dig Dis 1967;12:277–284.

22. Meshkinpour H, Dinoso VP, Lorber SH: Effect of intraduodenal administration of essential amino acids and sodium oleate on motor activity of the sigmoid colon. Gastroenterology 1974;66:373–377.

23. Holtmann G, Kelly DG, DiMagno EP: What is the preferred site of enteral nutrition in humans with a normal gut? Gastroenterology 1992;102:A558.

24. Valentine RJ, Turner WW Jr, Borman KR et al: Does nasoenteral feeding afford adequate gastroduodenal stress prophylaxis? Crit Care Med 1986;14:599–601.

25. Rigaud D, Chastre J, Accary JP et al: Intragastric pH profile during acute respiratory failure in patients with chronic obstructive pulmonary disease. Chest 1986;90:58–63.

26. Layon AJ, Florete OG, Day AL et al: The effect of duodenojejunal alimentation on gastric pH and hormones in intensive care unit patients. Chest 1991;99:695–702.

27. Go VLW, Hofmann AF, Summerskill WHJ: Pancreozymin bioassay in man based on pancreatic enzyme secretion: potency of specific amino acids and other digestive products. J Clin Invest 1970;49:1558–1564.

28. Holtmann G, Kelly DG, DiMagno EP: What regulates human pancreatic enzyme secretion during nutrient infusion into the stomach or duodenum? Gastroenterology 1992;102:A270.

29. Stabile BE, Borzatta M, Stubbs RS: Pancreatic secretory responses to intravenous hyperalimentation and intraduodenal elemental and full liquid diets. J Parenter Enter Nutr 1984;8:377–380.

30. Traverso LW, Abou-Zamzam AM, Maxwell DS et al: The effect of total parenteral nutrition or elemental diet on pancreatic proteolytic activity and ultrastructure. J Parenter Enter Nutr 1981;5:496–500.

31. Ragins H, Levenson SM, Signer R et al: Intrajejunal administration of an elemental diet at neutral pH avoids pancreatic stimulation. Am J Surg 1973;126:606–614.

32. Klein E, Shemesh E, Ben-Ari G et al: Effects of enteral nutrition on exocrine pancreatic secretion in dogs. Mt Sinai J Med 1988;55:362–364.

33. Grant JP, Davey-McCrae J, Snyder PJ: Effect of enteral nutrition on human pancreatic secretions. J Parenter Enter Nutr 1987;11:302–304.

34. Vidon N, Pfeiffer A, Franchisseur C et al: Effect of different caloric loads in human jejunum on meal-stimulated and nonstimulated biliopancreatic secretion. Am J Clin Nutr 1988;47:400–405.

35. Vidon N, Chaussade S, Merite F et al: Inhibitory effect of high caloric load of carbohydrates or lipids on human pancreatic secretions: a jejunal brake. Am J. Clin Nutr 1989;50:231–236.

36. de Angelis GL, Poitevin C, Cezard JP et al: Gastric pepsin and acid secretion during total parenteral nutrition and constant-rate enteral nutrition in infancy. J Parenter Enter Nutr 1988;12:505–508.

37. Moreau H, Laugier R, Gargouri Y et al: Human preduodenal lipase is entirely of gastric fundic origin. Gastroenterology 1988;95:1221–1226.

38. Triadou N, Bataille J, Schmitz J: Longitudinal study of the human intestinal brush border membrane proteins. Distribution of the disaccharidases and peptidases. Gastroenterology 1983;85:1326–1332.

39. Erickson RH, Kim YS: Digestion and absorption of dietary protein. Ann Rev Med 1990;41:133–139.

40. Jensen C, Buist NRM, Wilson T: Absorption of individual fatty acids from long chain or medium chain triglycerides in very small infants. Am J Clin Nutr 1986;43:745–751.

41. Caliari S, Benini L, Bonfante F et al: Pancreatic extracts are necessary for the absorption of elemental and polymeric enteral diets in severe pancreatic insufficiency. Scand J Gastroenterol 1993;28:749–752.

42. Semenza N, Kessler M, Schmidt U et al: The small-intestinal sodium-glucose cotransporter(s). Ann NY Acad Sci 1985;456:83–96.

43. Ghisan FK: The transport of electrolytes in the gut and the use of oral rehydration solutions. Pediatr Clin North Am 1988;35:35–51.

44. Camilleri M, Prather CM, Evans MA et al: Balance studies and polymeric glucose solution to optimize therapy after massive intestinal resection. Mayo Clin Proc 1992;67:755–760.

45. Levitt MD: Malabsorption of starch: a normal phenomenon. Gastroenterology 1983;85:769–770.

46. Kim YS, Erickson RH: Role of peptidases of the human small intestine in protein digestion. Gastroenterology 1985;88:1071–1073.

47. Levy E: Selected aspects of intraluminal and intracellular phases of intestinal fat absorption. Can J Physiol Pharmacol 1992;70:413–419.

48. Bronner F: Current concepts of calcium absorption. J Nutr 1992;122:641–643.

49. Sandström B: Dose dependence of zinc and manganese absorption in man. Proc Nutr Soc 1992;51:211–218.

50. Kayne LH, Lee DBN: Intestinal magnesium absorption. Miner Electrolyte Metab 1993;19:210–217.

51. Hardwick LL, Jones MR, Brautbar N et al: Magnesium absorption: mechanisms and the influence of vitamin D, calcium and phosphate. J Nutr 1991;121:13–23.

52. Karbach U: Cellular-mediated and diffusive magnesium transport across the descending colon of the rat. Gastroenterology 1989;96:1282–1289.

53. Donaldson RM: How does cobalamin (vitamin B_{12}) enter and traverse the ileal cell? Gastroenterology 1985;88:1069–1071.

54. Hagedorn CH, Alpers JH: Distribution of intrinsic factor-vitamin B_{12} receptors in human intestine. Gastroenterology 1977;73:1019–1022.

55. Lenz K: The effect of the site of lesion and extent of resection on duodenal bile acid concentration and vitamin B_{12} absorption in Crohn's disease. Scand J Gastroenterol 1975;10:241–248.

56. Steinberg WM, King CE, Toskes PP: Malabsorption of protein-bound cobalamin but not unbound cobalamin during cimetidine administration. Dig Dis Sci 1980;25:188–191.

57. Hofmann AF, Poley JR: Role of bile acid malabsorption in the pathogenesis of diarrhea and steatorrhea in patients with ileal resection. I. Response to cholestyramine or replacement of dietary long-chain triglycerides with medium-chain triglycerides. Gastroenterology 1972;62:918–934.

58. Heymsfield SB, Bleier J, Whitmire L et al: Nutrient bioavailability from nasojejunally administered enteral formulas: comparison to solid food. Am J Clin Nutr 1984;39:243–250.

59. Benya R, Zarling EJ, Monteagudo J et al: Protein and carbohydrate absorption efficiency of chronically malnourished and well-nourished patients during enteral feeding initiation. J Am Coll Nutr 1991;10:50–56.

60. Phillips SF: Diarrhea: a current view of pathophysiology. Gastroenterology 1972;63:495–518.

61. Debognie JC, Phillips SF: Capacity of the human colon to absorb fluid. Gastroenterology 1978;74:698–703.

62. Spiller RC, Jones BJM, Silk DBA: Jejunal water and electrolyte absorption from two proprietary enteral feeds in man: importance of sodium content. Gut 1987;28:681–687.

3

Enteral Nutrition and Protein Metabolism

PER-OLOF HASSELGREN
TORY A. MEYER

Trauma, sepsis, and other critical illnesses are associated with pronounced changes in whole body protein balance caused by specific changes in protein synthesis and breakdown rates in various organs and tissues.[1] Nutritional support is frequently an important component of the treatment of injured and septic patients. The role of enteral vs parenteral nutrition in critical illness has been the subject of a number of studies, both in experimental animals and patients. Most of those reports have focused on mortality rates, function of the immune system, infectious complications, and bacterial translocation in the gut; few studies have been published addressing specifically the effect of enteral feeding on protein turnover rates. In several reports, however, data have provided indirect evidence of changes in protein metabolism during enteral feeding, such as changes in nitrogen balance; concentrations of certain plasma proteins, including acute phase proteins; plasma amino acids; muscle weight; urinary excretion of 3-methylhistidine (3-MH); intestinal weight; and mucosal protein content.

This chapter will review changes in protein metabolism that have been ascribed to the ef-

fect of enteral nutrition during sepsis and following injury. Because catabolic hormones and cytokines are important mediators of altered protein metabolism in critical illness, we will also discuss how enteral feeding affects the release of these substances. Although the role of enteral nutrition has been examined in other conditions as well, such as starvation, cancer, gastrointestinal (GI) disease, and liver disease, this chapter will focus on enteral nutrition and protein metabolism following injury and sepsis, in part reflecting the research interest in our laboratory.

When considering the role of enteral feeding, three important aspects are crucial: route of administration (enteral vs parenteral), timing (early vs delayed nutritional support), and composition of the nutritional support. Most of this chapter will focus on route of administration, but the other aspects will be briefly discussed as well.

To give a better understanding of changes in protein metabolism induced by enteral feeding in critical illness, we will first summarize the response to sepsis and injury of protein turnover and the role of catabolic hormones and cytokines. A more detailed review of sepsis-related changes in protein metabolism was published recently.[1] We will then discuss results that have been generated in experimental ani-

Supported in part by NIH grants R01 DK37908 and R01 DK44201 and by grants #15851 and #15861 from the Shriners of North America.

23

mals and patients receiving enteral nutrition. Few studies have been reported in which the primary goal was to measure protein turnover rates following enteral feeding. Most information about protein metabolism, therefore, has been extracted from papers that were mainly designed to study morbidity and mortality rates. Results other than those related to protein metabolism, such as septic complications, bacterial translocation, and mortality rates, will only be discussed briefly. Those aspects of enteral feeding are reviewed in other chapters of this volume.

PROTEIN METABOLISM IN SEPSIS AND TRAUMA

The hypermetabolism that follows severe injury and infection represents a coordinated response to reprioritize synthetic capacity from peripheral to visceral tissues and to boost host defense against infection (Fig. 3–1).[1,2] Elevated circulating levels of glucocorticoids, catecholamines, and cytokines induce net protein breakdown in skeletal muscle by inhibiting amino acid uptake, decreasing protein syn-

thetic activity, and increasing the energy-ubiquitin-dependent pathway of muscle proteolysis.[3-8] Amino acids released from peripheral tissues, in particular alanine and glutamine, are taken up by the liver and intestine. Glutamine is a primary fuel in intestinal epithelial cells, and its metabolism produces alanine, which has direct access to the liver through the portal vein.[9] Increased intestinal protein synthesis has been demonstrated during sepsis and endotoxemia[10,11] and probably reflects a combination of increased epithelial cell turnover,[12] increased production of secreted gut hormones such as PYY and VIP,[13,14] and perhaps increased intestinal production of acute phase proteins and mucus glycoproteins.[15,16] The liver uses circulating amino acids both for gluconeogenesis and to produce acute phase proteins.[1,17] During the acute phase response, reprioritization of hepatic protein synthesis results in decreased production of constitutive carrier proteins, such as prealbumin, albumin, and transferrin, and increased synthesis of immunoactive proteins, such as C-reactive protein (CRP), complement factors C3 and C4, α_2-macroglobulin, and α_1-antitrypsin (AAT).[18,19]

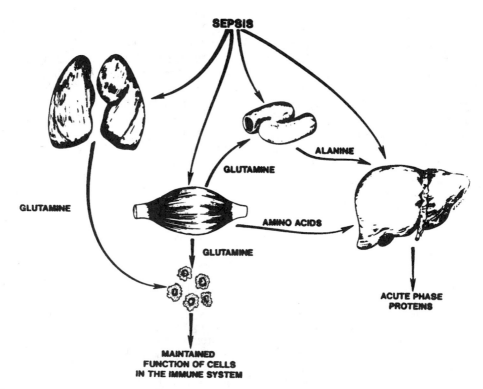

FIGURE 3-1   Integrated concept of sepsis-induced changes in protein metabolism. The function of cells in the immune system and the synthesis of acute phase proteins are supported by changes in skeletal muscle, liver, intestine, and lungs. (From Hasselgren PO: Protein metabolism in sepsis. Austin, TX: RG Landes Co., 1993. With permission.)

The importance of this integrated response to sepsis was documented in clinical studies in which sustained acute phase protein synthesis was essential for survival in septic patients.[20,21]

Although the beneficial effects of the hypermetabolic response to sepsis and injury are apparent in the short term, the cost to the body over the following days to weeks may be significant negative nitrogen balance, loss of muscle mass, and substantial depletion of visceral and circulating protein stores. Such depletion of lean tissue may be associated with decreased immune function, increased infection rates, poor wound healing, and diminished muscle function resulting in slower recovery and rehabilitation.[22] Many of the infectious and noninfectious complications seen in these patients are ascribed to sustained hypercatabolism.[2] In addition, the magnitude and duration of this metabolic activity may be prolonged if adequate nutrition is not provided to patients after severe trauma or infection. Therefore, one of the potential advantages of enteral nutrition is to provide adequate energy and substrates for increased protein synthesis and blunting of the hypercatabolic response.

ENTERAL FEEDING AND PROTEIN METABOLISM

Animal Studies

A relatively large number of studies have been published in which animal experiments were performed to assess the role of enteral feeding in various conditions characterized by metabolic stress, including injury and sepsis. In other reports, the influence of enteral nutrition was studied in unstressed animals. In the majority of studies, indirect evidence of changes in protein metabolism was reported, such as changes in nitrogen balance and concentrations of certain plasma proteins and amino acids. Measurements of actual protein turnover rates have been reported in only a few studies.

In one of those reports, Enrione and colleagues[23] randomly assigned rats to an orally fed group and three different groups receiving intravenous total parenteral nutrition (TPN) that provided 25 percent, 100 percent, or 175 percent of sufficient nutrients and calories for normal growth and development of rats. After a 5-day treatment period, whole body protein turnover and muscle and liver protein synthesis rates were determined following constant infusion of [^{15}N]-glycine. For the purpose of this review, comparisons between the orally fed rats and the TPN-100 percent group are of particular interest because nutritional intake was isocaloric and isonitrogenous in these groups. Results are summarized in Table 3–1. Nitrogen balance was positive and similar in the two groups of rats. Whole body protein turnover, the increase in body weight, and fractional synthesis rate of liver proteins were significantly higher in rats being fed orally than in rats receiving isocaloric and isonitrogenous TPN. The synthesis rate of muscle (gastrocnemius) protein was also higher in the enteral group than in the TPN group, although

TABLE 3–1 Calorie and Nitrogen Intake, Nitrogen Balance, Changes in Body Weight, and Protein Turnover Rates in Rats Fed Orally or by Intravenous Total Parenteral Nutrition (TPN)

	Oral Feeding	TPN
Calorie intake (kcal/day)	58.4 ± 7.7	55.7 ± 2.6
Nitrogen intake (mg N/day)	474.6 ± 62.9	445.8 ± 20.6
Nitrogen balance (mg N/day)	11.3 ± 3.0	10.9 ± 1.1
Body weight change (g/day)	4.6 ± 0.1	2.3 ± 0.7*
Whole body protein turnover (g N/kg/day)	10.4 ± 0.5	6.7 ± 0.3[†]
Whole body protein synthesis (g N/day)	1.7 ± 0.1	1.0 ± 0.5*
Whole body protein breakdown (g N/day)	1.5 ± 0.1	0.7 ± 0.02[†]
Liver FSR (%/day)	58.2 ± 6.1	43.3 ± 2.4*
Muscle FSR (%/day)	13.0 ± 2.5	7.2 ± 0.7

* $P < 0.05$.
[†] $P < 0.01$ vs oral feeding.
Rats were fed orally (n = 6) or received isocaloric and isonitrogenous intravenous TPN (n = 6) during 5 days, after which protein turnover rates were measured following constant infusion of [^{15}N]glycine. FSR, fractional synthesis rate.
Data from Enrione EB, Gelfand MJ, Morgan D et al: The effects of rate and route of nutrient intake on protein metabolism. J Surg Res 1986;40:320–325.

this difference did not reach statistical significance.

The study by Enrione and colleagues[23] is important because it is one of the few reports in which actual measurements of protein turnover rates were performed in specific tissues following enteral or parenteral nutrition. The results are consistent with the concept that protein synthesis, in particular visceral protein synthesis (liver), is better maintained in animals receiving their nutrition through the enteral route than intravenously. The results also illustrate that changes in protein turnover rates in specific organs and tissues are not necessarily reflected by changes in nitrogen balance. One potential drawback of the study is that it was done in unstressed animals and did not address the question whether protein synthesis rates are different between enterally and parenterally fed rats with sepsis or after injury.

In a series of studies by Kudsk and coworkers,[24-26] the effects of enteral and parenteral feeding were investigated in malnourished and septic rats. In one set of experiments,[25] rats were protein depleted for 2 weeks, whereafter

they were randomized into three groups to be refed for 12 days with a dextrose-amino acid solution orally, by gastrostomy, or intravenously. Because rats in the gastrostomy and intravenous groups were pair-fed with the group of rats that took the dextrose–amino acid solution orally, treatment in all three groups was isocaloric and isonitrogenous. Despite equal substrate intake in the three groups of rats, nitrogen balance was significantly higher in the orally fed rats than in the two other groups. Both groups of rats fed through the GI tract maintained mass and nitrogen content of the proximal small intestine better than the intravenously fed rats, suggesting that the mucosal protein balance was better maintained in enterally fed animals (Fig. 3–2). The influence of enteral feeding was less obvious in the distal small bowel, and no differences between the three experimental groups were noticed in the colon. Liver weight and protein content were not influenced by any of the feeding regimens. Thus, this study suggests that the whole body nitrogen balance and protein balance in the mucosa of small intestine, in par-

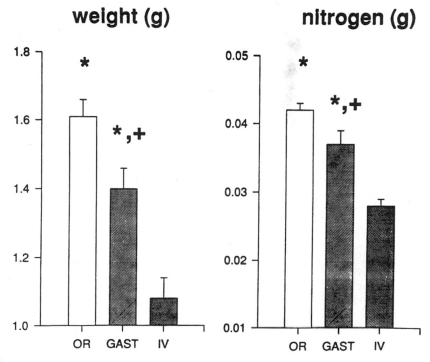

FIGURE 3–2   Weight (left panel) and nitrogen content (right panel) of proximal small intestine of rats that were first protein depleted for 2 weeks and then refed for 12 days with a dextrose–amino acid solution orally (OR), by gastrostomy (GAST), or intravenously (IV). Intestinal mass and nitrogen content were better maintained in both groups of rats fed enterally than in the intravenously fed rats. *$P < 0.05$ vs IV; $^+P < .05$ vs OR. (Data from Kudsk KA, Stone JM, Carpenter G, Sheldon GF: Effects of enteral and parenteral feeding in malnourished rats on body composition. J Trauma 1982;22:904–906.)

ticular in the proximal small intestine, are better maintained in malnourished rats that are refed through the gastrointestinal tract rather than intravenously. Because no specific measurements of protein turnover rates were performed, it is not known if the greater mass and protein content in the small intestine of the enterally fed rats reflected improved protein synthesis, reduced protein breakdown, or a combination of these changes. Alternatively, increased intestinal mass and nitrogen content may have reflected increased cellularity due to increased cell proliferation or reduced cell loss.

In another experiment from the same group of researchers,[24] *Escherichia coli*–hemoglobin adjuvant septic peritonitis was induced in malnourished rats that had been refed with equal amounts of a dextrose–amino acid solution enterally (orally) or parenterally. In this study, total body nitrogen balance was not influenced by the route of feeding. Survival during sepsis was significantly higher in rats that were fed enterally than in rats that received intravenous nutrition, but because protein content was not measured in the intestine or liver (or any other tissue), it is not known if the improved survival was associated with improved protein balance.

When normal (well nourished) rats were fed identical amounts of a dextrose–amino acid solution intravenously or by gastrostomy for 12 days, nitrogen balance was significantly higher in the enterally fed than in the intravenously fed animals,[26] again supporting the concept that enteral feeding is superior to parenteral feeding in maintaining whole body protein balance. In the same study, rats fed by gastrostomy had a significantly higher survival rate following induction of septic peritonitis than intravenously fed rats. Although the improved survival rate in enterally fed rats was associated with higher nitrogen balance, it is not known which specific organs or tissues benefited from enteral feeding.

Thus, in this series of reports by Kudsk and coworkers,[24-26] enteral feeding of normal or malnourished rats resulted in improved whole body nitrogen balance, maintained small bowel mass and protein content, and increased survival after a septic insult. The data do not allow for any conclusions regarding possible causative relationships between the improved nitrogen balance and survival, but it is tempting to speculate that improved protein balance in the small intestine may reflect improved integrity of small bowel mucosa. This in turn may result in decreased bacterial translocation and improved survival.[27] More work is needed, however, to elucidate the association (if any) between enteral feeding, improved protein balance (in particular in the intestine), and survival during sepsis.

Levine and associates[28] provided further evidence for better maintained intestinal mass and protein balance in gut mucosa following enteral feeding in an early study. Groups of rats received equal volumes of glucose–amino acid solution orally or intravenously for 7 days. After the treatment period, weight and protein content of small intestinal mucosa were higher in rats fed enterally than intravenously. Similar to the report by Kudsk and coworkers,[25] the effect of enteral feeding was most pronounced in the proximal segments of the intestine (Fig. 3–3). The higher mucosal weight and protein content in enterally fed rats at least in part reflected greater cell mass as illustrated by higher DNA content and higher villus height in the mucosa of enterally fed rats. It is possible, however, that the increased mucosal protein content also reflected improved protein balance in the individual enterocytes following enteral nutrition.

Secretory immunoglobulin A (IgA) is important for the mucosal defense system.[29] In rats, the majority of IgA found in the intestinal lumen is produced in the liver and secreted in the bile.[30] Alverdy and colleagues[31] reported that the secretion in bile of IgA was higher in rats fed enterally (by gastrostomy) than in rats receiving isocaloric and isonitrogenous intravenous feeding. These results are important because they suggest that the route of nutritional support may influence the synthesis and secretion of a specific protein. The data also offer a possible mechanism of reduced bacterial translocation in enterally fed individuals compared with parenterally fed subjects.

In a series of studies by Alexander and coworkers,[32,33] different aspects of enteral feeding were studied in guinea pigs with burn injury. In initial experiments, the effects of early vs delayed enteral feeding were examined.[32] A 30 percent total body surface area burn injury was inflicted in guinea pigs, whereafter groups of animals were fed 175 kcal/kg/day enterally through a gastrostomy tube starting 2 hours after burn (early feeding) or after an initial 3-day adaptation period. Metabolic studies were performed on postburn day 14, at which time point body weight, weight of gastrocnemius muscle, nitrogen content in liver, and serum concentrations of albumin, transferrin, and C3 were significantly higher in animals that received early feeding than in animals with delayed feeding (Table 3–2). Although no mea-

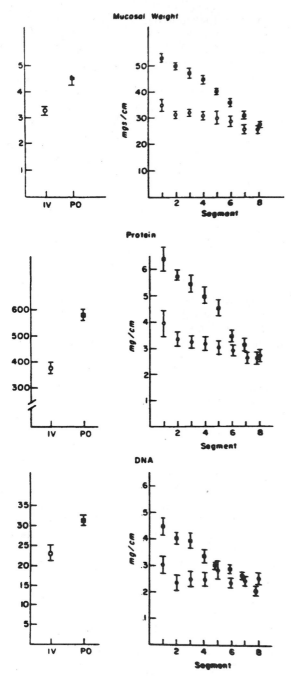

FIGURE 3–3 Small intestinal mucosal weight (upper), protein content (middle), and DNA content (lower) in groups of rats treated with equal volumes of glucose–amino acid solution intravenously (IV, open circles) or orally (PO, closed squares) for 7 days. Total mucosal weight, protein, and DNA in the entire small intestine are shown on the left. Mucosal weight, protein, and DNA per centimeter of each segment of the small bowel are shown in the panels on the right. (From Levine GM, Deren JJ, Steiger E, Zinno R: Role of oral intake in maintenance of gut mass and dissacharide activity. Gastroenterology 1974;67:975–982. With permission.)

surements of actual protein turnover rates were performed, the results suggest that early enteral feeding following burn injury is superior to delayed enteral feeding with respect to protein balance in muscle and liver. In addition to improving protein balance and serum concentrations of certain circulating proteins, early feeding significantly blunted the hypermetabolic response seen in burned animals that received delayed enteral feeding.

On postburn day 1 in the same study,[32] small bowel mucosal weight and nitrogen content were significantly higher in burned animals receiving early feeding than in animals with delayed feeding (only receiving lactated Ringer's solution during the initial 24 hours after burn injury). By postburn day 14, the differences in mucosal weight and nitrogen content between the groups of animals had disappeared. These results are consistent with the concept that early feeding following burn injury prevents early mucosal injury, which in turn may abolish subsequent negative effects on protein balance in muscle, liver, and perhaps other organs and tissues. One mechanism for this effect of early feeding may be a reduced release of catabolic hormones and other mediators of the catabolic response to burn injury (see below).

In a subsequent report, the same group of researchers[33] compared the effects of immediate enteral vs parenteral feeding after burn injury. After a 30 percent total body surface area burn injury in guinea pigs, the animals were randomly assigned to receive 175 kcal/kg/day by gastrostomy or by central venous catheter beginning 2 hours after burn. Although average daily nitrogen balance was significantly greater in enterally than in parenterally fed animals (Fig. 3–4), other measurements reflecting protein metabolism did not differ between groups. Thus, serum levels of albumin, transferrin, and C3 and muscle and liver weight were similar in burned animals receiving early enteral or intravenous nutrition. Small intestinal mucosal weight and thickness were better maintained in the enterally fed group, but this effect was seen only early after burn (on postburn day 1) and was not present on postburn day 14. Enterally fed guinea pigs tended to have a higher nitrogen content in intestinal mucosa than the intravenous group, but this difference was not statistically significant.

Although this review of animal experiments is only partial, the data seem to support the following conclusions: (1) enteral feeding, compared with parenteral feeding, results in improved whole body and visceral (intestine and

TABLE 3–2 Nutritional Measurements on Postburn Day 14 in Guinea Pigs Receiving Early Feeding or Delayed Feeding with 175 kcal/kg/day by Gastrostomy Tube

	Early Feeding	Delayed Feeding
Body weight (% of preburn)	95.2 ± 1.3	84.4 ± 1.7*
Carcass weight (% of preburn)	32.2 ± 0.5	26.0 ± 0.8*
Gastrocnemius weight (g)	1.12 ± 0.03	0.86 ± 0.03*
Nitrogen content in liver (mg)	528 ± 29	453 ± 22*
Serum albumin (g/dl)	3.0 ± 0.1	2.5 ± 0.2*
Serum transferrin (% of normal)	150 ± 9	129 ± 3*
C3 (% of normal)	150 ± 8	103 ± 9*

* $P < 0.05$ vs early feeding.
A 30% TBSA burn injury was inflicted in guinea pigs. Feeding (175 kcal/kg/day) through a gastrostomy tube was initiated 2 hours after burn (early feeding) or after a 72-hour adaptation period (delayed feeding).
Data from Mochizuki H, Trocki O, Dominioni L et al: Mechanism of prevention of postburn hypermetabolism and catabolism in early enteral feeding. Ann Surg 1984;200:297–310.

liver) protein balance; (2) the influence of enteral feeding on muscle protein turnover is less pronounced than the influence on visceral protein balance; and (3) early enteral feeding is superior to delayed enteral feeding following burn injury.

Because indirect evidence of altered protein metabolism was obtained in most previous reports, much work remains to be done to define the effect of enteral vs parenteral feeding on actual protein turnover rates in different organs and tissues. Of particular interest will be to test the influence of enteral feeding on protein synthesis and breakdown rates in liver, muscle, and intestine during sepsis and other catabolic conditions, such as major trauma, cancer, and starvation.

Human Studies

Similar to animal experiments, most human studies have reported indirect evidence of changes in protein metabolism following enteral feeding. Even in studies designed primarily to test the effect of enteral nutrition on protein metabolism, measurements of actual protein turnover rates have rarely been performed.

Enteral Feeding After Burn Injury

In a study by Alexander and coworkers[34] published almost 15 years ago, children with burn injury averaging 60 percent of total body surface area were randomized to receive normal oral diet providing 105 g protein/m²/day (control) or a diet supplemented with high protein content (134 g protein/m²/day). Approximately 15 percent of the calories were in the form of proteins or amino acids in the first group of patients; the corresponding figure for patients in the second group was 25 percent. In addition to higher protein intake, the patients in the second group had a lower caloric intake. Patients were studied serially for up to 6 weeks and were followed with respect to survival, complications, and a number of different parameters reflecting protein metabolism.

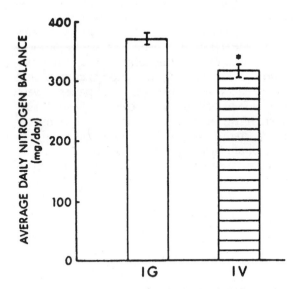

FIGURE 3–4 Average daily nitrogen balance in guinea pigs with a 30% total body surface area burn injury randomized to immediate enteral feeding by gastrostomy (IG) or to immediate isocaloric, isonitrogenous intravenous feeding (IV). (From Saito H, Trocki O, Alexander JW et al: The effect of route of nutrition administration on the nutritional state, catabolic hormone secretion, and gut mucosal integrity after burn injury. J Parenter Enter Nutr 1987;11:1–7. With permission.)

Nitrogen balance studies indicated better retention of nitrogen in patients receiving the high-protein diet, although the difference in nitrogen balance between the groups did not reach statistical significance. Most serum protein concentrations were significantly higher in the high-protein group than in the control group (Table 3–3). In general, proteins with short turnover (e.g., transferrin) showed the greatest differences between the groups during the early phase of the study, whereas proteins with relatively slow synthesis rates (e.g., IgG) and total serum protein showed the greatest differences 2 to 3 weeks into the study.

Plasma levels of several individual amino acids (valine, lysine, threonine, leucine, arginine, isoleucine, proline, serine, asparagine, tryptophan, and tyrosine) as well as total amino acids were significantly higher in the high-protein group than in the control group. Interpretation of these results is difficult, however, since they may represent changes in protein metabolism in various organs and tissues as well as the higher protein load in the GI tract. Most important, survival rate was significantly higher in the high-protein group than in the control group (9/9 vs 5/9, $P < 0.03$). The number of bacteremic days/total days at risk was 11 percent in the control group (27/254) and was significantly lower (23/281, 8 percent) in the high-protein group ($P < 0.005$).

The study by Alexander and colleagues[34] did not compare enteral vs parenteral nutrition; nevertheless, the results are important because they suggest that survival and metabolic response to burn injury can be modulated by more protein through the enteral route. Although increased plasma protein levels can be caused by a number of different mechanisms in addition to increased protein synthesis, such as reduced protein breakdown and altered distribution of plasma proteins, the results are consistent with stimulated acute phase protein synthesis by high-protein enteral feeding. The paper has become a classic in the field of enteral feeding of patients with burn injury.

Studies in Patients with Major Abdominal Trauma

In a series of papers, Moore and colleagues[35-39] reported the consequences of enteral feeding in patients with severe abdominal trauma. In an early study,[35] the feasibility of enteral feeding through a needle catheter jejunostomy was tested in a group of patients undergoing emergency laparotomy for abdominal trauma. Patients were randomized to a control group receiving conventional dextrose solution intravenously for 5 days followed by TPN by central vein if they did not tolerate a regular oral diet at that point. In the other group of patients, a needle catheter jejunostomy was placed just before abdominal closure and infusion of an elemental diet (Vivonex) was started 12 to 18 hours postoperatively. The enteral infusions were continued until the patients tolerated adequate oral intake. Not surprisingly, nitrogen balance was better maintained in the patients receiving enteral nutrition than in the control patients receiving dextrose alone for 5 days (Fig. 3–5). Despite this, there were no significant differences in serum levels of albumin and transferrin between the groups. Septic complications occurred less frequently (9 percent vs 29 percent, $P < 0.05$) and hospital cost was lower in the enteral than in the control group. Interpretation of the results in this study is complicated by the fact that the two groups of patients were not isonitrogenous or isocaloric. Results suggest, however, that the catabolic response to major trauma (negative nitrogen balance) can be blunted by early enteral feeding.

In a subsequent study from the same institution, patients with major trauma were randomized to receive isocaloric and isonitrogenous enteral vs parenteral nutrition.[36] The en-

TABLE 3–3 Selected Serum Proteins in Burned Children who Received Normal Diet or a Diet with a High Protein Content

	Control	High Protein	*P*
Total serum protein (g/dl)	5.5 ± 0.1	6.3 ± 0.2	< 0.0002
Albumin (g/dl)	2.93 ± 0.08	2.95 ± 0.08	NS
Transferrin (mg/dl)	200 ± 10	283 ± 18	< 0.0001
C3 (µg/ml)	1371 ± 55	1585 ± 64	< 0.01
IgG (mg/dl)	805 ± 52	975 ± 56	< 0.03

From Alexander JW, MacMillan BG, Stinnett JD et al: Beneficial effects of aggressive protein feeding in severely burned children. Ann Surg 1980;192:505–517. With permission.

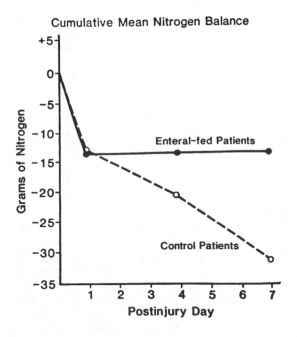

Cumulative Mean Nitrogen Balance

Enteral-fed Patients

Control Patients

FIGURE 3–5 Postoperative cumulative nitrogen balance in patients undergoing emergency laparotomy for abdominal trauma. Patients were randomized to receive conventional dextrose solution intravenously (control patients) or enteral infusion of an elemental diet through a needle catheter jejunostomy (enteral-fed patients) postoperatively. (From Moore EE, Jones TN: Benefits of immediate jejunostomy feeding after major abdominal trauma: a prospective, randomized study. J Trauma 1986;26:874–881. With permission.)

teral feeding was administered through a needle catheter jejunostomy and the parenteral feeding through a central venous catheter. There was no significant difference in nitrogen balance between the two groups of patients. Individual proteins, however, behaved differently in the two groups. Serum levels of total protein, albumin, transferrin, and retinol-binding protein decreased during the 10-day study period in patients receiving TPN, whereas the serum levels of the same proteins increased in patients receiving enteral nutrition (Fig. 3–6). On

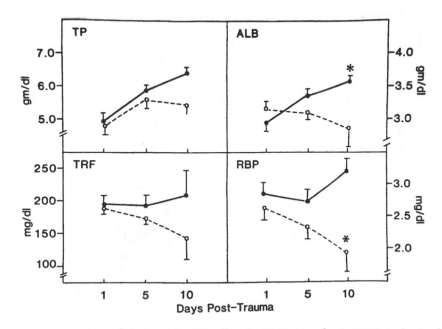

FIGURE 3–6 Serum concentrations of total protein (TP), albumin (ALB), transferrin (TRF), and retinol-binding protein (RBP) in patients who underwent laparotomy for major abdominal trauma and were randomized to receive postoperative TPN (o—o) or isocaloric, isonitrogenous total enteral nutrition (●—●). *$P < 0.05$ between groups. (From Peterson VM, Moore EE, Jones TN et al: Total enteral nutrition versus total parenteral nutrition after major torso injury: attenuation of hepatic protein reprioritization. Surgery 1988;104:199–207. With permission.)

posttrauma day 10, serum levels of albumin and retinol-binding protein were significantly higher in the enterally fed patients than in the TPN group. Thus enteral feeding prevented the fall in serum concentrations of "negative" acute phase proteins, in particular albumin. In contrast, the increase in serum levels of the acute phase proteins α_1-antitrypsin and α_1-antichymotrypsin seen in patients on TPN was blunted in patients receiving enteral nutrition (Fig. 3–7). These results suggest that enteral nutrition attenuates the reprioritization of hepatic protein synthesis typically seen during sepsis and after trauma.[18]

In an extension of the study described above, the authors continued to randomize patients with major abdominal trauma to receive enteral feeding or isocaloric and isonitrogenous TPN.[37] Again, there was no difference in nitrogen balance between enterally and parenterally fed patients. However, the decline in serum concentrations of albumin, transferrin, and retinol-binding protein noticed in patients receiving TPN was not seen in enterally fed patients, supporting the concept that enteral feeding attenuates the reprioritization of hepatic protein synthesis following major trauma.

Kudsk and coworkers[40,41] performed similar studies in patients with major injury and randomized patients who underwent laparotomy for abdominal trauma to early (within 24 hours) enteral feeding through a needle catheter jejunostomy or to early parenteral nutrition. There was no difference in nitrogen balance between the two groups on any of the study days. Serum concentrations of individual proteins, however, were affected differently by enteral and parenteral feeding. Prealbumin levels declined after injury, and this reduction in serum levels of prealbumin was blunted by early enteral nutrition. In contrast, the increase in serum levels of the acute phase proteins C-reactive protein and α_1-acid glycoprotein was reduced by enteral feeding. Thus, these results further support the concept that enteral feeding attenuates the reprioritization of hepatic protein synthesis seen after major trauma.

In an effort to study the role of infection and severity of injury on protein response, patients in the study by Kudsk and coworkers[41] were divided into infected vs noninfected groups and patients with early (< 10 days) vs late (> 10 days) exit from the protocol (patients in the early exit group had significantly lower trauma index and hospital stay than patients with a late exit from the protocol). Few significant differences in proteins were noted between noninfected enteral vs parenteral groups and between infected enteral vs parenteral groups. The authors therefore concluded that the most important mechanism of changes in protein levels induced by enteral feeding is the reduction of septic complications in the enterally fed group.

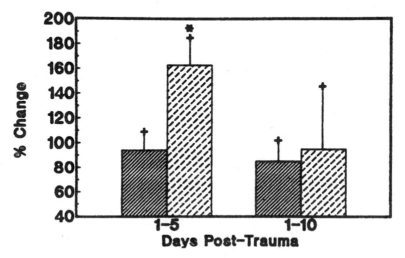

FIGURE 3–7   Changes in α_1-antichymotrypsin serum levels in patients randomized to receive TPN (bars with broken lines) or isocaloric, isonitrogenous total enteral nutrition (TEN, bars with unbroken lines) after laparotomy for major abdominal trauma. The early (days 1–5) postoperative rise in α_1-antichymotrypsin levels seen in patients receiving TPN was not seen in patients receiving TEN, consistent with attenuation of the reprioritization of hepatic protein synthesis. *P < 0.05 vs TEN. (From Peterson VM, Moore EE, Jones TN et al: Total enteral nutrition versus total parenteral nutrition after major torso injury: attenuation of hepatic protein reprioritization. Surgery 1988;104:199-207. With permission.)

When patients with early or late exit from the protocol were analyzed separately, no significant differences were noted between the enteral and parenteral groups in patients with late exit, i.e., in more severely injured patients. In contrast, prealbumin and transferrin levels were significantly higher and C-reactive protein levels were significantly lower in the enterally fed group than in the parenterally fed group among patients with less severe injuries (early exit group) (Fig. 3–8). Thus, the study by Kudsk and coworkers[41] suggests that enteral feeding blunts the acute phase protein response in injured patients by two mechanisms: (1) reducing septic complications; and (2) blunting the

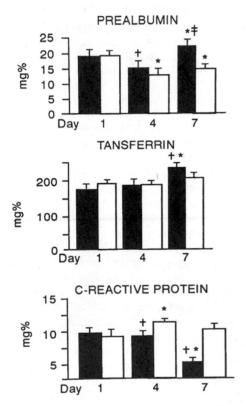

FIGURE 3–8 Serum concentrations of prealbumin, transferrin, and C-reactive protein in patients randomized to enteral (black bars) or parenteral (light bars) feeding following laparotomy for abdominal trauma. Results are from patients with less severe injury (early exit group). The postinjury fall in prealbumin levels and rise in C-reactive protein levels were attenuated by enteral nutrition. *P < 0.01 vs baseline; ^+P < 0.05 vs parenteral feeding; ^{++}P < 0.01 vs parenteral feeding. (Redrawn from Kudsk KA, Minard G, Wojtysiak SL et al: Visceral protein response to enteral versus parenteral nutrition and sepsis in patients with trauma. Surgery 1994;116: 516–523. With permission.)

acute phase protein synthesis in less severely injured patients, independent of the effect on infectious complications.

One important observation made in the studies described above is that unchanged nitrogen balance does not rule out changes in individual hepatic acute phase proteins (at least as reflected by changes in serum concentrations). Also note that the implication of a blunted acute phase response after enteral feeding is not clear. On one hand, it may reflect reduced release of metabolic mediators, in particular cytokines and catabolic hormones, perhaps secondary to improved integrity of gut mucosa, and may therefore reflect a beneficial response to enteral feeding. On the other hand, several studies suggest that the acute phase response is important for survival in patients with sepsis and other critical illness.[20,21] This also illustrates that the relationship between improved survival and reduced morbidity on one hand and changes in protein metabolism on the other hand in patients receiving enteral feeding remains unclear.

In addition to the reports described above, at least one additional prospective randomized study of patients receiving enteral vs parenteral nutritional support following laparotomy for trauma has been published.[42] In that study, no significant differences in serum concentrations of albumin, prealbumin, and transferrin or in nitrogen balance were noted between enterally and parenterally fed patients, although there was a trend to less negative nitrogen balance in patients receiving TPN. Other laboratory values and complication rates were also similar in both groups. In particular, the frequency of septic complications, including wound infection, pneumonia, and intra-abdominal infections, was similar between groups. Thus, this study did not confirm previous reports of beneficial effects of enteral vs parenteral nutrition following major abdominal trauma.

Enteral Feeding in Sepsis

Enteral feeding was compared with parenteral feeding in septic patients in a study by Cerra and coworkers.[43] Patients who had persistent hypermetabolism 4 to 6 days after onset of sepsis were randomized to isocaloric and isonitrogenous enteral vs parenteral nutrition. The enteral feeding was given through a naso-duodenal tube placed endoscopically or fluoroscopically or through a jejunostomy tube placed surgically. The study tested the hypothesis that the enteral feeding would reduce the incidence of multiple organ failure syndrome

(MOFS) and overall postsepsis mortality compared with parenteral nutrition control patients. In addition, certain parameters reflecting protein metabolism were monitored, i.e., nitrogen balance and serum concentrations of transferrin and prealbumin.

The route of nutritional support did not influence the incidence of MOFS or mortality in this group of septic patients. The incidence of MOFS was almost identical in the enterally and parenterally fed groups (22 percent vs 21 percent), and the death rate was also almost identical between the groups (22 percent vs 23 percent). The study also failed to show any major differences in parameters indicating protein metabolism between the enteral and parenteral groups. Mean nitrogen balance was -3.4 ± 10 g/day in the enterally fed group and 0.4 ± 3.8 g/day in the parenterally fed patients. This difference was not statistically significant. Serum transferrin levels increased significantly (from 127 ± 32 to 153 ± 55 mg/dl, $P < 0.05$) during the study period in patients receiving parenteral nutrition, whereas no significant changes in transferrin levels were noticed in the enterally fed patients. There were no significant differences in transferrin levels between the two groups of patients on any study day. Serum levels of prealbumin showed no significant changes within or between the groups.

Thus, this study did not provide evidence that enteral feeding improves protein metabolism in septic patients. Note, however, that only few (and indirect) measures of protein metabolism were studied. Because sepsis is associated with pronounced changes in protein metabolism in various organs and tissues, some of which may influence morbidity and mortality in septic patients (see earlier sections of this chapter), future studies must focus on protein metabolism in septic patients receiving enteral vs parenteral nutrition.

In another report by Cerra and coworkers,[44] septic patients were randomized to receive enteral feedings with a branched-chain amino acid (BCAA) enriched solution (44 percent BCAA) or an isonitrogenous, isocaloric standard amino acid solution containing 28 percent BCAA. A positive nitrogen balance was achieved in the patients receiving the BCAA-enriched solution but not in the patients receiving standard amino acid solution (fed enterally in both groups). Significantly more patients had a rise in serum levels of transferrin following the BCAA-enriched solution than following the standard amino acid solution. From that observation, the authors concluded that patients receiving BCAA-enriched solutions had enhanced visceral protein mass (although the data may not have fully supported this conclusion). Not surprisingly, plasma levels of leucine, isoleucine, and valine were increased in the patients receiving the BCAA-enriched solution. Plasma levels of phenylalanine rose during the study period in patients receiving standard amino acid solution but not in patients receiving BCAA-enriched solution, possibly reflecting a more severe muscle catabolism in patients receiving standard solution. Although this study did not compare enteral vs parenteral nutrition, the results are important because they suggest that modifying solutions used for enteral feeding may influence the metabolic response to sepsis.

Enteral Feeding in Postoperative Patients

Although supplementary nutrition is not normally required for patients undergoing elective surgery of moderate severity (such as cholecystectomy and gastric or bowel resection), these patients are ideal subjects for studies on the influence of enteral vs parenteral nutrition, since they display a predictable and reproducible catabolic response and since treatment of these patients is more or less standardized.

In an early study, Hoover and associates[45] reported nutritional benefits of immediate postoperative enteral feeding. Patients undergoing major upper GI operations were randomized to receive either intravenous therapy of isotonic glucose or enteral feeding started immediately postoperatively through a needle catheter jejunostomy. Thus, the study groups were not isocaloric or isonitrogenous, but the patients receiving enteral feeding had substantially greater intake of calories and nitrogen than the intravenous group. Not surprisingly, therefore, nitrogen balance was significantly greater in the enterally fed patients (Fig. 3–9). Because the study did not compare parenteral and enteral isonitrogenous and isocaloric feedings, it could not determine whether the enteral route of feeding was superior to parenteral nutrition. The study clearly demonstrated, however, that it was possible to provide sufficient enteral feeding in the early postoperative course, with nitrogen balance becoming positive after the fourth postoperative day.

Several subsequent studies compared patients receiving isocaloric and isonitrogenous feeding enterally or parenterally. In a matched prospective study, Muggia-Sullam and colleagues[46] compared enteral (provided by needle catheter jejunostomy) vs parenteral isocaloric

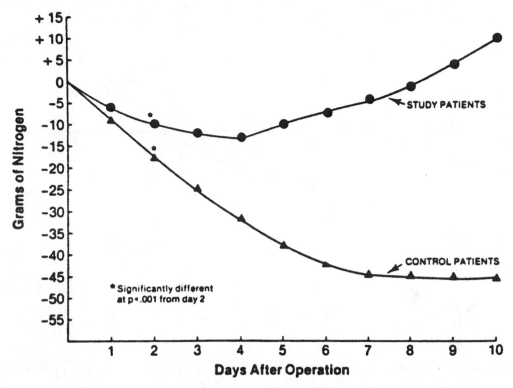

FIGURE 3–9 Postoperative cumulative nitrogen balance in patients who were randomized to receive isotonic intravenous glucose (control patients) or an elemental diet by needle catheter jejunostomy (study patients) after upper GI surgery. (Reprinted by permission of the publisher from Hoover HC, Ryan JA, Anderson EJ, Fischer JE: Nutritional benefits of immediate postoperative jejunal feeding of an elemental diet. Am J Surg 1980;139:153–159. Copyright 1980 by Excerpta Medica Inc.)

and isonitrogenous feeding in postoperative patients who had undergone various types of elective abdominal operations, including vagotomy and antrectomy, choledochojejunostomy, pancreaticojejunostomy, and bowel resections. The feeding regimens were started on the first postoperative day and continued for 7 to 10 days.

There were no significant differences in nitrogen balance between the two groups of patients, both of which achieved positive nitrogen balance by postoperative day 5 (Fig. 3–10). Urinary excretion of 3-MH, a measure of whole body myofibrillar protein breakdown and at least in part reflecting muscle catabolism,[47-49] increased after surgery and started to decline after 2 days. There were no differences in 3-MH excretion between enterally and parenterally fed patients (Fig. 3–11). Other parameters reflecting protein metabolism, including serum levels of albumin, transferrin, thyroxine-binding prealbumin, and retinol-binding protein, were also similar in both groups of patients. Thus, this study did not support the hypothesis that enteral feeding is superior to parenteral administration of calories and protein. Because the isocaloric and isonitroge-

nous formulae with which the study was carried out were limited by tolerance to the enteral feeding, the authors concluded that TPN may be more appropriate in patients in whom larger amounts of calories are needed immediately after operation. Note that the study was conducted in a group of patients with moderate metabolic stress, and it therefore does not rule out beneficial effects of enteral feeding in patients with more severe illness.

In a subsequent study from the same group of authors,[50] a somewhat larger number of patients were randomized to TPN or enteral nutrition administered by needle catheter jejunostomy. This study differed from the previous report in two important aspects: (1) the diet provided to the enterally fed group (Vivonex-TEN) differed from the previously used elemental diet (Vivonex-HN) in its amino acid composition, lower osmolality, addition of a small amount of fat, and a more favorable calorie/nitrogen ratio; the lower osmolality of the new elemental diet made it possible to advance the enteral feeding more rapidly than in the earlier report; and (2) a larger number of more exten-

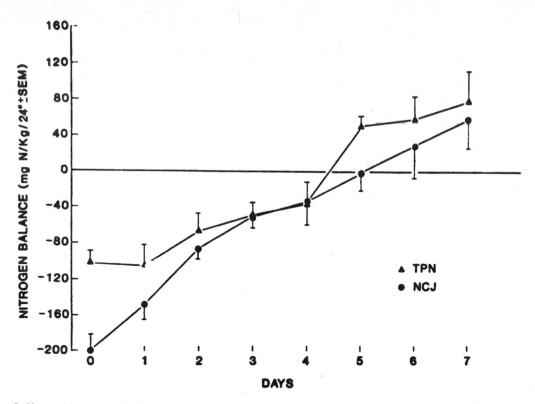

FIGURE 3–10 Daily nitrogen balance in patients receiving TPN or enteral feeding through a needle catheter jejunostomy (NCJ) after elective abdominal operations. (From Muggia-Sullam M, Bower RH, Murphy RF et al: Postoperative enteral versus parenteral nutritional support in gastrointestinal surgery. A matched prospective study. Am J Surg 1985;149:106–112. Reprinted with permission from *American Journal of Surgery*.)

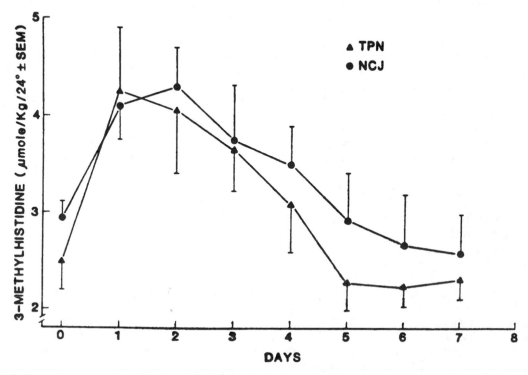

FIGURE 3–11 Urinary excretion of 3-methylhistidine in the same groups of patients shown in Fig. 3–10. TPN, total parenteral nutrition; NCJ, needle catheter jejunostomy. (From Muggia-Sullam M, Bower RH, Murphy RF et al: Postoperative enteral versus parenteral nutritional support in gastrointestinal surgery. A matched prospective study. Am J Surg 1985;149:106–112. Reprinted with permission from *American Journal of Surgery*.)

sive procedures were performed in the new study, such as pancreaticoduodenectomies, distal pancreatectomies, subtotal gastrectomies, and esophagectomy. Whereas in the preceding report[46] no differences were found in nitrogen balance or other parameters indicating protein metabolism, in the new study, involving patients with presumably more pronounced metabolic stress, some interesting differences were noted between the enterally and parenterally fed patients. Nitrogen balance was greater in the TPN group than in the enteral group on postoperative days 1, 2, and 4, and nitrogen balance was achieved earlier in the TPN group than in the enteral group (Fig. 3–12). Urinary excretion of 3-MH was greater in the enterally fed group than in the TPN group on day 2 (P < .05) but was similar between groups on the other study days (Fig. 3–13). There was a statistically significant fall in serum albumin concentrations (from 3.85 ± 0.15 to 3.20 ± 0.21 g/dl, P < .03) during the study period in the TPN group, whereas in the enterally fed group, albumin levels remained stable. There were no sig-

nificant intragroup or intergroup differences in serum levels of transferrin, prealbumin, retinol-binding protein, or C3.

Thus, this study also failed to support the hypothesis that enteral feeding is superior to parenteral nutrition with respect to protein metabolism. If anything, TPN was superior to enteral feeding in achieving positive nitrogen balance and reducing urinary 3-MH excretion. The only exception was serum levels of albumin, which were better maintained in the enteral group. Whether this finding reflected increased synthesis, reduced breakdown, or altered distribution of albumin is not known.

ENTERAL FEEDING AND MEDIATORS OF PROTEIN METABOLISM

Sepsis and severe injury activate both the neuroendocrine system and the immune system, and the two systems interact at several levels. The response to injury and sepsis of hormones and cytokines, as well as other inflammatory mediators, and their role in regulating

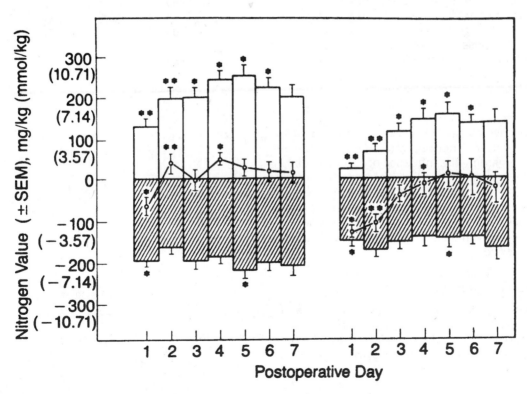

FIGURE 3–12 Nitrogen metabolism in patients undergoing major upper GI or pancreaticobiliary surgery and randomized to receive postoperative nutritional support by TPN (left) or needle catheter jejunostomy (NCJ, right). Nitrogen intake (open bars), nitrogen excretion (hatched bars), and nitrogen balance (open circles) are depicted for each postoperative day for both groups. *P < 0.05 TPN vs NCJ; **P < 0.01 TPN vs NCJ. (From Bower RH, Talamini MA, Sax HC et al: Postoperative enteral vs parenteral nutrition. A randomized controlled trial. Arch Surg 1986;121:1040–1045. Copyright 1986, American Medical Association.)

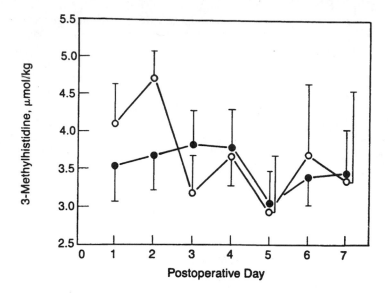

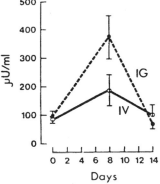

FIGURE 3–13 Daily urinary excretion of 3-MH in the same groups of patients shown in Fig. 3–12. TPN, filled circles; NCJ, open circles. (From Bower RH, Talamini MA, Sax HC et al: Postoperative enteral vs parenteral nutrition. A randomized controlled trial. Arch Surg 1986;121:1040–1045. Copyright 1986, American Medical Association.)

protein metabolism have been reviewed elsewhere.[51-53] In this segment of the chapter, we will discuss changes induced by enteral feeding in hormones important for regulating protein metabolism during metabolic stress, in particular the catabolic (counterregulatory) hormones cortisol, glucagon, and catecholamines. In addition, changes in the synthesis and release of proinflammatory cytokines, especially TNF, interleukin (IL)-1, and IL-6, will be reviewed.

Whereas the effects of enteral feeding on nitrogen balance, serum protein levels, and other parameters reflecting protein metabolism are not always consistent in the literature (as discussed above), there seems to be more agreement regarding the influence of enteral feeding on the release of catabolic hormones and cytokines. Thus, several studies, both in experimental animals and humans, support the concept that enteral feeding blunts the release of the metabolic mediators after injury and during sepsis/endotoxemia.

Catabolic Hormones

When normal rats were fed isocaloric and isonitrogenous diets enterally or intravenously for 14 days, serum glucagon levels rose in both groups of rats but significantly more so in the intravenous group (Fig. 3–14).[54] In the same study, serum insulin levels were higher in the enterally fed rats than in the intravenous group. The enterally fed animals gained more in body weight during the study period than the parenterally fed rats, which was interpreted as indicating that the release of insulin seen in

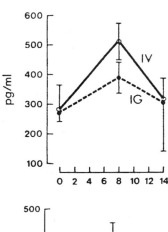

FIGURE 3–14 Serum concentrations of glucagon (upper) and insulin (lower) in rats receiving infusion of a glucose–amino acid solution intravenously (IV) or intragastrically (IG). Enteral feeding blunted the rise in glucagon levels and resulted in higher insulin concentrations. (From Lickley HLA, Track NS, Vranic M, Bury KD: Metabolic responses to enteral and parenteral nutrition. Am J Surg 1978;135:172–176. Reprinted with permission from *American Journal of Surgery*.)

rats receiving their nutrition through the GI tract contributed to a better disposal of nutrients. It is possible, however, that the results also reflected reduced catabolism due to lower levels of glucagon in the enterally fed rats.

The influence of enteral feeding on the release of catabolic hormones following burn injury was studied in a series of papers by Alexander and coworkers.[32,33] When guinea pigs were fed by gastrostomy tube or by central venous

catheter beginning early (2 hours) after burn injury, the catabolic response was less pronounced in the enterally fed animals.[33] Thus, the urinary excretion of vanillylmandelic acid (VMA) was higher in the intravenous group than in the intragastric group (Fig. 3–15), and the role of VMA excretion in the catabolic response was illustrated by the correlation between VMA excretion and loss of body weight (Fig. 3–16). The blunted catabolic response in the enterally

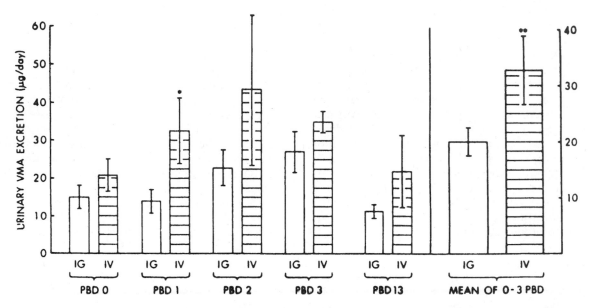

FIGURE 3–15 Urinary VMA excretion in burned guinea pigs fed by gastrostomy tube (IG) or by central venous catheter (IV) beginning early (2 hours) after injury. The animals fed intravenously excreted more VMA than the animals fed by gastrostomy. (From Saito H, Trocki O, Alexander JW et al: The effect of route of nutrient administration on the nutritional state, catabolic hormone secretion, and gut mucosal integrity after burn injury. J Parenter Enter Nutr 1987;11:1–7. With permission.)

FIGURE 3–16 Relationship between change in body weight and urinary VMA excretion in burned guinea pigs receiving enteral feeding by gastrostomy tube (IG) or intravenous feeding (IV). A greater weight loss was seen in animals with greater VMA excretion. (From Saito H, Trocki O, Alexander JW et al: The effect of route of nutrient administration on the nutritional state, catabolic hormone secretion, and gut mucosal integrity after burn injury. J Parenter Enter Nutr 1987;11:1–7. With permission.)

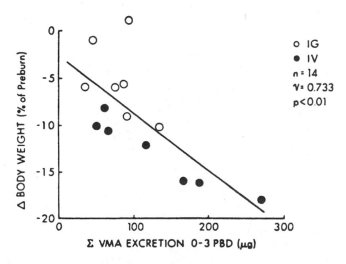

fed guinea pigs was further supported by lower plasma levels of both cortisol and glucagon noted on postburn day 1 and persisting throughout the study period to postburn day 14 (Fig. 3–17); the comparison with hormone levels in unburned guinea pigs suggested that enteral feeding completely blocked the burn-induced increase in plasma cortisol and glucagon levels. Because significant correlations were found between weight and protein content of small intestinal mucosa on one hand, and plasma levels of cortisol and glucagon on the other hand, it was speculated that loss of gut mucosal integrity during parenteral nutrition may be an important mechanism of catabolic hormone secretion after burn.

In another study from the same laboratory,[32] the influence of early vs delayed enteral feeding on the catabolic response to burn injury was studied. Groups of guinea pigs with a 30 percent total body surface area burn injury were fed enterally (through a gastrostomy tube) starting 2 hours after burn or after an initial 72-hour adaptation period designed to mimic the nutritional adaptation period often used to manage patients with burn injury. Twenty-four hours after burn, during which time the delayed group received only lactated Ringer's so-

lution through the gastric tube, plasma levels of cortisol and glucagon were significantly lower in the early feeding group than in the delayed feeding group (Table 3–4). These differences persisted throughout the study period and were noted on postburn day 14 as well. Urinary excretion of VMA was also blunted in the group of guinea pigs that received early enteral feeding.

Taken together, these studies[32,33] suggest that the release of catabolic hormones after burn injury is blunted by enteral feeding and that early enteral feeding is more effective than delayed enteral feeding. Reduced loss of body and carcass weight and improved nitrogen balance suggest that the inhibited release of catabolic hormones following early enteral feeding was associated with reduced muscle catabolism, although actual muscle protein turnover rates in similar groups of burned animals (and patients) remain to be determined. A more recent study from the same laboratory suggests that the inhibition of catabolic hormone release following enteral feeding is secondary to inhibited bacterial translocation across the intestinal mucosa.[55]

The role of enteral feeding for the release of catabolic hormones in humans was studied by Fong and associates.[56] Endotoxin was adminis-

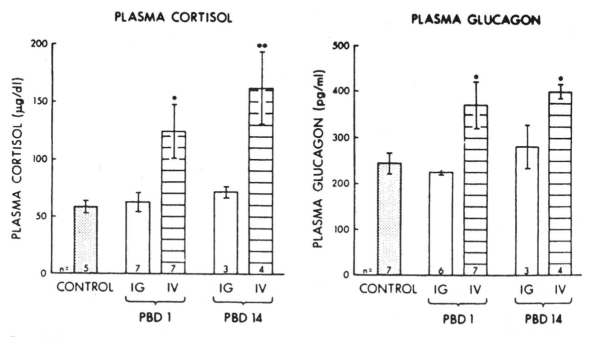

FIGURE 3–17   Plasma cortisol and glucagon levels in unburned controls and in burned guinea pigs receiving enteral feeding by gastrostomy tube (IG) or feeding intravenously (IV). The IV group had higher hormone levels than the IG group. (From Saito H, Trocki O, Alexander JW et al: The effect of route of nutrient administration on the nutritional state, catabolic hormone secretion, and gut mucosal integrity after burn injury. J Parenter Enter Nutr 1987;11:1–7. With permission.)

TABLE 3–4   Plasma Cortisol and Glucagon Levels in Guinea Pigs with a 30% Total Body Surface Area Burn Injury

	Preburn	Postburn Day 1		Postburn Day 14	
	Fed Ad Lib	**Early Feeding (2 Hours)**	**Delayed Feeding (72 Hours)**	**Early Feeding (2 Hours)**	**Delayed Feeding (72 Hours)**
Plasma cortisol (µg/dl)	48.1 ± 6.1	61.1 ± 2.5	122.8 ± 12.8*	59 ± 8.5	116.6 ± 17.9*
Plasma glucagon (pg/ml)	19.1 ± 2.8	26 ± 6.8	313.7 ± 60*	23 ± 5	101.8 ± 17.6*

* $P < 0.01$ vs early feeding.
Data from Mochizuki H, Trocki O, Dominioni L et al: Mechanism of prevention of postburn hypermetabolism and catabolism by early enteral feeding. Ann Surg 1984;200:297–310.

tered to healthy volunteers after 1 week of enteral feeding or 1 week of isocaloric parenteral feeding. The response of body temperature and heart rate to endotoxin was less pronounced in enterally than in parenterally fed subjects. In addition, the circulating levels of epinephrine and glucagon were significantly lower in the enterally fed subjects (Fig. 3–18), suggesting that the catabolic response to endotoxemia is blunted by enteral feeding in humans as well. Because in this study subjects receiving parenteral feeding had no oral intake for 1 week before endotoxin challenge, the difference between the two groups probably reflected impaired integrity of the intestinal mucosa (although no morphologic or other measurements of mucosal integrity were performed).

Proinflammatory Cytokines

Less is known about how enteral feeding affects the release of cytokines, but it may blunt the release of proinflammatory cytokines during endotoxemia, similar to the effect on catabolic hormones. In the same study described above, Fong and colleagues[56] measured arterial and hepatic venous TNF concentrations following administration of endotoxin to enterally or parenterally fed subjects. Circulating TNF levels were significantly higher at all time points in the parenteral than in the enteral group (Fig. 3–19), suggesting that the release of proinflammatory cytokines during sepsis/endotoxemia may be influenced by the route of nutritional support. The relationship between blunted release of TNF (and catabolic hormones; see above) and metabolic events following enteral feeding was illustrated by inhibited net efflux of amino acids (in particular alanine and glutamine) from the lower extremity and by reduced serum C-reactive protein levels

(Fig. 3–20) in the enterally fed subjects. These results suggest that the inhibited release of catabolic hormones and cytokines following enteral feeding translated into reduced muscle catabolism and blunted acute phase response in liver.

An important observation made in the paper by Fong and colleagues[56] was that hepatic venous levels of TNF were consistently higher than arterial levels (Fig. 3–19). This result suggests that the splanchnic bed is an important source of TNF (and probably other cytokines as well) during sepsis and endotoxemia. Although release of TNF from activated Kupffer cells may account for most of the difference in TNF levels between peripheral and hepatic venous blood, release of TNF by other (prehepatic) splanchnic tissues may have contributed. Interestingly, recent reports suggest that small intestinal mucosa may be an important source of proinflammatory cytokines during sepsis/endotoxemia and shock.[16,57] We recently found evidence that the enterocyte itself produces IL-6 in response to endotoxin.[58,59] These results support the concept that the gut is an important participant in the response to sepsis and endotoxemia and suggest that one mechanism of enteral feeding may be to exert a direct effect on the intestinal mucosa to inhibit the initial steps in the "cytokine cascade." This hypothesis needs further testing but is exciting both from the standpoint of understanding the role of the intestine in the response to sepsis/endotoxemia and from the standpoint of understanding the mechanism(s) of enteral feeding.

PROSPECTS FOR ADVANCES IN ENTERAL FEEDING

Several recent studies suggest that adding specific nutrients to enteral feeding, in particu-

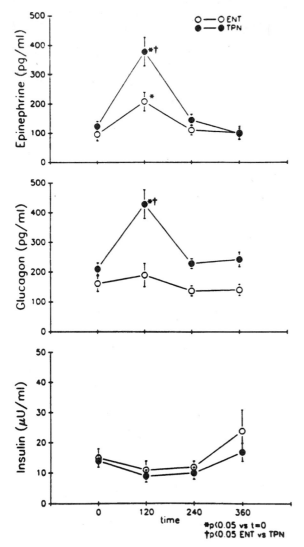

FIGURE 3–18 Plasma levels of epinephrine, glucagon, and insulin after intravenous injection of endotoxin (20 units/kg) in healthy volunteers who had received enteral feeding (ENT) or total parenteral feeding (TPN) for 7 days before injection of endotoxin. The endotoxin-induced rise in epinephrine and glucagon levels was blunted in subjects who had received enteral feeding. (From Fong Y, Marano MA, Barber A et al: Total parenteral nutrition and bowel rest modify the metabolic response to endotoxin in humans. Ann Surg 1989;210:449–457. With permission.)

lar glutamine, arginine, nucleotides, fish oil, and BCAA, may aid in attenuating catabolism and promoting immune function.[60-68] Welbourne and Joshi[60] demonstrated in acidotic rats that an enteral diet enriched with glutamine resulted in increased hepatic glutamine uptake and glutamate production and reduced muscle proteolysis compared with rats fed the same diet without glutamine supplementation. Other investigators have noted that oral glutamine administration affects gut integrity and function. Alexander and colleagues[61] found that oral glutamine decreased translocation of enteric bacteria and improved killing of bacteria that had passed through the mucosal barrier. These results support an important role of enteral glutamine in the maintenance of gut barrier and synthetic function and are consistent with in vitro experiments by Higashiguchi and colleagues[62] that showed a dose-dependent stimulation by glutamine of protein synthesis in isolated enterocytes. Further evidence for the important role of glutamine was reported by Ziegler and coworkers,[63] who found that TPN supplemented with glutamine decreased infectious episodes, improved nitrogen balance, and shortened hospital stay in patients undergoing bone marrow transplantation.

Arginine supplementation has also received attention recently, since it is known to have stimulatory effects on the release of pituitary growth hormone, insulinlike growth factor, and several other hormones[64] and in addition is a precursor for the immunologically active metabolite nitric oxide. Administration of arginine in pharmacologic doses has promoted wound healing and immune function.[64]

Several new "immune-enhancing" diets have been tested recently, and, at present, at least five prospective randomized trials have been reported. Gottschlich and coworkers[69] reported in 1990 the results of a trial in which patients with burn injury received a special formula enriched with arginine and ω-3 polyunsaturated fatty acids or one of two control formulas. No positive immune response was noted in that study, but patients receiving the special formula had fewer burn wound infections, and survivors had reduced length of hospital stay. In 1991, Cerra and colleagues[70] tested a diet enriched with ω-3 polyunsaturated fatty acids, arginine, and nucleotides (Impact, Sandoz Nutrition, Minneapolis, MN) vs an isonitrogenous control formula. No differences were noted between the study groups in nitrogen balance, visceral protein markers, or clinical outcome. Daly and associates[66] showed in 1992 that in patients undergoing upper GI surgery for malignancy, administration of Impact vs Osmolite-HN (Ross Laboratories, Columbus, OH) resulted in improved nitrogen balance, reduction in infectious complications, and decreased length of hospital stay. Note, however, that the treatment protocols

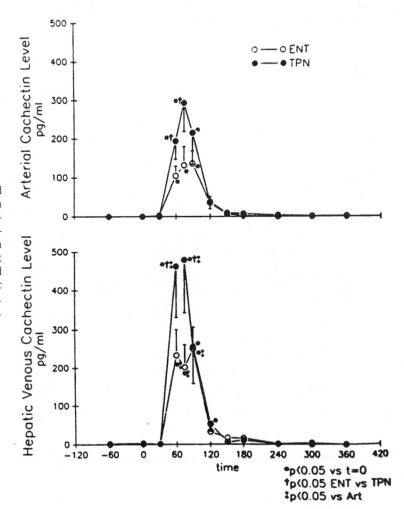

FIGURE 3–19 Arterial (upper) and hepatic venous (lower) cachectin (TNF) levels after injection of endotoxin in the same group of subjects shown in Fig. 3–18. (From Fong Y, Marano MA, Barber A et al: Total parenteral nutrition and bowel rest modify the metabolic response to endotoxin in humans. Ann Surg 1989;210:449–457. With permission.)

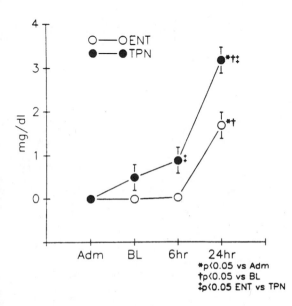

FIGURE 3–20 C-reactive protein concentrations in arterial blood on admission (Adm), immediately before (BL), 6 hours after, and 24 hours after endotoxin challenge in the same groups of subjects shown in Figs. 3–18 and 3–19. (From Fong Y, Marano MA, Barber A et al: Total parenteral nutrition and bowel rest modify the metabolic response to endotoxin in humans. Ann Surg 1989;210:449–457. With permission.)

were not isonitrogenous in that study. In 1993, Bower and colleagues[67] reported a prospective, randomized, double-blind, multicenter study of 326 intensive care unit patients and confirmed the beneficial effects of the same immune-enhancing diet (Impact) with lower rates of infection and a 7-day decrease in length of hospital stay compared with patients receiving isocaloric standard enteral therapy. Finally, in 1994, Moore and coworkers[68] combined a similar diet with a greater proportion of BCAA (Immun-Aid, McGaw Inc., Irvine, CA) in the treatment of trauma patients. The BCAA-enriched diet resulted in increased numbers of total circulating lymphocytes, T-lymphocytes, and T helper cells, compared with control nutrition (Vivonex TEN, Sandoz Nutrition, East Hanover, NJ). The modified enteral diet was also associated with significantly fewer septic complications. There were no significant differences between the groups in nitrogen balance, visceral protein markers, or acute phase reactants. Further studies are required to delineate the mechanism by which the "immune-enhancing" enteral feeding supplements act. In particular, it will be important to define the specific nutrient or combination of nutrients responsible for the beneficial effects of these diets. Further studies are also needed to examine the effects on protein metabolism in gut mucosa, liver, and muscle.

SUMMARY

The metabolic response to sepsis and injury is characterized by protein catabolism in muscle and lungs and increased protein synthesis in liver and intestine. Early enteral feeding has been shown to preserve intestinal integrity and function, to reduce the hepatic protein response, and to decrease the rate of infectious complications. New enteral formulas supplemented with arginine, glutamine, nucleotides, fish oil, and BCAA may have metabolic and immune supporting actions and appear to decrease patient morbidity.

The specific influence of enteral vs parenteral feeding and of different nutritional formulas on protein metabolism during critical illness is not completely understood, mainly because previous studies have only provided indirect measures of changes in protein metabolism, such as changes in nitrogen balance, plasma proteins, amino acids, and urinary excretion of nitrogen and 3-MH. When these changes were studied in postoperative patients and in patients with severe injury or sepsis, conflicting results were found, with unchanged, improved, and worsened nitrogen balance following enteral feeding. Future experiments, designed to specifically measure protein synthesis and breakdown rates in muscle, liver, gut mucosa, and other tissues, will be important to give a better understanding of the metabolic impact of enteral feeding.

Enteral feeding appears to blunt the release of cytokines and counterregulatory hormones during sepsis/endotoxemia and injury. Because these substances are important regulators of protein metabolism in critical illness, enteral feeding may prove beneficial in reversing muscle catabolism and preserving visceral proteins.

Acknowledgment

We are grateful to Drs. J.W. Alexander, R.H. Bower, and J.E. Fischer for reviewing the manuscript and providing valuable advice.

REFERENCES

1. Hasselgren PO: Protein Metabolism in Sepsis. Austin, TX: RG Landes Co, 1993.
2. Cerra FB: Hypermetabolism, organ failure, and metabolic support. Surgery 1987;101:1–14.
3. Hall-Angerås M, Angerås U, Zamir O et al: Effect of the glucocorticoid receptor antagonist RU 38486 on muscle protein breakdown in sepsis. Surgery 1991;109: 468–473.
4. Zamir O, Hasselgren PO, Higashiguchi T et al: Tumor necrosis factor (TNF) and interleukin-1 (IL-1) induce muscle proteolysis through different mechanisms. Mediat Inflam 1992;1:247–250.
5. Zamir O, Hasselgren PO, Kunkel SL et al: Evidence that tumor necrosis factor participates in the regulation of muscle proteolysis during sepsis. Arch Surg 1992; 127:170–174.
6. Zamir O, Hasselgren PO, O'Brien W et al: Muscle protein breakdown during endotoxemia in rats and after treatment with interleukin-1 receptor antagonist (IL-1ra). Ann Surg 1992;216:381–387.
7. Zamir O, O'Brien W, Thompson R et al: Reduced muscle protein breakdown in septic rats following treatment with interleukin-1 receptor antagonist. Int J Biochem 1994;26:943–950.
8. Tiao G, Fagan JM, Samuels N et al: Sepsis stimulates non-lysosomal energy-dependent proteolysis and increases ubiquitin mRNA levels in rat skeletal muscle. J Clin Invest 1994;94:2255–2264.
9. Souba WW, Klimberg VS, Plumley DA et al: The role of glutamine in maintaining a healthy gut and supporting the metabolic response to injury and infection. J Surg Res 1990;48:383–391.
10. von Allmen D, Hasselgren PO, Higashiguchi T et al: Increased intestinal protein synthesis during sepsis and following administration of tumor necrosis factor α (TNFα) or interleukin-1α (IL-1α). Biochem J 1992;286: 585–589.
11. Higashiguchi T, Noguchi Y, O'Brien W et al: Effect of sepsis in rats on mucosal protein synthesis in different parts of the gastrointestinal tract. Clin Sci 1994;87: 207–211.

12. Rafferty JA, Noguchi Y, Fischer JE et al: Sepsis in rats stimulates cellular proliferation in the mucosa of the small intestine. Gastroenterology 1994;107:121–127.

13. Zamir O, Hasselgren PO, Higashiguchi T et al: Effect of sepsis or cytokine administration on release of gut peptides. Am J Surg 1992;163:181–185.

14. Higashiguchi T, Noguchi Y, Noffsinger A et al: Sepsis increases production of total secreted proteins, vasoactive intestinal peptide (VIP), and peptide YY (PYY) in isolated rat enterocytes. Am J Surg 1994;168:251–256.

15. Molmenti EP, Ziambras T, Perlmutter DH: Evidence for an acute phase response in human intestinal epithelial cells. J Biol Chem 1993;268:14116–14124.

16. Mester M, Tomkins RG, Gelfand JA et al: Intestinal production of interleukin-1α during endotoxemia in the mouse. J Surg Res 1993;54:584–591.

17. Hasselgren PO, Jagenburg R, Karlstrom L et al: Changes of protein metabolism in liver and skeletal muscle following trauma complicated by sepsis. J Trauma 1984;24:224-228.

18. Sganga G, Siegel JH, Brown G et al: Reprioritization of hepatic plasma protein release in trauma and sepsis. Arch Surg 1985;120:187–189.

19. Gauldie J, Baumann H: Cytokines and acute phase protein expression. In Kimball ES (ed): Cytokines and Inflammation. Boca Raton: CRC Press, 1991:275–305.

20. Pearl RH, Clowes GHA, Hirsch EF et al: Prognosis and survival as determined by visceral amino acid clearance in severe trauma. J Trauma 1985;25:777–783.

21. Dominioni L, Dionigi H, Zanello M et al: Sepsis score and acute phase protein response as predictors of outcome in septic surgical patients. Arch Surg 1987;122:141–146.

22. Wilmore DW: Catabolic illness: strategies for enhancing recovery. N Engl J Med 1991;325:695–702.

23. Enrione ED, Gelfand MJ, Morgan D et al: The effects of rate and route of nutrient intake on protein metabolism. J Surg Res 1986;40:320–325.

24. Kudsk KA, Carpenter G, Peterson S et al: Effect of enteral and parenteral feeding on malnourished rats with *E. coli*-hemoglobin adjuvant peritonitis. J Surg Res 1981;31:105–110.

25. Kudsk KA, Stone JM, Carpenter G et al: Effects of enteral and parenteral feeding in malnourished rats on body composition. J Trauma 1982;22:904–906.

26. Kudsk KA, Stone JM, Carpenter G et al: Enteral and parenteral feeding influences mortality after hemoglobin-*E. coli* peritonitis in normal rats. J Trauma 1983;23:605–609.

27. Deitch EA: Bacterial translocation of the gut flora. J Trauma 1990;30:184–189.

28. Levine GM, Deren JJ, Steiger E et al: Role of oral intake in maintenance of gut mass and disaccharide activity. Gastroenterology 1974;67:975–982.

29. Clamp JR: The relationship between secretory immunoglobulin A and mucus. Biochem Soc Trans 1977;5:1579–1581.

30. Lemaitre-Coelho I, Jackson GDF, Vaerman JP: Relevance of biliary IgA antibodies in rat intestinal immunity. Scand J Immunol 1978;8:459–463.

31. Alverdy J, Chi HS, Sheldon GF: The effect of parenteral nutrition on gastrointestinal immunity. The importance of enteral stimulation. Ann Surg 1985;202:681–684.

32. Mochizuki H, Trocki O, Dominioni L et al: Mechanism of prevention of postburn hypermetabolism and catabolism by early enteral feeding. Ann Surg 1984;200:297–310.

33. Saito H, Trocki O, Alexander JW et al: The effect of route of nutrient administration on the nutritional state, catabolic hormone secretion, and gut mucosal integrity after burn injury. JPEN 1987;11:1–7.

34. Alexander JW, MacMillan BG, Stinnett JD et al: Beneficial effects of aggressive protein feeding in severely burned children. Ann Surg 1980;192:505–517.

35. Moore EE, Jones TN: Benefits of immediate jejunostomy feeding after major abdominal trauma: a prospective, randomized study. J Trauma 1986;26:874–881.

36. Peterson VM, Moore EE, Jones TN et al: Total enteral nutrition versus total parenteral nutrition after major torso injury: attenuation of hepatic protein reprioritization. Surgery 1988;104:199–207.

37. Moore FA, Moore EE, Jones TN et al: TEN versus TPN following major abdominal trauma: reduced septic morbidity. J Trauma 1989;29:916–923.

38. Moore FA, Feliciano DV, Andrassy RJ et al: Early enteral feeding, compared with parenteral, reduces postoperative septic complications. The results of a meta-analysis. Ann Surg 1992;216:172–183.

39. Moore EE, Moore FA: Immediate enteral nutrition following multisystem trauma: a decade perspective. J Am Coll Nutr 1991;10:633–648.

40. Kudsk KA, Croce MA, Fabian TC et al: Enteral versus parenteral feeding. Effects on septic morbidity after blunt and penetrating abdominal trauma. Ann Surg 1992;215:503–513.

41. Kudsk KA, Minard G, Wojtysiak SL et al: Visceral protein response to enteral versus parenteral nutrition and sepsis in patients with trauma. Surgery 1994;116:516–523.

42. Adams S, Dellinger EP, Wertz MJ et al: Enteral versus parenteral nutritional support following laparotomy for trauma: a randomized prospective trial. J Trauma 1986;26:882–891.

43. Cerra FB, McPherson JP, Konstantinides FN et al: Enteral nutrition does not prevent multiple organ failure syndrome (MOFS) after sepsis. Surgery 1988;104:727–733.

44. Cerra FB, Shronts EP, Konstantinides NN et al: Enteral feeding in sepsis: a prospective, randomized, double-blind trial. Surgery 1985;98:632–639.

45. Hoover HC, Ryan JA, Anderson EJ et al: Nutritional benefits of immediate postoperative jejunal feeding of an elemental diet. Am J Surg 1980;139:153–159.

46. Muggia-Sullam M, Bower RH, Murphy RF et al: Postoperative enteral versus parenteral nutritional support in gastrointestinal surgery. A matched prospective study. Am J Surg 1985;149:106–112.

47. Young VR, Munro HN: N-methylhistidine (3-methylhistidine) and muscle protein turnover: an overview. Fed Proc 1978;37:2291–2300.

48. Hasselgren PO, James JH, Benson DW et al: Total and myofibrillar protein breakdown in different types of rat skeletal muscle: effects of sepsis and regulation by insulin. Metabolism 1989;38:634–640.

49. Long CL, Birkhahn RH, Geiger JW et al: Urinary excretion of 3-methylhistidine: an assessment of muscle protein catabolism in adult normal subjects and during malnutrition, sepsis, and skeletal trauma. Metabolism 1981;30:765–776.

50. Bower RH, Talamini MA, Sax HC et al: Postoperative enteral vs parenteral nutrition. A randomized controlled trial. Arch Surg 1986;121:1040–1045.

51. Fong Y, Moldawer LL, Shires T et al: The biological characteristics of cytokines and their implication in surgical injury. Surg Gynecol Obstet 1990;170:363–378.

52. Fischer JE, Hasselgren PO: Cytokines and glucocorticoids in the regulation of the "hepato-skeletal muscle axis" in sepsis. Am J Surg 1991;161:266–271.

53. Hasselgren PO: Mediators, hormones, and control of metabolism. Regulation of protein, carbohydrate, and lipid metabolism in critical illness, in Fischer JE (ed): Surgical Nutrition, 2nd edition. Boston: Little, Brown & Co, in press.

54. Lickley HLA, Track NS, Vranic M et al: Metabolic responses to enteral and parenteral nutrition. Am J Surg 1978;135:172–176.

55. Gianotti L, Nelson JL, Alexander JW et al: Post injury hypermetabolic response and magnitude of translocation: prevention by early enteral nutrition. Nutrition 1994;10:225–231.

56. Fong Y, Marano MA, Barber A et al: Total parenteral nutrition and bowel rest modify the metabolic response to endotoxin in humans. Ann Surg 1989;210:449–457.

57. Deitch EA, Xu D, Franko L et al: Evidence favoring a role of the gut as a cytokine-generating organ in rats subjected to hemorrhagic shock. Shock 1994;1:141–146.

58. Meyer TA, Noguchi Y, Ogle CK et al: Endotoxin stimulates interleukin-6 production in intestinal epithelial cells: a synergistic effect with prostaglandin E_2. Arch Surg 1994;129:1290–1295.

59. Meyer TA, Tiao G, James JH et al: Nitric oxide inhibits LPS-induced IL-6 production in enterocytes. J Surg Res 1995;58:570–575.

60. Welbourne TC, Joshi S: Enteral glutamine spares endogenous glutamine in chronic acidosis. JPEN 1994;18:243–247.

61. Alexander JW: Immunoenhancement via enteral nutrition. Arch Surg 1993;128:1242–1245.

62. Higashiguchi T, Hasselgren PO, Wagner K et al: Effect of glutamine on protein synthesis in isolated intestinal epithelial cells. JPEN 1993;17:307–314.

63. Ziegler TR, Young LS, Benfell K et al: Clinical and metabolic efficacy of glutamine-supplemented parenteral nutrition after bone marrow transplantation: a randomized, double-blind, controlled study. Ann Intern Med 1992;116:821–828.

64. Kirk SJ, Barbul A: Role of arginine in trauma, sepsis, and immunity. JPEN 1990;14:226S–229S.

65. Darmaun D, Just B, Messing B et al: Glutamine metabolism in healthy adult men: response to enteral and intravenous feeding. Am J Clin Nutr 1994;59:1395–1402.

66. Daly JM, Lieberman MD, Goldfine J et al: Enteral nutrition with supplemental arginine, RNA, and omega-3 fatty acids in patients after operation: immunologic, metabolic, and clinical outcome. Surgery 1992;112:56–67.

67. Bower RH, Lavin PT, Licari JJ et al: A modified enteral formula reduces hospital length of stay in intensive care units. Crit Care Med 1993;21:S275. Abstract.

68. Moore FA, Moore EE, Kudsk KA et al: Clinical benefits of an immune-enhancing diet for early postinjury enteral feeding. J Trauma 1994;37:607–615.

69. Gottschlich MM, Jenkins M, Warden GD et al: Differential effects of three enteral dietary regimens on selected outcome variables in burn patients. JPEN 1990;14:225–236.

70. Cerra FB, Lehmann S, Konstandinides N et al: Improvement in immune function in ICU patients by enteral nutrition supplemented with arginine, RNA and menhaden oil is independent of nitrogen balance. Nutrition 1991;7:193–199.

4

Lipids and Enteral Nutrition

ROLANDO H. ROLANDELLI
JOAN R. ULLRICH

Lipids provide most of the energy in oral diets and in defined formula diets because of their high caloric density. With the realization that the body depends on the exogenous supply of linoleic and linolenic acids, oil sources with high concentrations of these essential fatty acids, such as corn oil or soybean oil, have become the standard fat source in enteral diets. In recent years, however, several questions have been raised regarding the wisdom of using long-chain triglycerides as a calorie source. Conversely, other fat sources have been noted to be beneficial in certain clinical conditions. Within the context of these controversies this chapter will review the biochemistry and physiology of lipids as well as the role of fat in enteral nutrition.

BODY LIPIDS

Fat accounts for approximately 15 percent of body weight. About half of the total body fat is in the subcutaneous tissue while the remaining half is distributed in other body tissues. Subcutaneous fat was once thought to serve only as a mechanical cushion and an insulating layer. In the 1950s, however, investigators demonstrated that the adipose tissue is also a reservoir of energy that can be mobilized in the form of nonesterified fatty acids (NEFA) to other tissues.[1,2]

Lipids circulate in the bloodstream in the form of lipoproteins. Lipoproteins are classified as very low density lipoproteins (VLDL), low density lipoproteins (LDL), high density lipoproteins (HDL), and chylomicrons depending on their centrifugation characteristics. Chylomicrons are the largest and lightest of the lipoproteins. They are made of triglycerides (80 to 95 percent of weight), cholesterol (2 to 7 percent), phospholipid (3 to 6 percent), and protein (1 to 2 percent). Chylomicrons transport dietary fat from the intestinal mucosa via the thoracic duct to most tissues and are ultimately cleared by the liver. VLDLs consist of triglycerides (55 to 65 percent), which derive from the liver, cholesterol (10 to 15 percent), phospholipid (15 to 20 percent), and protein (5 to 10 percent). LDLs originate, at least in part, from VLDL degradation and are made of 45 percent cholesterol, 22 percent phospholipid, 10 percent triglyceride, and 25 percent protein. HDLs originate in the liver, independently of VLDLs, and contain 45 to 50 percent protein, 30 percent phospholipid, and 20 percent cholesterol.

Lipids are also constituents of cell membranes. Singer and Nicholson[3] described the biomembranes as fluid-like phospholipid bilayers. Various proteins are scattered throughout the lipidic bilayer in the form of a mosaic (Fig. 4–1). The proportion of lipids and proteins varies from membrane to membrane within a cell and also from cell to cell. The outer mitochondrial membrane consists of 50 percent protein and 46 percent lipids, whereas the inner mitochondrial membrane consists of 75 percent protein and 23 percent lipids. Most cell membranes consist of approximately 50 percent lipids and 50 percent protein. Myelin is unique with a lipidic content of 75 percent, which includes glycosyl ceramides and sphingolipids in addition to phospholipids. The phospholipids present in membranes are 1,2-diacylphosphoglycerides, of which phosphatidylcholine predominates in humans. The acyl chains of phosphatidylcholine are occupied by even-numbered fatty acids. Whereas the n-1 position is occupied by saturated fatty acids, the n-2 position includes unsaturated fatty acids such as 18:1, 18:2, 18:3, and 20:4. The type of fatty acid incorporated into membrane phopholipids varies depending on the type of dietary fat. Increasing amounts of polyunsaturated fatty acids in the diet change the membrane fluidity, which in turn may affect cell function.[4,5]

LIPID BIOCHEMISTRY: CLASSIFICATION OF FATTY ACIDS

Fatty acids are classified according to their chain length and the position and number of double bonds. Several nomenclature systems are used to refer to fatty acids. One system uses the chain length followed by the number of double bonds in the same word, preceded by the type and position of double bonds. According to this system linoleic acid is expressed as 9,12-octadecadienoic acid. A simpler way to refer to fatty acids is by a numeric system in which the number of carbons is separated from the number of double bonds by a colon sign and then followed by a subscript with the position of the double bonds. In this system, linoleic acid is expressed as $18:2_{\Delta9,12}$. Many fatty acids have been given a name, such as arachidonic acid or linoleic acid, usually related to their metabolic characteristics or abundance in nature. Naturally occurring fatty acid double bonds are in the *cis* position. Unsaturation in the *trans* position occurs during hydrogenation or processing by intestinal bacteria.

In the aforementioned examples the carbon chain is numbered from the carboxyl group; 9 and 12 refer to the ninth and twelfth carbon counting from the carboxyl end of linoleic acid. Biochemists have introduced another classification system for fatty acids in which the numbering is begun from the methyl group end. According to this classification, fatty acids are divided in series (ω or n-) depending on the location of the first double bond: 3-ω or n-3 series. The 3, 6, 7, and 9 series' are common in humans. Figure 4–2 illustrates the basis for the different nomenclature systems of fatty acids.

Finally another classification divides fatty acids into three groups according to the length of the carbon chain: short, medium, and long fatty acids. The short-chain fatty acids (SCFAs) of interest in human physiology are acetate (2 carbon chain), propionate (3 carbon chain), and butyrate (4 carbon chain). The origin and metabolism of SCFAs are discussed elsewhere in this text. These fatty acids are unique because

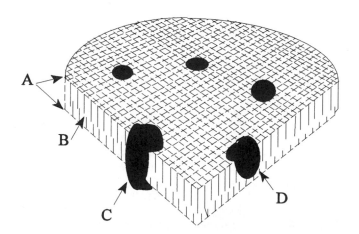

FIGURE 4–1 Mosaic model of cell membranes with lipidic bilayer and proteins scattered throughout (*black*). The polar head of phospholipids (*A*) is exposed to both surfaces—extracellular and intracellular. The nonpolar fatty acid tails (*B*) are hidden between the two layers. Proteins can be transmembrane proteins (*C*) or surface proteins (*D*).

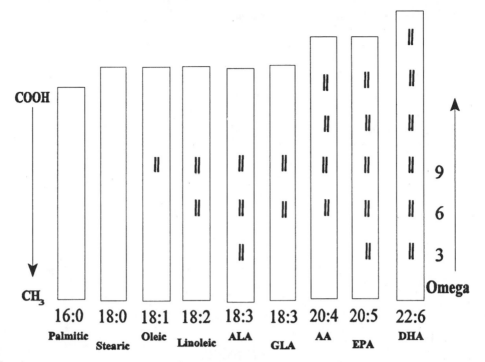

FIGURE 4–2 Schematic representation of fatty acids. Some of the key fatty acids are stacked together to demonstrate the basis for the different nomenclature systems used to classify fatty acids. The *arrow* on the left side of the graph indicates the direction of the chemical numbering of carbons from the carboxyl to the methyl group. The biologic classification numbers the carbons beginning in the methyl group (*arrow* on the right side of the graph). The vertical double lines within the rectangles indicate the position of double bonds. Fatty acids are grouped in series (*omega*) according to the position of the first double bond. Oleic acid belongs to the 9–ω series. Linoleic, γ–linolenic (GLA), and arachidonic (AA) acids are part of the 6–ω series whereas α–linolenic acid (ALA), eicosapentanoic acid (EPA), and docosahexanoic acid (DHA) are part of the 3–ω series.

they are produced by bacteria, usually from a carbohydrate source, and because their metabolism more closely resembles that of carbohydrates than of lipids. For instance, the respiratory quotient of SCFA oxidation is approximately 0.8 to 0.9 instead of the typical 0.7 of fat oxidation. The medium-chain fatty acids (MCFAs) are those with chains between 6 and 12 carbons. MCFAs are degraded by β oxidation yielding a low respiratory quotient. MCFAs enter the mitochondrium for oxidation independent of transporters. Long-chain fatty acids (LCFAs) are those with chains between 14 and 24 carbons. Because of their diverse effects on the body and their essential nature, LCFAs have been extensively studied. Contrary to MCFAs, LCFAs require a transporter to enter the mitochondrium for oxidation. This system depends on 1-carnitine—the acyl transferase system (Fig. 4–3).

Those fatty acids with more than two double bonds are called polyunsaturated fatty acids or PUFAs. PUFAs are precursors for the synthesis of eicosanoids, that is, prostaglandins, leukotrienes, and thromboxanes. These substances act on target cells at very low concentrations and for a brief period of time, indicating that they behave as autocrine or paracrine mediators rather than systemic hormones.

ESSENTIAL FATTY ACIDS

The essential fatty acids are linoleic and α-linolenic acids. Since the advent of parenteral nutrition it has become evident that deprivation of linoleic and α-linolenic acid in the diet or parenteral formulas leads to a deficiency syndrome characterized by scaly dermatitis, hair loss, thrombocytopenia, and poor wound healing.[6] This syndrome can be reversed by the exogenous administration of linoleic acid.

The body can synthesize fatty acids from glucose. For instance, palmitic (16:0) and

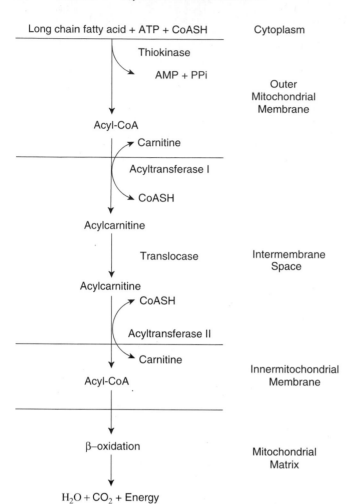

Long chain fatty acid + ATP + CoASH   Cytoplasm

Thiokinase

AMP + PPi

Outer
Mitochondrial
Membrane

Acyl-CoA

Carnitine

Acyltransferase I

CoASH

Acylcarnitine

Translocase   Intermembrane
Space

Acylcarnitine

CoASH

Acyltransferase II

Carnitine

Innermitochondrial
Membrane

Acyl-CoA

β–oxidation   Mitochondrial
Matrix

$H_2O + CO_2 +$ Energy

FIGURE 4–3 Carnitine-mediated transport of long-chain fatty acids into mitochondria. (From Tao RC, Yoshimura NN: Carnitine metabolism and its application in parenteral nutrition. J Parenter Enter Nutr 1980;4:469–486.)

stearic (18:0) acids can be synthesized from glucose via lipogenesis. These fatty acids are desaturated to produce palmitoleic (16:1 n-7) and oleic (18:1 n-9) acids by the Δ 9 desaturase. In turn, these fatty acids can be further elongated and desaturated, but the products will always remain within the 7 and 9 series (the first double bond in either the seventh or the ninth carbon) (Fig. 4–4).

There are two families of essential fatty acids, one within the n-6 series and the other within the n-3 series. The precursor of the n-6 series is linoleic acid (18:2 n-6) and the precursor of the n-3 series is α-linolenic acid (18:3 n-3). These fatty acids are desaturated by the Δ-6-desaturase to be converted into γ-linolenic (18:3 n-6) and stearidonic (18:4 n-3) acids, respectively. γ-Linolenic acid is then elongated to dihomo γ-linolenic acid (DHLA, 20:3 n-6) and desaturated to arachidonic acid (20:4 n-6). Stearidonic acid is elongated (20:4 n-3) and

then desaturated to produce eicosapentanoic acid (20:5 n-3).

In the absence of essential fatty acids the body tries to compensate for this deficit by overproducing metabolites of palmitic and stearic acid. The end products of metabolism of these nonessential fatty acids are eicosatrienoic acid (20:3 n-9) and docosatrienoic acid (22:3 n-9). Therefore, the diagnosis of essential fatty acid deficiency (EFAD) is made by calculating the ration of trienoic over tetranoic fatty acids in plasma. When this ratio is less than 0.4 a diagnosis of EFAD is established.[7] Clinical signs of EFAD are usually seen following 3 weeks of a diet devoid of long-chain triglycerides. The need for essential fatty acids is met by providing 1 to 2 percent of the total calories as linoleic acid. In an average weight adult this is equivalent to 2.5 to 5 g of linoleic acid per day.

Despite providing sufficient quantities of linoleic acid with formulas containing soybean

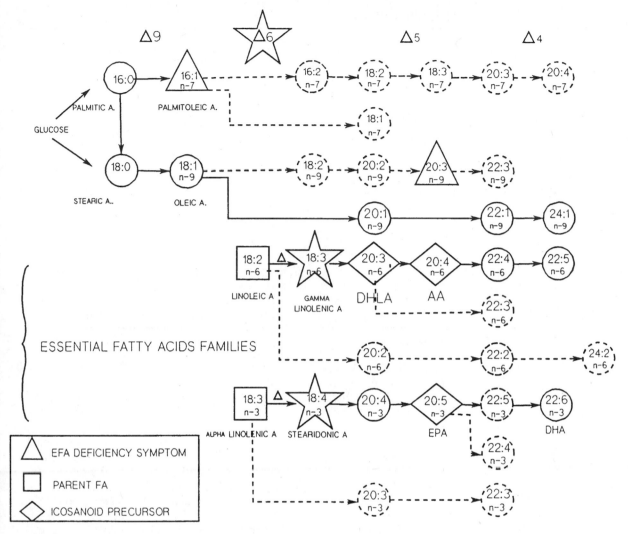

FIGURE 4–4 Biosynthesis of fatty acids. (From Halperin MJ [ed.]: Lipid Metabolism and Its Pathology. Amsterdam: Elsevier Science, 1986:213–223.)

oil, patients have developed EFAD.[8,9] This deficiency of α-linolenic acid results in scaly and hemorrhagic dermatitis, hemorrhagic folliculitis of the scalp, growth retardation, and delayed wound healing.[10]

α-Linolenic acid is a 3-ω fatty acid precursor of eicosapentanoic acid (EPA). The requirement for α-linolenic acid is even less than that of linoleic acid. This need is met by providing 0.5 to 0.6 percent of the total calories as α-linolenic acid or an equivalent of 2 to 3 g per day.

DIETARY FAT

Vegetable oils are rich in saturated fatty acids and derivatives of linoleic acid, the 6-ω series.

The only fatty acid of the 3-ω series present in vegetables is α-linolenic acid. Fatty acids of longer carbon chains in the 3-ω, such as EPA and docosahexanoic acid (DHA), are present only in cold-water fish, shellfish, and fish oils. Beef and dairy products also contain linoleic acid. The fatty acid composition of different oils is listed in Table 4–1. Medium-chain triglycerides are present in oils with high concentrations of saturated fat such as those obtained from the coconut and the palm kernel.

The liquid diets marketed by the pharmaceutical industry contain variable amounts of fatty acids. The early elemental diets provided sufficient amounts of long-chain triglycerides to prevent EFAD and used carbohydrates as a

TABLE 4–1　Fatty Acid Composition of Oils

Oil	Fatty Acids (%)			
	Linoleic	α-Linolenic	EPA	DHA
Safflower	76			
Sunflower	66			
Cottonseed	60			
Corn	56			
Soybean	47	7		
Sesame	42			
Peanut	32			
Canola	21	9		
Linseed	18	54		
Perilla	15	58		
Olive	7			
Palm	2			
Palm kernel	2			
Cod liver	2	2	9	9
Coconut	1			
MaxEPA	1	3	14	9
Herring			7	4
Menhaden			13	8

EPA = eicosapentanoic acid; DHA = docosahexanoic acid.

source of calories. This made elemental diets hyperosmolar, which resulted in tube feeding intolerance. As the ready-to-use liquid diets were being developed the side-effects of over-feeding carbohydrate calories became known. These side-effects were respiratory insufficiency from the excess of carbon dioxide produced from carbohydrate oxidation, and deposition of fat in the liver. To reduce the osmolality and also the side-effects of carbohydrate overfeeding, more and more fat was added to enteral diets. Diets with as much as 50 g/L of linoleic acid were developed and marketed as therapeutic for pulmonary diseases. As knowledge of lipid metabolism has evolved, two significant changes have been introduced in enteral diets. Many diets now include a proportion of MCTs and 3-ω fatty acids. The fat content of various enteral products is summarized in Table 4–2.

As already mentioned PUFAs such as linoleic and α-linolenic acids are the precursors for the synthesis of eicosanoids, that is, prosta-glandins, leukotrienes, and thromboxanes. The two major pathways of eicosanoid synthesis are the cyclooxygenase and the lipooxygenase pathways. While the cyclooxygenase pathway results in prostanoids, prostaglandins, and thromboxanes, the metabolites of the lipooxy-genase pathway are leukotrienes, hydroxyei-cosatrienoic acids, and lipoxins (Fig. 4–5).

The substrates for eicosanoid synthesis are arachidonic acid and EPA, and the main source of

the acids is the membrane phospholipids. Arachi-donic acid is released from phosphadyl choline by the action of phospholipase A2.[11] Eicosanoids de-rived from arachidonic acid are mainly the dienoic prostanoids and the tetraenoic leuko-trienes; the metabolism of EPA, however, yields trienoic prostanoids and pentanoic leuko-trienes.[12,13] In addition to being a substrate for dif-ferent eicosanoid production, 3-ω fatty acids di-rectly suppress the activity of cyclooxygenase.[14]

Eicosanoids influence cellular activity by al-tering the intracellular levels of the cyclic nu-cleotides adenosine 3':5' cyclic phosphate (cAMP) and cyclic guanosine monophosphate (cGMP). The ratio between these two nu-cleotides determines cell function rather than the absolute concentrations. For instance, PGE2, a product of cyclooxygenase metabo-lism, suppresses blastogenesis by lymphocytes through an increase in this ratio.[11]

Thromboxane A2 and leukotriene B4, both products of arachidonic acid via linoleic metab-olism, are potent vasoconstrictors and induce platelet aggregation while thromboxane A3 is only a mild vasoconstrictor and inhibits platelet aggregation.

Other PUFAs can be synthesized by conver-sion of linoleic and α-linolenic acids. One of the limiting steps in the conversion of linoleic and α-linolenic acids to their derivatives is the en-zyme Δ-6-desaturase. This enzyme is regulated by many factors. Whereas dietary protein and

TABLE 4–2   Fat Content (g/L) of Selected Enteral Products

Formula	Total	% Cal	LO#	MCT	O-3@	Oil Source
Alterna	15.6	38.1	0.5	0	0.1	Soy
Amin-Aid	46.2	21.2	10.2	0	0.92	Soy, lecithin, glycerides
Attain	35.0	30.0	7.2	17.3	0.2	Corn, MCT
Compleat Reg	42.8	36.0	17.5	0	0.43	Beef, corn
Compleat Mod	36.8	31.0	14.4	0	0.37	Beef, corn
Comply	60.0	36.0	26.2	0	0.72	Corn
Criticare HN	5.3	4.5	3.3	0	0.13	Safflower
Deliver 2.0	102.0	45.0	38.0	29.0	5.6	Soy, MCT
Ensure	37.1	31.5	20.0	0	0.46	Corn
Ensure Plus	53.2	32.0	28.6	0	0.7	Corn
Ensure with Fiber	37.1	30.5	20.0	0	0.46	Corn
Entera	34.0	30.0	19.1	4.0	0	Sunflower, MCT
Entera Iso	34.0	30.0	19.1	13.0	2.3	Soy, MCT
Entera OPD	26.0	22.0	19.1	14.3	0	Sunflower, MCT
Fibersource	51.6	30.0	5.2	25.8	2.06	Canola, MCT
Fibersource HN	51.6	30.0	5.2	25.8	2.06	Canola, MCT
Glucerna	55.7	50.0	11.0	0	0.75	Safflower, soy, oleic
Hepatic-Aid II	36.2	27.7	8.0	0	0.75	Soy, lecithin, glycerides
Immun-Aid	22.0	20.0	2.1	11.0	1.2	Canola, MCT
Impact	28.0	25.0	2.2	7.0	1.7	Menhaden, MCT, kernel/sunflower
Isocal	44.0	37.0	19.4	8.9	2.7	Soy, MCT
Isocal HN	45.0	37.0	14.4	17.8	2.3	Soy, MCT
Isosource	41.6	30.0	4.1	20.5	1.7	Canola, MCT
Isosource HN	41.6	30.0	4.1	20.5	1.7	Canola, MCT
Isotein HN	34.0	25.0	3.7	8.5	0.34	Soy, MCT
Jevity	36.8	30.0	12.3	18.5	0.33	Corn, soy, MCT
Lipisorb	48.0	48.0	3.9	41.0	<0.1	Corn, MCT
Magnacal	80.0	36.0	29.6	0	4.8	Soy
Newtrition HN	40.0	30.0	8.16	15.0	0.56	Corn, MCT
Newtrition Isofiber	40.0	29.0	10.88	20.0	0.56	Corn, MCT
Newtrition Iso	36.0	31.0	9.79	18.0	0.5	Corn, MCT
Newtrition 1 & 1/2	50.0	30.0	8.16	25.0	0.7	Corn, MCT
Nutren 1.0	38.0	33.0	14.7	9.0	0.38	Corn, MCT
Nutren 1.0 with Fiber	38.0	33.0	14.7	9.0	0.38	Corn, MCT
Nutren 1.5	67.5	39.0	17.4	32.7	0.56	Corn, MCT
Osmolite	38.5	31.4	12.9	19.25	0.34	Corn, soy, MCT
Osmolite HN	36.8	30.0	12.3	18.25	0.33	Corn, soy, MCT
Pediasure	50.0	44.5	11.4	9.9	1.1	Safflower, soy, MCT
Peptamen	39.0	33.0	4.8	27.0	0.21	Sunflower, MCT, lecithin
Pulmocare	92.0	55.2	52.0	0	1.2	Corn
Reabilan	39.0	35.0	12.5	15.4	0.56	Primrose, soy, MCT
Reabilan HN	51.9	35.0	15.4	19.95	1.0	Linoleic, MCT
Replena	95.0	43.0	19.9	0	0.85	Safflower (high oleic), soy
Replete	33.0	30.0	17.0	0	0.42	Corn
Resource Liquid	37.0	32.0	21.8	0	0.37	Corn
Resource Plus	53.1	32.0	31.3	0	0.53	Corn
Stresstein	27.3	20.0	4.09	16.9	0.55	Soy, MCT
Sustacal	23.0	21.0	8.7	0	0.4	Soy
Sustacal HC	58.0	34.0	35.0	0	0.3	Corn
Sustacal with Fiber	35.0	30.0	19.2	0	0.4	Corn
Tolerex	1.45	1.3	1.16	0	0	Safflower
Traum-Aid HBC	12.4	11.2	1.6	5.0	0.15	Soy, MCT
TraumaCal	68.0	40.0	27.0	20.0	4.3	Soy, MCT
Ultracal	45.0	37.0	13.1	18.2	2.2	Soy, MCT
Vital HN	10.7	9.4	4.1	4.8	0	Safflower, MCT
Vitaneed	40.0	36.0	22.1	0	0	Corn, beef
Vivonex TEN	2.8	2.5	2.17	0	0	Safflower

LO# = linoleic acids; O-3@ = omega-3 fatty acids; HN = high nitrogen; Iso = isotonic; MCT = medium-chain triglycerides.
Modified from Gottschlich MM: Selection of optimal lipid sources in enteral and parenteral nutrition. Nutr Clin Pract 1992;7:155–156.

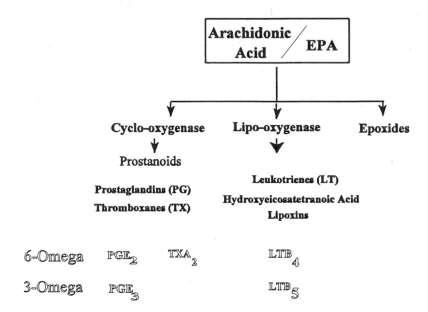

FIGURE 4–5   Eicosanoid synthesis. The two rows on the bottom illustrate the influence of dietary lipids on the synthesis of eicosanoids. Diets rich in 6–ω fatty acids result in the production of eicosanoids of the 2 or 4 series while diets enriched with 3–ω fatty acids result in the production of eicosanoids of the 3 and 5 series.

insulin levels activate the Δ-6-desaturase, starvation, carbohydrates, and counterregulatory hormones inhibit it.[15] A peculiar mode of regulation is by the presence of linoleic acid. Contrary to other chemical reactions where substrate stimulates an enzyme, the activity of Δ-6-desaturase is inhibited by an excess of linoleic acid. This phenomenon was elegantly demonstrated in rats receiving parenteral nutrition for 1 week with either no lipids or with a soybean emulsion. Analysis of the liver phosphatidylcholine of these animals revealed a decrease in all the upper derivatives of both linoleic and α-linolenic acids while high levels of linoleic acid were being supplied.[12] Similarly, in children receiving a short course of parenteral nutrition with a soybean emulsion, the liver phosphatidylcholine was deficient in the upper derivatives of the 3-ω and 6-ω families.[16]

An interesting study on the effects of various fat sources was published by Diboune and collaborators.[17] This group studied critically ill patients receiving three different types of enteral diets. Group A received an enteral diet with only LCFAs provided as soybean oil. Group B received the same enteral diet, but 50 percent of the fat was provided as LCFAs and 50 percent as MCFAs. Group C also received 50 percent LCFAs, but 42.5 percent was given as LCFAs and 7.5 percent was given as black-currant–seed oil. Black-currant–seed oil contains

14 percent γ-linolenic acid and 4 percent stearidonic acid, which are products of the 3-ω series beyond the step of the Δ-6-desaturase. To assess the metabolism of fatty acids, the group studied the lipid composition of circulating erythrocytes. They demonstrated that patients in Group A had an inhibition of the Δ-6-desaturase as demonstrated by an increase in linoleic acid without a corresponding increase in DHLA. Replacing 50 percent of fat calories with MCFAs reduced this inhibition, and adding black-currant–seed oil increased both DHLA and EPA. Further studies are needed to delineate the exact needs for fatty acids under different pathologic conditions.

FAT DIGESTION AND ABSORPTION

In the typical western diet, fat is present in the form of long-chain triglycerides (LCTs). When ingested fat reaches the duodenum it stimulates the release of cholecystokinin (CCK). CCK delays stomach emptying and produces both contraction of the gallbladder and pancreatic secretion. LCTs are then hydrolyzed by pancreatic lipase in the alkaline environment provided by pancreatic juice. Co-lipase is another substance present in pancreatic juice that produces adherence of lipase to the oil droplets. Fat hydrolysis is usually incomplete and results in glycerol, fatty acids, and monoglycerides. Monoglycerides and fatty acids are then incorporated into micelles, which are aggregates of bile salts with a hydrophilic and water soluble external surface and a hydrophobic internal core. These micelles allow the transport of fatty acids across the unstirred layer of water that overlies the villi. Once in proximity to the epithelial cells the micelles break up and the fatty acids are transported into the jejunal epithelium while bile salts return to the lumen to be absorbed later in the ileum. Within the epithelial cells of the jejunum LCTs are resynthesized and then combine with phospholipids, cholesterol, and protein to form chylomicrons. Chylomicrons are transported through lacteals and then through the thoracic duct into systemic circulation.

Fat not absorbed in the small intestine creates water secretion in the colon and steatorrhea. Steatorrhea is associated with large, greasy, and foul-smelling stools. Causes for steatorrhea include bile salt deficiency, pancreatic enzyme deficiency, or defects in lymphatic transport. A deficiency of bile salts in the intestinal lumen may be due to lack of excretion, such as in biliary obstruction, or excessive loss, as occurs with ileal resection. Pancreatic enzyme deficiency is typically seen in chronic pancreatitis or following extensive pancreatic resections. Disorders of lymphatic transport are more rare and include chylous fistulae due to injury of the thoracic duct in addition to congenital lymphangectasia and Whipple's disease.

FATTY ACIDS AS A FUEL SOURCE

The smaller molecular size of MCTs as compared to LCTs facilitates the action of pancreatic lipase. MCTs are hydrolyzed faster and more completely than LCTs. Studies in humans have demonstrated that MCTs do not stimulate pancreatic secretion while LCTs significantly increase pancreatic secretion.[18] Because their intraluminal hydrolysis is complete, MCTs are rapidly absorbed as free fatty acids. MCFAs are absorbed via the portal venous system. Once MCFAs reach the liver they undergo extensive metabolism with only a very small amount passing out of the liver.

Another major difference between MCFAs and LCFAs is their intracellular metabolism. MCFAs cross the double mitochondrial membrane rapidly and, once inside the mitochondria, are activated to acyl-CoA. LCFAs entering the cell are first activated by thiokinases with extramitochondrial CoASH at the expense of adenosine triphosphate (ATP). Activated LCFAs, in the form of acyl-CoA, are impermeable to the mitochondrial membrane. To traverse the mitochondrial membrane, acyl-CoA is converted to acyl carnitine by acyltransferase I. Another enzyme, translocase, transports the acyl carnitine through the intermembrane space. At the inner mitochondrial membrane acyltransferase II removes the carnitine and replaces the CoA to form acyl-CoA ready to enter β-oxidation.[19]

Carnitine is β-hydroxy-γ-trimethylaminobutyric acid. The carbon chain of carnitine derives from lysine which is methylated by S-adenosyl-methionine to produce ε-trimethyl-lysine. ε-Trimethyl-lysine first undergoes hydroxylation and later dehydrogenation requiring ascorbic acid, iron, and pyridoxal phosphate. While all these reactions normally maintain an adequate supply of carnitine, conditions such as uremia, cirrhosis, and sepsis can result in a relative deficiency of carnitine. Under these circumstances LCFAs cannot be oxidized and accumulate in muscle, resulting in lipid storage myopathy and cardiomyopathy.[20]

Under normal conditions the carnitine palmityl transferase is rather inactive. Therefore, LCFAs are preferentially redirected to lipogenesis instead of oxidation. MCFAs, however, are preferentially oxidized to acetyl-CoA. A fraction of the acetyl-CoA produced from MCFA oxidation enters the Krebs cycle for complete oxidation. Another fraction of acetyl-CoA is redirected toward the synthesis of ketone bodies, which explains the ketogenic capacity of MCTs.[21]

A single oral dose of MCTs results in slight hypoglycemia.[22] This is caused by a decrease in the hepatic output of glucose rather than an increase in peripheral utilization of glucose. Paradoxically, insulin levels increase at the same time, presumably due to stimulation of the islets of Langerhans by ketone bodies or by MCFAs. However, MCTs tend to improve carbohydrate tolerance.[23] Other side-effects reported with the use of MCTs are increased thermogenesis and a derangement in lipoproteins leading to a proatherogenic lipid profile.

In summary, the physicochemical properties of MCFAs make them a readily available source of calories. MCFAs are not stored in adipose tissue and do not produce hyperlipidemia; however, they are rapidly oxidized and are ketogenic. In addition, by replacing LCT calories with MCTs the immunosuppressive effects of linoleic acid, and its 6-ω derivatives, can be minimized.

STRUCTURED LIPIDS

It has now become apparent that neither LCTs nor MCTs alone can meet the body needs for fat, that is, prevention of EFAD and fuel for oxidation. Therefore, many commercial diets include various proportions of LCT and MCT oils. A novel approach is the combination of MCTs and LCTs within the same molecule creating a structured triglyceride or structured lipid.[24] These particles are made by hydrolysis and reesterification of LCTs and MCTs after random mixing in a process called transesterification. The final products are either two LCFAs with one MCFA or two MCFAs with one LCFA (Fig. 4–6). The proportions of structured triglycerides resulting from a mixture can be predicted depending on the starting proportions of the base oils.

The combination of LCFAs with MCFAs provides both the EFA and a readily available fuel source, and, in addition, seems to potentiate the effects of each. In a rat model of burn wound, structured triglycerides administered through a gastrostomy tube resulted in an increase in the protein fractional synthetic rate of the liver and improved nitrogen balance in animals that received structured triglycerides.[25] These structured triglycerides were made from 35 percent MCTs, 50 percent butter, and 15 percent safflower oil. Similar results were obtained in the rat model of burn wound using structured triglycerides made from palm kernel oil and sunflower oil[26] or from MCTs and fish oil.[27]

IMMUNE-MODULATION BY FATTY ACIDS

Long-chain unsaturated fatty acids are incorporated into the membranes of all mammalian cells where they influence fluidity and function. This is of particular importance in cell-to-cell interactions, particularly in antigen-presenting cells, in the cells' response to injury, and in cytolysis. For example, large amounts of arachidonic acid in the membrane phospholipids yield higher amounts of prostaglandin E2 (PGE2) and prostacyclin. PGE2 is a potent immunosuppressive agent. One of the mechanisms for the immunosuppressive effect is the stimulation of suppressor T-cell activity.[28] Other mechanisms for the immunosuppressive effects of 6-ω fatty acids are stimulation of macrophages to release superoxide,[29] decreased synthesis of fractions of complement,[30] and depression of delayed hypersensitivity responses.[1,31]

The immunosuppressive effect of 6-ω fatty acids has been exploited for therapeutic purposes. In rats supplementation with linoleic acid prolongs the life of skin allografts;[32] supplementation with linoleic acid in conjunction with a donor-specific transfusion prolongs survival of heart allografts.[33] Linoleic acid can also act synergistically with cyclosporin and transfusion to produce a permanent allograft survival.[34] Another demonstration of the role of fatty acids on the immune response is that the effects of donor-specific transfusion on allograft survival can be blocked by cyclooxygen-

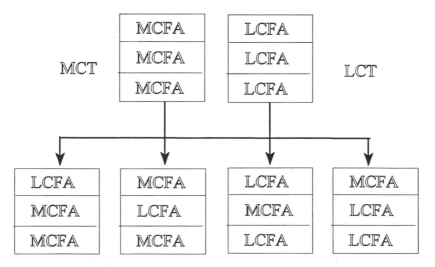

FIGURE 4–6 Structured triglycerides. Different proportions of structured triglycerides are constructed depending on the starting concentrations of long-chain triglycerides (LCTs) and medium-chain triglycerides (MCTs).

ase inhibition and enhanced by lipooxygenase inhibition.[35]

In other studies 6-ω fatty acids have been shown to alter the response to endotoxin. In rats with essential fatty acid deficiency (EFAD) the mortality following endotoxin challenge was 24 percent. However, when the EFAD was reversed by administration of arachidonic acid 2 days before the endotoxin challenge, the mortality was 100 percent.[36] The response to the endotoxin was improved when guinea pigs received a diet with 3-ω fatty acids (Menhaden oil) as compared with animals receiving safflower oil.[37]

Similarly, guinea pigs recovering from a major burn wound had improved immune function when they received the same amount of fat in the diet (10 percent of calories) but in the form of 3-ω fatty acids (EPA [18 percent] and docosahexanoic acid [17 percent]) as compared to animals that received 6-ω fatty acids (safflower oil [74 percent linoleic acid]) or 100 percent linoleic acid. Animals fed 3-ω fatty acids had better cell-mediated immune responses, better opsonic indexes, higher splenic weights, and lower serum C3 levels.[38]

One concern regarding the dietary supplementation of 3-ω fatty acids in the diet is the development of glucose intolerance. Glucose intolerance has been described as a side-effect in patients with non-insulin dependent diabetes when they received a supplement of 3-ω fatty acids. However, to our knowledge this has not been a problem in hospitalized patients receiving tube feedings.

CLINICAL APPLICATIONS OF ENTERAL FORMULAS MODIFIED IN FAT CONTENT

Respiratory Failure

The respiratory function is highly dependent on nutritional status and nutrient supply. The ventilatory function is accomplished by muscle work through the diaphragm and accessory muscles. Malnutrition can result in impaired muscle function and decreased immune function. Poor ventilation and poor immune response leads to pulmonary infections, which in turn can cause respiratory failure. Attempts at correcting malnutrition too quickly can result in overproduction of carbon dioxide and increased oxygen consumption, with greater dependency on mechanical ventilation. Therefore, nutritional support is an integral part of the treatment of patients in respiratory failure.[39]

The oxidation of fat calories produces less carbon dioxide per unit of oxygen consumed, that is, fat combustion has a low respiratory quotient.[40] Extrapolation of this concept to clinical practice has led to the development of enteral formulas with a high fat content for use in patients with respiratory failure.[41] A few studies have documented a benefit from using a high fat, low carbohydrate diet during the period of weaning from mechanical ventilation.[42] However, others have questioned its efficacy.

One of the problems of supplementing the diet with fat in critically ill patients is steatorrhea. Of all nutrients, fat requires the most complex mechanism of absorption. As mentioned, dietary LCTs need to be emulsified before absorption. Absorption takes place at the apex of the villi which becomes blunted with gut atrophy or injury. Therefore, it is not uncommon to see some degree of fat malabsorption in critically ill patients.

Burn Injury

Extensive burn wounds produce the greatest insult to the body's homeostasis. The importance of aggressive nutritional support has been well established in view of the high demand of energy and protein to meet metabolic demands, heal wounds, and resist infection in these wounds.[43] Following numerous studies in burn animals and patients, Alexander and collaborators at the Shriners Burn Institute in Cincinnati[44] tested a new modular diet. This diet included only 15 percent of the total calories as fat—50 percent in the form of fish oil and 50 percent from safflower oil. In addition, the diet was high in protein and supplemented in arginine, cysteine, histidine, and various micronutrients. Patients were randomized to receive this diet or one of two other diets. One diet was a standard tube feeding formula (Osmolite, Ross, Columbus, OH) supplemented with whey protein (ProMix R.D., Navaco, AZ), and the other diet was a commercial formula commonly used for trauma and burn patients (Traumacal, Mead Johnson, Evansville, IN). The study diet was associated with a significant reduction in the incidence of infections and in the length of stay/percent wound. Also, the patients who received this diet had improved glucose tolerance, less diarrhea, lower serum triglycerides, and better preservation of muscle mass.

Surgery for Cancer

Patients undergoing surgery for gastrointestinal malignancies are at high risk for postopera-

TABLE 4–3   Recommended Use of Fat Sources in Tube Feedings

	Clinical Conditions	
	Supplementation	Restriction
6-ω Fatty acids	Autoimmune disease, transplantation	Cancer, infection, wound healing
3-ω Fatty acids	Cancer, stress, cardiovascular disease	Bleeding diathesis
MCT	Malabsorption, liver dysfunction	Diabetes (?)

MCT = medium-chain triglycerides.

tive complications. Reasons for this increased risk of complications include decreased immune response due to the disease itself, malnutrition, systemic chemotherapy, or some combination of these effects, and impaired wound healing due to malnutrition, local radiation injury, or both. In an attempt to reduce these complications a diet was designed to restore the immune response. This diet, which is now commercially available, included 3-ω fatty acids, as well as a supplement of arginine and RNA. The use of this diet was reported by Daly and collaborators[45] who conducted a study in patients undergoing surgery for gastrointestinal malignancies. All patients received a needle jejunostomy catheter at surgery and were then randomized to receive either a standard tube feeding formula (Osmolite) or a formula supplemented in 3-ω fatty acids, arginine, and RNA (Impact, Sandoz, MN). The group of patients who received Impact showed improvement in immunologic parameters associated with a reduction in the incidence of postoperative complications and a reduction in length of hospital stay. One of the criticisms of this study was that both study groups did not receive isocaloric and isonitrogenous diets. This issue was addressed in a study by Senkal and collaborators[46] who used a control diet that was identical for both groups in all aspects except the three nutrients in question. The clinical outcome of these patients was assessed by calculating an APACHE II score through the postoperative period. Patients who received the dietary supplement of 3-ω fatty acids, arginine, and RNA had a lower APACHE II score on postoperative days 7 and 10; the score became significantly lower by day 16. In addition, the concentrations of cytokines in whole blood stimulated with phytohemagglutinin (PHA) or without stimulation were measured on postoperative days 1, 3, 7, 10, and 16.

SUMMARY AND CONCLUSIONS

In the early days of nutritional support a great deal of attention was paid to the nitrogen source in enteral diets. Presently, the interest of nutritionists has turned toward fat sources for enteral nutrition. Commercially available diets include very high proportions of 6-ω fatty acids, in particular linoleic acid. Recent investigations demonstrate that this is not beneficial in the acutely ill patient and is potentially deleterious. MCFAs are a much better source for calories without the immunosuppressive effects of 6-ω fatty acids. In addition, the physiologic role of 3-ω fatty acids is just being investigated. A summary of the potential applications of fat sources in clinical nutrition is presented in Table 4–3. Advances in technology can now custom-make triglycerides in the form of structured lipids. Research should continue to guide the industry in using this new technology to produce optimal fat sources for enteral nutrition that can improve patient outcome.

REFERENCES

1. Gordon RS: Unsterified fatty acid in human plasma. II. The transport function of unsterified fatty acid. J Clin Invest 1957;36:810–815.
2. Dole VP: A relation between non-sterified fatty acids in plasma and the metabolism of glucose. J Clin Invest 1956;35:150–154.
3. Singer SJ, Nicholson GL: The fluid mosaic model of the structure of cell membranes. Science 1972;175(23): 720–731.
4. Berlin E, Bhathena SJ, Judd JT: Dietary fat and hormonal effects on erythrocyte membrane fluidity and lipid composition in adult women. Metabolism 1989; 38(8):790–796.
5. Leger CL, Daveloose D, Christon R et al: Evidence for a structurally specific role of essential polyunsaturated fatty acids depending on their peculiar double-bond distribution in biomembranes. Biochemistry 1990; 29(31):7269–7275.
6. Caldwell MD, Jonsson HT, Othersen HB: Essential fatty acid deficiency in an infant receiving prolonged parenteral alimentation. J Pediatr 1972;81(5):894–898.
7. McCarthy MC, Cottam GL, Turner WW: Essential fatty acid deficiency in critically ill surgical patients. Am J Surg 1981;142(6):747–751.
8. Holman RT, Johnson SB, Hatch TF: A case of human linolenic acid deficiency involving neurological abnormalities. Am J Clin Nutr 1982;35:617–623.

9. Bjerve KS, Mostad IL, Thoresen L: Alpha-linolenic acid deficiency in patients on long term gastric tube feeding. Estimation of linolenic acid and long chain unsaturated n-3 fatty acid requirement in man. Am J Clin Nutr 1987;45(1):66–77.

10. Bjerve KS: n-3 fatty acid deficiency in man. J Intern Med Supp 1989;225(731):171–175.

11. Janniger CK, Racis SP: The arachidonic acid cascade: an immunologically based review. J Med 1987;18:69–80.

12. Needleman P, Raz A, Minkes MS et al: Triene prostaglandins: prostacyclin and thromboxane biosynthesis and unique biological properties. Proc Natl Acad Sci USA 1979;76(2):944–948.

13. Granstrom E: The arachidonic acid cascade: the prostaglandins, thromboxanes and leukotriene. Inflammation 1984;8:S15–S24.

14. Lokesh BR, Kinsella JE: Modulation of prostaglandin synthesis in mouse peritoneal macrophages by enrichment of lipids with either eicosapentanoic or docosahexaenoic acids in vitro. Immunobiology 1987;175(5):406–419.

15. Spielmann D, Bracco U, Traitler H et al: Alternative lipids to usual (6 PUFAs: (-linolenic acid, (-linolenic acid, stearidonic acid, EPA, Etc. J Parenter Enter Nutr 1988;12:111S–123S.

16. Martinez M, Ballabriga A: Effects of parenteral nutrition with high doses of linoleate on the developing human liver and brain. Lipids 1987;22:133–138.

17. Diboune M, Ferard G, Ingenbleek Y et al: Composition of phospholipid fatty acids in red blood cell membranes of patients in intensive care units: effects of different intakes of soybean oil, medium-chain triglycerides, and black-currant seed oil. J Parenter Enter Nutr 1992;16(2):136–141.

18. Mott CB, Sarles H, Tiscornia O: Action différente des triglycérides à chaines courtes, moyennes ou longues, sur la sécrétion pancréatique exocrine de l'homme. Biol Gastroenterol 1972;5:79–84.

19. Brosnan JT, Fritz IB: The permeability of mitochondria to carnitine and acyl carnitine. Biochem J 1971;125(4):94P–95P.

20. Tao RC, Yoshimura NN: Carnitine metabolism and its application in parenteral nutrition. J Parenter Enter Nutr 1980;4:469–486.

21. Bach A, Schirardin H, Weryha A et al: Ketogenic response to medium-chain triglyceride load in the rat. J Nutr 1977;107(10):1863–1870.

22. Bach A, Weryha A, Schirardin H: Influence of an oral MCT or LCT load on glycemia in Wistar and Zucker rats and guinea pigs. Ann Biol Anim Biochem Biophys 1979;19:625–635.

23. Tantibhedhyangkul P, Hashim SA, Van Itallie TB: Effects of ingestion of long-chain and medium-chain triglycerides on glucose tolerance in man. Diabetes 1967;16:766–769.

24. Babayan VK: Medium chain triglycerides and structured lipids. Lipids 1987;22(46):417–420.

25. DeMichele SJ, Karlstad MD, Babayan K et al: Enhanced skeletal muscle and liver protein synthesis with structured lipid in enterally fed burned rats. Metabolism 1988;37:787–795.

26. DeMichele SJ, Karlstad MD, Bistrian BR et al: Effect of total enteral nutrition with structured lipid on protein metabolism in thermally injured rats. Fed Proc 1987;46:1086.

27. Teo TC, DeMichele SJ, Selleck KM et al: Administration of structured lipid composed of MCT and fish oil reduces net protein catabolism in enterally fed burned rats. Ann Surg 1989;210:100–107.

28. Friend JV, Lock SO, Gurr MI et al: Effect of different dietary lipids on the immune responses of Hartley strain guinea pigs. Int Arch Allergy Immunol 1980;62:292–301.

29. Bromberg Y, Pick E: Unsaturated fatty acids as second messengers of superoxide generation by macrophages. Cell Immunol 1983;79(2):240–252.

30. Strunk RC, Kunke K, Nagle RB et al: Inhibition of in vitro synthesis of the second (C2) and fourth (C4) components of complement in guinea pig peritoneal macrophages by a soybean oil emulsion. Pediatr Res 1979;13(3):188–193.

31. Wagner WH, Silberman H: Lipid-based parenteral nutrition and the immunosuppression of protein malnutrition. Arch Surg 1984;19:809–810.

32. Ring J, Seifert J, Mertin J et al: Prolongation of skin allografts in rats by treatment with linoleic acid (Letter). Lancet 1974;2(7892):1331.

33. Perez RV, Munda R, Alexander JW: Dietary immunoregulation of transfusion-induced immunosuppression. Transplantation 1988;45:614–617.

34. Perez RV, Munda R, Alexander JW: Augmentation of donor-specific transfusion and cyclosporine effects with dietary linoleic acid. Transplantation 1989;47:937–940.

35. Perez RV, Babcock GF, Alexander JW: Immunoregulation of transfusion-induced immunosuppression with inhibitors of the arachidonic acid metabolism. Transplantation 1989;48(1):85–87.

36. Cook JA, Wise WC, Knapp DR et al: Essential fatty acid deficient rats: a new model for evaluating arachidonate metabolism in shock. Adv Shock Res 1981;6:93–105.

37. Mascioli EA, Iwasa Y, Trimbo S et al: Endotoxin challenge after menhaden oil diet: effects on survival of guinea pigs. Am J Clin Nutr 1989;49:277–282.

38. Alexander JW, Saito H, Trocki O et al: The importance of lipid type in the diet after burn injury. Ann Surg 1986;204(1):1–8.

39. Askanazi J, Weissman C, Rosenbaum SH et al: Nutrition and the respiratory system. Crit Care Med 1982;10(3):163–172.

40. Askanazi J, Nordenstrom J, Rosenbaum SH et al: Nutrition for the patient with respiratory failure: glucose vs. fat. Anesthesiology 1981;54(5):373–377.

41. Heymsfield SB, Head CA, McManus III CB et al: Respiratory, cardiovascular and metabolic effects of enteral hyperalimentation: influence of formula dose and composition. Am J Clin Nutr 1984;40:116–130.

42. Al-Saady NM, Blackmore CM, Bennet ED: High fat, low carbohydrate, enteral feeding lowers pCO2 and reduces the period of ventilation in artificially ventilated patients. Intensive Care Med 1989;15(5):290–295.

43. Alexander JW, MacMillan BG, Stinnett JO et al: Beneficial effects of aggressive protein feeding in severely burned children. Ann Surg 1980;192(4):505–517.

44. Gottschlich MM, Jenkins M, Warden GD et al: Differential effects of three enteral dietary regimens on selected outcome variables in burn patients. J Parenter Enter Nutr 1990;14:225–236.

45. Daly JM, Lieberman MD, Goldfine J et al: Enteral nutrition with supplemental arginine, RNA, and omega-3 fatty acids in patients after operation: immunologic, metabolic, and clinical outcome. Surgery 1992;112(10):56–67.

46. Senkal M, Kemen M, Homann HH et al: Modulation of postoperative immune response by enteral nutrition

with a diet enriched with arginine, RNA, and omega-3 fatty acids in patients with upper gastrointestinal cancer. Eur J Surg 1995;161:115–122.

47. Gottschlich MM: Selection of optimal lipid sources in enteral and parenteral nutrition. Nutr Clin Pract 1992; 7:152–165.

5

Glucose Metabolism

M. Burress Welborn, III
Lyle L. Moldawer

Glucose is the primary substrate for the generation of energy required for cellular metabolism. Although fatty acid oxidation can be used to provide fuel for most organs, glucose remains the primary source of adenosine triphosphate (ATP) for the most vital organ system: the brain and central nervous system. Glucose is also the primary fuel source for the adrenal medulla, erythrocytes, and white blood cells, and when a tissue is deprived of oxygen, glucose is the only source of ATP for cellular metabolism. Because glucose availability is essential for cellular function, it is not surprising that plasma glucose levels are maintained within a narrow normal range to (4 to 6 mM) and the control of glucose metabolism and the generation of new glucose by gluconeogenesis is tightly regulated. In those states of glucose dysregulation where glucose homeostasis is compromised, the organism's ability to survive environmental stress is reduced.

The primary organ involved in regulating glucose availability is the liver, which is the only organ with the ability to generate glucose de novo for use by those organ systems dependent solely on glucose. Glucose metabolism in the liver is under the control of several hormonal systems, primarily insulin, glucagon, catecholamines, growth hormone, corticosteroids, and proinflammatory cytokines. Tissue regulation of glucose metabolism occurs both immediately by altering enzyme function, primarily by phosphorylation, and additionally in a delayed fashion by altering DNA gene expression of enzymes required for glucose synthesis and catabolism. These regulatory mechanisms act together to ensure that an adequate supply of circulating glucose is available for metabolism by the organism at all times. In periods of metabolic stress, such as following operative trauma and during sepsis or inflammatory response syndromes, these controls are altered and changes in glucose homeostasis can occur. These changes in glucose metabolism that accompany surgical stress and systemic inflammatory response syndromes have both beneficial and ultimately adverse effects on the host. This altered regulation in glucose metabolism is due in part to release of several hormones and may also be due to overproduction of paracrine mediators, such as tumor necrosis factor-α (TNF-α) and interleukin-1 (IL-1), secreted primarily by macrophages during inflammatory states such as the sepsis syndrome.

Acute inflammation, due to either injury or infection, induces a variety of alterations in glucose metabolism that include enhanced peripheral glucose uptake and use, increased glucose production, decreased glycogenesis, glucose intolerance, hyperlactacidemia, and insulin resistance. In the flow phase of the hypermetabolic state, a hyperglycemic milieu is intended to meet the increased obligatory requirements for glucose as an energy substrate.

For the surgical patient, an adequate supply of glucose is necessary for recovery from the trauma associated with operative procedures. Meeting the patient's energy requirements is necessary for both wound healing and to augment host immunologic defense systems. The crucial role glucose plays in the immune response to infection cannot be overemphasized. Without an adequate supply of glucose the surgical patient will use tissue amino acids as the primary source of glucose. This loss of protein stores will deprive both the wound substrate for healing and the immune system vital substrate for host defenses.

GLYCOGEN

Glycogen is the primary storage form of glucose and acts as an easily accessible energy reservoir. Although found in various cell populations, the majority of glycogen is found in liver and skeletal muscle. In the liver, glycogen serves as a reservoir for the release of glucose for systemic use. When glucose is plentiful, the liver forms glycogen as a storage form which can then be broken down to release glucose when required. Skeletal muscle contains the majority of the stored glycogen but this energy reserve is generally unavailable to other tissues. Theoretically, 5 to 10 percent of the glucose stored as muscle glycogen could be released into the circulation during glycogen debranching as occurs in glycolysis; however, this pathway is not of physiologic significance.[1] Rather, skeletal muscle glycogen serves solely as a fuel for muscle and is not available for use by other organ systems.

Glycogen formation occurs in the liver and in skeletal muscle after glucose is transported into cells via facilitated diffusion by the transport proteins GLUT 1 to 5. Upon entrance into the cell, glucose is phosphorylated at the expense of ATP to become glucose-6-phosphate (P) by hexokinase in most cell populations and by glucokinase in the liver. Glucose is converted to glucose-6-P irreversibly, thus trapping glucose intracellulary. The conversion of glucose to glucose-6-P intracellularly is rapid and almost complete, resulting in essentially no free glucose within the cell. The absence of free intracellular glucose maintains a gradient from extracellular to intracellular pools allowing for glucose uptake even when circulating concentrations are low. The first step to the production of glycogen is the conversion of glucose-6-P to glucose-1-P by phosphoglucomutase.[1] Glucose-1-P is then joined to uridine diphosphate (UDP) to form UDP-glucose by UDP-glucose pyrophosphory-lase, which is the substrate for glycogen synthetase.[2] Glycogen synthetase then polymerizes glucose to form glycogen. Glycogen is an efficient storage form of glucose by virtue of the fact that it requires little hydration, thus taking up less cellular space. Thus, glycogen acts as a high-density energy storage system.

Glycogenolysis releases glucose for either local use as in skeletal muscle, or in the case of hepatic glycogenolysis for systemic use. The enzyme responsible for this is glycogen phosphorylase. This enzyme breaks glycogen down into glucose-1-P, which is then converted back to glucose-6-P by phosphoglucomutase as described above. At this step glucose-6-P can be used for glycolysis or it can be converted to glucose by glucose-6-phosphatase in the liver for release into the systemic circulation.

GLYCOLYSIS

Glycolysis was first described by Embden and Meyerhof. This pathway of glucose metabolism is used by all prokaryotic and eukaryotic cells for the generation of energy in the form of ATP for cellular metabolism. This reaction does not require oxygen and is used as a primary source of energy only in states of tissue hypoxia. As a primary source of energy this metabolic pathway is not efficient, generating only two molecules of ATP for each molecule of glucose. Of the energy that should be released by the conversion of glucose to lactate, only 43 percent is used to generate the two molecules of ATP. The rest of the energy released is lost in the form of heat.

Glycolysis is depicted in Figure 5–1. The first step in the glycolytic pathway is the generation of glucose-6-P as previously described, and requires the expenditure of one ATP. Glucose-6-P is then converted to fructose-6-P. The next step in glycolysis involves the conversion of fructose-6-P to fructose-1,6-P by phosphofructokinase which requires an additional ATP molecule. This step is a key regulatory step in glycolysis and gluconeogenesis. Fructose-1,6-P is then split into two molecules: glyceraldehyde-3-P and dihydroacetone phosphate. Dihydroacetone phosphate is then converted to glyceraldehyde-3-P. Glyceraldehyde-3-P is converted to 1,3-diphosphoglyceric acid, donating a total of 4 hydrogen ions to nicotinamide-adenine dinucleotide phosphate (NADP) to form the reduced form of NADP, NADPH. The next step is the formation of 3-phosphoglyceric acid. The two phosphate moieties that are released form two ATP molecules. 3-Phosphoglyceric acid is then converted

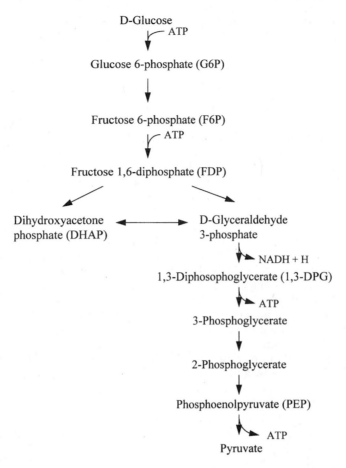

FIGURE 5–1 Glycolysis as depicted in two stages. Although the term glycolysis originally referred to the breakdown of glucose to lactate, it more loosely refers to the pathway leading to pyruvate. The first stage of glycolysis refers to the conversion of simple sugars into glyceraldehyde-3-phosphate and the input of ATP. The second stage refers to the conversion of glyceraldehyde-3-phosphate into lactate with conservation of ATP. The net yield of the two stages is 2 ATP molecules per molecule of glucose.

to 2-phosphoglyceric acid and then to phosphoenolpyruvic acid (PEP). The two PEP molecules are then converted to pyruvate, releasing another two reactive phosphate moieties that are used to form two more ATP molecules. In anoxic states pyruvate is converted to lactate at the expense of the previously released hydrogen ions used to reduce NADP to NADPH. The final reaction yields:

Glucose + 2 ADP + 2 P_i $\longleftrightarrow$ 2 lactate + 2 ATP + 2 H_2O

Lactate that is produced can be recycled in the liver to form pyruvate for further energy production or to act as the starting substrate for the generation of glucose via gluconeogenesis. When oxygen is abundant, the NADPH generated during glycolysis can be used to form ATP in the mitochondria by oxidative phosphoryla-

tion. The generated pyruvate can be used to form more ATP or as a substrate for fatty acid and amino acid generation (see below).

GLUCONEOGENESIS

The liver is the primary source of gluconeogenesis with a small contribution from the kidneys. The reactions involved in gluconeogenesis are the same as for glycolysis except at three key regulatory steps. These steps occur at the conversion of pyruvate to PEP, the conversion of fructose-1,6-P to fructose-1-P, and the conversion of glucose-6-P to glucose. Pyruvate is converted to oxaloacetate (OAA) which is then converted to PEP by the enzyme phosphoenolpyruvate carboxykinase. Fructose-1,6-P is converted to fructose-1-P by the enzyme fructose-1,6-biphosphatase. The last reaction involves the conversion of glucose-6-P to glucose by glucose-6-phosphatase to release free glucose, which can leave the cell for systemic use. The conversion of pyruvate to glucose requires the use of three high-energy phosphate bonds (ATP and guanosine triphosphate [GTP]) and the reduced form of nicotinamide-adenine dinucleotide, NADH.

The other reactions involved in gluconeogenesis are the same as for glycolysis and are substrate controlled. Therefore, the direction of this reaction is dictated by the concentration of the substrates involved. If the substrate concentrations favor a reaction proceeding toward gluconeogenesis then these reactions will occur in the direction of glucose production, assuming adequate ATP.

The conversion of pyruvate to PEP is the starting point for the reaction of gluconeogenesis, and it is at this point in the reaction that the liver uses diverse substrates for the generation of glucose. Lactate that is generated peripherally during anaerobic metabolism is converted to pyruvate and then proceeds to glucose production. The amino acids alanine and serine are directly converted to pyruvate to generate glucose. Aspartate is converted to OAA and then to PEP. Citrate, glutamate, histidine, proline, and arginine are converted to α-oxoglutarate and then to OAA after conversion to succinate, fumarate, and then malate. Valine, isoleucine, threonine, and proprionate follow a similar path to OAA via succinate, fumarate, and malate. Fatty acids cannot be converted to glucose; however, glycerol can be converted to glucose by entering the gluconeogenic pathway at the level of 3-phosphoglyceric acid.

KREBS CYCLE

A majority of the energy released to form ATP from glucose is produced by oxidative phosphorylation using NADH and $FADH_2$ generated by the Krebs cycle. This cycle of enzymatic reactions occurs in the inner matrix of the mitochondria and releases electrons that are used to generate ATP by reduction of oxygen with hydrogen to water. The net production of ATP achieved via this pathway is an additional 36 ATP molecules. Thus, catabolism of glucose in the presence of oxygen yields a total of 38 molecules of ATP as opposed to only 2 molecules generated by the breakdown of glucose to lactate in the absence of oxygen. This process converts 40 percent of the energy generated from the complete oxidation of glucose to ATP with the rest of the energy lost as heat.

The Krebs cycle begins with the generation of pyruvate (Fig. 5–2). Pyruvate is converted to acetyl-CoA by the pyruvate dehydrogenase complex, generating NADH in the mitochondria. Acetyl-CoA is then converted to citrate by citrate synthase by Claisen condensation with OAA. Citrate is then isomerized to isocitrate by a series of dehydration and hydration reactions. α-Ketoglutarate is produced from isocitrate by the enzyme isocitrate dehydrogenase, generating NADPH. Another NADH molecule is released by the conversion of α-ketoglutarate to succinyl-CoA by the α-ketoglutarate dehy-

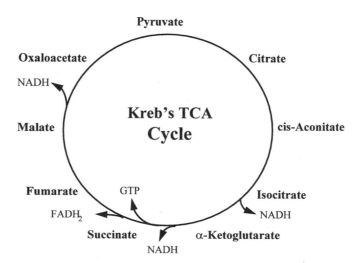

FIGURE 5–2 The Krebs tricarboxylic acid cycle. Intermediates are shown as free acids.

drogenase complex. Succinyl-CoA is then converted to succinate-releasing GTP, which is converted to ATP for cellular usage. Succinate is subsequently oxidized to fumarate, generating $FADH_2$. Fumarate is then converted to L-malate and then oxidized back to oxaloacetate, completing the cycle. The harvested electrons in the form of NADH, NADPH, and $FADH_2$ are then used to generate ATP by oxidative phosphorylation in the presence of oxygen.

The Krebs cycle acts not only to generate ATP but also to generate the carbon precursors for the production of amino acids, fatty acids, and porphyrins. Acetyl-CoA acts as the precursor for the generation of fatty acids. α-Ketoglutarate is the precursor for glutamate, which can then be converted to glutamine, proline, arginine, and the purines. Oxaloacetate can be modified to form aspartate and asparagine, which are the precursors for the synthesis of pyrimidines. By the conversion of oxaloacetate to PEP, serine, glycine, cysteine, phenylalanine, tyrosine, and tryptophan can be manufactured. And lastly, succinyl-CoA acts as the precursor for the production of porphyrins.

REGULATION OF GLUCOSE METABOLISM

Control over glucose metabolism is crucial to the survival of the organism. A common mechanism exists for fine control of glucose metabolism in the liver so that in times of plentiful glucose, glucose is used for the formation of glycogen and glycolysis is used for the generation of ATP. Glucose metabolism is primarily under the control of hormones. Glycogen formation and glycolysis are promoted by the actions of insulin on the hepatic cell, whereas glucagon, the catecholamine, vasopressin, and angiotensin II act to promote glycogen breakdown and gluconeogenesis. Glucagon and the β-adrenergic stimulation act to promote the increase of cellular adenosine $3':5'$-cyclic phosphate (cAMP) and cAMP-dependent protein kinases. These cAMP-dependent protein kinases exert their effects by phosphorylation of the enzymes crucial to the regulation of glycogen metabolism and glycolysis/gluconeogenesis. α-Adrenergic stimulation, vasopressin, and angiotensin II act via increasing intracellular Ca^{2+} concentration with activation of calmodulin-dependent protein kinases. Insulin exerts its effects by promoting dephosphorylation of the regulatory enzymes or by decreasing the cAMP effects. The hormonal signals themselves are regulated by allosteric molecules mainly comprised of nucleotides (AMP, ADP, ATP) acting at substrate

concentrations. These allosteric effectors act to refine hormonal control so that the energy needs of the hepatocyte are met in addition to the glucose requirements of other organ systems. This control by phosphorylation and allosteric molecules occurs at every rate-limiting step in glycogen metabolism and glycolysis/gluconeogenesis and, as will be described below, is very similar at each step. In addition to short-term control by phosphorylation, long-term control of glucose metabolism occurs by hormonal control of the expression of the genes encoding the enzymes responsible for glycogen metabolism and glycolysis/gluconeogenesis.

Regulation of Glycogen Metabolism

The primary storage form of glucose for organisms from yeast to humans is glycogen. The regulation of glycogen production and breakdown is highly controlled at the level of glycogen synthetase and glycogen phosphorylase. These enzymes represent the rate-limiting step of their respective reactions and, thus, are ideally suited for both substrate and allosteric control. While much has been uncovered about the regulation of glycogen phosphorylase, the regulatory mechanisms for glycogen synthetase are less well understood.

Short-term regulation of glycogen synthetase occurs by three mechanisms—phosphorylation, substrate control, and allosteric regulation. Glycogen synthetase has multiple phosphorylation sites for covalent modification of the enzyme, and these sites are under hormonal control. When the enzyme is phosphorylated it is converted from the I or *a* form to the D or *b* form.[3,4] The phosphorylated form of the enzyme is the less active form and is phosphorylated by a cAMP-dependent protein kinase and by Ca^{2+}-dependent calmodulin.[2] Glucagon and β-adrenergics induce glycogen synthetase phosphorylation by cAMP-dependent mechanisms, whereas angiotensin II, vasopressin, and the α-adrenergics operate through Ca^{2+} and calmodulin.[4] Glucocorticoids may act to decrease synthetase activity by increasing cAMP-dependent protein kinase activity independent of cAMP.[5] There are multiple kinases that act to phosphorylate the enzyme in response to different hormones.[2,6] This generates a graded inhibition of the enzyme. Glycogen synthetase is dephosphorylated to the I form in response to insulin via glycogen synthetase phosphatase.[2] This conversion is inhibited by the presence of Ca^{2+}; thus, insulin effects can be offset by the Ca^{2+}-

dependent hormonal control of the synthetase enzyme.[4] Inhibitor-1 controls glycogen synthetase phosphatase activity and when phosphorylated by the above cAMP kinases acts to inhibit glycogen synthetase phosphatase.[2] Insulin exerts its effects at this point by promoting the dephosphorylation of inhibitor-1 and thus disinhibiting glycogen synthetase phosphatase.[2] Insulin also increases synthetase activity by inhibiting those kinases responsible for synthetase phosphorylation.[2] The balance between phosphorylation and dephosphorylation determines the activity of the glycogen synthetase activity, and this balance is determined by the inhibitory effects of glucagon and the adrenergics acting against the disinhibitory actions of insulin. This balance of antagonist activities allows the organism to maintain very fine control over glycogen synthesis.

The substrates that play a pivotal role in the regulation of glycogen synthetase are glucose-6-P and UDP-glucose. When these substrates are plentiful the activity of glycogen synthetase increases. Thus, when glucose is readily available the reaction is driven toward glycogen formation.[7] Glucose-6-P, when present, allows the D or dependent form of the synthetase enzyme to carry out glycogen synthesis. When the synthetase enzyme is in the I form it will carry out glycogen synthesis independent of glucose-6-P.[2] In this manner inhibitory hormonal control can be overcome when glucose-6-P is plentiful. Glucose and glucose-6-P have also been found to increase glycogen synthetase phosphatase activity and thus upregulate glycogen synthetase activity.[8] Phosphorylation of the enzyme appears to increase the substrate effect of glucose-6-P and UDP-glucose. Therefore substrate control and control by phosphorylation are coordinated.[6] Glycogen synthetase activity is inhibited by the active or *a* form of phosphorylase. Glucose stimulates synthetase activity by promoting the conversion of phosphorylase to the *b* or inactive form thus releasing phosphorylase control over synthetase activity.[4] In addition, it is apparent that other substrates may control the rate of glycogen synthesis. Glucose itself represents only 40 percent of the precursor used to generate glycogen while the other 60 percent is generated by the gluconeogenic pathway.[8] Peripherally released lactate and glycogenic amino acids, when taken up by the liver, act to drive gluconeogenesis to form glucose-6-P, and in times of plentiful glucose the products of gluconeogenesis are stored as glycogen.[8] In this manner substrate release peripherally and glycogen formation are closely linked.

The primary allosteric effectors of glycogen synthetase are the nucleosides. ATP, AMP, ADP, UMP, and free phosphate all inhibit glycogen synthetase activity.[7] The allosteric inhibitors of synthetase activity are only active when the enzyme has been inhibited by phosphorylation to the D form.[2] As the enzyme acquires more phosphate groups by multiple phosphorylation the effects of these inhibitors increase.[2] This generates a graded control of synthetase activity. At present, no allosteric stimulators of glycogen synthetase have been identified. Some authors have reported that magnesium increases synthetase activity, but this has been disputed.[2,8] The search for allosteric activators continues based on the observation that glycogen synthesis in vivo is much greater than synthesis in vitro when stimulated by various metabolite mixtures including glucose-6-P and UDP-glucose.[8]

The regulation of glycogen phosphorylase and glycogenolysis is very similar to that of glycogen synthetase in that regulation is mediated by hormonal control, substrate control, and allosteric effectors. Hormonal control as in the case of glycogen synthetase is dependent on phosphorylation. Glycogen phosphorylase exists in two forms, the *a* or active form and the *b* or inactive form. The *b* form is converted to the *a* form by phosphorylation mediated by phosphorylase kinase. Phosphorylase kinase is itself controlled by phosphorylation by cAMP-dependent protein kinase in response to glucagon and β-adrenergic activation.[4] In a manner similar to glycogen synthetase, α-adrenergics, vasopressin, and angiotensin II can activate phosphorylase kinase by a cAMP-independent manner. These hormones act to increase cellular levels of inositol triphosphate (IP$_3$) by the activation of phosphodiesterase.[9] This release of IP$_3$ leads to a release of intracellular Ca^{2+}, which acts to increase the activity of phosphorylase in both the *a* and *b* forms.[4] Thus, cAMP-independent hormones can activate glycogenolysis independent of glucagon or β-adrenergic stimulation. However, the level of activation of phosphorylase is estimated to be only 60 percent of the maximal stimulation achieved through phosphorylation.[9] The roles of angiotensin II and vasopressin as glycogenolytic agents have been questioned. At low dose these hormones promote the activation of phosphodiesterases, which result in the degradation of cAMP and, thus, inhibit cAMP-mediated glycogen breakdown. This effect occurs at physiologic concentrations of these agents and may be more important in vivo.[4] Inhibitor-1 also plays a role in the regulation of phosphorylase as in the regulation of glycogen synthetase. When phosphorylated by cAMP, protein kinase inhibitor-1 acts to inhibit phosphorylase phosphatase.[4] In this manner glucagon and the β-adrenergics exert their effects via cAMP by promoting the phosphorylation of phosphorylase to the *a* form and inhibiting the conversion of the *a* form to the *b* form by phosphorylase. Glucocorticoids also act to increase phosphorylase activity by acting directly on cAMP-dependent protein kinase.[5] The control of glycogenolysis by insulin is exerted by dephosphorylation of phosphorylase, mirroring its control over glycogen synthetase. The binding of insulin to its receptor promotes dephosphorylation of inhibitor-1 which disinhibits phosphorylase phosphatase.[4] Phosphorylase phosphatase then proceeds to dephosphorylate phosphorylase converting the *a* to the *b* form. Insulin, by activating guanine nucleotide protein, may exert a direct inhibitory effect on the cAMP system and IP$_3$ stimulation of free Ca^{2+} release.[4] In this manner insulin can counteract both the cAMP-dependent and -independent stimulation of glycogenolysis.

Glucose, glucose-6-P, and glycogen itself act as substrate regulators of phosphorylase activity. Glucose binds to phosphorylase *a* which stimulates the conversion from the *a* to the *b* form by phosphorylase phosphatase.[3] As mentioned above, phosphorylase *a* inhibits glycogen synthetase activity by direct inhibition of synthetase phosphatase. Thus, glucose acts directly to inhibit phosphorylase and indirectly to increase synthetase.[3] Glucose-6-P acts to inhibit glycogenolysis by inhibition of phosphorylase *b* but has no effect on the activity of the *a* form of the enzyme.[10] A large percentage of phosphorylase is found associated with glycogen. Glycogen appears to stimulate phosphorylase activity in both the *a* and the *b* forms.[10] By these mechanisms glycogenolysis is inhibited when glucose and its derivative glucose-6-P are plentiful, augmenting the insulin response. When glycogen is plentiful phosphorylase activity is increased to supplement the actions of the glycogenolytic hormones.

As with glycogen synthetase, control of phosphorylase activity is mediated by nucleotides. AMP and IMP activate the *b* form of phosphorylase but have no effect on the *a* form of the enzyme. ATP, in contrast, inhibits the *b* form but like AMP has no effect on the *a* form.[11] In this manner when the cell has depleted its fuel sources, resulting in an increased AMP, glycogenolysis can be activated independent of hormonal control. This allows for finer control of glycogen metabolism at the molecular level. An example of this is the finding that skeletal muscle glycogenolysis in the rat hind limb occurs independent of phosphorylation during exercise.[5]

Regulation of Glycolysis and Gluconeogenesis

The balance of hepatic glycolysis and gluconeogenesis is controlled by two mechanisms. The first involves the binding of hormones to their receptors and immediate second messenger systems that lead to rapid regulation for the two pathways. Hormones also control the balance between glycolysis and gluconeogenesis by regulating the transcription of the genes coding for the enzymes crucial in controlling the flux of glucose to pyruvate and vice versa. This mechanism has been coined *long-term regulation* and is not an immediate response in that gene regulation is required. The control of glycolysis and gluconeogenesis occurs through three reaction pathways. These three reactions involve the conversion of glucose to glucose-6-P, the conversion of fructose-1,6-P to fructose-1-P, and the conversion of pyruvate to PEP.

Regulation of Glucose/Glucose-6-P

Short-term regulation of the conversion of glucose to glucose-6-P is not under direct hormonal control. Rather short-term control of this conversion is under substrate control. The uptake of glucose by the glucose transporters is facilitated by immediate phosphorylation of glucose to glucose-6-P. This is carried out in most cell populations by the enzyme hexokinase. In these cell populations, hexokinase activity is inhibited by the presence of glucose-6-P.[12] Thus, in these cell populations the uptake of glucose is inhibited by an overabundance of glucose-6-P. Glucose-6-P exerts this effect by decreasing hexokinase activity, thereby decreasing glucose concentration gradients across the cell membrane and inhibiting glucose transport. The other isoenzyme responsible for the conversion of glucose to glucose-6-P is glucokinase, which is located in hepatocytes and the β-cells of the pancreatic islets. Unlike hexokinase, glucokinase is not inhibited by glucose-6-P, but rather is controlled by the concentration of glucose. When glucose is abundant glucokinase activity increases and thus drives either the production of glycogen or glycolysis.[12] Fructose also plays a crucial role in the regulation of glucokinase. Glucokinase is inhibited by a regulatory protein that is stimulated by the presence of fructose-6-P, a metabolite of glycolysis.[12] Fructose is taken up by hepatocytes and is converted to fructose-1-P by fructose kinase and acts to block inhibition of glucokinase by the regulatory protein.[12] Therefore, when monosaccharides are ingested and glucose and fructose are plentiful, the availability of these substrates drives glucokinase and acts to pull more glucose into the hepatocyte.

Hormonal control of glucokinase is exerted at the DNA level. Glucagon exerts its control by decreasing the amount of mRNA of glucokinase that is transcribed.[13] This occurs via a cAMP mechanism.[14] Insulin on the other hand increases glucokinase gene transcription, but this effect can be blocked by the presence of cAMP.[13] There is also evidence that insulin may act by increasing phosphodiesterase levels to lower cAMP levels, which counteract glucagon's effects on the glucokinase gene transcription.[14] β-Adrenergics may exert an effect on glucokinase gene transcription in a manner similar to glucagon via cAMP. There is no evidence to date that the hormones that lead to increased Ca^{2+} levels act to control the transcription of the glucokinase gene.

The control of glucose-6-phosphatase is unknown at present. There is no evidence of substrate control or gene transcriptional control to date. However, some authors speculate that hormonal control of glucose-6-phosphatase transcription will be uncovered in the future.[13] It is logical to propose that control of glucose-6-phosphatase must be present to regulate release of free glucose into the circulation versus utilization of glucose-6-P for the formation of glycogen, although control of glycogen formation may serve the same function.

Regulation of Fructose-6-P/Fructose-1,6-P

The second control site for glycolysis and gluconeogenesis occurs at the conversion of fructose-6-P to fructose-1,6-P. Unlike the glucose/glucose-6-P cycle, direct short-term hormonal control is achieved by phosphorylation. The two enzymes involved in this cycle are phosphofructose kinase which converts fructose-6-P to fructose-1,6-P, and fructose-1,6-biphosphatase which carries out the reverse reaction. These two enzymes both have phosphorylation sites, and phosphorylation of these enzymes was initially felt to be the hormonal control mechanism.[15] Further investigation proved that a small effector molecule, fructose-2,6-P, may be responsible for control of these enzymes. Fructose-2,6-P acts to inhibit fructose-1,6-biphosphatase and thereby inhibits gluco-

neogenesis. In contrast, fructose-2,6-P acts to stimulate phosphofructokinase and drive glycolysis.[15] Hormonal control is exerted by phosphorylation of the two enzymes that convert fructose-6-P to the effector molecule fructose-2,6-P. 6-Phosphofructose-2-kinase converts fructose-6-P to fructose-2,6-P while fructose-2,6-biphosphatase converts the reaction back to fructose-6-P. These two enzymatic functions are carried out by the one bifunctional enzyme.[15] Glucagon and the β-adrenergics activate cAMP-dependent protein kinases which phosphorylate this bifunctional enzyme causing an increased biphosphatase activity. This decreases the concentration of fructose-2,6-P and drives the reaction toward fructose-6-P.[13] The α-adrenergics, vasopressin, and angiotensin II exert no control over the 6-phosphofructo-2-kinase/fructose-2,6-phosphatase complex.[15] Thus, changes in intracellular Ca^{2+} concentrations do not effect the function of this enzyme complex. Insulin on the other hand promotes dephosphorylation of the bifunctional enzyme, which leads to increased activity and higher concentrations of fructose-2,6-P.[13] Insulin may also act by increasing phosphodiester activity thus decreasing cAMP levels and offsetting the actions of glucagon and the β-adrenergics.[15]

As in the case of glycogen metabolism, the enzymes that mediate the conversion of fructose-1-P to fructose-1,6-biphosphate are under the control of small allosteric effectors. Phosphofructokinase is activated by the presence of AMP, ADP, and cAMP while it is inhibited by the presence of ATP.[15] Fructose-2,6-P and AMP act synergistically to activate phosphofructokinase and can overcome inhibition by ATP.[15] In addition, glycerol-3-phosphate, the product of the breakdown of fructose-1,6-P is an inhibitor of phosphofructokinase.[12] Fructose-1,6-biphosphatase, on the other hand, is inhibited by AMP and activated by glycerol-3-phosphate.[12,15] These allosteric effectors act to augment the hormonal response by inhibiting glycolysis and activating gluconeogenesis when cellular energy is plentiful. There does not appear to be allosteric control over the production of the enzymes regulating the concentration of the fructose-2,6-P.

Long-term hormonal control of fructose-1-P/fructose-1,6-P, as in the case of glucose/glucose-6-P metabolism, is carried out at the nuclear level by regulation of gene expression of mRNA for the involved enzymes. Glucagon controls the expression of the gene for phosphofructokinase via cAMP-mediated inhibition of gene transcription.[15] Insulin is known to increase the expression of this gene and may do so, again, by decreasing cellular levels of cAMP. The opposite effect is seen in the case of fructose-1,6-biphosphatase—mRNA levels for this enzyme increase after administration of cAMP and insulin decreases transcription.[15] The genes encoding the 6-phosphofructo-2-kinase/fructose-2,6-phosphatase complex are also regulated at the transcriptional level. Glucagon via cAMP inhibits transcription whereas insulin upregulates transcription.[14] In addition, the promoter for this enzyme complex is regulated by glucocorticoids. Glucocorticoids bind to a glucocorticoid-responsive unit that acts as an enhancer for the promoter controlling the 6-phosphofructo-2-kinase/fructose-2,6-phosphatase complex gene.[14] Thyroid hormones appear to effect transcription by potentiating the effects of glucocorticoid enhancement of transcription of this gene.[14]

Regulation of Pyruvate/Phosphoenolpyruvate

In a manner similar to the control mechanisms previously described, the flux of pyruvate to phosphoenolpyruvate is under hormonal and allosteric control mechanisms. Hormonal control is exerted via phosphorylation of pyruvate kinase, which decreases the activity of the enzyme. Glucagon and the β-adrenergics promote cAMP-dependent phosphorylation pyruvate kinase.[15] The α-adrenergics, vasopressin, and angiotensin II increase intracellular Ca^{2+}, which activates calmodulin-dependent protein kinases and leads to phosphorylation of pyruvate kinase.[13] In times of plentiful glucose, phosphorylation of pyruvate kinase is inhibited by the action of insulin. Insulin inhibits phosphorylation of pyruvate kinase by decreasing intracellular cAMP.[15] Insulin acts to inhibit Ca^{2+}-mediated phosphorylation of pyruvate kinase by inhibiting the activation of calmodulin by phosphorylation.[13]

Allosteric control of pyruvate kinase is exerted by alanine, ATP, and fructose-1,6-P. Pyruvate kinase is inhibited by ATP and alanine whereas fructose-1,6-P acts to increase pyruvate kinase activity.[15] The phosphorylated form of the enzyme is more readily inhibited by alanine and ATP, and the stimulatory effect of fructose-1,6-P is attenuated.[15] Additionally, these allosteric effectors exert control over the ability of cAMP-dependent kinases to phosphorylate the enzyme. Fructose-1,6-P decreases the ability of cAMP-dependent kinases to phosphorylate the enzyme, whereas alanine makes the enzyme a better substrate for phosphorylation.[15] Once again, as with the other reactions described there is an interplay between hormonal control and allosteric effectors so that

the pyruvate/phosphoenolpyruvate balance is under fine control.

Long-term control of the balance between pyruvate and phosphoenolpyruvate is exerted by regulation of gene expression. Insulin acts to increase the expression of pyruvate kinase in the liver. However, this occurs only in the presence of glucose or fructose, with neither insulin nor glucose having the ability to increase gene expression alone.[14] In addition, insulin and glucose will only upregulate expression of the pyruvate kinase gene in the presence of glucocorticoids and thyroid hormone.[13] Glucagon, as would be expected, exerts the opposite effect. Acting through cAMP glucagon decreases the transcription of the gene for pyruvate kinase and destabilized pyruvate kinase mRNA.[14] Additionally, long-term control of the balance between pyruvate and phosphoenolpyruvate is provided by the regulation of the expression of the gene encoding phosphoenolpyruvate carboxykinase (PEPCK) which acts to convert phosphoenolpyruvate back to pyruvate. Glucose acts to destabilize PEPCK mRNA and to directly decrease gene transcription.[14] Insulin also acts to decrease PEPCK gene expression directly and by decreasing intracellular levels of cAMP.[14] The opposite effect is seen in the presence of glucagon, which acts to increase gene expression via cAMP.[13] Glucocorticoids and thyroid hormone also act to increase the expression of the PEPCK gene.[14]

Substrate Cycling

All of the reactions that are under hormonal control exhibit substrate cycling. That is, both the reactions that promote glycolysis and gluconeogenesis are occurring at the same time with net movement of carbon atoms to form pyruvate or glucose governed by the hormonal or allosteric milieu of the cell. This flux of substrates has been termed *substrate cycling* or *futile cycling* and is present in the reaction interconverting glucose to glucose-6-P, fructose-1-P to fructose-1,6-P, and PEP and pyruvate. This substrate cycling occurs at the expense of energy (ATP) with no net formation of either pyruvate or glucose. Originally futile cycling was felt to function primarily to generate heat.[16] It is now known that, in addition to thermogenesis, substrate cycling acts to increase the organism's ability to change the direction of glycolysis or gluconeogenesis quickly and efficiently.[17] The more substrate cycling occurring in the hepatocyte the larger the flux of molecules in one direction when one reaction rate is decreased and the other increased. In this manner substrate cycling will amplify the net flux of molecules in one direction with an inverse change in both reaction rates.[16]

The primary hormone responsible for governing substrate cycling is glucagon. Glucagon increases substrate cycling while the catecholamines appear to exert only a minimal effect.[17-19] The glucocorticoids and insulin act to decrease futile cycling in response to glucagon. For the clinician, substrate cycling is felt to play a major role in the increased energy requirements in burn patients as well as in the increases in body temperature that accompany major burns.[17] In addition, substrate cycling may promote increased hepatic glucose production in diabetes due to overstimulation by glucagon without the counterregulatory effect of insulin.[19] Futile cycling may have more far-reaching ramifications for the trauma or septic patient because it may play a crucial role in thermogenesis and in promoting the changes in glucose metabolism that occur in these disease states.

GLUCOSE METABOLISM IN THE FASTED STATE

The adaptation to fasting is one in which the fuel usage by the host shifts from primarily using a mixed fuel system where carbohydrate metabolism predominates to one in which the primary fuel is fat. Carbohydrate metabolism changes profoundly during this period. An understanding of the changes in glucose metabolism that accompany starvation is essential to understanding the alterations in glucose metabolism that accompany injury, infection, or neoplastic disease. As is evident, the changes in glucose metabolism that accompany disease are often superimposed on altered nutrient intake, and an understanding of the adaptive changes in glucose metabolism that occur during inadequate nutrient intake is essential.

Mobilization of endogenous energy stores is an essential component of starvation. Most previously healthy adults can tolerate weight loss of 5 to 10 percent of body weight with relatively little functional consequence, whereas losses of body weight in excess of 25 to 30 percent are generally associated with significant morbidity. The root of the metabolic changes and adaptation that occurs during starvation is the need to replace exogenously provided calories with an endogenous supply of energy substrate. Glucose homeostasis and the sparing of proteins critical to survival are essential components of this re-

sponse. Key tissues, including the central and peripheral nervous system, red blood cells, phagocytic cells, and fibroblasts normally require glucose as the sole or major energy source. The brain oxidizes glucose entirely to carbon dioxide and water, whereas in other tissues glycolysis yields lactate that must be recycled into glucose by the liver and kidney via the Cori cycle. Provision of glucose to meet these needs is required.

Glycogen stores are relatively small and can provide only 600 to 1000 kcals of available energy. Furthermore, only the glycogen stored in liver is accessible to the circulation since blood glucose cannot be derived from muscle glycogen pools. Total body glycogen pools are depleted within the first 24 hours of fasting, and afterward contribute little to energy metabolism. Within 24 hours, as hepatic glycogen stores are depleted, gluconeogenesis from amino acids proceeds at a rapid rate and provides the main support for the maintenance of near-normal blood levels of glucose. During this early phase of starvation skeletal muscle and intestinal protein provide the major amount of substrate for gluconeogenesis. Early in starvation (initial 24 hours), before the transition to a fat-based fuel system that occurs later in prolonged starvation, glucose needs are on the order of 180 g/day. Glycogenolysis provides two thirds of that (or approximately 120 g/day) and gluconeogenesis from amino acids provides approximately one third (or 60 g/day). As starvation proceeds and organs shift from a carbohydrate-based to a fat-based fuel, the absolute need for glucose declines. Similarly, as starvation progresses, energy expenditure declines and thus total energy requirements also decrease.

In starvation, skeletal muscle is a major source of alanine and glutamine, the primary precursors for hepatic and renal gluconeogenesis. Muscle alanine is produced from several sources, including the direct release of alanine from muscle proteolysis as well as the transamination of pyruvate produced by glycolysis. As Felig and colleagues[20-23] originally proposed, glucose taken up by muscle undergoes glycolysis to pyruvate where it is transaminated to alanine and shuttled back to the liver for gluconeogenesis. It should be noted, however, that this glucose-alanine cycle does not account for a net flow of amino acid carbon to carbohydrate during fasting when the source of carbon molecules for alanine biosynthesis is from pyruvate released from glycolysis. Rather, the transport of carbon atoms from the periphery to the liver via the glucose-alanine cycle for hepatic gluconeogenesis and the net synthesis of glucose results only when the source of alanine is independent of glycolysis, and results from either protein degradation or the metabolic transformation of other glucogenic amino acids. Net synthesis of alanine can occur from cysteine, methionine, glycine, and serine.

Glutamine also plays the critical function of transporting amino nitrogen and carbon skeletons that can be used for gluconeogenesis.[24,25] From the quantitative standpoint, the release of glutamine from skeletal muscle equals or is greater than the release of alanine. In addition, the intestines and lungs are major sources of glutamine, especially during fasting and injury. In skeletal muscle, glutamine is formed from glutamate that originates from either net proteolysis or transamination of α-ketoglutarate derived from the Krebs cycle. α-Ketoglutarate is derived from the net synthesis of fatty acid oxidation which is increased in starvation, and from the carbon skeletons of some amino acids such as aspartate from the Krebs cycle.

Both glutamine, which is the primary substrate for renal gluconeogenesis, and alanine, the primary substrate for hepatic gluconeogenesis, are derived from amino acid metabolism in skeletal muscle. Glutamine metabolism is also significant in the intestines and lung. Therefore factors that regulate the protein balance in these organs will directly affect the rate of synthesis and release of these amino acids. Both skeletal muscle and the intestines are extremely catabolic during the early phases of starvation when gluconeogenesis rates are high. While the liver is the primary site of gluconeogenesis from alanine, the kidney is the primary source of gluconeogenesis from glutamine. In prolonged starvation, the kidney becomes a significant source of body glucose. Thus, as much as 90 percent of gluconeogenesis occurs in the liver and only 10 percent in the kidney early in starvation; later in starvation as much as 45 percent of gluconeogenesis occurs in the kidney and 55 percent in the liver.

GLUCOSE METABOLISM IN THE SEPTIC STATE

Glucose metabolism during injury and sepsis is complex and not well understood. The patient who has suffered injury or who has developed sepsis is often malnourished and receiving inadequate nutritional support. Despite this, the patient commonly exhibits a hypermetabolic state and accelerated protein catabolism.

The underlying processes that drive this hypermetabolism are not fully known. Historically, Stoner and his colleagues in the United Kingdom[26] have proposed that this response to injury can be characterized as being either a "push or pull" phenomenon. Increased energy demands may be "pushed" to increased levels by the neuroendocrine and proinflammatory cytokine milieu. Conversely, increased energy requirements may be due to (or "pulled" by) the metabolic demands imposed by healing tissues and an activated immune system. For example, Wannemacher[27] and Wilmore and Aulick[28] independently argued that the wounded tissue and distant immunologic tissues drive hypermetabolism through induction of a neuroendocrine and proinflammatory mediator response to meet the demands of the reparative process or induction of an antimicrobial state.

Evidence of hypermetabolism and increased energy demands was first described by Cuthbertson[29] in patients suffering from long bone fractures. Cuthbertson described two phases of metabolic response to injury termed the *ebb* and *flow* phases (Fig. 5–3). The ebb phase occurs immediately after the injury with the resultant hypotension, altered cardiac status, and/or shock from sepsis or hypovolemia. This stage is variable, lasting between 12 to 24 hours,[30] and is characterized by a decrease in oxygen consumption, energy expenditure, and body temperature.[31] With resolution of the ebb phase and restoration of normal hemodynamics, the flow phase, which is characterized by general catabolism, begins. During this period the patient's metabolic rate, energy expenditure, and temperature rise with breakdown of skeletal muscle and visceral proteins to manufacture the hepatic acute-phase proteins.[31] The flow phase may last for several weeks and with resolution, anabolism and rebuilding of skeletal and visceral protein stores commence. Glucose metabolism is altered in both of these phases through the actions of the glucoregulatory hormones, but it is different in the two phases.

During the ebb phase, changes in glucose metabolism result in hyperglycemia. This is the result of the release of the catecholamines, glucagon, vasopressin, angiotensin II, and the glucocorticoids. In the liver, glycogenolysis is driven by these hormones to enable the liver to release glucose for use by the glucose-dependent organs, most importantly the central nervous system. Of the hormones, the catecholamines acting via the β-adrenergic recep-

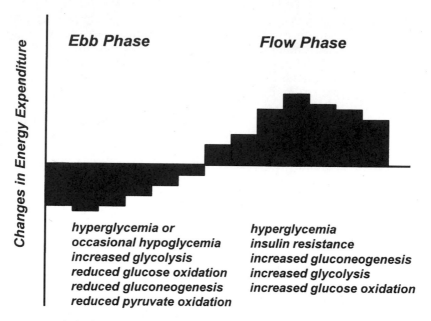

FIGURE 5–3   Changes in carbohydrate metabolism during the ebb and flow phases of injury. The ebb phase is characterized by declines in energy expenditure and decreases in glucose use, whereas the flow phase of injury is generally hyperdynamic and characterized by increases in gluconeogenesis and protein wasting.

tor appear to play the major role in promoting glycogenolysis since the resultant hyperglycemia parallels catecholamine release.[30] Glucagon release is promoted by the catecholamines, whereas insulin release is inhibited.[32] Glucagon, however, may not play a significant role in promoting glycogenolysis because circulating glucagon levels are not elevated.[30] The glucocorticoids are believed to play a permissive role in the mobilization of glycogen stores.[32] After hepatic glycogen stores are depleted, hyperglycemia is maintained by increased hepatic gluconeogenesis. The increase in hepatic gluconeogenesis is mediated primarily by β-adrenergic stimulation by the catecholamines.[30] While the liver is producing more glucose for systemic use, peripheral glucose oxidation decreases in part due to the hemodynamic changes associated with the shock state. In addition, glucose oxidation is decreased in the periphery by the induction of insulin resistance.[30] The mechanisms for the development of insulin resistance are poorly understood, but the effect is to maintain adequate circulating glucose for use by the glucose-dependent organs during trauma or sepsis. Thus, the ebb phase of injury is marked by hyperglycemia ensuring an adequate glucose supply for the central nervous system. The hyperglycemia is initiated by catecholamine-induced glycogenolysis and main-

tained by hepatic gluconeogenesis and peripheral insulin resistance.

The patient will either succumb during the ebb phase or will stabilize and then move on to the flow phase of injury. As opposed to the ebb phase of injury, carbohydrate metabolism during the flow or catabolic phase is characterized by normoglycemia or hyperglycemia, increased glucose turnover, and increased glucose oxidation.[32] Glucose oxidation increases compared to normal patients, but the fraction of glucose that is metabolized by oxidation is smaller in relation to the amount undergoing glycolysis.[31] During this phase, the patient exhibits elevated core body temperature that is believed to be due, in part, to the increased substrate cycling during glycolysis and the subsequent generation of heat.[32] During this catabolic phase, there is increased proteolysis with release of alanine, which is converted to glucose by gluconeogenesis in the liver. Hepatic glucose is released, and then converted from lactate back to glucose in the liver. The patient in the catabolic phase of injury has rates of gluconeogenesis that can be twice as high as normal fasted patients.[31] Despite the dramatic increases in gluconeogenesis at the expense of skeletal muscle, serum glucose levels often remain normal.

During the flow phase, patients exhibit elevated insulin levels despite normal serum glucose levels, and also exhibit a markedly decreased glucose-to-insulin ratio[30] (Fig. 5–4). Despite the elevated insulin levels, glycogen formation is suppressed and gluconeogenesis continues.[32] Additionally, the anabolic effects of insulin on skeletal muscle are diminished.[30] This change in the actions of insulin is believed to be due to the development of insulin resistance, most likely through changes in insulin receptor function and at the postreceptor level.[30,32] The development of insulin resistance has been linked to corticosteroid release in rat sepsis models.[32]

The neuroendocrine stimulus that is responsible for the increased gluconeogenesis, glucose turnover, and glucose oxidation is poorly understood. It was initially postulated that glucagon, the corticosteroids, growth hormone, and the catecholamines drive the hepatic gluconeogenesis and increased glucose oxidation. This hypothesis was based on the observation that infusion of these hormones into normal patients will produce the changes in glucose metabolism seen during the flow phase.[30] However, the levels of these hormones in trauma and sepsis patients during the flow phase are unlikely to explain the magnitude of the response.[30,31] In addition, animal models have failed to show an effect on the elevation of glucose metabolism by hormonal blockade.[33] Therefore, release of the stress hormones after injury only partly explains the alterations of glucose metabolism

during the flow phase. There is now evidence that the host immunologic response to injury may play a role in this phenomenon. A major consumer of glucose in the post-traumatic or septic patient may be effector cells of the inflammatory and reparative response.[30] Leukocytes, macrophages, and fibroblasts rely on glycolysis as the primary source of fuel and may be responsible for the increase in glucose turnover seen in this patient population. The wound may therefore be a privileged site, not unlike the central nervous system, able to drive glucose metabolism and gluconeogenesis at the expense of injured cellular protein.[30] This allows for the manufacture of large amounts of glucose to generate ATP for wound healing and host defense by glycolysis. At present the mechanisms for communication between the site of infection or the wound and the liver are poorly understood. Clearly the nervous system plays a role in this communication as is evidenced by the fact that epidural anesthesia will blunt the postoperative catabolic state.[32] However, there is new evidence that the reticuloendothelial cell system may play a role in this communication by the release of paracrine cytokines.

Cytokine Control of Glucose Metabolism

It has become clear that the changes in the concentrations of epinephrine, norepinephrine,

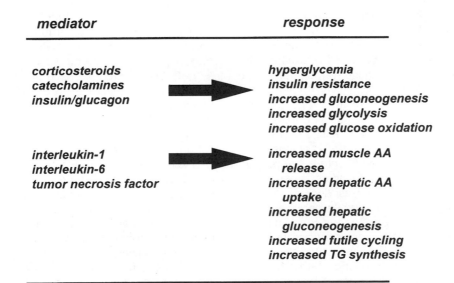

mediator	response
corticosteroids **catecholamines** **insulin/glucagon**	**hyperglycemia** **insulin resistance** **increased gluconeogenesis** **increased glycolysis** **increased glucose oxidation**

interleukin-1
interleukin-6
tumor necrosis factor
	increased muscle AA
	  release
	increased hepatic AA
	  uptake
	increased hepatic
	  gluconeogenesis
	increased futile cycling
	increased TG synthesis

FIGURE 5–4 Hormonal and inflammatory mediator changes during the flow phase of injury. Changes in carbohydrate metabolism are under regulatory control of insulin/glucagon, growth hormone, catecholamines, and corticosteroids, all of which contribute to the regulatory changes that accompany injury or infection. In addition, increases in proinflammatory cytokines alter not only precursor availability for gluconeogenesis but also glycogenolytic pathways.

glucagon, vasopressin, and glucocorticoids after trauma and during sepsis explain part but not all of the observed changes in glucose metabolism. Recently, interest has centered around the ability of the innate immune system to mediate these changes in metabolism through the expression of cytokines by macrophage and leukocyte population. Endotoxin, a primary stimulus for the release of cytokines by macrophage populations, has been shown to alter glucose metabolism possibly by virtue of this ability to promote cytokine release. The two cytokines that have been implicated in altering glucose metabolism are TNF-α and members of the IL-1 family. These cytokines appear to act both independently and via a neuroendocrine response. The ability of the remaining members of the cytokine family to alter glucose metabolism is only now being investigated.

Endotoxin or lipopolysaccharide (LPS) is a component of gram negative bacterial cell walls and is felt to be the mediator of the hemodynamic and metabolic alterations encountered in sepsis.[34] Endotoxin exerts these effects by promoting the release of cytokines from macrophage populations. As mentioned above, endotoxin is known to alter glucose metabolism during sepsis. In a model of endotoxemia in the rat, low-dose endotoxin increases hepatic glucose production either by stimulating glycogenolysis or gluconeogenesis depending on the nutritional state of the animal.[35] In addition to increasing the glucose production, administration of endotoxin increases peripheral usage of glucose, with the most dramatic increases in glucose usage noted in organs with large resident macrophage populations—the liver and the spleen.[35] In the liver 90 percent of the increased glucose use after LPS infusion was noted to be due to hepatic nonparenchymal cells, primarily Kupffer cells.[36] In a model of high-dose endotoxin infusion, glucose metabolism was noted to be affected. As opposed to the low-dose endotoxin studies, it was found that glucose production was decreased —resulting in hypoglycemia—while peripheral glucose use was once again increased.[37] The conclusion was that the hypoglycemia noted with the high-dose LPS study represented decreased endogenous glucose production rather than increased use.[37] Administration of high-dose endotoxin induced hemodynamic instability and shock, which led to the development of hypoglycemia as a result of decreased hepatic perfusion and decreased delivery of substrate to the liver.[37] The infusion of high doses of endotoxin recreates the ebb phase of injury that has been described in humans after trauma or during sepsis, while low-dose infusion of LPS more accurately recreates the catabolic or flow phase of injury.

The mechanisms by which endotoxin exerts its effects on glucose metabolism are in part due to the release of catecholamines and glucagon. α-Adrenergic and β-adrenergic blockade before endotoxin infusion abolishes the resultant hyperglycemia and attenuates increases in peripheral glucose use.[35] The changes in glucose concentrations and decreased glucose utilization are partially a result of increased insulin secretion after adrenergic blockade, but this does not explain the magnitude of the effect.[35] Additionally, adrenergic blockade decreases glucose use in the liver but not in the lungs, spleen, and intestines.[36] Thus, catecholamines are responsible for the hyperglycemia during endotoxemia but do not fully explain increased glucose use. Catecholamines appear to play a pivotal role in promoting hepatic glucose production in the early phase of endotoxin challenge and may be responsible for sustaining hepatic glucose production in the later phases.[36] Glucagon, like the adrenergics, also appears to play a pivotal role in promoting hepatic glucose production. Blunting the glucagon response to chronic infection with *Escherichia coli* in the rat with somatostatin while replacing the insulin will decrease hepatic gluconeogenesis.[38] Once again the magnitude of the response cannot be fully explained by the effects of glucagon alone, implicating the tissue responses to endotoxin challenge as the primary mediator of altered glucose metabolism.

TNF-α is secreted by macrophages after stimulation with endotoxin. This cytokine has many biologic functions including the inducement of shock, the killing of tumor cells, the induction of neutrophil adhesion molecules, neutrophil activation, and complement activation.[39] TNF-α also acts to alter glucose metabolism in a manner similar to that seen after the infusion of endotoxin. As with endotoxin, infusion of TNF-α increases hepatic glucose production by both glycogenolysis and gluconeogenesis, and TNF-α increases peripheral glucose use.[40-42] This response is, however, of a lesser magnitude than that demonstrated after endotoxin infusions.[43] This increase in glucose use occurs predominately in organs with large resident macrophage populations such as the spleen, liver, kidney, lungs, and skin.[41,44] The increase in glucose use shifts the organisms's primary source of energy from lipids to carbohydrates.[42] In contrast to what is known about glucose use in septic humans, the infusion of TNF-α in the dog increases glucose oxidation.[45] However, it is likely that TNF-α also increases nonoxidative glucose use by organs rich in leukocytes in a manner similar to endotoxin.

Much like the response to endotoxin, the glucoregulatory response to TNF-α is in part mediated by the counterregulatory hormones. Adrenergic blockade abolishes hepatic glucose release in response to TNF-α despite increases in glucagon and glucocorticoids.[43] Thus, the catecholamines play a primary role in mediating TNF-α–induced hepatic glucose production. In addition, the increase in peripheral glucose uptake and use by TNF-α in the spleen, liver, and skin can be blocked or attenuated by antiadrenergics.[43] However, adrenergic blockade had no effect on terminal ileum glucose use in the lung.[43] The administration of TNF-α leads to the development of insulin resistance in the periphery, particularly the skeletal muscle and skin.[46] The insulin resistance generated in skeletal muscle is under the control of the β-adrenergics, while insulin resistance in the skin and gut is under the control of adrenergics and possibly direct control by TNF-α.[40] This effect may be due to direct downregulation of the expression of the insulin-dependent GLUT 4 glucose transport molecule by TNF-α.[46] Therefore it can be concluded that most but not all of the effects of TNF-α on glucose metabolism are achieved by the actions of counterregulatory hormones.

Other Cytokines

While a large body of evidence demonstrating the effects of TNF-α and IL-1 in altering glucose metabolism exists, information about the role of the remaining cytokines is lacking. IL-6 is a cytokine released by macrophages in response to endotoxin and TNF-α. The primary effect of IL-6 is to alter hepatocyte protein synthesis patterns.[47] IL-6 induces the liver to decrease the synthesis of albumin and directs the cells to manufacture proteins making up the hepatic acute-phase response. The proteins include C-reactive protein, haptoglobin, α-1 antitrypsin, serum amyloid A, and others. The hepatic acute-phase response acts in a protective manner in part by enabling improved clearance of invasive organisms.[48] Clearly IL-6 exerts a direct effect on the hepatocyte by promoting the hepatic acute-phase response, and there is now evidence that it acts to alter glucose metabolism in vitro. Isolated rat hepatocytes have been shown to promote the release

of glucose from prelabeled glycogen stores, while TNF-α, IL-1, and interferon gamma (IFN-γ) had no effect.[49] This response was inhibited by coincubation with antibodies specific for IL-6. The authors concluded, based on the time course of these studies, that IL-6 may act by inhibiting glycogen synthetase thus allowing phosphorylase activity to predominate.[49] As mentioned above, the role of other cytokines in altering glucose metabolism is unknown. However, the cytokine cascade is a complex response in which one cytokine promotes the release of a cascade of other cytokines. This raises the question of whether TNF-α and the IL-1 may act independently to alter hepatic and systemic glucose metabolism or via this cascade effect.

GLUCOSE REQUIREMENTS: IMPLICATIONS FOR NUTRITIONAL SUPPORT IN HEALTHY MAN AND IN INJURY AND INFLAMMATION

It should be recognized that the ideal energy substrate formulation for hospitalized patients receiving enteral or parenteral nutrition support is not fully known. Regardless of the exact formulation, carbohydrate calories and, for parenteral formulations, glucose remain the primary energy sources. A general rule of thumb for the hospitalized patient is that maximal rates of glucose oxidation approximate 5 to 6 mg/kg body weight/min. In the patient with inadequate carbohydrate intake, ongoing gluconeogenesis, which is elevated in the injured or septic patient, will partially meet these requirements. Much of this increase in gluconeogenesis is related to an increased use of glucose for healing and in inflammatory tissues. Glucose intake will suppress gluconeogenesis in a dose-dependent fashion, but in the critically ill patient suppression is not complete. In critically ill patients, maximal suppression of gluconeogenesis occurs with approximately 600 g/day of glucose.[50]

In catabolic patients, low-dose (100 to 200 g/day) glucose infusions have little or no nitrogen-sparing effects and do not suppress either gluconeogenesis or ureagenesis.[51,52] However, when carbohydrate infusions progress from 200 to 500 to 600 g/day and crystalline amino acids are also provided, nitrogen balance improves progressively.[53-56] At that point, a plateau is reached, and further increases in glucose provision are not associated with any further increases in nitrogen retention. This plateau is reached when calorie intake approaches 100 to 120 percent of energy expenditure.[57] The use of supplemental insulin in this setting is controversial. In highly catabolic patients, insulin can improve nitrogen balance. However, the clinical usefulness of insulin infusions remains questionable because adding insulin to high-dose glucose infusions does not appear to further suppress hepatic gluconeogenesis when glucose uptake is already maximally stimulated.[58] In general, insulin infusions at a rate to maintain normal blood glucose levels (< 160 mg/dl) during moderate rates of glucose infusion (i.e., near or at predicted resting energy expenditures) can provide some improvement in nitrogen balance in catabolic patients.

However, potential adverse effects of glucose feeding include hyperglycemia, increased production of carbon dioxide, and hepatic steatosis. When administered parenterally, hypertonic glucose can also cause venous sclerosis. Osmotic diuresis also accompanies excessive enteral carbohydrate administration. However, the incidence and magnitude of these adverse effects can often be minimized when an understanding of their underlying pathogenesis is present.

Hyperglycemia can be a frequent occurrence with glucose administration, especially in critically ill patients, when given at rates that exceed maximal glucose uptake (4 to 6 mg/kg/min; 400 to 600 g/day). Insulin supplementation often has been recommended with glucose infusions, and regular monitoring of glycemic levels is required. Realize, however, that although supplemental insulin will often control hyperglycemic episodes during glucose infusions, insulin supplementation does not necessarily increase glucose oxidation and utilization as an energy source. Rather, increased glucose uptake in the presence of insulin often leads to enhanced glycogen synthesis rather than glucose oxidation and energy generation. However, if glucose levels are allowed to increase, nonketotic hyperosmolar syndrome and diabetic ketoacidosis can result. In critically ill patients with alterations in glucose uptake, hyperosmolarity, diuresis, and aggravation of central nervous system injury may occur even at moderate rates of glucose infusion (200 to 400 g/day).

When carbohydrates in general and glucose in particular are given in excess of energy requirements, lipogenesis will occur. If excessive glucose is administered, lipogenesis will occur even in the critically ill patient who is losing body nitrogen to urea. In the normal adult, administration of carbohydrate in excess of resting energy expenditure increases minute ventilation and the work of breathing in proportion to the increase in carbon dioxide production. The respiratory quotient (V_{CO_2}/V_{O_2}) for the oxidation of glucose is 1.0, whereas it is 8.0 for lipogenesis. Thus, lipogenesis from glucose will result in increased carbon dioxide production. In the 1980s Askanazi and colleagues[59,60] observed that overfeeding critically ill patients with glucose led to significant increases in energy expenditure, oxygen consumption, carbon dioxide production, and minute ventilation. Some investigators have reported that such increases in carbon dioxide production and minute ventilation have led to respiratory distress syndromes. However, the clinical significance of these findings has been questioned because, when respiratory distress has been reported, it has been limited primarily to patient populations with underlying pulmonary disease and marginal respiratory reserves.

Several approaches have been recommended to minimize the risk of hypercapnia-induced respiratory failure. These include reducing the absolute number of glucose calories administered as well as exchanging some carbohydrate calories for lipids. The most efficient means of reducing the risk of such complications is to prevent total calories, carbohydrate calories, or both from exceeding resting energy expenditure.

Finally, hepatic complications associated with excessive carbohydrate intake have been reported for several decades and range from hepatic steatosis to hepatic failure and death. There is some controversy whether the development of hepatic steatosis is the result of excess carbohydrate intake or rather is due to the hormonal milieu that is present. The incidence of hepatic steatosis is considerably higher in the critically ill patient in whom it often leads to intrahepatic cholestasis than in other patients receiving parenteral glucose. It has been proposed that the induction of hepatic steatosis is secondary to an inability to package and dispose of very low density lipoprotein particles rather than the result of increased hepatic lipogenesis per se. The former process is extremely sensitive to the insulin:glucagon ratio, which is dependent not only on the portal and systemic concentrations of glucose, but also upon the hormonal milieu of the critically ill patient.

Caution should be exercised when extending these data to individual clinical settings since there has been inadequate experimentation in humans to conclude that all of these processes are operative and biologically significant. Thus, although it is reasonable to assume that infusions of glucose in excess of resting energy requirements are associated with metabolic perturbations detrimental to the patient, definitive recommendations for individual patients require additional research. We can conclude, however, that glucose requirements in critically ill patients are not likely to exceed those necessary to meet energy requirements and that mixed fuel systems offer some theoretic advantages.

Alternative Glucose Fuels

In Europe, especially in Germany, carbohydrate energy sources other than glucose have not only been studied for their usefulness in partial peripheral and total parenteral nutrition, but are also available as a component of the clinical armamentarium. Although not commonly used in the United States, research interests remain high to evaluate the effectiveness of these nonglucose carbohydrate fuels in meeting energy needs and reducing protein catabolism in the stressed host. Among the alternative energy sources considered for parenteral nutrition are fructose and the polyols—sorbitol and xylitol. The desire to use nonglucose carbohydrate fuels stems from a better understanding of glucose metabolism in the injured or infected patient, and the desire to obtain an optimal fuel mixture that will be efficiently used and will reduce protein catabolism. This review will summarize our current knowledge concerning the use of these fuels in patients in whom glucose and lipid-based substrates are not well used.

Xylitol Metabolism

Xylitol is a five carbon polyol that differs structurally from glucose at the first three carbon atoms, suggesting that its transport into cells may not be facilitated by insulin. Xylitol is a normal intermediary in the glucuronic acid-xylulose cycle.

Compared to glucose, insulin secretion and hepatic lipogenesis are reduced significantly by xylitol administration.[61] Administration of xylitol to humans at a rate of 135 to 185 g/day is accompanied by a mobilization of endogenous fat sources and a rise in ketone body levels so that energy expenditure is partly met by oxidation of free fatty acids and ketone bodies.[61] Maximal disposal rates of xylitol in humans are approximately 600 g/day, but depending upon the magnitude of injury may actually increase to up to 1200 g/day.

During intravenous administration of xylitol at a rate of 200 to 400 g/day, blood glucose and insulin levels remain unchanged. In surgical patients who underwent gastric resection, insulin levels actually declined when glucose calories were replaced with xylitol.[62]

During periods of insulin resistance, as is seen during trauma, xylitol infusions reduce ketone body formation to a lesser extent than does glucose. Endogenous fat continues to be mobilized and oxidized more rapidly, thus contributing more to energy expenditure than during hypocaloric glucose infusions.[61,62] Gluconeogenesis is increased during injury and infection, but the use of xylitol can reduce gluconeogenesis and simultaneously increase fatty acid oxidation, thereby increasing the contribution of fat to overall energy expenditure.

Metabolic Responses to Xylitol Infusions. Xylitol infusions have been employed in rodent and clinical studies as either the sole carbohydrate source or as a replacement for some glucose calories. As expected, responses have varied from a beneficial effect on skeletal protein metabolism in septic rats treated with glucose/xylitol regimens to adverse protein metabolism in rats treated with xylitol alone.[62-65]

For example, Ardawi[63] recently reported that septic rats treated with xylitol-supplemented total parenteral nutrition had markedly improved outcome compared with rats not receiving caloric supplements or equicaloric glucose supplements. Not only was nitrogen balance improved in these animals, but protein and RNA content of the muscles were also markedly higher. Drews and Stein[65] were also able to show in rats with a cecal ligation and puncture that supplementation of total parenteral nutrition with xylitol improved nitrogen balance and reduced skeletal muscle protein degradation as measured by urinary 3-methylhistidine excretion. Similarly, Georgieff and colleagues[64] were able to show in burned rats that xylitol replacement of half the glucose calories resulted in reduced rates of hepatic gluconeogenesis. The investigators were able to confirm these rodent studies in surgical intensive care unit patients. Replacing half the glucose calories of total parenteral nutrition with xylitol resulted in a 45 percent reduction in urea production rates, measured isotopically.[62] Those authors recommend that during critical illness, a total parenteral nutrition formula be employed that uses glucose and xylitol in a 1:1 ratio with a total carbohydrate intake of 3 g/kg body weight/day.

However, other investigators have failed to show a superiority of xylitol over glucose as a component of total parenteral nutrition. In rats subjected to a thermal injury, Karlstad and colleagues[66] were unable to show any superiority of partial replacement of glucose calories with xylitol in terms of whole body amino acid kinetics, nitrogen balance, or energy expenditure. In fact, Drews and Stein[65] and Fried and colleagues[67] reported that in healthy, parenterally fed rats, providing all of the carbohydrate calories as xylitol resulted in less positive nitrogen balance and development of a fatty liver. The discrepancy between these latter studies where xylitol infusions were associated with either no improvement or worsening of protein status and earlier studies that demonstrated efficacy can be explained by the quantities of xylitol administered and the degree of metabolic stress. As discussed earlier, critical illness is often associated with increased xylitol utilization rates, and administration of xylitol in excess of utilization often results in excessive urinary losses and metabolic abnormalities. For these reasons, conservative estimates of xylitol requirements have been promulgated.

Sorbitol and Fructose

Studies delineating the mechanisms by which fructose and sorbitol spare body protein in the critically ill patient are much less well defined. This is due in large part to the decision of several regulatory groups in Europe to withdraw fructose and sorbitol from the market because of congenital fructose intolerance. This loss of commercialization has hampered studies on the metabolic basis for such therapies.

In contrast to glucose, fructose is primarily metabolized by the liver. In the liver cell, fructose is activated to fructose-1-phosphate by fructokinase, an insulin-independent enzyme with activities far greater than all of the glucose phosphorylating enzymes in the liver. Fructose-1-phosphate is then cleaved to two trioses by aldolases and enters the Emden-Meyerhoff pathway. The rapid turnover rate in the glycolytic pathway during fructose administration can thus lead to increased lactate production.

Adverse Effects

The major risk associated with fructose administration, and therefore associated with sorbitol infusions that are metabolized via fructose, is hereditary fructose intolerance. This congenital disorder is relatively rare (1 in 21,000), but before 1987 when fructose use was restricted in Europe, 12 lethal complications were reported. Toxicity appears to be associated with accumulation of hyperosmolar quantities of fructose in the circulation. Experi-

ence in Germany has demonstrated that it is almost impossible to identify a history of intolerance, and warning labels do not avoid this complication.

Toxicities associated with xylitol overdose have also been reported in the literature. The first detectable effect of a xylitol overdose is increased loss of a xylitol in the urine.[61] When given orally in excessive quantities to healthy volunteers, nausea, increased liver specific enzymes, and increased uric acid secretion have been reported. Oxalate deposits in the brain and kidney have also been reported in patients receiving xylitol infusions, although pathophysiology has only been reported when recommended dosages have been exceeded.

In general, the search for alternative carbohydrate fuels in the parenteral feeding regimen of critically ill patients has focused on reducing glucose intolerance and improving overall nitrogen metabolism. Three alternative carbohydrate fuels, xylitol, fructose, and sorbitol, have been used as insulin-independent fuels that may supplement glucose-based parenteral feeding regimens. Although fructose and sorbitol have now been removed from the market in Europe because of unexpected mortalities due to congenital fructose intolerance, xylitol infusions appear relatively safe and effective when used under closely controlled guidelines. Animal studies also suggest that when used in the critically ill, replacing approximately half of the glucose calories with xylitol leads to reduced gluconeogenesis, increased protein retention, and improved nitrogen balance. In preliminary studies of surgical intensive care unit patients, these results have been confirmed. However, these studies need to be confirmed in other clinical trials and guidelines for xylitol's use need to be refined.

SUMMARY AND CONCLUSIONS

A better understanding of the underlying mechanisms that alter carbohydrate metabolism in injury, infection, inflammation, or in neoplastic diseases should lead to a more rational approach to the provision of nutrient support. Although there recently has been a fair amount of direct investigation into alterations in carbohydrate metabolism in critically ill patients and the effects of glucose provision on carbohydrate and protein metabolism, there is no complete agreement to the optimal nutrient formulation or delivery system for the hospitalized patient. There are, however, some guidelines that can be generally accepted when considering the quantities and sources of carbohydrate to administer to hospitalized patients. Hyperglycemia during the flow phase of injury or inflammation is not an abnormal or pathologic response, and modest degrees of hyperglycemia ($< 160-180$ mg/dl) can be tolerated without efforts to lower blood glucose concentrations below 140 mg/dl. These modestly elevated levels of glucose promote glucose uptake but are below the concentrations that cause hyperosmolarity. In fact glucose concentrations in the range of 160 to 200 mg/dl maximally promote glucose uptake without a significant risk of complications associated with hyperglycemia.

In general, glucose administration can be used to meet a significant component of resting energy expenditure. Early speculations that in the critically ill patient glucose intakes less than resting energy expenditure were not as efficiently used for energy production have not been confirmed by recent isotopic studies. Rather, the consensus today is that the oxidative use of glucose below resting energy expenditure is unimpaired in the critically ill patient.

There are, however, some settings where alternative carbohydrate fuels and lipid emulsions may be indicated: lipid emulsions are beneficial when more concentrated sources of calories are required for volume-restricted patients or when prolonged nutritional support is anticipated and lipid emulsions are required to prevent fatty acid deficiency. The use of xylitol to replace glucose calories in the critically ill patient remains controversial. However, there are now experimental data to suggest that xylitol can replace some glucose calories in critically ill patients without adversely affecting either protein or carbohydrate homeostasis, although there is little evidence to suggest a significant benefit of xylitol.

Infusions of glucose in excess of resting energy expenditure appear to offer little benefit in terms of carbohydrate and protein metabolism and may, under some situations, pose adverse risks to the critically ill patients. Increased energy expenditure, carbon dioxide production and ventilatory work, increased risk of hepatic steatosis, and hyperglycemia can result from these excessive administrations of glucose and should be avoided.

REFERENCES

1. Butler PC, Rizza RA: Regulation of carbohydrate metabolism and response to hypoglycemia. Endocrinol Metab Clin North Am 1989;18:1–25.
2. Larner J: Insulin and the stimulation of glycogen synthesis. The road from glycogen structure to glycogen synthase to cyclic AMP-dependent protein kinase to insulin mediators. Adv Enzymol Relat Areas Mol Biol 1990;63:173–231.
3. Liu Z, Gardner LB, Barrett EJ: Insulin and glucose suppress hepatic glycogenolysis by distinct enzymatic mechanisms. Metabolism 1993;42:1546–1551.
4. van de Werve G, Jeanrenaud B: Liver glycogen metabolism: an overview. Diabetes Metab Rev 1987;3:47–78.
5. Coderre L, Srivastava AK, Chiasson JL: Role of glucocorticoid in the regulation of glycogen metabolism in skeletal muscle. Am J Physiol 1991;260:E927–E932.
6. Roach PJ, Cao Y, Corbett CA et al: Glycogen metabolism and signal transduction in mammals and yeast. Adv Enzyme Regul 1991;31:101–120.
7. Nuttall FQ, Gannon MC: Allosteric regulation of glycogen synthase in liver. A physiological dilemma. J Biol Chem 1993;268:13286–13290.
8. Radziuk J, Pye S, Zhang Z: Substrates and the regulation of hepatic glycogen metabolism. Adv Exp Med Biol 1993;334:235–252.
9. Keppens S, Vandekerckhove A, Moshage H et al: Regulation of glycogen phosphorylase activity in isolated human hepatocytes. Hepatology 1993;17:610–614.
10. Johnson LN: Glycogen phosphorylase: control by phosphorylation and allosteric effectors. FASEB J 1992; 6:2274–2282.
11. Preiss J, Romeo T: Molecular biology and regulatory aspects of glycogen biosynthesis in bacteria. Prog Nucleic Acid Res Mol Biol 1994;47:299–329.
12. Van Schaftingen E: Glycolysis revisited. Diabetologia 1993;36:581–588.
13. Pilkis SJ, Granner DK: Molecular physiology of the regulation of hepatic gluconeogenesis and glycolysis. Annu Rev Physiol 1992;54:885–909.
14. Lemaigre FP, Rousseau GG: Transcriptional control of genes that regulate glycolysis and gluconeogenesis in adult liver. Biochem J 1994;303:1–14.
15. Pilkis SJ, Claus TH: Hepatic gluconeogenesis/glycolysis: regulation and structure/function relationships of substrate cycle enzymes. Annu Rev Nutr 1991;11:465–515.
16. Wolfe RR, Klein S, Herndon DN et al: Substrate cycling in thermogenesis and amplification of net substrate flux in human volunteers and burned patients. J Trauma 1990;30:S6–S9.
17. Wolfe RR, Herndon DN, Jahoor F et al: Effect of severe burn injury on substrate cycling by glucose and fatty acids. N Engl J Med 1987;317:403–408.
18. Miyoshi H, Shulman GI, Peters EJ et al: Hormonal control of substrate cycling in humans. J Clin Invest 1988;81:1545–1555.
19. Lickley HL, Kemmer FW, el Tayeb KM et al: Importance of glucagon in the control of futile cycling as studied in alloxan-diabetic dogs. Diabetologia 1987; 30:175-182.
20. Felig P, Pozefsky T, Marliss E et al: Alanine: key role in gluconeogenesis. Science 1970;167:1003–1004.
21. Felig P, Marliss E, Owen OE et al: Blood glucose and gluconeogenesis in fasting man. Arch Intern Med 1969;123:293–298.
22. Felig P, Marliss E, Owen OE et al: Role of substrate in the regulation of hepatic gluconeogenesis in fasting man. Adv Enzyme Regul 1969;7:41–46.
23. Felig P, Owen OE, Wahren J et al: Amino acid metabolism during prolonged starvation. J Clin Invest 1969; 48:584–594.
24. Owen OE, Felig P, Morgan AP et al: Liver and kidney metabolism during prolonged starvation. J Clin Invest 1969;48:574–583.

25. Felig P, Owen OE, Morgan AP et al: Utilization of metabolic fuels in obese subjects. Am J Clin Nutr 1968;21: 1429–1433.

26. Stoner HB: Hypothalamic involvement in the response to injury. In Richards JR, Kinney JM (eds): Nutritional Aspects of Care in the Critically Ill. Edinburgh: Churchill Livingston, 1977:257–272.

27. Wannemacher RWJ: Protein metabolism: applied biochemistry. In Ghadimi H (ed): Total Parenteral Nutrition: Premises and Promises. New York: John Wiley & Sons, 1975:85–153.

28. Wilmore DW, Aulick LH: Metabolic changes in burned patients. Surg Clin North Am 1978;58:1173–1187.

29. Cuthbertson DP: Post-shock metabolic response. Lancet 1942;1:433–436.

30. Frayn KN: Hormonal control of metabolism in trauma and sepsis. Clin Endocrinol (Oxf) 1986;24:577–599.

31. Goldstein SA, Elwyn DH: The effects of injury and sepsis on fuel utilization. Annu Rev Nutr 1989;9:445–473.

32. Douglas RG, Shaw JH: Metabolic response to sepsis and trauma. Br J Surg 1989;76:115–122.

33. Spitzer JJ, Bagby GJ, Hargrove DM et al: Alterations in the metabolic control of carbohydrates in sepsis. Prog Clin Biol Res 1989;308:545–561.

34. Ulevitch RJ, Wolfson N, Virca GD et al: Macrophages regulate the host response to bacterial lipopolysaccharides. Prog Clin Biol Res 1989;299:193–202.

35. Meszaros K, Lang CH, Bojta J et al: Early changes in glucose utilization of individual tissues after endotoxin administration. Circ Shock 1989;29:107–114.

36. Ottlakan A, Spolarics Z, Lang CH et al: Adrenergic blockade attenuates endotoxin-induced hepatic glucose uptake. Circ Shock 1993;39:74–79.

37. Lang CH, Spolarics Z, Ottlakan A et al: Effect of high-dose endotoxin on glucose production and utilization. Metabolism 1993;42:1351–1358.

38. Lang CH, Bagby GJ, Blakesley HL et al: Importance of hyperglucagonemia in eliciting the sepsis-induced increase in glucose production. Circ Shock 1989;29: 181–191.

39. van der Poll T, Lowry SF: Tumor necrosis factor in sepsis: mediator of multiple organ failure or essential part of host defense? Shock 1995;3:1–12.

40. Lang CH: Beta-adrenergic blockade attenuates insulin resistance induced by tumor necrosis factor. Am J Physiol 1993;264:R984–R991.

41. Meszaros K, Lang CH, Bagby GJ et al: Tumor necrosis factor increases in vivo glucose utilization of macrophage-rich tissues. Biochem Biophys Res Commun 1987;149:1–6.

42. Sakurai Y, Zhang XJ, Wolfe RR: Effect of tumor necrosis factor on substrate and amino acid kinetics in conscious dogs. Am J Physiol 1994;266:E936–E945.

43. Bagby GJ, Lang CH, Skrepnik N et al: Attenuation of glucose metabolic changes resulting from TNF-alpha administration by adrenergic blockade. Am J Physiol 1992;262:R628–R635.

44. Spolarics Z, Schuler A, Bagby GJ et al: Tumor necrosis factor increases in vivo glucose uptake in hepatic non-parenchymal cells. J Leukoc Biol 1991;49:309–312.

45. Sakurai Y, Zhang XU, Wolfe RR: Short-term effects of tumor necrosis factor on energy and substrate metabolism in dogs. J Clin Invest 1993;91:2437–2445.

46. Lang CH, Dobrescu C, Bagby GJ: Tumor necrosis factor impairs insulin action on peripheral glucose disposal and hepatic glucose output. Endocrinology 1992;130: 43–52.

47. Hirano T, Akira S, Taga T et al: Biological and clinical aspects of interleukin 6. Immunol Today 1990;11: 443–449.

48. Powanda MC, Moyer ED: Plasma proteins and wound healing. Surg Gynecol Obstet 1981;153:749–755.

49. Ritchie DG: Interleukin 6 stimulates hepatic glucose release from prelabeled glycogen pools. Am J Physiol 1990;258:E57–E64.

50. Wolfe RR, Allsop JR, Burke JF et al: Glucose metabolism in man: response to intravenous glucose infusion. Metabolism 1979;28:210–220.

51. Shaw JHF, Klein S, Wolfe RR: Assessment of alanine, urea and glucose interrelationships in normal subjects and in patients with sepsis with stable isotopic tracers. Surgery 1985;97:557–568.

52. Wolfe BM, Culebras JM, Sim AJW et al: Substrate interaction in intravenous feeding: comparative effects of carbohydrate and fat on amino acid utilization in fasting man. Ann Surg 1977;186:518–540.

53. Elwyn DH, Gump FE, Iles M et al: Protein and energy sparing of glucose added in hypocaloric amounts to peripheral infusions of amino acids. Metabolism 1978; 27:325–331.

54. Askanazi J, Carpentier YA, Jeevanandam J et al: Energy expenditure, nitrogen balance, and norepinephrine excretion after injury. Surgery 1981;89:478–484.

55. Skillman JJ, Rosenoer VM, Pallotta JA et al: Effect of isocaloric fat or glucose on albumin synthesis and nitrogen balance in patients receiving amino acid infusion. Surgery 1981;89:168–174.

56. McDougal WS, Wilmore DW, Pruitt BA, Jr: Effect of intravenous near isoosmotic nutrient infusions on nitrogen balance in critically ill injured patients. Surg Gynecol Obstet 1977;145:408–414.

57. Iapichino G, Gattinoni L, Solca M et al: Protein sparing and protein replacement in acutely injured patients during TPN with and without amino acid supply. Intensive Care Med 1982;8:25–31.

58. Brooks DC, Bessey PQ, Black PR et al: Insulin stimulates branched chain amino acid uptake and diminishes nitrogen flux from skeletal muscle of injured patients. J Surg Res 1986;40:395–405.

59. Askanazi J, Rosenbaum SH, Hyman AI et al: Respiratory changes induced by the large glucose loads of total parenteral nutrition. JAMA 1980;243:1444–1447.

60. Askanazi J, Elwyn DH, Silverberg PA et al: Respiratory distress secondary to a high carbohydrate load: a case report. Surgery 1980;87:596–598.

61. Georgieff M, Moldawer LL, Bistrian BR et al: Xylitol: an energy source for intravenous nutrition after trauma. J Parenter Enter Nutr 1985;9:199–209.

62. Georgieff M, Pscheidl E, Gotz H et al: The mechanism of the reduction of protein catabolism following trauma and during sepsis using xylitol. Anaesthesist 1991;40:85–91.

63. Ardawi MS: Effects of xylitol and/or glutamine supplemented parenteral nutrition on septic rats. Clin Sci 1992;82:419–427.

64. Georgieff M, Pscheidl E, Moldawer LL et al: Mechanisms of protein conservation during xylitol infusion after burn injury in rats: isotope kinetics and indirect calorimetry. Eur J Clin Invest 1991;21:249–258.

65. Drews D, Stein TP: Effect of excess xylitol on nitrogen and glucose metabolism in parenterally fed rats. J Parenter Enter Nutr 1992;16:521–524.

66. Karlstad MD, DeMichele SJ, Bistrian BR et al: Effect of total parenteral nutrition with xylitol and protein and energy metabolism in thermally injured rats. J Parenter Enter Nutr 1991;15:445–449.

67. Fried RC, Mullen JL, Blackburn GL et al: Effects of nonglucose substrates and carnitine on nitrogen metabolism in stressed rats. J Parenter Enter Nutr 1990; 14:134–138.

6

Dietary Fiber and Its Clinical Applications to Enteral Nutrition

CHARLENE COMPHER
RENÉE W. SETO
JOHN I. LEW
JOHN L. ROMBEAU

During the 1990s, dietary fiber has been widely accepted as an important component of human nutrition. Several epidemiologic studies have shown that the lack of dietary fiber intake is associated with the development of certain diseases such as colon cancer, atherosclerosis, diverticular disease, and obesity that are found predominantly in Western countries. Since Burkitt's observations more than 2 decades ago that demonstrated a low incidence of these "Western diseases" in the African population accustomed to a high-fiber diet, there has been considerable interest in the potential benefits of fiber to human health.[1] Consequently, considerable research has shown dietary fiber to possess several physiologic effects and functions essential to maintaining the gastrointestinal (GI) tract.

For a complete description of liquid formula diets (LFDs), please refer to Chapter 13. Briefly, commercially produced LFDs are known nutritional formulations with balanced carbohydrate, protein, fat, mineral, and vitamin contents. In such liquid diets, macronutrients and micronutrients are included in purified form. Macronutrients included as polymers in such diets are known as low-residue

diets, whereas macronutrients included as monomers in elemental diets are considered residue-free diets. These LFDs, however, are fiber free. Although current fiber-free enteral diets have a role in hospitalized patients with intestinal dysfunction, current research indicates that adding fiber to LFDs may be more clinically efficacious. This chapter reviews the physiologic effects of dietary fiber on the GI tract, emphasizing clinical trials with fiber-supplemented LFDs. Accordingly, clinical recommendations for use of fiber-supplemented enteral formulas in hospitalized patients are provided.

DEFINITION OF DIETARY FIBER

Dietary fiber has traditionally been defined as carbohydrate of plant origin that escapes enzymatic digestion in the small intestine to enter the colon. This definition, however, is not entirely accurate, since it includes malabsorbed starch that may resemble dietary fiber in the colon. Dietary fiber, therefore, is best described chemically as nonstarch polysaccharide (NSP) with the addition of lignin. Nonstarchy polysaccharides that comprise a major component of fiber are classified into two major classes: cellulosic and noncellulosic.[2] Lignin, a polyphenol that provides rigidity to the plant structure, is a minor component of fiber, but its presence may significantly affect the properties of polysaccharides. Table 6–1 includes a summary of dietary fiber components.

Cellulosic Polysaccharides

Cellulosic polysaccharides are long, linear polymers of $\beta 1$->4 glucans. These high-molecular-weight chains found within plant cell walls are arranged such that strong hydrogen bonding occurs between these parallel glucose strands. These structural chains, which ultimately form microfibrils, confer the characteristic stability and low reactivity of these molecules. The best-known cellulosic polysaccha-

ride, cellulose, is resistant to colonic bacterial degradation and excreted intact to a great extent. In plant cell walls, cellulose is embedded in a matrix of noncellulosic polysaccharide and lignin. Fibers rich in cellulose (e.g., wheat bran) greatly contribute to fecal mass by increasing its water-holding capacity in the colon. Therefore, these fibers increase wet and dry stool weights and reduce stool mean transit time by eliciting peristalsis.

Noncellulosic Polysaccharides

Noncellulosic polysaccharides (NCPs), most commonly represented in the form of hemicelluloses and pectic substances, constitute the cell wall matrix. Hemicelluloses are composed of branched chains and pyranoside sugars whereas pectic substances (i.e., pectin) are composed primarily of D-galacturonic acid with

TABLE 6–1   Chemical Classification of Fiber Types

Fiber	Main Chain	Side Chain	Description	Bacterial Degradation
Nonstarch Polysaccharides				
Cellulosic	Glucose	None	Main structural component of plant cell wall. Insoluble in concentrated alkali; soluble in concentrated acid.	No
Noncellulosic				
Hemicelluloses	Xylose Mannose Galactose Glucose	Arabinose Galactose Glucuronic acid	Cell wall polysaccharides containing backbone of 1,4--linked pyranoside sugars. Vary in degree of branching and uronic acid content. Soluble in dilute alkali.	No
Pectic substances	Galacturonic acid	Rhamnose Arabinose Xylose Fucose	Components of primary cell wall and middle lamella vary in methyl-ester content. Generally water soluble and gel forming.	Yes
Mucilages	Galactose-mannose Glucose-mannose Arabinose-xylose Galacturonic acid–rhamnose	Galactose	Synthesized by plant secretory cells; prevent dessication of seed endosperm. Food industry use, hydrophilic, stabilizer (e.g., guar).	Yes
Gums	Galactose Glucuronic acid–mannose Galacturonic acid–rhamnose	Xylose Fucose Galactose	Secreted at site of plant injury by specialized secretory cells. Food and pharmaceutical use (e.g., Karaya gum).	Yes
Algal polysaccharides	Mannose Xylose Glucuronic acid	Galactose	Derived from algae and seaweed. Vary in uronic acid content and presence of sulfate groups. Food and pharmaceutical use (e.g., carrageenan, agar).	Yes
Lignin	Sinapyl alcohol Coniferyl alcohol p-Coumaryl alcohol	3-D structure	Noncarbohydrate cell wall component. Complex cross-linked phenyl propane polymer. Insoluble in 72% sulfuric acid.	No

Adapted with permission from McPherson R: Classification of fiber types. In Clinical Role of Fibre. Mississauga, Ontario: Medical Education Services, 1985:13.

partially methylated carboxyl and acetylated hydroxyl groups. Fibers rich in hemicelluloses, pectin, or other NCPs (e.g., gums and mucilages) are degraded rapidly by anaerobic microflora of the cecum and colon. This process of bacterial fermentation leads to the formation of short-chain fatty acids (SCFAs) of which acetate, propionate, and butyrate are the most important. The SCFAs play a key role in the maintenance of the colonic milieu. Fiber-supplemented LFDs are perhaps beneficial because SCFA production occurs when these fermentable substrates are provided to colonic bacteria.

The analysis of the fiber content of liquid formula diets is most frequently determined by the Association of Official Analytic Chemists (AOAC) method.[3] The liquid diet is dried, defatted, and deproteinized before being separated into filtrate and residue portions (Fig. 6–1). The filtrate is solvent-extracted in ethanol and hence termed "soluble (alcohol-soluble) dietary fiber" (SDF) after protein and ash are removed. Pectins and gums are rich in soluble fiber. The residue portion is not alcohol soluble and hence termed "insoluble dietary fiber" (IDF) after protein and ash are removed. Cellulose, wheat bran, and soy polysaccharide are rich in insoluble dietary fiber. Table 6–2 lists the SDF, IDF, and total dietary fiber (TDF) content of liquid formula diets commercially available in the United States as of January 1996.

PHYSIOLOGIC EFFECTS OF DIETARY FIBER ON THE GI TRACT

Dietary fiber profoundly affects GI tract structure and function. The small intestine and colon are anatomic regions most pertinent to fiber and enteral nutrition (EN); therefore, the other areas of the GI tract will not be discussed. Although minimal digestion and absorption of dietary fiber may occur in the small bowel, the major site of NSP degradation is the colon.[13-15] In humans, no intestinal enzymes capable of NSP degradation have been identified. Conversely, there is little doubt that colonic bacterial enzymes play a key role in the anaerobic breakdown of fiber. As mentioned, this process of fermentation generates end products, of which SCFAs are the most important. Although colonic microflora produces some extracellular polysaccharidases, most of these enzymes are bound to bacterial cell walls. Of importance to dietary fiber and EN, many of these polysaccharide degrading enzymes are inducible.[16,17] Most of the physiologic effects of dietary fiber are mediated by SCFAs, which result from the bacterial enzymatic degradation of NSP.

Fecal Weight

The fermentation of dietary fiber components increases fecal weight. This effect is not due to water-holding properties characteristic of cellulosic polysaccharides, since colonic bacterial degradation of NCP is almost complete. Rather,

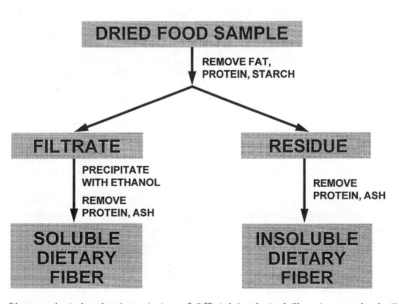

FIGURE 6–1 Dietary fiber analysis by the Association of Official Analytical Chemists method. (Data from Lee S et al: Determination of total, soluble, and insoluable dietary fiber in foods. Enzymetric-gravimetric method, MES-TRIS buffer: collaborative study. J Assoc Off Anal Chem 1992;75:395.)

TABLE 6–2 Fiber-Supplemented Liquid Formula Diets: Dietary Fiber Content and Analysis by AOAC Method

Product	Manufacturer	Fiber Source	TDF (g/L)[†]	IDF (g)[*]	SDF (g)[*]	Published Clinical Trial
Advera	Ross	Soy polysaccharide	8.4	[††]	[††]	No
Compleat	Sandoz	Fruits and vegetables	4.4	1.6	1.2	No
Compleat Modified	Sandoz	Fruits and vegetables	4.4	2	1.2	No
Ensure with Fiber	Ross	Soy polysaccharide	14.4	16	3.2	Yes[a]
Fiberlan	Elan	Soy polysaccharide	14	[††]	[††]	No
Fibersource	Sandoz	Soy polysaccharide	10	9.2	0.8	No
Fibersource HN	Sandoz	Soy polysaccharide	6.8	6.4	0.4	No
Glucema	Ross	Soy polysaccharide	13.6	14.4	2.4	Yes[b]
Glytrol	Clintec	Gum arabic, soy polysaccharide, and pectin	15	5[†]	10[†]	No
Impact with Fiber	Sandoz	Soy polysaccharide and guar	10	5	5	No
Isofiber	O'Brien	Soy polysaccharide	14	11.6	3.2	No
Isosource VHN	Sandoz	Soy polysaccharide and guar	10	4.8	5.2	No
Jevity	Ross	Soy polysaccharide	14.4	14.4	2.8	Yes[c]
Nutren 1.0 with Fiber	Clintec	Soy polysaccharide	14	[††]	[††]	No
PediaSure with Fiber	Ross	Soy polysaccharide	4.8	[††]	[††]	No
ProBalance	Clintec	Soy polysaccharide and gum arabic	10	7.5[†]	2.5[†]	No
Promote with Fiber	Ross	Soy polysaccharide and oat hull	13.6	[††]	[††]	No
Profiber	Sherwood	Soy polysaccharide	12	11.2	3.6	No
Protain XL	Sherwood	Soy polysaccharide	8	[††]	[††]	No
Replete with Fiber	Clintec	Soy polysaccharide	14	[††]	[††]	No
Sustacal with Fiber	Mead-Johnson	Soy polysaccharide, acacia, and microcrystalline cellulose	10	7[†]	3[†]	No
Ultracal	Mead-Johnson	Soy polysaccharide and oat	13.6	12.9[†]	0.7[†]	No
Vitaneed	Sherwood	Soy polysaccharide, fruits, and vegetables	8	6	4.8	No

AOAC = Association of Official Analytical chemists; TDF = total dietary fiber; IDF = insoluble dietary fiber; SDF = soluble dietary fiber.
*Unless otherwise indicated, data from Fredstrom SB et al: J Parenter Enter Nutr 1991;15(4):450.
†Manufacturer data, 1995.
††Information not available.
[a]Data from Dobb GJ et al: Int Care Med 1990;16(4):252; Frankenfield DC et al: Am J Clin Nutr 1989;50:533; Liebl BH et al: J Parenter Enter Nutr 1990;14(4):371; Shankardass K et al: J Parenter Enter Nutr 1990;14(5):508; Shinnick FL et al: Am J Clin Nutr 1989;49:471; Slavin JL et al: J Parenter Enter Nutr 1985;9(3):317; Thomas BL et al: Am J Clin Nutr 1988;48:1048; Peters AL et al: J Parenter Enter Nutr 1992;16(1):69.
[b]Data from Peters AL et al: J Parenter Enter Nutr 1992;16(1):69.
[c]Data from Guenter PA et al: J Parenter Enter Nutr 1991;15(3):277.

this rise in stool weight occurs from an increase of fecal bacterial mass.[18] As colonic bacteria anaerobically degrade NCP-rich fiber, they use the energy generated from this catabolism for maintenance and proliferation. Therefore, the bacterial cell population in the colon is enlarged. By raising fecal weight, dietary fiber reduces mean stool transit time by stimulating peristalsis.

Short-Chain Fatty Acids

SCFAs are fermentation end products of bacterial polysaccharidase degradation of dietary fiber in the colon. These SCFAs are either used as energy for bacterial maintenance and proliferation or absorbed by the colonic epithelium. In general, SCFAs are products of pyruvate metabolism that are essential for the metabolic welfare of colonocytes. The physiologic effects of SCFA include (1) enhanced sodium absorption, (2) increased colonocyte proliferation, (3) metabolic energy production, (4) enhanced colonic blood flow, (5) stimulation of the autonomic nervous system, and (6) increased GI hormone production. These effects all influence the maintenance of the colonic milieu. Acetate, propionate, and N-butyrate account for about 85 percent of all SCFAs produced in the human colon.[19,20] Of the SCFAs, butyrate is preferentially oxidized by normal colonocytes.[21,22]

SCFA and Sodium Absorption

Rapid absorption of SCFAs from the colonic lumen is principally a nonsaturable, transcellular process (Fig. 6–2). Protonated SCFAs cross into colonocytes apically by nonionic diffusion in a concentration-dependent manner.[23-25] For nonionized diffusion to occur, SCFA anions must be protonated. Protons are obtained at the apical colonocyte membrane by Na^+-H^+ exchange.[25] SCFA absorption is coupled to sodium absorption by this way of H^+ recycling. After entering the colonic mucosal cells, protonated SCFAs dissociate and release hydrogen ions. These hydrogen ions, in turn, are transported back into the colonic lumen in exchange for sodium. This overall process leads to increased sodium, and consequently water, absorption by colonocytes. Interestingly, in this case, SCFAs derived from the dietary fiber may have an antidiarrheal effect for potential use in EN.

SCFA and Colonocyte Proliferation

Dietary fiber is the substrate precursor of SCFAs that increases colonocyte proliferation. Studies with radiolabelled thymidine show increased colonic crypt cell turnover and migration in animals fed fiber-supplemented diets.[26] In rats given separate guar gum and pectin-supplemented diets, colonocyte proliferation increases more than in those fed cellulose or fiber-free diets. Low-fiber diets produce colonic atrophy characterized by mucosal hypoplasia and decreased colonocyte proliferation.[27] Dietary components such as cellulose may sustain the colonic mucosa, but the trophic effects in the colon are generally believed to be mediated by SCFAs.[28,29] Although the precise mechanism is unknown, SCFAs may exert their trophic effect by providing energy to colonocytes or by stimulating GI hormone release.[28,30,31]

Of the primary SCFAs, butyrate plays a major role in colonocyte proliferation and consequent colonic mucosal growth. SCFAs have a

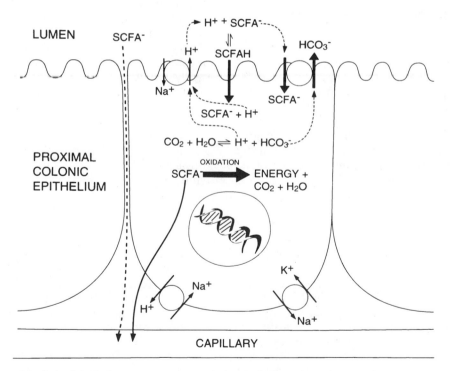

FIGURE 6–2 Simplified model of absorption and metabolism of short-chain fatty acids (SCFA) in the proximal colonic epithelium of composite animal species. SCFA⁻ is the dissociated form; SCFAH is the undissociated form. (Adapted with permission from Engelhardt WV: Absorption of short-chain fatty acids from the large intestine. In Cummings JH, Rombeau JL, Sakata T (eds): Physiological and Clinical Aspects of Short-Chain Fatty Acids. Cambridge: Cambridge University Press, 1995:149. Copyright 1995. Reprinted with the permission of Cambridge University Press.)

dose-dependent stimulatory effect on crypt cell proliferation in the following order of effectiveness: butyrate > propionate > acetate.[22,28] When less dietary fiber is delivered to the colonic lumen, butyrate production diminishes, resulting in mucosal atrophy.[32,33] Accordingly, butyrate infusions into the colonic lumen promote mucosal growth characterized by increased mucosal mass, DNA content, and mitotic indexes.[28,34] In rats, intraluminal perfusion of butyrate concentrations of 20 mM, 40 mM, and 150 mM into cecectomized colon increase segmental DNA by 100 percent, 100 percent, and 50 percent, respectively. Butyrate infusions of 20 mM stimulate colonic mucosal growth similar to physiologic concentrations of butyrate, proprionate, and acetate combined. However, butyrate concentrations 7.5 times the normal colonic concentration (20 mM) do not significantly increase colonocyte proliferation and mucosal growth.[35] The trophic effect of SCFAs, especially butyrate, on colonocyte proliferation is of interest because of the potential to enhance intestinal adaptation in postoperative surgical patients by fiber supplemented LFDs.

SCFA and Metabolic Energy Production

As the preferred metabolic fuels for the colonic mucosa, SCFAs provide approximately 70 percent of the energy supply to the colonic mucosa. Of the three principal SCFAs, butyrate is the preferred metabolic fuel of normal rat colonocytes.[21,22] When compared with other common fuels, butyrate is again the principal respiratory fuel for rat colonocytes with acetoacetate, L-glutamine, and D-glucose following in sequential order of importance.[22,36] Regional differences demonstrate that butyrate oxidation predominates in the distal colon whereas glucose and glutamine oxidation are more pronounced in the proximal colon. In humans, colonocyte preference for metabolic fuels is similar to that found in rats.[21,22]

Since SCFAs are not endogenously synthesized, the colonic mucosa can only obtain these metabolic fuels from bacterial fermentation. Thus, in states of SCFA deprivation such as decreased dietary fiber ingestion or colonic microflora reduction, diminished SCFA oxidation leading to reduced adenosine 5′ triphosphate (ATP) production may severely impair colonocyte function and mucosal breakdown. Indeed, such conditions of energy starvation may increase the risk of ulcerative colitis.[37]

SCFA and Colonic Blood Flow

The trophic effects of SCFAs on the colonic mucosa are probably mediated partially by enhanced mesenteric blood flow.[38,39] Intraluminal infusion of SCFA produces a 24 percent increase of colonic blood flow, which suggests SCFAs directly dilate the colonic vasculature. Of the main SCFAs, acetate produces the greatest increase of blood flow.[38] SCFAs individually and combined produce a significant concentration-dependent dilatation of resistant arteries in resected human colon.[40] This vasodilatory effect suggests SCFAs may improve colonic microcirculation in vivo, thereby having a trophic effect on colonic mucosa. These results may explain why modest doses of SCFA have trophic effects on intestinal mucosa even after parenteral administration.[40-42]

SCFA and the Autonomic Nervous System

Accumulating evidence suggests that the autonomic nervous system (ANS) has a role in mediating the enterotrophic effects of SCFAs. In rats, SCFAs rapidly perfused into the colon increase the mitotic and labeling indexes of colonocytes.[43] This trophic effect is abolished by preceding surgical vagotomy or chemical sympathectomy with guanethidine sulfate.[34,43-44] Furthermore, acute SCFA infusions significantly increase crypt cell production rate in both normally innervated and extrinsically denervated jejunal segments.[45] These results indicate SCFAs can stimulate jejunal enterocyte proliferation systemically without requiring efferent autonomic nerve connections.

Findings from studies of chronic infusions, however, differ from the aforementioned acute study. Administration of SCFAs for 10 days into normally innervated rat cecum out of continuity produce trophic changes in jejunum.[46] When extrinsic denervation of rat ceca is performed, the jejunotrophic effects of SCFA infused through the ceca are abolished. This chronic study suggests that afferent innervation is essential for the jejunotrophic effects of cecally infused SCFAs, whereas the previous acute study suggests transection of efferent innervation does not alter the trophic effects of SCFAs.

In a recent study to determine which component of the ANS (i.e., parasympathetic or sympathetic) is responsible for jejunotrophism, rats received cecal infusions of either SCFAs or saline for 10 days after surgical vagotomy, chemical sympathectomy, or sham operation.[47] In such rats, both parasympathetic and sympathetic systems mediate the trophic effects of cecal SCFA on jejunum. However, only disrupted parasympathetic connections fully block these effects on jejunal function such as glucose absorption.[47] When considered together, these findings suggest autonomic receptors play an important role in SCFA-induced regulation of enterocyte proliferation.

SCFA and GI Hormones

SCFAs may produce their enterotrophic effects by enhanced production of GI hormones. Gastrin, enteroglucagon, and peptide tyrosine tyrosine (PYY) are most often implicated in the mediation of intestinal proliferation and mucosal growth. Increased colonocyte proliferation stimulated by fermentable fiber, the substrate precursor for SCFA, is closely associated with increased plasma enteroglucagon levels throughout the GI tract and elevated PYY levels in the colon only. There is no significant correlation with levels of plasma gastrin.[48] In rats with normally innervated ceca, however, SCFA infusions have a systemic jejunotrophic effect associated with increased levels of jejunal tissue gastrin.[46] In denervated rat ceca, SCFAs do not elevate tissue gastrin levels or promote a jejunotrophic effect. Jejunal PYY levels do not increase significantly with innervated or denervated cecal infusions of SCFA.[44] Clearly, more studies are needed to clarify the relationship between SCFA and GI hormones.

DIETARY FIBER AND ENTERAL NUTRITION

There is significant physiologic rationale to support adding dietary fiber to LFD. Dietary fiber normalizes colonic function by increasing fecal weight and bowel frequency. Furthermore, as the precursor to SCFA, dietary fiber is essential in maintaining small bowel and colon mucosal structure and function. This overall effect of dietary fiber prevents bacteria from penetrating the small bowel and, more important, the colonic wall by preserving the mucosal barrier. Conversely, as a fuel for anaerobic bacteria, dietary fiber maintains the colon's normal microflora.

Several animal studies demonstrate that fiber-supplemented diets significantly improve intestinal structure and function when compared with fiber-free diets. Rats fed fiber-free diets or cellulose-supplemented diets have slowed villus maturation that is reversed by ingestion of pectin or regular chow.[49] Furthermore, adult rats fed cellulose or pectin have significant increases in villous height and

width when compared with rats fed fiber-free diets.[50] Additionally, chronic pectin supplementation significantly increases small bowel length and weight, jejunal and ileal villous height, crypt depth, and crypt cell proliferation rate when compared with cellulose or fiber-free supplementation.[51-53] Finally, both guar gum and pectin diets increase crypt cell migration rate when compared with oat bran or fiber-free diets. This effect depends on the water-solubility and viscosity of the fiber source.[54]

Potential Clinical Applications of Dietary Fiber in Liquid Formula Diets

Since 1983, the number of commercially available fiber-supplemented LFDs has grown (Table 6–2). Their efficacy, however, has been proved only in a few controlled clinical trials. Potential clinical applications for fiber-supplemented LFDs include (1) alleviating constipation in chronically institutionalized patients, (2) reducing diarrhea associated with enteral nutrition, (3) enhancing mucosal healing in inflammatory bowel disease (IBD), (4) maintaining the gut barrier in critically ill patients, and (5) enhancing intestinal adaptation in short-bowel syndrome (SBS).

Constipation

Constipation occurs most commonly in chronically hospitalized or institutionalized elderly patients. Current medical management for these individuals involves laxatives, which are often expensive and ineffective. Additionally, many of these patients receive fiber-free LFDs that decrease fecal bulk. The most important clinical application of fiber-supplemented LFDs is found in this patient population. When fiber-supplemented LFDs are given to healthy human subjects, stool weight and frequency are increased.[55,56] Cellulosic fibers, especially wheat bran, are more beneficial to patients with constipation than are noncellulosic fibers.[57,58] Furthermore, larger bran particles are considered more effective than smaller particles in treating constipation.[59,60]

Soy polysaccharide as a supplement to LFDs has also been studied for its effect on constipation. In healthy humans, chronically administered soy polysaccharide–supplemented LFDs decrease laxative use without increasing the daily number of defecations.[7] Although small particle size may limit its clinical effectiveness, soy polysaccharide–supplemented LFD may improve stool consistency and decrease laxative use in some constipated patients.

Diarrhea

Diarrhea occurs in 30 percent of critically ill patients receiving enteral feeding.[12] Because colonic function includes water and electrolyte absorption, which ultimately determines fecal composition, diarrhea associated with enteral feeding may result from alterations of the colonic milieu. The possible causes of diarrhea in such patients include fiber-free diets and broad-spectrum antibiotics.[61] In such conditions, decreased fiber intake leads to reduced production of SCFAs by decimated colonic bacteria, which may decrease sodium and water absorption to produce osmotic diarrhea. Interestingly, in healthy subjects with high fiber intakes, a sudden change to a fiber-free diet may cause diarrhea.[62,63]

In healthy humans, fiber-free LFDs significantly increase liquid stool output compared with regular diets. Fiber-free LFDs decrease sodium and SCFA concentrations and increase the osmotic gap in colonic fluid. Pectin-supplemented LFDs, however, decrease the number of liquid stools and promote SCFA production compared with fiber-free LFDs.[63] Pectin-supplemented LFDs may increase the production of SCFAs, which enhance sodium absorption by colonocytes. This physiologic effect may then increase water absorption and thereby reduce the fluidity of the colonic lumen and prevent liquid stool formation.

Fiber supplementation may be beneficial in selected conditions following the use of antimicrobial agents that disrupt the normal fecal flora. Antibiotics depress bacterial fermentation of carbohydrate, possibly producing antibiotic-related diarrhea and overgrowth of *Clostridium difficile*.[64,65] Of the 30 percent of critically ill patients who develop diarrhea while receiving enteral feedings, approximately one half are *C. difficile* toxin positive.[12] Adding soy fiber to a liquid diet delays disease onset and prolongs survival in *C. difficile*–induced ileocecitis in hamsters. Increased colonic water absorption decreases diarrhea, and the faster intestinal transit time leads to less exposure to the toxin.[66] Randomized controlled human trials are needed to evaluate the effects of fiber supplementation in *C. difficile* diarrhea incidence and treatment in hospitalized patients.

Inflammatory Bowel Disease

Despite the common practice of bowel rest adjunctive treatment for patients with acute inflammatory bowel disease (IBD), there is little evidence to support its efficacy. Conversely, recent studies suggest that patients with IBD may actually benefit from LFDs similarly to total parenteral nutrition (TPN).[67] The pathogenesis of IBD, particularly ulcerative colitis, has been linked with impaired production of SCFAs.[37,68,69] The potential clinical use of fiber-supplemented LFDs is based on the premise that colonocyte energy deficiency may contribute to the pathogenesis of IBD and that SCFAs generated from such fiber diets may ameliorate this condition and promote mucosal healing.

In rats with chemically induced transmural colitis, pectin-supplemented LFDs reduce the degree of colonic inflammation, independent of nutritional status.[70] Additionally, in a model of mucosal ulcerative colitis, guinea pigs receiving pectin-supplemented diets showed significant increases in mucosal DNA, RNA, protein and weight, and positive nitrogen balance compared with guinea pigs receiving fiber-free diets.[71] These studies suggest that fiber may provide SCFAs for the colonic mucosa, which may improve mucosal healing in IBD patients.

Gut Barrier

Disruption of the gut barrier followed by translocation of bacteria and their endotoxins into the portal and lymphatic systems may encourage development of systemic inflammatory response syndrome (SIRS) in critically ill patients. Several studies suggest that compromised gut barrier function leading to bacterial translocation and other detrimental sequelae is possibly due to lack of enteral feeding.[72,73] Since most critically ill patients are unable to eat voluntarily, TPN is frequently given. TPN, however, does not directly stimulate the intestinal lumen and deprives the gut of essential nutrients. Consequently, such conditions promote mucosal atrophy and impair gut barrier function. If fiber-supplemented LFDs are provided to prevent the mucosal atrophy associated with fiber-free LFDs and TPN, the gut barrier may be preserved.

In rats, bacterial translocation increases with LFDs compared with regular chow diets.[74-76] With cellulose-supplemented LFDs, however, bacterial translocation decreases. In burned mice, soy polysaccharide–supplemented LFDs reduce bacterial translocation compared with LFDs alone.[77] Although these animal studies suggest that fiber-supplemented LFDs may preserve gut barrier function, studies in hospitalized patients are needed to determine the clinical significance of these findings.

Short-Bowel Syndrome

Short-bowel syndrome (SBS) is characterized by decreased mucosal surface area that results in malabsorption, diarrhea, nitrogen depletion, and weight loss. After significant small bowel resection, the remaining intestine lengthens and dilates to compensate for this loss of absorptive area. The delivery of enteral nutrients, therefore, may play an important role in short-bowel adaptation. Fiber-supplemented LFDs may enhance small bowel and colonic adaptation. In rat models of massive small bowel resection, pectin-supplemented elemental diets promote small bowel and colonic adaptation (measured by mucosal weight, DNA, RNA, and protein content) more significantly than elemental diets alone.[78,79]

Fiber-supplemented LFDs may also affect other mechanisms of intestinal adaptation. Rats with SBS do not have impaired fat absorption when pectin is added to defined formula diets.[80] Furthermore, pectin-supplemented LFDs increase water absorption in rats with SBS, thereby decreasing diarrhea.[79,81] Finally, sucrase, maltase, and lactase activities are significantly greater in resected rats fed pectin-supplemented elemental diets compared with resected rats fed elemental diets alone. These studies strongly suggest that fiber-supplemented LFDs improve intestinal surface area and functional capacity.

Clinical Trials with Fiber-Supplemented Liquid Formula Diets

Published randomized controlled clinical trials with fiber-supplemented LFDs are listed in Table 6–3. Eighteen published reports include eight performed in healthy subjects. Although these latter studies undoubtedly provide important physiologic and metabolic information, their relevance to hospitalized patients is unknown. This section, therefore, focuses only on clinical trials conducted on hospitalized patients. These trials are arbitrarily listed in one of the following categories: chronic central nervous system (CNS) disorders, critical illness, and clinically stable patients.

Chronic CNS Disorders

The severe and chronic constipation that often exists in patients with significant neurologic impairment may be ameliorated by increased fiber intake. Because of swallowing deficits, these patients are often prescribed varied diets ranging from liquid formula to pureed or blended foods, which all have limited fiber content. Other factors prolonging constipation include muscle paralysis, lack of ambulation, and narcotics.

In a short-term clinical trial, the effects of soy polysaccharide–supplemented LFDs were studied in 28 nonambulatory and mentally retarded youths with chronic constipation.[82] The subjects received fiber-free LFDs for 4 weeks followed by soy fiber–supplemented LFDs for 2 weeks. In this short time, the addition of soy fiber to an LFD did not significantly change wet stool weight, stool frequency, or transit time. Subsequently, the effects of long-term (1 year) soy polysaccharide on bowel function were investigated in 11 nonambulatory, mentally retarded youths (aged 7 to 17).[6] These severely constipated patients were fed a fiber-free LFD and a soy polysaccharide–supplemented LFD by gastrostomy. The addition of soy fiber to the LFD significantly increased wet stool weight and mean daily stool frequency. With the fiber-free LFD, wet stool weight was measured at 30 ± 13 g/day. This weight increased significantly to 87 ± 45 g/day after soy fiber administration. Furthermore, mean daily stool frequencies increased from 0.6 ± 0.2 to 1.1 ± 0.5 after soy fiber supplementation. This clinical trial concluded that soy polysaccharide dosages of 18 to 25 g/day significantly improved bowel function in these nonambulatory and mentally disabled patients.

The effects of fiber-supplemented enteral formulas were studied in 28 patients with neurologically based swallowing dysfunction.[7] In this randomized crossover trial, patients received fiber-free and soy polysaccharide–supplemented enteral formulas in two consecutive 6-week periods. The mean amount of fiber ingested was 22 g/day. Although fiber-supplemented enteral formulas significantly decreased laxative use, wet stool weight and stool frequency were not significantly different between the study groups.

Although only soy polysaccharide has been studied in this population, these clinical trials show that fiber-supplemented LFDs may be efficacious in certain patients with constipation. Furthermore, these studies demonstrate that longer periods of administration may be required to show the effects of fiber-supplemented LFDs on bowel function.

Critical Illness

Critically ill patients requiring intensive care have a greater incidence of diarrhea (30

TABLE 6–3   Controlled Clinical Trials Fiber-Supplemented Liquid Formula Diets

Year, Investigator	Patient Group	Number of Subjects	Diet Groups	Duration of Diet (days)	Conclusions
1985, Fischer[82]	Mentally retarded youths	28	Fiber free + 20–22 g SP	14 14	↑ Stool weight; softer stool; no change in transit time.
1985, Matzkies[83]	Controls	8	Fiber free + 30 g SP	7 14	SP ↑ stool weight, ↓ transit time; no change in urinary K, Na, Mg, Ca.
1985, Patil[84]	Malnourished, GI-diseased patients	5	Fiber free + 12 g carrot fiber	5 5	No difference in stool weight, breath hydrogen, glucose tolerance, diarrhea, stool frequency, or amino acid profile.
1985, Slavin[9]	Controls	16	Fiber free + 30 g SP + 60 g SP	10 10 10	+ 60 g SP ↑ defecation frequency, ↑ stool wet weight to normal and produced softer stool.
1988, Hart[85]	ICU	68	+ 7 g ispaghula Placebo cereal	4–18 4–18	No difference in incidence of diarrhea.
1988, Heymsfield[86]	Malnourished patients	8	Fiber free + 12 g SP + 39 g SP	7–14 7–14 7–14	SP ↑ fecal wet and dry weights, nitrogen, fat, water and minerals; need increased mineral intake with SP.
1988, Taper[87]	Students	16	Fiber free + 20 g SP + 30 g SP + 40 g SP	11 11 11 11	SP ↑ Cu, Fe intake; slight negative Fe, Cu balance with + 40 g SP through normal serum levels.
1989, Frankenfield[5]	Head injury	9	Fiber free + 21 g SP	4–6 4–6	No change in fecal weight, consistency or nitrogen. All improved over time.
1989, Zimmaro[63]	Controls	14	Fiber free Self-selected + 14.5 g pectin	8 8 7	Pectin ↓ liquids stools to normal; fiber free ↑ colonic pH and ↓ SCFA levels; pectin normalized pH and SCFA.
1990, Dobb[4]	ICU	91	Fiber free + 14 g SP	3–18 3–18	No difference in diarrhea or constipation.
1990, Guenter[12]	Hospitalized, malnourished patients	100	Fiber free + 14 g SP/L	mean of 15.8	30% incidence of patients with diarrhea; no difference in *C. difficile* (+) or antidiarrheal treatments.
1990, Liebl[6]	Mentally retarded, non-ambulatory males	11	#1 fiber free #2 + 12–20 g SP #3 + 18–25 g SP	60 240 60	Stool frequency ↑ with #3 vs #1; stool water and wet weight ↑ with #2 vs #1; stool wet weight ↑ with #3 vs #2 and #1; stool dry weight ↑ with #3 vs #1; no difference in suppository use.
1990, Shankardass[7]	Neurologic dysfunction	28	Fiber free + 12 g SP	28 28	No change in stool frequency or weight; transit time ↑ with + 12 g SP; laxative use ↑ and diarrhea ↓ with + 12 g SP.
1992, Lampe[88]	Controls	11	Self-selected Fiber free + 15 g GG + 15 g SP	5 18 18 18	GG and fiber free ↑ transit time; all LFDs ↓ fecal weight, nitrogen, and stool frequency and ↑ pH vs self-selected diet.
1993, Kapadia[89]	Controls	6	Fiber free Self-selected + 40 g SP	7 7 7	LFD ↑ transit time, ↓ stool wet weight and bowel frequency; + 40 g SP normalized transit time, stool wet weight, and bowel frequency.
1993, Meier[90]	Controls	12	Fiber free Self-selected + 20 g GG	7 7 7	GG ↑ colonic transit time; no effects on stool frequency.
1994, Homann[91]	Stable med-surg patients	30	Fiber free + 20 g GG	≥5 ≥5	GG ↑ breath hydrogen; ↓ diarrhea; ↑ flatulence.
1995, Kapadia[92]	Controls	11	Fiber free Self-selected + 15 g total dietary fiber as SO, SP, or oat fiber	4–7 4–7 4–7	No difference in transit time, stool weight, or frequency; SO and SP ↑ stool SCFA, SO > SP.

SP = soy polysaccharide; SCFA = short-chain fatty acids; LFD = liquid formula diet; GG = guar gum; SO = soy oligosaccharide; ↑ = increase; ↓ = decrease.

percent) than the general hospital population.[12] The use of fiber-supplemented LFDs to control or prevent diarrhea in these patients has been studied in several controlled clinical trials.

The effects of soy polysaccharide–supplemented LFDs were examined in 100 critically ill patients who received tube feedings for an average of 15.8 days.[12] There were no significant differences between the days with diarrhea and the presence of *C. difficile* diarrhea between the fiber-supplemented and fiber-free groups. The incidence of diarrhea, however, was strongly associated with antibiotic usage. In another clinical trial, 68 critically ill patients were randomly given LFDs with or without ispaghula husk (7 g/day).[85] The duration of enteral feeding ranged from 3 to 18 days. There were no significant differences between the groups. Again, however, a strong correlation between diarrhea and antibiotic administration was found.

In a comparison of soy polysaccharide–supplemented and fiber-free LFDs in nine patients with acute brain injury, no significant differences in bowel function were seen. The incidence of diarrhea did not differ significantly between groups. Patients received either fiber-supplemented or fiber-free diets in 4- to 6-day periods.[5] Finally, the effects of fiber-supplemented LFDs were compared with fiber-free LFDs in 30 burn patients for 16 days.[93] Although stool weight and frequency did not differ significantly between groups, burn patients receiving fiber-supplemented formulas ingested more calories without developing diarrhea compared with patients receiving fiber-free formulas.

These studies suggest that fiber-supplemented LFDs have a limited therapeutic role in managing diarrhea in critically ill patients. Antibiotic administration and the effects of stress on the gut complicate the enteral feeding of these patients and may decrease the effectiveness of fiber-supplemented LFDs for diarrhea.

Clinically Stable Patients

The effects of fiber-supplemented LFDs in malnourished hospitalized patients with heterogeneous diagnoses were studied in three controlled trials. In the first study, five patients with abdominal pain or decreased frequency of bowel action received either fiber-free polymeric diets or carrot fiber–supplemented polymeric diets by nasogastric infusion for two 15-day periods.[84] There were no significant differences in GI symptoms, glucose intolerance, or

plasma amino acid profile between the two enteral groups. In the second trial, the effects of soy polysaccharide–supplemented liquid formulas were investigated in eight malnourished patients with various diagnoses.[86] After 1 to 2 weeks of enteral feeding, there were no significant differences in clinical outcome or stool measurement between fiber-free and fiber-supplemented groups. In the third study, the effects of guar gum–supplemented LFDs were studied in 100 clinically stable hospitalized patients.[91] In this randomized, double-blind trial, patients fed fiber-supplemented LFDs were less likely to develop diarrhea than patients fed LFDs alone (12 percent vs 30 percent). However, the fiber-supplemented group had more flatulence than did the fiber-free group (22 percent vs 8 percent).

Problems in Interpreting Data from Clinical Trials

There are several problems in data interpretation as shown by the aforementioned clinical trials. Because most of the published studies are short term (7–10 days), the full physiologic effects of fiber may not become apparent during this brief investigative period. Additionally, most of these published trials have been conducted in small groups of patients. These studies, with limited numbers of patients, use crossover study designs that limit data interpretation because of possible cumulative effects of sequential feeding periods. Another problem relates to the methodology of fiber measurement. Since various fibers affect the GI tract differently, appropriate methods to differentiate the specific physicochemical characteristics and composition of these fibers are needed to interpret more clearly the results of clinical trials. Finally, because of its commercial availability, most studies have been performed with soy polysaccharide. As more studies are conducted with different fiber sources, additional clinical benefits may be discovered.

Complications and Their Prevention

Feeding tube patency is of practical concern with fiber-supplemented LFDs. Fiber formulas should be infused with feeding tubes greater than 10 F internal diameter. Smaller tubes preclude use of fiber-supplemented LFDs. Most patients requiring fiber-supplemented LFDs are fed with the aid of a feeding pump; however, these diets can also be delivered with reasonable success by intragastric bolus drip feeding. If fiber supplements are delivered by feeding catheter separately from LFDs (as with medications), the tube is flushed with 60 ml of water after each dose. Flushing the tube with 120 to 240 ml of water three times daily is also recommended when additional fluid intake is indicated. This approach may prevent formula, medications, and fiber from adhering to the walls of the feeding tube, thereby avoiding occlusion.

Additional complications of fiber-supplemented LFDs are bezoar formation, fecal impaction, bloating, and flatulence. Although bezoar formation is extremely rare with fiber-supplemented diets, careful monitoring for stool output (particularly in patients with significant sedation or neurologic impairment), gradual increase in fiber dose, and adequate fluid intake should reduce the likelihood of this problem. Fecal impaction is easily prevented by ensuring adequate fluid intake and avoiding excessive fiber doses. Daily abdominal examination and monitoring for stool production are advised for all enterally fed patients. Although some patients experience bloating and flatulence with fiber-supplemented LFDs, reduced fiber doses should be tried before administering fiber-free LFDs. Significant abdominal distention is a contraindication to fiber-supplemented LFD. Ileus, obstruction, impaction, or other serious GI problems should be treated before reinstituting feeding. In summary, if a standardized feeding and monitoring protocol is followed, fiber-supplemented LFDs can be administered to hospitalized patients with very few complications.

CLINICAL RECOMMENDATIONS

Fiber-supplemented LFDs are indicated in patients with chronic constipation or diarrhea or diverticular disease. For patients with constipation, soy polysaccharide as a supplement to LFDs at an intake level of 25 to 30 g/day is generally well tolerated. If constipation is severe, 60 ml of prune juice administered daily through the feeding tube provides vegetable fiber that may be efficacious. Unless a patient's clinical status demands fluid restriction, 35 to 45 ml free water/kg body weight is provided with fiber-supplemented diets, and daily stool production is carefully monitored. If required, additional water can be easily flushed through the feeding tube. However, soy polysaccharide intake greater than 35 g/day should be avoided, since such amounts may decrease mineral absorption and cause GI complaints.

Patients with diarrhea may benefit from pectin 5 g given three times daily through the feeding tube or from soy polysaccharide–supplemented LFD at total doses of 25 to 30 g/day. In patients with *C. difficile*–associated diarrhea, soy polysaccharide–supplemented LFDs are well tolerated and ameliorate diarrhea. Patients with uncomplicated diverticular disease should receive cellulosic fiber-supplemented LFD to decrease intraluminal colonic pressure. Although soy polysaccharide–supplemented LFDs are well tolerated, fiber supplementation during acute phases of bowel inflammation is not advised.

CONCLUSION

Fiber-supplemented diets are commercially available and in widespread clinical use. Surprisingly, very little data justify their use in hospitalized patients. Most studies have been conducted in healthy subjects for short periods. The use of fiber-supplemented enteral feedings in long-term patients may be substantiated in future trials. There is sufficient physiologic rationale to justify adding dietary fiber to LFDs in selected patients. The routine addition of fiber (soy polysaccharide, 15–25 g/day) to LFDs is recommended for nonambulatory patients predisposed to severe constipation and in need of long-term enteral nutrition and for those with quiescent IBD. A trial of fiber-supplemented diets is also recommended for malnourished patients with diarrhea.

REFERENCES

1. Burkitt DP: Epidemiology of cancer of the colon and rectum. Cancer 1971;28(1):3.
2. Palacio JC, Rolandelli RH, Settle RG et al: Dietary fiber's physiologic effects and potential applications to enteral nutrition. In Rombeau JL, Caldwell M (eds): Clinical Nutrition: Enteral and Tube Feeding, 2nd edition, vol 2. Philadelphia: WB Saunders, 1990:556.
3. Lee S, Prosky L, DeVries J: Determination of total, soluble, and insoluble dietary fiber in foods. Enzymetric-gravimetric method, MES-TRIS buffer: collaborative study. J Assoc Off Anal Chem 1992;75:395.
4. Dobb GJ, Towler SC: Diarrhoea during enteral feeding in the critically ill: a comparison of feeds with and without fibre. Int Care Med 1990;16(4):252.
5. Frankenfield DC, Beyer PL: Soy-polysaccharide fiber: effect on diarrhea in tube-fed, head-injured patients. Am J Clin Nutr 1989;50:533.
6. Liebl BH, Fischer MH, Van Calcar SC et al: Dietary fiber and long-term large bowel responses in enterally nourished nonambulatory profoundly retarded youth. J Parenter Enter Nutr 1990;14(4):371.
7. Shankardass K, Chuchmach S, Chelswick K et al: Bowel function of long-term tube-fed patients consuming formulae with and without dietary fiber. J Parenter Enter Nutr 1990;14(5):508.

8. Shinnick FL, Hess RL, Fischer MH et al: Apparent nutrient absorption and upper gastrointestinal transit with fiber-containing enteral feedings. Am J Clin Nutr 1989;49:471.

9. Slavin JL, Nelson NL, McNamara EA et al: Bowel function of healthy men consuming liquid diets with and without dietary fiber. J Parenter Enter Nutr 1985; 9(3):317.

10. Thomas BL, Laine DC, Goetz FC: Glucose and insulin response in diabetic subjects: acute effect of carbohydrate level and the addition of soy polysaccharide in defined-formula diets. Am J Clin Nutr 1988;48:1048.

11. Peters AL, Davidson MB: Effects of various enteral feeding products on postprandial blood glucose response in patients with type I diabetes. J Parenter Enter Nutr 1992;16(1):69.

12. Guenter PA, Settle G, Perlmutter S et al: Tube feeding-related diarrhea in acutely ill patients. J Parenter Enter Nutr 1991;15(3):277.

13. Sandberg A-S, Hasselblad C, Hasselblad K: The effect of wheat bran on the absorption of minerals in the small intestine. Br J Nutr 1982;48(2):185.

14. Holloway WD, Tasman-Jones C, Maher K: Pectin digestion in humans. Am J Clin Nutr 1983;37:253.

15. Cummings JH, Englyst HN: Fermentation in the human large intestine and the available substrates. Am J Clin Nutr 1987;45(5S):1243.

16. Salyers AA, Leedle JAZ: Carbohydrate metabolism in the human colon. In Hentges DJ (ed): Human Intestinal Microflora in Health and Disease. New York: Academic Press, 1983:129.

17. Salyers AA, Palmer JK, Wilkins TD: Degradation of polysaccharides by intestinal bacterial enzymes. Am J Clin Nutr 1978;31(suppl 10):5128.

18. Stephan AM, Cummings JH: The microbial contribution to human fecal mass. J Med Microbiol 1980; 13(1):45.

19. Cummings JH: Colonic absorption: the importance of short-chain fatty acids in man. Scand J Gastroenterol 1984;19(S93):89.

20. Cummings JH, Branch WJ: Fermentation and the production of short chain fatty acids in the large intestine. In Vahouny GV, Kritchevsky D (eds): Basic and Medical Aspects of Dietary Fiber, 1st edition. New York: Plenum Press, 1986:131.

21. Roediger WEW: Role of anaerobic bacteria in the metabolic welfare of the colonic mucosa in man. Gut 1980;21(9):793.

22. Roediger WEW: Utilization of nutrients by isolated epithelial cells of the rat colon. Gastroenterology 1982;83(2):424.

23. Ruppin H, Bar-Meir S, Sorgel KH: Absorption of short-chain fatty acids by the colon. Gastroenterology 1980; 78:1500.

24. Rechkemmer G, Engelhardt WV: Concentration and pH-dependence of short-chain fatty acid absorption in the proximal and distal colon of guinea pig (cavia porcellus). Comp Biochem Phys 1988;91A:659.

25. Engelhardt WV: Absorption of short-chain fatty acids from the large intestine. In Cummings JH, Rombeau JL, Sakata T (eds): Physiological and Clinical Aspects of Short-Chain Fatty Acids. Cambridge: Cambridge University Press, 1995:149.

26. Vahouny GV, Cassidy MM: Dietary fiber and intestinal adaptation. In Vahouny GV, Kritchevsky D (eds): Basic and Medical Aspects of Dietary Fiber, 1st edition. New York: Plenum Press, 1986:181.

27. Bristol JB, Williamson CN: Large bowel growth. Scand J Gastroenterol 1984;19(S93):25.

28. Sakata T: Stimulatory effect of short chain fatty acids on epithelial cell proliferation in the rat intestine: a possible explanation for trophic effects of fermentable fibre, gut microbes and luminal trophic factors. Br J Nutr 1987;58(1):95.

29. Cameron IL, Ord VA, Hunter KE et al: Quantitative contribution factors regulating rat colonic crypt epithelium: role of parenteral and enteral feeding, caloric intake, dietary cellulose level and the colon carcinogen DMH. Cell Tissue Kinet 1990;23(3):227.

30. Clarke RM: "Luminal nutrition" versus "functional work-load" as controllers of mucosal morphology and epithelial replacement in the rat small intestine. Digestion 1974;15:411.

31. Chinery R, Goodlad RA, Wright NA: Soy polysaccharide in an enteral diet: effects on rat intestinal cell proliferation, morphology and metabolic function. Clin Nutr 1992;11:277.

32. Goodlad RA, Wright NA: Effects of addition of kaolin or cellulose to an elemental diet on intestinal cell proliferation in the rat. Br J Nutr 1983;50(1):91.

33. Sakata T: Depression of intestinal epithelial cell production rate by hindgut bypass in rats. Scand J Gastroenterol 1988;23(10):1200.

34. Sakata T, Yajima T: Influence of short chain fatty acids on the epithelial cell division of the digestive tract. Quant J Exp Physiol 1984;69(3):639.

35. Kripke SA, Fox AD, Berman JM et al: Stimulation of intestinal mucosal growth with intracolonic infusion of short chain fatty acids. J Parenter Enter Nutr 1989; 13(2):109.

36. Ardawi MSM, Newsholme EA: Fuel utilization on colonocytes of the rat. Biochem J 1985;231(3):713.

37. Roediger WEW: The starved colon-diminished mucosal nutrition, diminished absorption, and colitis. Dis Colon Rectum 1990;33(10):8582.

38. Kvietys PR, Granger DN: Effect of volatile fatty acids on blood flow and oxygen uptake by the dog colon. Gastroenterol 1981;80(5Pt1):962.

39. Demigné C, Remesy C: Stimulation of absorption of volatile fatty acids and minerals in the cecum of rats adapted to a very high fiber diet. J Nutr 1985;115(1):53.

40. Mortensen FV, Nielsen H, Mulvany MJ et al: Short-chain fatty acids dilate isolated human colonic resistance arteries. Gut 1990;31(12):1391.

41. Koruda MJ, Rolandelli RH, Zimmaro-Bliss D et al: Parenteral nutrition supplemented with short-chain fatty acids: effect on the small bowel mucosa in normal rats. Am J Clin Nutr 1990;51:685.

42. Karlstad MD, Killeffer JA, Bailey JW et al: Parenteral nutrition with short and long-chain triglycerides: triacetin reduces atrophy of small and large bowel mucosa and improves protein metabolism in burned rats. Am J Clin Nutr 1992;55:1005.

43. Sakata T, Engelhardt WV: Stimulatory effect of short-chain fatty acids on the epithelial cell proliferation in the rat large intestine. Comp Biochem Physiol 1983; 74A(2):459.

44. Reilly KJ, Frankel WL, Bain A et al: The autonomic nervous system mediates both structural and functional effects of cecal short-chain fatty acids (SCFA) in rat jejunum. J Parenter Enter Nutr. In press.

45. Sakata T: Stimulatory effect of short-chain fatty acids on the epithelial cell proliferation of isolated and denervated jejunal segment of the rat. Scand J Gastroenterol 1989;24(7):886.

46. Frankel WL, Zhang W, Singh A et al: Stimulation of the autonomic nervous system mediates short-chain fatty acid induced jejunotrophism. Surg Forum 1992;43:24.

47. Reilly K, Frankel W, Klurfeld D et al: The parasympathetic (PSNS) and sympathetic (SNS) nervous systems mediate the systemic effects of short-chain fatty acids (SCFA) on jejunal structure and function. Surg Forum 1993;44:20.

48. Goodlad RA, Lerton W, Ghatei MA et al: Effects of an elemental diet, inert bulk, and different types of dietary fiber on the response of the intestinal epithelium to refeeding in the rat and relationship to plasma gastrin, enteroglucagon, and PYY concentrations. Gut 1987;28:171.

49. Tasman-Jones C, Owen RL, Jones AL: Semipurified dietary fiber and small bowel morphology in rats. Dig Dis Sci 1982;27(6):519.

50. Cassidy HH, Lightfoot FG, Grau LE et al: Effect of chronic intake of dietary fibers on the ultrastructural topography of rat jejunum and colon: a scanning electron microscopy study. Am J Clin Nutr 1981;37:954.

51. Brown RC, Kelleher J, Losowsky MS: The effect of pectin on the structure and function of the rat small intestine. Br J Nutr 1979;42(3):357.

52. Johnson IT, Mahoney RR: Effect of dietary supplements of guar gum and cellulose on intestinal cell proliferation, enzyme levels, and sugar transport in the rat. Br J Nutr 1984;52:477.

53. Chun W, Bamba T, Hosoda S: Effect of pectin, a soluble dietary fiber, on functional and morphological parameters of the small intestine in rats. Digestion 1989; 42:22.

54. Jacobs LR: Effects of dietary fiber on mucosal growth and cell proliferation in the small intestine of the rat: a comparison of oat bran, pectin, and guar with total fiber deprivation. Am J Clin Nutr 1983;37:954.

55. Hill C, Greco RS, Brooks DL: Alleviation of constipation in the elderly by dietary fiber supplementation. J Am Geriatr Soc 1980;28(9):410.

56. Bowen PE: The role of fiber in liquid formula diets. In The Clinical Role of Fiber. Montreal: Ross Laboratories, 1985:53.

57. Cummings JH, Southgate DA, Branch WJ et al: The digestion of pectin in the human gut and its effect on calcium absorption and large bowel function. Brit J Nutr 1979;41:477.

58. Jenkins DJA, Peterson D, Thorne MJ et al: Wheat fiber and laxation: dose response and equilibration time. Am J Gastroenterol 1987;82(12):1259.

59. Brodribb AJM, Groves C: Effect of bran particle size on stool weight. Gut 1978;19:60.

60. Heller SN, Hackler LR, Rivers JM: Dietary fiber: the effect of particle size of wheat bran on colonic function in young adult men. Am J Clin Nutr 1980;33:1734.

61. Dickerson RN, Melnik G: Osmolality of oral drug solutions and suspensions. Am J Hosp Pharm 1988;45:832.

62. Peaston MJT: External metabolic balance studies during nasogastric feeding in serious illness requiring intensive care. Br J Med 1966;2(256):1367.

63. Zimmaro DM, Rolandelli RH, Koruda MJ: Isotonic tube feeding formula induces liquid stool in normal subjects: reversal by pectin. J Parenter Enter Nutr 1989; 13(2):117.

64. Rao SSC, Holdsworth CD, Read NW: Symptoms and stool patterns in patients with ulcerative colitis. Gut 1988;29:342.

65. Bjorneklett A, Midtvedt T: Influence of three antimicrobial agents—penicillin, metronidazole, and doxycyclin—on the intestinal microflora of healthy humans. Scand J Gastroenterol 1981;16:473.

66. Frankel WL, Choi DM, Zhang W et al: Soy fiber delays disease onset and prolongs survival in experimental *Clostridium difficile* ileocecitis. J Parenter Enter Nutr 1994;18(1):55.

67. Alun Jones V: Comparison of total parenteral nutrition and elemental diet in induction of remission of Crohn's disease. Long-term maintenance of remission by personalized food exclusion diets. Dig Dis Sci 1987;32S:117.

68. Roediger WEW: What sequence of pathogenic events leads to acute ulcerative colitis? Dis Colon Rectum 1988;31:482.

69. Roediger WEW: The place of short-chain fatty acids in colonocyte metabolism in health and ulcerative colitis: the impaired colonocyte barrier. In Cummings JH, Rombeau JL, Sakata T (eds): Physiologic and Clinical Aspects of Short-chain Fatty Acids. Cambridge: Cambridge University Press, 1995:337.

70. Rolandelli RH, Saul SH, Settle RG et al: Comparison of parenteral nutrition and enteral feeding with pectin in experimental colitis in the rat. Am J Clin Nutr 1988; 47(4):715.

71. Palacio JC, Barbera CF, DePaula JA: Fermentable fiber stimulates colonic mucosal cell proliferation in an experimental model of mucosal ulcerative colitis. Surg Forum 1989;XL:13.

72. Border JR, Hassett J, LaDuca J: The gut origin septic states in blunt multiple trauma (ISS + 40) in the ICU. Ann Surg 1987;206(4):427.

73. Alexander JW: Nutrition and translocation. J Parenter Enter Nutr 1990;14(5):170S.

74. Alverdy JC, Aoys E, Moss GS: Effect of commercially available chemically defined liquid diets on the intestinal microflora and bacterial translocation from the gut. J Parenter Enter Nutr 1990;14(1):1.

75. Barber AE, Jones WG, Minei JP et al: Glutamine or fiber supplementation of a defined formula diet: impact on bacterial translocation, tissue composition, and response to endotoxin. J Parenter Enter Nutr 1990;14(4): 335.

76. Spaeth G, Berg RD, Specian RD: Food without fiber promotes bacterial translocation from the gut. Surgery 1990;108(2):240.

77. Zapata-Sirvent RL, Hansbrough JF, Ohara MM et al: Bacterial translocation in burned mice after administration of various diets including fiber- and glutamine-enriched enteral formulas. Crit Care Med 1994;22(4): 690.

78. Koruda MJ, Rolandelli RH, Settle RG: The effect of a pectin-supplemented elemental diet on intestinal adaptation to massive small bowel resection. J Parenter Enter Nutr 1986;10(4):343.

79. Roth J, Frankel WL, Zhang W et al: Pectin improves colonic function in rat short bowel syndrome. J Surg Res 1995;58:240.

80. Toki A, Todani T, Watanabe Y et al: Effects of pectin and cellulose on fat absorption after massive small bowel resection in weaning rats. J Parenter Enter Nutr 1992;16(3):255.

81. Zhang W, Roth L, Sasaki K et al: Calcium-chelated pectate polymer improves pectin-induced gut trophism and function in short bowel syndrome. J Parenter Enter Nutr 1995;19(1):18S.

82. Fischer M, Adkins W, Hall L et al: Effects of dietary fiber in a liquid diet on bowel function of mentally retarded individuals. J Ment Def Res 1985;29(4):373.

83. Matzkies F, Webs B: Wirkung einer neuen sondennahrung auf den stoffwechsel, die urinelektrolyte und den gastrointestinaltrakt beim gesunden Erwachsenen mit und ohne zulage eines ballastoffes aus sojakleie. Z Ernahrungswissenschaft 1985;24:105.

84. Patil DH, Grimble GK, Keohane P et al: Do fibre containing enteral diets have advantages over existing low residue diets? Clin Nutr 1985;4:67.

85. Hart GK, Dobb GJ: Effect of fecal bulking agent on diarrhea during enteral feeding in the critically ill. J Parenter Enter Nutr 1988;12(5):465.

86. Heymsfield SB, Roongspisuthipong C, Evert M: Fiber supplementation of enteral formulas: effects on the bioavailability of major nutrients and gastrointestinal tolerance. J Parenter Enter Nutr 1988;12(3):265.

87. Taper LJ, Milam RS, McCallister MS et al: Mineral retention in young men consuming soy-fiber-augmented liquid-formula diets. Am J Clin Nutr 1988;48:305.

88. Lampe JW, Effertz ME, Larson JL et al: Gastrointestinal effects of modified guar gum and soy polysaccharide as part of an enteral formula diet. J Parenter Enter Nutr 1992;16(6):538.

89. Kapadia SA, Raimundo AH, Silk DBA: The effect of a fibre free and fibre supplemented polymeric enteral diet on normal human bowel function. Clin Nutr 1993;12:272.

90. Meier R, Beglinger C, Schneider H et al: Effect of a liquid formula diet with and without soluble fiber supplementation on intestinal transit and cholecystokinin release in volunteers. J Parenter Enter Nutr 1993;17(3):231.

91. Homann H-H, Kemen M, Fuessenich C et al: Reduction in diarrhea incidence by soluble fiber in patients receiving total of supplemental enteral nutrition. J Parenter Enter Nutr 1994;18(6):486.

92. Kapadia SA, Raimundo AH, Grimble GK et al: Influence of three different fiber-supplemented enteral diets on bowel function and short-chain fatty acid production. J Parenter Enter Nutr 1995;19(1):63.

93. Heimbach DM, Williamson J, Marvin J: The Gastrointestinal Tolerance of Fibre-Supplemented Tube Feeding Formula in Burn Patients. The Clinical Role of Fibre. Toronto: Medical Educational Services, 1985:67.

7

Micronutrients

ALAN SHENKIN

CLINICAL DEFICIENCY SYNDROMES AND SUBCLINICAL DEFICIENCY STATES

After many years of micronutrients being regarded as esoteric and of minor importance relative to the major energy and protein nutrients, there recently has been a surge of interest in nutritional and metabolic requirements of trace elements and vitamins. It is now recognized that micronutrients not only prevent deficiency syndromes but also may have a subtle role in metabolic processes. This role may not be immediately obvious, but it may contribute to overall well-being.

"Classic" nutritional deficiency usually results in a complex syndrome of typical signs and symptoms, and these have been fully characterized for each vitamin and trace element. These syndromes were the basis on which the essential micronutrients were initially identified, and careful dietary studies on both animals and humans have permitted a reasonable understanding of the nutritional consequences of severe deficiency and the intake necessary to prevent clinically obvious deficiency from developing.

On the other hand, it is now clear that as an individual develops progressively more severe depletion of micronutrient status, he or she will pass through a series of stages with biochemical or physiologic consequences. The metabolic or physiologic penalty of such suboptimal nutritional status is usually not clear, but this impaired metabolism is likely to result in detri-

mental effects. Alternatively, although the concentration of a micronutrient may be adequate in the blood or most tissues, specific and localized tissue deficiencies can occur and can lead to pathological changes.[1] For instance, folic acid may be locally deficient in bronchopulmonary, esophageal, or cervical tissue,[2] and vitamin A may be deficient only in lung tissue.[3] Such situations can be defined as subclinical deficiency.[4]

The time for development of a subclinical deficiency state varies for the individual micronutrients and depends on the nature and extent of any tissue or body stores of particular micronutrients. Moreover, the extent of depletion necessary before there are significant changes in biochemistry, physiology, or histology is poorly characterized. It is tempting to speculate that there might be a linear relationship between rate of depletion of a micronutrient and reduction in function of that micronutrient. However, as has been pointed out for most nutrients, it is probable that the early period of depletion of nutrients will result in compensatory mechanisms that will protect the organism; only with severe depletion will these subclinical effects become apparent (Fig. 7–1).

The consequences of an inadequate intake are more clearly delineated in Figure 7–2. This figure demonstrates the progression from optimal tissue status through a period of initial depletion to subclinical deficiency, with a variety of biochemical and nonspecific physiologic deficits and, for certain micronutrients, non-

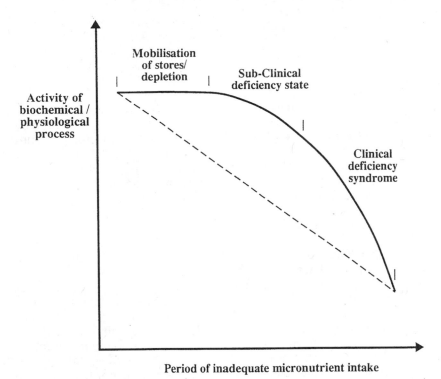

FIGURE 7–1   Relationship between period of inadequate micronutrient intake and activity of biochemical and physiologic processes. The dotted line shows linear reduction in function, which would probably only occur in in vitro reactions. In vivo, the solid line is expected.

specific histologic changes, until finally the full-blown clinical deficiency state can be recognized.

A subclinical deficiency state can be either absolute or relative. Thus an intake less than the requirement in normal health will ultimately lead to subclinical deficiency, or to a typical clinical deficiency state, even in otherwise healthy individuals. However, certain patients have significantly increased requirements as a result of their disease process, and hence an intake normally regarded as adequate may be relatively insufficient and lead to a subclinical deficiency state. Indeed, even changes in lifestyle such as increased cigarette smoking may increase the requirement for particular micronutrients, such as vitamin C. The recommended daily allowance (RDA) suggested by the U.S. National Research Council is 100 mg/day for regular cigarette smokers and 60 mg/day for nonsmokers.[5] One of the major challenges in clinical nutrition is to clarify the extent of this increased need for each micronutrient in particular disease states, possibly through better laboratory methods, and hence ensure optimal intake to meet the body's requirement.

FUNCTIONS OF MICRONUTRIENTS

Micronutrients can be classified as having two main types of function. First, they are required for optimal enzyme activity. Thus many trace elements are essential as activators of particular enzyme systems (e.g., zinc or manganese) or indeed may be part of the prosthetic group of particular enzymes (e.g., selenium or molybdenum). Similarly, most vitamins are, or are part of, coenzymes, which are essential for enzyme activity (e.g., the coenzymes of the electron transport chain). Second, certain micronutrients are involved directly in metabolic or regulatory activities. Thus vitamin E and vitamin A (and β-carotene) take part directly in antioxidant activities, whereas vitamin D, vitamin A, and zinc (as "zinc fingers") are involved directly in controlling DNA transcription.

The functions of these micronutrients can also be classified into those involved in control of metabolism (as cofactors or coenzymes), those involved in control of DNA transcription, and those taking part in free radical scavenging systems. There is, however, no simple system for classifying the increasingly wide range of reactions in which micronutrients are directly involved.

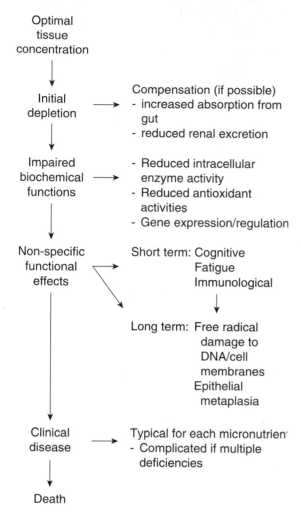

FIGURE 7–2 The consequences of inadequate micronutrient intake.

Those micronutrients especially important in free radical metabolism are vitamin A (β-carotene) and vitamin E, which being fat soluble help protect cell membranes, and vitamin C, superoxide dismutase (zinc/copper), and glutathione peroxidase (selenium), which protect the aqueous phase of the cell.[6,7]

Given the range of function of micronutrients, and especially the fact that most micronutrients take part in more than one mechanism, it is inevitable that an intake that achieves adequate function in one mechanism may not be optimal for another (e.g., the intake of vitamin A necessary to prevent night blindness may not be ideal to prevent epithelial metaplasia).[3] Similarly, because zinc binds to prosthetic groups of many enzymes and to cross-linking sites of other proteins, the concentration of free zinc in the cytoplasm ($10^{-9} - 10^{-10}$M) required to bind to cytoplasmic enzymes is much lower than the concentration in cell vesicles (e.g., 10^{-4}M) necessary to bind proteins such as insulin.[8] Even if the reactions are similar, concentrations necessary to achieve optimal effect might be different. For example, vitamin K is necessary to achieve gamma carboxylation of glutamic acid in the synthesis of certain proteins, such as blood coagulation proteins, and osteocalcin in the bone matrix.[9] A different concentration of vitamin K may well be necessary to optimize these reactions in different tissues.[10]

An even more complex situation exists for selenium. Severe selenium deficiency can lead to myopathy, either cardiomyopathy in endemic deficiency,[11] or skeletal[12,13] or cardiomyopathy[14] in artificial nutrition. However, only a relatively small proportion of all those with biochemically proven selenium deficiency, receiving long-term selenium-deficient artificial nutrition or in population studies, develop clinical signs of deficiency.[15] Whether this depends on the requirement for some precipitating agent (e.g., a viral infection or some other stress) is not known. There may also be an interaction with vitamin E, which has similar antioxidant activity and which can compensate for selenium in some animal conditions.[16] The effect of selenium in this situation has been found to be due to the selenoenzyme glutathione peroxidase. A recently identified function for selenium is as part of the enzyme tyrosine deiodinase, which is required for triiodothyronine biosynthesis.[17] The interaction of selenium and iodine in sustaining thyroid metabolism is an area of special interest.[18] Thus the optimal intake of selenium may depend not only on selenium status, but also on vitamin E and iodine status and upon physiologic or pathologic factors.

RECOMMENDED DAILY ALLOWANCES OR DIETARY REFERENCE VALUES

Overview

How much of a particular micronutrient does an individual require in normal health? The approach to this problem in the United States (Food and Nutrition Board, 1989)[5] and in the United Kingdom (Department of Health, 1991)[19] have differed, and different recommendations have thus emerged. A closer examination of these two reports merits further discussion, since it helps to identify the problems in reaching recommendations in this area.

In the report *Recommended Dietary Allowances,* the U.S. National Research Council (1989)[5] defines the RDA as the level of intake of essential nutrients that, on the basis of scientific knowledge, is judged by the Food and Nutrition Board to be adequate to meet the known nutrient needs of practically all healthy persons. This definition has remained essentially unchanged since 1984. Many individuals have smaller requirements than the RDA value, but the recommendation is made to ensure that it meets the requirements of individuals with a particularly high requirement.

On the other hand, the most recent tables issued by the Department of Health in the United Kingdom[19] summarize dietary reference values (DRVs), which are a range of intakes based on the distribution of requirements for each nutrient in the population. On this basis, an estimated average requirement (EAR) for the population can be defined; a point in the distribution curve at two standard deviations above the EAR is defined as the reference nutrient intake (RNI), and a point two standard deviations below the mean is the lower reference nutrient intake (LRNI). It is thus possible that 2.5 percent of the population will not be covered by taking the RNI amount, but it seems unlikely that intake at the RNI would be inadequate for many of the population.

Thus the RDA in the U.S. and the RNI in the U.K. should be approximately equivalent. The criteria used in reaching these values are summarized in Table 7–1 and have been rearranged to demonstrate the equivalence of these criteria. Given the apparent similarity in these criteria, and the discussion above, it is therefore surprising that there are such large differences between the RDA and the RNI, as summarized in Tables 7–2 and 7–3.

A number of problems further complicate applying these tables of requirements and recommendations, which have been reached from population studies, to an individual's immediate requirements. First, population studies have demonstrated that there is significant interindividual variation in nutrient intake, but this does not necessarily relate directly to the variation in requirements of that individual. An individual's intake may therefore not be identical to his or her requirement. On the other hand there is likely to be some correlation between intake and requirement although this may vary significantly from micronutrient to micronutrient. Hence increased intakes of

TABLE 7–1 Criteria for Reaching RDA (United States) and RNI (United Kingdom)

United States	United Kingdom
Studies of subjects maintained on a diet containing low artificial levels of a nutrient, followed by correction of the deficit with measured amounts of nutrient.	Intakes of a nutrient needed to cure clinical signs of deficiency.
Nutrient balance studies that measure nutrient status in relation to intake.	Intakes of nutrient needed to maintain balance, noting that the period over which such balance must be measured differs for different nutrients and between individuals.
Biochemical measurements of tissue saturation or adequacy of molecular function in relation to nutrient intake.	The intakes of nutrients needed to maintain a given circulating level or whole body saturation or tissue concentration.
Nutrient intakes of fully breast-fed infants and of apparently healthy people from their food supply.	Intakes of a nutrient by individuals and by groups that are associated with the absence of any signs of deficiency diseases.
Epidemiologic alterations of nutrient status in populations in relation to intake.	Intakes of a nutrient associated with an appropriate biologic marker of nutritional adequacy.
Extrapolation of data from animal experiments.	

RDA = recommended daily allowance; RNI = reference nutrient intake.

energy and protein in relation to body size may also lead to increased intakes of micronutrients.

Thus, the main conclusion is that to meet the requirements of an individual with confidence, especially in situations of artificial nutrition by the enteral route, an intake at least as high as the RDA should be provided. This will be significantly greater than the RNI, and hence should be adequate for most stable patients who do not have special needs.

TABLE 7–2   Essential Inorganic Micronutrients (Trace Elements)

	Function(s)	Biochemical Modes of Action	Effects of Deficiency	Dietary Factors Affecting Absorption
Zinc	Protein synthesis Control of differentiation Many enzymes	Enzyme cofactor "Zinc fingers" in DNA[71]	Growth ↓[39] Hair loss Skin rash[42] Immune function ↓[72]	Reduced when oral Cu ↑, non-heme Fe↑, or phytate/fiber↑[28,73]
Iron	O₂ transport Electron transport	Heme/myoglobin Cytochromes	Hypochromic anemia Possibly increased resistance to infection	Increased with heme Fe[20] Non-heme Fe absorption ↑ with vitamin C[73]
Copper	Collagen/elastin synthesis Antioxidant	Lysyl oxidase Zn/Cu superoxide dismutase Ceruloplasmin	Subperiosteal bleeding[74] Cardiac arrythmia Anemia Neutropenia[75]	Reduced when oral Zn ↑[30] or Fe↑[32] ? Reduced by high vitamin C intake[73]
Selenium	Antioxidant Immune function	Glutathione peroxidase Tyrosine deiodinase[17] T-lymphocyte-receptor expression	Cardiomyopathy[11,14] Skeletal myopathy[12,13] Nail abnormalities Macrocytosis[76] Neoplastic risk↑	Selenite may be reduced to Se by vitamin C at acid pH
Manganese	Not clear Some antioxidant	Enzyme cofactor Mitochondrial superoxide dismutase	Lipid abnormalities[77] Anemia Possibly mucopolysaccharide abnormalities	
Chromium	Carbohydrate metabolism	Insulin activity Lipoprotein metabolism Gene expression	Glucose intolerance[78] Weight loss Peripheral neuropathy[79]	Organic Cr better absorbed
Molybdenum	Amino acid metabolism Purine metabolism	Sulfite oxidase Xanthine oxidase	Intolerance to S amino acids:[80] tachycardia, visual upset	Reduced by Cu
Iodine	Energy metabolism	Thyroid hormones	Hypothyroidism	
Fluoride	Bone/tooth mineralization	Calcium fluorapatite	Dental caries	

Cu = copper; Fe = iron; Zn = zinc; IBC = iron-binding capacity; CRP = c-reactive protein; Se = selenium; Mn = manganese; Cr = chromium; S = sulfur; Mo = molybdenum; T₄ = thyroxine; T₃ = triodothyronine; TSH = thyroid stimulating hormone; NR = not recorded.

Bioavailability

In reaching recommendations regarding intake, the bioavailability of each micronutrient must always be taken into account;[19a,27] this factor was considered in the recommendations of the UK and USA expert bodies. Bioavailability is defined as the efficiency (usually expressed as a percent) with which any dietary nutrient is used in the body. Bioavailability is a combination of two key features of a micronutrient's physiology and biochemistry, absorption from the gut and utilization by the tissues.

The difficulty in defining suitable physiologic and biochemical markers of an end point for utilization has often resulted in the term *bioavailability* being used only to express efficiency of absorption, which has led to some uncertainty in the literature.

To discuss the bioavailability of micronutrients, we must consider (1) dietary composition, (2) changes to the diet occurring in the gut lumen, (3) mucosal effects within the gut, and (4) systemic factors altering use. Each of these factors may be relevant in the patient requiring enteral nutrition, especially since many such

Recommended Oral Intake (adult male)		Amount/2000 Kcal Tube Feed*	Assessment of Status	Comments
United States	**United Kingdom**			
15 mg	9.5 mg	13–36 mg	Plasma Zn—alone;[c] with albumin and C-reactive protein[a] Leukocyte[b] Alkaline phosphatase[c] Hair Zn[c]	Plasma Zn falls in acute-phase reaction
10 mg	8.7 mg	18–27 mg	Serum Fe/IBC[c] Serum ferritin with CRP[a] Bone marrow Fe[a]	Serum Fe falls in acute-phase—care needed not to exceed IBC
1.5–3 mg	1.2 mg	2–3.4 mg	Plasma Cu or ceruloplasmin with CRP[a] Liver Cu[b] Cu, Zn superoxide dismutase	Plasma Cu increases in acute-phase reaction
70 µg	75 µg	30–130 µg	Plasma Se[a] RBC glutathione peroxidase[a] Urine Se[b] Whole blood Se[b] Platelet glutathione peroxidase[b]	Preillness Se status varies depending on total Se intake Se depletion may be asymptomatic
2–5 mg	1.4 mg	2.4–8 mg	Plasma Mn[b] Whole blood Mn[b] Mitochondrial superoxide dismutase	Deficiency state not confirmed in humans
50–200 µg	> 25 µg	30–200 µg	Plasma Cr[b] Glucose tolerance[c]	Contamination free blood sampling
75–250 µg	50–400 µg	74–240 µg	Urine xanthine[b] Hypoxanthine[b] Sulfite[b] Plasma Mo[b]	Rarely measured
150 µg	140 µg	120–220 µg	Serum T$_4$[a] Serum T$_3$[a] Serum TSH[a]	
1.5–4 mg	0.05 mg/kg (infants)	NR–1.6 mg	Urine excretion[b]	Provision in nutritional support is controversial

[a]Widely available and clinically useful tests.
[b]Good markers of status but of limited availability.
[c]Tests of little value in assessing status.
* The range of amounts present in various tube feeds, including Ensure (Abbott), Nutrison (Cow & Gate), Fresubin (Fresenius), Clinifeed (Roussel), Flexical (Squibb), and Elemental 028 (Scientific Hospitals Supplies).

patients receive a normal oral diet plus supplementary enteral nutrition. Even in patients receiving 100 percent of their nutrition by artificial tube feeding, the variety of components now used in preparing such feeds (e.g., the proportion of peptides or amino acids, the presence or absence of fiber, and the specific objectives of particular preparations) helps to explain at least part of the variability between the content of micronutrients in such preparation. On the other hand, it is not always clear why different manufacturers have chosen different levels of micronutrients. Most enteral preparations do, however, meet either U.S. or U.K. recommendations (Tables 7–2 and 7–3).

Factors Affecting Bioavailability

The main factors affecting bioavailability are discussed below.

Dietary Factors

Chemical Form of the Nutrient. Elements in the form of organometal compounds (e.g., iron and heme,[20] or selenium in selenomethionine[21]) are significantly better absorbed than the re-

TABLE 7–3   Essential Organic Micronutrients (Vitamins)

	Function(s)	Biochemical Modes of Action	Effects of Deficiency	Dietary Factors Affecting Absorption
Vitamin A	Visual acuity Antioxidant (as β-carotene) Growth and development Immune function	Rhodopsin in retina Free radical scavenger Induces DNA transcription	Xerophthalmia[81] Night blindness[82] Increased risk of some neoplasms[4]	Requires fat absorption
Vitamin D	Calcium absorption Differentiation of macrophages	Receptor-mediated transcription	Osteomalacia (adults) Rickets (children) Immune status ↓[83]	Requires fat absorption Mainly synthesized in skin under ultraviolet light
Vitamin E	Antioxidant in membranes	Free radical scavenger	Hemolytic anemia in infants[84] Central/peripheral neuropathy[85] Myopathy[86] Increased risk of athero-sclerosis, certain neoplasia[4]	Requires fat absorption
Vitamin K	Blood coagulation Bone calcification	γ-glutamyl carboxylation Coagulation proteins and osteocalcin[9]	Bleeding disorders ? Bone disorders[10]	Requires fat absorption Mainly synthesized in bowel
B_1 (thiamin)	Carbohydrate and fat metabolism	Decarboxylation reactions as TPP	Beri-beri with neurologic or cardiac effects[87] Wernicke-Korsakoff syndrome[88] Immune function ↓[89]	
B_2 (riboflavin)	Oxidative metabolism	Coenzyme as FAD or FMN	Lesions of lips, tongue, skin[90] Possibly immune function ↓[89]	
B_6 (pyridoxine)	Amino acid metabolism	Transamination reactions	Anemia (children) Lesions of lips and skin Premenstrual symptoms[91] Carpal tunnel syndrome	Certain drugs alter bioavailability or metabolism
Niacin	Oxidative metabolism	Coenzyme as NAD/NADP	Pellagra—rash, weakness, diarrhea	Bioavailability in cereals may be poor
B_{12}	DNA metabolism	Recycling folate coenzymes Valine metabolism	Megaloblastic anemia Demyelination of neurons	
Folate	Purine/pyrimidine metabolism	Single carbon transfer—methylation reactions	Megaloblastic anemia Growth retardation Pancytopenia[92] Bronchial, colonic metaplastic change Neural tube defects in pregnancy[93]	Bioavailibility from food 50% of crystalline folate Interaction with Zn[25]
Biotin	Lipogenesis/gluconeogenesis	Carboxylase reactions	Scaly dermatitis[94] Hair loss	Poor availability in wheat
Vitamin C (ascorbic acid)	Collagen synthesis Antioxidant Absorption of iron	OH proline/OH lysine synthesis Reduction reactions $Fe^{3+} \rightarrow Fe^{2+}$	Scurvy, impaired wound healing ? Impaired immune function[57] ? Oxidative damage	

PUFA = Polyunsaturated fatty acids; Ca = calcium; P = phosphorus; TPP = thiamin pyrophosphate; RBC = red blood cell; FAD = flavin adenine dinucleotide; FMN = flavin mononucleotide; NAD/NADP = nicotinamide adenine dinucleotide/nicotinamide adenine dinucleotide phosphate; Fe = iron; Zn = Zinc.

Recommended Oral Intake (adult male)		Amount/2000 Kcal Tube Feed*	Assessment of Status	Comments
United States	United Kingdom			
1000 µg	700 µg	1000–2160 µg	Plasma retinol[c] Plasma retinol-binding protein[c] Liver biopsy retinol[b]	Fall in retinol during acute-phase response due to fall in retinol-binding protein
5 µg	—	8.5–14.6 µg	Serum Ca/P/alkaline phosphatase[a] Serum 25-hydroxy vitamin D[a] (Rarely, 1,25 dihydroxy vitamin D)[b]	
10 mg	> 4 mg	20–64 mg	Plasma tocopherol/cholesterol[a] Hydrogen peroxide hemolysis[b]	Vitamin E is transported in low density lipoproteins
80 µg	1 µg/kg/day	100–200 µg	Prothrombin time[a] Plasma phylloquinone[b] Results should be expressed per mmol triglyceride	Time-consuming assay
1.2 mg	0.9 mg	1.4–3.4 mg	RBC transketolase[a] Blood thiamine[b] Urine thiamine/creatinine[b]	Deficiency may occur and is reversed rapidly
1.4 mg	1.3 mg	2–6 mg	RBC glutathione reductase[a] Blood FAD[b] Urine riboflavin/creatinine[a]	
2 mg	1.4 mg	2–13.8 mg	RBC transaminase[a] Blood pyridoxal phosphate[b] Urine 4 pyridoxic acid[b]	Less interference by disease than for transaminase
15 mg	16 mg	18–45 mg	Urine N-methyl nicotinamide[b] Blood niacin[b]	Rarely measured
2 µg	1.5 µg	3–15 µg	Serum vitamin B_{12}[a] Methyl malonic acid[b]	
200 µg	200 µg	340–880 µg	Serum folate[a] RBC folate[a] Serum homocysteine[b]	Recent intake Whole body status
30–100 µg	10–200 µg	100–660 µg	Serum biotin[b] Urine biotin[b]	Rarely assayed
60 mg	40 mg	100–300 mg	Leucocyte vitamin C[b] Plasma vitamin C[c]	Plasma vitamin falls in injury or infection

*The range of amounts present in various tube feeds, including Ensure (Abbott), Nutrison (Cow & Gate), Fresubin (Fresenius), Clinifeed (Roussel), Flexical (Squibb), and Elemental 028 (Scientific Hospitals Supplies).
[a]Widely available and clinically useful tests.
[b]Good markers of status but of limited availability.
[c]Tests of little value in assessing status.

spective inorganic form of the element. Similarly, the organic complex of chromium is better absorbed than ionic chromium.[22] The valency of the element may also be important: Fe^{2+} is better absorbed than Fe^{3+}.[23] Different organic forms of the same nutrient may have different absorption; for instance, the polyglutamate form of folic acid is the naturally occurring form, but it must first be converted to the monoglutamate form before absorption. Pyridoxine glycoside, which is present in many vegetables, is relatively unavailable compared with free pyridoxine.

Antagonistic Ligand. A number of substances in the diet may complex micronutrients to prevent their absorption. For example, phytate may complex zinc (helping to explain the reduced zinc absorption from soy products)[24] and iron, as well as the macroelements calcium and magnesium; polyphenols may complex iron; avidin will complex biotin to prevent its absorption; and folic acid supplements may reduce zinc absorption, possibly by forming insoluble complexes,[25] but do not alter iron or copper absorption. Fiber in the form of hemicellulose, pectin, or lignin may complex many elements, especially zinc and iron,[26] and most commercial enteral feeding preparations containing fiber therefore have a higher content of trace elements than the otherwise identical fiber-free preparations.

Facilitatory Ligands. Certain acids such as picolinic acid and citric acid aid the absorption of zinc; ascorbic acid aids absorption of iron (but reduces that of copper).[27]

Competitive Interactions. A number of elements interact by competition for similar absorption mechanisms. For example, iron and zinc compete directly for absorption, and hence iron supplements may reduce zinc absorption.[28] However, the effect of iron may depend on whether the zinc is provided as an aqueous solution or as part of the meal.[29] Similarly, a high zinc intake can inhibit absorption of copper.[30] We have seen at least one patient receiving long-term intravenous nutrition plus a small amount of oral nutrition in whom oral copper supplements precipitated clinical zinc deficiency.[31]

Luminal Factors

Certain events occurring in the lumen are vital for absorption.

Effect of Redox State. In an acid environment, reduction of Fe^{3+} to Fe^{2+} is more likely.

Dietary Hydrolysis. Dietary hydrolysis may also be important in releasing trace elements complexed within carbohydrate or protein molecules.

Complexation with Amino Acids. A key part of the absorption process for copper and zinc is to complex with free histidine and cysteine molecules released by digestion of protein, with the metal amino acid complex being readily absorbed.[32]

Mucosal Factors

Mechanisms exist within mucosal cells to assist uptake of elements and transfer them to the portal circulation. Transferrin is necessary to bind iron and transfer it to the bloodstream, this being increased in iron deficiency. Metallothionein similarly complexes zinc and transfers it to albumin.[33] Mucosal uptake is the net effect of several processes. For zinc there are two main processes, only one of which is saturable and stimulated by zinc depletion.[34] If dietary zinc is low, there is low secretion of zinc into the lumen and hence reduced excretion of zinc in the feces, together with higher absorption into the bloodstream.

Systemic Factors

The above factors influence the extent of absorption of individual elements, but the distribution of elements to tissues and their subsequent use is also an important part of bioavailability. These post-absorption aspects depend on body status and physiologic state. Anabolic demands of growth in childhood, or in recovery from a catabolic illness, increase the requirement and retention of elements, whereas hepatic and renal disease or infection lead to mobilization of micronutrients from tissues, such as muscle and liver, and redistribution of these elements to other tissues.[35] This redistribution complicates testing for adequacy of micronutrient provision in certain patients.

Summary

Bioavailability of micronutrients varies according to the chemical state of the nutrient, its absorption mechanism, and any physiologic adaptation processes at the gut, as well as functional effects after absorption. In the absence of better information regarding status in an individual patient, the best practical advice is to provide elements in a readily absorbed chemical form, in an appropriate balance to minimize competition for absorption mechanisms, and in an amount that meets the basal requirements of most healthy individuals. Status should be monitored, especially in complicated patients (see below), who may have increased or decreased requirements (if excretion is altered) or abnormal utilization.

FACTORS AFFECTING THE MICRONUTRIENT REQUIREMENT OF INDIVIDUAL PATIENTS

Although it is possible to suggest an intake for each trace element and vitamin that is likely to meet most patients' requirements, clinicians must be aware of circumstances that lead to an increased requirement, so that specific individual or multiple supplements can be considered.

Micronutrient Status at Onset of Disease or on Admission to Hospital

The typical diet or lifestyle of a patient in relative health may already have compromised his or her micronutrient status. Since many individuals have poor dietary habits, with an excessive intake of refined carbohydrates, inadequate fiber, and variably inadequate intake of fruit, vegetables, and milk, they are already at risk of inadequate intake, especially of B vitamins and iron. This is particularly the case in adolescence, when the anabolism associated with rapid growth puts demands on the provision of all nutrients. At the same time, such individuals frequently have food fads or undergo atypical reducing diets, further exacerbating the situation. Studies have suggested that this group is particularly at risk of inadequate folate and vitamin A intake.[36,37]

Elderly individuals also have a high frequency of nutritional problems, relating to the inadequacy of their diet, dental problems, interactions of drugs with nutrient metabolism, chronic illness, and economic factors. It is therefore not surprising that there is a high incidence of abnormalities, especially in micronutrient status, and studies have shown a high prevalence of vitamin C, iron, zinc, and folate deficiency.[38]

Too much alcohol or cigarette smoke also alters micronutrient status. Individuals who derive a high proportion of their energy from alcohol are likely to have inadequate intake of most water-soluble vitamins as well as phosphate and magnesium. Moreover, there may be impaired metabolism of vitamin A in cirrhosis, possibly related to inadequate zinc status.[39] Vitamin B_1 deficiency should be particularly sought in this group of individuals.

Smokers appear to require additional vitamin C, possibly due to altered metabolic turnover.[40]

Similarly, both β-carotene and vitamin E status are impaired compared with nonsmokers, suggesting a link with free radical production and oxidative damage.[41]

Effects of the Underlying Disease Process

Micronutrient status at presentation may also be impaired due to effects of the disease process. Any condition causing malabsorption will affect absorption of trace elements and vitamins. Inflammatory bowel disease (IBD), celiac disease, chronic pancreatitis, biliary cirrhosis, and other forms of small bowel disease will affect all micronutrients, but particularly the fat-soluble vitamins. When considering the possibility of malabsorption, it should be remembered that individual supplements of iron, zinc, or copper may cause reduced absorption of other trace elements.

Similarly, underlying disease may cause increased loss of elements in body fluids, especially in chronic diarrhea. Although this mainly affects the major minerals of sodium, potassium, and magnesium, patients with chronic diarrhea will lose large amounts of zinc and other water-soluble trace elements.

Moreover, the disease state itself may cause an inflammatory or acute-phase response with increased protein turnover in tissues such as skeletal muscle, leading to release of intracellular elements, especially zinc, which are then excreted in the urine.[42] Such a deficit must be corrected during recovery from illness.

Increased Requirements due to Illness or the Effect of Treatment or Surgery

Effects of Illness

The increase in metabolic rate and in protein turnover associated with an illness, infection, or trauma inevitably lead to increased involvement of micronutrients as cofactors of the metabolic processes. If patients receive this increased intake within a balanced regimen, when the amount of micronutrient provided increases proportionally with protein and energy substrates, metabolic requirements should be adequately met. This is especially so in patients receiving enteral nutrition, where the formulation of a single proprietary preparation ensures that as the total volume of feed is increased, the ratio of protein/energy to micronutrients remains constant. This is, of course, not necessarily the same in patients receiving some of their nutrition by the parenteral route. Moreover, if hypermetabolic patients receive a high carbohydrate intake as part of their energy requirement, there is an increased likelihood of water-soluble vitamin deficiency, especially vitamin B_1.[43]

Effects of Surgery

Complications of surgery frequently alter micronutrient status. Most obviously, short-bowel syndrome reduces absorption of most micronutrients, although some may be absorbed throughout the whole length of the small bowel. Hence the total length of gut remaining is critical in determining how much micronutrient intake can be absorbed. Special care is necessary if the terminal ileum has been resected, since vitamin B_{12} is absorbed from this region.

Small bowel or pancreatic fistula losses have a high content of micronutrients, especially zinc, whereas biliary fistula fluid is rich in copper and manganese.

There is also a theoretical risk of loss of water-soluble vitamins and trace elements in patients who require peritoneal dialysis or hemodialysis. Somewhat surprisingly, this is usually not a major problem, with folic acid deficiency being most prevalent.[44]

Patients with severe burns lose micronutrients through the damaged skin. The loss of zinc, copper, and selenium, and probably also other micronutrients, are much greater in burn exudate fluid than the losses in urine or feces.[45,46] These elements can become depleted quickly, and the best way to replace such elements, and the amounts required, are currently not known. Some studies have suggested that increasing trace elements by a factor of about four to six may be beneficial,[47] although many factors are not clear including whether such additional micronutrients should be provided intravenously or enterally, what is the optimal amount, and what is the mechanism of the beneficial effects.

Effects of Anabolism

Patients who have lost a significant amount of lean body mass due to catabolic illness may develop an acute deficiency state when there is a change to net anabolism and tissue regeneration. This point in a patient's progress generally occurs when the stimulus to the release of catabolic mediators (interleukins and tumor necrosis factor) and of catabolic hormones (especially catecholamines and cortisol) has been resolved (e.g., by drainage of an abscess or coverage of a burn area). Deficiency states are therefore more likely to occur during the anabolic phase that follows resolution of a catabolic illness.[48] Well-recognized examples are a zinc deficiency rash[42] or skeletal muscle myopathy due to selenium deficiency.[13]

Optimal Intake of Micronutrients

Defining the optimal intake of micronutrients is therefore far from ideal. On the one hand, it is possible to assess an individual's requirements based on requirements in health, likely underlying nutritional state at presentation, and ongoing effects of the disease process. However, providing micronutrients to ensure the best possible tissue function remains a distant goal. Two possible methods of trying to optimize such provision relate to the free radical scavenging system and to the immune system.

The role of micronutrients to limit the oxidative damage caused by free radicals is now well established. A major issue is whether increased provision of free radical scavengers such as β-carotene or vitamin E, or of micronutrients directly involved in free radical metabolic pathways, such as vitamin C, selenium, zinc, or copper, or of the metalloenzyme superoxide dismutase may influence outcome.[1,4] Increased provision of these substances alters the fatty acid content of cell membranes, and also the production of end products of oxidative metabolism, such as malonyl dialdehyde. Correlations between these biochemical markers and outcome, however, tend to be tenuous and may be more coincidental than "cause and effect." Free radical damage has been especially related to pancreatitis. There is clear biochemical evidence of oxidative stress in experimental models of acute pancreatitis,[49,50] although pretreatment with antioxidants seems necessary to achieve a clinically beneficial effect.[49,51] Biochemical benefit of a cocktail of antioxidant nutrients has also been shown in recurrent pancreatitis.[52] Well-controlled clinical trials will help clarify situations where increased provision of these micronutrients is or is not helpful, both in reducing the biochemical effects of free radicals and in altering complication rates and outcome in serious illness.

Micronutrient deficiencies have been associated with impairment of various aspects of immune function. However, controlled evidence of efficacy in vivo is limited. A study of the effect of a mixture of vitamins and trace elements in free living, healthy, elderly individuals demonstrated a marked reduction in episodes of infection over a 1-year period.[38] This was found to correlate with an increase in T4-lymphocyte cell numbers, improved lymphocyte responsiveness to phytohemagglutinin (PHA), and an increase in natural killer (NK) cells. A small but variable proportion of patients was found to have biochemical evidence of deficiency for individual or multiple micronutrients at the start of the trial, and supplementation improved biochemical status for these nutrients.

Supplementation with zinc alone in elderly individuals with mild zinc deficiency has been shown to increase lymphocyte nucleotidase activity and serum thymulin, together with an improved response to skin test antigens.[53] Improved taste acuity was also observed. Similarly, zinc supplements in patients with Crohn's disease lead to increased plasma thymulin.[54]

There has been a longstanding interest in the potential value of vitamin A supplementation in infectious diseases, and a recent meta-analysis of 20 trials has confirmed that such supplements to children in developing countries do have anti-infective properties. There is a significant reduction in specific mortality from diarrheal disease in community studies and in respiratory disease in children with measles.[55]

Many studies have been performed on the value of intakes higher than Recommended Daily Allowances (RDAs), but few have had a convincing overall effect. Thus despite considerable enthusiasm for the use of high-dose vitamin C in treatment of the common cold[56] and other disease states, clear-cut benefit has not been proved.[57]

A number of studies have suggested that large doses of vitamin E might improve immunity in the elderly. Various aspects of cell-mediated immunity, including skin tests, mitogenic responses, and interleukin (IL)-2 production, have been shown to respond to vitamin E alone or with vitamin C and vitamin A.[58]

An interesting recent study on university students has shown that a selenium intake of 200 μg/day in individuals with an apparently healthy diet led to an increase in markers of immune function.[59,60] These included increased IL-2 receptor expression and improved T-lymphocyte function.

A major challenge to nutritionists is to determine whether all individuals benefit from this type of supplementation, or whether only those who are depleted benefit. The magnitude of the improvement, in laboratory tests and clinical outcome, must be investigated in relation to initial nutritional status for the micronutrient in question.

MONITORING MICRONUTRIENT STATUS IN PATIENTS RECEIVING ENTERAL NUTRITION

Ideally, micronutrient provision would be matched to requirements by monitoring with laboratory tests. Unfortunately, the accuracy of such tests in reflecting nutritional state, the sensitivity to small changes in status, and the specificity in terms of being affected only by nutritional status, and not by other effects of disease, are generally fairly poor. Hence at best laboratory tests can only be used as a guide toward substantial underprovision or overprovision of particular nutrients; they probably cannot be used to "fine tune" the provision to meet individual patients' requirements.

Measuring micronutrient concentration in plasma or serum provides a reasonable index of status for only a few nutrients (e.g., vitamin B_{12}) and also may reflect adequacy of recent intake for certain other micronutrients (e.g., folate or selenium). An excess provision of elements such as manganese and chromium may also be reflected in high serum concentration.

For most other micronutrients, serum measurement is seriously limited in value. On the one hand, this reflects the lack of correlation between the plasma compartment and the state of the nutrient within the intracellular compartment in most body tissues. For example, there may be substantial stores of particular nutrients in individual tissues (e.g., vitamin A or vitamin B_{12} in the liver), but their mobilization into the plasma may be affected by an availability of appropriate binding proteins or by metabolism. Alternatively, there may be differences in the content of individual micronutrients between different tissues, and hence the serum concentrations in all tissues of the body.

Furthermore, the concentration in plasma can alter rapidly when an acute-phase response to trauma or infection redistributes metals between body compartments.[61] For example, during an acute-phase response, there is increased synthesis of metallothionein, leading to increased uptake of zinc into the liver,[62] and increased synthesis of ferritin causing increased uptake of iron,[63] leading to a fall in the plasma concentration of both these elements. These changes in plasma concentration clearly do not reflect changes in whole body status.[35] Moreover, there may be changes in the binding proteins in plasma due to disease process. Serum albumin concentration falls in association with any acute illness,[64] which inevitably leads to a fall in plasma zinc concentration. Similarly, reduction in retinol binding protein concentration as part of the acute-phase response or protein malnutrition will also lead to a fall in serum retinol, whatever the content of retinol stores within the liver.[65]

On the other hand, patients receiving long-term nutritional support, especially by the enteral route, may well be sufficiently stable for there to be relatively little acute-phase response to injury, infection, or other inflammation. If this is so, then it may be possible to interpret the plasma concentrations of elements such as zinc, copper, and iron. A low plasma concentration in a patient with no evidence of an acute-phase reaction probably indicates poor status. Of particular relevance is to follow the trend in concentration of the trace element in relation to changes in the magnitude of the acute-phase response. Repeated measurements of a short-acting acute-phase protein, such as C-reactive protein, may therefore help in assessing changes in size of the acute-phase response and the validity of some of these plasma measurements.[66,67]

Increasingly, attempts are being made to relate blood cell concentrations to requirements for micronutrients. It is well established that the concentration of certain intracellular enzymes gives a good index of micronutrient provision (e.g., red blood cell [RBC] transketolase as an index of thiamine status or RBC glutathione peroxidase as an indication of selenium status).[68] Alternatively, whole blood thiamine or selenium analysis probably yields better precision for comparative studies. Similarly, RBC folate is widely used as a good index of whole body folate status. Because the acute-phase response causes significant alterations in the distribution of vitamin C and zinc between body compartments, leukocyte studies have been attempted, and these provide a better index of body status for the nutrients.[69,70] Preparation of white blood cells (WBCs) is more difficult, and such techniques are likely to be used only in the research environment.

There is increasing interest in methods of detecting disturbances in intracellular metabolism due to impaired activity of enzymes requiring trace elements or vitamins as cofactors. For example, in molybdenum deficiency, there is increased urinary excretion of sulfite and hypoxanthine, due to reduced activity of the molybdenum dependent enzymes, sulfite oxi-

dase and xanthine oxidase.[80] Similarly methylmalonic acid may be increased in vitamin B_{12} depletion, due to reduced conversion of methylmalonyl CoA to succinyl CoA,[95] and homocysteine may be increased in folate depletion due to reduced methylation to methionine.[96] Supplements of vitamin B_{12} and folate may reduce the concentration of these metabolites despite normal concentrations of vitamin B_{12} and folate in plasma.[97] However specific biochemical indicators are available for only a few of the micronutrients.[98]

Tests commonly used to assess micronutrients are summarized in Tables 7–2 and 7–3. Because of limitations in interpreting these data, it is common practice, especially in patients receiving enteral nutrition, only to assess on a regular basis the status of zinc, copper, selenium (mainly in long-term nutritional problems), iron, and folic acid. Laboratory tests available to assess other micronutrients are usually only used when a particular clinical problem necessitates confirmation of micronutrient deficiency. When such tests are not available and a deficiency is suspected, it is common practice to add a multimineral or multivitamin supplement to the regimen to seek clinical benefit in the short term. A 2-week course of a well-balance micronutrient supplement is unlikely to cause any harm and may occasionally be beneficial. Documentation of patients who benefit clinically in this way could in the long term help clarify the increased micronutrient requirements of certain types of patients.

SUMMARY

Providing adequate amounts of vitamins and trace elements involves more than just preventing clinical deficiency states. Inadequate supply may lead to subclinical yet important effects with long-lasting consequences to health (e.g., free radical damage or failure or delay of tissue repair). An adequate intake is therefore necessary both in patients admitted to hospital who are already malnourished as well as in patients with increased requirements for protein-energy nutrition. Most enteral nutrition preparations currently available have adequate amounts of all essential vitamins and trace elements. Clinicians should, however, take care to ensure that the composition is indeed complete and contains adequate amounts of the less commonly provided trace elements, such as selenium, chromium, and molybdenum, especially in patients requiring long-term artificial nutritional support.

Controversy exists regarding whether providing larger amounts of individual micronutrients will improve outcome, particularly for those micronutrients known to affect the free radical scavenging mechanisms or immune function. It also remains to be established whether providing large amounts of these micronutrients will improve outcome more than providing an adequate amount of all micronutrients within a well-balanced diet. Controlled clinical trials of different amounts of micronutrients in different diseases are required, in both short- and long-term studies, and preferably relating outcome to the best available markers of micronutrient status. Such studies should ultimately lead to the better matching of nutritional provision to patient requirements.

REFERENCES

1. Sauberlich HE, Machlin LJ: Beyond deficiency. New views on the function and health effects of vitamins. Ann NY Acad Sci 1992;669:1–404.

2. Heimberger DC: Localised deficiencies of folic acid in aerodigestive tissues. Ann NY Acad Sci 1992;669: 87–96.

3. Biesalski HK, Stofft E: Biochemical, morphological and functional aspects of systemic and local vitamin A deficiency in the respiratory tract. Ann NY Acad Sci 1992;669:325–331.

4. Gaby SK, Bendich A, Singh VN et al: Vitamin Intake and Health — A Scientific Review. New York: Marcel Dekker,1991:1–217.

5. Food and Nutrition Board, National Research Council: Recommended Dietary Allowances. 10th edition. National Academy Press, Washington, DC, 1989.

6. Dreosti IE: The physiological biochemistry and antioxidant activity of the trace elements copper, manganese, selenium and zinc. Clin Biochem Rev 1991; 12:127–129.

7. Halliwell B, Gutteridge JMC: Free Radicals in Biology and Medicine. 2nd edition. Oxford: Clarendon Press, 1989.

8. Williams RJP: An introduction to the biochemistry of zinc. In Mills CF (ed): Zinc in Human Biology. London: Springer-Verlag, 1989:15–31.

9. Shearer MJ: Vitamin K metabolism and nutriture. Blood Rev 1992;6:92–104.

10. Vermeer C, Knapen MHJ, Jie K-SG et al: Physiological importance of extra hepatic vitamin-K dependent carboxylation reactions. Ann NY Acad Sci 1992;669: 21–33.

11. Diplock AT: Metabolic and functional defects in selenium deficiency. Phil Trans Royal Soc Lond 1981;294: 105–117.

12. Mansell PI, Rawlings J, Allison SP et al: Reversal of skeletal myopathy with selenium supplementation in a patient on home parenteral nutrition. Clin Nutr 1987;6:179–183.

13. Van Rij AM, Thompson CD, McKenzie JM et al: Selenium deficiency in total parenteral nutrition. Am J Clin Nutr 1979;32:2076–2085.

14. Johnson RA, Baker SS, Fallon JT et al: An occidental case of cardiomyopathy and selenium deficiency. N Engl J Med 1981;304:1210–1212.

15. Shenkin A, Fell GS, Halls DJ et al: Essential trace element provision to patients receiving home intravenous nutrition in the United Kingdom. Clin Nutr 1986;5:91–97.

16. Combs GF, Combs SB: Biochemical functions of selenium. In The Role of Selenium in Nutrition. London: Academic Press, 1986:205–263.

17. Arthur JR, Nicol F, Beckett GJ: Selenium deficiency, thyroid hormone metabolism, and thyroid hormone deiodinases. Am J Clin Nutr 1993;57(suppl):236S–239S.

18. Vanderpas JB, Contempre B, Duale NL et al: Selenium deficiency mitigates hypothyroxinemia in iodine-deficient subjects. Am J Clin Nutr 1993;57(2):271S–275S.

19. Panel on Dietary Reference Values, Department of Health: Dietary Reference Values for Food Energy and Nutrients for the United Kingdom. London: HMSO, 1991.

19a. O'Dell BL: Bioavailability of trace elements. Nutr Rev 1984;42:301–308.

20. Lynch SR, Dassenko SA, Morck TA et al: Soy protein products and heme iron absorption in humans. Am J Clin Nutr 1985;41:13–20.

21. Thomson CD, Robinson MF, Campbell DR et al: Effect of prolonged supplementation with daily supplements of selenomethionine and sodium selenite on glutathione peroxidase in blood of New Zealand residents. Am J Clin Nutr 1982;36:24–31.

22. Anderson M, Riley D, Rotruck J: Chromium (III) trisacetylacetonate: an absorbable, bioactive source of chromium. Fed Proc 1980;39:787.

23. Linder MC, Munro HN: The mechanism of iron absorption and its regulation. Fed Proc 1977;36:2017–2023.

24. Lonnerdal B, Cederblad A, Davidsson L et al: The effect of individual components of soy formula and cow's milk on zinc bioavailability. Am J Clin 1984;40:1064–1070.

25. Milne DB, Canfield WK, Mahalko JR et al: Effect of oral folic acid supplements on zinc, copper and iron absorption and excretion. Am J Clin Nutr 1984;39:535–539.

26. Drews LM, Kies HM, Fox HM: Effect of dietary fibre on copper, zinc and magnesium utilisation by adolescent boys. Am J Clin Nutr 1979;32:1893–1897.

27. Burk RF, Solomons NW: Trace elements and vitamins and bioavailability as related to wheat and wheat foods. Am J Clin Nutr 1985;41:1091–1102.

28. Solomons NW: Competitive interaction of iron and zinc in the diet: consequences for human nutrition. J Nutr 1986;116:927–935.

29. Sandstrom B, Davidsson L, Cederblad A et al: Oral iron, dietary ligands and zinc absorption. J Nutr 1985; 115:411–414.

30. Brewer GJ: Interactions of zinc and molybdenum with copper in therapy of Wilson's disease. Nutrition 1995;11:114–116.

31. de Caestecker JS, Shenkin A, Fell GS et al: Hazards and benefits in a patient on long-term total parenteral nutrition. Proc Nutr Soc 1986;45:15a.

32. Snedeker SM, Greger JL: Metabolism of zinc, copper and iron is affected by dietary protein, cysteine and histidine. J Nutr 1983;113:644.

33. Steel L, Cousins RJ: Kinetics of zinc absorption by luminally and vascularly perfused rat intestine. Am J Physiol 1985;248:G46–53.

34. Hoadley JE, Leinart AS, Cousins RJ: Kinetic analysis of zinc uptake and serosal transfer by vascularly perfused rat intestine. Am J Physiol 1987;252:G825–831.

35. Fraser WD, Taggart DP, Fell GS et al: Changes in iron, zinc and copper concentrations in serum and in their binding to transport proteins after cholecystectomy and cardiac surgery. Clin Chem 1989;35:2243–2247.

36. Clark AJ, Mossholder S, Gates R: Folinic status in adolescent females. Am J Clin Nutr 1987;46:302–306.

37. Sumner SK, Liebman M, Wakefield LM: Vitamin A status of adolescent girls. Nutr Rep Inter 1987;35:423–431.

38. Chandra RK: Effect of vitamin and trace element supplementation on immune response and infection in elderly subjects. Lancet 1992;340:1124–1127.

39. Aggett PJ: Severe zinc deficiency. In Mills CF (ed): Zinc in Human Biology. London: Springer-Verlag, 1989:259–279.

40. Kallner AB, Hartmann D, Hornig DH: On the requirements of ascorbic acid in man: steady state turnover and body pool in smokers. Am J Clin Nutr 1981;34:1347–1355.

41. Stryker WS, Kaplan LA, Stein EA et al: The relation of diet, cigarette smoking, and alcohol consumption to plasma β-carotene and α-tocopherol levels. Am J Epidemiol 1988;127:283–296.

42. Kay RG, Tasman-Jones C, Pybus J et al: A syndrome of acute zinc deficiency during total parenteral alimentation in man. Ann Surg 1976;183:331–340.

43. Cruickshank AM, Telfer ABM, Shenkin A: Thiamine deficiency in the critically ill. Intensive Care Med 1988;14:384–387.

44. Kopple JD: Nutrition, diet and the kidney. In Shils ME, Young VR (eds): Modern Nutrition in Health and Disease, 7th edition. Philadelphia: Lea & Febiger, 1988:1230–1268.

45. Berger MM, Cavadini C, Bart A et al: Cutaneous copper and zinc loses in burns. Burns 1992;18:373–380.

46. Berger MM, Cavadini C, Bart A et al: Selenium losses in 10 burned patients. Clin Nutr 1992;11:75–82.

47. Berger MM, Cavadini C, Chiolero R et al: Influence of large intakes of trace elements on recovery after major burns. Nutrition 1994;10:327–334.

48. Tasman-Jones C, Kay RG, Lee SP: Zinc and copper deficiency with particular reference to parenteral nutrition. In Nybus LM (ed): Surgery Annual. New York: Appleton, 1978:23–52.

49. Niederau C, Niederau M, Borchard F et al: Effects of antioxidants and free radical scavengers in three different models of acute pancreatitis. Pancreas 1992;7(4):486–496.

50. Schulz HU, Niederau C: Oxidative stress-induced changes in pancreatic acinar cells: insights from in vitro studies. Hepatogastroenterology 1994;41(4):309–312.

51. Schoenberg MH, Buchler M, Younes M et al: Effect of antioxidant treatment in rats with acute hemorrhagic pancreatitis. Dig Dis Sci 1994;39(5):1034–1040.

52. Uden S, Schofield D, Miller PF et al: Antioxidant therapy for recurrent pancreatitis: biochemical profiles in a placebo-controlled trial. Aliment Pharmacol Ther 1992;6(2):229–240.

53. Prasad AS, Fitzgerald JT, Hess JW et al: Zinc deficiency in elderly patients. Nutrition 1993;9:218–224.

54. Brignola C, Belloli C, De-Simone G et al: Zinc supplementation restores plasma concentrations of zinc and thymulin in patients with Crohn's disease. Aliment Pharmacol Ther 1993;7:275–280.

55. Glasziou PP, Mackerras DEM: Vitamin A supplementation in infectious diseases; a meta-analysis. Br Med J 1989;306:366–370.

56. Hemila H, Herman ZS: Vitamin C and the common cold: a retrospective analysis of Chalmers' review. J Am Coll Nutr 1995;14:116–123.

57. Gaby SK, Singh VN: Vitamin C. In Gaby SK, Bendich A, Singh VN et al (eds): Vitamin Intake and Health. New York: Marcel Dekker, 1991:103–161.

58. Meydani SN, Hayek M, Coleman L: Influence of vitamin E and B₆ on immune response. Ann NY Acad Sci 1992;669:125–140.

59. Kiremidjian-Schumacher L, Roy M, Wishe HI et al: Supplementation with selenium and human immune cell functions — effect on cytotoxic lymphocytes and natural killer cells. Biol Trace Elem Res 1994;41:115–127.

60. Roy M, Kiremidjian-Schumacher L, Wishe HI et al: Supplementation with selenium and human immune cell functions — effect on lymphocyte proliferation and interleukin 2 receptor expression. Biol Trace Elem Res 1994;41:103–114.

61. Shenkin A: Trace elements and inflammatory response: implications for nutritional support. Nutrition 1995;11:100–105.

62. Schroeder JJ, Cousins RJ: Interleukin 6 regulates metallothionein gene expression and zinc metabolism in hepatocyte monolayer cultures. Proc Nat Acad Sci USA 1990;87:3137–3141.

63. Konjin AM, Carmel N, Levy R et al: Ferritin snythesis in inflammation. II. Mechanisms of increased ferritin synthesis. Br J Haematol 1981;49:361–370.

64. Fleck A: Plasma proteins as nutritional indicators in the perioperative period. Br J Clin Pract 1988;42(suppl 63):20–24.

65. Olson JA: New approaches to methods for the assessment of nutritional status of the individual. Am J Clin Nutr 1982;36:1160–1168.

66. Malone M, Shenkin A, Fell GS et al: Evaluation of a trace element preparation in patients receiving home intravenous nutrition. Clin Nutr 1989;8:307–312.

67. Louw JA, Werbeck A, Louw MEJ et al: Blood vitamin concentrations during the acute phase response. Crit Care Med 1992;20:934–937.

68. Fidanza F: Nutritional Status Assessment. London: Chapman & Hall, 1991.

69. Goode HF, Kelleher J, Walker BE: The effects of acute infection on indices of zinc status. Clin Nutr 1991;10:55–59.

70. Schorah CJ, Habibzadeh N, Hancock M et al: Changes in plasma and buffy layer vitamin C concentration following major surgery: what do they reflect? Ann Clin Biochem 1986;23:566–570.

71. Klug A, Rhodes D: Zinc fingers. Trends Biochem Sci 1987;121:464–469.

72. Fraker PJ, Gershwin ME, Good RA et al: Interrelationship between zinc and immune function. Fed Proc 1986;45:1474–1479.

73. Rosenberg IH, Solomons NW: Biological availability of minerals and trace elements: a nutritional overview. Am J Clin Nutr 1982;35:781–782.

74. Karpel JT, Peden VH: Copper deficiency in long-term parenteral nutrition. J Pediatr 1972;80:32–36.

75. Dunlap WM, James GW, Hume DM: Anaemia and neutropenia caused by copper deficiency. Ann Intern Med 1974;80:470–476.

76. Vinton N, Dahlstrom K, Strobel C et al: Macrocytosis and pseudoalbinism: manifestations of selenium deficiency. J Pediatr 1988;111:711–717.

77. Friedman BJ, Freeland-Graves JH, Bales CW et al: Manganese balance and clinical observations in young men fed a manganese deficient diet. J Nutr 1987;117:133–343.

78. Anderson RA: Recent advances in the role of chromium in human health and disease. In Prasad AS (ed): Essential and Toxic Trace Elements in Human Health and Disease. New York: Alan R. Liss, 1988:189–197.

79. Jeejeebhoy KN, Chu RC, Marliss EB et al: Chromium deficiency, glucose intolerance and neuropathy reversed by chromium supplementation in a patient receiving long-term parenteral nutrition. Am J Clin Nutr 1977;30:531–538.

80. Abumrad NN, Schneider AJ, Steel D et al: Amino acid intolerance reversed by molybdate therapy. Am J Clin Nutr 1981;34:2551–2559.

81. Watson NJ, Hutchinson CH, Atta HR: Vitamin A deficiency and xerophthalmia in the United Kingdom. Br Med J 1995;310:1050–1051.

82. Main ANH, Mills PR, Russell RI et al: Vitamin A deficiency in Crohn's disease. Gut 1983;24:1169–1175.

83. Manolagas SC, Hustmeyer FG, Yu XP: 1,25 dihydroxy vitamin D_3 and the immune system. Proc Soc Exp Biol Med 1989;191:238–245.

84. Ritchie JH, Fish MB, McMasters V et al: Edema and haemolytic anemia in premature infants: a vitamin E deficiency syndrome. N Engl J Med 1968;279:1185–1190.

85. Howard L, Oversen L, Satya-Marti S et al: Reversible neurological symptoms caused by vitamin E deficiency in a patient with short bowel syndrome. Am J Clin Nutr 1982;36:1243–1249.

86. Bieri JG, Farrell PM: Vitamin E. Vit Horm 1976;34:31–75.

87. La Selve P, Demolin P, Holzapfel L et al: Shoshin beriberi: an unusual complication of prolonged parenteral nutrition. J Parenter Ent Nutr 1986;10:102–103.

88. Nadel AM, Burger PC: Wernicke encephalopathy following prolonged intravenous therapy. JAMA 1976;235:2403–2405.

89. Chandra RK: Immunology of Nutritional Disorders. London: Edward Arnold, 1980:1–110.

90. Duhamel JF, Ricour C, Dufier JL et al: Deficit en vitamin B_2 et nutrition parenteral exclusive. Arch Fr Pediat 1979;36:342–346.

91. Gaby SK: Vitamin B_6. In Gaby SK, Bendich A, Singh VN et al (eds): Vitamin Intake and Health. New York: Marcel Dekker, 1991:163–174.

92. Tennant GB, Smith RC, Leinster SJ et al: Amino acid infusion induced depression of serum folate after cholecystectomy. Scand J Hematol 1981;27:333–338.

93. Czeizel AE, Dudas I: Prevention of the first occurrence of neural-tube defects by periconceptional vitamin supplementation. N Engl J Med 1992;327:1832–1835.

94. Innis SM, Allardyce DB: Possible biotin deficiency in adults receiving long-term total parenteral nutrition. Am J Clin Nutr 1983;37:185–187.

95. Stabler SP, Marcell PD, Podell ER et al: Assay of methylmalonic acid in the serum of patients with cobalamin deficiency using capillary gas chromatography-mass spectrometry. J Clin Invest 1986;7:1606–1612.

96. Stabler SP, Marcell PD, Podell ER et al: Elevation of total homocysteine in the serum of patients with cobalamin or folate deficiency detected by capillary gas chromatography mass spectrometry. J Clin Invest 1988;81:466–474.

97. Naurath HJ, Joosten E, Riezler R et al: Effects of vitamin B_{12}, folate, and vitamin B_6 supplements in elderly people with normal serum vitamin concentrations. Lancet 1995;346:85–89.

98. Fidanza F: Nutritional Status Assessment. London: Chapman & Hall, 1991.

8

Therapeutic Effects of Specific Nutrients

THOMAS R. ZIEGLER
LORRAINE S. YOUNG

Specialized enteral and parenteral nutrition support is now routine in pediatric and adult clinical care. Providing adequate calories, proteins, fats, and micronutrients in currently available nutrient solutions clearly benefits patients with severe protein-energy malnutrition (PEM), prolonged catabolic illness, and specific micronutrient deficiency states. Classic nutrient deficiencies in patients receiving appropriate enteral or parenteral nutrition are now rare. Further, body protein losses are attenuated with nutrition support compared with responses in patients receiving limited or no dietary intake.[1] The beneficial effects of enteral feeding documented in animal models and in selected patient groups have led to a marked increase in the use of enteral nutrient products and tube feedings in hospitalized patients.[2-4]

An increasing number of therapeutic strategies designed to enhance the efficacy of enteral and parenteral nutritional support are undergoing clinical investigation. These include studies on the potential use of early enteral feeding in critically ill patients, use of recombinant growth factors and conditionally essential amino acids, administration of biologic response modifiers, provision of nutrient antioxidants, and combinations of these strategies. Many of these approaches are specifically designed to maintain or improve intestinal ab-

sorptive, digestive, immunologic, and barrier function. The list of specific nutrients and metabolites being evaluated in recent clinical nutrition studies is growing (Table 8–1). Many of the published clinical trials have provided these nutrients in parenteral nutrition solutions; however, a number of studies have investigated enteral products enriched with one or more specific nutrients. Although data are limited, the use of enteral diets enriched in the specific nutrients outlined in Table 8–1 may be more efficacious than use of enriched parenteral formulas. Compared with parenteral feedings, enteral feedings are associated with improved intestinal mucosal cellularity, increased number of immune cells, and augmented gut barrier function. Enteral diets also may provide a more "balanced" nutrient mix and contain potentially important gut-trophic substrates such as fiber, polyamines, and small peptides.

The metabolic and clinical effects of specific nutrient administration are undoubtedly affected by multiple variables in individual patients, including age, sex, underlying illnesses, general nutritional status, degree of whole-body nutrient deficiency, and the quantity and quality of substrate and micronutrient provision. This chapter will focus primarily on important clinical findings from studies in adults evaluating diets enriched with arginine, gluta-

TABLE 8–1 Specific Nutrients and Metabolites Evaluated in Recent Clinical Nutrition Research

Amino Acids
Arginine
Branched-chain amino acids
Cysteine
Dipeptides (e.g., L-alanyl-L-glutamine)
Glutamine
Glutathione

Lipids
Fish oils (omega-3 fatty acids)
Short-chain fatty acids
Short- and medium-chain triglycerides
Structured lipids

Carbohydrates
Xylitol and other alternative carbohydrate sources

Micronutrients
Nutrient antioxidants
Zinc

Miscellaneous
Ornithine-alpha ketoglutarate
α-ketoglutarate
Nucleotides
Soluble and insoluble dietary fibers

mine, and specific lipid products. Data on other selected nutrient metabolites currently undergoing clinical investigation will be briefly highlighted.

SPECIFIC AMINO ACIDS

Arginine

Arginine, originally classified by Rose as a semiessential amino acid,[5] is an intermediary metabolite in the urea cycle, where it is hydrolyzed to urea and ornithine by the enzyme arginase. As a component of the urea cycle, arginine is indirectly linked to the citric acid cycle and the oxidation of fuel molecules for energy. Conversion to ornithine explains arginine's role in the production of polyamines, which are key molecules involved in cellular growth and differentiation. In addition, L-arginine is a critical substrate for in vivo and in vitro nitric oxide (NO) production through conversion to citrulline by the arginine deaminase pathway.[6] Endogenous arginine is thus involved in key pathways of nitrogen and fuel metabolism and nitrogen excretion from the body. Arginine's role in NO production is apparently critical to the body's homeostatic mechanisms, because NO appears to be a major regulator of the vascular endothelium as a vasodilator and is involved in macrophage physiology, among other cellular functions.[7] Arginine is a known secretagogue for several peptide hormones, including growth hormone (GH), insulin, prolactin, and glucagon, although the magnitude and importance of this effect in normal physiology is unclear.

A large number of animal studies suggest that the arginine-supplemented enteral feeding has trophic effects on immune cell number or function. In addition to these immunostimulatory effects, arginine-enriched diets attenuate thymic atrophy,[8] improve animal survival to septic challenge,[9] and enhance wound healing (Table 8–2).[10,11] However, several studies of oral arginine supplementation in rodents have failed to demonstrate significant effects on animal survival after experimental burn injury or peritonitis.[12,13]

Human data on arginine's potential benefits are limited; however, several published studies suggest that arginine may be an important dietary component in catabolic patients, primarily as an immune-stimulating agent and also in wound healing (Table 8–3). Data in animals suggested that arginine was required for optimal nitrogen balance in young, more rapidly growing rats but nonessential for nitrogen retention in adult rats.[5] In 1978, Elsair and colleagues described a 60 percent reduction in nitrogen excretion with intravenous arginine administration (15 g/day) after cholecystectomy compared with control subjects not receiving arginine.[14] Modest improvements in nitrogen retention (≈ 2 to 3 g/day difference) in postop-

TABLE 8–2 Some Beneficial Effects of Arginine-Enriched Enteral Diets Observed in Animal Models

Reduced mortality after bacterial/septic challenge
Increased survival of tumor-bearing animals, associated with reduced tumor size
Increased survival after thermal burn injury; improved local bacterial containment with subcutaneous bacterial inoculation
Enhanced bacterial killing after bacterial translocation in burn/septic states
Improved delayed cutaneous hypersensitivity reactions
Increased thymic size and cellularity
Increased natural killer cell and macrophage lysis of tumor targets
Increased lymphocyte interleukin-2 production
Enhanced lymphocyte proliferation to mitogens and alloantigens
Moderate improvement in nitrogen retention

TABLE 8–3   Effects of Oral Arginine Supplements in Healthy, Elderly Subjects in a Randomized, Double-Blind Trial

	Arginine Aspartate (30 g/day × 14 days)	Placebo (Excipient × 14 days)
Number of subjects	30	15
Age (yrs)	74.3 ± 0.8	72.2 ± 0.8
Wound hydroxyproline (nmol/cm)	26 ± 2	17 ± 2†
Wound protein content (µg/cm)	43 ± 4	22 ± 2‡
Wound DNA content (µg/cm)	25 ± 3	30 ± 4
Wound epithelialization (days)	12.6 ± 0.4	12.5 ± 0.6
Lymphocyte ConA response (cpm)	70,000 ± 10,000	40,000 ± 3000*
Blood urea nitrogen (mg/dl)	24 ± 1	18 ± 1†
Serum IGF-I (ng/ml)	203 ± 18	140 ± 18*

IGF-I = insulin-like growth factor-I.
Mean ± SE.
*$P < 0.05$.
†$P < 0.03$.
‡$P < 0.01$.
Data from Kirk SJ, Hurson M, Regan MC et al: Arginine stimulates wound healing and immune function in elderly human subjects. Surgery 1993;114:155–160.

erative patients were observed when jejunal tube feedings were supplemented with L-arginine (25 g/day) vs isonitrogenous supplementation with oral L-glycine.[15]

Consistent improvement in immune function tests and wound healing has been noted with enteral arginine administration in humans. In 1981, Barbul and coworkers reported that normal volunteers given 30 g of arginine HCl orally for 7 days demonstrated a significant increase in peripheral blood lymphocyte blastogenic responses to concanavalin A (Con A) by 3.7-fold and phytohemagglutinin (PHA) by 3.6-fold.[16] No effect of L-arginine was noted on total circulating lymphocyte counts or on B- and T-cell ratios in this study.[16]

In a randomized, double-blind, prospective trial, Daly and coworkers evaluated the immune and metabolic effects of L-arginine (25 g/day) or isonitrogenous L-glycine added to enteral feeding solutions given by needle-catheter jejunostomy for 7 days postoperatively in 30 elderly patients with gastrointestinal (GI) malignancies.[15] Immune parameters were measured preoperatively and on days 1, 4, and 7 postoperatively. The L-arginine-supplemented group demonstrated significantly increased plasma arginine levels by day 7 (from a preoperative value of 87 µM to 213 µM postoperatively). In addition, enteral arginine administration significantly increased plasma ornithine levels (≈ fourfold). No differences in infection rates were noted in this short-term trial; however, supplemental arginine significantly enhanced mean T-lymphocyte responses to the mitogens PHA

and Con-A vs control group responses on postoperative days 4 and 7.[15]

Arginine supplementation also increased the CD-4 phenotype 1.7-fold by postoperative day 7, compared with no CD-4 response over time in the controls. Arginine administration had no effect on other phenotype subsets, including total T-cells, CD-8 cells, or the CD-4:CD-8 ratio. Insulinlike growth factor-I (IGF-I) levels were approximately 50 percent higher in the arginine group by day 7.[15] The increase in serum IGF-I reflects arginine's known effects as a growth hormone (GH) secretagogue. GH, IGF-I, and prolactin appear to mediate beneficial anabolic and immune responses in humans;[17] thus, arginine's secretagogue effect on secretion of these peptide hormones may represent an important mechanism of immunostimulation by this amino acid.

In a study focusing on the effects of oral arginine on experimental wound healing, Barbul and coworkers studied healthy adults with subcutaneously implanted polytetrafluoroethylene tubing inserted into the deltoid region.[18] The subjects were randomized into three groups and given either 30 g of arginine HCl (24.8 g of free arginine); 30 g of arginine aspartate (17 g of free arginine), or placebo daily for 2 weeks at home with an uncontrolled ad libitum diet. Mitogenic responses of peripheral blood lymphocytes to PHA and ConA were assessed at baseline and after 2 weeks. The hydroxyproline content in the polytetrafluoroethylene tubes was assessed after 2 weeks as an index of collagen formation and wound healing.[18] Both arginine-supplemented groups demonstrated significantly enhanced hydroxyproline concentrations in the experimental wounds, and a greater response occurred with oral arginine HCl (control 10.1 ± 2.3 nmol/cm vs arginine aspartate 17.6 ± 2.2 and vs 23.8 ± 2.2 with arginine HCl; both P < 0.03 vs control). Both arginine regimens significantly increased lymphocyte blastogenic responses to PHA and ConA vs the controls.[18]

A similar randomized, double-blind protocol was performed by Kirk and colleagues in healthy elderly adults.[19] The experimental subjects (15 men and 15 women, mean age 74 years) were given 30 g of arginine aspartate (17 g of free arginine) dissolved in 60 ml of aromatic syrup daily for 14 days; age-matched control patients (9 men and 6 women, mean age 72 years) received placebo consisting of the excipient syrup. Subcutaneously placed deltoid polytetrafluoroethylene tubes were assessed for nitrogen, DNA, and hydroxyproline content; 2- × 2-cm split-thickness wounds were also created on the upper thigh to evaluate skin reepithelialization. Peripheral blood mitogenic responses were also assessed before and after the 14 days of treatment.[19]

In these elderly, healthy subjects, oral arginine supplementation significantly enhanced wound catheter hydroxyproline content (an index of collagen deposition) and protein content but did not significantly alter cellularity as measured by DNA content in the tubing. Furthermore, arginine supplementation did not significantly influence wound epithelialization (Table 8–3). The blastogenic response to a panel of lymphocyte mitogens was significantly enhanced with arginine compared with control group responses, and this group also demonstrated a significant increase in the mixed lymphocyte response to allogeneic stimulation by donor lymphocytes. As in previous studies, oral arginine increased plasma IGF-I levels (Table 8–3). The arginine-treated patients demonstrated a slight but significant rise in blood urea nitrogen and a slight fall in serum potassium levels but no adverse clinical effects to arginine. Thus, in this trial, oral arginine specifically enhanced wound collagen synthesis (fibroblast mediated) and protein content but not wound cellularity or reepithelialization.[19] The upregulation of mitogenic T-cell responses and IGF-I levels is consistent with arginine's effects in young healthy patients, and suggest potentially beneficial roles for arginine supplementation in the elderly, who demonstrate decreased T-cell number and function and reduced serum IGF-I levels.[17,19]

Several animal studies indicate that arginine-supplemented intravenous (IV) solutions also improve immune cell responses and indexes of wound healing.[20,21] In the only study reported to date on immune effects of IV arginine in humans, Sigal and colleagues gave 30 patients either 20 g/day of parenteral arginine or a mixed isonitrogenous amino acid solution (providing 3.7 g of arginine/day) for 7 days to cancer patients after major GI operations.[22] A small amount of dextrose calories (40 g/day) was also administered in each group. No differences in nitrogen balance were observed, and each group demonstrated marked nitrogen loss (≈ 9 g/day). The mononuclear cell response to mitogens decreased in each of the groups on day 1 postoperatively but returned to baseline levels by day 7. The mitogenic response to PHA and IL-2 was greater in the mixed amino acid group on day 4 after operation; however, the mean total number of circulating T-cells increased in the arginine group on day 7. In general, this study did not document improved indexes of immunity in these patients with IV arginine vs a more balanced amino acid mixture.[22] Thus, it is possible that arginine must be administered with an adequate substrate background to exert beneficial effects. Arginine may interact with other nutrients provided in an otherwise balanced diet to affect immune responses (see discussion on use in combination therapy below).

Arginine supplementation has been well tolerated in humans at doses up to 30 g/day for several weeks. In our hospital, we occasionally supplement enteral feedings or dietary liquids with L-arginine powder (10 to 30 g/day) in patients with large wounds or those with severe immunosuppression. However, no controlled data are available to define the efficacy of diets supplemented with arginine as a single nutrient in catabolic patients. One potential complication of arginine administration is its known competition with the essential amino acid lysine for tubular reabsorption.[23] Thus, large doses of arginine may induce lysine deficiency by increasing the renal excretion of this amino acid. An additional potential complication relates to the risk of worsening metabolic acidosis in patients receiving the acidic arginine salts enterally (intravenous amino acid solutions are routinely buffered by acetate). As a contribution to the total amino acid load, supplemental arginine may contribute to azotemia in individuals with compromised renal function. Although L-arginine is required for NO synthesis[6,7] and thus may potentially affect vascular tone, no adverse effects on blood pressure or hemodynamic stability have been reported in humans with enteral or parenteral arginine administration in nutrient infusions to date.

Branched-Chain Amino Acids

Branched-chain amino acids (BCAAs) comprise about 35 percent of the total essential amino acids and 14 percent of skeletal muscle amino acids in humans. In the postabsorptive state a significant proportion of skeletal muscle amino acid uptake is accounted for by BCAAs.[24] Interest in BCAAs in nutrition initially derived from studies performed in vitro or in animal models suggesting that BCAAs (especially leucine) or their ketoacids have a regulatory and anabolic role in protein metabolism by increasing rates of skeletal muscle protein synthesis or decreasing rates of protein degradation. Also, patients with hepatic failure demonstrate decreased circulating BCAA and accumulation of aromatic amino acids (phenylalanine, tyrosine, and tryptophan) and methionine in the blood. An increased aromatic amino acid:BCAA ratio may increase tryptophan uptake across the blood-brain barrier and contribute to increased cerebral serotonin levels, precipitating or worsening encephalopathy. Thus, providing amino acid solutions designed to correct this imbalance was suggested as a method to improve hepatic encephalopathy and enhance nitrogen balance.[24,25]

Although enteral products enriched with BCAAs are used routinely in hospital settings, little human data on the efficacy of these diets are available.[13] Mochozuki and associates published a trial in burned guinea pigs indicating no beneficial effect of enteral BCAA on protein metabolism but worsened animal survival.[26] Two Japanese trials of oral BCAA supplements in patients with hepatic cirrhosis indicated improved nitrogen balance and increased circulating proteins with BCAA, in association with increased plasma BCAA levels.[27,28] Recently, Ferrando and coworkers[29] studied the acute effects on protein metabolism in healthy volunteers with oral BCAA taken as a one-time drink (5.2 g of leucine, 2.6 g of isoleucine, and 3.2 g of valine with 50 g of carbohydrate) vs controls ingesting an isonitrogenous, isocaloric amount of essential amino acids (threonine, histidine, and methionine with carbohydrate). No changes in protein synthesis or breakdown occurred with oral BCAAs, and net leg balance of phenylalanine was unchanged. However, whole-body phenylalanine flux was slightly, but significantly, reduced with the oral BCAAs (by 27 percent vs 15 percent with the control drink). Thus, oral BCAAs acutely suppressed whole-body proteolysis in tissues other than skeletal muscle.[29] Nonetheless, due to the paucity of efficacy data and randomized, controlled trials, the role of BCAA-supplemented enteral nutrition in catabolic patients and in other clinical settings remains unclear.

BCAA-enriched parenteral nutrition has been fairly extensively investigated as a method to improve nitrogen retention in critical illness and as therapy in patients with hepatic encephalopathy. Standard amino acid solutions provide 18 to 23 percent of amino acids as BCAAs, and the BCAA-enriched formulations provide 36 to 46 percent of total protein as BCAAs. Initial studies showed decreased hepatic encephalopathy in cirrhosis[24,25] and improved nitrogen retention in sepsis[30] with BCAA-enriched parenteral solutions (35 to 45 percent of AA as BCAA). The results of a meta-analysis of randomized clinical trials of BCAA-enriched parenteral nutrition in hepatic encephalopathy (up to 1988) were published by Naylor and colleagues in 1989.[31] The authors concluded that slight, but significant, improvements in hepatic encephalopathy may occur in cirrhotic patients given parenteral BCAA-enriched solutions, which may thus allow larger amounts of protein to be administered.

However, effects on mortality are discrepant among the trials, which were primarily short-term studies.[31] The recently published clinical guidelines of the American Society for Parenteral and Enteral Nutrition suggest that BCAA-enriched enteral or parenteral formulas should be used in patients with hepatic encephalopathy only when, despite standard medical care (lactulose or neomycin), the encephalopathy makes it impossible to provide adequate protein to the patient.[2]

Recent, randomized trials in catabolic and critically ill patients without hepatic disease comparing BCAA-enriched parenteral nutrition vs standard parenteral formulas showed no significant clinical outcome or metabolic differences.[32-34] The American Society for Parenteral and Enteral Nutrition clinical guidelines state that because proven effects on clinical outcomes are lacking, BCAA-supplemented diets cannot be routinely advocated during critical illness.[2] No adverse effects specifically attributable to the BCAA component of enteral or parenteral diets have been described in the adult studies published to date.

Glutamine

Glutamine (GLN), which has classically been considered a nonessential amino acid, has received increasing attention as a potentially beneficial amino acid during various catabolic states.[35] Data are now available to support the concept that GLN is conditionally essential in certain catabolic states.[36,37] Thus, GLN may expand the list of several other amino acids believed to be semiessential or conditionally essential in human nutrition, including histidine, arginine, taurine, and cysteine.[38,39]

GLN is the most abundant free amino acid in plasma, skeletal muscle, and the human body as a whole.[40] GLN exhibits dynamic interorgan metabolism, particularly between skeletal muscle and the splanchnic bed and kidney,[41,42] and plays an important physiologic role in several key metabolic processes (Table 8–4). The small intestine extracts 25 to 30 percent of circulating GLN in the postabsorptive state; thus intestinal tissues are perhaps the major user of circulating GLN.[41]

The intestinal uptake of GLN increases with operative trauma and corticosteroid administration, but gut GLN uptake in animals and in humans is inhibited during sepsis or endotoxemia.[43] Numerous studies have described a state consistent with relative GLN depletion during catabolic illness. GLN concentrations in plasma, and especially skeletal muscle pools, may decrease markedly during various catabolic states, including sepsis, burns, or trauma.[43-45] Glutamine efflux from skeletal muscle and lung increases during stress and illness. In animal models and postoperative humans, a relationship exists between GLN concentrations and rates of muscle protein synthesis and breakdown.[46,47] In addition, it is now recognized that GLN is a major fuel of the intestinal mucosa and other rapidly replicating cells, and its use appears to be concentration dependent.[48-50]

Dietary GLN requirements appear to increase markedly during certain catabolic states because cellular requirements of the primary GLN-utilizing tissues (intestinal and immune cells, kidney, and perhaps other tissues such as wounds) are increased.[35-37] GLN use by body tissues apparently exceeds endogenous GLN production from skeletal muscle and liver during catabolic illness, even during provision of standard enteral and parenteral feeding. GLN deficiency may develop if the increased GLN requirements of GLN-utilizing tissues are not met by adequate dietary provision of GLN; however, standard parenteral feedings do not contain GLN, and only a few enteral products are GLN enriched. Reduced GLN concentration in intracellular and plasma pools appears to be coupled with altered structure and function of the key tissues that synthesize or use GLN (e.g., skeletal muscle breakdown and weakness, gut mucosal atrophy, and immune cell dysfunction may develop).[35-37] Net catabolism of skeletal muscle with GLN efflux may increase, in part, to provide increased quantities of GLN for certain tissues.

Numerous factors other than the dietary content or tissue bioavailability of GLN interact during catabolic states to induce tissue damage and facilitate tissue repair. However, if GLN is conditionally essential, then dietary supplementation of GLN during catabolic states may improve structure and function of organs and tissues that are able to use GLN for important metabolic processes.

Animal Studies of GLN-Enriched Feeding

The potential use of GLN-enriched nutrition has been defined by a large number of studies in animals performed over the past decade. Although several negative studies of both enteral and parenteral GLN therapy have been published,[51-54] at least 80 percent of the reported data in animal models demonstrate positive effects of GLN-enriched feeding (Table 8–5). Beneficial effects on protein metabolism, intestinal and pancreatic growth, repair, and regeneration, nutrient absorption, gut barrier function, systemic and intestinal immune cell number and function, and animal survival occurred with GLN-supplemented nutrition compared with isonitrogenous, isocaloric control diets containing little or no GLN.[35] GLN has been provided at doses equivalent to about 25 percent or more of administered amino acid nitrogen; thus GLN has been supplemented in rela-

TABLE 8–4 Important Metabolic Functions of Glutamine

Major substrate for gluconeogenesis
Interorgan nitrogen and carbon transport
Essential precursor for nucleotide synthesis
Constituent amino acid in synthesis of body
  proteins
Substrate for renal ammoniagenesis
Stimulation of glycogen synthesis
Regulator of protein synthetic and breakdown rates
Important metabolic fuel source for rapidly
  replicating cells

TABLE 8–5 Beneficial Effects Reported with Enteral or Parenteral Glutamine Supplementation in Animal Models

Enteral GLN Supplementation

Improved nitrogen retention

Reduced skeletal muscle protein breakdown during chronic acidosis

Enhanced intestinal mucosal cellularity, decreased pancreatic atrophy, and reduced hepatic steatosis during elemental enteral feeding

Improved gut mucosal repair and decreased bacterial translocation after irradiation or chemotherapy

Maintained gut mucosal cellularity and decreased bacterial translocation in experimental sepsis

Improved survival after chemotherapy, irradiation, or experimental sepsis

Reduced ulceration and enhanced mucosal repair in experimental colitis

Increased intestinal adaptation in experimental short-bowel syndrome

Enhanced growth and nutrient absorption in transplanted small intestine

Enhanced water and electrolyte absorption across inflamed small bowel

Increased gastric healing in acetylsalicylate-induced mucosal injury

Upregulated hepatic IGF-I mRNA content in experimental short-bowel syndrome

Parenteral GLN Supplementation

Improved nitrogen retention, increased protein synthesis, and reduced protein degradation in catabolic illness models

Maintenance of intracellular GLN concentrations (muscle, intestine)

Enhanced intestinal mucosal cellularity, decreased pancreatic atrophy, and reduced hepatic steatosis during parenteral feeding

Improved gut mucosal repair and decreased bacterial translocation after irradiation or chemotherapy

Maintained gut mucosal cellularity and decreased bacterial translocation in experimental sepsis

Improved survival after chemotherapy, irradiation, or experimental sepsis

Maintained or improved intestinal and systemic immune functions during parenteral feeding

---

tively large amounts to achieve beneficial effects.

Human Studies of GLN-Enriched Feeding: Enteral Route

Despite the large number of animal trials published concerning benefits of GLN-enriched enteral and parenteral feeding, relatively little human data are available on the efficacy of GLN in human nutrition. Several trials in patients have reported positive metabolic or clin-

ical effects with parenteral administration of GLN or GLN dipeptides. However, surprisingly little data on the clinical effects of enteral diets enriched in GLN have been published to date, although a number of trials are in progress. Multiple methods are now available for GLN supplementation in human nutrition (Table 8–6). Thus, the efficacy and cost effectiveness of both enteral and parenteral GLN in specific patient groups will likely become defined within the next several years.

L-glutamine-enriched nutrient formulas for enteral use are now commercially available. These products appear to be very well tolerated under a variety of clinical conditions. They offer a theoretical advantage over parenteral GLN-containing diets because they provide GLN directly to the gut mucosa and splanchnic tissue and, in animal models, exert similar metabolic and clinical effects as intravenous GLN. Enteral GLN administration may confer other advantages related to use of enteral vs intravenous feeding, including better gut mucosal structure and function due to trophic effects of enteral diets per se. Disadvantages of enteral L-GLN products relates to their instability in solution, which necessitates storage in powder form with reconstitution into solution just before delivery. In addition, there are little human efficacy data published, and the current enteral products remain very expensive at present (five to 10 times the cost of standard enteral formulations).

The safety and metabolic effects of enteral L-GLN administration in healthy adults has been documented.[55] In addition, no untoward effects of L-GLN-enriched tube feedings (which provide up to 28 percent of protein intake as L-GLN) have been described. In healthy male subjects, L-GLN doses of 0.1 and 0.3 g/kg were given as an oral bolus, without objective or sub-

TABLE 8–6 Methods of Glutamine Provision in Nutrition Support

---

Parenteral L-GLN-enriched amino acid solutions

Parenteral GLN-dipeptide enriched amino acid solutions

Enteral L-GLN-supplemented liquid formulas

L-GLN powder as a dietary supplement in drinks or in enteral nutrient solutions

Parenteral or enteral provision of GLN analogs or substrates for GLN synthesis (ornithine α-ketoglutarate, α-ketoglutarate)

Future development of GLN-containing peptides for enteral use

---

jective evidence of toxicity. Whole blood concentrations of GLN rose in proportion to the administered oral GLN load (Table 8–7). Blood GLN levels peaked 30 to 45 minutes following GLN ingestion (to approximately double the baseline values with 0.3 g/kg) and then steadily declined to the normal range within 90 to 120 minutes (low dose) or 180 to 240 minutes (high dose).[55] Whole blood levels of glutamate and ammonia tended to rise in proportion to GLN dose, but these values were not significantly different from those with water ingestion alone.

Administration of oral GLN resulted in a significant dose-related increase in known amino acid end products of intestinal GLN metabolism in blood, including alanine, citrulline, and arginine (Table 8–7). It is known that arginine is produced through conversion of citrulline in the kidney, and integrated responses of citrulline and arginine after oral L-GLN bolus were highly correlated (r = 0.697; $P < 0.001$). Interestingly, total and individual plasma BCAAs fell significantly, possibly due to insulin release with oral GLN.[55] The basal to peak concentrations of glucagon were positively correlated to the oral L-GLN dose (r = 0.593; $P < 0.01$). Plasma peak growth hormone levels also rose with increasing oral L-GLN doses (zero GLN 11 ± 4 ng/ml vs 0.1 g of GLN 15 ± 6 vs 0.3 g GLN 26 ± 7; $P < 0.085$). The estimated splanchnic uptake of oral GLN in the high dose study was approximately 84 percent of the oral load, vs extraction of approximately 57 percent with the 0.1 g/kg dose, suggesting induction of splanchnic bed glutaminase with increasing oral GLN loads in humans.[55]

Jensen and associates recently published a preliminary report on metabolic effects of a commercially available elemental L-GLN-enriched tube feeding formula in critically ill patients.[56] Arterial and venous amino acids and lymphocyte subsets in peripheral blood were assessed in 28 ICU patients randomized to receive 10 days of isocaloric, isonitrogenous tube feeds that differed sixfold in GLN content. Nasojejunal feeds were begun in a double-blind fashion within 48 hours after ICU admission. Plasma GLN was below normal in both groups on beginning tube feeding and tended to rise (NS) in the group receiving GLN-enriched enteral nutrition. The phenylalanine:tyrosine ratio, an indicator of the protein catabolic response, was elevated in both groups at entry (1.3 to 1.4), but this ratio fell significantly by day 5 of feeding only in the L-GLN supplemented group (control 1.4 vs GLN 1.1; $P < 0.05$).[56] Further, the patients receiving GLN-supplemented tube feeding demonstrated a significantly greater rise in the helper T-cell (CD-4)/suppressor T-cell (CD-8) ratio from day 1 to day 5 than the control patients (controls 3.3 vs GLN 2.6 on day 1; controls 3.8 vs GLN 6.0 on day 5; $P < 0.05$).[56] Thus, it is possible that L-GLN-enriched tube feedings decreased body protein catabolism, as evidenced by altered plasma amino acid profiles, and favorably improved immune cell parameters in this trial. No clinical outcome data were reported in this short-term trial.

In another recent preliminary report, Buchman and colleagues studied eight healthy adults who received standard central venous parenteral nutrition for 14 days followed by 5 days of nasogastric tube feedings.[57] Four subjects received a commercially available elemental L-GLN-enriched tube feeding and the other four a standard polymeric tube feeding. Small-bowel biopsies were obtained on day 1 (before PN), day 14, and day 17, after the 5 days of tube feeds. Intestinal permeability was measured after the parenteral and enteral feeding periods. Parenteral nutrition was associated with decreased small-bowel mucosal thickness and abnormally elevated gut permeability; these changes were reversed to normal with 5

TABLE 8–7 Integrated Responses for Whole Blood Amino Acids After Oral L-GLN Bolus Ingestion in Healthy Adult Subjects

GLN Dose	GLN	Alanine	Citrulline	Arginine	Total BCAA
Zero g/kg	4.4 ± 5.2	−2.2 ± 2.1	−0.2 ± 0.4	−0.1 ± 0.2	0.5 ± 1.1
0.1 g/kg	36.3 ± 6.8	2.5 ± 4.1	1.1 ± 0.3	1.5 ± 0.3	−1.7 ± 1.6
0.3 g/kg	72.6 ± 12.7	9.0 ± 3.3	1.9 ± 0.4	2.1 ± 0.2	−6.0 ± 1.3
P value	0.001	0.025	0.001	0.001	0.013

Mean ± SE as $\mu M \times 4$ hour $\times 10^3$.
Data from Ziegler TR, Benfell K, Smith RJ et al: Safety and metabolic effects of L-glutamine administration in humans. J Parenter Enter Nutr 1990;14(suppl 4):137S–146S.

days of enteral refeeding. However, no additional benefit of GLN-enriched enteral feeding was observed.[57] Increased circulating immunoglobulins IgA, IgG, and IgM occurred with parenteral feeding, without a change in gut mucosal production of these immunoglobulin produced by histochemistry. Enteral feeding had no effect on immunoglobulin levels in blood or gut mucosal, and no differences were noted between the two types of enteral formulas.[57] It is likely that the small sample sizes in this trial lacked sufficient power to detect differences, if any exist, in the types of enteral feeds provided. Also, the metabolic and gut use of GLN in these healthy individuals may differ from catabolic states in which GLN may become conditionally essential.

In a novel trial of GLN administration, Wischmeyer and colleagues studied the efficacy of L-glutamine-containing suppositories on mucosal healing in patients with chronic pouchitis after ileal-anal anastomosis.[58] In this unblinded trial patients with chronic pouchitis were removed from conventional therapy (antibiotics, corticosteroids, anti-inflammatory agents). They were then treated with suppositories containing L-GLN (1 g of L-GLN in a polyethylene glycol base) or 40 mmol of sodium butyrate twice daily for 21 days. During treatment, six of 10 patients treated with L-GLN suppositories had no recurrence of symptoms, but only three of nine patients receiving butyrate suppositories responded similarly.[58] This interesting pilot study suggests that administration of GLN locally to the mucosa may exert beneficial effects in states of intestinal inflammation in humans. Further investigation to determine the potential metabolic and clinical efficacy of GLN given enterally (or by other routes such as enema or suppository) is warranted in well-defined patient subsets.

Human Studies of GLN-Enriched Feeding: Parenteral Route

An increasing number of studies have documented benefits of parenteral nutrient solutions enriched with either free L-GLN or various GLN-dipeptides, which are now commercially available in Europe (Table 8–8). There are a number of potential advantages and disadvantages of parenteral nutrient solutions enriched in L-GLN or GLN-dipeptide, respectively. Advantages of L-GLN-containing parenteral nutrient solutions include the low cost of L-GLN powder, the fact that nutrient solutions made with L-GLN are stable in solution at 4°C for up to several weeks,[35,55] and the availability of human

TABLE 8–8   Beneficial Effects of Dietary Supplementation with Intravenous L-GLN or GLN-Dipeptide in Clinical Settings

Maintained plasma GLN levels in catabolic stress (L-GLN and GLN dipeptide)

Maintained skeletal muscle intracellular GLN levels after operation or trauma (GLN dipeptide)

Improved nitrogen balance in catabolic states (L-GLN and GLN dipeptide)

Attenuated 3-methylhistidine excretion after BMT (L-GLN)

Enhanced skeletal muscle protein synthetic rates (GLN dipeptide)

Attenuated extracellular fluid expansion after BMT (L-GLN)

Increased D-xylose absorption in critical illness (GLN dipeptide)

Improved intestinal nutrient absorption in severe short-bowel syndrome, combined with a modified diet and growth hormone (L-GLN)

Reduced microbial colonization and clinical infection after BMT (L-GLN)

Enhanced lymphocyte recovery after BMT (L-GLN)

Shortened hospital length of stay after allogeneic or autologous BMT (L-GLN)

BMT = bone marrow transplantation.

safety and efficacy data. Disadvantages of L-GLN include the generation of pyroglutamic acid, ammonia, and glutamate with heat sterilization (necessitating cold sterilization methods using filters) and poor solubility in solution. Thus, L-GLN-containing nutrient solutions cannot be stored for long periods and manufacture requires special procedures with added personnel costs.[59] These potential problems may be obviated by use of cold sterilization and proper storage methods. However, there is an extra cost associated with adding L-GLN to amino acid solutions that are rich in essential amino acids, because these are generally more expensive than standard amino acid solutions. Future development of commercially available L-GLN-containing solutions with large-scale production may reduce the extra costs associated with manufacture of L-GLN-containing TPN solutions.

The metabolic and clinical effects with GLN-dipeptides are generally similar to those observed with L-GLN supplementation.[60-62] These compounds are heat stable and are very soluble in solution; thus the sterilized product also has a long shelf-life. At present, the only apparent disadvantage of GLN-dipeptides relates to their potential expense due, in part, to the complex process required for their manufacture.

Administration of L-GLN- or GLN-dipeptide-enriched IV formulas for up to several weeks has been shown to be safe in healthy adults and in hospitalized patients.[55,60,61] However, patients with significant organ dysfunction, especially those with renal or hepatic dysfunction, often tolerate amino acid solutions poorly. It is important to consider the possibility that individuals with kidney or liver failure may develop azotemia or other metabolic complications with the administration of nutrient solutions enriched in GLN or GLN dipeptides. Dysfunction of these organs may compromise the patient's ability to use GLN efficiently and could potentially lead to increased concentrations of end products of GLN metabolism in blood and tissues (e.g., glutamate or ammonia). Although GLN toxicity in these patient groups has not been demonstrated, reasonable exclusion criteria for GLN-enriched parenteral (and enteral) nutrition include patients with moderate or severe renal or hepatic function. Patients with CNS dysfunction (e.g., hepatic encephalopathy) may theoretically not tolerate elevations in blood GLN and may be predisposed to increased blood ammonia levels; therefore large doses of GLN are probably contraindicated in these individuals.

It is also possible that GLN is used as a growth factor or fuel for malignant cells. However, animal studies have not confirmed dietary GLN as a potential tumor growth factor,[35,43] and available human data do not suggest that GLN supplementation enhances or induces tumor growth in vivo. Further study of clinical tolerance to GLN supplementation is indicated to complement the safety data available to date in small patient groups; however, published clinical studies have not described complications unique to GLN administration.

The original clinical trials of GLN-enriched nutrition primarily focused on nitrogen and amino acid metabolism. Improved nitrogen retention and maintenance of plasma GLN concentrations were observed by Stehle and colleagues and by Furst and associates, who studied patients receiving ALA-GLN dipeptide-enriched TPN following major abdominal operations[62] or trauma.[63] In one study, cumulative 5-day nitrogen balance was improved with GLN dipeptide-enriched TPN compared with a GLN-free TPN solution (-7.1 ± 2.2 g/day vs -18.1 ± 1.7; $P < 0.001$).[62] Subsequent studies in trauma patients comparing ALA-GLN enriched solutions (providing ≈ 20 g of L-alanine-L-GLN dipeptide, equivalent to $\approx$ 13 g GLN) with standard GLN-free nutrient solutions demonstrated improved cumulative 4-day nitrogen balance with dipeptide therapy. However, intracellular muscle GLN concentrations were not affected with this dose of GLN.[63]

Several studies evaluated nitrogen balance and blood and intracellular muscle amino acid concentrations in patients receiving several experimental amino acids in balanced TPN solutions following elective cholecystectomy.[47,60,64] Isocaloric (≈ 32 kcal/kg/day) and isonitrogenous (≈ 1.25 g/kg/day) intravenous diets contained either a commercially available amino acid solution (without GLN) or a reduced amount of this solution to which either GLN (0.285 g/kg/day) or ALA-GLN dipeptide (0.325 g/kg/day) was added.

Compared with the standard amino acid solution (and an isonitrogenous BCAA-enriched solution), the GLN-containing experimental solutions resulted in significantly improved nitrogen balance.[47,60,64] The experimental solutions attenuated skeletal muscle intracellular GLN losses and preserved muscle protein synthesis compared with the GLN-free standard or BCAA-enriched TPN solutions. Significant positive correlations were noted between changes in postoperative muscle GLN concentration and muscle protein synthesis and cumulative nitrogen balance.[47] A portion of the improved nitrogen balance may be accounted for by an increase in the free GLN pool within skeletal muscle (i.e., nonprotein nitrogen balance).[65] It is likely, based on available human data, that the GLN requirement increases as patients are more critically ill, in terms of GLN supplementation's ability to improve nitrogen retention and muscle GLN concentrations. This may relate to increased GLN use and requirements in tissues such as the gut mucosa or immune cells.[35]

Two recent studies demonstrated gut-trophic effects of GLN-containing dipeptides in humans.[66,67] Van Der Hulst and colleagues studied the use of glycyl-L-GLN dipeptide-enriched parenteral feeding given for 10 to 14 days to patients with stable underlying intestinal disease requiring TPN.[66] With glycyl-L-GLN supplementation (0.23 g of GLN/kg/day), villus height was slightly but significantly greater and intestinal permeability significantly less than in the control patients receiving standard TPN.[66] Tremel and colleagues studied critically ill patients receiving L-alanyl-L-GLN dipeptide in TPN or similar GLN-free TPN solutions for 8 days.[67] Patients receiving L-alanyl-L-GLN dipeptide (0.3 g/kg/day) had significantly enhanced absorption of oral D-xylose, indicating improved small-bowel mucosa functional capacity compared with controls.[67]

Two randomized, double-blind, controlled studies in catabolic adult bone marrow transplant (BMT) patients have recently been published.[68,69] In the first trial, patients undergoing allogenic BMT for hematologic malignancy received standard GLN-free TPN per usual protocols (n = 21) or isocaloric, isonitrogenous, GLN-supplemented TPN, providing 0.57 g L-GLN/kg/day (n = 24). Following multidrug chemotherapy and total body irradiation, intravenous nutrient solutions were started on the day following BMT. Energy needs were calculated as 1.5 times basal energy requirements; these were provided as dextrose (70 percent of nonprotein energy) and fat emulsion (30 percent of nonprotein energy). Protein intake was calculated to provide 1.5 g/kg/day. The amino acid solutions were prepared by adding varying amounts of GLN, alanine, and glycine to a commercially available solution enriched in essential amino acids and then filter sterilized.[68] The parenteral diets provided adequate amounts of essential amino acids (EAA) for stressed patients; however, the GLN-containing solution contained approximately 30 percent less EAA than the control solution (33 percent of total AA vs 45 percent) and thus proportionally more nonessential amino acids (NEAA), including L-GLN. The solutions contained equivalent amounts of BCAA, but the control diet contained twice the amount of arginine as the experimental L-GLN-containing diet.[68]

Clinical, nutritional and treatment indexes were similar in both treatment groups at entry. GLN levels rose approximately 40 percent with L-GLN-enriched parenteral nutrition, but plasma glutamate, ammonia, and pyroglutamic acid levels were unrelated to dietary GLN administration. Nitrogen balance was significantly improved by ≈ 2.8 g/day with GLN treatment (GLN −1.4 ± 0.5 g/day vs control −4.2 ± 1.2 g/day; P = 0.002). The 3-MH/creatinine excretion ratio was reduced significantly (10.9 ± 0.4 vs 13.3 ± 0.9; P = 0.03), suggesting, for the first time in humans, that L-GLN diminished rates of protein breakdown.[68]

In addition, post-BMT morbidity was diminished with GLN supplementation (Table 8–9). The incidence of clinical infection, total and site-specific microbial colonization, and length of hospital stay were significantly reduced vs the controls.[68] Significantly more standard TPN than GLN-supplemented patients developed one or more positive throat cultures (86 percent vs 54 percent, P < 0.05) and stool cultures (75 percent vs 42 percent, P < 0.05). No clinical or biochemical evidence of toxicity to GLN-enriched feeding was noted during the duration of TPN in the experimental group (26 ± 2 days).

These represent the first data demonstrating reduced hospital morbidity with L-GLN-enriched parenteral nutrition.[68] Additional blinded studies in a subgroup of this patient population demonstrated that GLN-enriched parenteral feeding attenuated the expansion of extracellular and total body water seen in controls receiving standard, GLN-free TPN following BMT.[70]

TABLE 8–9 Outcome Variables in a Double-Blind, Randomized Trial of L-GLN Enriched TPN in Adult Bone Marrow Transplantation

Variable	Standard TPN	L-GLN-Supplemented TPN
Number of subjects	21	24
Cumulative mucositis score	2.2 ± 0.5	2.1 ± 0.4
Total days receiving antibiotics	15 ± 2	13 ± 2
Patients with AGVHD	10	11
Patients with no positive cultures	1	10*
Patients with clinical infectious foci	9	3†
Length of hospital stay (days)	36 ± 2	29 ± 1‡

AGVHD = acute graft-versus-host disease.
Data as mean ± SE.
Mucositis graded on a 1 to 5 scale.
*P = .005.
†P = .041.
‡P = .017.
Data from Ziegler TR, Young LS, Benfell K et al: Clinical and metabolic efficacy of glutamine-supplemented parenteral nutrition after bone marrow transplantation. A randomized, double-blind, controlled study. Ann Intern Med 1992;116: 821–828.

The latter finding suggests that GLN may influence cell membrane function or other factors related to alterations in body water compartments.

The reduction in hospital stay in the BMT study markedly reduced hospital costs (by ≈ $21,000/patient), primarily due to reduced charges for room and board.[71] The mechanisms of GLN action that resulted in reduced infection and length of hospital stay in the bone marrow study are unclear. GLN supplementation may exert a number of effects that may be interrelated. Thus, enhanced protein synthetic rates and reduced protein-catabolic rates may have improved nitrogen retention. Improved resistance to colonization and clinical infection may have been due to improved protein sparing combined with enhanced number or function of fixed or circulating immune cells,[35] maintenance of gut mucosal barrier defenses,[66,67] or improved tissue antioxidant (glutathione) stores,[72,73] compared with the group not receiving L-GLN.

In a subgroup of patients from the parent BMT trial,[68] we recently found circulating total lymphocyte, total T-lymphocyte, T-helper (CD-4), and T-suppressor (CD-8) cell recovery to be enhanced in the L-GLN supplemented group.[74] Because no effects of L-GLN were observed in total leukocyte or neutrophil engraftment, this finding suggests that dietary GLN may predominately influence lymphocyte metabolism.[74] Consistent with this observation, O'Riordain and coworkers demonstrated that glycyl-glutamine dipeptide-enriched TPN significantly enhances postoperative T-lymphocyte DNA synthesis compared with patients receiving GLN-free TPN.[75] Further data on immune effects of GLN in vivo are clearly needed in catabolic patient groups.

In the other trial of L-GLN-supplemented TPN in BMT, Schloerb and Amare studied adult patients with hematologic (n = 16) or solid tumors (n = 13) in a double-blind, randomized format.[69] All patients received high-dose chemotherapy, and a subset with acute myelogenous leukemia also received total body radiation. Patients undergoing both autologous (n = 15) or allogeneic BMT (n = 14) were studied. All subjects received ad libitum low-bacteria oral diet and gut decontamination. L-GLN-enriched TPN (similar to the previous trial[68]) or GLN-free, isonitrogenous, isocaloric TPN was initiated on the day following BMT.

TPN was given for approximately 30 days in each group, and oral food intake was similar. There were no differences between groups in mucositis, fever, engraftment, antibiotic requirements, clinical infections, or microbial colonization.[69] However, in the allogeneic BMT subset, two of six controls had bacteremia vs zero of seven in the L-GLN group ($P < 0.05$). The change in total body water during hospitalization was significantly less in the L-GLN group (control + 3.1 ± 1.5 L vs L-GLN – 3.4 ± 1.3 L). Further, the length of hospital stay was significantly less in the L-GLN group (33 ± 2 days vs 27 ± 1 days; $P < 0.05$).[69] No complications of L-GLN administration were noted. Infection rates were not reduced in the latter trial.[69] The patient populations studied, clinical conditions, and cancer treatment protocols were different between the two BMT studies, which may have influenced the effect of GLN on infection and colonization.

Several published papers suggest that dietary GLN may have beneficial psychotrophic effects, possibly due to direct effects of GLN or its metabolites in the CNS.[35] In the double-blind BMT study,[68,76] we found several indexes of patient mood and attitude to improve with L-GLN supplementation, and these psychological effects may have influenced the primary physicians as to the date of patient discharge from the hospital.[76]

In contrast to these generally favorable results, a recent study was published evaluating alanyl-GLN dipeptide (40 g/day or 26 g of free GLN) in non-BMT patients undergoing chemotherapy for hematologic malignancy.[77] Use of GLN dipeptide was not associated with improvement in clinical outcome, infection rates, mucositis, diarrhea, or in neutrophil engraftment.[77] Thus, further trials to determine which patient groups may benefit from dietary GLN appear indicated in patients receiving cancer chemotherapy. Further studies on the clinical efficacy and the molecular basis for GLN effects are necessary, as are additional controlled, double-blind trials to determine the clinical efficacy and cost effectiveness of enteral or parenteral GLN supplementation in selected patients. Based on data available to date, GLN should be considered an important dietary amino acid in a number of clinical settings (Table 8–10). However, additional randomized, double-blind controlled trials are needed to define further which patient subgroups may benefit from glutamine supplementation. Data on GLN combined with other nutrients and growth factors are covered below.

Therapeutic Effects of Other Amino Acids

A number of other amino acids may have therapeutic effects in patients requiring spe-

TABLE 8–10 Patient Groups Who May Benefit from Enteral or Parenteral Glutamine Supplementation

Severe Catabolic Illness
Burn, trauma, major operation
Acute or chronic infection
Bone marrow transplantation

Intestinal Dysfunction
Inflammatory bowel disease
Infectious enteritis
Short-bowel syndrome
Mucosal structural and functional damage following chemotherapy or irradiation and in critical illness

Immunodeficiency States
Immune system dysfunction associated with critical illness or bone marrow transplantation
AIDS

AIDS = acquired immunodeficiency syndrome.

cialized feeding. Patients may have a specific amino acid deficiency due to increased illness-related requirements, abnormal metabolism of the amino acid, or an insufficient parenteral or enteral diet. Individual amino acids may have specific effects on certain tissues or metabolic pathways when provided in larger amounts than usual in catabolic stress. Unfortunately, other than the arginine and glutamine studies noted above, little human data are available on effects of enterally administered diets enriched in single amino acids during catabolic states.

Synthetic L-amino acid combinations available for IV use or in standard elemental or polymeric enteral liquid formulas should provide estimated daily requirements of the eight classic essential amino acids (isoleucine, leucine, lysine, methionine, phenylalanine, threonine, tryptophan, and valine). All the intravenous solutions available in the United States also contain L-histidine, which is essential for infants and may be semiessential for older children and adults.[2] Standard IV amino acid solutions provide 40 to 50 percent of total protein as a mixture of all eight EAA. The proportion of EAA is greater in the solutions modified for pediatrics and patients with hepatic or renal failure (primarily due to greater percentage of BCAA).

In enteral solutions used as meal supplements or for tube feeding, amino acids are provided in the form of intact proteins (e.g., milk, egg white solids), partially hydrolyzed proteins (e.g., whey, casein, lactalbumin), dipeptides, or crystalline amino acids. These protein sources are combined in many complete enteral formulas. These formulations provide known ade-

quate amounts of EAA for stressed patients; however, because the amino acid composition is usually derived directly from high-biologic value proteins such as egg, the overall amino acid pattern (especially the NEAA pattern) of enteral formulas may be more complete or "balanced" than parenteral amino acid solutions. The possible clinical implications of these differences between parenteral and enteral amino acid pattern are unclear at present and require further clinical study.

Children's protein requirements are more complex than adults' and are altered by age and growth phase (e.g., infancy, puberty) as well as by the underlying illness and its severity. Neonates, especially those with low birth weight or prematurity, appear to require cysteine and taurine,[79] while infants require additional histidine and tyrosine.[2,38] Immaturity of enzyme systems in low-birth-weight infants inhibits the normal conversion of methionine to cysteine and taurine and the conversion of phenylalanine to tyrosine.[2,78,79] L-cysteine HCL is available as a single amino acid supplement for neonates and preterm infants that can be mixed with IV solutions containing mixed amino acids or used to supplement enterally fed patients.

Taurine is beginning to receive more attention as a potentially important amino acid in nutrition and metabolic support in adults. It is the most abundant intracellular free amino acid in the human body but is not incorporated into body protein.[78] Taurine is important in bile acid conjugation, cell volume regulation, neural and retinal function, platelet aggregation, and as an antioxidant, among other functions.[80,81] Several studies have reported low plasma and urinary taurine levels in adults with catabolic illnesses such as cancer,[81] after operative injury,[81] with burns,[82] and after chemotherapy/irradiation,[83] suggesting total body taurine depletion in these conditions. The rate-limiting enzyme for taurine synthesis from methionine or cysteine, cysteine sulfinic acid decarboxylase, may be inhibited during catabolic illness.[84] In one study by Mequid and colleagues, intravenous taurine supplementation (8.6 mg/kg/day) in otherwise balanced TPN corrected low plasma taurine levels in 12 malnourished patients after 10 days of infusion.[81] Many of the newer enteral feeding formulations designed for adults are now supplemented with taurine. Further study is needed on taurine's metabolism in catabolic illness and the effects of taurine supplementation in adults. Although apparently important in infants, to date no studies have defined specific beneficial effects of taurine supplementation in adults.

As reviewed by Furst and Stehle, current IV amino acid formulas may provide limited or excessive amounts of certain amino acids and therefore may be unbalanced in certain patient subgroups.[38] However, it is difficult to determine amino acid requirements or to diagnose amino acid "deficiency" as measured by plasma levels or free amino acid levels in tissues. Amino acid levels are in a dynamic state of flux and are influenced by prior nutritional status, amino acid and energy intake, underlying diseases, severity of illness, and patient age and sex.[38] Low plasma or intracellular free histidine, serine, taurine, tyrosine, valine, and threonine levels occur in uremic patients, and low cysteine, taurine, and tyrosine levels have been documented in cirrhotic patients receiving TPN, suggesting possible conditional deficiency of these amino acids.[38,39,78] To our knowledge, altered clinical outcomes with enteral or parenteral repletion of these amino acids individually have not been reported (amino acid administration in patients with renal or hepatic insufficiency is covered in Chapters 24 and 26). Some amino acids are currently totally lacking in standard parenteral amino acid formulations (taurine, cysteine, and glutamine) or are present in very small amounts (tyrosine).[38] Poor solubility (in the case of cystine, tyrosine, and glutamine) or instability in solution (with cysteine) may limit their use in the free form in parenteral diets.

Gazzaniga and colleagues studied the effects of a pediatric amino acid formula administered as part of balanced TPN on plasma amino acids and nitrogen balance in stable adult patients requiring TPN.[85] The formula contained 33 percent BCAA (intermediate between adult standard and BCAA-enriched solutions), increased amounts of histidine, tyrosine and arginine, and taurine. Patients received the solution with or without added cysteine HCl (0.5 mmol/kg/day) and a total protein dose of 1.5 g/kg/day for at least 6 days. Positive nitrogen balance was achieved in each group of adult patients (cysteine supplemented, +3.21 ± 0.70 g/day vs no cysteine, +1.75 ± 0.70 g/day, not statistically significant) and plasma tyrosine levels normalized in each group.[85] A significant positive correlation between the increase in taurine levels in plasma and improved nitrogen balance occurred, but only in the group receiving cysteine supplementation.[85] Positive correlation was also noted between improved nitrogen balance and

plasma levels of cystine, total cysteine + cystine, tyrosine, and ornithine.[85] Although a control group receiving standard adult solutions was not studied, these findings suggest possible benefits in adults with amino acid solutions tailored initially for infants and children. Further clinical study is needed on the efficacy of new enteral and parenteral amino acid formulations in patients with organ failure and other clinical conditions.

ORNITHINE α-KETOGLUTARATE AND α-KETOGLUTARATE

The use of ornithine α-ketoglutarate (OKG) and α-ketoglutarate (AKG) in enteral and parenteral nutrition has received considerable research attention, especially in Europe.[86-96] OKG is a salt formed of one AKG molecule and two ornithine molecules. After IV or enteral administration, OKG dissociates readily into ornithine and AKG.[86-89] Both substances serve as GLN biosynthetic precursors, through conversion to glutamate in the body and then metabolism to GLN by the enzyme GLN synthetase.[86] AKG is also a key intermediary in the Krebs cycle and ornithine is a central amino acid in the urea cycle. OKG in particular has been shown to stimulate GH and insulin release, and ornithine is important in polyamine synthesis.[86,89] Both OKG and AKG have been shown to be safe when provided in both enteral and parenteral feedings, and no adverse side-effects have been described to date.

A number of trials evaluated enteral administration of OKG.[86-89,92-94] Enteral OKG administration improved nitrogen retention and protein synthesis in postoperative patients,[88] burns,[89,93] and sepsis.[86] OKG given at a dose of 20 g/day vs isonitrogenous placebo significantly improved wound healing, nitrogen balance, and serum proteins in patients with moderate-sized burns.[93] In another study, trauma patients were given enteral tube feedings supplemented with OKG (≈ 16 g/day).[94] Enteral OKG enhanced nitrogen balance, in association with increased GLN, GH, and IGF-I levels vs matched patients receiving OAK-free isonitrogenous tube feedings.[94]

Intravenous OKG and AKG administration in postoperative and critically ill patients induces metabolic and protein-sparing effects very similar to those produced by L-GLN and GLN dipeptide administration.[64,89,95,96] In general, effects on nitrogen retention with GLN-, GLN-dipeptide-, OKG-, or AKG-enriched solutions have been similar. Both IV OKG and AKG-enriched nutrient solutions attenuate the loss of skeletal muscle intracellular GLN and preserve muscle protein synthesis (measured by skeletal muscle polyribosome concentration). In a study in children with growth retardation secondary to short-bowel syndrome, OKG (15 g/day) added to TPN was associated with increased height velocity and increased GLN and IGF-I levels.[91] Both OKG and AKG are likely to be evaluated extensively in future clinical nutrition studies to determine whether other clinical outcomes are improved with their use. A list of beneficial effects reported in patients receiving enteral OKG is provided in Table 8–11.

MICRONUTRIENTS AND ANTIOXIDANTS

A number of micronutrients and antioxidant nutrients are considered to be important in human nutrition. Trace elements such as selenium, copper, and zinc are totally depleted during catabolic illness in humans.[2,97] Depletion of major antioxidants, such as glutathione, or nutrient substrates for glutathione synthesis or metabolism such as GLN, vitamin C, vitamin E, zinc, and selenium are believed to be common in patients with critical illness and with multiple organ failure.[73,98-104] Antioxidant capacity is important to prevent peroxidation of cell membranes and cell damage during catabolic states and appears to be critical for immune function. Although data in humans are limited, emerging evidence suggests that antioxidant nutrients[105] or compounds such as glutathione[106] should be considered to be important components of enteral and parenteral nutrition support.

Several studies indicated that supplemental vitamin A improves immune function[98] and wound healing in burns and other catabolic states.[99] In one study, adult burn patients exhibited total body depletion of copper, selenium, and zinc. A subgroup received supplements of these trace elements and demonstrated increased plasma levels associated with improved immune function and reduced length of hospital stay.[97] β-carotene is a precursor to vitamin A in the body and may be important in immunomodulation.[100] Other studies indicate that supplemental vitamin E or combinations of antioxidant nutrients upregulate antioxidant capacity and improve immune function after trauma,[101,102] and in the elderly.[103,104] Chandra found that elderly subjects commonly exhibit low circulating levels of antioxidant nutrients.[105] In a double-blind, randomized trial, simple daily administration of a multivitamin-mineral tablet rich in antioxidants significantly reduced infections and hospitalization rates over a 1-year period in this group.[105]

It is now recognized that the tripeptide glutathione (cysteine-glutamate-glycine) is critical for immune cell function and for antioxidant protection of many cell types and tissues of the body, including GI epithelial cells.[106] GLN-enriched parenteral nutrition maintains plasma, hepatic, and intestinal glutathione levels and improves survival in animal models of glutathione depletion following chemotherapy[72] or acetaminophen toxicity.[73] Additional studies on the efficacy of enteral GLN in this regard are needed.

Other than the Recommended Dietary Allowances,[2] it is not possible to recommend additional doses of micronutrients and antioxidants for patient subgroups receiving nutrition support pending additional data on dose responses. One problem is that assessment of total body nutrient stores and body antioxidant capacity is an uncertain but emerging science in humans. Many of the most reliable assays for micronutrients are not available or too expensive for routine use in clinical care. However, many clinicians provide additional doses of selected vitamins and trace elements during critical illness, when net body loss of micronutrients is likely, or when serum and urine levels are low, indicating possible deficiency (e.g., zinc, selenium, glutamine, vitamin C, vitamin E). Supplemental antioxidant nutrients are usually provided in combination, because of their multiple interactions (e.g., selenium is critical for glutathione peroxidase and vitamin C is important in regeneration of reduced vitamin E). Further, some antioxidants may become prooxidants under certain conditions and induce negative effects.[97,105] For example, additional intravenous zinc (5 to 15 mg/day), vitamin C (0.5 to 1 g/day), selenium (60 to 120 µg/day), with enteral vitamin E (400 IU/day), or enteral glutamine (10 to 30 g/day) may be prescribed

TABLE 8–11 Effects Reported in Patients Receiving Enteral Ornithine α-Ketoglutarate (OKG)

Improved nitrogen balance
Enhanced protein synthesis
Increased serum insulin, growth hormone, and IGF-I levels
Increased plasma glutamine levels
Increased serum proteins (prealbumin, retinol-binding protein)
Enhanced wound healing in burn patients

in selected septic or critically ill patients. This practice has been well tolerated, but further safety data and double-blind, randomized trials are indicated to determine efficacy in defined, at-risk patient subgroups.

NEW LIPID SOURCES IN NUTRITION SUPPORT

Scientific research over the past decade has provided exciting developments in the field of alternative lipid sources for use in enteral or parenteral nutrition. Historically, the use of fat in nutrition support had focused on providing a calorically dense (9 kcal/g) and isotonic fuel source, as well as supplying the essential fatty acid, linoleic acid. Lipids have important biochemical, structural, and regulatory functions, in addition to being a calorically dense nutrient substrate. It is now clear that fat sources are used differently depending on the underlying disease; that the source of fat may actually modulate the inflammatory response to stress and disease; and that fat can be easily overused in nutrition support, which in some cases may be detrimental to recovery. Predominantly, lipids in enteral and tube feedings are supplied as vegetable oils with primarily long chain fatty acids (LCFAs) (14 to 24 carbons). Specialized enteral formulas developed for patients with digestive or absorptive problems include medium-chain triglycerides (MCTs, 6 to 12 carbons), and short-chain fatty acids (SCFAs, which have carbon lengths of two to four). Several commercially available tube-feeding formulas are enriched in MCT oil. More recently, a group of polyunsaturated fatty acids called omega-3 has become an ingredient in specialized formulas designed to enhance immune and metabolic function in the stressed, critically ill patient. This section will focus on some of the newer fat sources, namely, omega-3 fatty acids and structured lipids, and will provide an overview on the use of MCT oil in nutrition support.

Fatty Acid Metabolism and Nomenclature

Fatty acids are characterized according to their carbon chain length, presence and number of double bonds, and the double bond position. Polyunsaturated fatty acids (PUFAs) have two or more double bonds per fatty acid. Monosaturated acids contain one double bond, and saturated fatty acids have no double bonds. PUFAs are further divided into four groups depending on the location of the first double bond in relation to the terminal methyl group of the carbon chain. These include n-3, n-6, n-7, and n-9 lipids. Linoleic acid, an essential fatty acid, is an example of an n-6 fatty acid with the chemical nomenclature 18:2 n-6. This means there are 18 carbons, two double bonds, with the first double bond on the sixth carbon from the methyl end (Table 8–12). The n-3 and n-6 are both considered essential because they are not synthesized by mammals. Linoleic acid, an n-6 fatty acid, is ubiquitous in the American diet. Its sources include all plant and seed oils except palm, coconut, and cocoa oils. α-Linolenic acid, an n-3 fatty acid, is found in the chloroplasts of green leafy vegetables and certain oils, such as soybean, rapeseed, and flaxseed oil.[107-109]

Other sources of omega-3 fatty acids (with longer carbon chains) include fish oils, which

TABLE 8–12 Nomenclature of Some Common Dietary Fatty Acids

Symbol	Systematic Name	Common Name
Saturated Fatty Acids		
8:0	Octanoic	Caprylic
10:0	Decanoic	Capric
12:0	Dodecanoic	Lauric
14:0	Tetradecanoic	Myristic
16:0	Hexadecanoic	Palmitic
18:0	Octadecanoic	Stearic
Unsaturated Fatty Acids		
18:1 n-9	9-Octadecanoic	Oleic
18:2 n-6	6,9,12-Octadecadienoic	Linoleic
18:3 n-3	9,12,15-Octadecatrienoic	Linolenic
20:4 n-6	5,8,11,14-Eicosatetraenoic	Arachidonic
20:5 n-3	5,8,11,14,17-Eicosapentaenoic	EPA, timnodonic
22:6 n-3	4,7,10,13,16,19-Docosahexaenoic	DHA, cervonic

contain abundant amounts of eicosapentaenoic acid (EPA) and docosahexaenoic acid (DHA). These fatty acids are also synthesized endogenously in the body by elongation and desaturation from α-linolenic acid substrate. Arachidonic acid (AA) and EPA are both precursors to various classes of prostanoids and leukotrienes, which have important cellular functions, including vascular and hemostatic actions[110,111] and involvement in critical inflammatory, allergic, and immune responses in humans.[112]

The fatty acid content of the diet is a major determinant of the type of lipid incorporated into cell membranes. The lipid composition of the cell membrane determines its structure, fluidity, and receptor function. Depending on the fatty acid ratio of AA to EPA within cell membranes, different families of eicosanoids may be formed, which ultimately exert different effects on metabolism.

The proportion of arachidonic acid, EPA, and DHA endogenously synthesized vs that derived from the diet is unknown. Synthesis of omega-3 fatty acids is slow in humans[113] and slower with aging and in certain disease states.[114] Additionally, since n-3 and n-6 fatty acids compete for desaturase and elongase enzymes,[115] the n-6-rich diet of western society interferes with the formation of EPA and DHA from α-linolenic acid.[108]

The prostanoids and leukotrienes synthesized from AA are of the series 2 and 4, respectively. These molecules are potent regulators of immune function. High concentrations are immunosuppressive because of their many effects on lymphocytes and macrophages. EPA and DHA, on the other hand, when incorporated in the phospholipid fraction of the cell membrane, produce series 3 prostanoids and series 5 leukotrienes, which are generally less metabolically active than the AA metabolites. The n-3 fatty acids are thought to exert their anti-inflammatory and immunomodulatory effects by this effect.[107,112,114]

The therapeutic benefits of the n-3 polyunsaturated fatty acids (PUFAs) have been well documented and are quite varied. They include effects on the cardiovascular and immunologic systems, as well as effects on cytokine metabolic cascades during critical illness.[107] Epidemiologic studies have attributed the low incidence of cardiovascular disease in Eskimos,[116] and inflammatory diseases, such as Type I diabetes and asthma in the Japanese and Dutch,[117] to the high dietary intake of n-3 fatty acids in these populations. Fish oil administration has been shown to lower blood pressure in patients with mild hypertension[118] and to decrease serum triglyceride and cholesterol levels in hyperlipidemic states.[119] Additionally, clinical studies demonstrate that dietary supplementation with n-3 PUFAs reduces inflammation and disease activity in chronic immunologically mediated disease, including rheumatoid arthritis, psoriasis, and atopic dermatitis.[120,121]

Dietary Omega-3 Fatty Acids in Catabolic Illness

Eicosanoids regulate production of several cytokines, which function in part as protein mediators of communication between cells. Cytokines appear to contribute to the pathogenesis of chronic illnesses such as atherosclerosis and inflammatory diseases and are also primary mediators of the acute metabolic response to illness.[121] An increase in n-3 PUFA intake appears to affect cytokine production and function. The production of several cytokines, namely, interleukin (IL)-1, tumor necrosis factor (TNF), and interleukin-2, is under negative control by PGE2, and because PGE2 synthesis is decreased after consumption of n-3 PUFA, investigators have studied how increased intake of these fatty acids affects cytokine production.

Endres[122] gave 18 g of fish oil concentrate per day to nine healthy volunteers as a supplement to their normal diet and measured IL-1-α and -β and TNF produced in vitro by endotoxin-stimulated peripheral blood mononuclear cells. After 6 weeks of supplementation, there was a 43 percent reduction in IL-1-β synthesis, which decreased to 40 percent of control baseline 10 weeks after n-3 supplementation was discontinued.[122] IL-1-α and TNF production responded similarly to fish oil, and the AA:EPA ratio in phospholipid cell membrane of mononuclear cells also decreased.[122] These effects on IL-1 and TNF production appear to be responsible, in part, for the anti-inflammatory effects of omega-3 fatty acids.

Effects of omega-3 fatty acids on the immune system have been demonstrated in patients following the Step 2 National Cholesterol Education Panel.[123] Twenty-two patients were randomized to one of two diets to follow for 24 weeks.[123] Both diets were low in total fat, saturated fat, and cholesterol; one was enriched with fish (1.23 g of EPA + DHA) and one was not. The low-fish diet increased IL-1-β, TNF, and blood mononuclear cell mitogenic response to Con A, while the high-fish diet significantly decreased the percentage of helper T-cells while increasing suppressor T-cells. Changing diet composition (without fish oil supplements) can alter the immune response; however, it takes much longer.[123]

When to incorporate EPA into cell membranes may be more important in critical illness than in chronic disease; therefore, anti-inflammatory or immune response to supplementation with omega-3 fatty acids in enteral nutrient formulas or in structured lipids for parenteral administration has been evaluated. EPA is incorporated rapidly (3 to 4 days) into hepatic Kupffer's and endothelial cell phospholipid membranes in animals receiving a fish oil–enriched liquid diet by gastrostomy.[124] Omega-3 fatty acids as part of enteral formulas containing additional specialized nutrients have also been studied in surgical patients, burn patients, and individuals with human immunodeficiency virus (HIV) (see below).

The use of omega-3 fatty acids either alone or with other conditionally essential nutrients may yet prove useful in the nutritional support of the critically ill patient. Further definitive work in humans is needed to evaluate omega-3 fatty acids as specific modulators of immune response and to test their effects on clinical outcome during critical illness. Several commercially available nutrient formulas for tube feeding are now enriched with omega-3 fatty acids. However, in light of data that indicate potential deleterious effects of omega-3 PUFAs, additional safety and outcome data are warrented.[125] For example, experimental data indicate that the long-chain PUFAs in fish oil are prone to autooxidation, which theoretically can damage cells through free radical formation and increased lipid peroxidation.[125] This effect increases vitamin E use and requirements during omega-3 fatty acid administration.[126] Omega-3 PUFA also may potentially prolong bleeding time by effects on platelet aggregation.[125] A study in surgical patients receiving an enteral formula containing 16.5 g of fish oil/1500 ml solution for 7 days did not show abnormal platelet aggregation or abnormal bleeding tendencies.[127]

Clinical Use of MCTs

MCTs are derived from the fractionation of coconut oil and consist of triglycerides containing 6 to 12 carbons, predominantly C8 (octanoic) and C10 (decanoic). They have been in use since the 1950s as treatment for patients with disorders of lipid absorption.[128] Pure MCT oil provides no essential fatty acids and has a caloric density of 8.3 calories/g. Data on possible immunosuppressive effects of high linoleic vegetable oil–based parenteral lipid emulsions are conflicting at present;[129] however, alternative lipid sources are being investigated. MCTs have been studied as part of blended or structured lipids for use parenterally, but discussion of this is beyond the scope of this chapter.

The use of MCTs in enteral feedings is advantageous for many reasons. MCTs are more water soluble than LCTs and are rapidly hydrolyzed in the intestinal lumen.[128] MCTs do not require pancreatic lipase or bile to be digested or absorbed, and they are transported into the blood through the portal system, bypassing the lymphatic system.[130] Compared with equimolar concentrations of LCTs infused intraduodenally, MCTs resulted in accelerated small-bowel transit time, and this effect may account for some of the GI symptoms that can occur with large amounts of MCTs.[131] MCTs also do not require carnitine for transport into the cell mitochondria; they enter mitochondria directly and are rapidly oxidized as a fuel source.[128] MCTs are not stored in adipose tissue,[132] nor do they accumulate in the liver.[128]

The clinical conditions whereby MCTs prove beneficial include defects in fat digestion, specifically hydrolysis of fat due to insufficient bile salts or pancreatic enzymes.[133] These disorders include pancreatitis, pancreatic insufficiency, liver disease, blind-loop syndrome, cystic fibrosis, and biliary atresia.[133] Enteral MCTs are also beneficial in short-bowel syndrome and in states of mucosal disease such as celiac sprue or Crohn's disease.[134] Finally, patients with disorders of lipid transport through the lymphatic system, as with deficient chylomicron synthesis, chylous ascites, or chylothorax, benefit from MCTs.[135] Since MCTs do not stimulate lymph flow, they may also be useful as therapy in healing enteric fistulas.

Many commercially available enteral formulas contain MCTs in various amounts, usually with long chain polyunsaturated fatty acids (LCTs), to provide the essential fatty acid linoleic acid.[130] In most cases, MCTs are added to enhance formula digestion or absorption.

MCTs as part of structured lipids (physical mixtures of MCTs and LCTs) have been studied, primarily as parenteral infusions, but a few studies have evaluated the effects of enterally fed structured lipids in animals. Structured lipid-enriched enteral diets promoted a higher cumulative nitrogen balance and higher muscle and liver fractional protein synthetic rates compared with rats fed MCT or LCT alone after burn injury.[136,137] Human studies are clearly needed on the specific effects of these novel lipid compounds, and data in catabolic patients are forthcoming.

DIETARY NUCLEOTIDES

Nucleotides are low-molecular-weight biologic compounds that play major roles in almost all biochemical processes.[138] Nucleotides consist of purines and pyrimidines, which are the building blocks of DNA and RNA. They are essential for cellular energetics (as part of adenosine triphosphate [ATP]); play a major role as physiologic mediators (as cyclic adenosine monophosphate [cAMP]); and are part of many coenzymes involved in the synthesis of glycogen and glycoproteins, among other functions.[138]

Nucleotides are ubiquitous in cells but are present as a small component of the normal diet (adults ingest approximately 1 to 2 g/day).[139] Nucleotides make up a large component (about 5 percent) of the total nitrogen in human milk, which may be important in the development and maturation of the human intestine and immune system. The endogenous supply of nucleotides is maintained through de novo synthesis and by salvage of preformed bases and interconversion to the desired compound.[140] Amino acids are the main sources of purine and pyrimidine synthesis. These processes have a high metabolic cost and may not provide sufficient amounts of nucleotides during critical illness. All parenteral and most enteral feedings are devoid of dietary nucleotides; thus their supplementation may prove beneficial in patients who are unable to consume an oral diet.[139,140]

Research performed in organ transplantation has suggested that exogenous nucleotide administration is important in the maintenance of host immunity to the allogeneic tissues.[140] The first observations on the potential role of the immunoenhancing effects of nucleotides were made with renal transplant patients in the early 1980s. It was noted that patients maintained on parenteral nutrition after renal transplantation had fewer rejection episodes despite reduced immunosuppression. When the patients resumed a normal diet, their immunosuppression requirements increased.[141]

These observations promoted research on the effects of a nucleotide-deficient diet to enhance immunosuppression necessary after organ transplantation. In animal models, rejec-tion of cardiac transplants, graft-vs-host disease, delayed cutaneous hypersensitivity, and in vitro mitogen-stimulated lymphocyte proliferation are all suppressed by a diet deficient in nucleotides.[138,140] Patients receiving diets supplemented with an additional 0.25 percent of RNA will maintain normal immune responses under these conditions. Animals fed nucleotide-deficient diets who are innoculated with *Candida albicans*[142] or *Staphylococcus aureus*[143] have markedly increased mortality. When the diets are supplemented with RNA or uracil, survival improves significantly.[142,143] Adenine supplements, on the other hand, do not appear to prevent the immunosuppressive effects of a nucleotide-free diet. Thus it appears that RNA or pyrimidine bases not only maintain cellular immunity but may improve survival after an infectious challenge.[140]

Nucleotides are known to have important effects on the GI tract.[144-146] Dietary nucleotides are broken down by proteases and pancreatic nucleases in the gut lumen to a mixture of nucleosides and N bases; these are then absorbed through efficient Na^+-dependent transport mechanisms.[144] Most of the absorbed purines are oxidized to uric acid in the intestine, whereas the pyrimidine bases are absorbed intact and incorporated into liver nucleic acids.[144] Nucleotides enhance the growth of bifidobacteria in the human intestinal tract, similar to the effects of breast-feeding. Bifidobacteria lower the colonic pH, thereby inhibiting the growth of enterobacteria and other pathogenic bacteria that are acid tolerant and may cause diarrhea.[145]

Nucleotides also appear to stimulate intestinal growth and maturation in young rats. Weanling rats fed a nucleoside-supplemented diet vs a nucleotide-free diet had greater intestinal villus height, crypt depth, and total protein and DNA content primarily in the proximal gut.[146] Enteral nucleotide supplementation has been studied in weanling rats during recovery from diarrheal illness.[140,141] Rats were given 2 weeks of lactose feeding to induce diarrhea, then randomized to receive a purified nucleotide-free diet or one containing 0.5 percent of nucleotides. After 4 weeks of feeding, rats receiving enteral nucleotides had higher disaccharidase (maltase, lactase, sucrase) activities than controls. They also had an improvement in villous height:crypt depth ratio compared with rats receiving the nucleotide-free diet. These data suggest that dietary nucleotides may modulate intestinal repair after injury.[140,144]

CLINICAL EFFICACY OF SPECIFIC NUTRIENT COMBINATIONS

A number of recent trials in animals and in specific patient groups evaluated the effects of specific enteral nutrient combinations and use of growth factors (GH, IGF-I) combined with GLN-enriched enteral feeding.[147,148] GH administration to postoperative patients was shown to maintain intracellular GLN concentrations in muscle.[149] In a rat model of short-bowel syndrome, both GLN-enriched enteral tube feedings alone and subcutaneous IGF-I administration alone (with standard GLN-free tube feedings) enhanced intestinal cellularity and adaptation.[150] However, combined enteral GLN and subcutaneous IGF-I had a synergistic effect on small intestinal protein synthesis and increased plasma IGF-I and plasma GLN to levels greater than with GLN or IGF-I alone.[150] Use of GH combined with GLN-enriched enteral or parenteral diets appears to have additive or synergistic effects on nitrogen retention in humans.[151,152] These data suggest that the GH-IGF-I and GLN action pathways have important metabolic interactions.[147,148]

We recently completed unblinded, pilot studies to evaluate combined effects of enteral/parenteral GLN (0.45 to 0.6 g/kg/day), subcutaneous GH (0.14 mg/kg/day), and a modified enteral diet in adult SBS patients dependent on parenteral nutrition.[151,152] During an initial control week, eight patients received their usual diet and IV prescription after which combined GLN-GH-diet therapy was started and continued for 3 weeks. The components of the enteral diet used are listed in Table 8–13. Near isotonic, commercially available, oral rehydration fluids (e.g., Pedialyte, Gatorade) were used as the primary source of enteral hydration, and hypoosmolar or hyperosmolar fluids were eliminated or severely restricted. Enteral glutamine powder (20 to 30 g/day) was mixed in the rehydration fluid, which patients sipped throughout the day. The diet was restricted simple sugars, lactose free, high in complex carbohydrate sources ($\approx$ 60 percent of enteral kilocalories as pasta, rice, potatoes, etc.), high in protein ($\approx$ 20 percent of enteral kilocalories), and low in dietary fat ($\approx$ 20 to 25 percent of enteral kilocalories).[151] Adequate enteral vitamins and minerals and calcium supplementation were provided, and small frequent feedings were instituted (six feedings throughout the day as three meals and three snacks). Finally, patients received intensive education on dietary choice and modification by a registered dietitian.[151,152]

TABLE 8–13 Components of Enteral Diet Used in Intestinal Rehabilitation in Adult Short-Bowel Syndrome

Near-isotonic, commercially available, oral rehydration fluids as primary source of enteral hydration (elimination of hypo- or hyperosmolar fluids)
Enteral fluids taken throughout waking hours
Restricted simple sugars, lactose free
Increased complex carbohydrate sources ($\approx$ 60% of enteral kilocalories)
High protein intake ($\approx$ 20% of enteral kilocalories)
Low-moderate fat intake ($\approx$ 20–25% of enteral kilocalories)
Adequate enteral vitamins and minerals, calcium supplementation
Enteral glutamine powder, mixed in rehydration fluid (20–30 g/day)
Smaller, more frequent feedings (six feedings throughout the day as three meals and three snacks)
Intensive education program by registered dietitian

Enteral nutrient absorption studies were performed during the control week and the last week of combined nutrient-growth factor therapy. Calorie and protein intake in the treatment period were matched to control week intake. With combined therapy, markedly improved intestinal absorption of protein (38 percent) and a $\approx$ 30 percent reduction in stool weight occurred (both $P < 0.05$). Sodium absorption was also enhanced by 37 percent with GLN/GH/diet therapy (not statistically significant).[151] The use of the modified diet alone, GLN-enriched modified diet alone, and GH alone was also studied in smaller groups of similar patients (two to four in a group). Both GLN supplementation and GH administration tended to enhance gut nutrient absorption; however, the combined therapy appeared to have synergistic effects, since nutrient absorption was significantly greater in this group.[152]

Data derived from a total of 47 SBS patients treated with combined therapy for 3 to 4 weeks demonstrated that at the end of the treatment period, 57 percent of the subjects were able to have all parenteral feedings discontinued, and an additional 30 percent had reduced parenteral requirements.[152] Prospective follow-up data are available in these individuals, who were discharged from the treatment center on both the modified diet and enteral GLN supplementation (Table 8–13). At approximately 1 year of follow-up, 40 percent of patients remain off of all parenteral feedings and an additional 40 percent maintain hydration and nutritional status with reduced parenteral requirements.[152] Additional, double-blind trials in adults and children are clearly indicated to determine the potentially beneficial effects of GLN-enriched feeding and GH alone, when combined with an appropriate modified diet, in patients with short-bowel syndrome. In addition, studies on the physiologic and molecular mechanisms of GLN and GH effects on the human intestine are needed.

In another trial of combined enteral therapy, Gottschlich and colleagues tested a modular tube feeding enriched in specific nutrients vs two separate, commercial enteral formulas (made to be isocaloric and isonitrogenous to the test diet), in 50 children with 10 to 89 percent body surface area burns.[153] The modular enteral formula was high in dietary protein (23 percent of total energy) and contained whey (87 percent of total protein intake), supplemental arginine (9 percent of protein or 6.1 g/L), and additional histidine and cysteine (2 percent of protein intake, respectively). Fat provided 15 percent of total energy in the diet, 50 percent as fish oil and 50 percent as safflower oil (5 g/L omega-3 fatty acids). Matched patients were fed for 3 to 4 weeks after the burn injury. Patients receiving the experimental formula had a significant reduction in wound infections ($P = 0.03$) and reduced length of hospital stay due to percentage of burn size ($P = 0.02$). In addition, the modular diet was associated with trends toward reduced pneumonia ($P = 0.06$) and total infection ($P = 0.07$) and reduced mortality.[153]

A number of recent trials have evaluated the effects of a commercial enteral tube feeding supplemented with L-arginine (12.5 g/L), omega-3 fish oils (as menhaden oil; 1.7 g/L of EPA and DHA), chemically structured lipid (palm kernel oil + sunflower oil; 17 g/L), and nucleotides (yeast RNA; 1.25 g/L).[154-157] In a pilot blinded, randomized study, Cerra and colleagues studied critically ill, septic patients given the arginine/lipid/RNA-enriched experimental formula vs isonitrogenous, isocaloric feeding as a standard, nonelemental commercially available enteral formula. After 7 to 8 days, patients receiving the enriched formula demonstrated significantly enhanced in vitro peripheral blood blastogenic responses to mitogens and to tetanus, suggesting upregulated immune functions induced by diet.[154] In a subsequent study in a small group of trauma patients with a similar study design, Cerra and coworkers found administration of the arginine/modified lipid/RNA-enriched diet to improve in vitro tests of immune function but not nitrogen retention, infection rates, or length of hospital stay.[155]

Daly and associates[156] evaluated this enteral diet in adult patients following surgery for upper GI malignancy. Patients were randomized into a standard enteral feeding group (N = 44) or a group administered the arginine/modified lipid/RNA-enriched diet (N = 41). The clinical characteristics and caloric intake of the two groups were similar; however, the experimental group received significantly more dietary nitrogen than the control group (15.6 vs 9.0 g/day). The experimental group thus had greater nitrogen balance than patients receiving the standard formula (-2.2 vs -6.6 g/day).[156]

Peripheral lymphocyte mitogenesis, measured by thymidine incorporation after stimulation with Con A or PHA, fell postoperatively in both groups but increased to normal by day 7 only in the experimental patients. There was no difference in other immune function tests, including CD-4, CD-8, and CD-3 counts and an opsonic index.[156] Patients receiving the experimental formula demonstrated no differences in infectious morbidity or wound healing complications vs the controls; however, the experimental patients had significantly less total complications (wound + infectious) than the controls (11 percent vs 37 percent; $P = 0.02$). In addition, hospital length of stay was reduced in the experimental group compared with the control patients (15.8 ± 5.1 days vs 20.2 ± 9.4 days; $P = 0.01$).[156]

Finally Bower and colleagues recently published the results of a large randomized, double-blind, and controlled trial using the same experimental and control enteral diets as the previous studies noted above.[157] Critically ill adult patients (N = 326) were randomized to receive the arginine/modified lipid/RNA-enriched diet or a control, nonelemental enteral diet within 48 hours after ICU admission. Enteral tube feedings were advanced to a target goal of 60 ml/hour by 96 hours after the primary event (trauma, operation, sepsis). Patients (substratifed as septic or inflamed and by amount of feeding actually administered) generally received significantly more nitrogen in the experimental subgroups than in the control subgroups, yet nitrogen balances were not different. There were no effects of diet on patient mortality; however, mortality in both study groups was significantly less than predicted by admission illness severity scores,[157] an effect possibly due to benefits of early enteral feeding.[3,4]

In patients receiving at least 821 ml/day of tube feeding ($\approx$ 34 ml/hour), the hospital median length of stay was significantly less with the experimental formula. In the subgroup of patients classified as septic on ICU admission, administration of the arginine/modified lipid/RNA-enriched diet was associated with statistically significant reductions in acquired infections ($P < 0.01$) and in length of hospital stay ($P < 0.05$).[157] In the septic subgroup, patients receiving the experimental diet at a dose of at least 821 ml/day had a median length of stay 11.5 days less than the comparable control patients ($P < 0.05$).[157]

CONCLUSION

Further studies to define which specific nutrient additives are responsible for the immunologic, metabolic, and clinical effects observed in these and other clinical trials are indicated. Taken together, however, emerging data both in animal studies and in catabolic patients[147-157] suggest that significant improvements in clinical outcome are possible with combinations of growth factors and specific nutrients in nutrition and metabolic support. The true clinical efficacy and cost effectiveness of these factors will undoubtedly emerge over the next several years on the basis of current and future randomized, double-blind, and controlled trials.

REFERENCES

1. Souba WW, Wilmore DW: Diet and nutrition in the care of the patient with surgery, trauma, and sepsis. In Shils ME, Olson JA, Shike M (eds): Modern Nutrition in Health and Disease, 8th edition. Philadelphia, Lea & Febiger, 1994:1207–1240.
2. American Society for Parenteral and Enteral Nutrition Board of Directors: Guidelines for the use of parenteral and enteral nutrition in adult and pediatric patients. J Parenter Enter Nutr 1993;14(suppl 4):1SA–52SA.
3. Kudsk KA, Croce MA, Fabian A et al: Enteral vs parenteral feeding: effects on septic morbidity following blunt and penetrating trauma. Ann Surg 1992;215:503–513.
4. Moore FA, Feliciano DV, Andrassy RJ et al: Early enteral feeding, compared with parenteral reduces postoperative septic complications. The results of a meta-analysis. Ann Surg 1992;216:172–183.
5. Rose WC: The nutritive significance of the amino acids and certain related compounds. Science 1937;86:298–300.
6. Moncada S, Palmer RMJ, Higgs EA: Biosynthesis of nitric oxide from L-arginine. A pathway for the regulation of cell function and communication. Biochem Pharmacol 1989;38:1709–1715.
7. Hibbs JB, Westenfelder C, Taintor R et al: Evidence for cytokine inducible nitric oxide synthesis from L-arginine in patients receiving interleukin-2 therapy. J Clin Invest 1992;89:867–877.
8. Barbul A: Arginine: biochemistry, physiology and therapeutic implications. J Parenter Enter Nutr 1986;10:227–238.
9. Gianotti L, Alexander JW, Payles T et al: Arginine-supplemented diets improve survival in gut-derived sepsis and peritonitis by modulating bacterial clearance—The role of nitric oxide. Ann Surg 1993;217:644–654.
10. Barbul A, Rettura G, Levenson S et al: Wound healing and thymotrophic effects of arginine: a pituitary mechanism of action. Am J Clin Nutr 1983;37:786–794.
11. Kirk SJ, Barbul A: Role of arginine in trauma, sepsis and immunity. J Parenter Enter Nutr 1990;14:226S–229S.
12. Gonce SJ, Peck MD, Alexander JW et al: Arginine supplementation and its effect on established peritonitis in guinea pigs. J Parenter Enter Nutr 1990;14:237–244.
13. Heyland DK, Cook DJ, Guyatt GH: Does the formulation of enteral feeding products influence infectious morbidity and mortality rates in the critically ill patient? A critical review of the evidence. Crit Care Med 1994;22:1192–1202.
14. Elsair J, Poey J, Isaad H et al: Effect of arginine chlorhydrate on nitrogen balance during the three days following routine surgery in man. Biomed Press 1978;29:312–317.
15. Daly JM, Reynolds J, Thom A et al: Immune and metabolic effects of arginine in the surgical patient. Ann Surg 1988;208:512–523.
16. Barbul A, Rettura G, Wasserkrug HL et al: Arginine stimulates lymphocyte immune responses in healthy humans. Surgery 1981;90:244–251.
17. Ziegler TR, Leader I: Adjunctive recombinant human growth hormone therapy in nutrition support: potential to limit septic complications in ICU patients. Semin Resp Infect 1994;9:240–247.
18. Barbul A, Lazarou S, Efron DT et al: Arginine enhances wound healing in humans. Surgery 1990;108:331–337.
19. Kirk SJ, Hurson M, Regan MC et al: Arginine stimulates wound healing and immune function in elderly human subjects. Surgery 1993;114:155–160.
20. Barbul A, Wasserkrug HL, Penberthy LT et al: Optimal levels of arginine in maintenance intravenous hyperalimentation. J Parenter Enter Nutr 1984;8:281–284.
21. Barbul A, Fishel RS, Shimazu S et al: Intravenous hyperalimentation with high arginine levels improves wound healing and immune function. J Surg Res 1985;38:328–334.
22. Sigal RK, Shou J, Daly JM: Parenteral arginine infusion in humans: nutrient substrate or pharmacologic agent? J Parenter Enter Nutr 1992;16:423–428.
23. Vinnars E, Furst P, Hallgren B et al: The nutritive effect in man of nonessential amino acids infused intravenously together with essential ones. I. Individual nonessential amino acids. Acta Anaesth Scand 1970;14:147–172.
24. Freund HR, Dienstag J, Lehrich et al: Infusion of branched-chain amino acid solution in patients with hepatic encephalopathy. Ann Surg 1982;196:209–220.
25. Cerra FB, Chung NK, Fischer JE et al: Disease-specific amino acid infusion (F080) in hepatic encephalopathy: a prospective, randomized, double-blind controlled trial. J Parenter Enter Nutr 1985;9:288–295.

26. Mochizuki H, Trocki O, Dominioni L et al: Effect of a diet rich in branched-chain amino acids on severely burned guinea pigs. J Trauma 1986;26:1077–1085.

27. Yoshida T, Muto Y, Moriwaki H et al: Effect of long-term supplementation with branched-chain amino acid granules on the prognosis of liver cirrhosis. Gastroenterol Jpn 1989;24:692–698.

28. Watanabe A, Shiota T, Okita M et al: Effect of a branched-chain amino acid-enriched nutritional product on the pathophysiology of the liver and nutritional state of patients with liver cirrhosis. Acta Med Okayama 1983;37:321–323.

29. Ferrando AA, Williams BD, Stuart CA et al: Oral branched-chain amino acids decrease whole-body proteolysis. J Parenter Enter Nutr 1995;19:47–54.

30. Cerra FB, Hirsch J, Mullen K et al: The effect of stress level, amino acid formula, and nitrogen dose on nitrogen retention in traumatic and septic stress. Ann Surg 1987;205:282–287.

31. Naylor CD, O'Rourke K, Detsky AS et al: Parenteral nutrition with branched-chain amino acids in hepatic encephalopathy: a meta-analysis. Gastroenterology 1989;97:1033–1042.

32. Lenssen P, Cheney CL, Aker SN et al: Intravenous branched chain amino acid trial in marrow transplant patients. J Parenter Enter Nutr 1987;11:112–118.

33. Hammarqvist F, Wernerman J, von der Decken A et al: The effects of branched chain amino-acids upon postoperative muscle protein synthesis and nitrogen balance. Clin Nutr 1988;7:171–175.

34. Jimenez FJJ, Leyba CO, Mendez SM et al: Prospective study of the efficacy of branched-chain amino acids in septic patients. J Parenter Enter Nutr 1991;15:252–261.

35. Ziegler TR, Smith RJ, Byrne TA et al: Potential role of glutamine supplementation in nutrition support. Clin Nutr 1993;12(suppl 1):S82–S90.

36. Souba WW, Klimberg VS, Plumley DA et al: The role of glutamine in maintaining a healthy gut and supporting the metabolic response to injury and infection. J Surg Res 1990;48:383–391.

37. Lacey JM, Wilmore DW: Is glutamine a conditionally essential amino acid? Nutr Rev 1990;48:297–304.

38. Furst P, Stehle P: Are we giving unbalanced amino acid solutions? In Wilmore DW, Carpentier YA (eds): Metabolic Support of the Critically Ill Patient. Berlin: Springer-Verlag, 1993;119–136.

39. Rudman D, Williams PJ: Nutrient deficiencies during total parenteral nutrition. Nutr Rev 1985;43:1–7.

40. Krebs H: Glutamine metabolism in the animal body. In Mora J, Palacios R (eds): Glutamine: Metabolism, Enzymology, and Regulation. New York: Academic Press, 1980;1–40.

41. Souba WW, Smith RJ, Wilmore DW: Glutamine metabolism by the intestinal tract. J Parenter Enter Nutr 1985;9:608–617.

42. Smith RJ: Glutamine metabolism and its physiologic importance. J Parenter Enter Nutr 1990;14(suppl 4):40S–44S.

43. Souba WW: Glutamine: a key substrate for the splanchnic bed. Annu Rev Nutr 1991;11:285–308.

44. Askanazi J, Furst P, Michelsen CB et al: Muscle and plasma amino acids after injury: hypocaloric glucose vs amino acids after injury. Ann Surg 1980;191:465–472.

45. Parry-Billings M, Evans J, Calder PC et al: Does glutamine contribute to immunosuppression after major burns? Lancet 1990;336:523–525.

46. MacLennan PA, Smith K, Weryk B et al: Inhibition of protein breakdown by glutamine in perfused rat skeletal muscle. FEBS Lett 1988;237:133–136.

47. Vinnars E, Hammarqvist F, von der Decken A et al: Role of glutamine and its analogs in posttraumatic muscle protein and amino acid metabolism. J Parenter Enter Nutr 1990;14:125S–129S.

48. Windmueller HG: Glutamine utilization by the small intestine. Adv Enzymol 1982;53:210.

49. Beaulieu JF, Calver R: Permissive effect of glutamine on the differentiation of fetal mouse small intestine in organ culture. Differentiation 1985;29:50–55.

50. Alverdy JC: Effects of glutamine-supplemented diets on immunology of the gut. J Parenter Enter Nutr 1990;14:109S–113S.

51. Wusteman M, Elia M: Effect of glutamine infusions on glutamine concentration and protein synthetic rate in rat muscle. J Parenter Enter Nutr 1991;15:521–525.

52. Scott T, Moellman J: Intravenous glutamine supplementation fails to accelerate gut mucosal recovery following 10 Gy abdominal radiation. Abstract. J Parenter Enter Nutr 1992;16:19S.

53. Bark T, Svenberg T, Theodorsson E et al: Glutamine supplementation does not prevent small bowel mucosal atrophy after total parenteral nutrition. Clin Nutr 1994;13:79–84.

54. Wusteman M, Tate H, Weaver L et al: The effect of glutamine deprivation and supplementation on the structure of rat small intestinal mucosa during a systemic injury response. J Parenter Enter Nutr 1995;19:22–27.

55. Ziegler TR, Benfell K, Smith RJ et al: Safety and metabolic effects of L-glutamine administration in humans. J Parenter Enter Nutr 1990;14(suppl 4):137S–146S.

56. Jensen GL, Miller RH, Talabiska D et al: A double-blind, prospective, randomized study of glutamine-enriched versus standard peptide-based feeding in the critically ill. Abstract. J Parenter Enter Nutr 1993;17:11S.

57. Buchman AL, Moukarzel AA, Ament ME et al: Parenteral nutrition leads to a decrease in intestinal mucosal thickness and an increase in intestinal permeability in man. Abstract. Gastroenterology 1993;104:A612.

58. Wischmeyer P, Pemberton JH, Phillips SF. Chronic pouchitis after ileal-anal anastomosis: responses to butyrate and glutamine suppositories in a pilot study. Mayo Clin Proc 1993;68:978–981.

59. Ziegler TR: Glutamine-supplemented nutrition in injury and infection. In Cynober L, Furst P, Lawin P (eds): Pharmacological Nutrition-Immune Nutrition. Munich: W. Zuckschwerdt Verlag, 1995:135–144.

60. Hammarqvist F, Wernerman J, Ali R et al: Addition of glutamine to total parenteral nutrition after elective abdominal surgery spares free glutamine in muscle, counteracts the fall in muscle protein synthesis, and improves nitrogen balance. Ann Surg 1989;209:455–461.

61. Ziegler TR, Gatzen C, Wilmore DW: Strategies for attenuating protein-catabolic responses in the critically ill. Ann Rev Med 1994;45:459–480.

62. Stehle P, Mertes N, Puchstein CH et al: Effect of parenteral glutamine peptide supplements on muscle glutamine loss and nitrogen balance after major surgery. Lancet 1989;1:231–234.

63. Furst P, Albers S, Stehle P: Glutamine-containing dipeptides in parenteral nutrition. J Parenter Enter Nutr 1990;14(suppl 4):118S–124S.

64. Wernerman J, Hammarqvist F, Ali MR et al: Glutamine and ornithine-alpha-ketoglutarate but not branched chain amino acids reduce the loss of muscle glutamine after surgical trauma. Metabolism 1989;38:63–66.

65. Walser M: Misinterpretation of nitrogen balances when glutamine stores fall or are replenished. Am J Clin Nutr 1991;53:1337–1338.

66. Van Der Hulst RRW, Van Kreel BK et al: Glutamine and the preservation of gut integrity. Lancet 1993; 341:1363–1365.

67. Tremel H, Kienle B, Weilemann LS et al: Glutamine dipeptide supplemented TPN maintains intestinal function in the critically ill. Gastroenterology 1994;107:1595–1601.

68. Ziegler TR, Young LS, Benfell K et al: Clinical and metabolic efficacy of glutamine-supplemented parenteral nutrition after bone marrow transplantation. A randomized, double-blind, controlled study. Ann Intern Med 1992;116:821–828.

69. Schloerb PR, Amare M: Total parenteral nutrition with glutamine in bone marrow transplantation and other clinical applications (A randomized, double-blind study). J Parenter Enter Nutr 1993;17:407–413.

70. Scheltinga M, Young LS, Benfell K et al: Glutamine-enriched intravenous feedings attenuate extracellular fluid expansion after a standard stress. Ann Surg 1991;214:385–395.

71. McBurney M, Young LS, Ziegler TR et al: A cost-evaluation of glutamine-supplemented parenteral nutrition in adult bone marrow transplantation. J Am Diet Assoc 1994;94:1263–1266.

72. Hong RW, Helton WS, Rounds JD et al: Glutamine-supplemented TPN preserves hepatic glutathione and improves survival following chemotherapy. Surg Forum 1990;41:9–11.

73. Hong RW, Rounds JD, Helton WS et al: Glutamine preserves liver glutathione after lethal hepatic injury. Ann Surg 1992;215:114–119.

74. Ziegler TR, Bye RL, Persinger RL et al: Glutamine-enriched parenteral nutrition increases circulating lymphocytes after bone marrow transplantation. Abstract. J Parenter Enter Nutr 1994;18:17S.

75. O'Riordain MG, Fearon KCH, Ross JA et al: Glutamine-supplemented total parenteral nutrition enhances T-lymphocyte response in surgical patients undergoing colorectal resection. Ann Surg 1994;220: 212–221.

76. Young LS, Bye R, Scheltinga M et al: Patients receiving glutamine supplemented intravenous feedings report an improvement in mood. J Parenter Enter Nutr 1993;17:422–427.

77. van Zaanen HCT, van der Lelie H, Timmer JG et al: Parenteral glutamine dipeptide supplementation does not ameliorate chemotherapy-induced toxicity. Cancer 1994;74:2879–2884.

78. Laidlaw SA, Kopple JD: Newer concepts of the indispensable amino acids. Am J Clin Nutr 1987;46: 593–605.

79. Zelikovic I, Chesney RW, Friedman AL et al: Taurine depletion in very low birthweight infants receiving prolonged total parenteral nutrition: role of renal immaturity. J Pediatr 1990;116:301–306.

80. Wright CE, Tallan HH, Lin YY: Taurine: biological update. Annu Rev Biochem 1986;55:427–436.

81. Gray GE, Landel AM, Mequid MM: Taurine-supplemented total parenteral nutrition and taurine status of malnourished cancer patients. Nutrition 1994;10: 11–15.

82. Paauw JD, Davis AT: Taurine concentrations in serum of critically injured patients and age- and sex-matched healthy control subjects. Am J Clin Nutr 1990;52:657–660.

83. Desai TK, Maliakkal J, Kinzie JL et al: Taurine deficiency after intensive chemotherapy and/or radiation. Am J Clin Nutr 1992;55:708–711.

84. Martensson J, Larson J, Schildt BO: Metabolic effects of amino acid solutions in burned patients: with emphasis on sulfur amino acid metabolism and protein breakdown. J Trauma 1985;25:427–432.

85. Gazzaniga AB, Waxman K, Day AT et al: Nitrogen balance in adult hospitalized patients with the use of a pediatric amino acid model. Arch Surg 1988;123: 1275–1281.

86. Cynober L. Ornithine alpha-ketoglutarate in nutritional support. Nutrition 1991;7:313–322.

87. Cynober L, Saizy R, Nguyen DF et al: Effect of enterally administered ornithine alpha-ketoglutarate on plasma and urinary levels after burn injury. J Trauma 1984;24:590–596.

88. Leander U, Furst P, Vesterberg K et al: Nitrogen sparing effect of Ornicetil in the immediate postoperative state: clinical biochemistry and nitrogen balance. Clin Nutr 1985;4:43–51.

89. Cynober L, Lioret N, Coudray-Lucas C et al: Action of ornithine alpha-ketoglutarate on protein metabolism in burn patients. Nutrition 1987;3:187–191.

90. Wernerman J, Hammarqvist F, Von der Decken A et al: Ornithine-alpha-ketoglutarate improves skeletal muscle protein synthesis as assessed by ribosome analysis and nitrogen use after surgery. Ann Surg 1987;206:674–678.

91. Moukarzel A, Gorski AM, Boya I et al: Growth retardation in children on long term total parenteral nutrition (TPN): effects of ornithine alpha-ketoglutarate. Abstract. Clin Nutr 1988;7(suppl):13.

92. Cynober L, Coudray-Lucas C, deBrandt J-P et al: Action of ornithine alpha-ketoglutarate, ornithine hydrochloride, and calcium alpha-ketoglutarate on plasma amino acid and hormonal patterns in healthy subjects. J Am Coll Nutr 1990;9:2–12.

93. Donati L, Signorini M: Nutritional effects of ornithine alpha ketoglutarate in burn patients. Abstract. Clin Nutr 1992;11(suppl):25.

94. Jeevanandam M, Ali MR, Peterson SR: Substrate and hormonal changes due to dietary supplementation with ornithine alpha ketoglutarate in critically ill trauma victims. Abstract. Clin Nutr 1992;11(suppl): 26.

95. Wernerman J, Hammarqvist F, Vinnars E: Alpha-ketoglutarate and postoperative muscle catabolism. Lancet 1990;335:701–703.

96. Petersson B, Gamrin L, Hammarqvist F et al: Alpha-ketoglutarate given together with TPN improves the free glutamine-levels in glutamine-depleted intensive care patients. Abstract. Clin Nutr 1992;11(suppl):26.

97. Berger MM, Cavadini C, Chiolero R et al: Influence of larger intakes of trace elements on recovery after major burns. Nutrition 1994;10:327–334.

98. Fusi S, Kupper TS, Green DR et al: Reversal of postburn immunosuppression by the administration of vitamin A. Surgery 1984;96:330–335.

99. Levenson SM, Gruber CA, Rettura G et al: Supplemental vitamin A prevents the acute radiation-induced defect on wound healing. Ann Surg 1984;200: 494–512.

100. Warson RR, Prabhala RH, Plezia PM et al: Effects of beta-carotene on lymphocyte subpopulations in el-

derly humans: evidence for a dose-response relationship. Am J Clin Nutr 1991;53:90–94.

101. Madrerazo EG, Woronick CL, Hickingbotham N et al: A randomized trial of replacement antioxidant vitamin therapy for neutrophil locomotory dysfunction in blunt trauma. J Trauma 1991;31:1142–1150.

102. Haberal M, Hamaloglu E, Bora S et al: The effects of vitamin E on immune regulation after thermal injury. Burns 1988;14:388–393.

103. Penn ND, Purkins L, Kelleher J et al: The effects of dietary supplementation with vitamins A, C, and E on cell-mediated immune function in elderly long-stay patients: a randomized controlled trial. Age Ageing 1991;20:169–174.

104. Sies H, Stahl W, Sundquist AR: Antioxidant functions of vitamins: vitamins E and C, beta-carotene, and other carotenoids. Ann NY Acad Sci 1992;669:7–20.

105. Chandra RK: Effects of vitamin and trace element supplementation on immune response and infection in elderly subjects. Lancet 1992;340:1124–1127.

106. Lash LH, Hagan TM, Jones DP: Exogenous glutathione protects intestinal epithelial cells from oxidative injury. Proc Natl Acad Sci USA 1986;83:4461–4465.

107. Seidner DL: Clinical uses for omega-3 polyunsaturated fatty acids and structured triglycerides. Support Line 1994;16:7–10.

108. Leaf A, Weber PC: Cardiovascular effects of n-3 fatty acids. N Engl J Med 1988;318:549–557.

109. Hepburn FN, Exler J, Weihrauch JL: Provisional tables on the content of omega-3 fatty acids and other fat components of selected foods. J Am Diet Assoc 1986;86:788–793.

110. Dyerberg J, Bang HO, Stofferson E et al: Eicosopentaenoic acid and prevention of thrombosis and atherosclerosis? Lancet 1978;2:117–119.

111. Goodnight SH, Harris WS, Connor WE: The effects of dietary omega-3 fatty acids on platelet composition and function in man: a prospective, controlled study. Blood 1981;58:880–885.

112. Samuelsson B: Leukotrienes: mediators of immediate hypersensitivity reactions and inflammation. Science 1983;220:568–575.

113. Tinoco J: Dietary requirements and functions of alpha-linolenic acid in animals. Prog Lipid Res 1982;21:1–45.

114. Lands WEM: Fish and human health. Orlando, FL: Academic Press, 1986;103–106.

115. Holman RT: Nutritional and metabolic interrelationships between fatty acids. Fed Proc 1964;23:1062–1067.

116. Bang HO, Dyerberg J: Plasma lipids and lipoproteins in Greenlandic west coast Eskimos. Acta Med Scan 1972;192:85–94.

117. Kromann N, Green A: Epidemiologic studies in the Upernavik district, Greenland: incidence of some chronic diseases 1950-1974. Acta Med Scand 1980;208:401–406.

118. Radack K, Deck C, Huster G: The effects of low doses of n-3 fatty acid supplementation on blood pressure in hypertensive subjects. Arch Intern Med 1991;151:1173–1180.

119. Sirtori CR, Gatti E, Tremoli E et al: Olive oil, corn oil, and n-3 fatty acids differently affect lipids, lipoproteins, platelets, and superoxide formation in Type II hypercholesterolemia. Am J Clin Nutr 1992;56:113–122.

120. Yetiv JK: Clinical applications of fish oil. JAMA 1988;260:665–670.

121. Meydani SN, Dinarello CA: Influence of dietary fatty acids on cytokine production and its clinical implications. Nutr Clin Pract 1993; 8:65–72.

122. Endres S, Ghorbani R, Kelley VE et al: The effect of dietary supplementation with n-3 polyunsaturated fatty acids on the synthesis of interleukin-1 and tumor necrosis factor by mononuclear cells. N Engl J Med 1989;320:265–271.

123. Meydani SN, Lichtenstein AH, Cornwall S et al: Immunologic effects of National Cholesterol Education Panel Step-2b diets with and without fish-derived N-3 fatty acid enrichment. J Clin Invest 1993;92:105–113.

124. Palombo JD, Bistrian BR, Fechner KD et al: Rapid incorporation of fish or olive oil fatty acids into rat hepatic sinusoidal cell phospholipids after continuous enteral feeding during endotoxemia. Am J Clin Nutr 1993;57:643–649.

125. Peck MD: Omega-3 polyunsaturated fatty acids: benefit or harm during sepsis? New Horizons 1994;2:230–236.

126. Meydani M, Natiello F, Goldin B et al: Effect of long-term fish oil supplementation on vitamin E status and lipid peroxidation. J Nutr 1991;121:484–491.

127. Swails WS, Bell SJ, Bistrian BR et al: Fish-oil containing diet and platelet aggregation. Nutrition 1993;9:211–217.

128. Bach AC, Babayan VK: Medium- chain triglycerides: an update. Am J Clin Nutr 1982;36:950–962.

129. Pomposelli JJ, Bistrian BR: Is total parenteral nutrition immunosuppressive? New Horizons 1994;2:224–229.

130. Gottschlich MM: Selection of optimal lipid sources in enteral and parenteral nutrition. Nutr Clin Pract 1992;7:152–165.

131. Ledeboer M, Masclee AAM, Jansen JBMJ et al: Effect of equimolar amounts of long-chain triglycerides and medium-chain triglycerides on small-bowel transit time in humans. J Parenter Enter Nutr 1995;19:5–8.

132. Baba N, Bracco EF, Hashim SA: Enhanced thermogenesis and diminished deposition of fat in response to overfeeding with diet containing medium chain triglyceride. Am J Clin Nutr 1982;35:678–682.

133. Holt PR: Medium chain triglycerides: their absorption, metabolism and clinical application. Prog Gastroenterol 1968;1:277–298.

134. Zurier RB, Campbell RG, Hashim SA et al: Use of medium chain triglyceride in management of patients with massive resection of the small intestine. N Engl J Med 1966;274:490–493.

135. Hashim SA, Roholt HB, Babayan VK et al: Treatment of chyluria and chylothorax with medium-chain triglyceride. N Engl J Med 1964;270:756–761.

136. DeMichele SJ, Karlstad MD, Babayan YK et al: Enhanced skeletal muscle and liver protein synthesis with structured lipid in enterally fed burned rats. Metabolism 1988;37:787–795.

137. Teo TC, DeMichele SJ, Selleck KM et al: Administration of structured lipid composed of MCT and fish oil reduces net protein catabolism in enterally fed burned rats. Ann Surg 1989;210:100–107.

138. Rudolph FB: The biochemistry and physiology of nucleotides. J Nutr 1994;124:124s–127s.

139. Kulkarni AD, Rudolph FB, Van Buren CT: The role of dietary sources of nucleotides in immune function: a review. J Nutr 1994;124:1442s–1446s.

140. Van Buren CT, Kulkarni AD, Rudolph FB: The role of nucleotides in adult nutrition. J Nutr 1994;124:160s–164s.

141. Van Buren CT, Kulkarni AD, Schandle VB et al: The influence of dietary nucleotides on cell-mediated immunity. Transplantation 1983;36:350–352.

142. Fanslow WC, Kulkarni AD, Van Buren CT et al: Effect of nucleotide restriction and supplementation on re-

sistance to experimental murine candidiasis. J Parenter Enter Nutr 1988;12:49–52.

143. Kulkarni AD, Fanslow WC, Rudolph FB et al: Effect of dietary nucleotides on response to bacterial infections. J Parenter Enter Nutr 1986;10:169–171.

144. Uauy R, Quan R, Gil A: Role of nucleotides in intestinal development and repair: implications for infant nutrition. J Nutr 1994;124:1436s–1441s.

145. Braun CH: Effect of consumption of human milk and other formulas on intestinal bacterial flora in infants. In Lebenthal E (ed): Textbook of Gastroenterology and Nutrition in Infancy Volume 1. New York: Raven Press, 1981;247–253.

146. Uauy R, Stringel G, Thomas R et al: Effect of dietary nucleosides on growth and maturation of the developing gut in the rat. J Pediatr Gastroenterol Nutr 1990;10:497–503.

147. Ziegler TR: Growth hormone administration during nutritional support: what is to be gained? New Horizons 1994;2:244–256.

148. Ziegler TR, Jacobs DO: Anabolic hormones in nutritional support. In Torosian MH (ed): Nutrition for the Hospitalized Patient: Basic Science and Principles of Practice. New York: Marcel-Dekker, 1995;11:207–232.

149. Hammarqvist F, Stromberg C, Decken von der A et al: Biosynthetic human growth hormone preserves both muscle protein synthesis and the decrease in muscle free glutamine, and improves whole-body nitrogen economy after operation. Ann Surg 1922;216:184–191.

150. Ziegler TR, Mantell MP, Rombeau JL et al: Effects of glutamine and IGF-I administration on intestinal growth and the IGF pathway after partial small bowel resection. Abstract. J Parenter Enter Nutr 1994;18 (suppl 1):20S.

151. Byrne TA, Morrissey TB, Nattakom TV et al: Growth hormone, glutamine and a modified diet enhance nutrient absorption in patients with the severe short bowel syndrome. J Parenter Enter Nutr 1995;19: 296–302.

152. Wilmore DW, Byrne TA, Persinger RL et al: A new treatment for patients with the short bowel syndrome: growth hormone, glutamine and a modified diet. Ann Surg 1995;222:243–255.

153. Gottschlich MM, Jenkins M, Warden GD, et al: Differential effects of three dietary regimens on selected outcome variables in burn patients. J Parenter Enter Nutr 1990;14:225–236.

154. Cerra FB, Lehman S, Konstantinides N et al: Effect of enteral nutrients on *in vitro* tests of immune function in ICU patients: a preliminary report. Nutrition 1990;6:84–87.

155. Cerra F, Lehmann S, Konstantinides N et al: Improvement in immune function in ICU patients by enteral nutrition supplemented with arginine, RNA, and menhaden oil is independent of nitrogen balance. Nutrition 1991;17:193–199.

156. Daly JM, Lieberman MD, Goldfine J et al: Enteral nutrition with supplemental arginine, RNA, and omega-3 fatty acids in patients after operation: immunologic, metabolic, and clinical outcome. Surgery 1992; 112:56–67.

157. Bower RH, Cerra FB, Bershadsky B et al: Early enteral administration of a formula (Impact®) supplemented with arginine, nucleotides, and fish oil in intensive care unit patients: results of a multicenter, prospective, randomized, clinical trial. Crit Care Med 1995; 23:436–449.

9

The Molecular Biology of Enteral Nutrition and the Gut

ROBERT J. SMITH
JESSE C. CHOW

Dietary nutrient content has important effects on gene expression in multiple body tissues. Specific macronutrients, minerals, and vitamins initiate processes of gene regulation that alter levels of metabolic enzymes, transport proteins, and structural proteins. Resulting changes in metabolism provide a basis for adaptation to diets of varying composition and quantity. When enteral nutrients are digested and absorbed, the gastrointestinal (GI) tract represents an important tissue site of gene regulation in response to dietary components. In addition, the GI tract's digestive, metabolic, and absorptive functions are critical determinants of the specific dietary components or derivatives that reach and exert regulatory effects on other tissues.

Although applying molecular biologic methods to the investigation of relationships between enteral nutrients and gene regulation is a relatively new science, progress in this field has already led to significant advances in our understanding of the effects of enteral nutrients on metabolic processes. In the next few years, a far greater amount of important information on the molecular biology of enteral nutrition will most likely emerge. This chapter will provide an overview of molecular biologic methods with applications in nutrition, a brief review of current knowledge on enteral nutri-

ents as specific modifiers of gene expression in nonintestinal tissues, and an introduction to the nutritional molecular biology of the intestine.

APPLICATIONS OF MOLECULAR BIOLOGY IN NUTRITION

Information Transfer from Genes to Proteins

Molecular biologic methods developed over the past 2 decades have provided powerful tools for probing gene structure, defining the steps involved in the conversion of gene sequence to protein sequence, and investigating the structure and function of specific proteins.[1] Ultimately, the levels of individual proteins in a tissue determine its fundamental differentiated properties and its adaptation to different levels of nutrient intake or otherwise altered metabolic conditions.

Figure 9–1 outlines the steps involved in the transfer of information from genes to proteins. After a specific gene is activated, for example, by the association of a transcriptional activator with the promoter region of the gene, the nucleotide sequence of one of the two strands of the genomic DNA is transcribed into a matching messenger RNA (mRNA) sequence. This initial

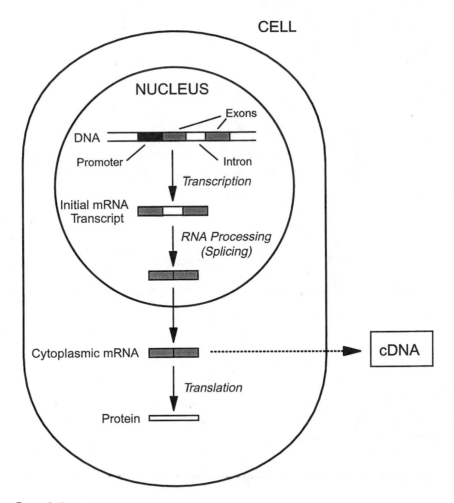

FIGURE 9–1   Steps involved in the transfer of information from genes to proteins.

mRNA transcript is next processed in the nucleus by removing strings of nucleotides termed *introns* and linking together the remaining segments of mRNA termed *exons.* The final mRNA transcript then moves from the nucleus to the cytoplasm, where it is used as a template to form proteins. The conversion of the mRNA sequence into the amino acid sequence of a protein, a process termed *translation,* involves the alignment and linking together of amino acids in a specific order determined by groups of three nucleotides (codons) in the mRNA.

The series of reactions illustrated in Figure 9–1 includes multiple steps at which regulatory events can determine the level or ultimate structure of individual proteins. Regulated changes in promoter activity, as well as the overall activity of the transcriptional apparatus, are important determinants of the rate of formation of initial mRNA transcripts from specific genes. As mRNA processing occurs under dif-

ferent physiologic conditions, the pattern of excluded introns and included exons can be modified for some genes (alternative mRNA splicing). Even though the same gene is being read, this changes the sequence of the final mRNA transcript and thus the primary structure of the protein product. Regulation of factors that determine mRNA stability can lead to changes in levels of specific mRNAs independent of actual transcription rates, and the overall activity of the translational apparatus can influence the rate of protein synthesis independent of the level of mRNA. Although knowledge of nutrient-mediated regulatory events is still quite limited, nutrient-related regulation probably has important effects on each of these steps.

Nutrition and Protein Translation

The synthesis of a new protein requires the association of an mRNA transcript with ribosomes, initiation factors, and a number of proteins that catalyze assembly of the amino acid chain of the protein.[2,3] As the synthesis of a peptide chain progresses, the ribosome moves along the mRNA strand, and a second ribosomal structure can become associated with the mRNA at the same time. As this process continues, a large complex (designated a polysome or polyribosome) is formed, consisting of a single mRNA strand, multiple ribosomes, and multiple nascent peptide chains of different lengths. Polysomes are large enough that they can be isolated from cell or tissue samples by density gradient centrifugation or other methods, and the total quantity of RNA in polysomes can be determined.[4] The amount of RNA in polysomes in a sample of tissue thus can be used to provide an index of the overall rate of protein synthesis occurring in the tissue in vivo.

The data in Figure 9–2 illustrate the application of polysome analysis to the investigation of protein synthesis rates in human skeletal muscle during fasting. In this study, healthy subjects fasted for 3 days, and needle biopsy samples were obtained each day from the quadriceps femoris muscle for ribosome analysis.[5] A decrease in ribosomal RNA in polysomes as a percentage of total ribosomes was evident after 2 days of fasting (Fig. 9–2A), and there was a more gradually developing decrease in the total content of ribosomes (Fig.

9–2B). Thus, there was a progressive decline in the total muscle content of polysomes, as well as the percentage of ribosomes in polysome structures due to fasting. In a more recent study using similar methods to analyze muscle biopsy tissue, adding the amino acid glutamine to a total parenteral nutrition (TPN) formula was shown in postoperative patients to increase the total amount of skeletal muscle RNA in polysomes and, in parallel, to improve total body nitrogen balance.[6] Polysome analysis has not been used extensively in other nutritional studies, but, when tissue samples are available, it represents a useful method to assess nutrient effects on protein synthesis rates in vivo.

cDNA Cloning and Amplification

Most current molecular biology methods make use of complementary DNA (cDNA) or experimental tools that have been developed through the use of cDNA. The generation of cDNA starts with the isolation of mRNA from a tissue of interest (Fig. 9–3). This RNA consists of a single strand of ribonucleotides that usually ends in a string of adenines (> 90 percent of mRNAs end with a poly-A tail). Using a synthetic string of thymines (oligo-dT primer) to provide a starting point for the enzyme reverse transcriptase, a strand of DNA complementary to the mRNA sequence is formed along the mRNA strand. The resulting double-stranded

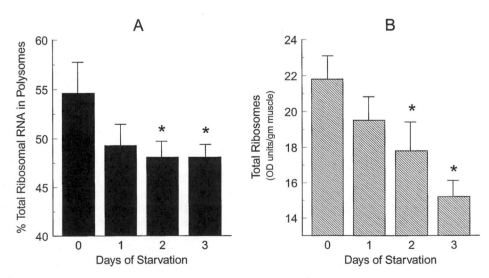

FIGURE 9–2 Effects of starvation on polysome profiles in skeletal muscle biopsies from healthy male volunteers. *A,* Polysome RNA as percent of total ribosomal RNA. *B,* Total ribosome content per unit muscle wet weight. *P < 0.05 vs day 0. (Redrawn with permission from Wernerman J, von der Decken A, Vinnars E: Size distribution of ribosomes in biopsy specimens of human skeletal muscle during starvation. Metabolism 1985;34:665.)

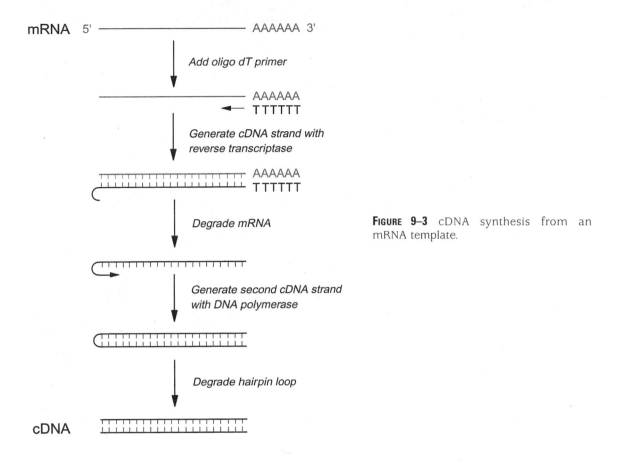

FIGURE 9–3 cDNA synthesis from an mRNA template.

RNA-DNA structure is not unlike newly formed, double-stranded DNA generated during normal cellular DNA synthesis. The strands are separated by adding appropriate salts and raising the temperature, and the relatively unstable mRNA is easily destroyed simply by raising the pH. The remaining DNA is then used as a template (with DNA polymerase rather than reverse transcriptase) to form a double-stranded cDNA molecule that contains the sequence originally present in the mRNA.

In contrast to mRNA, which is unstable and difficult to manipulate experimentally, cDNA is resistant to degradation. There also are an enormous number of widely available experimental tools for analyzing, modifying, amplifying, and otherwise making use of cDNA. Of particular importance, once a double-stranded cDNA fragment has been generated, it can readily be inserted into a plasmid vector and greatly amplified (Fig. 9–4). The plasmid, which is most often an engineered circular DNA molecule, is cut by digestion with a restriction enzyme, the cDNA is inserted through a process termed *ligation,* and the plasmid is introduced into a special host strain of bacteria where it is replicated to produce millions of identical copies. The newly formed plasmids can then be separated from the bacteria, the cDNA fragments excised by digestion with a restriction enzyme, and an essentially unlimited quantity of the original DNA segment can thus be obtained for study.

Applications of cDNA Technology

A number of uses of cDNA that have application in the field of nutrition are summarized in Table 9–1. Rapid and reliable methods are available for obtaining the nucleotide sequence of cloned cDNA fragments. This can be done manually with a small amount of specialized equipment or even more rapidly with an automated DNA sequencer. Since cDNA is generated from an mRNA template after the excision of introns as described in Figure 9–1, its nucleotide sequence can be used to deduce the amino acid sequence of the corresponding protein. Once the translation start codon has been identified or the reading frame established by other methods, the series of complementary triplet codons that make up the mRNA strand

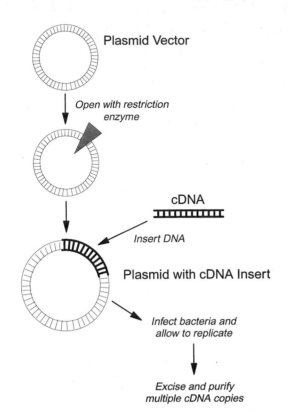

FIGURE 9–4   Basic steps in cDNA cloning and amplification.

can be determined. The specific amino acid associated with each of these codons is known, and it is thus possible to define the protein sequence without ever actually analyzing the protein itself. With the power of DNA amplification methods, this can be accomplished with cDNA derived from a small amount of mRNA. By contrast, analysis of proteins themselves usually requires laborious and difficult purification procedures, large amounts of starting material to accommodate losses during purification, and much slower and more complicated sequencing methods. Selected examples of nutrition relevant protein sequences derived form cDNA sequences are listed in Table 9–2. For many of

TABLE 9–1   cDNA Applications in the Field of Nutrition

Determination of protein sequences
mRNA quantitation
mRNA cell type localization
Recombinant protein production
Investigation of protein function
Gene therapy

TABLE 9–2   Protein Sequences Derived from cDNA

Function	Examples
Carbohydrate metabolism	Phosphoenolpyruvate carboxykinase
	Pyruvate kinase
	Insulin receptor
	Glucose transporters
Lipid metabolism	Intenstinal fatty acid–binding protein (FABPI)
	Low density lipoprotein receptor
	Apolipoproteins
Growth control	Growth hormone
	Insulinlike growth factors (IGFs)
	IGF receptors
	IGF-binding proteins
Micronutrient metabolism	Retinol-binding protein
	Transferrin
	Transferrin receptors
	Ferritin

these proteins, the amino acid sequence would not be known if we had to depend on traditional protein purification and analysis methods, and we would thus have significantly less knowledge of their structure, function, regulation, and roles in human disease states.

Northern Blotting and Other Methods of mRNA Analysis

Through the same process of nucleotide base-pairing that correctly aligns complementary nucleotides along an mRNA strand during cDNA synthesis, intact complementary strands of DNA or RNA will associate to form a double-stranded complex under appropriate conditions of temperature, pH, and salt concentration. Because the formation of these complexes requires correct matching of nucleotide pairs along the length of the two strands, a specific cDNA will associate only with its corresponding mRNA, even though many other mRNA sequences may be present. With techniques for detecting cDNA (using incorporated radioactive nucleotides or other nonradioactive methods), it is possible to use the specific pairing of cDNA and mRNA strands to identify and quantify individual mRNAs in tissue extracts.

This is most often accomplished by the method of Northern blotting. RNA is isolated from a tissue of interest, and, by gel electrophoresis, the individual RNAs are separated according to size (i.e., number of nucleotides).

The RNA is transferred or blotted to a nitrocellulose or nylon membrane (hence the term *blotting*), and this membrane is incubated with a specific labeled cDNA probe under conditions where the probe will anneal with high specificity to mRNA strands with correct complementary sequence. If ^{32}P labeling of cDNA is used as a detection method, a sheet of x-ray film is simply laid over the blotting membrane. The position of exposed bands on the film can be used to determine the size of mRNA transcripts interacting with the cDNA probe, and the density of the bands can be used to determine the quantity of mRNA present in the tissue extract.

An example of the use of Northern blotting to determine the effects of fasting and refeeding on the levels of mRNA for insulin-like growth factor-I (IGF-I) receptors and insulin receptors in rat jejunum is shown in Figure 9–5. The IGF-I receptor mRNA transcript is a single species of approximately 11,000 bases long. Its content in the jejunum is not significantly altered by 72 hours of fasting, but it is increased during refeeding. By contrast, insulin-receptor mRNA, which consists of two species of 9600 and 7400 bases, is markedly increased during fasting and decreased to control levels with refeeding. These Northern blotting results demonstrate independent patterns of regulation of insulin and IGF-I receptors in the intestine, even though these two receptors are very closely related in structure. Insulin receptor gene expression correlates inversely with plasma insulin levels during fasting and refeeding (low plasma insulin and high mRNA with fasting, high plasma insulin and low mRNA with refeeding), consistent with down-regulation of receptor gene expression by the hormone. IGF-I receptor gene expression, on the other hand, correlates with tissue growth rate during fasting and refeeding, such that both receptor mRNA and the plasma level of IGF-I are high during refeeding.[7]

The Northern blotting technique has been used to determine the content of specific mRNAs in samples of human tissue obtained by needle biopsy. For example, levels of mRNA for myosin heavy chain in skeletal muscle biopsy samples have been determined to investigate factors that influence protein synthetic rates and tissue nitrogen balance.[8] Other methods, including dot blotting, solution hybridization, RNase protection, and quantitative PCR (polymerase chain reaction) have been developed that use the same principal of selective base pairing to detect and quantify specific mRNAs.[9] These methods can define mRNA content in tissues with higher speed, accuracy, or sensitivity.

Recombinant Protein Products

Once a cDNA fragment has been cloned into a plasmid, multiple copies can be produced in a host strain of bacteria as discussed above and illustrated in Figure 9–4. With biologically engineered plasmids that contain a promoter adjacent to the inserted cDNA in the plasmid, bacteria can be induced not only to make copies of the plasmid DNA, but also to transcribe multiple copies of the cDNA itself into bacterial mRNA. These mRNAs are then translated into protein by the bacterial ribosomal apparatus in the same way that normal bacterial proteins are formed. The net result is the conversion of the bacteria into protein-producing biologic factories. With the combined use of specialized plasmids termed *expression vectors,* bacterial strains optimized for protein production, and biochemical methods to obtain purified proteins from the bacteria, it is possible to produce large quantities of human proteins.

Examples of proteins with relevance to the field of nutrition that have been produced by recombinant DNA technology are listed in Table 9–3. For some of these proteins, such as insulin, large quantities of the hormone were previously obtained from animal sources. Recombinant human insulin has largely replaced the animal-derived insulins with a human protein that has low antigenicity, lower production costs, and a supply that does not depend on the availability of pancreatic tissue from slaughter houses. The production of recombinant human growth hormone has not only provided much larger quantities of the hormone than could be obtained from human sources, but it has made it possible to avoid the serious problem of pathologic viral contamination of human pituitary-derived growth hormone.[10] For most of the proteins listed in Table 9–3, levels in human and animal tissues are so low that they never could be obtained in adequate quantities from natural sources. The availability of these recombinant proteins for research and therapeutic purposes has opened a new era in the field of nutrition support. Multiple studies with recombinant hormones, for example, have demonstrated that administered trophic hormones and nutrients can have additive or synergistic anabolic effects.[11,12] As our knowledge of these interactions progresses, it is likely that optimal nutrition support for many patients in the future will involve the coordinated administration of

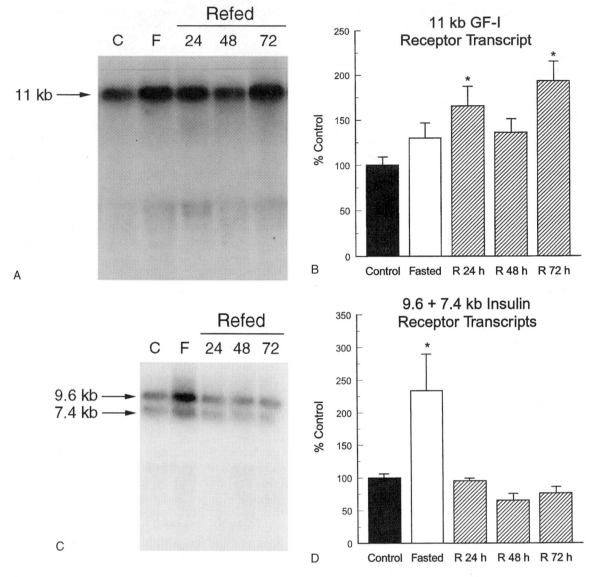

FIGURE 9–5 Effects of fasting and refeeding on IGF-I and insulin receptor mRNA in rat jejunum. *A,* Representative IGF-I receptor Northern blot. *B,* Quantitation of IGF-I receptor transcripts in multiple experiments. *C,* Representative insulin receptor Northern blot. *D,* Quantitation of 9.6 and 7.4 kb insulin receptor transcripts (combined). Data represent mean ± SEM; *$P < 0.05$ vs control. (Redrawn with permission from Ziegler TR, Almahfouz A, Pedrini MT et al: A comparison of rat small intestinal insulin and IGF I receptors during fasting and refeeding. Endocrinology 1995;136:5148. © The Endocrine Society.)

nutrients and recombinant, tissue-specific trophic hormones.

Recombinant Protein Expression in Cultured Mammalian Cells

Using methods fundamentally similar to those that generate recombinant proteins in bacteria, cloned cDNA can be introduced into cultured human and animal cells, and recombinant proteins expressed at high levels.[13] Sev-

TABLE 9–3   Proteins with Relevance to Nutrition Produced from Recombinant DNA

Insulin
IGF-I
IGF-binding proteins
Growth hormone
Epidermal growth factor
Tumor necrosis factor
Interleukins

eral different experimental approaches are available, but mammalian expression vectors are most often introduced into cells by a method termed *transfection,* and the introduced cDNA, linked to a promoter, becomes permanently incorporated into the cellular DNA. The promoter causes the cDNA to be transcribed into mRNA at a high rate, and the cell produces the new protein. By comparing transfected cells with normal cells, the properties of the expressed protein can be studied. For example, the consequences of high expression of cell surface receptors involved in nutritionally important pathways, such as insulin receptors,[14] IGF-I receptors,[15] and low density lipoprotein receptors,[16] have been assessed in transfected cells. In other studies, the functional properties of intracellular proteins, such as the uncoupling protein of brown adipose tissue,[17] have been studied in a similar manner.

It is possible to modify the amino acid sequences of expressed proteins by site-directed mutagenesis of the cDNAs before transfection,[18] and the functional consequences of the engineered structural changes in the proteins can then be investigated.[19] Alternatively, naturally occurring abnormal cDNAs isolated from patients with inherited metabolic disorders can be transfected into cultured cells, and the effects of the mutation on protein function can be assessed.[20] As the specific genetic origins of inherited risk for nutritionally related disorders, such as obesity, hyperlipidemias, and digestive diseases, are defined in coming years, studies with transfection methods in cultured cells undoubtedly will continue to provide information about the functional properties of the abnormal proteins and thus the molecular basis for the clinical disease.

Genetic Modification and Protein Expression in Intact Organisms

One of the most rapidly progressing areas of applied molecular biology involves introducing cDNAs into intact organisms. This is most often accomplished using laboratory mice as a model system. The desired cDNA is introduced into embryonic stem cells maintained in culture, where it becomes incorporated into the cellular genome. The stem cells are then implanted into the uterus of a hormonally primed pseudopregnant mouse, where they develop into complete embryos. If the introduced gene does not produce changes incompatible with survival, progeny transgenic mice are obtained that will demonstrate the effects of the introduced gene. If these mice are fertile, they can

be used by backcross breeding to obtain a strain of animals homozygous for the newly acquired trait.

In the simplest construct, the in vivo properties of an introduced gene can be investigated through its overexpression in multiple body tissues. For example, the photograph in Figure 9–6 demonstrates increased somatic growth of a transgenic mouse expressing multiple copies of the growth hormone gene. This was accomplished by introducing growth hormone cDNA linked to a metallothionein promoter that resulted in high expression in many tissues.[21] In current studies, introduced genes often are linked to regulated or tissue-specific promoters, so that expression of the introduced protein can be turned on and off, or restricted to target tissues, such as skeletal muscle, liver, or fat.[22] The use of intestine-specific promoters in transgenic animals is an active area of research that will be discussed in a subsequent section of this chapter.

In addition to introducing new genes into a recipient organism, methods have been developed to exchange portions of an endogenous gene with an introduced cDNA sequence through a process termed homologous recombination.[23] Using this technique in embryonic stem cells, it has become a relatively simple undertaking to replace small portions of genes with nonsense sequence, such that the protein product of the gene can no longer be produced, so-called *gene knockout.* By implanting the embryonic stem cells into pseudopregnant mice and studying the progeny, the effects of elimination of specific genes can be investigated.

These and other methods for introducing or modifying genes in intact organisms currently have great power as research tools. However, it can readily be envisioned that similar methods also could become part of a practical strategy for gene therapy. Using modified viruses or other methods to introduce DNA into target cells of intact organisms, it is possible to insert, knockout, or modify specific genes. The results of pilot studies in cystic fibrosis and other genetic disorders have recently been reported,[24] and genetic modification will most likely become part of the approach to the management of nutritional disorders.

ENTERAL NUTRIENTS AS SPECIFIC MODIFIERS OF GENE EXPRESSION

Nutrient regulation of gene expression in body tissues occurs as an adaptive response to diets of altered composition. Such adaptation is

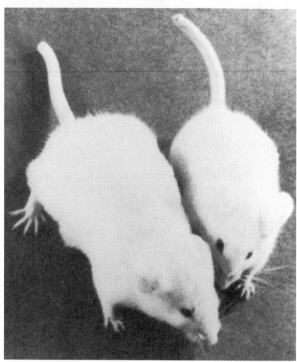

FIGURE 9–6 Sibling male mice at approximately 10 weeks of age that are genetically identical except for multiple copies of the growth hormone gene introduced into the animal on the left. (Photograph from Dr. Ralph Brinster, with permission.)

essential for coordinating tissue growth with nutrient availability and regulating metabolic pathways important for fuel use and maintenance of homeostasis. In addition, regulation of pathways responsible for balancing tissue nutrient availability with changes in dietary nutrient intake helps prevent malnutrition or toxicity.

Nutrient Regulation of Growth Factor Expression

Growth factors have a major role in stimulating tissue anabolism, but tissue growth rates ultimately depend on the availability of both growth factors and nutrients. Regulation of growth factor expression by nutrients provides a mechanism for coordinating overall tissue growth responses with nutrient availability. For example, synthesis and secretion of the peptide growth factor IGF-I in the liver is controlled by growth hormone during states of adequate nutrient intake.[25] As a consequence, there is a close relationship between growth hormone levels, plasma IGF-I levels, and tissue growth responses mediated by IGF-I. However, this regulatory mechanism uncouples when dietary nutrient intake is inadequate. When experimental animals are fasted or given a diet low in protein, hepatic IGF-I mRNA and circulating IGF-I levels dramati-

cally decrease. Exogenous growth hormone administration does not reverse the effects of fasting or caloric dietary protein restriction on IGF-I gene expression, but refeeding or dietary protein repletion leads to rapid normalization of IGF-I levels.[26]

Although the molecular mechanisms involved in nutrient regulation of IGF-I gene expression are not well defined, there is evidence that the largest of three IGF-I mRNA transcripts (~7.7 kb) is markedly decreased compared with two shorter transcripts (~1.8 and 0.9 kb) in protein- and energy-restricted animals.[27,28] This difference in regulation for the 7.7 and 0.9 kb transcript is illustrated in Figure 9–7. It has been postulated that nutritionally sensitive regulatory elements in the 3'-untranslated region of the 7.7 kb transcript of IGF-I mRNA may influence its stability when protein is limiting.[28] Studies in cultured cells have demonstrated that reduced provision of amino acids to hepatocytes decreases IGF-I gene expression,[29] suggesting that amino acids may be directly responsible for regulating IGF-I gene expression during protein restriction. The resistance to growth hormone effects on IGF-I synthesis and secretion induced through these mechanisms may have adaptive value by decreasing tissue growth during a period when nutrient supply is limited. At the same time, the lipolytic effects of sustained growth hormone levels are pre-

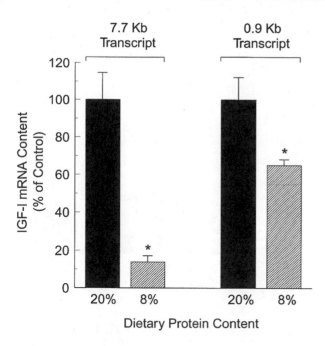

FIGURE 9–7 Differential effects of dietary protein restriction on 7.7 kb and 0.9 kb IGF-I mRNA transcripts in rat liver. Mean ± SEM; *$P < 0.05$ vs 20 percent protein diet. (Redrawn with permission from Straus DS, Takemoto CD: Effect of dietary protein deprivation on insulin-like growth factor (IGF) -I and -II, IGF binding protein-2, and serum albumin gene expression in rat. Endocrinology 1990;127:1849. © The Endocrine Society.)

served and have an important role in mobilizing alternative fuel sources.

Nutrient Regulation of Metabolic Pathways

Dietary intake may vary greatly in both overall quantity and content of specific nutrients. Alterations in the metabolism of individual nutrients in accordance with changes in their intake is made possible in part by rapid modulation of the expression of tissue enzymes. This can function as a negative feedback system, in which increased dietary supply of a nutrient suppresses endogenous pathways leading to synthesis of the same nutrient.

For example, dietary cholesterol regulates 3-hydroxy-3-methyglutaryl coenzyme A (HMG-CoA) reductase, an enzyme that catalyzes the rate-limiting step of HMG-CoA conversion to mevalonate, which is a precursor for cholesterol biosynthesis. Within hours after experimental animals are fed a diet high in cholesterol, the activity and protein levels of HMG-CoA reductase in the liver are markedly reduced.[30,31] This regulatory effect of cholesterol on HMG-CoA reductase occurs at the level of mRNA transcription in rat liver and in cultured cells (Fig. 9–8).[32,33] When cells are incubated in the absence of cholesterol, HMG-CoA reductase mRNA levels are high in accordance with the need for endogenous cholesterol biosynthesis. Adding cholesterol to the culture medium rapidly suppresses mRNA levels for

HMG-CoA reductase, a response that is appropriate when maximal cholesterol biosynthesis is not required.[34] This suppression occurs through the action of cis-acting elements in the reductase promoter region, referred to as sterol regulatory elements (SREs).[35] Analysis of the HMG-CoA reductase promoter has provided evidence for a complicated mechanism involving several DNA-binding proteins and overlapping recognition sequences within the promoter. To date, three proteins that bind to the sterol regulatory region have been isolated and identified: cellular nucleic–binding protein (CNBP),[35] SRE-binding factor (SREBF)[36] and Red 25.[37] The integrated action of these proteins is thought to result in potent and specific regulation of HMG-CoA expression that balances endogenous synthesis of cholesterol with its availability from the diet.

In addition to simple negative feedback mechanisms, nutrients can modify gene expression of enzymes that catalyze reactions involved in the metabolism of other nutrients. This can help to provide an overall balance of nutrient flux through alternative pathways. For example, polyunsaturated fatty acids (PUFA) regulate the expression of genes encoding proteins involved in nonessential fatty acid biosynthetic pathways.[38] When rats are fed a diet containing PUFA, hepatic expression of the rate-limiting enzyme fatty acid synthase and the putative lipogenic protein S14 is decreased.[39] These effects are specific for PUFA as evident from a lack of inhibition by other fatty acids on

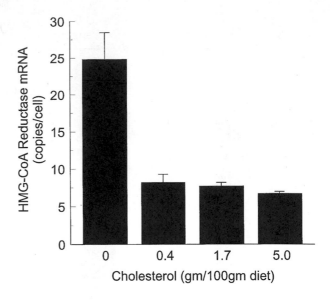

FIGURE 9–8   Effects of dietary cholesterol on HMG-CoA reductase mRNA abundance in rat liver. (Redrawn with permission from Rudling M: Hepatic mRNA levels for the LDL receptor and HMG-CoA reductase show coordinate regulation in vivo. J Lipid Res 1992;33:493.)

expression of these lipogenic proteins. The decreased levels of fatty acid synthase and S14 correlate with lower levels of gene transcription and a decrease in their tissue mRNA content (Fig. 9–9).[40] The changes in mRNA levels occur rapidly after dietary PUFA administration and are rapidly reversible, supporting the hypothesis that PUFA action is at the level of mRNA transcription. DNA promoter analysis of the fatty acid synthase and S14 genes has revealed cis-acting elements that confer PUFA responsiveness,[41] and it is thought that PUFA-regulated transacting factors or transcription factors that interact with these sequences ultimately will be identified. The physiologic importance of the inhibitory effects of PUFA on gene expression of lipogenic enzymes is not fully understood, but it may be part of a mechanism that favors incorporating these fatty acids into cell membranes. Inhibition of endogenous fatty acid synthesis at times when PUFA are available may decrease nonessential fatty acid competition for membrane incorporation.

Regulation of Pathways that Balance Micronutrient Availability

Marked alterations in the intake of specific micronutrients can cause micronutrient deficiency at times of decreased intake or toxicity from excess micronutrient intake. As a protective mechanism, complex gene regulatory

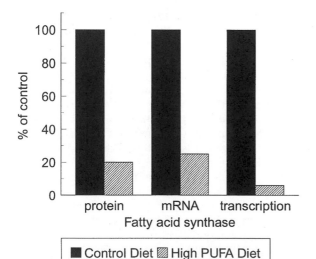

FIGURE 9–9   Effects of dietary polyunsaturated fatty acids (PUFAs) on fatty acid synthase protein, mRNA and RNA transcription rate in rat liver. (Reprinted with permission from Clarke SD, Jump DB: Regulation of hepatic gene expression by dietary fats: a unique role for polyunsaturated fatty acids. In Berdanier CD, Hargrove JL (eds): Nutrition and Gene Expression. Boca Raton, FL: CRC Press, 1993. Copyright © 1993 CRC Press, Boca Raton, Florida.)

pathways balance micronutrient availability with changes in dietary intake. This type of regulation is illustrated by the effects of iron on gene expression of two molecules: ferritin, which functions as an intracellular iron storage protein, and the transferrin receptor, which binds and takes up transferrin, an important protein that transports iron in the blood. When cellular iron levels are low, transferrin receptor mRNA is stabilized by aconitase, an iron-responsive regulatory protein (Fig. 9–10).[42,43]

Aconitase association with a stem-and-loop structure or iron response element in the transferrin receptor mRNA results in stabilization of the RNA, increased translation of transferrin receptors, and thus increased transport of iron into cells. At the same time, aconitase inhibits translation of ferritin mRNA by binding to an iron response element that blocks ribosomal binding and ferritin translation.[44] This appropriately decreases the pathway of cellular iron sequestration and storage when

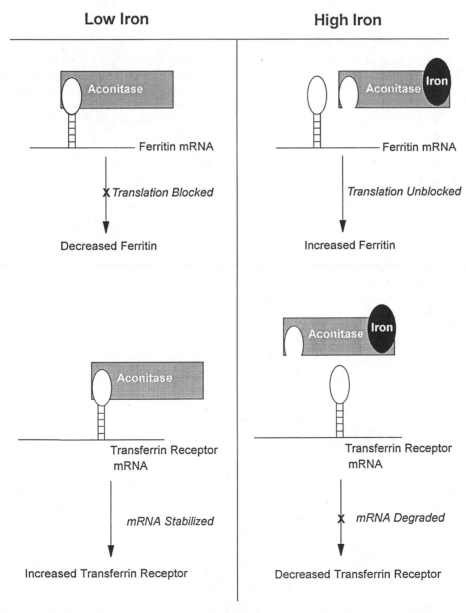

FIGURE 9–10 Regulation of cellular iron availability through iron-mediated changes in aconitase interaction with ferritin and transferrin receptor mRNA.

iron levels are low. Conversely, when cellular iron levels are excessive, iron binds to aconitase and causes it to dissociate from the transferrin receptor mRNA. This exposes the stem-and-loop structure to endonucleases that degrade the mRNA, and less transferrin receptor protein is synthesized.[43] Aconitase also dissociates from ferritin mRNA when it is bound to iron, and this releases the inhibition of ribosomal binding and promotes the translation of ferritin mRNA.[44] Decreased transferrin receptors and increased ferritin levels result in less iron imported into the cell and increased binding and storage of iron within the cell. By altering the stability of transferrin receptor mRNA and translation of ferritin mRNA in this coordinated manner, cellular levels of iron are increased during times of dietary iron depletion and decreased when dietary iron is in excess. The net effect is a buffering of cellular iron levels, which serves as an important mechanism for preventing iron deficiency or toxicity.

DIETARY CONSTITUENTS AS MODIFIERS OF INTESTINAL GENE EXPRESSION

The GI tract is not only an important portal of entry for nutrients that can affect gene expression in other body tissues, but the intestine itself is also an important site of regulated gene expression in response to specific nutrients. Adaptive changes in intestinal enzymes and cellular structure that occur with alterations in diet or partial loss of intestinal tissue provide clear evidence of a dynamic local regulation of gene expression by nutrients. At present, however, there is only limited information on inter-

actions between nutrients and specific intestinal genes at the molecular level.

One of the most extensively studied examples is the gene for intestinal fatty acid–binding protein (FABPI). The product of this gene is a cytoplasmic protein that is predominantly expressed in villus enterocytes and believed to function in the uptake, metabolism, or transport of long chain fatty acids. In mice, FABPI expression has been shown to be tightly regulated. It first appears in late fetal life and persists through adulthood, is limited to differentiated intestinal enterocytes, exhibits an increasing gradient of expression from the proximal to the distal small intestine, and is expressed at increased levels in response to a low-fat diet.[45,46] By linking different fragments of the promoter of the FABPI gene to the growth hormone gene and then studying growth hormone expression in intestinal tissue of transgenic mice, it has been possible to assign regulatory functions to distinct regions of the promoter, as illustrated in Figure 9–11. Although nutrient regulation of FABPI is quite marked, the region of the promoter mediating the effects of low dietary fat on gene expression (i.e., transcriptional induction by low-fat diet or repression by high-fat diet) has not yet been identified. Ultimately, an understanding of the molecular basis for the regulation of FABPI expression by changes in diet is likely to be of great interest, both for increasing understanding of the mechanism of dietary regulation of fat metabolism and also for providing insight into mechanisms of nutrient regulation that are likely to affect other genes.

Dietary regulation of several other genes in the intestine has been demonstrated, although

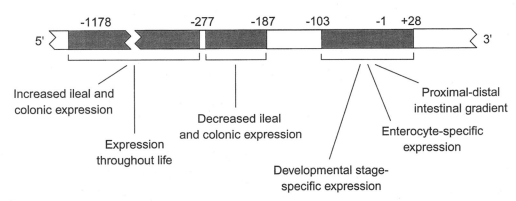

FIGURE 9–11   Regulatory regions of the intestinal fatty acid–binding protein (FABPI) gene. (Redrawn with permission from Knapp JR, Kopchick JJ: The use of transgenic mice in nutrition research. © J Nutr 1994;124:461, American Institute of Nutrition.)

less is known about their promoter structure and the specific mechanisms of transcriptional regulation. For example, high-fiber diets have been shown to decrease mRNA levels of apolipoprotein (apo) A-I in the jejunum and ileum and also to decrease apo A-IV mRNA in the ileum (Fig. 9–12).[47] The molecular basis for this regulatory response is still not defined but is of considerable interest, since high-fiber diets lead to decreased plasma cholesterol. Apo A-I and apo A-IV levels affect intestinal lipoprotein synthesis and thus have an important role in determining the rate of entry of lipids to the plasma from the intestine. It is likely that decreased intestinal apo A-I and apo A-IV gene expression induced by dietary fiber is an important factor in lowering cholesterol. Other examples of nutrient-sensitive genes in the intestine include the enzyme 3-hydroxy-3-methylglutaryl-CoA synthase, which is present during the postweaning period in rat jejunum with high-fat feeding and absent with high-carbohydrate feeding.[48] As for the apolipoprotein genes, Northern blotting studies have documented diet-induced changes in 3-hydroxy-3-methylglutaryl-CoA synthase mRNA content, but the gene promoter has not yet been investigated.

MOLECULAR MARKERS OF NUTRIENT EFFECTS ON THE INTESTINE

Even though there is only a limited amount of information available about nutrient regulation of specific genes in the intestine, there is abundant evidence that intestinal tissues are markedly responsive to nutrients. With fasting, there is rapid atrophy of the intestinal mucosa, associated with a reduction in villus enterocyte content.[49] Following partial loss of intestinal tissue and development of short-bowel syndrome, there is marked villus hypertrophy and enterocyte hyperplasia.[50] Specific nutrients (e.g., the amino acid glutamine[51]) and hormones such as IGF-I[52] can significantly increase this adaptive hyperplastic response. Nutrient-responsive cell types include not only the enterocytes, but also lymphoid cells, which are abundant and sensitive to both overall nutritional state and the effects of specific nutrients.[53]

Increased knowledge of the mechanisms through which nutritional state and specific nutrients modulate the proliferation, differentiation, and turnover of cells in the intestine will undoubtedly help to guide efforts to optimize nutritional formulas and to modify intestinal function through other interventions, such as providing growth factors. Even without yet understanding the specific mechanisms of intestinal cell growth control, currently available molecular markers can be used to monitor growth responses. For example, rapid changes in small intestinal mRNA levels of the proto-oncogenes c-fos and c-jun during refeeding after a 4-day fast in laboratory rats have been shown to anticipate the cell proliferation that will follow (Fig. 9–13).[54]

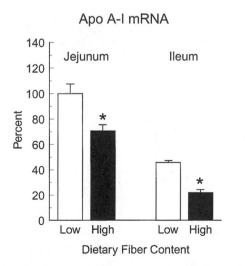

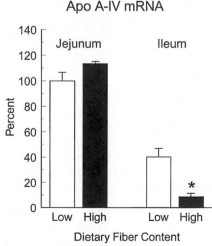

FIGURE 9–12 Effects of low fiber (fiber free) and high fiber (30 percent sugar beet fiber) diets on intestinal apolipoprotein A-I and A-IV mRNA levels. Data normalized to low fiber jejunum values; mean ± SEM; *P <0.05 vs low-fiber diet. (Redrawn with permission from Felgines C, Mazur A, Remesy C et al: The effect of dietary fiber on apolipoprotein A-I and A-IV gene expression in rat intestine. Cell Mol Biol 1993;39:371.)

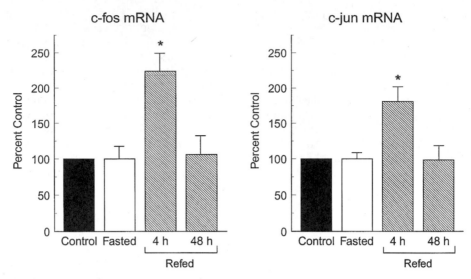

FIGURE 9–13   Effects of fasting (4 days) and refeeding on c-fos and c-jun mRNA content in rat ileum. Data represent mean ± SEM; *P < 0.01 vs fasted. (Redrawn with permission from Hodin RA, Graham JR, Meng S et al: Temporal pattern of rat small intestinal gene expression with refeeding. Am J Physiol 1994;266:G83.)

Expression of other genes appears to correlate temporally with intestinal growth rather than precede it. As an example, the Northern blotting data in Figure 9–14 demonstrate a specific increase in mRNA content for glucagon in the ileum that is temporally associated with postresection adaptive hyperplasia.[55] Levels of control tubulin mRNA and 18S ribosomal RNA are unchanged in the ileum under the same conditions, and regulated glucagon expression is specific for the ileum (not evident in liver and kidney). If similar markers of cell proliferation were measured in human intestine (e.g., in endoscopic biopsy samples), this could make possible rapid assessment of individual patient responses to specific nutrient support formulas and other therapeutic interventions.

INTESTINAL EXPRESSION OF TRANSGENES

As genes specifically expressed in the intestine are identified and the promoters responsible for this expression are characterized, these same promoters will be available as tools to direct the expression of novel genes introduced by transgenic techniques. For example, the growth hormone gene can be expressed specifically in the intestinal enterocytes of transgenic mice, if it is coupled to the intestinal FABPI promoter.[56] Similar experiments with the promoter for the sucrase-isomaltase gene have demonstrated that it also can be used to direct

the expression of introduced genes to intestinal cells.[57]

With even less tissue specificity than achievable with these FABPI and disaccharidase promoters, it already has been shown that intestinal expression of transgenes can be used to induce favorable changes in systemic substrate

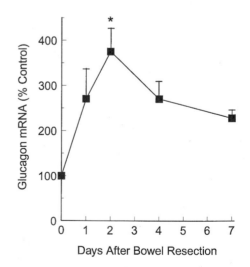

FIGURE 9–14   Time course of increase in ileal glucagon mRNA following extensive (80 percent) small bowel resection. Data represent mean ± SEM; *P < 0.05 vs control. (Redrawn with permission from Taylor RG, Verity K, Fuller PJ: Ileal glucagon gene expression: ontogeny and response to massive small bowel resection. Gastroenterology 1990;99:724.)

metabolism. Transgenic mice have been generated that overexpress apo E under the control of the metallothionein promoter, which does not specifically direct gene expression to the intestine.[58] From progeny mice with different levels of apo E expression in various tissues, lines of mice were isolated that expressed, by chance, high levels of apo E in the intestine. These animals exhibited markedly increased chylomicron clearance from the plasma, presumably due to incorporation of increased quantities of apo E into chylomicrons formed in the intestine. Although not yet extensively studied, such changes in chylomicron kinetics would be expected to result in decreased levels of cholesterol and triglycerides and a less atherogenic state. With a similar approach to the generation of transgenic animals, but with the use of promoters from intestine-specific genes, it should be possible to explore even more easily the functional effects of introducing novel genes or altering the expression of endogenous genes in the intestine.

THE FUTURE

Compared with knowledge of gene regulation by nutrients in the liver and other tissues, there is still relatively little known about nutrient regulation of gene expression in the intestine. With the application of current methods to studies on GI tissues, however, and continued advances in the power of molecular biologic tools, our understanding of the nutritional molecular biology of the GI tract will advance rapidly in the next few years. Standard molecular biologic techniques will provide new information about the regulatory events that determine intestinal and systemic responses to specific nutrients. It is highly likely that the genetic basis for susceptibility to common nutritional disorders, such as obesity and diet-induced atherogenesis, will be defined. This will mandate efforts to reduce disease risk by changes in nutrient intake developed through applying the knowledge of underlying mechanisms. It is also likely that the intestine will be evaluated as a major route for the introduction of novel genetic material, whether the goal of gene therapy is correction of a primary intestinal disorder or a systemic disorder. As knowledge of the specific mechanisms responsible for nutrient regulation of intestinal genes advances, we can anticipate the development of new research areas within the field of nutrition including, for example, efforts directed to the controlled modulation of transgenes by specific enteral nutrients. These are tangible and exciting prospects that undoubtedly will require cooperative efforts of molecular biologists and clinicians specializing in enteral nutrition.

REFERENCES

1. Lewin B: Genes, vol V. New York: Oxford University Press, 1994.
2. Lewin B: Genes, vol V. New York: Oxford University Press, 1994:163–195.
3. Altmann M, Trachsel H: Regulation of translation initiation and modulation of cellular physiology. Trends Biochem Sci 1993;18:429.
4. Wernerman J, von der Decken A, Vinnars E: The interpretation of ribosome determination to assess protein synthesis in human skeletal muscle. Infusionstherapie 1986;13:162.
5. Wernerman J, von der Decken A, Vinnars E: Size distribution of ribosomes in biopsy specimens of human skeletal muscle during starvation. Metabolism 1985; 34:665.
6. Hammarqvist F, Wernerman J, Ali R et al: Addition of glutamine to total parenteral nutrition after elective abdominal surgery spares free glutamine in muscle, counteracts the fall in muscle protein synthesis, and improves nitrogen balance. Ann Surg 1989;209:455.
7. Ziegler TR, Almahfouz A, Pedrini MT et al: A comparison of rat small intestinal insulin and IGF-I receptors during fasting and refeeding. Endocrinology 1995; 136:5148.
8. Fong Y, Minei JP, Marano MA et al: Skeletal muscle amino acid and myofibrillar protein mRNA response to thermal injury and infection. Am J Physiol 1991;261:R536.
9. Sambrook J, Fritsch EF, Maniatis T: Molecular Cloning: A Laboratory Manual, 2nd edition. Cold Spring Harbor, NY: Cold Spring Harbor Laboratory Press, 1989.
10. Tintner R, Brown P, Hedley-Whyte ET et al: Neuropathologic verification of Creutzfeldt-Jakob disease in the exhumed American recipient of human pituitary growth hormone: epidemiologic and pathogenetic implications. Neurology 1986;36:932.
11. Jacobs DO, Evans DA, Mealy K et al: Combined effects of glutamine and epidermal growth factor on the rat intestine. Surgery 1988;104:358.
12. Ziegler TR, Mantell MP, Rombeau JL et al: Effects of glutamine and IGF-I administration on intestinal growth and the IGF pathway after partial small bowel resection. J Parenter Enter Nutr 1994;18(suppl):20S.
13. Scangos G, Ruddle FH: Mechanisms and applications of DNA mediated gene transfer in mammalian cells; a review. Gene 1981;14:1.
14. Ebina Y, Edery M, Ellis L et al: Expression of a functional human insulin receptor from a cloned cDNA in Chinese hamster ovary cells. Proc Natl Acad Sci USA 1985;82:8014.
15. Steele-Perkins G, Turner J, Edman JC et al: Expression and characterization of functional human insulin-like growth factor I receptor. J Biol Chem 1988;263: 11486.
16. Myanohara A, Sharkey MF, Witztum JL et al: Efficient expression of retroviral vector-transduced human low density lipoprotein (LDL) receptor in LDL receptor-deficient rabbit fibroblasts in vitro. Proc Natl Acad Sci USA 1988;85:6538.
17. Casteilla L, Blondel O, Klaus S et al: Stable expression of functional mitochondrial uncoupling protein in Chi-

nese hamster ovary cells. Proc Natl Acad Sci USA 1990;87:5124.

18. Harris T: In vitro mutagenesis. Nature 1982;299:298.

19. Ellis L, Clauser E, Morgan DO: Replacement of insulin receptor tyrosine residues 1162 and 1163 compromises insulin-stimulated kinase activity and uptake of 2-deoxyglucose. Cell 1986;45:721.

20. Moller DE, Flier JS: Mechanisms of disease. Insulin resistance-mechanisms, syndromes, and implications. N Engl J Med 1991;325:938.

21. Palmiter RD, Brinster RL: Germ-line transformation of mice. Annu Rev Genet 1986;20:465.

22. Knapp JR, Kopchick JJ: The use of transgenic mice in nutrition research. J Nutr 1994;124:461.

23. Waldman AS: Targeted homologous recombination in mammalian cells. Crit Rev Oncol Hematol 1992;12:49.

24. Wilson JM: Cystic fibrosis. Vehicles for gene therapy [news]. Nature 1993;365:691.

25. Roberts CT, Jr, Brown AL, Graham DE et al: Growth hormone regulates the abundance of insulin-like growth factor I RNA in adult rat liver. J Biol Chem 1986;261:10025.

26. Thissen J-P, Ketelslegers J-M, Underwood LE: Nutritional regulation of the insulin-like growth factors. Endocrine Rev 1994;15:80.

27. Emler CA, Schalch DS: Nutritionally-induced changes in hepatic insulin-like growth factor I (IGF-I) gene expression in rats. Endocrinology 1987;120:832.

28. Straus DS, Takemoto CD: Effect of dietary protein deprivation on insulin-like growth factor (IGF) -I and -II, IGF binding protein-2, and serum albumin gene expression in rat. Endocrinology 1990;127:1849.

29. Pao C-I, Farmer PK, Begovic S: Regulation of insulin-like growth factor-I (IGF-I) and IGF-binding protein 1 gene transcription by hormones and provision of amino acids in rat hepatocytes. Molec Endocrinol 1993;7:1561.

30. Jenke HS, Lowel M, Berndt J: In vivo effect of cholesterol feeding on the short term regulation of hepatic hydroxymethylglutaryl coenzyme A reductase during the diurnal cycle. J Biol Chem 1981;256:9622.

31. Ness GC, Eales S, Lopez D et al: Regulation of 3-hydroxy-3-methylglutaryl coenzyme A reductase gene expression by sterols and nonsterols in rat liver. Arch Biochem Biophys 1994;308:420.

32. Goldstein JL, Brown MS: Regulation of the mevalonate pathway. Nature 1990;343:425.

33. Rudling M: Hepatic mRNA levels for the LDL receptor and HMG-CoA reductase show coordinate regulation in vivo. J Lipid Res 1992;33:493.

34. Brown MS, Faust JR, Goldstein JL: Induction of 3-hydroxy-3-methylglutaryl coenzyme A reductase activity in human fibroblasts incubated with compactin (ML-236B), a competitive inhibitor of the reductase. J Biol Chem 1978;253:1121.

35. Rajavashisth TB, Taylor AK, Andalibi A: Identification of a zinc finger protein that binds to the sterol regulatory element. Science 1989;245:640.

36. Stark HC, Weinberger O, Weinberger J: Common double- and single-stranded DNA binding factor for a sterol regulatory element. Proc Natl Acad Sci 1992;89:2180.

37. Osborne TF, Bennett M, Rhee K: Red 25, a protein that binds specifically to the sterol regulatory region in the promoter for 3-hydroxy-3-methylglutaryl-coenzyme A reductase. J Biol Chem 1992;267:18973.

38. Clarke SD, Jump DB: Regulation of hepatic gene expression by dietary fats: a unique role for polyunsaturated fatty acids. In Berdanier CD, Hargrove JL (eds): CRC Press Reviews. Boca Raton, FL: CRC Press, 1993.

39. Clarke SD, Armstrong MK, Jump DB: Dietary polyunsaturated fats uniquely suppress rat liver fatty acid synthase and S14 mRNA content. J Nutr 1990;120:225.

40. Blake WL, Clarke SD: Suppression of hepatic fatty acid synthase and S14 gene transcription by dietary polyunsaturated fat. J Nutr 1990;120:1727.

41. Amy CM, Williams-Ahlf B, Naggert J et al: Molecular cloning of the mammalian fatty acid synthase gene and identification of the promoter region. Biochem J 1990;271:675.

42. Alberts B, Bray D, Lewis J et al: Molecular Biology of the Cell, 3rd edition. New York: Garland Publishing, Inc., 1994:464–465.

43. Casey JL, Hentze MW, Koeller DM et al: Iron-responsive elements: regulatory RNA sequences that control mRNA levels and translation. Science 1988;240:924.

44. Hentze MW, Caughman SW, Rouault TA et al: Identification of the iron-responsive element for the translational regulation of human ferritin mRNA. Science 1987;238:1570.

45. Green RP, Cohn SM, Sacchettini JC et al: The mouse intestinal fatty acid binding protein genes: nucleotide sequence, pattern of developmental and regional expression, and proposed structure of its protein product. DNA Cell Biol 1992;11:31.

46. Graham S, Dayal H, Swanson M et al: Diet in the epidemiology of cancer of the colon and rectum. J Natl Cancer Inst 1978;61:709.

47. Felgines C, Mazur A, Remesy C et al: The effect of dietary fiber on apolipoprotein A-I and A-IV gene expression in rat intestine. Cell Mol Biol 1993;39:371.

48. Thumelin S, Forestier M, Girard J et al: Developmental changes in mitochondrial 3-hydroxy-3-methylglutaryl-CoA synthase gene expression in rat liver, intestine and kidney. Biochem J 1993;292:493.

49. Johnson LR: Regulation of gastrointestinal mucosal growth. Physiol Rev 1988;68:456.

50. Williams RCN, Bauer FLR: Evidence for an enterotropic hormone: compensatory hyperplasia in defunctioned bowel. Br J Surg 1978;65:736.

51. Smith RJ, Wilmore DW: Glutamine nutrition and requirements. J Parenter Enter Nutr 1990;14:94S.

52. Vanderhoof JA, McCusker RH, Clark R et al: Truncated and native insulinlike growth factor I enhances mucosal adaptation after jejunoileal resection. Gastroenterology 1992;102:1949.

53. Chandra RK: Cellular and molecular basis of nutrition-immunity interactions. Adv Exp Med Biol 1990;262:13.

54. Hodin RA, Graham JR, Meng S et al: Temporal pattern of rat small intestinal gene expression with refeeding. Am J Physiol 1994;266:G83.

55. Taylor RG, Verity K, Fuller PJ: Ileal glucagon gene expression: ontogeny and response to massive small bowel resection. Gastroenterology 1990;99:724.

56. Cohn SM, Simon TC, Roth KA et al: Use of transgenic mice to map cis-acting elements in the intestinal fatty acid binding protein gene (FABPI) that control its cell lineage-specific and regional patterns of expression along the duodenal-colonic and crypt-villus axes of the gut epithelium. J Cell Biol 1992;119:27.

57. Markowitz AJ, Wu GD, Birkenmeier EH et al: The human sucrase-isomaltase gene directs complex patterns of gene expression in transgenic mice. Am J Physiol 1993;265:G526.

58. Shimano H, Namba Y, Ohsuga J et al: Metabolism of chylomicron remnants in transgenic mice expressing apolipoprotein E in the intestine. Biochem Biophys Res Comm 1994;200:716.

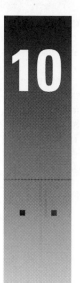

10

Assessment of Nutritional Status and Body Composition

Patients with disease frequently lose weight and become malnourished. The manifestations of malnutrition are varied and do not produce a common clinical or biochemical picture.[1] The changes in tissue and body function produced by malnutrition may be difficult to distinguish from those produced by other factors such as immobility, age, and disease. Furthermore, generalized malnutrition is usually associated with depletion or deficiency of multiple nutrients. For example, the loss of protein and energy stores in chronic protein-energy undernutrition is frequently associated with depletion of one or more minerals, vitamins, or trace elements. In addition, there is a complex interdependence of nutrients, since a deficiency of an intracellular constituent may lead to loss of other intracellular constituents. For example, potassium or phosphate deficiency produce loss of protein (negative N balance).[2]

Attempts to assess nutritional status, and attempts to decide whether nutritional support is required on the basis of a single biochemical or anthropometric measurement (or a single prognostic "nutritional" index based on biochemical or anthropometric measurements), are simplistic and of limited value. Indeed, the uncritical use of such measurements may be misleading or inappropriate in some circumstances. This is partly because of the failure to

appreciate the sensitivity and specificity of the tests and partly because of the difficulties in demonstrating benefits of nutritional support in some groups of patients with such abnormalities (see below).

The clinician must use a variety of methods to obtain a reasonable estimate of nutritional status in sick patients. This task begins with the clinical history and examination.

CLINICAL ASSESSMENT

The clinical approach is the oldest and probably the most important method for assessing both nutritional status and the requirement for nutritional support. A well-structured history will often throw light on the likelihood of malnutrition. For example, a history that indicates a loss of body weight (e.g., ≥20 percent) in association with anorexia is particularly important. A history of painful mouth conditions or chewing difficulties is also important. Table 10-1 lists examples of some of the risk factors associated with malnutrition in elderly subjects without serious inflammatory disease.

Another important aspect of the history is the diet history (with or without written dietary records). However, such information is either qualitative or semiquantitative, partly because the information the patient provides may not

TABLE 10–1   Some Factors Predisposing to Malnutrition in Elderly Individuals Without Serious Inflammatory Disease

Medical Conditions
Difficulties in chewing or swallowing (e.g., poorly fitting dentures)
Esophageal strictures
Previous gastric surgery
Recent surgery
Alcoholism

Psychosocial Conditions
Institutionalization
Housebound
Low social class
Difficulties in preparing meals
Recent loss of spouse
Use of multiple drugs

be accurate, and partly because the dietitian must interpret the size of food portions eaten. The weighed food intake method, which involves weighing all food items eaten, is theoretically the most accurate method, but this requires patient compliance and reliability, and the procedure itself may alter eating habits. Other methods that attempt to assess daily food intake (24-hour recall or dietary records) may fail to give representative information about food intake that varies from day to day. The number of days required to obtain representative intake data (e.g., ±10 percent of average intake) varies with the nutrient (Table 10–2), being greatest for vitamins and minerals (10 to 36 days), intermediate for protein, fat, and carbohydrate (6 to 10 days), and shortest for total energy intake (5 days).[3,4]

These considerations are less important with the dietary history, which aims to assess usual intake over time. Although the method is at best semiquantitative, it has two particular clinical values. First, the patient may clearly identify changes in food intake. For example, anorexia coupled with a loss of 10 percent or more of body weight is clinically important because it is associated with deterioration in body function.[5] Second, the dietary history may alert the clinician to specific nutrient deficiencies. For example, house bound patients who do not eat margarine, fatty fish, or eggs are prone to vitamin D deficiency. The typical Asian diet may predispose individuals to vitamin D deficiency. Vegans are at risk of vitamin B_{12} deficiency. The less efficient absorption of iron in vegetarian diets means that vegetarians are more prone to iron deficiency (especially if they are women with large menstrual losses). Furthermore, some patients eat unusual or unbalanced diets, which may predispose to a variety of specific deficiencies. For example, individuals ingesting "junk" food may be prone to zinc deficiency,[6] which has been implicated in growth failure.

Patients with gastrointestinal (GI) diseases are particularly prone to generalized malnutrition, but the pattern of nutrient deficiencies varies with the condition (Table 10–3). The

TABLE 10–2   Daily Variation in the Intake of Various Dietary Components Expressed as Percent Coefficient Variation, and the Number of Days Necessary to Obtain Estimates Within 10% of Average Intake

Dietary Component	Within Person Coefficient of Variation (CV)(%)	% Standard Error (SE) of Average 7-day Record	Number of Days Required to be Within ±10% of Average Intake
Energy	23	9	5
Carbohydrate	25	9	6
Protein	27	10	7
Fat	31	12	10
Dietary fiber	31	12	10
Calcium	32	12	10
Iron	35	13	12
Thiamin	39	15	15
Riboflavin	44	17	19
Cholesterol	52	20	27
Vitamin C	60	23	36

Calculated from $\% \text{ SE} = \dfrac{\text{CV}\%}{\sqrt{n}}$ and $n = \dfrac{\text{CV}^2}{\%\,\text{SE}}$; n = number of days.

Data from Bingham SA: Nutrition Abstracts and Reviews (Series A) 1987;57(10):705–742, and Balogh M et al: Am J Clin Nutr 1971;24:304–310.

TABLE 10–3 Mineral and Vitamin Deficiencies Associated with Gastrointestinal Diseases

Disorder	Mineral/Vitamin Deficiency
Gastric surgery	Iron, vitamin B_{12}, vitamin D
Crohn's disease	Iron (blood loss and malabsorption), folic acid
Celiac disease	Iron, folic acid
Tropical sprue	Folic acid
Ulcerative colitis	Iron
Short-bowel syndrome	Many nutrients and trace elements (e.g., sodium, potassium, magnesium, zinc, chromium, iron)

drug history may also alert the clinician to the possibility of specific nutritional problems.[7] For instance, isoniazid, penicillamine, and L-dopa may lead to vitamin B_6 deficiency; corticosteroids may cause sodium retention and loss of potassium and result in hypertension, hyperglycemia, and osteoporosis. Many cytotoxic drugs are folate antagonists, and anticonvulsants may increase the requirement for folate and vitamin D.

In general, it is difficult to establish a diagnosis of specific nutrient deficiencies from the history alone because the symptoms are usually nonspecific. The physical signs associated with individual nutrient deficiencies (Tables 10–4 and 10–5) may also be nonspecific and often appear late, but they are useful because they can alert the clinician to the possible existence of a variety of deficiencies, including trace element deficiencies (Table 10–6).

Generalized signs of undernutrition are particularly important for assessing chronic protein-energy malnutrition. These include muscle wasting, especially of the quadriceps, deltoids and temporalis, and loss of subcutaneous fat (e.g., in the arm and chest). The obese individ-

TABLE 10–4 Clinical Signs Associated with Nutrient Deficiencies

Skin

Easy bruising	Vitamin C (positive Hess test)
	Vitamin K (negative Hess test)
	May also occur with steroids and anticoagulants
Dry scaly skin	Essential fatty acid deficiency, but much more commonly it is a nonspecific feature of other conditions
Depigmented, thin hair (easily plucked), and skin depigmentation	Kwashiorkor
Peristomal and perianal pustular eruption	Zinc

Nails

Koilonychia	Iron, but occasionally genetic in origin
Leukonychia	Protein, but may occur with many chronic diseases (reduced synthesis of protein—keratin—in nails)
Light blue sclera	Iron deficiency but may occur in osteogenesis imperfecta

Tongue

Atrophic tongue	Iron, vitamin B_{12}, folic acid, other B vitamins, but also occurs after administration of broad-spectrum antibiotics

Mouth

Angular stomatitis	Iron and vitamin B but commonly occurs in patients with ill-fitting dentures
Aphthous ulcers	Usually nonspecific but a feature of inflammatory bowel disease and celiac disease; in some cases may improve with iron and folic acid
Varicose venules under tongue	Vitamin C

Skeleton

Painful swelling around end of long bones (e.g., wrists and knees) muscle weakness	Rickets; muscle weakness occurs with many clinical conditions
Kyphosis	Osteoporosis, lack of calcium and vitamin D

Other

Postural hypotension	Lack of sodium but may occur in patients taking antihypertensive drugs and in those with autonomic neuropathy and Addison's disease

TABLE 10–5   Physical Signs of Specific Nutrient Deficiencies

Nutrient	Sign
Vitamins	
Vitamin B$_{12}$	Anemia (megaloblastic and macrocytic), atrophic tongue, peripheral neuropathy and subacute combined degeneration of the cord (e.g., absent ankle jerks and upgoing toes)
Folic acid	Anemia (megaloblastic), atrophic tongue
Vitamin A	Xerophthalmia, hyperkeratosis of the skin, Bitot's spots
Vitamin C	Easy bruising, ecchymosis (positive Hess test)
Vitamin K	Easy bruising (negative Hess test)
Vitamin D	Rickets (swollen wrists, rickety rosary, knock knees), tetany, and positive Trousseau's sign (hypocalcemia), proximal myopathy
Vitamin E	Myelopathy, ataxia, loss of position sense in legs, retinopathy/blindness
Thiamine	Peripheral neuropathy (dry beriberi), edema (wet beriberi), ophthalmoplegia, Wernicke-Korsakoff syndrome
Minerals	
Iron	Anemia (microcytic hypochromic), koilonychia, angular stomatitis, atrophic tongue
Zinc	Bulbous-pustular peristomal and acral dermatitis, loss of hair
Magnesium	Tetany, positive Trousseau's sign, cardiac arrhythmias
Sodium	Postural hypotension
Potassium	Cardiac arrhythmias
Essential Fatty Acids	
	Diffuse scaly dermatitis

TABLE 10–6   Features Produced by Trace Element Deficiencies

Iron	Hypochromic anemia, angular stomatitis, koilonychia
Chromium	Hyperglycemia, peripheral neuropathy, confusion
Cobalt (vitamin B$_{12}$)	Megaloblastic anemia, peripheral neuropathy, subacute combined degeneration of the spinal cord
Copper	Anemia (with megaloblastic features), neutropenia
Iodine	Goiter, hypothyroidism
Manganese	Dermatitis, changes of hair color, hypoprothrombinemia
Molybdenum	Decreased level of consciousness, intolerance to sulfite and amino acids, hypouricemia
Selenium	Myopathy, cardiomyopathy
Zinc	Rash, alopecia, loss of taste sensation, diarrhea

ual may pose particular problems, since the excessive fat may prevent detection of underlying muscle wasting. The patient with a neurologic disorder may also pose problems because it can be difficult to assess the extent to which muscle wasting is due to nerve denervation or immobility as opposed to inadequate nutrition.

A variety of bedside body composition techniques may help the clinician to confirm these suspicions and quantitate some impressions. Many of the bedside techniques of body composition are indirect, since they aim to predict measurements obtained by reference methods (e.g., hydrodensitometry, water dilution techniques, total body potassium, and neutron activation). These are not widely available and have little place in routine clinical practice. The

advantages and disadvantages of these reference techniques when used alone or together are discussed elsewhere both from a theoretical and practical point of view.[8-11] Here only the bedside techniques and reference methods that are finding increasing use in clinical practice will be discussed.

BEDSIDE BODY COMPOSITION TECHNIQUES

Anthropometry

Weight and Height

Evidence of chronic protein-energy malnutrition can be provided by relating weight to height (Fig. 10–1). However, the "ideal range"

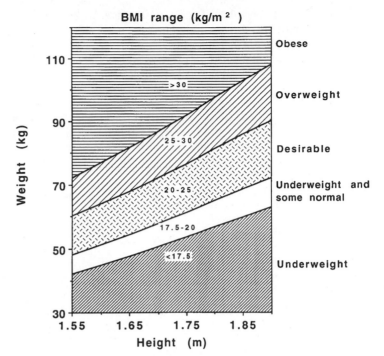

FIGURE 10–1 Weight and height for different ranges of body mass index (BMI).

is large, and therefore it is possible for individuals to lose (or gain) a substantial amount of weight and remain within the body mass index range of 20 to 25 kg/m². Nevertheless, values of body mass index (BMI) outside the ideal range may alert the clinician to the presence of chronic protein-energy undernutrition (e.g., BMI <17.5 kg/m²) and possibly 17.5 to 20 kg/m², or overnutrition (e.g., BMI 25 to 30 kg/m² suggests that individuals are overweight and > 30 kg/m² suggests obesity) (Fig. 10–1).

The trend for the BMI to increase in many developed countries[12] is a cause for concern with respect to overnutrition, while the high prevalence of a low BMI in patients admitted to the hospital is a cause for concern with respect to undernutrition.[13] For example, in one recent study, 20 to 30 percent of adult patients admitted to a British hospital had a BMI less than 20 kg/m² (compared with ~5 to 10 percent in the general population). Furthermore, two thirds of patients lost weight while in the hospital, suggesting that many patients may leave the hospital more malnourished than when they were admitted.[13] However, in some circumstances, changes in weight may be difficult to interpret, especially in patients with edema. Indeed, large acute changes in body weight (e.g., over 24 hours) are more likely to reflect changes in fluid balance than changes in protein and energy balances.

The BMI can be used to estimate the proportion of fat and fat-free tissue in individual subjects, but equations derived from the use of different reference methods (e.g., densitometry and water-dilution techniques) in different populations may give somewhat different results.[8] In subjects in whom measurement of standing height is not possible, predictions can be made from lying height, demispan, or knee height. The relationship between height (centimeters) and knee height obtained between the condyles of the femur and the foot which is placed on a broad blade caliper (with the knee bent at a 90-degree angle while pressure is applied) is given by the following equations:[14,15]

$$\text{Height (men)} = 64.19 - 0.04 \text{ age} + 2.03 \text{ knee height}$$

$$\text{Height (women)} = 84.88 - 0.24 \text{ age} + 1.83 \text{ knee height}$$

Height can be estimated from the demispan,[12] since the ratio of height/demispan is 2.12 ± 0.005 (SEM) for men (range 2.13 ± 0.005 for 16 to 24 years to 2.11 ± 0.003 for >75 years) and 2.15 ± 0.006 for women (ranging from 2.16 ± 0.008 for 16 to 20 years to 2.14 ± 0.008 for >75 years). The demispan is defined as the distance between sternal notch and the finger roots with the arm outstretched laterally. Measurement of weight may also be difficult in some circumstances, but special weighing scales are available for patients who are bed bound (e.g., in intensive care units) or in wheelchairs.

In children the relationship between weight and height varies with age, and care must be taken not to extrapolate from the adult ranges of BMI to children who show complex changes in BMI during growth and development.[16] Centile charts of weight for height or weight for age or height for age[17] can be invaluable to those involved in pediatric practice. Again, changes in weight and height are much more useful than single measurements, although gross abnormalities can be detected from single measurements (severe malnutrition), which often fall well outside the normal range.

Skinfold Thicknesses

Body composition (fat and fat-free mass) can be assessed from skinfold thicknesses, which are typically measured at multiple sites (e.g., biceps, triceps, subscapular, and suprailiac)[18] to overcome some of the problems associated with variations in fat distribution. Generally this method is superior to the BMI (or equations that depend on weight and height alone).[8,19-22] However, there is a learning curve associated with the accurate and reproducible measurement of skinfold thickness. Furthermore, the between-observer variability is larger with this method than with some other bedside methods (see below). Changes in hydration may greatly affect the measurements and their interpretation,[8] which are ultimately based on hydrodensitometry measurements in healthy subjects. Sequential measurements of skinfold thicknesses are yet again of greater value than single measurements, especially when carried out by the same observer.

Limb Anthropometry

Measurements of limb circumferences and skinfold thickness can be used to estimate the amount of muscle and fat within limbs (Table 10–7).[23] As with body weight, the range of normality is large (Fig. 10–2), and sequential measurements are of more general value. However, a result outside the normal range (obtained in the absence of disturbances in hydration status), indicates chronic protein-energy malnutrition, although immobility and neurologic diseases (e.g., motor neuron disease) can cause substantial muscle wasting independent of nutritional status.

Impedance or Resistance Measurements

This technique depends on the principle that lean tissue conducts electricity much better than fat. Therefore, measurement of whole body resistance indicates the amount of lean tissue[24,25]: the smaller the resistance, the greater the lean body mass. The basic principles can be readily used and understood by considering the resistance (R) of a wire of uniform cross-sectional area (A) and length (L):

The resistance $R \propto L/A$, which when multiplied by L/L gives $R \propto L^2/V$ (V is the volume of the wire).

By analogy the resistance of the body is given by:

$$R \propto ht^2/V \text{ or } R \propto ht^2/M$$

where V and M represent the volume and mass of the fat free body respectively. The equations assume that the conducting length (typically between wrist and ankle) is proportional to height and that the density (d) fat-free mass is fixed ($M = dV$).

The technique has gained some popularity because the measurements are easy, quick to perform, and reproducible. The recent increase in the popularity of bioelectrical resistance or impedance, which has been referred as the

---

Table 10–7 Estimating Cross-Sectional Area of Muscular and Nonmuscular Tissues in Limbs*

1. Limb muscle circumference = limb muscle circumference – $\pi \times$ skinfold thickness

2. Limb muscle cross-sectional area = $\dfrac{[\text{limb circumference} - \pi \times \text{skinfold thickness}]^2}{4\pi}$

3. Nonmuscle limb area (adipose tissue + skin) = limb cross-sectional area – muscle cross-sectional area

4. Limb cross-sectional area = $\dfrac{(\text{limb circumference})^2}{4\pi}$

* The formulas assume circular limb and muscle configurations. A correction can be made to take into account the cross-sectional area for bone, which for the mid-upper arm is 10 cm^2 for men and 6.5 cm^2 for women.

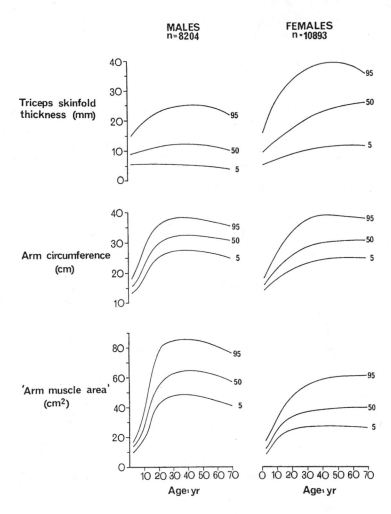

MALES
n=8204

FEMALES
n=10893

FIGURE 10–2 Centiles of arm circumference, triceps, skinfold thicknesses, and arm muscle area in men and women. The numbers 5, 50, and 95 refer to the centiles.

"bioimpedance craze,"[26] has led to at least 30 identifiable commercial machines worldwide. These use different equations, but some manufacturers do not release their equations and do not specify which reference method was used to establish the prediction equation.

The various prediction equations may give widely different results (Table 10–8), which are almost certainly due to a combination of biologic factors (Table 10–9). One important biologic factor variable concerns the contribution of different body segments to whole body impedance.[19] Figure 10–3 shows that the arm, which accounts for only 4 percent of body weight, is responsible for about 46 percent of whole body impedance measured between wrist and ankle. This is due to the arm's relatively small cross-sectional area, which offers a high resistance to an electrical current compared with other body segments.

In contrast the trunk, which has a large cross-sectional area, accounts for 46 percent

body weight and only 10 percent of whole body impedance. The leg is similar to the arm because the leg's larger cross-sectional area, which reduces impedance, is balanced by its greater length, which increases impedance.

The disproportionate effects of different body segments have important clinical implications. For example, the hope that the same impedance equations might predict body composition throughout growth and development as well as in individuals with disease is ill founded. The relative length of individual body segments varies during growth and development (e.g., sitting to standing height decreases by 8 percent between the ages of 2 and 12 years), and it varies between races (e.g., sitting to standing height is lower in blacks than in whites or Mexicans),[38] and in individuals of the same race. Interestingly, the differences between races are greatest for the distal limbs (forearm, lower leg), which account for up to three quarters of the imped-

TABLE 10–8   Prediction of Body Compostition in Men Using Different Bioimpedance/Resistance Equations*

Source		Predicted Fat as % Body Weight in 40-year-old Man 173.2 cm	
		60kg, 550Ω	120kg, 450Ω
Hoffer et al[27]*†	$TBW(L) = 0.586H^2/R + 1.988$	22.5	50.5
Holtain[19]††	$TBW(kg) = 0.585H^2/R + 1.825$	23.0	50.8
Lukaski et al[28]†	$TBW(L) = 0.63H^2/R + 2.03$	16.9	46.9
Kushner & Schoeller[29]†	$TBW(kg) = 0.396H^2/R + 0.143W + 8.399$	11.9	38.9
RJL[30]	$FFM(kg) = 0.4936H^2/R + 0.332W + 6.493$	11.1	32.4
Segal et al[30]	$FFM(kg) = 0.00132H^2/R - 0.04394R + 0.30520W$ $- 0.1676A + 22.6687$	17.15	38.7
Gray et al[31]	$FFM(kg) = 0.00139H^2/R - 0.0801R + 0.187W + 39.83$		
Deurenberg et al[32]	$FFM(kg) = 0.698H^2/R + 12.9$	15.0	48.2
Lukaski et al[33]	$FFM(kg) = 0.827H^2/R + 5.214$	16.1	47.0
Lohman[34]	$FFM(kg) = 0.485H^2/R + 0.338W + 5.32$	13.2	33.2
Valhalla†§	$\% Fat = 9.07 + 0.603W - 0.581H^2/R$	13.6	40.4

* W = weight in kg; H = height in cm; A = age in years; R = whole body resistance in Ω; TBW = total body water (kg or l see equation); FFM = fat free mass in kg. Calculated using published data sets.
† In these equations R represents impedance rather than resistance, but in practice the two are only about ~1% different (making ~1% difference to the estimation of % fat). The Holtain equation applies to both males and females. The Hoffer equation was derived using individuals of unstated sex. All other equations are specific for male subjects.
† Fat-free mass was calculated from total body water assuming that the hydration fraction of fat-free mass is 0.73 (wt/wt). For the purposes of these calculations it was assumed that numerically, kg water = l water (at the temperature of measurement). The error from this source at 20°C is considered to be very small (~0.2%).
§ The prediction formula was established from the Valhalla package by feeding different values of W and H^2/R into the software of the machine (Valhalla Scientific, San Diego, CA).
Data from Elia M: Clin Nutr 1992;11:114–127.

ance of the limbs due to their smaller cross-sectional area.

In view of the trunk's small contribution to whole body impedance, it is not surprising that several studies have reported that total body water estimated by the standard impedance techniques and equations is substantially underestimated in patients with ascites. Accumulation of large amounts of fluid in abdominal or thoracic fluid produces very little change in whole body impedance or resistance.

Several studies have also drawn attention to the limitations of using impedance to measure changes in fluid volume, for instance, in subjects undergoing dialysis for chronic renal failure[39] or receiving diuretics[40] or after removal of ascitic fluid in patients with cirrhosis[41] and after abdominal surgery.[42] One study[39] reported that in individual patients there is a good relationship between the amount of fluid removed during renal dialysis and the change in height[2]/R. However, the amount of fluid that had to be removed (up to 3 L) to produce the same change in height[2]/R in different subjects differed threefold.[39] This variability may be partly due to the site of fluid removal (see above) as well as to the resistivity of the fluid removed, which may differ among subjects.

Finally, several studies in normal subjects have shown little or no advantage of whole body impedance over skinfold thicknesses in predicting body fat and lean tissue mass, measured using classic two-compartment methods (fat and fat-free mass as measured by densitometry[19] or water-dilution techniques),[22] three-compartment methods (measured by densitometry and water-dilution techniques),[21] or four-compartment methods (fat, water, protein, and mineral, measured by densitometry, water-dilution techniques, and dual energy absorptiometry for estimation of the mineral content of the body).[21] What then are the advantages of the bioimpedance/resistance techniques?

First, in adults the technique is precise and gives more reproducible interindividual observer results than other bedside techniques such as skinfold thicknesses and near infrared and interactance. This is illustrated in Tables 10–10 and 10–11, which also indicate the precision of some reference methods. The reproducibility of impedance is not only good in adults but also in toddlers and infants.[49] There-

TABLE 10–9 Methodologic and Biologic Reasons for the Existence of Different Bioimpedance/Bioresistance (R) Equations for Predicting Body Composition

Methodologic Differences

1. Reference methods. Different reference methods have been used to establish the bioimpedance prediction equations (e.g., densitometry, water-dilution techniques, or a combination of reference methods).
2. Electrodes
    - The position of the electrodes has not been the same in all studies or is unspecified.
    - The age of the electrodes may alter contact resistance.
    - Cleaning the skin may alter the measured resistance.
3. Variability between machines
    - By different manufacturers[†]
    - By the same manufacturer[*]

Biologic Differences

4. Different variables. In some equations the only variable in height^2/R, while others also depend on weight, age, and gender. The impedance measurement may offer only a small additional advantage over the anthropometric variables.[35]
5. Obesity. Some equations were based on measurements in lean individuals, others in obese, and yet others in lean and obese. Extrapolation from one age group to another may lead to errors.
6. Body segments. Disproportionate effects of body segments and the associated variability between individuals and races (see text).
7. Resistivity of body fluids. Varies among subjects but is assumed to be constant in the equations.
8. Variable penetration into intracellular compartment (see text).

[*] In one study[36] a 17Ω difference was observed in the same individuals (corresponding to ~1.0 to 1.5 kg fat).
[†] In one study[37] a 50Ω difference was observed between four commercial bioimpedance machines (corresponding to ~3.0 to 4.5 kg fat). The difference was ascribed to the difficulty in the machines produced by some manufacturers to maintain the correct current in the presence of contact resistance between skin and sending electrode. The result is a lower current and underestimation of bioresistance.

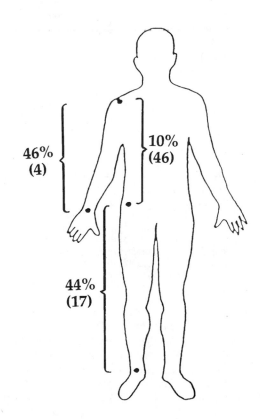

FIGURE 10–3 Contribution of different body segments to whole body impedance or resistance. The numbers show the percentage individual segments contribute, and the numbers in parenthesis show the percentage the same segment contributes to the body weight of the reference man. The values in obese subjects are similar to lean subjects. (From Fuller NJ, Elia M: Potential use of bioelectrical impedance of the whole body and of body segments for the assessment of body composition: comparison with densitometry and anthropometry. Eur J Clin Nutr 1989;43:779–791.)

TABLE 10–10 Interobserver Measurement Variability for Bedside Body Composition Techniques

Method	Residual CV (%)	
	Raw Measurement	**Calculated Body Fat (kg)**
Weight (kg)	0.001	0.8*
Height (cm)	0.4	0.8*
Skinfold thicknesses (mm)		
Triceps	11	4.6[†]
Biceps	16	
Subscapula	13	
Suprailiac	18	
Resistance (Ω)	1.2	2.6[†]
Near infrared interactance		
Optical density 1	5.6	4.2[§]
Optical density 2	6.2	4.2[§]

CV = coefficient of variation.
*Calculated from equation of Black et al,[43] which uses the body mass index.
[†]Calculated from Durnin and Wormersley.[18]
[‡]Calculated from manufacturers' equations (Valhalla equation):
  (% fat = 9.07 + [0.603 × weight (kg)] = [0.581 height²/resistance(Ω)].
[§]Calculated from manufacturers' equations provided at the time (Futrex 5000):
  % fat (men) = 54.172 – 4.2 od2 + 0.1232 weight (kg) – 0.11693 (cm) – 14.9 od1 – 139.4 activity score.
  % (women) = 60.228 – 4.2 od2 + 0.1232 weight (kg) – 0.11693 height (cm) – 14.9 od1 – 139.4 activity score.
Adapted from Fuller NJ, Jebb SA, Goldberg GR et al: Interobserver variability in the measurement of body composition. Eur J Clin Nutr 1991;45:43–49.

TABLE 10–11 Precision in the Basic Measurement and Estimates of Body Fat

Method	Precision		
	Raw Measurement (% CV)	**Body Fat* (kg)**	**Reference**
Reference methods			
Density	0.21–0.23	0.73–0.79	44,45
Total body water	1.0–2.0	0.55–1.10	21,46
Total body potassium	2.0–3.0	1.1–4.7	47,48
DEXA	—	0.45	21
Bedside techniques			
BMI[†]	0.8	0.15	20
Skinfold thickness[‡]	9.0	0.65	20
Resistance[§]	1.2	0.35	20
NIRI[||]	5.9	0.60	20

CV = coefficient of variation; DEXA = dual-energy x-ray absorptiometry; BMI = body mass index; NIRI = near infrared interactance.
*Assuming 20% fat in a 70-kg reference man.
[†]Calculated from equation of Black et al,[43] which uses the body mass index.
[‡]Calculated from Durnin and Wormersely.[18]
[§]Calculated from manufacturers' equations (Valhalla equation):
  (% fat = 9.07 + [0.603 × weight (kg)] = [0.581 Height²/Resistance(Ω)].
[||]Calculated from manufacturers' equations provided at the time (Futrex 5000) (see footnote to Table 10–10).
Data from Elia M: Clin Nutr 1992;11:114–127.

fore in studies in which measurements are made by multiple observers, as in multicenter trials, there is an advantage in using impedance. This was the case in the National Health and Nutrition Examination Survey (NHANES) III survey, a national study in the United States.[50] Furthermore, in grossly obese individuals in whom skinfold thickness measurement may vary or be difficult or impossible to obtain due to the limited "jaw" width of the skinfold calipers, other bedside techniques have an advantage.

Second, it may be possible to use bioelectrical impedance to assess the composition of individual limbs, especially their fat and muscle content,[51] which change during malnutrition and repletion. The bioimpedance measurements are quick to make, and the results obtained in at least one study are particularly encouraging, since they were found to be as good if not better than those based on anthropometry. In this study computed tomography (CT) scanning was the reference method.[51]

Third, the bioimpedance technique, unlike other methods, can estimate the distribution of water between intracellular and extracellular space,[25,52,53] which would be of particular value in certain clinical situations, especially those associated with fluid overload. This is based on the principles of multifrequency or swept-frequency impedance. At low frequencies the current cannot penetrate the capacitative resistance of the cell membrane, and therefore the resistance/impedance measurements depend on the properties and mass of the extracellular fluid. With increasing frequency the current increasingly penetrates the cell, and the resistance/impedance depends on the properties and mass of the extracellular plus intracellular fluid. Therefore, by comparing results obtained at different frequencies it is possible to estimate the distribution of water between the intracellular and extracellular fluid. However, the measurements do not overcome the problems associated with the disproportionate effect of individual body segments. For example, large fluid volumes in the abdomen (ascites) or chest (pleural effusion) will have relatively little effect on the swept-frequency results of the whole body because the trunk contributes little to whole body impedance/resistance (see above).

Fourth, the impedance technique could have an important future in diagnostic medicine (e.g., using microimpedance techniques, in which needles that can measure tissue impedance are inserted into tumors to distinguish malignant from benign tumors[54]) and in bioimpedance tomography,[55] which gives images of tissues based on composition and their electrical properties. An increase in resolution is required before three-dimensional imaging is attempted.

Near Infrared Interactance

The bedside technique of near infrared interactance (NIRI) depends on irradiating a limb (typically the anterior aspect of the mid-upper arm) with at least two frequencies of near infrared radiation.[56-59] The amount and ratio of reflected radiation are influenced by underlying tissue composition. The technique is quick and easy to perform and has intermediate precision between skinfold and impedance measurements (Tables 10–10 and 10–11). A disadvantage of making measurements only at one site is that they may not reflect body composition as a whole. However, attempts to obtain better estimates by combining measurements obtained from two or three sites (biceps, triceps, and anterior quadriceps areas) have not been successful.[56]

Another potential problem with this technique is that the radiation may fail to adequately penetrate the muscles of grossly obese individuals. The technique has not yet been found to be superior to skinfold thicknesses or certain impedance techniques in predicting body composition obtained by densitometry[56] or four-compartment models of body composition[21] (assessed by a combination of hydrodensitometry, water-dilution techniques and dual-energy x-ray absorptiometry [DEXA]). NIRI was found to underestimate fat in the obese and to greatly underestimate it in the grossly obese.[56] The equations provided by one commercial system (Futrex 5000) have been changed. These equations (Table 10–10) depend not only on the near infrared measurements of optical density but also on weight, height, and a subjective assessment of activity score, which in themselves can provide a reasonable estimate of body composition.[21,56] The additional improvement provided by incorporating the optical density measurement is probably small. One study based on stepwise regression analysis concluded that near infrared optical density readings did not predict additional variance in percent body fat beyond the variables already used.[59]

Measuring Muscle Mass

Muscle wasting, a common and frequently early finding in protein-energy malnutrition, is associated with functional consequences. Muscle mass may be assessed by a variety of techniques ranging from clinical examination, anthropometry, bioelectrical impedance, biochemical methods, and various scanning techniques (magnetic resistance imaging, CT scans, and DEXA). Here only the urinary creatinine and DEXA methods will be discussed. DEXA is briefly discussed partly because hospitals are increasingly acquiring such machines for this purpose, and partly because of its multiple potential uses in body composition.

Creatinine Excretion

Creatinine is an end product of N metabolism that is formed nonenzymatically from creatine and creatine phosphate, which are found almost exclusively in muscle. If the intramuscular concentrations of creatine and creatine phosphate are constant (some variability is known to occur),[60] then the spontaneous formation of creatinine is expected to be constant provided intramuscular pH and temperature are maintained within the normal narrow physiologic range. It is generally believed that a daily creatinine excretion of 1 g (8.85 mmol) arises from about 18 kg of muscle. Creatinine excretion has been related to height to take into account differences in body build. Separate tables are available for men and women because the contribution of muscle to lean body mass is lower in women than men. The creatinine height index of a subject is the 24-hour excretion of creatinine relative to a reference value obtained from groups of healthy subjects of the same height and gender. Malnutrition is expected to reduce the creatinine height index (e.g., to ≤0.8). However, a variety of factors can affect creatinine excretion independently of muscle mass (Table 10–12), and it is necessary to obtain complete 24-hour urine collections for the measurement to be of value.

The first study to use a marker to assess the completeness of 24-hour urine collection in patients receiving parenteral nutrition in general medical and surgical wards[69] suggested that the completeness varied, with the average collection being only about three quarters complete. In view of these factors, many clinicians do not routinely use the creatinine height index, although it is of value in stable patients involved in research studies in whom urine collections are more likely to be complete and in whom major changes in renal function are not likely to occur.

Dual Energy X-ray Absorptiometry

This method, which has been increasingly used in some hospitals, involves irradiating the body with x-ray films containing two different energies. The dose of radiation is small and corresponds to about 1 day's natural background radiation. The differential absorption of these x-ray films by fat and fat-free soft tissue and by bone mineral and soft tissue allows the body and its segments to be divided into three components: bone mineral, fat, and fat-free soft tissue. In the limbs the fat-free soft tissue consists largely of muscle, which accounts for approximately 70 percent of the total muscle mass in the whole body. More sophisticated equations for predicting limb muscle mass that take into account the amount of skin, the water content of adipose tissue, and the fat content of muscle have been produced,[71] but all methods give erroneous estimates in the presence of edema, which is a component of fat-free soft tissue. DEXA also gives information about whole body fat mass, lean body mass, and mineral content, which is of particular value for assessing osteoporosis. However, there is still some concern about the accuracy of DEXA and about the discrepancy in results obtained by different commercial machines.

TABLE 10–12 Factors Affecting the "Apparent" Creatinine Excretion Independent of Muscle Mass

Pathophysiologic
Normal daily variation (approximately 10%)[62,63]
Meat in diet (up to approximately 25%)[64,65]
Menstrual cycle (up to approximately 10%)[66]
Pyrexial/traumatic conditions (?0–50%)[67]
Changing renal function
Chronic and stable renal function[68]
Incomplete urine collection[69]

Biochemical
Temperature (i.e., pyrexia/hypothermia)[67]
pH[67]
Intramuscular concentration of creatine and creatine phosphate[60,67]
Ratio of intramuscular creatine (fractional conversion to creatinine approximately 1.3%/day at pH 7, 37°C)
   to creatine phosphate (fractional conversion to creatinine approximately 2.3%/day at pH 7, 37°C)[67]
Interference with assay—ketone bodies, certain drugs, and chromagens interfere with Jaffé's reaction[70]
Creatine/creatinine conversions in urine[67]

Data from Elia M, Jebb SA: South African J Clin Nutr 1990;3:21–26.

Measuring the Status of Specific Nutrients

The diagnosis or confirmation of specific nutrient deficiencies strongly depends on the laboratory. Iron deficiency anemia produces microcytic hypochronic blood cells, low serum concentrations of iron and ferritin, and high concentrations of transferrin. Folate and vitamin B_{12} deficiencies are associated with a macrocytic (apparent on blood examination) and megaloblastic anemia (apparent on bone marrow examination) and low circulating concentrations of folate or B_{12}. Vitamin D deficiency is associated with low plasma calcium, alkaline phosphatase (bone isoenzyme), and low plasma 25-hydroxy vitamin D. Vitamin C deficiency is associated with low plasma and leukocyte ascorbic acid levels. The diagnosis of many trace element deficiencies also depends on the laboratory.

The clinician should be aware of the specificity and sensitivity of these tests. For example, a microcytic hypochronic anemia may occur in thalassemia or renal failure, while a macrocytic anemia may occur in hypothyroidism or alcoholism. The plasma concentration of several minerals or trace elements is often affected by the concentration of the proteins that bind them. For example, an acute-phase response reduces the plasma calcium concentration because it reduces the plasma albumin concentration, which binds about 60 percent of the plasma calcium. It also reduces the plasma iron (decreases transferrin concentration) and zinc concentrations (bound to albumin and α_2-macroglobulin). Additional causes of low plasma zinc concentrations after injury are the increased uptake of zinc in the liver and the high corticosteroid concentrations. Paradoxically, the plasma zinc concentration increases during starvation[72] (and is associated with a marked increase in urinary zinc excretion) due to the zinc released directly into the circulation during the breakdown of lean tissues. The associated changes in circulating albumin and α_2-macroglobulin concentrations are small.

Plasma ferritin concentrations have been increasingly used to assess iron status, particularly since they relate to the iron stores even within the iron replete range. Thus the circulating ferritin concentration frequently changes before the development of anemia or other biochemical or hematologic indexes of iron deficiency. However, the circulating ferritin concentration increases during inflammatory reactions. It is also affected by liver disease. The interpretation of many of the above measurements can be made easier if measurements of acute-phase proteins (indicating inflammatory reactions) are made at the same time.

Functional Tests

Body structure and composition are frequently poor indicators of function. An international group classified five areas of body function that may be affected by malnutrition[73]: cognitive ability, disease response, reproductive competence, physical activity, and social and social/behavioral performance. Although the importance of these functions are widely recognized, a systematic and reliable assessment linked to clinical outcome has not been widely used. However, some of these functions are assessed as part of normal clinical assessment, but nonnutritional components may limit their usefulness. Additionally, although some tests can measure certain functions, some of the measurements are unsuitable for sick patients (e.g., ability to perform strenuous [maximal] exercise on an ergometer).

Maximal Voluntary Muscle Strength

Hand dynamometry has been used to assess maximal voluntary grip strength. The results correlate with muscle mass[74] and, in some cases, clinical outcome.[75,76] The range of normality is large,[67] and therefore changes in grip strength are of more value than single measurements. In addition to muscle mass, the results depend on the following[74,77]: subject's level of consciousness and cooperation, presence of arthritis and other neuromuscular conditions, whether dynamometry induces pain (even abdominal incisions can cause pain during hand dynamometry), and whether the subject is receiving muscle relaxants or sedatives.

Peak expiratory or inspiratory flows have been used to assess respiratory muscle function, and these are again attractive to the clinician, especially when linked to clinical outcome. However, these tests are also influenced by nonnutritional factors, including many indicated above.

Muscle Stimulation Tests

Muscle stimulation tests have the advantage over classic hand dynamometry in that they do not depend on volition.[78-82] Typically the adductor pollicis muscle is stimulated, and force frequency relationships are established. Some studies have shown a good relationship between muscle stimulation tests and the outcome of elective surgery[78] and have documented important changes during starvation.

One such study concluded that the change in relaxation rate following muscle stimulation was a good index of the change in nutritional status during starvation,[79] and another[80] considered it to be more specific and sensitive in predicting complications after surgery than a variety of other indexes (hand grip strength, arm circumference, and circulating concentrations of transferrin and albumin).

Yet another study[81] considered that a variety of indexes including the relaxation rate of adductor pollicis were better predictors of surgical outcome than of weight loss. One of the interesting observations made with this technique concerns the muscular fatigue that occurs during undernutrition: the changes are large and are corrected before changes in N balance.[78] However, the tests can be uncomfortable and are not well-tolerated by some subjects. A modification of the test to make it less invasive while retaining its reproducibility may be possible. So far, muscle stimulation tests have only been used for research purposes but it appears that they can be affected by nonnutritional factors.

Hepatic Secretory Function

The circulating concentration of various proteins secreted by the liver have been used to assess visceral nutritional function. The principle is that protein-energy malnutrition reduces production of these proteins, while repletion increases their production.[83] Interpretation may be difficult for a variety of reasons. First, the circulating concentrations of proteins are influenced not only by the rate of production but also by the rate of removal. Second, concentration is also influenced by a variety of nonnutritional factors (Table 10–13; 1; Clinical and Laboratory of Assessment of Nutritional Status IFRC, unpublished) such as state of hydration and the presence of an acute inflammatory response. The albumin concentration, for example, is a nonspecific marker of inflammatory disease rather than of undernutrition. In the absence of disease, starvation,[77] even if prolonged,[5,84] produces little change in the circulating albumin concentration, and values within the normal range are seen in patients with anorexia nervosa.[85] Furthermore, within about 1 hour after posture is changed from erect to lying, the circulating albumin concentration decreases by about 10 percent in both well-nourished and malnourished individuals.[86] Presumably the muscle pump, which affects the transcapillary escape of albumin between the intravascular space (containing about 60 percent of the albumin in healthy subjects) and extravascular space (containing about 40 percent) is less active in the lying position. A major increase in the transcapillary escape rate after injury and sepsis (normally about 5 percent of the circulating albumin passes into the extravascular space each hour) is a major cause of hypoalbuminemia in these states.[87]

Many other proteins that are affected by nutritional status or recent food intake are also influenced by the acute inflammatory response, renal function, hepatic function, estrogens, and other factors (Table 10–13). Therefore care should be exercised in using these measurements as nutritional indexes, especially some of the recently suggested indexes, for which there is relatively little information.[88] Interpretation is easier when complicating factors such as an inflammatory reaction (e.g., an acute protein response) are absent. However, the presence of normal circulating concentrations of most of these proteins in anorexia nervosa (uncomplicated by inflammatory or infective disease),[74,85] even when associated with substantial depletion, raises questions about their value.

Some of the proteins respond to recent changes in nutrient intake (starvation or recent weight reduction), especially the proteins with a short half-life (e.g., weight stability in patients with anorexia nervosa). Therefore, in some situations they may be better indicators of recent weight loss or recent dietary intake than of nutritional status. Finally, a general relationship between many of these proteins and nutritional status may exist because inflammatory disease, which reduces their circulating concentration, also reduces food intake, which eventually leads to malnutrition.

Immunologic Tests

Undernutrition may depress immune function. An antigenic extract (e.g., mumps, *Candida* antigens) injected subcutaneously elicits a delayed hypersensitivity response in healthy subjects, producing an area of erythema and swelling. Several antigens are frequently injected, since 5 to 10 percent of the population may not react to individual ones. Undernourished individuals may show an attenuated or absent response (anergy). This anergy has been related to clinical outcome after surgery in some studies,[89] but not others,[90] possibly because of the nonspecific nature of the response. It appears to be affected by age, drugs (e.g., steroids, immunosuppressants and possibly amefidine, warfarin, and aspirin) and dis-

TABLE 10–13 Nonnutritional Factors Affecting the Circulating Concentration of Specific Proteins

Protein	Molecular Weight (daltons)	Half-life (days)	Conditions That Alter Concentration		Adult Range	Comments
			Increases	Decreases		
Albumin	66,500	20	Dehydration	Overhydration Inflammatory disease Protein loss, nephrotic syndrome, protein-losing enteropathy, burns Liver disease	40 ± 3 g/L	Nonspecific indicator of inflammatory disease
Prealbumin	55,000	2	Dehydration Renal failure	Overhydration Inflammatory reaction Nephrotic syndrome Hyperthroidism Liver disease	315 ± 53 mg/L (men) 283 ± 48 mg/L (women)	Responds to recent dietary intake Normal range increases throughout childhood; antisera vary in specificity and sensitivity
Retinol-binding protein (RBP)	21,000	0.5	Dehydration Renal failure Alcoholism	Overhydration Inflammatory reaction Nephrotic syndrome Chronic liver disease Zinc deficiency Vitamin A deficiency	63 ± 11 mg/L (men) 56 ± 14 mg/L (women)	Responds to recent dietary intake Concentration increases throughout childhood
Transferrin	80,000	9	Dehydration Iron deficiency Pregnancy Estrogen 17 α-alkylated steroids Acute hepatitis	Overhydration Inflammatory reaction Nephrotic syndrome and other-protein losing states Severe/chronic liver disease	2–4 g/L	
Insulin-like growth factor	7400	0.12	Dehydration	Hypothroidism Estrogens	600–1400 IU/L	Responds rapidly to fasting; limited information available
Fibronectin	450,000	0.5	Dehydration Acute-phase reaction	Overhydration	2.9 ± 0.2 g/L (plasma) 1.8 ± 0.2 g/L (serum)	Limited information available; tentative normal ranges

169

ease (e.g., viral and bacterial infections and liver and renal disease, trauma, and burns) after surgery. The tests, which may cause discomfort when they are positive, have not found routine clinical use.

The circulating lymphocyte count (normally 1500 to 4000 cells/mm^3) is reduced in malnutrition, but the decrease can occur in a variety of hematological inflammatory conditions and after administration of certain drugs (e.g., cytotoxic drugs).

Prognostic Indexes Based on Multiple Variables

The lack of a simple reference indicator to predict morbidity and mortality in various clinical situations (e.g., after elective surgery) has led some workers to combine several measurements to obtain a single prognostic index. For example, some prognostic indexes[91] have combined anthropometry (triceps, skinfold thickness), biochemical measurements (albumin, transferrin, or total iron-binding capacity), and in some cases immunologic tests such as delayed cutaneous hypersensitivity to establish an overall prognostic index. Because inflammatory disease influences many of these parameters (either directly or indirectly by reducing food intake and causing depletion), it is not surprising that a relationship has been obtained between prognostic indexes and clinical outcome (e.g., complication rate after elective abdominal surgery). However, because a variety of factors affect the measurements including constitutional differences, hydration status, and other specific factors (Table 10–13), and because complication rates are affected by nonnutritional factors such as the skill of the surgeon and the quality of nursing care provided, it is not surprising that this method has met with variable success in different circumstances.

Furthermore, because circulating protein concentrations change rapidly after trauma, the prognostic indexes will depend on when the measurements are made in relation to the trauma and the elective procedure or series of procedures that may follow the initial injury. In addition, ischemic heart disease and increasing age, which increase the risk of surgery, are not included in these prognostic indexes. Therefore, it is not surprising that prognostic indexes have met with variable enthusiasm in different clinical specialties. Interpretation must be made with caution in some circumstances. For example, the practice of delaying surgery in an attempt to improve a prognostic index by providing nutritional support, may have detrimental effects, as in a patient with abscess requiring a simple drainage procedure. There is no replacement for good clinical judgment.

Subjective Global Assessment

Attempts to predict clinical outcome on the basis of nutritionally mediated factors[92-97] have led to the development of a measure called "subjective global assessment." One scoring system[95] relies on five features: (1) weight loss in the preceding 6 months, (2) a change in dietary intake (dietary history), (3) significant GI symptoms (anorexia, nausea, vomiting, and diarrhea) persisting for more than 2 weeks (vomiting occurring daily or secondary to obstruction is considered significant, while short-term diarrhea or intermittent vomiting is not), (4) functional capacity or energy level (e.g., bedridden or normal capacity), and (5) disease and its activity (no stress, low stress, or high stress). The physical examination depends on a subjective assessment of loss of subcutaneous fat and muscle wasting (mild, moderate, or severe) at specific sites and the presence of sacral and ankle edema. Overall, the patient is ranked into one of three categories: well nourished, moderately (or suspected of being) malnourished, or severely malnourished.

Control studies have shown that the results obtained by this method are reproducible. Results obtained by two independent observers were found to agree with each other in 81 percent of patients in one study and 91 percent in another.[92,96] The prediction of complications after surgery by subjective global assessment[78] has been reported to be better than single objective parameters such as delayed cutaneous hypersensitivity, and equal to predictions based on plasma protein measurements. In addition, subjective global assessment adequately predicted the outcome of patients who were involved in a perioperative feeding study.[98]

The success of subjective global assessment to predict outcome in several situations may partly depend on the influence of nonnutritional factors. For example, ankle and sacral edema may be the result of cardiac failure or cor pulmonale, which increase the risk of surgery irrespective of whether malnutrition is present. In contrast, other important nonnutritional factors such as age and the presence of ischemic heart disease or respiratory disease are again not included in the index. A list indicating all conditions responding to nutritional support and improving outcome (decreased morbidity, decreased mortality, improvement in well-being, reduced hospital stay) would be useful. Unfortunately, situations where such information is available are still limited due to the complex nature of disease and malnutrition and their interaction. Therefore, clinicians must use a variety of skills based on knowledge of the likely progression of the underlying disease and the patient's age and nutritional status to decide on the best course of action to follow.

CONCLUSION

Nutritional assessment is of considerable importance in the nutritional care of patients with acute and chronic illnesses, particularly those who require artificial nutritional support. However, the protean nature of malnutrition means that it is difficult to use single measurements to predict its presence and its outcome. General nutritional care of the malnourished patient depends on good bedside judgment and management. Although this is probably more important than a large range of laboratory tests for assessing generalized malnutrition, the tests can be useful for documenting sequential changes in body composition and function. Furthermore, the clinician relies heavily on the laboratory for diagnosis of specific nutrient deficiencies (e.g., folate, B_{12}, iron, vitamin D), although in some circumstances treatment is given without laboratory evidence of specific nutrient deficiencies (e.g., administration of intravenous thiamine in alcoholic patients suspected of having Wernicke-Korsakoff syndrome).

REFERENCES

1. Neale G, Elia M: Nutritional assessment. In Heatley RV, Losowsky MS, Kelleher J (eds): Clinical Nutrition in Gastroenterology. New York: Churchill Livingstone, 1986:48–71.
2. Rudman D, Millikan WJ, Richardson TJ et al: Elemental balances during intravenous hyperalimentation of underweight adult subjects. J Clin Invest 1975;55:94–104.
3. Bingham SA: The dietary assessment of individuals; methods, accuracy, new techniques and recommendations. Nutr Abstr Rev 1987;57(10):705–742.
4. Balogh M, Kahn HA, Medalie JH: Random repeat 24 hour dietary recall. Am J Clin Nutr 1971;24:304–310.
5. Keys A, Brozek J, Henschel A et al: The Biology of Human Starvation. Minneapolis: University of Minnesota Press, 1950.
6. Hambridge KM, Walravens PA, Brown RM et al: Zinc nutrition of preschool children in the Denver Head Start Program. Am J Clin Nutr 1976;29:734–738.
7. Winick M: Nutrition and Drugs. New York: John Wiley & Sons, 1983.
8. Elia M: Body composition analysis: an evaluation of two component models, multicomponent models and bedside techniques. Clin Nutr 1992;11:114–127.
9. Jebb SA, Elia M: Measurement of body composition in clinical practice. In Heatley RV, Greeg JH, Losowsky MS (eds): Consensus in Clinical Nutrition. Cambridge: Cambridge University Press, 1994:1–21.
10. Jebb SA, Elia M: Techniques for the measurement of body composition: a practical guide. Int J Obes 1993;17:611–621.
11. Elia M, Jebb SA: Assessment of body composition: research techniques and bedside methods. South African J Clin Nutr 1990;3:21–26.
12. White A, Nicholaas G, Foster K et al: Health Survey for England 1991. London: Her Majesty's Stationary Office, 1993.
13. McWhirter JP, Pennington CR: Incidence and recognition of malnutrition in hospital. Br Med J 1994;308:945–948.
14. Chumlea WC: Methods of nutritional anthropometric assessment for special groups. In Lohman TG, Roche AF, Martorell R (eds): Anthropometric Standardization Reference Manual, Champaign, IL: Human Kinetic Books, 1988.
15. Chumlea WC, Roche AF, Steinbaugh ML: Estimating stature from knee height for persons 60 to 90 years of age. J Am Geriatr Soc 1985;33:116–120.
16. Rolland-Cachera MF, Sempe M, Guilloud-Bataille M et al: Adiposity indices in children. Am J Clin Nutr 1982;36:178–184.
17. Waterlow JC: Protein energy malnutrition. London: Edward Arnold, 1992.
18. Durnin JVGA, Womersley J: Body fat assessed from total body density and its estimation from skinfold thickness: measurements on 481 men and women aged 16 to 72 years. Br J Nutr 1974;32:77–97.
19. Fuller NJ, Elia M: Potential use of bioelectrical impedance of the whole body and of body segments for the assessment of body composition: comparison with densitometry and anthropometry. Eur J Clin Nutr 1989;43:779–791.
20. Fuller NJ, Jebb SA, Goldberg GR et al: Inter-observer variability in the measurement of body composition. Eur J Clin Nutr 1991;45:43–49.
21. Fuller NJ, Jebb SA, Laskey MA et al: Four-component model for the assessment of body composition in humans: comparison with alternative methods and evaluation of the density and hydration of fat-free mass. Clin Sci 1992;82:687–693.
22. Pullicino E, Coward WA, Stubbs RJ et al: Bedside and field methods for assessing body composition: comparison with the deuterium dilution technique. Eur J Clin Invest 1990;44:753–762.
23. Frisancho AR: New norms of upper limb fat and muscle areas for assessment of nutritional status. Am J Clin Nutr 1981;34:2540–2545.
24. Kushner RF: Bioelectrical impedance analysis: a review of principles and applications. J Am Coll Nutr 1992;11:199–209.
25. Thomas BJ, Cornish BH, Ward LC: Bioelectrical impedance analysis for measurement of body fluid volumes: a review. J Clin Eng 1992;17:505–510.
26. Elia M: The bioimpedance "craze." Eur J Clin Nutr 1993;47:825–827.
27. Hoffer EC, Meador CK, Simpson DC: Correlation of whole body impedance with total body water volume. J Appl Physiol 1989;27:231–234.
28. Lukaski HC, Johnson PE, Bolonchuk WW et al: Assessment of fat free mass using bioelectrical impedance

measurements of the human body. Am J Clin Nutr 1985;47:810–817.

29. Kushner RF, Schoeller DA: Estimation of total body water by bioelectrical impedance analysis. Am J Clin Nutr 1986;44:417–424.

30. Segal KR, van Loan M, Fitzgerald PI et al: Lean body mass estimation by bioelectrical impedance analysis: a four-site cross validation study. Am J Clin Nutr 1988;47:7–14.

31. Gray DS, Bray GA, Gemayel N et al: Effect of obesity on bioelectrical impedance. Am J Clin Nutr 1989; 50:255–260.

32. Deurenberg P, Westrate JA, Hautvast JG: Changes in fat free mass during weight loss measured by bioelectrical impedance and densitometry. Am J Clin Nutr 1989;49:33–36.

33. Lukaski HC, Bolonchuk WW, Hall CB et al: Validation of tetrapolar bioelectrical impedance method to assess human body composition. J Appl Physiol 1986; 60:1327–1332.

34. Graves JE, Pollock ML, Colvin A et al: Comparison of different bioelectrical impedance analysers in the prediction of body composition. Am J Hum Biol 1989;1: 603–611.

35. Diaz EA, Villar J, Immink M et al: Bioimpedance or anthropometry? Eur J Clin Nutr 1989;43:129–137.

36. Deurenberg P, Kooy K van de, Leenen R: Differences in body impedance when measured by different instruments. Eur J Clin Nutr 1989;43:885–886.

37. Smye SW, Sutcliffe J, Pitt E: A comparison of four commercial systems used to measure whole body electrical impedance. Phys Meas 1993;14:473–478.

38. Martorell R, Malina RM, Costillo RL et al: Body proportions in three ethnic groups: children and youths 2-17 years in NHANES II and HHANES. Hum Biol 1988; 60:205–222.

39. Jebb SA, Elia M: Assessment of changes in total body water in patients undergoing renal dialysis using bioelectrical impedance analysis. Clin Nutr 1991;10: 81–84.

40. Cin SD, Braga M, Molinari M et al: Role of bioelectrical impedance analysis in acutely dehydrated subjects. Clin Nutr 1992;11:128–133.

41. Zillikens MC, Berg JWO van den, Wilson JHP et al: Whole body and sequential bioelectrical impedance analysis in patients with cirrhosis of the liver: changes after treatment of ascites. Am J Clin Nutr 1992;55:621–625.

42. Carlson GL, Visvanathan R, Pannarate OC et al: Change in bioelectrical impedance following laparoscopic and open abdominal surgery. Clin Nutr 1194; 13:171–176.

43. Black D, James WPT, Besser GM et al: Obesity. A report of the Royal College of Physicians. J Royal Coll Phys 1983;17:5–65.

44. Siri WB: Body composition from fluid spaces and density. In Brozek J, Henschel H (eds): Techniques for Measuring Body Composition. Washington, DC: Nat Acad Sci, 223–244.

45. Durnin JVGA, Taylor A: Replication of measurement of density of the human body as determined by underwater weighing. J Appl Physiol 1960;15:142–144.

46. Murgatroyd PW, Coward WA: An improved method for estimating changes in whole-body fat and protein mass in man. Br J Nutr 1989;62:311–314.

47. Shukla KK, Ellis KJ, Dombrowski CS et al: Physiological variation of total body potassium in man. Am J Physiol 1973;224:271–274.

48. Forbes GB, Shultz F, Cafarreli C et al: Effect of body size on potassium-40 measurement in the whole body counter (lift chair technique). Health Phys 1968;15: 435–442.

49. Vettorazzi C, Smits E, Solomons NW: The inter-observer reproducibility of bioelectrical impedance analysis measurements in infants and toddlers. J Pediatr Gastro 1994;19:277–282.

50. Woteki CE, Briesel RR, Kuczmarski R: Contributions of the National Centre for Health Statistics. Am J Clin Nutr 1988;471:320–328.

51. Brown BH, Karatzas T, Nakielny R et al: Determination of upper arm muscle and fat areas using electrical impedance measurements. Clin Phys Physiol Meas 1988; 9:47–55.

52. Cornish BH, Thomas BJ, Ward LC: Improved prediction of extracellular and total body water using impedance generated by bioelectrical impedance analysis. Phys Med Biol 1993;337–346.

53. Van Loan MD, Mayclin PL: Use of multifrequency bioelectrical impedance analysis for the estimation of extracellular fluid. Eur J Clin Nutr 1992;46:117–124.

54. Morimoto T, Kinouchi Y, Iritani T et al: Measurement of the electrical bioimpedance of breast tumors. Eur Surg Res 1990;22:86–92.

55. Barber DC, Brown BH: Electrical impedance tomography. Phys Meas 1994;(suppl 2A):A1–A224.

56. Elia M, Parkinson SA, Diaz EO: Evaluation of near infra-red reactance as a method for predicting body composition. Eur J Clin Nutr 1990;44:113–121.

57. Heyward VH, Jenkins KA, Cook KL et al: Validity of single-site and multi-site models for estimating body composition of women using near infra-red interactance. Am J Hum Biol 1992;4:579–593.

58. Conway JM, Norris KH, Bodwell CE: A new approach for the estimation of body composition: infra-red interactance. Am J Clin Nutr 1984;40:1123–1130.

59. Hortobagyi T, Israel RG, Houmard JA et al: Comparison of body composition assessment by hydrodensitometry, skinfolds and multiple site near infra-red spectroscopy. Eur J Clin Nutr 1992;46:205–211.

60. Reeds PJ, Jackson AA, Picou D et al: Muscle mass and composition in malnourished infants and changes seen after recovery. Pediatr Res 1978;12:613–618.

61. Elia M, Jebb SA: Assessment of body composition: research techniques and bedside methods. South African J Clin Nutr 1990;3:21–26.

62. Greenhalt DE, Rausil BJ, Harmatz et al: Variability of 24 hour urinary creatinine in normal subjects. J Clin Pharmacol 1976;10:321–328.

63. Waterlow JC: Observations on the variability of creatinine excreiton. Hum Nutr Clin Nutr 1986;40C: 125–129.

64. Beiler RE, Schedl HP: Creatinine excretion: variability and relationship to diet and body size. J Lab Clin Med 1972;59:945–953.

65. Crim MC, Calloway DH, Margen S: Creatinine metabolism in men: urinary creatinine excretions with creatine feeding. J Nutr 1975;105:428–438.

66. Smith OW: Creatinine excretion in women, data collected in the course of urine analysis for female sex hormones. J Clin Endocrinol 1942;2:1–12.

67. Fuller NJ, Elia M: Factors affecting the production of creatinine: implications for the determination and determination of urinary creatinine and creatinine in man. Clin Chim Acta 1988;175:199–200.

68. Mitch WE, Collier VW, Walser M: Creatinine metabolism in chronic renal failure. Clin Sci 1980;58:327–335.

69. Elia M, Fuller NJ, Fotherby K et al: The use of sodium para-amino-hippurate (PAH) as a marker of the completeness of urine collections: studies in patients re-

ceiving total parenteral nutrition. Clin Nutr 1987; 6:267–275.

70. Spencer K: Analytical reviews in clinical biochemistry: the estimation of creatinine. Ann Clin Biochem 1986; 23:1–25.

71. Fuller NJ, Laskey MA, Elia M: Assessment of major body regions by dual energy X-ray absorptiometry (DEXA), with special reference to limb muscle mass. Clin Physiol 1992;12:1–15.

72. Elia M, Crozier C, Neale G: Mineral metabolism during short term starvation in man. Clin Chim Acta 1984; 139:37–45.

73. Solomons NW, Allen LH: The functional assessment of nutritional status: principles, practice and potential. Nutr Rev 1983;41:33–50.

74. Martin S, Neale G, Elia M: Factors affecting maximal voluntary grip strength. Hum Nutr Clin Nutr 1985; 39C:137–147.

75. Klidjian AM, Archer TJ, Foster KJ et al: Detection of dangerous malnutrition. J Parenter Enter Nutr 1982; 6:119–121.

76. Klidjian AM, Foster KJ, Kammerling RM et al: Relation of anthopometric and dynamometric variables of serious post-operative complications. Br Med J 1980; 281:899–901.

77. Elia M, Martin S, Price C et al: Effect of starvation and elective surgery on hand dynamometry and circulating concentrations of various proteins. Clin Nutr 1984; 2:173–179.

78. Jeejeebhoy KN. Clinical and functional assessments. In Shils ME, Olson JA, Shike M (eds): Modern Nutrition in Health and Disease, 8th edition. Philadelphia: Lea & Febiger, 1994:805–811.

79. Lennmarken C, Sandstedt S, Schenck HV et al: The effect of starvation on skeletal muscle function in man. Clin Nutr 1986;5:99–103.

80. Zeiderman MR, MacMahon MJ: The role of objective measurements of skeletal muscle function in the preoperative patient. Clin Nutr 1989;8:161–166.

81. Windsor JA, Hill CL: Weight loss with physiologic impairment. A basic indication of surgical risk. Ann Surg 1988;207:290–296.

82. Zeiderman MR, Wilson IJ, Price R: An objective test of muscle function using the BBC microcomputer. J Microcomp Appl 1984;7:309–317.

83. Ingenbleek Y, Van den Schreich HG, De Nayer P et al: Albumin transferrin and thyroxin-binding prealbumin/retinol-binding proteins (TBPA-RPB) complex in assessment of malnutrition. Clin Chim Acta 1975;63: 61–67.

84. Ballentyne FC, Smith J, Fleck A: Albumin metabolism in fasting obese subjects. Br J Nutr 1973;30:585–592.

85. Dowd PS, Kelleher J, Walker BE et al: Nutritional and immunological assessment of patients with anorexia nervosa. Clin Nutr 1983;2:79–83.

86. Medical Research Council Special Report No. 275: Studies of Undernutrition. Wuppental 1946-9. London: HMSO, 1951:165–174, 204–206.

87. Fleck A, Hawker F, Wallace PI et al: Increased vascular permeability: a major cause of hypoalbuminaemia in disease and injury. Lancet 1985;781–784.

88. McWhirter JP, Ryan MF, Pennington CR: An evaluation of insulin like growth factor-1 as an indicator of nutritional status. Clin Nutr 1995;14:74–80.

89. Christou NV, Meakins JL, Maclean LD: The predictive role of delayed hypersensitivity in pre-operative patients. Surg Gynecol Obstet 1981;152:297–301.

90. Bancewicz J, Brown R, Hamid J et al: In Wesdrop RIC, Soeters PB (eds): Clinical Nutrition. Edinburgh: Churchill Livingstone, 1989:265–274.

91. Buzby GP, Mullen JL, Matthews DC et al: Prognostic nutritional index in gastrointestinal surgery. Am J Surg 1980;139:160–167.

92. Baker JP, Detsky AS, Weeson DE et al: Nutritional assessment: a comparison of clinical judgement and objective measurements. N Engl J Med 1982;306: 969–972.

93. Baker JP, Detsky AS, Whitwell J et al: A comparison of the predictive value of nutritional assessment techniques. Hum Nutr Clin Nutr 1982;36C:233–241.

94. Detsky AS, Baker JP, Mendelson RA et al: Evaluating the accuracy of nutritional assessment techniques applied to hospitalized patients; methodology and comparisons. J Parenter Enter Nutr 1984;8:153–159.

95. Detsky AS, MacLaughlin JR, Baker JP et al: What is subjective global assessment of nutritional status? J Parenter Enter Nutr 1987;11:8–13.

96. Detsky AS, Baker JP, O'Rourke K et al: Predicting nutrition-associated complications for patients undergoing gastrointestinal surgery. J Parenter Enter Nutr 1987;11:440–446.

97. Detsky AS, Smalley PS, Chang J. Is the patient malnourished? JAMA 1994;271:54–58.

98. The Veterans Affairs Total Parenteral Nutrition Cooperative Study Group: Perioperative nutrition in surgical patients. N Engl J Med 1991;325:525–532.

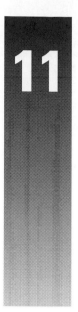

Minimally Invasive Access to the Gastrointestinal Tract

ROBERT C. GORMAN
JON B. MORRIS

All hospitalized patients need adequate nutrition. This is particularly true for critically ill patients who, for any number of reasons, cannot maintain their nutritional status. Recent advances in techniques for long-term vascular and enteral access provide the clinician with many options for providing nutritional support to patients who are unable to maintain themselves completely with normal oral alimentation.

This chapter will present currently available minimally invasive techniques including endoscopic, laparoscopic, and radiologically assisted modalities for obtaining access to the gastrointestinal (GI) tract to provide enteral nutritional support. Each procedure's indications, contraindications, complications, and relative benefits will be discussed.

HISTORICAL PERSPECTIVE

Advances in techniques for providing adequate enteral alimentation to patients unable to maintain nutrition orally have paralleled advances in GI surgery. Attempts to provide enteral nutrition by mechanical means date back to the ancient Egyptians, who used emetics and nutrient enemas to preserve health.[1] The use of nutrient enemas continued and in the late 19th century were considered by some the method of choice for providing nutrition to patients unable to eat.[2]

Technical problems with rectal alimentation included the tendency to induce evacuation, poor absorption, and mucosal irritation. These problems, combined with increasing knowledge about normal digestion, caused Einhorn in 1910 to propose gastric and duodenal feedings as an alternative to nutrient enemas.[1] A similar technique had been employed by John Hunter, who in 1790 treated a 50-year-old patient who was rendered unable to swallow due to recent stroke. Hunter recommended that a hollow flexible tube be passed into the patient's stomach so that medicines and nourishment could be provided to sustain the patient. Treatment continued for 5 weeks until the patient could swallow normally.[1]

Success with nasoenteric feedings continued throughout the early 20th century. In 1939, Stengel and Ravdin[3] used a nasogastric-jejunal tube placed at surgery to provide jejunal feedings as well as gastric decompression.

Surgical access to the GI tract for tube feedings was a logical extension of previously described nasoenteric methods for nutrient delivery. Advances in surgical technique stimulated development of this type of enteral feeding access. The forerunners of surgical enteral access were gastrocutaneous fistulas resulting from trauma. The best-known case of traumatic gastric fistula is that of Alexis St. Martin, who sustained a gunshot wound to the abdomen in 1822.[4] Beaumont's detailed study of this patient led to further understanding of gastric physiology and demonstrated the feasibility of feeding through surgical gastrostomy.[4]

Gastrostomy as a planned surgical procedure was proposed first by Egeberg[5,6] in 1837 and performed initially by Sedillot[5,7] in 1849 and 1853. The first gastrostomy resulting in survival was performed by Jones[5,8] in 1875. The chronologic development of surgical gastrostomies is presented in Figure 11–1. Gauderer and colleagues described an endoscopic-assisted technique for gastrostomy without laparotomy.[9] This technique offered the advantage of decreased procedure time, local anesthesia, lack of wound complications, and a decreased incidence of postoperative ileus. Since its initial description, the percutaneous endoscopic gastrostomy has been widely adopted and has largely replaced surgical gastrostomy at most institutions.

The introduction of the laparoscopic cholecystectomy in the late 1980s has stimulated the use of laparoscopic modalities in many aspects of GI surgery. Innovative surgeons have developed laparoscopic techniques for gaining access to the upper GI tract to provide enteral nutrition. These procedures, although still evolving, may ultimately provide alternatives to standard open surgical procedures in patients who are not candidates for endoscopic procedures.

Surgical jejunostomies for feeding were initially constructed to palliate patients with esophageal and gastric cancers in the late 19th century. In 1912, W.T. Mayo proposed the extensive use of surgical jejunostomy in patients with esophageal obstruction and severe peptic ulcer disease.[10] Intraoperative placement of feeding jejunostomies in patients with gastric outlet obstruction was described by Andersen in 1918.[4] In 1952, Bowles and Zollinger reported on 103 patients who had been fed by a surgically placed jejunostomy during abdominal exploration. A Stamm technique was employed, and feedings were typically begun within 12 hours of surgery.[11]

Recent studies have demonstrated the efficacy of jejunal feedings in patients at risk of aspiration and as an adjunct in patients undergoing major hepatobiliary, pancreatic, and gastric surgery.[12,13] Alternatives to standard surgical options for jejunal access have paralleled ad-

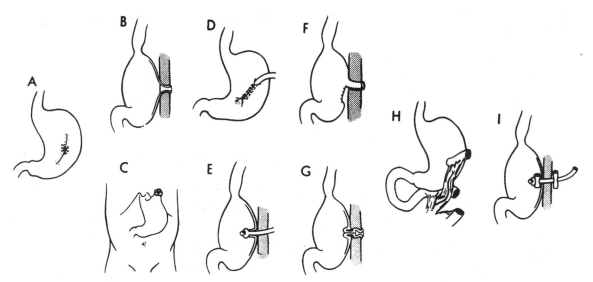

FIGURE 11–1. The six basic types of gastrostomies arranged chronologically in order of development. Type 1: *A,* Gastric fistula secondary to trauma (1635). Type 2: Formation of a gastric cone—*B,* through the incision (1846) and *C,* through a counterincision (1890). Type 3: Formation of a channel from the anterior gastric wall—*D,* catheter parallel to stomach (1891) and *E,* catheter perpendicular to stomach (1894). Type 4: Formation of a tube from the gastric wall *F,* without valve (1899) and *G,* with valve (1901). Type 5: *H,* Formation of a tube from small or large bowel (1906). Type 6: *I,* Gastrostomy without celiotomy (percutaneous endoscopic) (1980). (From Gauderer MW, Stellato TA: Gastrostomies: evolution, techniques, indications and complications. Curr Prob Surg 1986;23:661–719.)

vances in endoscopic and laparoscopic procedures. In the late 1980s and early 1990s various techniques for laparoscopic jejunostomies and endoscopic conversion of gastrostomies to jejunostomies were developed and described. These "minimally invasive" options for providing safe and effective enteral feeding access are the focus of the chapter.

PATIENT SELECTION FOR ENTERAL NUTRITIONAL SUPPORT

Presented in this section is a brief review of the indication for enteral feeding access. An algorithm for determining the best means of enteral access for the individual patient is also discussed.

The patient must take in a sufficient diet to maintain normal body composition and function. This equilibrium may be disturbed by decreased intake, increased requirements, or alteration in the body's normal milieu that prevents nutrients from being used effectively for tissue repair. A detailed presentation on nutritional assessment can be found in Chapter 10; however, to establish the need for supplementary feedings, a careful evaluation of the patients' nutritional status should demonstrate that the patient's current dietary intake is insufficient to meet nutrient needs. Once volitional oral intake is found to be inadequate, the route for forced feeding must be selected.

It is generally accepted that in patients with a functional GI tract, enteral feedings are superior to the parenteral route. Increased safety is a major factor in support of enteral feeding. Although complications of enteral feeding do occur, they are usually more easily managed and are not life threatening. Common complications are related to the catheter (occlusion, migration, granulation tissue, persistent fistula) or the enteral infusions (nausea, vomiting, and diarrhea).[1] The potentially life-threatening complications of pneumothorax, hemothorax, arterial puncture, catheter or air embolism, electrolyte abnormalities, and line sepsis associated with central venous cannulation and feedings are avoided.

Another benefit of enteral feedings over venous feedings is reduced cost. Most of this benefit is a result of a lower cost for enteral feeding formulas compared with comparable parenteral formulas. Parenteral formulas can be 2 to 10 times more expensive than enteral formulas that provide a similar amount of nutrients.[14] Finally, enteral feedings are superior to parenteral nutrition in sustaining intestinal structure and function.[14]

As mentioned previously, patients who require nutritional support and have a functioning GI tract should receive feedings enterally. Common indications for enteral feedings include neurologic disorders, trauma, critical illness, head or neck surgery, upper GI surgery, and prolonged respiratory failure (Table 11–1).

Enteral nutrients may be delivered intragastrically (prepylorically) or postpylorically. There is considerable debate over which of these two basic yet physiologically different techniques is most appropriate. A primary concern is the risk of aspiration of enteral contents, particularly in neurologically impaired patients, who frequently require enteral nutrition. We favor postpyloric feedings for patients judged to be at risk for aspiration, an approach that substantially reduces episodes of feeding-related aspiration.[12]

Risk factors for aspiration of enteral feeds are many (Table 11–2). After a thorough history and physical examination, which sometimes necessitates direct and indirect laryngoscopy, tests that help assess aspiration risk are barium studies, fluoroscopy, manometry, and scintigraphy.[16] Evaluation of the patient by a neurologist or speech pathologist may also help to assess the patient at risk for aspiration.[17]

Once enteral supplementation has been decided on, the clinician must choose among the many available delivery techniques for enteral feedings. Possible access techniques include surgical (open or laparoscopic), endoscopic, and radiologic intervention, which may be performed with either local or general anesthesia. The type of technique employed often varies

TABLE 11–1   Indications for Enteral Nutritional Support

Neurologic and muscular diseases
Cerebrovascular accidents
Dementia
Head trauma
Brain neoplasms
Parkinson's disease
Myopathy
Critical illness/trauma
Cancer of the head and neck or gastrointestinal tract
Respiratory failure with prolonged intubation
Inflammatory bowel disease
Enterocutaneous fistula
Anorexia nervosa

TABLE 11–2 Risk Factors for Aspiration

Altered mental status
Swallowing dysfunction
    Central (cerebrovascular accident)
    Local (vagal disruption, trauma)
History of aspiration
Severe gastroesophageal reflux
Gastric outlet obstruction
Gastroparesis

From Nance ML, Morris JB: Enteral nutritional support: techniques and common complications. Hosp Phys 1992; 28:24–29. Copyright Turner White Communications, Inc. With permission.

among institutions and clinicians, but each choice should be based on the patient's nutritional goals, the patient's ability to tolerate the procedure, and the expected duration of therapy. An algorithm for determining the most appropriate means of enteral access is presented in Figure 11–2.

ENDOSCOPIC TECHNIQUES

Percutaneous Endoscopic Gastrostomy

Percutaneous endoscopic gastrostomy (PEG), which Gauderer and coworkers first described

in 1980,[9] has been a major advance in long-term nutritional support and has nearly supplanted the open gastrostomy. Its rapid acceptance and popularity as a means of enteral access are due largely to its time and cost effectiveness. Many variations on Gauderer's initial technique have been described. The initial steps are, however, similar for all methods and will be described before the various options for completing the procedure.

The patient is kept nil per os (NPO) for at least 8 hours before the procedure. Prophylactic antibiotics, usually a cephalosporin, are recommended preoperatively. The patient lies supine on the operating room table, and intravenous (IV) sedation as well as local pharyngeal anesthesia is administered. Before placing a gastrostomy tube, perform a full diagnostic esophagogastroduodenoscopy (EGD) to rule out any luminal pathologic condition in the esophagus, stomach, or duodenum.

Introduce the gastroscope into the stomach; insufflate air to distend the stomach. Adequate air insufflation opposes the stomach to the anterior abdominal wall and displaces the transverse colon caudally to avoid injury to this organ. Transilluminate the abdominal wall with the gastroscope. Watch as the assistant indents

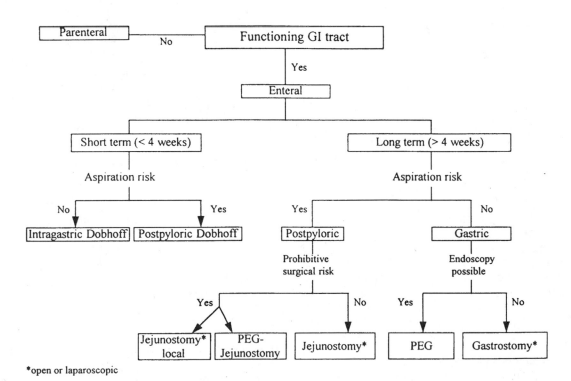

FIGURE 11–2 Enteral access algorithm for selecting the most appropriate technique for an individual patient.

the abdominal wall at the point of the proposed gastrostomy. This position should be at least 2 cm below the costal margin to avoid painful contact between the tube and the rib. It is at this point that the various techniques differ (Fig. 11–3).

Pull Technique of Gauderer and Ponsky

This is the classic technique as originally described.[9] At the point where the assistant's finger indents the abdominal wall and stomach, make a small skin incision after local anesthesia is given. Introduce an angiocatheter through the incision. The endoscopist verifies entry of the needle into the stomach. Pass a biopsy snare through the endoscope and maneuver it around the catheter. Remove the needle and place a long suture, or guidewire, through the catheter into the stomach. The biopsy snare grasps the suture; then withdraw the endoscope and suture through the mouth. Secure the suture to the gastrostomy tube, and with gentle but firm traction pull the tube through the esophagus into the stomach. Pass the gastroscope again while pulling the tube against the anterior stomach wall. The endoscopist verifies tube position to ensure that adequate traction is applied without creating ischemia on the gastric wall (Fig. 11–4). Remove the scope and apply a bolster to the outside of the tube and suture it to the abdominal wall.

Push Technique of Sachs and Vine

This technique is identical to the method of Gauderer and Ponsky, except that a long flexible guidewire is placed into the stomach through the angiocatheter. Using the gastroscope and biopsy snare, pull the wire through the esophagus and out of the patient's mouth. Advance ("push") the gastrostomy tube over the wire by a technique similar to the Seldinger technique used to place intravascular devices. Commercially available tubes have a tapered end that facilitates tube advancement. One of the potential problems with this technique is the coiling of the guidewire and tube within the esophagus. To avoid this problem, keep the guidewire taut by gentle traction at both ends while advancing the tube over it. Just as in the Gauderer/Ponsky technique, pass the gastroscope a second time to verify tube location against the anterior stomach wall. Complete the procedure as described above (Fig. 11–5).[19]

Single Endoscopic Technique

Newer PEG tubes include markings forming a ruler along the length of the tube that indicates the distance to the end of the tube. This allows calculation of the distance between the stomach and the skin and, consequently, estimation of the degree of approximation of the stomach to the anterior abdominal wall. Although this method is not infallible, it is sufficiently accurate to avoid the passing of the gastroscope a second time to verify the position of the tube.

Grant[20] reported his results using this technique in 598 patients. The significance of the patient's illness was graded by the American Society of Anesthesiologists (ASA) scoring system (1 = no systemic disease, 5 = imminent danger of death) as assessed by the anesthesiologist on each patient. Of the 598 patients, 287 were assigned an ASA of 3 and 150 patients were assigned a score of 4, indicating a severe degree of illness in most patients. Thirty-three patients were obese, and 74 patients required general anesthesia. All these procedures were performed in the operating room in an average time of 34 minutes. Complications were noted in 29 patients: 10 cases of leakage around the tube site, 5 cases of peritonitis, 5 site infections, 3 failures of placement, 3 aspirations from the EGD, 2 episodes of bleeding at the PEG site, 1 alveolar ridge fracture, and 1 esophageal laceration. Only one patient died due to peritonitis, which resulted in a mortality rate of only 0.16 percent.

Introducer Technique of Russell

This technique differs from the standard pull and push methods in that it requires passing the gastroscope only once (only one endoscopy). The gastrostomy tube is not passed (pulled) through the mouth but instead is placed directly across the abdominal wall. This has the theoretical advantage of reducing the possibility of wound infection due to contamination with oral bacteria. Using the previously described procedure, pass the gastroscope into the stomach and identify the site of the proposed gastrostomy. Make a small skin incision and place the angiocatheter in the stomach through the abdominal wall. Pass a flexible guidewire through the catheter and, using the Seldinger method, pass a #16 F dilator with a peel-away introducer over the guidewire (Fig. 11–6). The endoscopist must verify the entrance of the dilator and introducer into the stomach. Remove the dilator. Place a well-lubricated #14 F Foley catheter through the introducer as it is peeled away. Inflate the Foley catheter balloon and secure it to the anterior abdominal wall. The endoscopist verifies adequate device position (Fig. 11–7).[21]

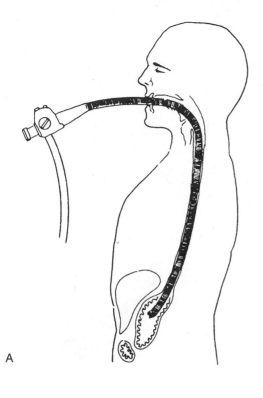

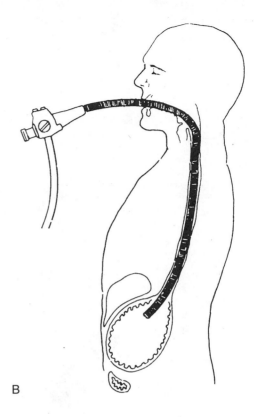

A

B

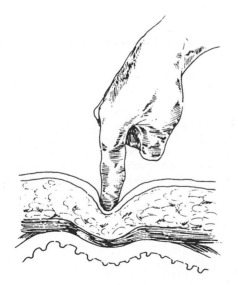

C

FIGURE 11–3 Initial steps common to all percutaneous endoscopic gastrostomy (PEG) techniques. *A,* The gastroscope is inserted into the esophagus and the stomach is intubated. *B,* Air insufflation distends the stomach to ensure opposition with the anterior abdominal wall and caudad displacement of the transverse colon. *C,* Endoscopic gastric transillumination at the proposed incision site is confirmed by digital palpation.

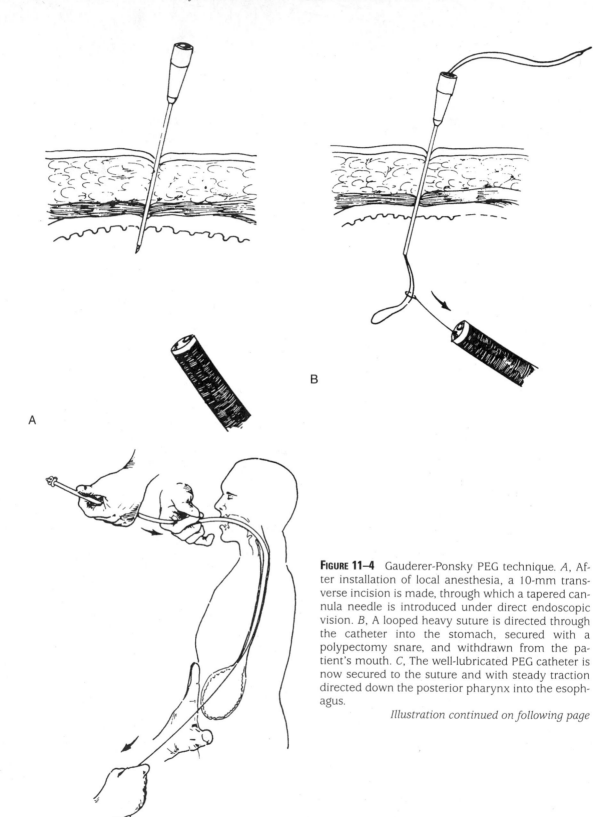

FIGURE 11–4 Gauderer-Ponsky PEG technique. *A*, After installation of local anesthesia, a 10-mm transverse incision is made, through which a tapered cannula needle is introduced under direct endoscopic vision. *B*, A looped heavy suture is directed through the catheter into the stomach, secured with a polypectomy snare, and withdrawn from the patient's mouth. *C*, The well-lubricated PEG catheter is now secured to the suture and with steady traction directed down the posterior pharynx into the esophagus.

Illustration continued on following page

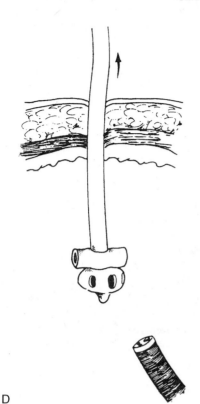

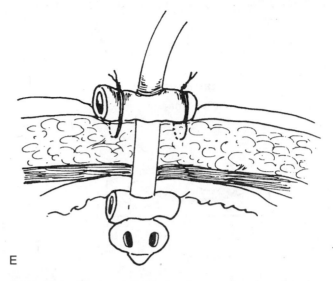

D

E

FIGURE 11–4 *Continued D*, The endoscope is reintroduced, and under direct vision the catheter is pulled across the gastroesophageal junction and then approximated to the anterior gastric wall. It is imperative that the inner crossbar gently approximate the mucosa without excess tension to avoid ischemic necrosis. The stomach is decompressed by aspiration and the gastroscope withdrawn. *E*, The outer crossbar is gently approximated to the skin level and secured with two 0-0 Prolene sutures.

The drawback of this procedure is that the permanence of the tube in the stomach depends on balloon integrity. If the ballon is deflated, intentionally or unintentionally, within the first 24 to 72 hours, the stomach will retract away from the anterior abdominal wall, and the gastrostomy becomes a perforation free in the peritoneal cavity. This then becomes a surgical emergency to prevent peritonitis. The advantage of this technique is tube replacement is done merely by deflating the balloon.

One-Step Placement of Percutaneous Endoscopic Gastrostomy Button

Another, newer type of gastrostomy tube is the low-profile or gastrostomy "button." These devices are very convenient for the young, active individual who prefers to wear tight clothing. Until recently these devices only existed for replacement of previously created gastrostomies. Usually, 3 months is allowed for proper adhesion of the stomach to the anterior abdominal wall before exchanging the gastrostomy tube. Recently, an ingenious kit has been introduced to the market that allows for the endoscopic placement of a gastrostomy button. This kit includes a trochar with stylet and a grading of distances marked on the needle. Once the trocar is introduced into the stomach,

Malencot-type wings can be opened at the end so the trochar is pulled back holding the stomach to the Malencot wings. This maneuver allows for a precise measurement of the distance between stomach and the skin and selection of the button by length. Then perform the procedure by the Gauderer-Ponsky method, using a tube with a Silastic button that has been folded and squeezed within a carrier tube. After deploying the button inside the stomach, peel the carrier tube away from the button.

Indications, Contraindications, and Complications

The indications for PEG are the same as those for standard surgical gastrostomy. The procedure is most often performed to provide enteral feeding access in the patient who is unable to eat and is not at risk for aspiration. Occasionally a PEG is performed to provide gastric decompression in patients with chronic small-bowel obstruction due to malignancy and in patients with proximal enterocutaneous fistulae.[22]

The only absolute contraindications to PEG are an inability to pass the endoscope, usually due to malignant obstruction of the pharynx or esophagus, and failure to transilluminate the abdominal wall adequately due to obesity.

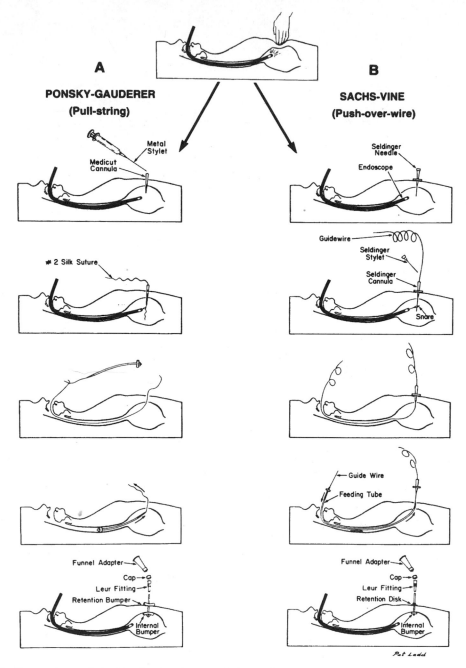

FIGURE 11–5 Comparison of the Ponsky-Gauderer and the Sachs-Vine PEG techniques. (From Hogan RB, De-Marco DC, Hamilton JK et al: Percutaneous endoscopic gastrostomy: to push or pull? Gastrointest Endosc 1986;32:253–258. With permission.)

Ascites and previous abdominal surgery at one time were considered contraindications to PEG; however, as experience with the procedure has grown, several authors have demonstrated acceptable results in these two groups of patients.[23,24] Ascites remains a relative contraindication, with the ascitic leak rate reported to be approximately 25 percent in some studies.[24] The incidence of ascitic leak is reportedly greatly reduced by preoperative paracentesis.[24]

Several large studies have demonstrated the relative ease and safety with which the PEG procedure can be performed.[22,23,25,26] Major

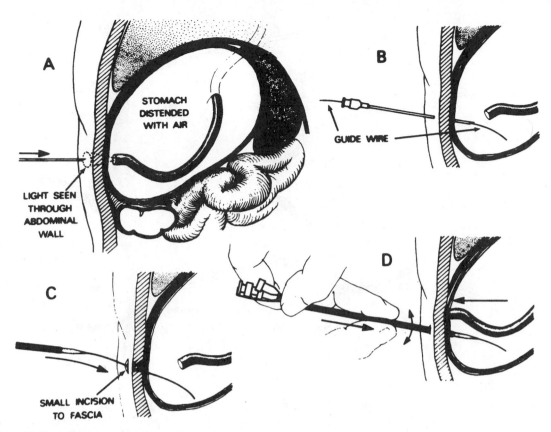

FIGURE 11–6 Russell techniques for PEG. *A*, Gastric distension with needle directed at light source. *B*, The guidewire is passed through the needle into the stomach. *C* and *D*, The introducer is passed over the wire into the stomach. (Reprinted by permission of the publisher from Russell TR, Brotman M, Norris F: Percutaneous gastrostomy: a new simplified and cost effective technique. Am J Surg 1984;142:132–137. Copyright 1984 by Excerpta Medica Inc.)

complications are rare (< 10 percent) and are often the result of aspiration, which could seemingly be minimized by proper patient selection. Extrusion of the gastrostomy is a serious complication that occurs in 1 to 11 percent of patients and is the result of excessive tightness between the inner and outer bolster that leads to pressure necrosis of the abdominal wall. Minor complications occur in 24 to 43 percent of patients[22,23,25,27] and typically include wound infections, peristomal leaks, cellulitis, and clogged tubes.

Studies comparing the PEG to open gastrostomy have demonstrated similar morbidity and mortality for patients undergoing either technique. Most studies indicate that the PEG procedures can be performed slightly faster than open gastrostomy at 50 to 75 percent of the cost.[27-29]

Comparison between the various techniques for performing PEGs has demonstrated similar safety and efficacy for all available methods. There is no clear advantage of one percuta-neous technique over another.[19,30] The advantages and disadvantages of the different methods are shown in Table 11–3.

Percutaneous Endoscopic Jejunostomy

A significant number of patients who require enteral access for feeding have substantial risk factors for aspiration and are best served by a feeding jejunostomy.[12] This fact, combined with the ease and efficacy with which percutaneous access to the stomach can be performed, has stimulated several innovative techniques for obtaining postpyloric enteral access through endoscopically assisted percutaneous methods.[25,31-36]

Two basic techniques for percutaneous endoscopic jejunostomy have been described. The most common method involves the placement of a transpyloric (postpyloric) feeding tube through a previously placed PEG using endoscopic guidance (transpyloric PEJ).[25,31-33] More recently, techniques for direct PEJ have

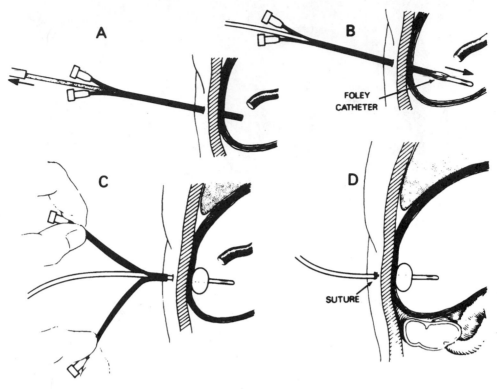

FIGURE 11–7   Russell techniques for PEG. *A,* The dilator is removed from the introducer. *B,* A Foley catheter is passed through the introducer into the stomach. *C,* The introducer is peeled away. *D,* The Foley balloon is inflated and secured against the abdominal wall. (Reprinted by permission of the publisher from Russell TR, Brotman M, Norris F: Percutaneous gastrostomy: a new simplified and cost effective technique. Am J Surg 1984; 142:132–137. Copyright 1984 by Excerpta Medica Inc..)

TABLE 11–3   Comparison of Methods for Percutaneous Endoscopic Gastrostomy

	Gauderer-Ponsky	Sachs-Vine	Russell
Passage of gastroscope	Twice	Twice	Twice
Trauma to the esophagus	+ +	+ +	+
Contamination by oral flora	Possible	Possible	Not possible
Accidental removal	Unlikely	Unlikely	Possible
Replacement	Difficult	Difficult	Easy

+ + = moderate chance of esophageal trauma; + = minimal chance of esophageal trauma.

been reported.[34-36] Both procedures will be described in the following sections.

Jejunal Access via Transpyloric PEJ

The principle underlying this technique is simple and is illustrated in Figure 11–8. Pass a small feeding tube with a heavy suture tied to the weighted tip through a previously placed gastrostomy. Then pass a gastroscope and grasp the suture with a biopsy forceps. Guide the tube as far as possible into the duodenum. Hold the biopsy forcep in place and withdraw the gastroscope alone to prevent inadvertent dislodgment of the feeding tube. Leave an excess amount of tubing within the stomach to allow peristalsis to pull the tip of the feeding tube past the ligament of Trietz.

Several studies have documented the relative ease of performing PEG with a jejunal extension as well as the short-term efficacy of the procedure.[25,31-33] Most authors report that the addition of a transpyloric PEJ to a PEG procedure only increases the procedure time from 10 to 15 minutes.[25,31-33,37]

Studies evaluating the long-term efficacy of transpyloric PEJ have not been as positive.[38,39]

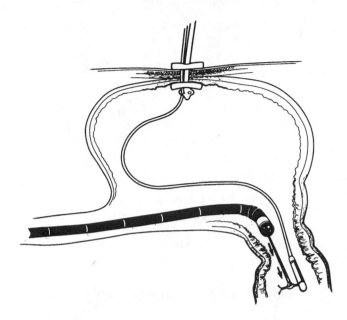

Figure 11–8 Technique for transpyloric PEJ. The endoscope guides the weighted tip of the feeding tube into the duodenum. (Reprinted by permission of the publisher from Ponsky JL, Gauderer MWL, Stellato TA et al: Percutaneous approaches to enteral nutrition. Am J Surg 1985;149:102–105. Copyright 1985 by Excerpta Medica Inc..)

Kaplan and colleagues followed 23 patients undergoing transpyloric PEJ over a 2-year period. They found that 84 percent of the tubes failed and were functional for an average of only 39.5 days. The reason for tube failures were (1) separation of the inner PEJ tube from the outer gastrostomy tubes, resulting in tube dislodgment (59 percent), (2) clogging due to small PEJ diameter (32 percent), and (3) kinking and knotting of the tube (9 percent). In addition, the authors did not demonstrate a significant decrease in the risk of aspiration pneumonia in patients fed through transpyloric PEJ. The failure of transpyloric PEJ to prevent aspiration is thought to be due to frequent retrograde migration of the tube into the stomach. The transpyloric nature of this type of enteral access also decreases the ability of the pyloric sphincter mechanisms to perform effectively, therefore pre-disposing to duodenogastric reflux and subsequent aspiration.

Direct PEJ

To avoid the mechanical and physiologic complications associated with transpyloric PEJ, methods for direct PEJ have recently been described by several authors.[34-36] These techniques all require advancement of an endoscope into the lumen of the small bowel to direct placement of the feeding tube. Initial reports of direct PEJ procedures were confined to patients who had undergone previous partial gastrectomies with Billroth II reconstruction and had had previous jejunostomies. Success with such procedures led to the development of

direct PEJ procedures for patients with intact foreguts. This section will present the available techniques for direct PEJ.

Direct PEJ After Gastrojejunostomy and Feeding Jejunostomy. In the patient who has had a previous Billroth II procedure with a concomitant feeding jejunostomy, pass an endoscope through the gastric remnant into the jejunum. Identify the site of the previous jejunostomy and transilluminate the abdominal wall. Cannulate the jejunum percutaneously with a peel-away plastic sheath using a Seldinger technique. Maintain endoscopic visualization continually. Place a #12 F feeding catheter through the sheath and, using the endoscope, advance it distally into the small intestine. After removing the sheath, confirm catheter position by contrast study (Fig. 11–9).[36]

Direct PEJ Without Previous Jejunostomy. Direct PEJ in patients without previous jejunostomy with and without intact foreguts has been described by Adams[34] and by Shike and colleagues.[35] Pass a 160-cm colonoscope into the jejunum approximately 20 cm distal to the ligament of Trietz. Transilluminate the abdominal wall, marking the site of opposition of the small bowel to the abdominal wall. After this point in the procedure, two alternate techniques have been described. The first method is a modification of the Gauderer-Ponsky PEG procedure. Under endoscopic visualization, cannulate the jejunum with a small-gauge needle. Once the intraluminal portion of the needle is confirmed, pass a heavy thread through the nee-

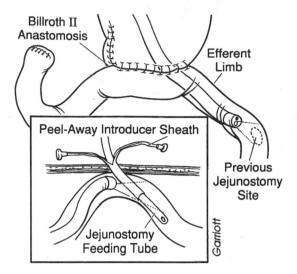

FIGURE 11–9   Technique for direct PEJ after Billroth II. The site of the previous jejunostomy is visualized. Inset: The jejunum is cannulated over a wire. A feeding tube is placed through a peel-away introducer. (From Pritchard TJ, Bloom AD: A technique of direct percutaneous jejunostomy tube placement. Surg Gynecol Obstet 1994;178:173–174. By permission of Surgery, Gynecology & Obstetrics, now known as the Journal of the American College of Surgeons.)

dle, grasp it with biopsy forceps, and withdraw it through the mouth. Tie the thread to a mushroom-tipped feeding tube and pull it into position under endoscopic guidance.[35]

An alternative approach requires a 3- to 4-cm incision in the left upper quadrant. Endoscopic intubation of the proximal jejunum is evident by transillumination of the intestines and palpation of the endoscope. Grasp the proximal end of the jejunum with a Babcock clamp, and eviscerate a short segment of small bowel (10 to 15 cm) into the operative field. Place the feeding tube using a Witzel technique. After placing the feeding tube, return the jejunum to the abdominal cavity, fixing the proximal and distal ends of the jejunum to the abdominal wall (Fig. 11–10).[34]

The techniques for direct PEJ appear to address the problems associated with transpyloric PEJ (tube migration, clogging, and aspiration); however, experience with these endoscopically demanding procedures is limited, and the final evaluation of their usefulness awaits further investigation.

LAPAROSCOPIC TECHNIQUES

The recent introduction of high-resolution video cameras to the established techniques of laparoscopy has ushered in an era of minimally invasive surgery.[40] A dramatic reduction in postoperative pain and recovery time coupled with excellent cosmetic results has led to the rapid development of many new and innovative procedures employing laparoscopy. Several techniques for obtaining enteral feeding access by laparoscopic means have recently been described.[41-48] Experiences with these new procedures is limited, and indications for their use continue to evolve. It appears that these techniques are best suited for patients who cannot undergo endoscopically assisted procedures but who would be best served by a minimally invasive approach. Presented in this section are several techniques for performing both laparoscopic gastrostomies and jejunostomies.

LAPAROSCOPIC GASTROSTOMIES

Laparoscopic gastrostomy is indicated when gastric enteral access is required and PEG cannot be performed. This may be particularly true when the patient is obese and a large incision would be required to perform a safe surgical gastrostomy. The most straightforward approach to laparoscopic gastrostomy is a modification of the Russell introducer technique for PEG placement.[41,42]

Create pneumoperitoneum in the usual manner through a Verres needle inserted through a small supraumbilical incision. Place the camera port through this incision and place a 5-mm port in the epigastrum. Grasp the stomach with an atraumatic instrument and identify the site of the proposed gastrostomy in the left upper quadrant. Place a 7-cm 18-gauge angiocatheter through the anterior abdominal wall into the stomach at the site chosen for the gastrostomy. Remove the needle and pass a soft J-wire through the catheter into the stomach. Pass a #12 F dilator followed by a #14 F dilator into the stomach. Then pass a #16 F peel-away catheter over a dilator into the stomach. Place a #16 F Foley catheter through the sheath as it is peeled away. Inflate the balloon and secure it snugly to the anterior abdominal wall. This procedure may be performed using either local or general anesthesia.

A modification of this technique using T-fasteners to secure the stomach more effectively to the anterior abdominal wall has been described by Duh and Way (Fig. 11–11).[43]

Laparoscopic Jejunostomy

Several methods for performing laparoscopic feeding jejunostomy have been described.[44-49]

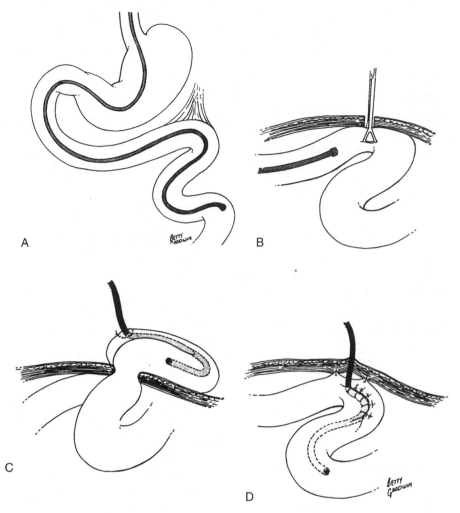

FIGURE 11–10 A technique for direct PEJ. *A*, A colonscope is passed beyond the ligament of Trietz to identify the site of the jejunostomy. *B*, The site of the jejunostomy is identified by transillumination. A small incision is made and the jejunum is grasped with a Babcock clamp. *C*, A small amount of jejunum is moved into the operative field, and a Witzel jejunostomy is performed. *D*, The jejunum is sutured to the anterior abdominal wall and to the skin. (From Adams DB: Feeding jejunostomy with endoscopic guidance. Surg Gynecol Obstet 1991;172:239–241. By permission of Surgery, Gynecology & Obstetrics, now known as the Journal of the American College of Surgeons.)

The indication for these procedures is currently evolving; however, laparoscopic jejunostomies may represent a minimally invasive alternative to PEJ techniques. Further experiences with both PEJ and laparoscopic jejunostomy are needed to determine their usefulness for providing safe, effective, and reliable postpyloric feeding access. The principal advantage of the minimally invasive laparoscopic approaches is a reduction in postoperative pain and rehabilitation time while achieving optional cosmetic results. Other theoretical advantages include reduction in wound infection rates and subsequent incisional herniation, as well as contact between the surgeon and the patient's blood.[50]

The cost of the procedures remains a drawback. In one recent study[47] comparing the cost of various forms of postpyloric feeding access, the laparoscopic jejunostomy was found to be almost three times more expensive than PEJ and two times more expensive than standard surgical jejunostomy. Two techniques for performing laparoscopically guided feeding jejunostomies will be presented in this section. The first technique was developed by J.B. Morris and involves extracorporeal placement of the feeding tube.[44] The second method is a jejunal modification of the T-fastener techniques previously described for laparoscopic gastrostomy.[45]

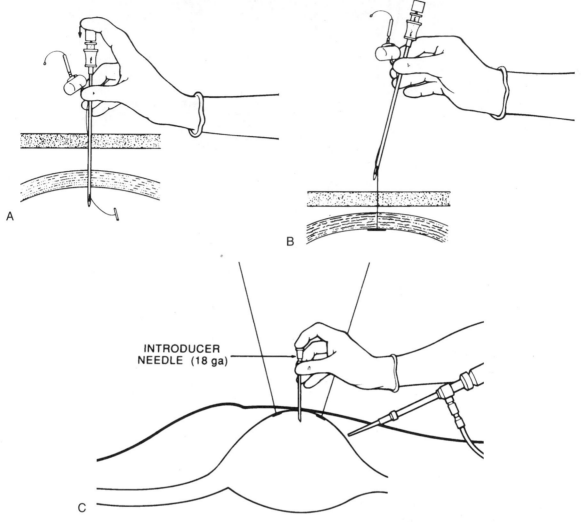

INTRODUCER
NEEDLE (18 ga)

FIGURE 11–11 T-fastener technique of laparoscopic gastrostomy. *A*, The metal T-bar with attached nylon suture is introduced through a slotted needle through the abdominal and stomach walls under laparoscopic guidance. The T-bar is dislodged inside the stomach lumen by the stylet. *B*, The stomach wall is approximated to the abdominal wall by traction on the suture. *C*, A wire is passed through an 18 gauge needle into the stomach, and the procedure is completed using a Russell PEG technique. (From Duh QY, Way LW: Laparoscopic gastrostomy using T-fasteners as retractors and anchors. Surg Endosc 1993;7:60–63. With permission.)

Laparoscopic Jejunostomy and the Extracorporeal Tube Placement

After general endotracheal anesthesia is induced, establish pneumoperitoneum using a Verres needle placed through a small incision just above the umbilicus. Insert a 12-mm trocar and introduce the laparoscope. Under laparoscopic guidance, place an accessory 10-mm trocar in the left anterior axillary line approximately 5 cm above the anterior superior iliac spine. Move the operating camera to the accessory port, inspect the abdomen, and identify the ligament of Treitz. Grasp the jejunum on the antimesenteric border at a point 25 cm distal to the ligament of Treitz and withdraw it through the umbilical wound, incising the fascial edges slightly if necessary. Introduce a #12 F straight red rubber catheter through an enterotomy within two concentric silk pursestring sutures, or use a Witzel tunnel. Secure the bowel to the fascial edge around the tube with four seromuscular 3-0 silk sutures and then return it to the abdominal cavity. Close the fascia and skin in a standard fashion and reestablish pneumoperitoneum. Under direct vision, distend the bowel with saline injected through the catheter to confirm the absence of leak and aboral tube positioning. The red rubber catheter is tunneled subcutaneously and brought externally through the lateral trocar site (Fig. 11–12).[44]

Laparoscopic Jejunostomy with T-Fasteners

This technique for laparoscopic jejunostomy employs so-called T-fasteners to anchor and retract the jejunum. The initial part of the procedure is similar to that described for the previous laparoscopic jejunostomy technique. Once the approximate area of jejunum is identified, grasp and hold it while passing a special slotted needle (commercially available) with previous-load T-fasteners through the abdominal wall into the jejunal lumen. Remove the needle, leaving the T-fasteners within the lumen. Repeat this maneuver three times so that four fasteners are arranged in a 3-cm diameter circle that is used to draw the bowel close to the anterior abdominal wall. After placing the four fasteners, position the jejunostomy tube using an introducer method similar to the Russell PEG technique. After tube placement, draw the T-fasteners taut against the abdominal wall with enough tension to oppose the jejunum to the posterior rectus sheath (Fig. 11–13).[45]

RADIOLOGICALLY ASSISTED TECHNIQUES

Recent advances in the field of interventional radiology have led to the development of methods for percutaneous radiologically assisted gastrostomies and jejunostomies. These techniques are seldom considered a first-line approach for enteral access, but they do provide attractive alternatives for patients for whom surgery is a prohibitive risk and in whom endoscopic procedures are impossible for anatomic reasons.

Percutaneous Radiologically Assisted Gastrostomy

An option for achieving access to the stomach using fluoroscopy has been described by Willis and Oglesby.[51] Before the procedure, obtain an ultrasound of the left upper quadrant to evaluate the relationship of the left lobe of the liver to the stomach. This ensures that the gastrostomy will not pass through the liver before entering the stomach. Place the patient supine and distend the stomach with insufflation of air through a nasogastric tube.

Determine stomach and transverse colon position through fluoroscopy. Determine the distance from the anterior stomach wall to the abdominal wall with a cross-table view. After placing local anesthesia and under fluoroscopic guidance, insert a long 18-gauge needle with a Teflon sheath to the desired depth and remove the needle. Verify intragastric location by injecting water-soluble contrast. Pass a guidewire and dilate the tract using progressively larger dilators until a #10 to 12 F pigtail catheter can be passed. Secure the catheter to the skin. The pigtail catheter prevents inadvertent removal.

Percutaneous Radiologically Assisted Jejunostomy

Techniques similar to those described for radiologically assisted access to the stomach have been described for the jejunum.[52] Experience with these techniques is limited, but they may provide a viable option for patients who cannot undergo surgery.

Achieve radiologically assisted percutaneous access to the stomach as described previously. Pass a guidewire through the duodenum into the proximal jejunum. Pass a #8 F balloon occluder catheter over a wire into the jejunum, and inflate the balloon with 30 ml of air and 10 ml of water-soluble contrast. Confirm the balloon's intrajejunal location and position adjacent to the abdominal wall by fluoroscopy. In thin patients, the balloon may also be palpated. Under fluoroscopic guidance, pass an 18-gauge needle into the jejunum. Confirm successful jejunal puncture by both palpable and fluoroscopic evidence of balloon puncture. Pass a guidewire and dilate the tract to approximately a #10 F. Place a pigtail catheter with or without an introducer. Remove the balloon occluder catheter and secure the feeding catheter to the skin.

SUMMARY

PEG and PEJ are quick, cost-effective, and well-tested techniques for obtaining enteral feeding access to the upper GI tract. The more recently developed laparoscopic and direct percutaneous jejunostomy procedures have been successful when applied by a select group of physicians. More widespread application of these approaches awaits trials that will more fully evaluate the safety, efficacy, patient satisfaction, and cost effectiveness of these new procedures.

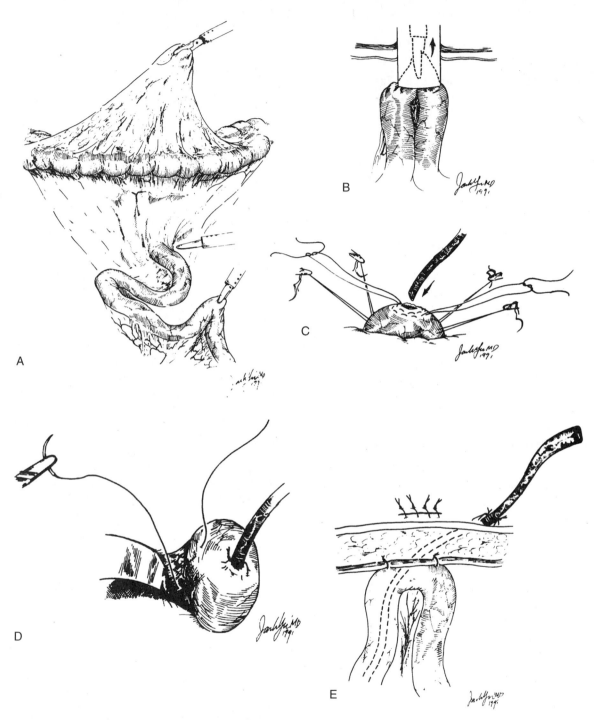

FIGURE 11–12 Laparoscopic jejunostomy. *A*, The proximal bowel is traced 25 cm distal to the ligament of Trietz. *B*, The bowel is grasped at its antimesenteric border and withdrawn into the umbilical port. *C*, The feeding tube is placed through two pursestring sutures. *D* and *E*, The bowel is secured to the fascial edges and brought out through the abdominal wall. (From Morris JB, Mullen JL, Yu JC et al: Laparoscopic-guided jejunostomy. Surgery 1992;112:96–99. With permission.)

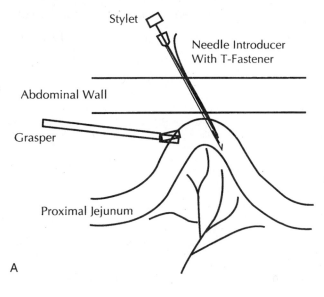

Stylet

Needle Introducer With T-Fastener

Abdominal Wall

Grasper

Proximal Jejunum

A

FIGURE 11–13 Laparoscopic jejunostomy with T-fasteners. *A*, The jejunum is grasped and stabilized. The T-fastener is inserted through a needle. *B*, Four T-fasteners are placed and used to retract the bowel against the abdominal wall. *C*, A guidewire is passed into the jejunum, and the feeding tube is placed using a Russell PEG technique. (From Duh QY, Way LW: Laparoscopic jejunostomy using T-fasteners as retractors and anchors. Arch Surg 1993;128:105–108. Copyright 1993, American Medical Association.)

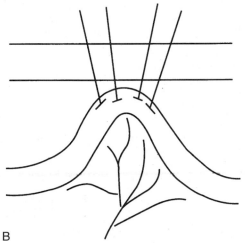

B

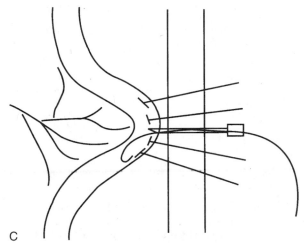

C

REFERENCES

1. Randall HT: Enteral nutrition: tube feedings in acute and chronic illness. J Parenter Enter Nutr 1984;8: 113–136.
2. Brown-Seguard CE: Feedings per rectum in nervous affections. Lancet 1978;1:144.
3. Stengel A, Ravdin IS: Maintenance of nutrition in surgical patients with description of an orojejunal method of feeding. Surgery 1939;6:511–519.
4. Andersen AFR: Immediate jejunal feedings after gastroenterostomy. Ann Surg 1918;67:565–566.
5. Gauderer MW, Stellato TA: Gastrostomies: evolution, techniques, indications and complications. Curr Prob Surg 1986;23:661–719.
6. Egeberg CA: Christianana med gessellsch. Om behandlingen af impenetrable strecturer: madroevect. Norsk Mag Laegevidensk 1841;2:97–105.
7. Sedillot O: DeLaGastrostomie fistulenge. Compt Mend Acad Sci 1846;23:222–230.
8. Jones S: Gastrostomy for stricture of the esophagus; death from bronchitis forty days after operation. Lancet 1875;1:678–681.
9. Gauderer MW, Ponsky JL, Izant RJ: Gastrostomy without laparostomy: a percutaneous endoscopic technique. J Pediatr Surg 1980;15:872–875.
10. Torosian MH, Rombeau JL: Feeding tube enterostomy. Surg Gynecol Obstet 1980;150:918–927.
11. Bowles T, Zollinger RM: Critical evaluation of jejunostomy. Arch Surg 1952;65:358–366.
12. Weltz CR, Morris JB, Mullen JL: Surgical jejunostomy in aspiration risk patients. Ann Surg 1992;215:140–145.
13. Ryan JA, Page CP: Intrajejunal feeding: development and current status. J Parenter Enter Nutr 1984;8: 187–198.
14. Steinberg EP, Andersons GF: Implication of Medicare's prospective payment system for special nutrition services. Nutr Clin Pract 1986;1:12–28.
15. Eastwood GL: Small bowel morphology and epithelial proliferation in intravenously alimented rabbits. Surgery 1977;82:612–620.
16. Sonies BC, Baum BJ: Evaluation of swallowing pathology. Otolaryngol Clin North Am 1988;21:637–648.
17. Nance ML, Morris JB: Enteral nutritional support: techniques and common complications. Hosp Phys 1992;28:24–29.

18. Jain NK, Larson DE, Shroeder KW et al: Does antibiotic prophylaxis reduce peristomal shunt infections after percutaneous endoscopic gastrostomy: a prospective randomized clinical trial. Gastrointest Endosc 1986; 32:139–145.

19. Hogan RB, DeMarco DC, Hamilton JK et al: Percutaneous endoscopic gastrostomy: to push or pull? Gastrointest Endosc 1986;32:253–258.

20. Grant JP: Percutaneous endoscopic gastrostomy. Ann Surg 1993;217:168–174.

21. Russell TR, Brotman M, Norris F: Percutaneous gastrostomy: a new simplified and cost effective technique. Am J Surg 1984;142:132–137.

22. Stellato TA, Gauderer MWL: Percutaneous endoscopic gastrostomy for gastrointestinal decompression. Ann Surg 1987;205:115–126.

23. Stellato TA, Gauderer MWL, Ponsky JL: Percutaneous endoscopic gastrostomy following previous abdominal surgery. Ann Surg 1984;200:46–51.

24. Lee MJ, Saini S, Brink JA et al: Malignant small bowel obstruction and ascites: not a contraindication to percutaneous endoscopic gastrostomy. Clin Radiol 1991; 44:332–374.

25. Ponksy JL, Gauderer MWL, Stellato TA et al: Percutaneous approaches to enteral nutrition. Am J Surg 1985;149:102–105.

26. Miller RE, Kummer BA, Kotler DP et al: Percutaneous endoscopic gastrostomy: procedure of choice. Ann Surg 1986;204:543–547.

27. Kirby DE, Craig RM, Tsang TK et al: Percutaneous endoscopic gastrostomy: a prospective evaluation and review of the literature. J Parenter Enter Nutr 1986;10: 155–159.

28. Tanker MS, Scheinfeldt BD, Steerman PH et al: A prospective randomized study comparing surgical gastrostomy and percutaneous endoscopic gastrostomy. Gastrointest Endosc 1986;32:144–148.

29. Stiegmann G, Goff J, VanWay C et al: Operative versus endoscopic gastrostomy preliminary results of a prospective randomized trial. Am J Surg 1988;155: 89–92.

30. Kozarek RA, Ball TJ, Ryan RJ: When push comes to shove: a comparison between two methods of percutaneous endoscopic gastrostomy. Am J Gastroenterol 1986;81:642–647.

31. Ponsky JL, Agzodi A: Percutaneous endoscopic jejunostomy. Am J Gastroenterol 1984;79:113–116.

32. McFadyen BV, Catalno MF, Raijman I et al: Percutaneous gastrostomy with jejunal extension: a new technique. Am J Gastroenterol 1992;87:725–728.

33. Bumpers HL, Luchette CA, Doerr RJ et al: A simple technique for insertion of PEJ via PEG. Surg Endosc 1994;8:121–123.

34. Adams DB: Feeding Jejunostomy with endoscopic guidance. Surg Gynecol Obstet 1991;172:239–241.

35. Shike M, Wallach C, Likier H: Direct percutaneous jejunostomies. Gastrointest Endosc 1991;37:62–65.

36. Pritchard TJ, Bloom AD: A technique of direct percutaneous jejunostomy tube placement. Surg Gynecol Obstet 1994;178:173–174.

37. Patterson DJ, Kozavek RA, Ball TJ et al: Comparison of percutaneous endoscopic gastrostomy alone versus PEG with jejunal extension. Gstrointest Endosc 1987; 33:176.

38. Kaplan DS, Murthy UK, Linscheer WH: Percutaneous endoscopic jejunostomy: long-term follow-up of 23 patients. Gastrointest Endosc 1989;35:403–406.

39. Disario JA, Foutch PG, Sanowski PA: Poor results with percutaneous endoscopic jejunostomy. Gastrointest Endosc 1990;36:257–260.

40. Dent TL, Ponsky JL, Berci G: Minimal access general surgery: the dawn of a new era. Am J Surg 1991;161: 323–326.

41. Edelman DS, Unger SW: Laparoscopic gastrostomy. Surg Gynecol Obstet 1991;173:410.

42. Edelman DS, Unber SW, Russin DR: Laparoscopic gastrostomy. Surg Lapar Endosc 1991;1:251–253.

43. Duh QY, Way LW: Laparoscopic gastrostomy using T-fasteners as retraction and anchors. Surg Endosc 1993;7:60–63.

44. Morris JB, Mullen JL, Yu JC et al: Laparoscopic-guided jejunostomy. Surgery 1992;112:96–99.

45. Duh QY, Way LW: Laparoscopic jejunostomy using T-fasteners as retractors and anchors. Arch Surg 1993; 128:105–108.

46. Reed DN: Percutaneous peritonendoscopic jejunostomy. Surg Gynecol Obstet 1992;174:527–529.

47. Sangster W, Swanstrom L: Laparoscopic-guided feeding jejunostomy. Surg Endosc 1993;7:308–310.

48. O'Regan PJ, Scarrow GD: Laparoscopic jejunostomy endoscopy 1990;22:39–40.

49. Eltringham WK, Roe AM, Galloway SW et al: A laparoscopic technique for full thickness intestinal biopsy and feeding jejunostomy. Gut 1993;34:122–124.

50. Cuschieria A: Minimal access surgery and the future of interventional laparoscopy. Am J Surg 1991;161: 404–407.

51. Willis JS, Oglesby DF: Percutaneous gastrostomy. Radiology 1987;149:449–453.

52. Rosenblum J, Taylor FC, Lu CT et al: A new technique for direct percutaneous jejunostomy tube placement. Am J Gastroenterol 1990;85:1165–1167.

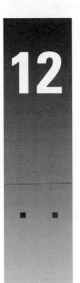

12

Radiologic Techniques for Enteral Access

SCOTT CRAIG GOODWIN
STAN LIU

Enteral access was originally achieved either transorally, transnasally, or surgically without fluoroscopic assistance. The earliest role for the radiologist was to assess the patient's anatomy prior to a procedure or to assess the locations of tubes that had been placed at the bedside or in the operating room.[1]

Investigators began describing fluoroscopically-guided transoral and transnasal enteric intubations as early as the 1930s. In the subsequent decades, fluoroscopically-guided percutaneous gastrostomy, gastrojejunostomy, and jejunostomy were developed and refined. The details of these developments are provided in the relevant subsections of this chapter.

TRANSNASAL AND TRANSORAL INTUBATION

Duodenal intubation under fluoroscopy using a standard duodenal tube and a stiffening wire was first described in 1933.[2] In 1967, rapid transnasal duodenal intubation using fluoroscopic control and a directable stylet was introduced by Gianturco.[3] In that same year, Hanafee and Weiner used a Muller handle, a deflecting piloguide wire, and a Dacron catheter to achieve intestinal intubation.[4] A flexible guiding wire to assist in the placement of duodenal tubes under fluoroscopic control to perform hy-

potonic duodenography was also developed in 1967.[5] Two years later, Cantor tube insertion under fluoroscopic control using a stiffening teflon-coated guidewire was described.[6] The use of a heavy angiographic guidewire and a Cantor-type single lumen tube for the rapid placement of enteric tubes appeared in the literature in 1978.[7] Multiple fluoroscopic techniques have subsequently been described and an assortment of tubes has been developed.[8-14]

Nasogastric Tube Placement

Informed consent should be obtained before the placement because intubation injuries are common.[15-19] In one study, 60 percent of patients had an esophageal or hypopharyngeal injury although only 2 percent were clinically apparent.[15] Other problems include tube malpositioning, aspiration, bowel perforation, and cardiac arrest, respiratory arrest, or both. Fortunately, the major complication rate is low. In one study, the major complication rate in 882 feeding tube placements was 0.4 percent.[10]

Anxiolysis and analgesia, although not necessary, will make the procedure more comfortable for the patient. We start with 1 mg of midazolam and 25 µg of fentanyl. These drugs, if not well tolerated, are fairly short-acting and are easily reversible. Additional doses can be given as necessary during the procedure. Local anesthesia is obtained in the pharynx with Cetacaine spray. It is also more comfortable for the patient if Xylocaine 2 % Jelly is introduced into the nares that will be used. Prior to placement, the nose should be examined to evaluate for deviated septum. The tube should be placed on the side which has the larger channel.

For placement, if possible, it is most helpful if the patient is in a sitting position with the neck flexed. The patient should be instructed to swallow the tube once he or she feels the tube in the back of the throat. This can best be achieved with small amounts of water sipped through a straw while the tube is being placed. Once the tube has passed into the proximal esophagus, the patient can then be placed in the supine position and fluoroscopy performed for final gastric intubation. In patients with esophageal anatomic abnormalities, it may be necessary to use an angiographic selective catheter such as a 5-F Glidecath with an angled taper shape, (manufactured by Terumo, Tokyo, Japan, distributed by Medi-tech, Boston Scientific, Watertown, MA) and a selective steerable wire such as the 0.035 in Glidewire (Medi-tech) (Fig. 12–1). Once the obstruction has been crossed using standard angiographic techniques and the catheter has been introduced into the stomach, an exchange wire can be placed and the final tube placed over the exchange wire. Because there is frequently a large amount of friction between the standard tubes and the guidewire, it is useful to use a hydrophilic exchange wire such as the Glidewire.

Some patients may not tolerate a large amount of manipulation through the nose; in these patients, the initial intubation can be performed transorally in the same fashion as described. Once intubation of the stomach, duodenum, or jejunum has been achieved, an exchange wire can be placed. Following this, an angiographic catheter is introduced through the nose and brought out through the mouth. The back end of the wire is then fed through the angiographic catheter and brought out through the nose. The catheter and wire are then pulled as a unit, straightening out the loop within the mouth (Fig. 12–2). The final tube can then be passed over this wire to the appropriate location. Thus, the amount of manipulation within the nose itself is kept to a minimum.

On occasion, it may be useful to elucidate the anatomy by injecting contrast. Although it is relatively expensive, nonionic contrast has the advantage of being relatively harmless both within the lungs and the mediastinum. In pa-

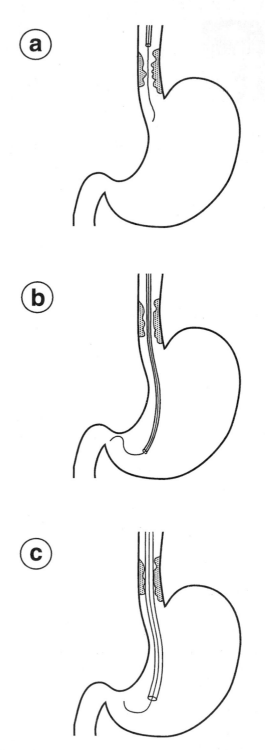

FIGURE 12–1 Nasoenteric tube placement in patients with esophageal stenosis. *A,* The stenosis is crossed with a selective guidewire. *B,* The selective catheter is advanced through the stenosis over the selective guidewire. *C,* The selective guidewire is removed. An exchange wire is placed. The selective catheter is removed. A nasogastric tube is then placed over the exchange wire and the exchange wire removed.

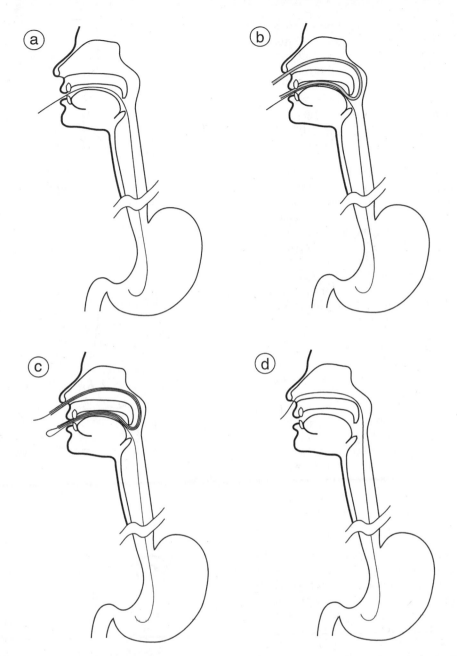

FIGURE 12–2 Conversion of orogastric tube to nasogastric tube. *A,* A transoral gastric exchange wire is placed. *B,* A selective catheter is brought through the nose into the pharynx and then out through the mouth. *C,* The back end of the exchange wire is placed through the leading end of the catheter and advanced all the way through the catheter. *D,* The wire and catheter are pulled as a unit until the loop is pulled out, and the catheter is removed. Subsequent catheters can then be placed transnasally over the wire.

tients with esophageal obstructing lesions, the risk of aspiration and perforation is present.

Duodenal and Jejunal Intubation

Many investigators have described duodenal and jejunal intubation using nasoenteric tubes and stiffening guidewires.[3-10,12,13] Following nasogastric intubation as described above, the tube is advanced into the distal antrum. The stiffening wire or stylet is placed at or near the end of the tube. The tube-wire/stylet assembly is then advanced, or the tube is fed off the wire or stylet, through the pylorus into the small bowel. This maneuver is facilitated by having the patient in the right lateral decubitus position. In some patients, the opposite position (left lateral decubitus) may help straighten out the pylorus. The tube-wire/stylet assembly can then be advanced, or the wire or stylet can then be readvanced, if it is not at the end of the tube, and the tube again fed off the wire or stylet to achieve distal duodenal or proximal jejunal intubation.

In many cases, instead of primary placement of nasoenteric tubes, we prefer the initial placement of an angiographic catheter followed by an exchange wire over which the nasoenteric catheter is placed. Nasogastric or orogastric intubation is achieved with a 5-F angled taper Glidecath as described above. The catheter is then advanced so that the tip lies within the antrum. At this point, the catheter tip should be directed superiorly and slightly posteriorly and the area of the pylorus probed with a selective guidewire such as the 0.035 in angled Glidewire. Once the pylorus is crossed with the wire, the catheter is advanced over the wire (Fig. 12–3). After the catheter and guidewire system has been placed in the duodenum, the tip of the guidewire and catheter will frequently engage the recesses of the valvulae. In some cases, the guidewire and catheter combination can be advanced by twirling the guidewire as it is being pushed forward and then following the guidewire with the catheter. In other cases, when the tip of the guidewire engages the recess of one of the valvulae, the wire can simply be buckled over and advanced as a large J wire through the bowel (Fig. 12–4). Usually this J wire configuration will hang up at areas of sharp angulation such as at the junction of the second and third parts of the duodenum and also at the ligament of Treitz. At these locations, the catheter tip should be advanced to the area of angulation and then the tip turned toward the direction of the outgoing bowel loop. The wire can then be advanced out of the turn into the subsequent bowel loop. Next the catheter is pushed over the wire until the desired location has been reached (Fig. 12–5). The wire is then exchanged for an exchange wire (preferably a hydrophilic wire such as the Glidewire). Last, the final feeding tube is passed over the exchange wire. In some patients, the valvulae may be particularly troublesome and it may be useful to exchange the selective wire for a J wire. The J wire will usually pass along the surface of the valvulae without entering one of the intervening recesses. However, J wires, as mentioned above, will frequently get hung up in ar-

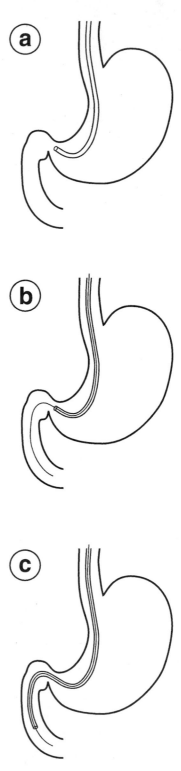

FIGURE 12–3 Crossing the pylorus. *A,* The selective catheter tip is brought to the antrum and the tip is directed superiorly and slightly posteriorly. *B,* The selective guidewire is then maneuvered through the pylorus into the duodenum. *C,* The selective catheter is advanced over the wire into the duodenum.

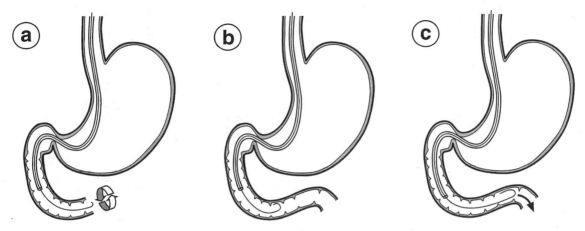

FIGURE 12–4 Advancing the catheter and wire through the small bowel. *A*, The selective wire can be advanced by twirling the wire, followed by advancement of the catheter. *B*, The tip of the wire can be engaged in the recess of one of the valvulae and a **J** wire configuration formed. *C*, The wire is then advanced with the **J** wire configuration followed by the catheter.

eas of sharp angulation and it may be necessary at these locations to exchange back to the steerable guidewire.

Many feeding tubes have weighted ends and do not have an end hole at the end of the catheter. In many cases, the wire can be placed successfully through the most distal side hole. In these cases, the catheter will buckle over on itself with the side hole serving as the apex of the buckle. These buckles in the catheter can typically be straightened out using a push-pull motion on the catheter. If this is not successful, the weight can be cut off and the catheter introduced over the wire using the end hole that has been created. However, if the weight is removed, the catheter tip is more likely to recoil into the stomach over time.

In patients with very large stomachs, the techniques described above may not work. The catheter coils in the stomach, resulting in very little control of the tip of the catheter. This lack of control, in combination with the relative size of the stomach compared to the size of the pylorus, makes cannulation of the pylorus very difficult. In these cases, it may be useful to use a stiffer selective catheter. This can be achieved by using a larger French-size catheter. It also may be useful to use the oral approach and to introduce a long stiff sheath such as those available from Cook, Incorporated (Bloomington, IN).

Jejunal Intubation in Patients with Gastrojejunostomies

From a nasal or oral starting point, it is usually easier to enter a gastrojejunostomy along the greater curvature of the stomach than it is to enter the pylorus, unless there is a stricture. If previous studies are available, they should be reviewed to understand the location of the anastomosis. The area of the anastomosis can be identified by injecting a small amount of contrast. The anastomosis is then probed with the angiographic catheter–guidewire combination until the gastrojejunostomy is crossed. Once having entered the bowel, it is important to pull out the guidewire and inject a small amount of contrast to ensure that the catheter is within the efferent loop. Inasmuch as the afferent and efferent loops are often projected over each other in the anteroposterior projection, it may be useful to use an oblique projection to separate these loops under fluoroscopy. Once the position has been secured in the jejunum, the same exchange technique as described above is used to place the final nasoenteric tube.

PERCUTANEOUS GASTROSTOMY AND GASTROJEJUNOSTOMY TUBE PLACEMENT

The percutaneous reestablishment of feeding gastrostomies in patients who had previously undergone surgical gastropexy was introduced by Sacks and Glotzer in 1979.[20] In 1980, Gauderer and colleagues introduced percutaneous endoscopic gastrostomy tube placement.[21] Preshaw went on to describe a percutaneous method for inserting gastrostomy tubes without endoscopic assistance using a one-step technique with a Stamey percuta-

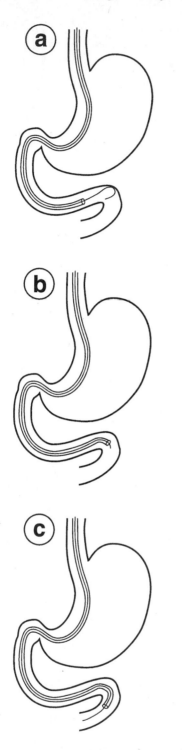

FIGURE 12–5 Advancing through the small bowel at points of acute angulation. *A*, The wire is looped back at the ligament of Treitz and will not advance. *B*, The wire is pulled back and the catheter is advanced with the tip directed toward the outgoing loop. *C*, The wire is then advanced followed by the catheter.

neous cystostomy catheter in 1981.[22] Jejunal intubation through a gastrostomy tube without fluoroscopic assistance was introduced in 1942.[23] In 1982, transgastrostomy jejunal intubation under fluoroscopic control appeared in the literature.[24] In 1983, several investigators described placement of percutaneous gastrostomy tubes using the Seldinger technique.[25-27] Finally, in 1987, direct percutaneous jejunostomy was introduced.[28]

Gastrostomy Tube Placement

The advantages of percutaneous gastrostomy tube placement include (1) the ability to place tubes in the presence of esophageal or pharyngeal obstruction; (2) the relative ease of catheter exchanges; (3) the preprocedural establishment of the location of the colon, the liver, ascites, and tumor; and (4) decreased morbidity when compared with surgical gastrostomy.[29]

Prior to the procedure, patients should be assessed for a variety of contraindications. Patients with large varices, sepsis, left upper quadrant burns, or malignant or infectious disease involving the left upper quadrant, anterior abdominal wall, or the anterior wall of the stomach should be excluded. Some investigators will also exclude patients with massive ascites. However, Lee and coworkers have described the safe use of percutaneous gastrostomy in patients with massive ascites who underwent paracentesis before the procedure.[30] Patients who are at risk for aspiration should not have a gastrostomy tube. These patients include those with gastric outlet obstruction, atonic stomachs, gastroesophageal reflux, and a known history of aspiration. Patients who aspirate may be candidates for gastrojejunostomy, which is discussed below. Laboratory tests given before the procedure, at a minimum, should include hematocrit, platelets, prothrombin time and partial thromboplastin time. Coagulopathy must be corrected before the procedure. Candidates for gastrostomy tube placement should then be evaluated for location of the left lobe of the liver and also for the location of the transverse colon. The relationship of the stomach to the left lobe of the liver can be established either with ultrasound or with computed tomography.[31] A spot below the margin of the left lobe is marked for the puncture site. The transverse colon is positively identified during the puncture process. If air within the colon is inadequate for visualization, contrast can be given orally the night before or can be given at the time of the procedure from below—either per rectum or through an ostomy. Before the procedure, informed consent is obtained. The patient is advised of the risks, which include transcolonic placement,[32] aspiration, peritoneal dislodgement of the catheter, peritonitis, sepsis, and hemorrhage. Fortunately, these complications are unusual.[29,33-36]

Adult patients are kept nil per os (NPO) past midnight. Pediatric patients can be held NPO for as little as 4 hours. Conscious sedation is used. Intravenous midazolam and fentanyl are good choices. Usually a one-time dose of a first generation cephalosporin is also given. Also, if peristalsis is a problem, 1 mg of glucagon can be administered intravenously.

The left upper quadrant is prepped and draped in the usual fashion. The puncture site selected is usually approximately 1 cm lateral to the rectus muscle and 1 cm inferior to the costal margin. The exact border of the rectus should be avoided so as not to traverse the superior epigastric artery. In some cases, it is necessary to go directly through the rectus or through a far lateral, even intercostal, approach to avoid the left lobe of the liver and the transverse colon. This is particularly true in patients who have had prior partial gastric resections. Local anesthesia is administered at the puncture site.

It is very helpful to have a nasogastric or orogastric tube in place to insufflate the stomach with air prior to the procedure. If, for a variety of reasons, it is not possible or not easy to place a nasogastric or orogastric tube, the stomach can be punctured with a 21-gauge Chiba needle (Cook) and the stomach inflated through this needle.[37] It is also useful to administer a small amount of nonionic contrast (10 to 20 ml) to outline the rugal folds.

In our practice, we are currently performing gastropexy using retention devices. The most commonly used devices are the Brown/Mueller T-fasteners (Medi-tech) and the Cope suture anchor (Cook).[36,38,39] Percutaneous gastropexy facilitates the placement of large or soft (Silastic) catheters, makes reinsertion easier, and also ensures that if the tract is lost because of failure of the balloon or other retention device, the gastric contents will leak directly out onto the skin rather than into the peritoneal cavity.[40] Deutsch and colleagues as well as other investigators do not routinely perform gastropexy, and their reported incidence of peritonitis is no greater than that experienced by investigators

using retention devices.[35,37] However, in general, investigators who are not using retention devices are placing locking pigtail-type catheters that are 16-F or smaller in size.

We place two to four Brown/Mueller T-fasteners (Medi-tech) at a distance of 1 to 2 cm apart. Each fastener is introduced by puncturing the stomach with the needle and then pushing the T-fastener out into the stomach. The T-fastener is then pulled back, bringing the anterior wall of the stomach to the anterior abdominal wall (Fig. 12–6). In patients with previous surgeries, this maneuver is performed gently rather than with force to avoid tearing the gastric wall (Rolandelli RH, personal communication). Rather than tying off the T-fastener at this point, it is better to just crimp the metal fasteners in place, saving the suture for later to secure the T-fastener directly to the gastrostomy tube. Once the T-fasteners are placed, a puncture is made with a 19-gauge thin wall needle through the anterior abdominal wall into the stomach. An intragastric location is confirmed by freely aspirating air. A stiff guidewire, either a Coon's interventional wire (Cook) or an Amplatz superstiff wire (Medi-tech) is then introduced. If the safety of the tract is in question, the puncture can be made with a nonionic contrast-filled syringe attached to the needle with the contrast under positive pressure. When the stomach is entered, injection will become markedly easier and the rugal folds will be outlined. If small or large bowel is entered, it will be apparent after contrast injection. Once the needle seems to be in the stomach, air can be aspirated as final confirmation of needle placement as modified from Foutch and coworkers.[41] Another method of proving tract safety is to use a 22-gauge needle for the initial puncture through which an 0.018 in wire is passed followed by placement of an Accustick system (Medi-tech). The inner stylet and catheter of the Accustick are then removed and a hemostatic valve attached. Contrast is then injected as the 6-F outer catheter is removed over the wire delineating the tract. If the tract does not pass through bowel or liver, the Accustick is reassembled and reintroduced followed by placement of a 0.035 in or 0.038 in stiff wire. This technique is modified from that which we use to check the safety of percutaneous transhepatic biliary drainage tracts.[42] Once the stiff wire has been placed, the tract is then dilated either with fascial dilators or with the balloon angioplasty catheter. We prefer the balloon angioplasty catheter because there is

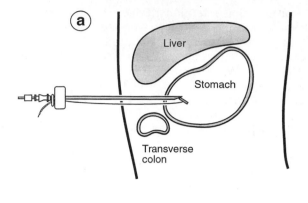

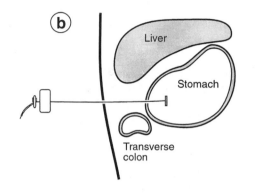

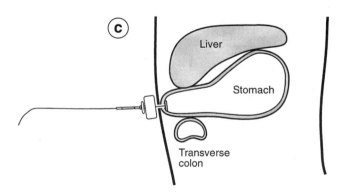

FIGURE 12–6 Percutaneous gastropexy. *A,* The needle is advanced into the stomach and the T-fastener is then deposited in the stomach. *B,* The needle is removed. *C,* Gentle tension is put on the string, pulling the anterior wall of the stomach up to the abdominal wall. The metal fasteners are crimped in place.

less shear damage along the tract and because balloon dilatation is a one-step procedure vs a multiple-step procedure when using fascial dilators.[43] In addition, using a balloon rather than dilators avoids putting a large amount of stress against the retention devices, thus reducing the risk of gastric wall laceration. Also, if a balloon is used, the catheter or peel-away sheath can be loaded onto the balloon and introduced into the stomach behind the balloon as the balloon is deflated, similar to the technique originally described for placement of stainless steel Greenfield IVC filter (Medi-tech)

delivery sheaths in the common femoral vein. If the tract is short, gastrostomy tubes, even Silastic tubes, can frequently be placed through a fresh tract without the use of a peel-away sheath. However, if the tubes are placed primarily without a peel-away sheath, they need to be stiffened internally either over the balloon as described or with a fascial dilator. If the tract is relatively long, a peel-away sheath of an appropriate size should be placed routinely (Fig. 12–7). Following tube placement over the wire, the catheter is either pigtailed or the balloon inflated depending on the type of catheter

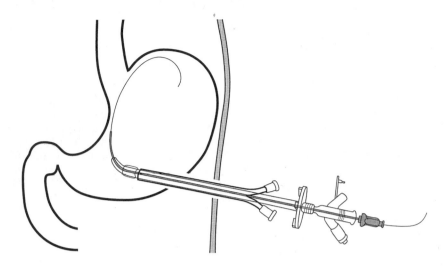

FIGURE 12–7 Gastrostomy tube placement. In this example, a silicone tube with an internal stiffening dilator has been placed over the wire through a peel-away sheath.

used. The wire and the peel-away, if one has been used, are then removed.

Contrast is then injected to verify location. Locking pigtail catheters are sometimes placed with the tip in the fundus if the tube will be used for aspiration purposes only and if there is no future possibility of gastroenterostomy conversion. However, for the most part, catheters are placed in the body with the tip directed toward the antrum. Balloon catheters are pulled back and the outside retention device brought down to the skin so that there is approximately 1 cm of slack. The sutures attached to the T-fasteners can then be tied to the outside retention device on balloon catheters. If the catheter is a locking pigtail type of catheter without an external retention device, these sutures can be tied to one another. A separate suture can then be introduced into the skin and tied to the catheter to afford additional safety. Patients can generally be fed through a percutaneously placed tube within 24 hours. T-fastener sutures are cut at the skin 7 to 10 days after the procedure.

Gastrojejunostomy Tube Placement

This procedure is the same as that for gastrostomy tubes except that once the wire is introduced, an 8-F vascular sheath is placed over the wire and the wire is left in place. An angiographic selective catheter such as the 5-F angled taper Glidecath is introduced adjacent to the wire, along with a selective guidewire such as the Glidewire (Fig. 12–8). It is important that the original puncture be directed toward the antrum rather than toward the fundus to facilitate passage through the pylorus. The same technique as described for nasojejunal tubes earlier in this chapter is used to cross the pylorus and advance around past the ligament of Treitz. Once the angiographic catheter is in position, the wire is removed and a stiff wire (stiff Glidewire) is introduced. The catheter is then introduced over this wire, usually through a peel-away sheath as described above under gastrostomy tube placement. In some cases, there is a large amount of friction between the wire and the Silastic catheter. The wire and catheter can be lubricated with a water-soluble lubricant or a hemostatic valve can be placed over the wire onto the back of the catheter, allowing for flushing between the catheter and wire.

Conversion of Gastrostomy Tube to Gastrojejunostomy Tube

If the tract is fresh (less than 7 days),[44] it is worthwhile to attempt the procedure through a previously placed gastrostomy tube without removing it to decrease the possibility of peritoneal spill. A 5-F angled taper Glidecath can be introduced through many gastrostomy tubes and brought out an end hole if there is one, or out a side hole. Using the same technique as described above, the angiographic catheter and wire are brought out into the jejunum. A stiff wire is then placed. Several manufacturers now make jejunostomy tubes that are made to fit coaxially within their gastrostomy tube. Some of

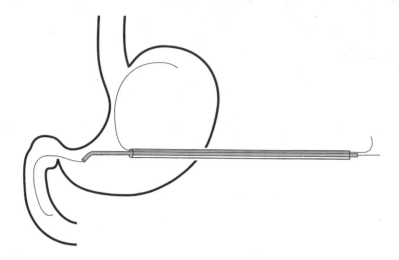

FIGURE 12–8 Gastrojejunostomy tube placement. An 8-F vascular sheath has been placed over the safety wire. Through this, a 5-F selective catheter has been introduced. The selective guidewire has been passed through the pylorus out into the duodenum.

these systems do not have end holes but they can be introduced over the most distal side hole and the catheter introduced into the jejunum using a push-pull maneuver to work out the loop that invariably forms at the end of the catheter if a side hole is used. If this is not successful, the distal tip can be severed, resulting in formation of an end hole, which will facilitate placement.

If the tract is mature (greater than 7 days),[44] it is useful to remove the previously placed gastrostomy tube over a wire and place a sheath. The procedure can then proceed in the same way as for initial placement of a gastrojejunostomy tube.

There are two problem situations that may occur when converting a gastrostomy to a gastrojejunostomy. The first of these occurs when the initial gastrostomy tube is placed in such a way that it points directly at the fundus.[45] The second of these occurs when the patient has a surgical gastrojejunostomy and the tube needs to enter the efferent limb.

When the gastrostomy tube has been placed pointing directly toward the fundus, it is often possible to redirect a wire from the fundus into the antrum using a Simmons-type catheter (Fig. 12–9). In some cases it may be necessary

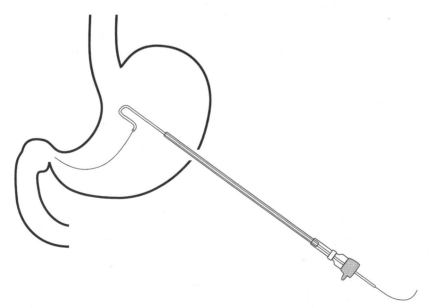

FIGURE 12–9 Gastrostomy to gastrojejunostomy tube conversion when the original tube is pointed toward the fundus. An 8-F vascular sheath is placed over a safety wire. A Simmons-type catheter is then introduced to redirect the selective guidewire into the antrum and out through the pylorus.

to place a very stiff fascial dilator which can be manually directed into the antrum[24] (Fig. 12–10). Through this, an angiographic catheter can be placed and the procedure can then proceed in the normal fashion.

When a patient has a gastrojejunostomy and requires conversion of a gastrostomy tube to a gastrojejunostomy tube, the efferent limb may lie immediately inferior or even infero-lateral to the entrance site of the gastrostomy tube. It is then necessary to use a backward-seeking catheter such as a Simmons-type catheter to probe the area of the anastomosis (Fig. 12–11). Once the wire has passed through the anastomosis, the Simmons-type catheter can be with-

drawn, an angled catheter can be introduced, and the procedure can proceed in the usual fashion as described above.

INTUBATION OF FISTULAS AND OSTOMIES

It is possible to place tubes through fistulas and ostomies using angiographic technique. A 5-F angled taper catheter and a selective wire are used to reach the area of the bowel where the tip of the catheter is needed. A stiff wire is then placed and the final tube placed over the wire. In some cases, it is not possible to secure the catheter in the normal fashion. Balloon

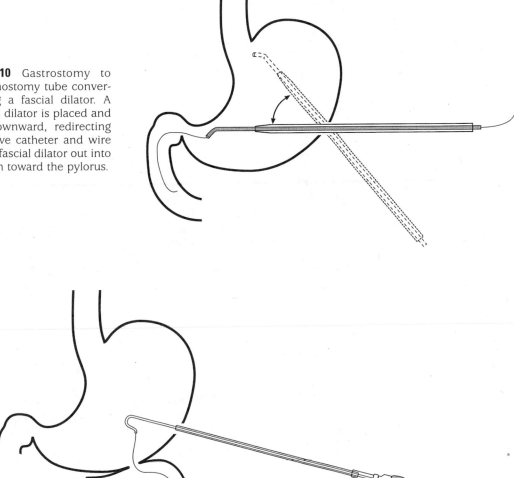

FIGURE 12–10 Gastrostomy to gastrojejunostomy tube conversion using a fascial dilator. A stiff fascial dilator is placed and rotated downward, redirecting the selective catheter and wire inside the fascial dilator out into the antrum toward the pylorus.

FIGURE 12–11 Gastrostomy to gastrojejunostomy tube conversion in a patient with surgical gastrojejunostomy. An 8-F vascular sheath is placed. Through this, a Simmons-type catheter is introduced pointing backward and downward into the anastomosis. The selective guidewire is then passed into the jejunum.

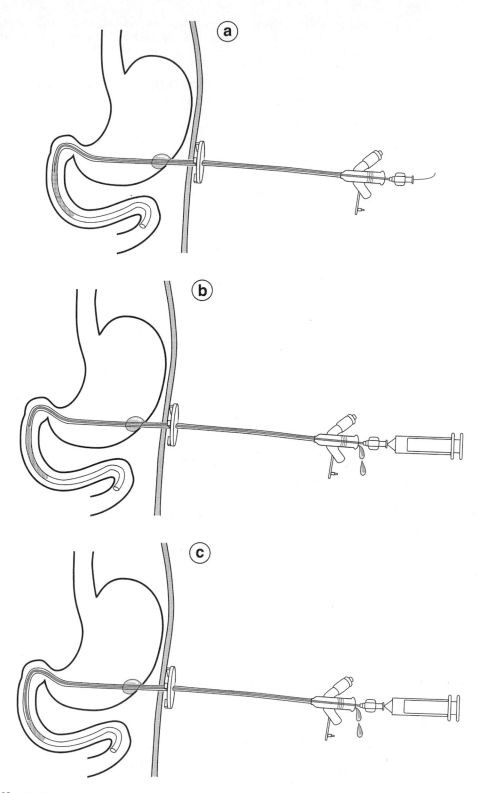

FIGURE 12–12 Unclogging obstructed gastrojejunostomy tubes. *A*, A hydrophilic catheter is introduced into the lumen and advanced to the point of the obstruction. A guidewire is then passed as far as possible into the obstruction. *B*, The wire is removed and saline injected, flushing the obstructing material out of the back of the gastrojejunostomy tube. *C*, The catheter is readvanced over the wire. The wire is passed as far as possible into the obstructing material. The wire is removed and the catheter flushed. The process is repeated until the tube injects freely.

catheters may not stay in place because of poor or reverse peristalsis. It also may not be possible to fix the catheter to the skin immediately adjacent to the entrance site because of breakdown of the wound or because of infection. In this case, a fascial dilator can be placed across the wound such that each end is sewn to normal skin on either side of the wound. The catheter can then be fixed directly to the fascial dilator.

UNCLOGGING OBSTRUCTED TUBES

The radiologist is frequently called upon to assist in the unclogging of obstructed tubes. In many cases, it is possible to clear the tube by injecting or by passing a guidewire. If this does not work and the catheter lumen is large enough, a hydrophilic catheter such as a straight Glidecath and a hydrophilic wire such as the angled or straight Glidewire can be introduced into the clogged catheter. The guidewire and catheter can be pushed forward until they meet the area of the obstruction. The wire is then removed and forceful injection of saline is made to back-flush the obstructing material out of the proximal end of the catheter. Once the flush is relatively clear, the wire is reintroduced and the wire-catheter combination readvanced until obstruction is again met. The wire is then removed and flushing repeated. The process is repeated several cycles until the catheter is cleared (Fig. 12–12). In our experience, this procedure results in the successful clearance of nearly 100 percent of obstructed tubes.

REFERENCES

1. Cantor MO: Intestinal intubation. Springfield, IL: Charles C. Thomas Publishing, 1949.
2. Rousselet LM, Bauman L: Cholesterol crystals and "calcium bilirubinate" granules: their significance in bile obtained through the duodenal tube. JAMA 1933;100: 254–256.
3. Gianturco C: Rapid fluoroscopic duodenal intubation. Radiology 1967;88:1165–1166.
4. Hanafee WN, Weiner M: External guided passage of an intestinal intubation tube. Radiology 1967;89: 1100–1102.
5. Bilbao MK, Frische LH, Dotter CT et al: Hypotonic duodenography. Radiology 1967;89:438–443.
6. Sargent EN, Meyers HL: Wire guide and technique for Cantor tube insertion: rapid small bowel intubation. Am J Roentgenol 1969;107:150–155.
7. Gelfand DW: An easy method for passing an intestinal intubation tube under fluoroscopic guidance. Radiology 1978;129:532.
8. Frederick PR, Miller MH, Morrison WJ: Feeding tube for fluoroscopic placement. Radiology 1982;145:847.
9. Grant JP, Curtas MS, Kelvin FM: Fluoroscopic placement of nasojejunal feeding tubes with immediate feeding using a nonelemental diet. J Parenter Enter Nutr 1983;7:299–303.
10. Gutierrez ED, Balfe DM: Fluoroscopically guided nasoenteric feeding tube placement: results of a 1-year study. Radiology 1991;178:759–762.
11. Lewis BS, Mauer K, Bush A: The rapid placement of jejunal feeding tubes: the Seldinger technique applied to the gut. Gastrointest Endosc 1990;36:139–141.
12. Ott DJ, Maddox HE, Gelfand DW et al: Enteral feeding tubes: placement by using fluoroscopy and endoscopy. Am J Roentgenol 1991;157:769–771.
13. Prager R, Laboy V, Venus B et al: Value of fluoroscopic assistance during transpyloric intubation. Crit Care Med 1986;14:151–152.
14. Ramos SM, Lindine P: Inexpensive, safe and simple nasoenteral intubation: an alternative for the cost conscious. J Parenter Enter Nutr 1986;10:78–81.
15. Ghahremani GG, Turner MA, Port RB: Iatrogenic intubation injuries of the upper gastrointestinal tract in adults. Gastrointest Radiol 1980;5:1–10.
16. Harris MR, Huseby JS: Pulmonary complications from nasoenteral feeding tube insertion in an intensive care unit: incidence and prevention. Crit Care Med 1989;17:917–919.
17. Hunter TB, Fon GT, Silverstein ME: Complications of intestinal tubes. Am J Gastroenterol 1981;76:256–261.
18. McWey RE, Curry NS, Schabel SI et al: Complications of nasoenteric feeding tubes. Am J Surg 1988;155: 253–257.
19. Siegle RL, Rabinowitz JG, Sarasohn C: Intestinal perforation secondary to nasojejunal feeding tubes. Am J Roentgenol 1976;126:1229–1232.
20. Sacks BA, Glotzer DJ: Percutaneous reestablishment of feeding gastrostomies. Surgery 1979;85:575–576.
21. Gauderer MWL, Ponsky JL, Izant RJ: Gastrostomy without laparotomy: a percutaneous endoscopic technique. J Pediatr Surg 1980;15:872–875.
22. Preshaw RM: A percutaneous method for inserting a feeding gastrostomy tube. Surg Gynecol Obstet 1981; 152:659–660.
23. Bisgard JD: Gastrostomy-jejunal intubation. Surg Gynecol Obstet 1942;74:239–241.
24. McLean GK, Rombeau JL, Caldwell MD et al: Transgastrostomy jejunal intubation for enteric alimentation. Am J Roentgenol 1982;139:1129–1133.
25. Ho CS: Percutaneous gastrostomy for jejunal feeding. Radiology 1983;149:595–596.
26. Tao HH, Gillies RR: Percutaneous feeding gastrostomy. Am J Roentgenol 1983;141:793–794.
27. Wills JS, Oglesby JT: Percutaneous gastrostomy. Radiology 1983;149:449–453.
28. Gray RR, Ho CS, Yee A et al: Direct percutaneous jejunostomy. Am J Roentgenol 1987;149:931–932.
29. Ho CS, Yee ACN, McPherson R: Complications of surgical and percutaneous nonendoscopic gastrostomy: review of 233 patients. Gastroenterology 1988;95: 1206–1210.
30. Lee MJ, Saini S, Brink JA et al: Malignant small bowel obstruction and ascites: not a contraindication to percutaneous gastrostomy. Clin Radiol 1991;44:332–334.
31. Sanchez RB, van Sonnenberg E, D'Agostino HB et al: CT guidance for percutaneous gastrostomy and gastroenterostomy. Radiology 1992;184:201–205.
32. Ponsky JL, Gauderer MWL, Stellato TA: Percutaneous endoscopic gastrostomy: review of 150 cases. Arch Surg 1983;118:913–914.
33. Halkier BK, Ho CS, Yee AC: Percutaneous feeding gastrostomy with the Seldinger technique: review of 252 patients. Radiology 1989;171:359–362.
34. Hicks ME, Surratt RS, Picus D et al: Fluoroscopically guided percutaneous gastrostomy and gastroenteros-

tomy: analysis of 158 consecutive cases. Am J Roentgenol 1990;154:725–728.

35. O'Keeffe F, Carrasco CH, Charnsangavej C et al: Percutaneous drainage and feeding gastrostomies in 100 patients. Radiology 1989;172:341–343.

36. Saini S, Mueller PR, Gaa J et al: Percutaneous gastrostomy with gastropexy: experience in 125 patients. Am J Roentgenol 1990;154:1003–1006.

37. Deutsch LS, Kannegieter L, Vanson DT et al: Simplified percutaneous gastrostomy. Radiology 1992;184:181–183.

38. Brown AS, Mueller PR, Ferrucci JT: Controlled percutaneous gastrostomy: nylon T-fastener for fixation of the anterior gastric wall. Radiology 1986;158:543–545.

39. Coleman CC, Coons HG, Cope C et al: Percutaneous enterostomy with the Cope suture anchor. Radiology 1990;174:889–891.

40. Cope C: Suture anchor for visceral drainage. Am J Roentgenol 1986;146:160–162.

41. Foutch PG, Talbert GA, Waring JP et al: Percutaneous endoscopic gastrostomy in patients with prior abdominal surgery: virtues of the safe tract. Am J Gastroenterol 1988;83:147–150.

42. Goodwin SC, Stainken BF, McNamara TO et al: Prevention of significant hemobilia when placing transhepatic biliary drainage catheters. J Vasc Interv Radiol. 1995;6:229–232.

43. McLean GK, LeVeen RF: Shear stress in the performance of esophageal dilation: comparison of balloon dilation and bougienage. Radiology 1989;172:983–986.

44. van Sonnenberg E, Wittich GR, Brown LK et al: Percutaneous gastrostomy and gastroenterostomy, I. Techniques derived from laboratory evaluation. Am J Roentgenol 1986;146:577–580.

45. Lu DS, Mueller PR, Lee MJ et al: Gastrostomy conversion to transgastric jejunostomy: technical problems, causes of failure, and proposed solutions in 63 patients. Radiology 1993;187:679–683.

13

Defined Formula Diets

MICHELE M. GOTTSCHLICH
EVA POLITZER SHRONTS
ANDREA M. HUTCHINS

Nutrition support has advanced well beyond simply providing protein and calories (Fig. 13–1). We have entered the era of nutritional pharmacology, and the importance of providing specialized enteral support in the dietary management of patients with specific diseases and medical conditions is widely accepted. A vast and ever-expanding array of enteral feeding products is currently available. Many are designed for use in specific disease states. However, the science of enteral nutrition has frequently lagged behind the marketplace, often making appropriate formula selection difficult to discern.

This chapter first reviews various nutrient substrates presently used in defined enteral formulas and considers both theoretical and scientific principles pertinent to their application, emphasizing the enteral literature. Additionally, we discuss the potential therapeutic use of administering specific fuels or immunomodulators. Next, we review the physical characteristics of enteral formulas and the various categories of available products to aid the clinician in selecting a formula. Particular attention is given to specialty products. Improved understanding of nutrient requirements during stress and disease will most likely provide further rationale for the use of enteral nutrients in the critically ill.

NUTRIENT COMPONENTS

Carbohydrate

Carbohydrate supplies 40 to 90 percent of the calories in most enteral solutions, making it the primary energy source. Contributing to the osmolality and sweetness of enteral solutions, the available forms of carbohydrate include monosaccharides, disaccharides, oligosaccharides/polysaccharides, and starch.[1,2]

The monosaccharide most commonly used is glucose. The small size of the glucose molecule increases the osmolality of the solutions, resulting in hypertonicity. Enteral solutions that use glucose taste sweet, and their tolerance is limited by the small bowel's absorptive capacity.[2,3]

Sucrose, lactose, and maltose comprise the disaccharides, which require specific enzyme activity in the intestinal mucosa for hydrolysis. Disaccharidase production can be decreased during illness, but the digestion of sucrose and maltose is usually not affected because they are rapidly hydrolyzed in the small intestine. Since lactose is hydrolyzed more slowly, a decrease in lactase production can result in lactose intolerance. Many of the enteral solutions on the market are lactose free to avoid this problem.

Oligosaccharides contain 2 to 10 glucose units, and polysaccharides contain more than

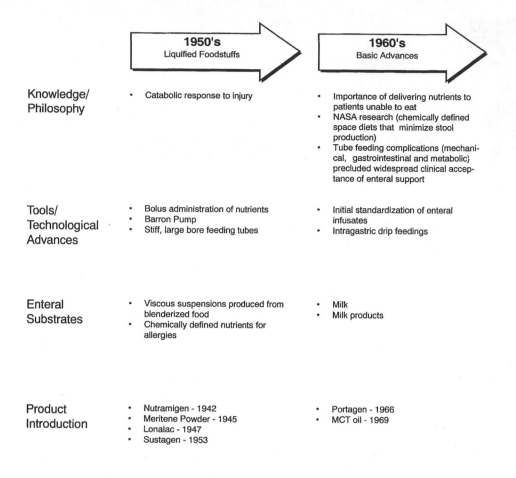

FIGURE 13–1   The evolution of enteral nutrition support.

10 glucose units. Contributing less to osmolality than glucose alone, they are more soluble than starch and rarely cause intolerance. Primary sources used in enteral solutions include glucose oligosaccharides, glucose polysaccharides, maltodextrins, corn syrup, and corn syrup solids (Table 13–1).

Starch contributes little to the osmolality of enteral solutions and is usually well tolerated and easily digested. However, its insolubility makes it difficult to use in enteral solutions. The sources currently used include hydrolyzed cornstarch, cereal solids, and blenderized fruits and vegetables.[1,2]

1970's Advent of Synthetic Diets	1980's Disease/Age Specific Compounds for Tailored Support	1990's Nutritional Approaches to Anatomic and Physiologic Modulation
• High incidence of malnutrition recognized in hospital populations • Broad nutritional assessment guidelines exist • IV hyperalimentation accepted as single-most effective means of preventing nutrient deficits in patients unable to eat	• Resurgence of interest in enteral nutrition. "If the gut works, use it." • Advances in metabolic assessment • Energy and macronutrient intake guidelines available for the critically ill	• Known pharmacologic effects of nutrient enhancing capabilities on the immune system, anabolic repair, recovery from disease, GI integrity and outcome • Elucidation of nutrient metabolism in disease • Clarification of micronutrient requirements • Early and intraoperative enteral support • FDA definition of medical foods
• Advances in food technology such as ability to isolate fractions of natural food and recombine to create new product • Small bore feeding tubes marketed	• Proliferation of commercial enteral products • Evolution of multidisciplinary nutrition support teams and home care • Improvements in feeding tube design and enteral infusion delivery systems • Endoscopic/Fluoroscopic/Surgical tube placement capabilities	• Sophisticated measures of nutritional status • Generic commercialization of products • Decentralization of nutrition support with interdisciplinary approach
• Lactose free products • Low residue products • Range of osmolalities • Intact nutrients as well as elemental • L-amino acids • Amino acid modified products for renal failure, hepatic disease, PKU • Chemically defined, low fat diets for malabsorption, pancreatic dysfunction	• Calorically dense products • Di and tri-peptides • Specialty products for trauma, stress, pulmonary compromise, glucose intolerance, pediatrics • Fiber fortification • Modular tube feeding production for disease/patient specific support	• Omega-3 fatty acids • Structured lipids • Short chain fatty acids • Growth factors and hormones • Product enrichment with specialty nitrogen sources such as glutamine, arginine, cysteine, histidine, taurine, nucleotides
• Sustacal - 1971 • Controlyte - 1971 • Citrotein - 1971 • Meritene Liquid - 1972 • Ensure - 1973 • Precision HN - 1973 • Vivonex - 1973 • Polycose - 1974 • Precision Isotonic - 1974 • Isocal - 1974 • Compleat B - 1975 • Amin Aid - 1976 • Ensure Plus - 1977 • Microlipid - 1977 • Vital HN - 1978 • Osmolite - 1978 • Hepatic Aid - 1979 • Magnacal - 1979	• Isocal HCN-1981 • Compleat Modified - 1981 • Travasorb Hepatic - 1981 • Travasorb Renal - 1981 • Criticare HN - 1981 • Isotein HN - 1982 • Sumacal - 1982 • Traumacal - 1983 • Osmolite HN - 1983 • Traum Aid - 1983 • Ross SLD - 1984 • Enrich - 1984 • Two Cal HN - 1984 • Nutrasource Modular System - 1984 • Pulmocare - 1985 • Resource - 1985 • Stresstein - 1986 • Isocal HN - 1987 • Pediasure - 1987 • Peptamen - 1987 • Reabllan - 1987 • Sustacal with Fiber - 1988 • Jevity - 1988 • Glucerna - 1989	• Impact - 1990 • Immun-Aid - 1990 • Suplena - 1990 • Ultracal - 1990 • Replete - 1991 • Citrosource - 1991 • Nepro - 1991 • Promote - 1992 • Alitrag - 1992 • Perative - 1992 • Advera - 1993 • Pediasure with Fiber - 1993 • Respalor - 1993 • Vivonex Plus - 1993 • Ensure with Fiber - 1993 • Impact with Fiber - 1994 • Isosource VHN - 1994 • Crucial - 1994 • L-Emental - 1994 • Nutri Hep - 1994 • Peptamen VHP - 1994 • Promote with Fiber - 1994 • Sandosource Peptide - 1995 • Diabetisource - 1995 • Peptamen Junior - 1995 • ProBalance - 1995 • Kindercal - 1995

FIGURE 13–1 *Continued*

Fiber

The advantage of using fiber in enteral solutions is controversial, although it is beneficial in a normal diet. When comparing fiber-containing enteral formulas (Table 13–2), it is important to differentiate between the amount of the fiber source itself compared with a standard-ized chemical measurement technique[4] that quantitates total dietary fiber (TDF) content. Soy polysaccharide is 75 percent TDF. Therefore, if a product contains 20 g of soy polysaccharide, it actually contains 15 g TDF.

When examining the fiber in enteral formulas, the clinician must consider the actual

TABLE 13–1   Categories and Macronutrient Sources for Various Types of Defined Formulas*

Type of Formula	Protein Sources	Carbohydrate Sources
Intact (polymeric)	Calcium and magnesium caseinates Sodium and calcium caseinates Soy protein isolate Calcium-potassium caseinate Delactosed lactalbumin Egg white solids Beef Nonfat milk	Maltodextrin Corn syrup solids Sucrose Cornstarch Glucose polymers Sugar Vegetables Fruits Nonfat milk
Hydrolyzed (oligomeric or monomeric)	Enzymatically hydrolyzed whey or casein Soybean or lactalbumin hydrolysate Whey protein Free amino acids Soy protein hydrolysate	Hydrolyzed cornstarch Sucrose Fructose Maltodextrin Tapioca starch Glucose oligosaccharides
Modular Protein	Low-lactose whey and casein Calcium caseinate Free amino acids	—
Carbohydrate	—	Maltodextrin Hydrolyzed cornstarch
Fat	—	—

*Information obtained from manufacturers' product information.
CM = ChroniMed, C = Clintec, CP = Corpak, EP = Elan Pharma, MG = McGaw, MJ = Mead Johnson, R = Ross, RPS = R.P. Scherer, SA = Sandoz, S = Sherwood, SHS = SHS North America.

source of the dietary fiber. With regard to gastrointestinal (GI) effects, dietary fiber substances can be divided into two categories: insoluble and soluble fibers. Insoluble fibers rich in cellulose and lignin (hydrophilic fibers found in wheat bran, psyllium seed, and ispaghula husk) increase fecal mass by holding water.[5,6] They are also believed to improve GI function,[6,7] prevent constipation,[8,9] and help regulate GI transit time in noncritically ill patients.[5-8] Soy polysaccharide is the fiber source most commonly used in fiber-containing formulas.[6] In addition to its potentially positive effects on bowel function, it has a minimal effect on formula viscosity and contains fiber that is partially digested by colonic bacterial flora.[5]

Soluble fibers such as pectin, mucilages, and gums are rapidly and completely fermented in the cecum by anaerobic microflora and represent important substrates for maintaining colonic structure and function. Studies have

Fat Sources	Kcal/ml	Protein Content	Nonprotein Calorie: Nitrogen Ratio	Examples
Medium-chain triglycerides Canola oil Corn oil Lecithin Soybean oil Partially hydrogenated soybean oil High-oleic safflower oil Beef fat	1–2	30–84 g/L	75–177:1	Compleat Regular (SA) Compleat Modified (SA) Fibersource (SA) Isocal (MJ) Isosource (SA) Jevity (R) Magnacal (S) Nepro (R) NutrAssist (CM) Nutren 1.0 (C) Osmolite (R) Resource Plus (SA) Suplena (R) TwoCal HN (R) Ultracal (MJ)
Medium-chain triglycerides Sunflower oil Lecithin Soybean oil Safflower oil Corn oil Coconut oil Canola oil Sardine oil	1–1.33	21–52.5 g/L	67–282:1	Advera (R) AlitraQ (R) Criticare HN (MJ) Neocate One+ (SHS) Peptamen (C) PeptiCal (CM) Perative (R) Reabilan (EP) Tolerex (SA) Vital HN (R)
—	Per 100 g 370–424	Per 100 g 75–88.5	—	Casec (MJ) Elementa (C) ProMod (R) Propac (S) ProMix (CP)
—	380–386	—	—	Moducal (MJ) Polycose Powder (R) Sumacal (SA)
Safflower oil Polyglycerol esters of fatty acids Soybean oil Lecithin Medium-chain triglycerides Fish oil	Per 1 Tbsp 67.5–115	—	—	MCT Oil (MJ) Microlipid (SA) MaxEPA (RPS)

shown that soluble fiber can prevent atrophy of the ileal and colonic mucosa,[6,8,10] stimulate mucosal proliferation,[6,8] provide fuel for colonic bacteria through short-chain fatty acid generation,[5,6,8] and possibly lower serum cholesterol[11] and improve glucose tolerance.[12] In the past, pectin and guar gum were not used much in enteral formulas because they form gels. However, recent advances in fiber technology have made it possible to add guar to formulas (Table 13–2).

A detailed review of the metabolism and clinical applications of dietary fiber can be found in Chapter 6. Briefly, soluble, fermentable fibers may be indicated for patients recovering from bowel surgery. Patients requiring long-term tube feeding as well as those patients presenting with diverticulosis or constipation may experience some normalization of stool patterns with the use of insoluble fiber bulking agents. When fiber is added to any nutrition support care plan, patient tolerance

TABLE 13–2   Total Dietary Fiber Content of Selected Enteral Formulas*

Product	Manufacturer[†]	Fiber Source	TDF[‡] (g/L)	kcal/ml	NPC:N[§]	vol USRDA[∥] (ml)
Advera	Ross	Soy polysaccharide	8.9	1.28	108:1	1184
Compleat	Sandoz	Vegetables, fruits	4.4	1.07	131:1	1500
Compleat Modified	Sandoz	Vegetables, fruits	4.4	1.07	131:1	1500
Ensure with Fiber	Ross	Soy polysaccharide	14.4	1.10	148:1	1391
Entralife HN-Fiber	Corpak	Soy polysaccharide	14.4	1.00	125:1	1250
Fiberlan	Elan Pharma	Soy polysaccharide	14.3	1.17	104:1	1250
Fibersource	Sandoz	Soy polysaccharide	10.0	1.20	151:1	1500
Fibersource HN	Sandoz	Soy polysaccharide	6.8	1.20	118:1	1500
Glucerna	Ross	Soy polysaccharide	14.4	1.00	125:1	1422
Impact with Fiber	Sandoz	Soy polysaccharide, modified guar	10.0	1.00	71:1	1500
IsoSource VHN	Sandoz	Soy polysaccharide, modified guar	10.0	1.00	77:1	1250
Jevity	Ross	Soy polysaccharide	14.4	1.06	125:1	1321
Nutren 1.0 with Fiber	Clintec	Soy polysaccharide	14.0	1.00	121:1	1500
PediaSure with Fiber	Ross	Soy polysaccharide	5.0	1.00	185:1	1000¶
Profiber	Sherwood Medical	Soy polysaccharide	12.0	1.00	134:1	1250
Promote with Fiber	Ross	Oat fiber, soy polysaccharide	14.4	1.00	75:1	1000
ProBalance	Clintec	Soy polysaccharide, gum arabic	10.0	1.20	117:1	1000
Replete with Fiber	Clintec	Soy polysaccharide, accacia, cellulose	14.0	1.00	75:1	1000
Sustacal with Fiber	Mead Johnson	Soy polysaccharide	10.6	1.06	120:1	1420
Ultracal	Mead Johnson	Oat fiber, soy polysaccharide	14.4	1.06	128:1	1180
Vitaneed	Sherwood Medical	Vegetables, fruits, soy polysaccharide	8.0	1.00	134:1	1500

*Product information verified by manufacturers 1/95.
[†]Location of manufacturers: Sandoz Nutrition, Minneapolis, MN; Ross Products Division, Abbott Laboratories, Columbus, OH; Corpak/Thermedics, Wheeling, IL; Elan Pharma, Cambridge, MA; Clintec Nutrition, Deerfield, IL; Sherwood Medical, St. Louis, MO; Mead Johnson, Evansville, IN.
[†]TDF = total dietary fiber.
[§]NPC:N = nonprotein calorie: nitrogen (g) ratio.
[∥]vol USRDA = volume of formula required to meet 100% of the U.S. RDA.
[¶]1000 ml for children 1–6 years; 1300 ml for children 7–10 years.

must be monitored frequently. Fluid-restricted patients or those with gastroparesis are at increased risk for bezoar formation and are not candidates for fiber supplementation.[6]

Because of the current popularity of dietary fiber, many manufacturers are adding purified sources of fiber to enteral formulas in quantities ranging from 5 to 14.4 g of TDF per liter. Blenderized formulas made from whole foods contain a natural source of fiber. The amount of TDF in commercial blenderized products averages 4.4 g/L. However, existing research does not clearly prove efficacy nor define the opti-

mal levels of fiber needed in various chronic and acute care conditions. The current popularity of fiber appears to be ahead of its scientific basis. After more precise guidelines for optimal fiber supplementation are established, product labeling to include grams of TDF as well as soluble fiber and insoluble fiber would be very useful to clinicians.

Lipids

Lipids represent a concentrated, secondary energy source. Because lipids are isotonic and not water soluble, they help lower the osmolality of enteral formulas. They also provide a source of essential fatty acids, carry the fat-soluble vitamins, and enhance substrate flavor and palatability.[13,14] Common sources of lipid for enteral formulas include corn oil, soybean oil, safflower oil, sunflower oil, coconut oil, lecithin, and whole milk (Table 13–1), and studies have shown that manipulating the type of lipid ingested can enhance or inhibit immune function, maintain or promote gut integrity, affect physiologic function, and alter clinical outcome.[14]

The classic categorization of the various types of fats separates them as saturates, monounsaturates, and polyunsaturates (Fig. 13–2). They can be further subdivided by structural and physiochemical functions. In the saturated group, fatty acids with two to four carbon atoms are considered short chain fatty acids (SCFAs); medium-chain fatty acids (MCFAs) consist of 6 to 12 carbon atoms, and long-chain fatty acids (LCFAs) have 14 to 24 carbon atoms. The monounsaturated fatty acids can be classified into two independent families, for which the initial precursors are palmitoleic (16:1, n-7) and oleic (18:1, n-9). Polyunsaturates can be divided into the omega-6 and omega-3 fatty acid families according to the location of the first double bond from the terminal methyl end of the carbon chain, whereby the precursors are linoleic (18:2) and α-linolenic (18:3) acid, respectively.

Similar to the diversity characterized by the categorization of fats is the varied lipid content evident in commercial enteral products. Tables 13–3 and 13–4 illustrate the fact that several hydrolyzed and dipeptide formulas are relatively low in fat and linoleic acid, whereas some intact protein products contain extremely high levels of fat in the upper range of 55 percent of total calories. There is little apparent justification for providing such high levels of fat. Because the absolute requirement for linoleate is only 2 to 4 percent of calories, and because large quantities of fat have numerous detrimental effects, use such products judiciously. The clinician should note the content and source of omega-3, omega-6, and MCFAs contained therein (Table 13–3), as well as keep abreast of future sources of enteral lipid substrates such as the availability of commercial products containing SCFAs and structured lipids.

Long-Chain Fatty Acids

LCFAs consist of carbon chains that are between 14 and 24 units long (Fig. 13–2). Cleared slowly from the bloodstream, LCFAs are preferentially reesterified and stored as triglyceride.[14-17] LCFAs require carnitine to aid in their transport across the mitochondrial membrane, where they are used for energy.[14,17-20] Some studies have shown that carnitine availability is decreased in critically ill patients, impairing the cells' ability to use LCFAs.[14]

Included in the category of LCFAs is the essential fatty acid linoleic acid and the possibly essential fatty acid α-linolenic acid. Linoleic acid, an omega-6 fatty acid, is metabolized to arachidonic acid (Fig. 13–3), which is the precursor of the eicosanoids series 2 prostanoids and series 4 leukotrienes.[14,18,19,21] Series 2 prostanoids induce inflammation and increase immunosuppression.[14,18-20,22,23] Although immunosuppression is desirable in some patients (e.g., transplant patients), it is undesirable in the critically ill population. Series 4 leukotrienes act as bronchoconstrictors and stimulate tracheal mucus secretions,[20] another undesirable effect in critically ill populations.

α-Linolenic acid, an omega-3 fatty acid, is the parent of eicosapentaenoic acid (EPA), the precursor of the eicosanoids series 3 prostanoids and series 5 leukotrienes[14,24] (Fig. 13–3). Series 3 prostanoids and series 5 leukotrienes have been shown to have anti-inflammatory and immune-enhancing properties. The omega-3 products also inhibit the formation of the omega-6 products.[1,14,18-20,23]

Medium-Chain Fatty Acids

MCFAs, the first alternative lipid source developed, consist of carbon chains between 6 and 12 units long (Fig. 13–2). Coconut and palm kernel oil are sources of MCFAs. They are primarily used in patients with impaired fat digestion, absorption, or transport.[14] MCFAs do not require bile salts or pancreatic lipase, so they are more rapidly and easily absorbed by the intestinal mucosa and directly enter the portal circulation.[14,18]

MCFAs are more readily used for energy than LCFAs because they can enter the mitochondria without undergoing biochemical transformation to a transport form. Their entry is considered independent of carnitine,[19,20] although some data suggest that carnitine stimulates β-oxidation of MCFAs in some tissues. In addition, MCFAs are not as readily used for deposit in adipose tissue or to synthesize triglyceride as are LCFAs.[14,16,17,25]

The disadvantages of the enteral administration of MCFAs are the lack of essential fatty acids, increased formula osmolality because

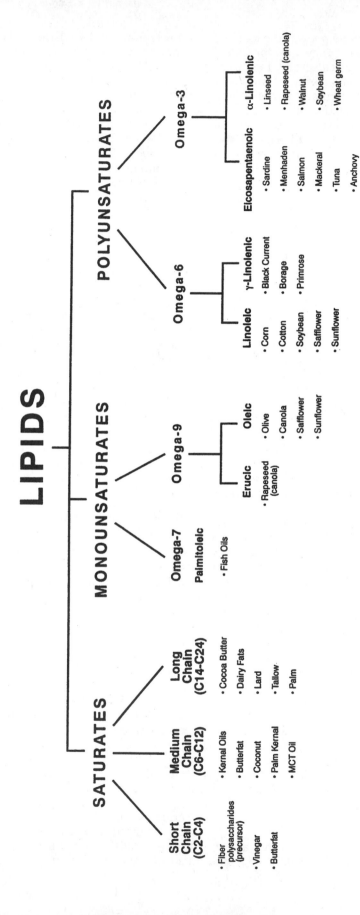

FIGURE 13–2   Classification of lipids.

TABLE 13–3 Fat Content of Selected Enteral Products*

Formula	Fat (g/L)	Fat (source)	Fat (% kcal)	Linoleic Acid (g/L)	MCT (g/L)	Omega-3 fatty acids (g/L)
Enteral						
Advera	22.8	Canola oil, MCT, sardine oil	15.8	3.4	4.0	1.16
AlitraQ	15.5	MCT, safflower oil	13.0	6.6	6.5	1.55
Alterna	15.6	Soybean oil	38.1	0.5	0.0	0.10
Amin-Aid	46.2	Soybean oil, lecithin, monoglycerides and diglycerides	21.2	10.2	0.0	0.92
Attain	35.0	Corn oil, MCT	30.0	10.9	18.2	0.35
Compleat Regular	42.7	Beef, corn oil	36.0	20.9	0.0	0.38
Compleat Modified	36.7	Beef, corn oil	31.0	6.24	0.0	1.84
Comply	60.0	Corn oil	36.0	26.2	0.0	0.72
Criticare HN	5.3	Safflower oil, emulsifiers	4.5	3.4	0.0	0.15
Crucial	67.6	MCT, fish oil, soybean oil, lecithin	39.0	7.7	33.8	3.80
Deliver 2.0	102.0	Soybean oil, MCT	45.0	38.0	29.0	5.60
DiabetiSource	48.7	Sunflower oil, canola oil, beef fat	44.0	4.8	0.0	2.10
Ensure	37.2	Corn oil	31.5	20.0	0.07	0.46
Ensure HN	35.5	Corn oil	30.1	19.1	0.07	0.44
Ensure Plus	53.3	Corn oil	32.0	28.6	0.10	0.66
Ensure Plus HN	50.0	Corn oil	30.0	26.8	0.07	0.62
Ensure with Fiber	37.2	Corn oil	30.5	20.0	0.03	0.46
Entéra	34.0	MCT, sunflower oil	30.0	19.1	4.0	0.00
Entéra Isotonic	34.0	MCT, soybean oil	30.0	19.1	13.0	2.30
Entéra OPD	26.0	MCT, sunflower oil	22.0	19.1	14.3	0.00
Fibersource	41.3	MCT, canola oil	30.0	4.1	21.7	1.73
Fibersource HN	41.3	MCT, canola oil	30.0	4.1	21.7	1.73
Glucerna	55.7	High-oleic safflower oil, soybean oil	50.0	13.2	0.18	0.74
Hepatic-Aid II	36.2	Soybean oil, lecithin, monoglyceride and diglycerides	27.7	8.0	0.0	0.72
Immun-Aid	22.0	Canola oil, MCT	20.0	2.1	11.0	1.20
Impact	28.0	Refined menhaden oil, MCT, structured lipid (from palm kernel/sunflower oils)	25.0	2.5	7.6	1.80
Introlite	18.4	MCT, corn oil, soybean oil	30.0	5.8	7.15	0.16
Isocal	44.0	Soybean oil, MCT	37.0	19.4	8.9	2.70
Isocal HN	45.0	Soybean oil, MCT	37.0	14.4	17.3	2.30
Isocal HCN	102.0	Soybean oil, MCT	45.0	38.0	29.0	5.60
Isosource	41.3	MCT, canola oil	30.0	4.1	21.6	1.70
Isosource HN	41.3	MCT, canola oil	30.0	4.1	21.6	1.70
Isotein HN	34.0	Soybean oil, MCT	25.0	3.7	8.5	0.34
Jevity	34.7	High-oleic safflower oil, canola oil, MCT	29.0	5.2	7.05	1.10
Lipisorb Liquid	57.0	MCT, soy oil	35.0	3.6	48.0	<0.50
Magnacal	80.0	Soybean oil	36.0	29.6	0.0	5.50
Nepro	95.6	High-oleic safflower oil, soy oil	43.0	18.9	Trace	0.80
Newtrition High Nitrogen	40.0	MCT, corn oil	30.0	8.16	15.0	0.56
Newtrition Isofiber	40.0	MCT, corn oil	29.0	10.88	20.0	0.56
Newtrition Isotonic	36.0	MCT, corn oil	31.0	9.79	18.0	0.50
Newtrition One and a Half	50.0	MCT, corn oil	30.0	8.16	25.0	0.70
Nutren 1.0	38.0	Canola oil, MCT, corn oil, lecithin	33.0	8.7	9.0	2.03

*Product information verified by manufacturers 12/94.

Adapted with permission from Gottschlich MM: Selection of optimal lipid sources in enteral and parenteral nutrition. Nutr Clin Prac 1992;7(4):152–165.

Table continued on following page

TABLE 13–3   Fat Content of Selected Enteral Products* *Continued*

Formula	Fat (g/L)	Fat (source)	Fat (% kcal)	Linoleic Acid (g/L)	MCT (g/L)	Omega-3 fatty acids (g/L)
Nutren 1.0 with Fiber	38.0	Canola oil, MCT corn oil, lecithin	33.0	8.7	9.0	2.03
Nutren 1.5	67.5	MCT, canola oil, corn oil, lecithin	39.0	10.5	32.7	2.43
Nutren 2.0	106	MCT, canola oil, lecithin, corn oil	45.0	8.04	77.6	1.84
Nutren VHP	34.0	Canola oil, MCT, corn oil, lecithin	30.0	5.3	8.5	1.70
NutriHep	21.0	MCT, canola oil, lecithin, corn oil	12.0	1.6	14	0.40
NutriVent	94.8	Canola oil, MCT, corn oil, lecithin	55.0	16.1	39.6	4.20
Osmolite	34.7	High-oleic safflower oil, canola oil, MCT	29.0	4.9	6.6	1.00
Osmolite HN	34.7	High-oleic safflower oil, canola oil, MCT	29.0	4.9	6.6	1.00
Pediasure	50.0	Safflower oil, MCT, soybean oil	44.1	10.7	9.5	1.00
Pediasure with Fiber	50.0	Safflower oil, MCT, soybean oil	44.1	10.7	9.5	1.00
Peptamen	39.0	MCT, sunflower oil, lecithin	33.0	5.1	27.0	0.20
Peptamen Junior	38.5	MCT, soybean oil, lecithin, canola oil	33.0	4.7	23.1	0.90
Peptamen VHP	39.0	MCT, soybean oil, lecithin	33.0	3.7	27	0.50
Perative	37.4	Canola oil, MCT, corn oil	25.0	7.48	15.0	1.60
ProBalance	33.8	Canola oil, MCT, corn oil, lecithin	30.0	8.68	6.77	2.15
Promote	26.0	High-oleic safflower oil, canola oil, MCT	23.0	3.9	4.5	0.72
Promote with Fiber	28.2	High-oleic safflower oil, canola oil, MCT	25.0	4.2	5.2	0.78
Pulmocare	93.3	Canola oil, MCT, corn oil, high-oleic safflower oil	55.1	21.4	18.5	5.30
Reabilan	40.5	MCT, soybean oil, canola oil, lecithin	35.0	6.7	20.0	1.20
Reabilan HN	51.9	MCT, soybean oil, canola oil, lecithin	35.0	9.1	26.5	1.60
Replena	95.6	High-oleic safflower oil, soybean oil	43.0	18.9	0.0	0.80
Replete	34.0	Canola oil, MCT, lecithin	30.0	5.54	8.5	2.18
Replete with Fiber	34.0	Canola oil, MCT, lecithin	30.0	5.54	8.5	2.18
Resource Liquid	37.0	Corn oil	32.0	21.8	0.0	0.41
Resource Plus	54.3	Corn oil	32.0	32.0	0.0	0.60
Suplena	95.6	High-oleic safflower oil, soy oil	43.0	18.9	Trace	0.80
Sustacal	23.0	Soybean oil	21.0	8.7	0.0	0.40
Sustacal Plus	58.0	Corn oil	34.0	34.0	0.0	0.30
Sustacal with Fiber	35.0	Corn oil	30.0	21.0	0.0	0.40
Tolerex	1.5	Safflower oil	1.3	1.13	0.0	0.00
TraumaCal	68.0	Soybean oil, MCT	40.0	27.0	20.0	4.30
TwoCal	90.9	Corn oil, MCT	40.1	39.5	17.3	1.21
Ultracal	45.0	Canola oil, MCT	37.0	5.7	18.2	2.40
Vital High Nitrogen	10.8	Safflower oil, MCT	9.4	4.0	3.5	0.08
Vitaneed	40.0	Corn oil, pureed beef	36.0	22.1	0.0	0.60
Vivonex Pediatric	24.0	MCT, soybean oil	25.0	3.84	16.3	0.50
Vivonex TEN	2.8	Safflower oil	3.0	2.8	0.0	0.00
Modules						
MCT	930.0	Coconut oil	100.0	0.0	930.0	0.00
Microlipid	500.0	Safflower oil	100.0	387	0.0	2.50
MaxEPA	930.0	Fish oil	100.0	35.0	0.0	300.00

MCFAs are partially water soluble, and the possibility of nausea, vomiting, abdominal distention, and diarrhea.[18,26] Because MCFAs are metabolized to ketones by the liver, their use is limited in patients prone to ketosis (e.g., diabetic or acidotic patients).[14,16,18]

Short-Chain Fatty Acids

SCFAs include acetate, propionate, and butyrate. Commonly referred to as the volatile fatty acids, they can be produced in the colon as fermentation end products of enzymatic breakdown of dietary fiber and undigested starch. SCFAs are readily absorbed by the GI mucosa and serve as the principal source of fuel for the colon.[6] Studies have shown SCFAs to enhance intestinal blood flow, stimulate mucosal proliferation, and increase colonic sodium, chloride, and water absorption.[6,27-29]

Theoretically, SCFAs may help prevent some of the functional and structural alterations frequently observed in both the small and large bowel following critical illness. At present, commercial tube feeding products do not contain SCFAs as such, perhaps in part because the therapeutic benefit incurred through the enteral route is in doubt; SCFAs are quickly and completely absorbed in the jejunum and therefore do not reach the colon. Consequently, providing fiber is an indirect means of providing SCFAs. Of recent interest is a report by Lynch and colleagues[29] demonstrating that 30 days of orally administered short-chain triglyceride triacetin to rats resulted in significantly elevated DNA concentration in the jejunum and colon compared with animals consuming the long-chain triglyceride diet. Certainly SCFAs and their precursors deserve further investigation to establish their safety and efficacy as enteral substrates during critical care.

Structured Lipids

Structured lipids are formed by the transesterification of MCFAs with LCFAs. Altering the MCFA:LCFA ratio allows a lipid of desired composition to be formed.[14,17,18] This chemical mixture of both MCFA and LCFA on the same glycerol backbone differs distinctly from a simple physical mixture of MCFA and LCFA. The advantages of structured lipids include the ability to provide both an efficient energy substrate in MCFAs along with essential LCFA. For example, structured lipids that combine MCFAs and fish oils have been shown to optimize whole-body protein synthesis and serum albumin levels in burn injury and cancer animal models.[30] Structured lipids have also been shown to decrease infection rates and increase survival rates when compared with conventional triglycerides, since they provide fewer inflammatory and immunosuppressive eicosanoids than conventional lipid emulsions. Their clinical usefulness in enteral support is currently under investigation.

Proteins

Protein provides amino acids and nitrogen for use in tissue repair, immune function, blood clotting, and fluid balance.[31] The protein composition of an enteral substrate is thus an important consideration. In addition to ensuring during product selection that the overall quantity of protein adequately addresses the patient's requirements, protein quality is an additional factor to evaluate. Two commonly used methods of assessing protein quality are determination of chemical score and biologic value (BV) (Table 13-5).[32-35] Chemical score compares the amino acid composition of a food with that of a specific, high-quality protein such as egg albumin. Chemical scores published for a variety of enteral feeding products have revealed some low (range 10 to 72 percent) protein values.[35] BV is the percent of absorbed nitrogen retained for growth or maintenance. In general, proteins with a low chemical score or BV have a higher nonessential amino acid content. The lower the protein's chemical score or BV, the greater the amount of protein required to achieve nitrogen equilibrium.

The forms of protein used in enteral solutions include intact proteins, hydrolyzed proteins, and crystalline amino acids (Table 13-1). How each form of protein affects efficacy and tolerance has been a controversial issue for many years.

Intact proteins are in their original natural form. Some examples are eggs, milk, and meat proteins. Intact proteins separated from the original food are termed "isolates." Some examples are soy protein isolate, lactalbumin, casein or whey from milk, and albumin from egg white. Because of their size, they do not have a significant impact on the formula's osmolality, but they do require normal levels of pancreatic enzymes for complete digestion.[2,3]

The form of protein becomes important when a patient's digestive or absorptive capacity is compromised. Hydrolyzed proteins have been enzymatically broken down to smaller peptide fragments (e.g., oligopeptides, tripeptides, dipeptides) and free amino acids. The smaller particles increase the formula's osmo-

TABLE 13–4   Hypermetabolic/Stress Formulas*

Formula	Source	g/1000 kcal	% kcal
	Intact Protein		
Immun-Aid	Lactalbumin, free amino acids	80	32
Impact	Caseinates, L-arginine	56	22
IsoSource VHN	Caseinates	62	25
Isotein HN	Lactalbumin	57	23
Nitrolan	Caseinates	60	19.1
ProBalance	Caseinates	45	18
Promote	Caseinates, soy protein isolates	62.5	25
Protain XL	Caseinates	55	22
Replete	Caseinates	62.5	25
Sustacal	Casein, soy	60	24
TraumaCal	Caseinates	55	22
	Hydrolyzed Protein/Amino Acids		
Accupep HPF	Hydrolyzed lactalbumin	40	16
Advera	Soy protein hydrolysate, casein	46.9	18.7
AlitraQ	Hydrolyzed soy and lactalbumin, whey, free amino acids, including L-arginine and glutamine	52.5	21
Crucial	Hydrolyzed casein, L-arginine	62.5	25
Peptamen	Hydrolyzed whey	40	16
Peptamen VHP	Hydrolyzed whey	62.5	25
Perative	Partially hydrolyzed caseinate, lactalbumin hydrolysate, L-arginine	51.2	20.5
Reabilan HN	Whey peptides, casein peptides	44	17.5
Sandosource Peptide	Casein hydrolysate, free amino acids, casein	50.0	20.0
Tolerex	Free amino acids including L-arginine and glutamine	45	18
Vital HN	Partially hydrolyzed whey, meat and soy, free essential amino acids	41.7	16.7

*Product information verified by manufacturers 12/94.

Fat			Carbohydrate			Energy	
Source	g/1000 kcal	% kcal	Source	g/1000 kcal	% kcal	NPC:N	kcal/ml
Canola oil, MCT	22	20	Maltodextrin	120	48	52.3:1	1.0
Structured lipid from palm kernel oil and sunflower menhaden oil	28	25	Hydrolyzed corn starch	132	53	71:1	1.0
Canola oil, MCT	29	25	Hydrolyzed corn starch, soy polysaccharide, modified guar	130	50	77:1	1.0
Soybean oil, MCT	29	25	Hydrolyzed corn starch, fructose	133	52	86:1	1.19
Corn oil, MCT	32	29	Maltodextrin	129	52	104:1	1.24
Canola oil, MCT, corn oil, lecithin	33.9	30	Maltrodextrin	130	52	114:1	1.2
Safflower oil, canola, MCT	26	23	Hydrolyzed corn starch, sucrose	130	52	75:1	1.0
MCT, corn oil	30	27	Maltodextrin	138	51	89:1	1.0
Canola oil, MCT	34	30	Maltodextrin, corn syrup	113	45	75:1	1.0
Soy oil	23	21	Corn syrup, sucrose	138	55	78:1	1.0
Soy oil, MCT	46	40	Corn syrup, sucrose	95	38	91:1	1.5
MCT, corn oil	10	8.5	Maltodextrin	188.8	75.5	134:1	1.0
Canola oil, MCT, sardine oil	17.8	15.8	Hydrolyzed corn starch, sucrose, soy polysaccharide	168.6	65.5	108:1	1.28
MCT, safflower oil	15.5	13	Hydrolyzed corn starch, sucrose, fructose	165	66	94:1	1.0
MCT, fish oil, soy, lecithin	45	39	Maltodextrin, starch	90	36	67:1	1.5
MCT, sunflower oil	39	33	Maltodextrin, starch	127	51	131:1	1.0
MCT, soy oil, lecithin	39	33	Maltrodextrin, corn starch	104	42	76:1	1.0
Canola oil, MCT, corn oil	28.8	25	Maltodextrin	136.3	54.5	97:1	1.3
MCT, soybean oil, canola oil, lecithin	40.5	35	Maltodextrin, tapioca starch	119	47.5	117:1	1.33
Soybean oil, MCT	17.6	15	Hydrolyzed corn starch	163.2	65.0	100:1	1.0
Safflower oil	6.7	6	Glucose, oligosaccharides	190	76	282:1	1.0
Safflower oil, MCT	10.8	9.4	Hydrolyzed corn-starch, sucrose, lactose	185	73.9	125:1	1.0

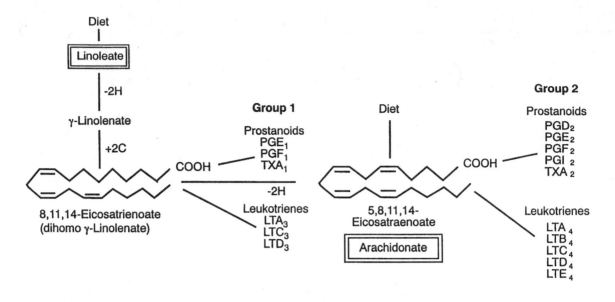

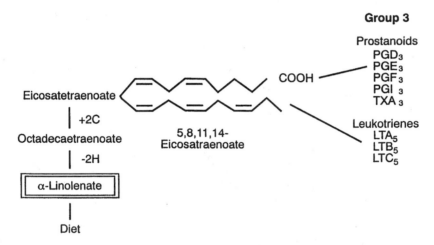

FIGURE 13–3 Pathways of eicosanoid synthesis from long-chain fatty acids. (Adapted with permission from Mayes PA: Metabolism of unsaturated fatty acids and eicosanoids. In Murray RK, Mayes PA, Granner DK (eds): Harper's Biochemistry. Norwalk, CT: Appleton & Lange, 1990:218–225.)

TABLE 13–5 Formulas for Determining Protein Quality

Chemical Score (CS)

$$CS = \frac{\text{Essential/total essential amino acids (product)}}{\text{Essential/total essential amino acids (egg)}} \times 100$$

Biologic Value (BV)

$$BV = \frac{\text{Dietary nitrogen} - (\text{urinary nitrogen} + \text{fecal nitrogen})}{\text{Dietary nitrogen} - \text{fecal nitrogen}} \times 100$$

---

lality. Although the larger peptides are broken down to smaller peptides and amino acids before absorption, the small peptides have specific carrier systems and can be absorbed intact. Formulas that contain protein hydrolysates frequently have free amino acids (e.g., methionine, tyrosine, and tryptophan) added to enhance their protein quality.[2,3]

Crystalline amino acids are available commercially through a fermentation process developed in Japan. Because the body uses the L-forms of crystalline amino acids, they are added to these formulas. Crystalline amino acids are about 10 times more expensive than their equivalent protein counterparts and contribute significantly to increased osmolality of enteral formulas due to their small size. They also may adversely affect taste. They need no further digestion but require the presence of sodium for absorption.[2,3]

Peptides

Current evidence supports the existence of separate transport systems for free amino acids and peptides. The promotion of peptide-containing formulas for patients with impaired digestion or absorption is based on research demonstrating a more rapid and efficient absorption of nitrogen in the form of peptides than free amino acid preparations by both the healthy and diseased gut.[36-38] A study by Silk and colleagues[36] used an intestinal perfusion technique in healthy volunteers to compare the absorption of peptide hydrolysates and their respective equimolar free amino acid mixtures. The results indicated that more nitrogen was absorbed from the hydrolysates than the respective free amino acid mixture and that improved absorption of specific amino acids occurred with the hydrolysates. An increase in serum visceral proteins was noted by Feller and coworkers[39] when they compared a peptide-based formula with an amino acid–based formula. Although the serum visceral proteins increased with the use of the peptide-containing formula, no change in the anthropometrics of the patients occurred.

Many of the comparative data published on peptide formulas to date serve only to confirm their superiority over free amino acids, over intravenous nutrition, or over starvation.[36,39,40] In fact, preliminary data indicate that peptides do not offer any advantages over standard enteral formulas in terms of tolerance or outcome in acutely injured.[41] To date, their initial promise has not been realized, and it is possible that hydrolysate-based diets are unnecessary in an optimally managed enteral feeding regimen. It is important to recognize that chemically defined diets offer less trophic stimulation to the bowel and are immunosuppressive[42,43]; consequently their use should be reserved for conditions that clearly warrant predigested products. Hydrolysate formulas are commonly prescribed for patients with impaired digestion, short-bowel syndrome, chronic intractable diarrhea, and inflammatory bowel disease (IBD) as well as for hypoalbuminemic or undernourished patients with or without intestinal diseases, conditions for which clinical trials providing evidence of superior efficiency of these products have not been adequate. There could be a number of disorders for which these substrates may be important, but their applications require closer scrutiny.

Branched-Chain Amino Acids

Branched-chain amino acids (BCAAs) — valine, leucine, and isoleucine — are essential amino acids that are mobilized from skeletal muscle during metabolic stress. It has been proposed that providing formulas with high percentages of BCAAs to severely catabolic, stressed, or traumatized patients may help preserve muscle, thus possibly improving outcome. In addition, for the patient with hepatic insufficiency, regimens with high ratios of BCAAs to aromatic amino acids have been recommended. In both the critically ill or liver-failure patient, numerous groups have assessed enteral BCAA therapy. Table 13–6 reviews the percentage of protein contributed by BCAAs in commercial products. Several enteral studies have found supplemental BCAAs to decrease the endogenous breakdown of somatic and visceral proteins, resulting in improved nitrogen retention and metabolic management.[44-46] However the use of products fortified with BCAAs at levels greater than those typically inherent in protein has not consistently demonstrated clinical benefit.[47-52] It is disappointing that thus far much of the success reported with parenteral BCAAs[53] has not been replicated using the enteral route. Evaluation of the current efficacy trials of enteral BCAA therapy is difficult because many of the investigations have not controlled for the degree of stress, encephalopathy, or presence of sepsis. Furthermore, small patient samples have been employed and different amounts of BCAAs and control diets used.

Glutamine

Glutamine classically has been considered a nonessential amino acid, but recent studies indicate that it may be conditionally essential during stress and starvation.[54,55] The most abundant free amino acid in plasma and body tissues, glutamine comprises approximately half the whole body pool of amino acids.[2,55] Glutamine is the principal carrier of nitrogen from skeletal muscle to visceral organs because

TABLE 13–6   Total Glutamine, Arginine, and Branched-Chain Amino Acid Content of Selected Enteral Formulas*

Formula	Manufacturer	Protein Source	Glutamine (g/L)	Arginine (g/L)	% BCAA Protein
AlitraQ	Ross	Lactalbumin and soy hydrolysates, free amino acids	14.2–15.5	4.5	18.5
Advera	Ross	Soy protein hydrolysate, casein	5.4–6.4	4.1	15.4
Citrosource	Sandoz	Whey	3.2	0.8	23.8
Citrotein	Sandoz	Egg white solids	2.6	2.4	21.2
Compleat Modified	Sandoz	Beef, casein	4.3	2.3	19.5
Compleat Regular	Sandoz	Beef, nonfat milk	4.1	2.5	19.4
Criticare HN	Mead Johnson	Casein hydrolysate, amino acids	1.6–2.4	1.5	23.7
Crucial	Clintec	Hydrolyzed casein, L-arginine	7.2	15.0	17.6
DiabetiSource	Sandoz	Casein, beef	4.9	1.9	19.1
Deliver 2.0	Mead Johnson	Casein	6.5–9.6	3	22.8
Ensure with Fiber	Ross	Casein, soy protein isolate	3.57–4.96	1.55	18.8
Ensure	Ross	Casein, soy protein isolate	3.34–4.65	1.45	18.8
Ensure HN	Ross	Casein, soy protein isolate	4–5.6	1.73	18.8
Ensure Plus	Ross	Casein, soy protein isolate	4.94–6.87	2.1	18.8
Ensure Plus HN	Ross	Casein, soy protein isolate	5.63–7.83	2.4	18.8
Entrition HN Diet	Clintec	Casein	3.84–5.49	1.6	21.0
Fibersource	Sandoz	Casein	4.8	1.6	20.8
Fibersource HN	Sandoz	Casein	5.9	2.0	20.9
Glucerna	Ross	Casein	3.8–5.4	1.5	19.0
Immun-Aid	McGaw	Lactalbumin, amino acids	12.5	15.4	36.1
Impact	Sandoz	Casein, L-arginine	5.9	14.0	17.1
Introlite	Ross	Casein	2–2.77	0.86	18.8
Isocal	Mead Johnson	Casein, soy	3–4.1	1.3	22.1
Isocal HN	Mead Johnson	Casein, soy	3.9	1.7	22.0
Isosource	Sandoz	Casein, soy	4.7	1.8	20.6
Isosource HN	Sandoz	Casein, soy	5.8	2.3	20.6
Isotein HN	Sandoz	Delactosed lactalbumin	6.0	1.9	22.4
Jevity	Ross	Casein	4–5.77	1.46	19.0
Lipisorb Liquid	Mead Johnson	Casein	7.3	2.3	22.8
Meritene	Sandoz	Nonfat milk, whole milk	7.3	2.5	22.2
Nepro	Ross	Casein	6.3–9.1	2.5	20.7
Nutren 1.0	Clintec	Casein	3.47–5.11	1.5	21.4
Nutren 1.5	Clintec	Casein	5.21–7.67	2.2	21.0
Nutren 2.0	Clintec	Casein	6.94–10.22	3.0	21.0
Nutren 1.0 with Fiber	Clintec	Casein	3.47–5.11	1.5	21.4
Nutren Junior	Clintec	Casein, whey	1.81–2.67	0.9	21.0
NutriVent Diet	Clintec	Casein	5.9–8.69	2.5	21.0
Osmolite	Ross	Casein, soy protein isolate	3.35–4.66	1.45	18.8
Osmolite HN	Ross	Casein, soy protein isolate	4–5.6	1.73	18.8
Pediasure	Ross	Casein, low-lactose whey	2.48–3.47	0.96	20.3
Pediasure with Fiber	Ross	Casein, low-lactose whey	2.48–3.47	0.96	20.3
Peptamen	Clintec	Hydrolyzed whey	3.0	1.2	21.0
Peptamen Junior	Clintec	Hydrolyzed whey	2.2	0.9	21.0
Peptamen VHP	Clintec	Whey	4.6	1.9	21.0
Perative	Ross	Casein and lactalbumin hydrolysate, L-arginine	5.4	14.7	18.2

*Product information verified by manufacturers 12/94; compiled by Michele Gottschlich, PhD, RD, and Theresa Mayes, RD. Glutamine content of some products for which data were not available per pharmaceutical company was thereby mathematically derived using methods described by Swails WS, Bell SJ, Borlase BC et al: Glutamine content of whole proteins: implications for enteral formulas. Nutr Clin Prac 1992;7(2):77–80.

TABLE 13–6 Total Glutamine, Arginine, and Branched-Chain Amino Acid Content of Selected Enteral Formulas* *Continued*

Formula	Manufacturer	Protein Source	Glutamine (g/L)	Arginine (g/L)	% BCAA Protein
ProBalance	Clintec	Casein	4.69–6.91	2.04	21.0
Promote	Ross	Casein, soy protein isolate	5.6–8.0	2.4	20.16
Promote with Fiber	Ross	Casein	5.6–8.0	2.1	19.0
Protain	Sherwood	Casein	5.5	1.98	21.0
Pulmocare	Ross	Casein	5.0	3.3	19.0
Reabilan	Clintec	Hydrolyzed whey	5.0	1.0	21.0
Reabilan HN	Clintec	Hydrolyzed casein and whey	9.3	1.9	21.0
Replete	Clintec	Casein	5.43–7.99	2.4	21.0
Replete with Fiber	Clintec	Casein	5.43–7.99	2.4	21.0
Resource	Sandoz	Casein, soy	4.4	1.5	21.4
Resource Plus	Sandoz	Casein, soy	6.1	2.1	20.3
Respalor	Mead Johnson	Casein	6.6–9.7	3.1	22.8
Sandosource Peptide	Sandoz	Casein hydrolysate, free amino acids	4.7	5.0	30
Suplena	Ross	Casein	2.6–8.9	1.1	20.7
Sustacal Basic	Mead Johnson	Casein, soy	3.2–4.6	1.3	19.8
Sustacal Plus	Mead Johnson	Casein	5.3–7.8	2.5	23.3
Sustacal	Mead Johnson	Casein, soy	5.4–7.3	2.6	20.9
Tolerex	Sandoz	Free amino acids	3.5	1.8	16.8
Traumacal	Mead Johnson	Casein	7.2–10.60	3.3	22.8
TwoCal HN	Ross	Casein	7.5–10.9	2.76	19.0
Ultracal	Mead Johnson	Casein	3.8–5.6	1.8	22.8
Vital HN	Ross	Partially hydrolyzed whey, meat, and soy; free essential amino acids	1.8–2.2	2.1	17.9
Vivonex Pediatric	Sandoz	Free amino acids	3.1	1.5	21.6
Vivonex Plus	Sandoz	Free amino acids	10	5.0	30

of its two amino groups.[54,55] In addition, it helps regulate acid-base balance by producing ammonia,[54] is a precursor of nucleic acids, nucleotides, amino sugars, and proteins,[6,54] and is the preferred respiratory fuel for rapidly proliferating cells such as enterocytes, macrophages, and lymphocytes.[54,55] Some studies indicate that supplemental glutamine prevents deterioration in gut permeability and preserves mucosal structure and function.[55-56] The therapeutic effects of glutamine are presented in more detail in Chapter 8.

Currently it is unclear whether glutamine must be in a free form to exert a beneficial effect or whether glutamine in any form will help the gut maintain its integrity. Most enteral formulas contain some protein-bound glutamine, and some tube-feeding products contain glutamine as a free amino acid (Table 13–4). If the glutamine in the formula is in the form of a free amino acid, then the amount is usually listed on the label. If the glutamine is protein bound,

then the amount may have to be estimated.[57] The amount of glutamine present will depend on the protein source, the amount of protein in the formula, and the processing conditions. Partially hydrolyzed protein will have a lower glutamine content when compared with the protein source because hydrolysis leads to the degradation of some glutamine. Table 13–6 compares the glutamine content of various tube-feeding products.

The optimal levels of glutamine supplementation for different disease states is still being determined. In enterally fed rats after small bowel resection, the maximal effect of glutamine supplementation occurred when glutamine was 25 percent of the total amino acids.[58] Glutamine supplementation of 20 to 40 g/day (23 to 44 percent of total amino acids or 0.29 to 0.57 g/kg of body weight/day) in healthy subjects and postsurgery patients has been well tolerated without evidence of toxicity such as abnormalities in hepatic function, mental status, or blood ammonia levels.[59] Administration of glutamine may be contraindicated in patients with hyperammonemia, hepatic encephalopathy, and renal failure because of its high ammonigenic potential. Glutamine is also considered a preferred fuel for many tumors, which may limit its use in patients with actively growing cancers who are not receiving any antiproliferative treatment.[60] However, a study by Klimberg and associates demonstrated that glutamine supplementation during methotrexate administration in a sarcoma rat model enhanced the drug's tumoricidal effectiveness while reducing morbidity and mortality.[61] Other studies that used the same model showed that glutamine-enriched enteral or parenteral diets repleted host glutamine stores and supported muscle glutamine metabolism without stimulating tumor growth.[62,63] More prospective, randomized human studies are needed to establish safe and effective doses of glutamine and to document its effects on nutrition and disease outcomes.

Arginine

Arginine, once thought to be a nonessential amino acid, is now considered semiessential in times of metabolic stress.[64] Arginine promotes the release of pituitary growth factor, prolactin, insulin, growth hormone, and insulinlike growth factor.[65-67] Arginine supplementation also improves nitrogen balance in stressed individuals,[68,69] enhances reparative collagen synthesis in animals and humans,[65,69,70] and improves immune function.[65,68,69,71,72] A thorough review of arginine can be found in Chapter 8.

In the past, enteral formulas have always contained small amounts of arginine (approximately 1 to 2 g/L), although recently several arginine-enriched products (14 to 15 g/L) have entered the market (Table 13–6). The effects of arginine on immune function and wound healing show exciting promise. However, sufficient studies delineating optimal intake guidelines are still lacking; therefore, selection of a product based solely on its arginine content is unwarranted at this time.

Taurine

Taurine is considered essential for infants and children. It therefore should be a component of pediatric tube-feeding programs. Taurine is important for normal retinal development. It is involved in a wide variety of metabolic processes (e.g., conjugation of bile acids, which is instrumental to micellar formation

and fat absorption).[73] Taurine also helps regulate cell volume, reduces platelet aggregation, serves as a neuromodulator, aids in the function of neutrophils, and is an antioxidant.[73-76] Requirements for taurine during metabolic stress have not been determined. However, taurine is synthesized from cysteine, and some studies indicate that the conversion of methionine to cysteine may be limited during metabolic stress.[77-80] Further investigation is warranted to delineate the role of taurine in enteral support.

Carnitine

Carnitine is a dipeptide produced primarily in the kidney and liver from lysine and methionine.[81] It is required by carnitine acyltransferase, the enzyme necessary to transport LCFAs into the mitochondria. A carnitine deficiency can be due to malnutrition, antibiotic therapy, carnitine-free parenteral or enteral feeding, or impairment of carnitine metabolism as a result of burns, hypermetabolism, or liver disease. Clinical signs of carnitine deficiency include hypoglycemia, progressive muscle weakness, and lipid accumulation in muscle fibers, which can produce skeletal myopathy, cardiomyopathy, or hypertriglyceridemia. Carnitine is currently available in a few enteral products, and L-carnitine is available in tablet or liquid form for supplementation.

Nucleotides

Nucleosides are composed of a sugar (usually D-ribose and 2-deoxy-D-ribose) attached to a purine or pyrimidine. Nucleotides are nucleosides with a phosphate group added to the sugar. They serve as cofactors, regulators, energy sources, and precursors for nucleic acid synthesis. When carbohydrate, protein, phosphate, and vitamin intake is adequate, de novo nucleotide synthesis is sufficient to meet the needs of an unstressed organism. Therefore, extrinsic supplementation of nucleotides has long been considered unnecessary. However, recent findings suggest they may play important roles in enhancing immune function[82-85] and intestinal development[86] as well as in the recovery of small intestine function and morphology after chronic diarrhea.[87] Thus, an exogenous source of purines and pyrimidines may be beneficial under certain conditions. Studies are not, however, consistently positive about the benefits of or necessity for dietary nucleotides,[52] and it appears that enteral supplementation is less effective than intravenous or intraperitoneal administration.[82,88] Their potential role therefore remains investigational.

Micronutrients

Carbohydrate, protein, fat, and energy cannot be efficiently used if essential cofactors and coenzymes are inadequate. Vitamin, mineral, and trace element supplementation should take into consideration the patient's nutritional status at the onset of the illness as well as the metabolic impact of stress and disease, although the effect of critical illness on micronutrient requirements is not precisely known. In general, at least 100 percent of the U.S. Recommended Daily Allowance (RDA) should be provided when the prescribed daily volume of enteral formula is administered. Deficient intake in cases such as low-calorie regimens or diluted formulas requires supplementation. Supplementation is likewise indicated for patients presenting with heightened needs or losses or for those individuals whose nutritional status was suboptimal before the onset of illness. Furthermore, enrichment with certain micronutrients may help boost immune function, accelerate wound healing, and minimize some of the negative metabolic effects associated with critical illness (Chapter 7).

Physical Characteristics

The physical characteristics of an enteral formula such as osmolality, renal solute load, pH, residue, viscosity, and caloric density could play important roles in a patient's response to a specific formula. Complications such as diarrhea, nausea, vomiting, abdominal distention, and aspiration pneumonia may be related to physical characteristics. In this section, these factors will be discussed with consideration given as to how they influence selection of an enteral formula.

Osmolality

Osmolality represents the number of osmoles of the particles (solutes) in a kilogram of solvent. Osmolarity refers to the number of osmoles per liter of solution (solvent plus solute). Osmolarity is thus influenced by the volumes of all the solutes contained in the solution as well as temperature, while osmolality is not. Although there are only small clinical differences between the terms osmolality and osmolarity, osmolality is generally considered the correct term for enteral products.

In the 1970s and 1980s it was suggested that high osmolality in enteral formulas was the primary cause of tube-feeding-related diarrhea. Consequently it has become a widespread practice to initiate tube feeding using diluted formulas or isotonic products in an effort to avoid diarrhea. More recent findings in healthy and sick patients do not support the notion that diet tonicity is significantly related to incidence of diarrhea.[89-92] Although osmolality of a formula may affect its tolerance, more important factors may include inappropriate formula selection and the absence of fiber.

Any dietary component that is soluble in water contributes to the osmolality of a solution. Osmolality is inversely related to the molecular size of the nutrients in solution. The smaller the particle size, the greater the effect on osmolality. Major determinants of enteral product osmolality are amino acids, small peptides, electrolytes, and simple carbohydrates. Solution concentration also affects osmolality. Therefore, calorically dense formulas with hydrolyzed nutrients are significantly more hyperosmolar than standard intact nutrient products. The osmolality of enteral formulas currently ranges from 270 to 700 mOsm/kg and should be considered during product selection.

Renal Solute Load

The renal solute load of an enteral formula is determined primarily by the content of protein and the electrolytes sodium, potassium, and chloride. The greater the renal solute load, the greater the obligatory water loss through the kidneys. If this water is not provided, the patient will become dehydrated. This is of particular concern with high-protein feeding regimens used in pediatric or geriatric populations. The renal solute load should also be considered in patients with impaired renal function or those with increased fluid losses from fever, diarrhea, vomiting, or burn injuries.

pH

Solutions with a pH of less than 3.5 will reduce gastric motility.[93] This does not appear to be a major concern with most commercial products,[2] because the pH levels generally exceed this.

Residue

Many formulas contain little or no residue. Diets that are low in residue result in decreased stool mass. In addition, stool passage is less frequent. This may be indicated before certain diagnostic procedures or in the management of specific GI disorders. On the other hand, low-residue diets may cause constipation, and fiber-containing products may be helpful in regulating bowel function.

Viscosity

Formulas containing fiber and products that have a higher caloric content per unit volume tend to be more viscous. More viscous formulas require a larger-bore feeding tube; however, larger tubes are generally less comfortable for the patient.

Caloric Density

The amount of energy per unit volume of formula is its caloric density, measured in kcal/ml. Most tube feedings yield 1 kcal/ml; however, 1.5 and 2 kcal/ml products are also available. More calorically dense formulas also have higher osmolality and renal solute loads. Therefore, the patient must be monitored carefully to prevent dehydration.

DEFINITIONS AND CATEGORIZATION OF DEFINED FORMULAS

In general, the selection of an enteral formula diet is based on an assessment of the patient as well as of the formula (Table 13–7). Considerations include pertinent medical conditions as well as the patient's ability to digest and absorb nutrients, total nutrient requirements or restrictions, and an objective evaluation of the physical, molecular, and physiologic characteristics of the enteral products under deliberation.

Formulas used for enteral feeding have been classified according to various criteria. The names given to different classes of solutions have not always been consistent and often overlap, thus leading to lack of clarity and confusion. The general term "medical foods" has been used since 1989 by the Food and Drug Administration (FDA) to define enteral nutrition products. Further characterization of medical foods and regulatory aspects of enteral substrates have been recently reviewed.[48,94,95]

The key to alimenting a patient successfully with a tube-feeding regimen is centered on appropriate product selection. Although there are more than 100 commercially available defined formulas, they can be classified into relatively few categories to assist in product selection decisions.

Three basic classification systems exist for enteral formulas. The simplest way to group formulas is to classify them as either "complete" or "incomplete" depending on their essential nutrient profile. Complete formulas contain all necessary nutrients in sufficient quantities to maintain the nutritional status of a normal, healthy individual receiving no other source of nourishment. Incomplete formulas lack one or more essential nutrients and may need supplementation if used for long-term feeding.

Another system of enteral diet categorization subdivides formulas according to the molecular form of the nutrients they contain, as either intact (polymeric), semielemental (oligomeric), or elemental (monomeric). Intact formulas (Table 13–1) contain carbohydrate, protein, and fat in large molecular form. They require normal digestion and absorption and supply all of the necessary nutrients for complete nutrition when a total daily prescription of, on average, 2 L is administered. Additional characteristics of

TABLE 13–7 Factors To Consider In Formula Selection

Assessment of Patient	Assessment of Formula
Past medical history and present problems	Composition of carbohydrate, protein, and fat
Age	Calorie:nitrogen ratio
Calorie and nutrient requirements	Electrolyte, vitamin, mineral, and trace element content
Hydration status	Osmolality
GI function	Renal solute load
Hepatic function	pH
Renal function	Residue/fiber content
Pulmonary status	Viscosity
	Caloric density
	Convenience of administration
	Bacteriologic safety
	Cost

polymeric formulas include the fact that they are usually lactose free and caseinate or soy protein isolate based. Protein content and caloric density ranges from standard (40 g protein/L; 1.0 kcal/mL) to high (84 g protein/L; 2.0 kcal/mL). Although most formulas are low residue, some are supplemented with fiber (5 to 14.4 g/L), usually as soy polysaccharide, although formulas with oat and guar fiber are also available. Many are palatable so that they may be used for oral supplements.

Oligomeric or semielemental formulas contain macronutrients that have been hydrolyzed by enzymatic action to varying degrees. Products in this category with the protein source as larger peptides are isotonic, whereas those formulas containing a portion of the protein source as free amino acids are hypertonic. Monomeric formula implies that all the nutrients are in their monomeric form. In general, oligomeric and monomeric formulas are lactose free and contain minimal residue. They vary in their fat content, ranging from 1 to 35 percent of the calories as fat. Those formulas containing few calories from fat may be limited in essential fatty acids, which restricts their long-term use. Because hydrolyzed formulas (Tables 13–1 and 13–4) require minimal digestion and absorption, they may be appropriate for patients with compromised digestive and absorptive capacity.

A third means of grouping, the descriptive method of classification, is based on the formula's overall characteristics. Using this system, formulas are categorized as blenderized, milk-based, standard, chemically defined and free amino acids, specialized, or feeding modules.[96]

Blenderized Products

Blenderized products are either kitchen-blenderized or commercially prepared liquids. The commercial formulas are nutritionally complete, contain high-quality proteins (usually meat or milk), and have moderate to high residue levels. The advantages of these products are that they are readily available, include micronutrients, fiber and undefined nutrients normally found in regular table food, and usually restore or maintain normal bowel movements. Contamination of these formulas during home or hospital preparation procedures is not uncommon. Other disadvantages include a high viscosity, making passage through small-bore feeding tubes problematic, difficulty in quality control because they are made from natural foods, and a need for complete digestive capabilities. Finally, many of these formulas contain lactose, which may be contraindicated in some patients.

Milk-Based Products

Milk-based products contain milk as a primary source of protein. These high-residue formulas are indicated for patients unable to consume a regular diet adequately. Patients require normal GI function as well as the ability to digest lactose. Formulas in this group are generally more palatable than milk-free products. They are well accepted as oral supplements and are also relatively inexpensive. The chief disadvantage is that they contain lactose. It is now widely recognized that many adults, especially blacks, Chinese, and persons of Mediterranean descent, have insufficient lactase concentrations in their intestinal brush borders. As much as 15 percent of the adult, white population has this same problem.[97] The critically ill patient is also prone to lactase deficiency secondary to brush border atrophy. Classic symptoms of lactose intolerance such as diarrhea, abdominal bloating, and cramping are often confused with more serious pathologic states and can inhibit adequate enteral support.

Standard Products

Products in this category are most often considered to represent "standard" tube feeding regimens because they are nutritionally complete, low in cost, create few osmolar problems, are lactose free, and include a wide range of choices relative to protein source, fat, and carbohydrate content.

Chemically Defined and Free Amino Acid Formulas

Chemically defined and free amino acid formulas require little or no digestion for their absorption. Frequently referred to as "elemental diets," this term is actually a misnomer because they are not composed of chemical elements in the strictest sense (e.g., carbon, nitrogen), but recently it has become increasingly misrepresentative. Originally, this term was used to describe monomeric elements of normal food such as free amino acids, simple carbohydrates, and virtually no fat. Later on, elemental diets began to accrue longer carbohydrate moieties, then peptides were included, and finally some products designated elemental contained fat substrates comparable to those of standard formulas, although usually with substantial proportions of medium-chain triglycerides.

The original prototype for this class of formulas consisted of free amino acids, oligosaccharides and glucose, and a small amount of safflower oil. Several partially hydrolyzed formulas consisting of short-chain polypeptides, hydrolyzed starches or maltodextrin, and moderate quantities of fat were subsequently developed. More recently, products containing a high proportion of protein as dipeptides and tripeptides have become available (Table 13–4).

Specialty Products

Specialized enteral formulas are designed for use by patients with organ failure, metabolic dysfunction, or heightened or restricted nutrient requirements and include both intact

TABLE 13–8 Considerations In Evaluating Specialized Enteral Formulas

- Nutrient profile is appropriate based on the known metabolic abnormalities and nutrient requirements of the given condition.
- Look for prospective, randomized, controlled, double-blind studies (not case reports).
- Data obtained using animal models may have limited applicability to humans. Extrapolation from animal models to humans must be done carefully, with the fullest possible understanding of the biochemical and physiologic differences between the two species.
- Product-specific research applies to that product only.
- Product-specific research sometimes cannot be generalized to a different population (e.g., results from studies with burn patients may not necessarily apply to trauma patients).
- When evaluating a specific formula, develop critieria by which to judge the product.

TABLE 13–10 Calorically Dense and Renal Failure Enteral Formula Comparison*

	AminAid (McGaw)	Deliver 2.0 (Mead Johson)	Magnacal (Sherwood)
Carbohydrate	187	100	125
g/1000 kcal	74.8	40	50
% kcal Source	Maltodextrin, sucrose	Corn syrup	Maltodextrin, sucrose
Protein	10	38	35
g/1000 kcal	4	15	14
% kcal Source	Essential amino acids plus histidine	Sodium and calcium caseinate	Sodium, calcium caseinates
Fat	24	51	40
g/1000 kcal	21.2	45	36
% kcal Source	Soybean oil, lecithin, monoglycerides, diglycerides	Soy oil, MCT	Soy oil
NPC:N	800:1	145:1	157:1
Caloric density (kcal/ml)	2.0	2.0	2.0
Sodium			
mg/1000 kcal	<177 mg	400	500
mEq/1000 kcal	<7.7 mEq	17.4	21.8
Potassium			
mg/1000 kcal	<118 mg	850	625
mEq/1000 kcal	<3 mEq	22	16
Calcium mg/1000 kcal	0	510	500
Magnesium mg/1000 kcal	0	200	200
Phosphorus mg/1000 kcal	0	510	500
Water-soluble vitamins	No	Yes	Yes
Fat-soluble vitamins	No	Yes	Yes

NPC:N = nonprotein calorie: nitrogen (g) ratio.
*Product information verified by manufacturers 12/94.

TABLE 13–9   Liver Failure Enteral Formula Product Comparison*

	NutriHep (Clintec Nutrition Company)		Hepatic Aid II (McGaw Laboratories)	
	Source	**per 1000 kcal**	**Source**	**per 1000 kcal**
Carbohydrate	Maltodextrin Modified cornstarch	193 g	Maltodextrins	143 g
Amino acids	L-amino acids Whey protein 50% BCAA 2.4% AAA	26.7 g protein 31 g amino acids	L-amino acids 46% BCAA 1.87% AAA	44.1 g
Fat	MCT (66%) Canola oil Soy lecithin Corn oil	14 g	Soybean oil Lecithin Monoglycerides and diglycerides	36.2 g
Sodium		213.3 mg 9.3 mEq		<345 mg <15 mEq
Potassium		880 mg 22.6 mEq		<230 mg <6 mEq
Caloric density (kcal/ml)	1.5		1.2	

BCAA = Branched chain amino acids; AAA = Aromatic amino acids; MCT = Medium-chain triglycerides.
*Information obtained from manufacturer's and product information 12/94.

Nepro (Ross)	Nutren 2.0 (Clintec)	Renalcal (Clintec)	Suplena (Ross Labs)	Two Cal HN (Ross)
107.6	98	145.2	127.6	109
43	39	58	51	43.2
Hydrolyzed cornstarch, sucrose	Corn syrup solids, maltodextrins, sucrose	Maltodextrins, modified corn starch	Hydrolyzed cornstarch, sucrose	Hydrolyzed cornstarch, sucrose
34.9	40	17.2	14.9	42
14	16	6.9	6	16.7
Calcium, magnesium, sodium caseinates	Casein	Whey protein concentrate	Sodium and calcium caseinates	Sodium and calcium caseinates
47.8	53	41.2	47.8	45
43	45	35	43	40.1
High-oleic safflower oil, soy oil	MCT, canola oil, lecithin	MCT, canola oil	High-oleic safflower oil, soy oil	Corn and MCT oils
154:1	131:1	338:1	393:1	125:1
2.0	2.0	2.0	2.0	2.0
415	650	<40 mg	392	655
18.1	28.3	<1.74	17.0	28.4
528	960	<40 mg	558	122.1
13.5	24.6	<1.02	14.3	31.2
686	670	<30	693	526
105	268	<10	105	210
343	670	<60	364	526
Yes	Yes	Yes	Yes	Yes
Yes	Yes	No	Yes	Yes

and hydrolyzed nutrients. A wide spectrum of specialty products are available and include medical foods that attempt to address the unique needs of the hypermetabolic or stressed individual, patients with hepatic or renal failure, GI dysfunction, pulmonary insufficiency, and diabetic and pediatric patients.

When considering specialty formulas, one should critically evaluate the formula composition and studies supporting its use (Table 13–8). Manufacturer claims for a product's intended use may not always equate with sound scientific principles. In addition to asking if the formula nutrient profile is appropriate based on the known metabolic abnormalities and nutrient requirements of a given condition, one should ask if the formula was designed and field tested using well-designed studies.[47,96,98]

Hypermetabolism/Stress Formulas

Catabolic processes predominate in hypermetabolic patients, increasing calorie and protein requirements (Chapters 18 and 19). A number of enteral products are available for use in patients with metabolic stress (Table 13–4). Most of these formulas are nutritionally complete with a high protein content to deliver 1.5 to 2 g/kg/day or have a nonprotein calorie to nitrogen ratio less than 125:1 needed for critically ill patients. Caution must be maintained when using the more calorically dense products, since their high osmolality without additional free water could lead to dehydration and azotemia.

Several enteral solutions designed for use in hypermetabolic patients contain high concentrations of BCAAs (Table 13–6), although there have been no significant demonstrable benefits with BCAAs on morbidity, length of hospital stay, or mortality in the critically ill.[47,52] Therefore, the use of these products should be restricted to the highly catabolic patient with markedly negative nitrogen balance, increasing blood urea nitrogen, or intolerance to standard diets.

More recently, other unique nutrients have been included in enteral formulas for use in critically ill patients. Formulas containing free amino acids and peptides were developed for use in patients with marginally functioning GI tracts. These formulas contain a limited amount of fat and provide a large percentage of total calories as carbohydrate. Formulas containing peptides as the nitrogen source provide protein as small molecular weight peptides or a mixture of peptides and free amino acids. Most of the peptide formulas contain fat as a mixture of long-chain and medium-chain triglycerides. Fiber has also been added to some of these formulas. The newest enteral formulas for use in critically ill patients contain glutamine, arginine, omega-3 fatty acids, and nucleotides as single agents or in combination. Several studies have been published documenting a significant effect on outcome parameters with the use of these formulas,[72,99-106] although additional well-designed, prospective, randomized, controlled studies are needed to substantiate their true clinical efficacy.[47]

Hepatic Failure Formulas

The Fischer and Baldessarini hypothesis of encephalopathy has been used in the formulation of enteral formulas for liver failure.[107] Such patients usually present with an abnormal plasma amino acid pattern characterized by an elevated concentration of methionine and aromatic amino acids (phenylalanine, tyrosine, tryptophan) and subnormal levels of BCAAs. Two modified amino acid products (Table 13–9) have been designed specifically to normalize plasma amino acid concentrations to ameliorate the encephalopathy supposedly induced when aromatic amino acids act as false neurotransmitters. One enteral formula contains virtually no electrolytes or vitamins and must be supplemented with appropriate amounts of each when used as the patient's primary source of nutrition. The other formula is ready to use and provides 100 percent of the RDA for vitamins and minerals. The effectiveness of these products on outcome, however, presently remains controversial,[47-49] although it appears that some patients with liver failure tolerate larger amounts of the modified amino acid mixtures while not worsening; hepatic encephalopathy may even improve.[45,46] Until further studies clarify whether BCAAs given in higher than normal amounts are useful to achieve the desired metabolic and pharmacologic effects, enteral hepatic failure formulas should be reserved for those patients who have a functional GI tract, exhibit encephalopathy, and do not respond to the administration of standard formulations. They should not be used in patients with nonencephalopathic manifestations of liver disease.

Renal Failure Formulas

Patients with acute renal failure are generally hypercatabolic and hypermetabolic. Stable predialysis patients need calorically dense, low-protein feedings, while patients undergoing dialysis require a protein- and calorie-dense regimen.

The provision of essential amino acids (EAAs) and hypertonic dextrose has been proposed as a method to deliver adequate calories without providing excessive protein, thereby minimizing the accumulation of nitrogenous compounds;[108] however, subsequent trials have not demonstrated any clear benefit of parenteral EAA alone vs mixtures of EAA and nonessential amino acids.[109,110] No studies comparing the efficacy of enteral EAA to standard formulas have been published at this time. Because of the lack of demonstrable clinical efficacy, renal failure formulas should be used only during the course of acute renal failure when attempting to avoid dialysis or to decrease dialysis requirements.

With renal dysfunction, metabolism of folic acid, pyridoxine, and vitamins A, C, and D may be altered and excretion of phosphorus, magnesium, and potassium impaired. Modification of intake of these nutrients should be based on renal function.

The clinician must be aware that the composition of commercial enteral formulas designed for renal failure patients varies (Table 13–10). Some products contain only essential amino acids and histidine, with few or no vitamins, minerals, or electrolytes, and are designed strictly for short-term use (when dialysis is not possible). Other formulas are low in protein (standard EAAs and nonessential amino acids), potassium, phosphorus, vitamins A and D, and enriched with vitamins B_6 and folate. Several of the newer formulas also have added histidine, arginine, taurine, and carnitine. The nonprotein calorie to nitrogen ratios vary, and all the renal failure formulas are calorically concentrated to facilitate fluid management. Standard calorically dense formulas are also frequently appropriate for renal failure patients.

Gastrointestinal Dysfunction Formulas

Patients with acute GI tract dysfunction causing maldigestion may benefit from easily digested and absorbed nutrients. Hydrolysate formulas or products containing peptides may be indicated (Table 13–4). GI recovery and gut health may be improved by providing glutamine or SCFA precursors such as soluble, fermentable fiber. Patients with IBD, diverticulosis or constipation may experience normalization of stool patterns with the use of insoluble fiber (Table 13–2).

TABLE 13–11   Pulmonary Enteral Formula Product Comparison*

	NutriVent (Clintec)	Pulmocare (Ross)	Respalor (Mead Johnson)
Kcal/ml	1.5	1.5	1.52
g Protein/1000 kcal	45	41.7	50
% kcal	18	16.7	20
Source	Calcium and potassium caseinates	Sodium and calcium caseinates	Sodium and calcium caseinates
g Carbohydrate/1000 kcal	67	70.5	97
% kcal	27	28.2	39
Source	Maltodextrin, sucrose	Maltodextrin, sucrose	Corn syrup, sucrose
g Fat/1000 kcal	63	62.2	47.0
% kcal	55	55.1	41
Source	40% MCT 42% Canola oil 13% Corn oil Lecithin	55.8% Canola oil 20% MCT 14% Corn oil 7% High-oleic safflower oil 3.2% soy lecithin	30% MCT 70% canola oil
Omega-6:Omega-3	4:1	4:1	2.4:1
Osmolality (mOsm/kg)	450	475	580
ml to meet 100% RDA	1000	1420	1420
NPC:N	116:1	125:1	102:1
Sodium mg/1000 kcal	780	873	830
Phosphorus mg/1000 kcal	800	704	460

MCT = medium-chain triglycerides; NPC:N = nonprotein calorie: nitrogen (g) ratio.
*Product information verified by manufacturers 12/94.

Pulmonary Insufficiency Formulas

Patients with pulmonary insufficiency characteristically retain CO_2 and experience O_2 depletion. When these patients are nutritionally supported, calories of any type are associated with an increase in total CO_2 production and O_2 consumption, placing an increased metabolic demand on the compromised respiratory system. The goal of therapy centers around diminishing or avoiding this metabolic demand. Two possible means are available from the nutrition standpoint — decreasing or discontinuing feeding or altering the proportions of carbohydrate and fat in the enteral formula. Before any substrate modifications are implemented, it is important to ensure that overfeeding is not the

TABLE 13–12 Selected Reduced-Carbohydrate (CHO) Enteral Formulas*

Moderate CHO Content (≤45 % of kcal)		Low CHO Content (≤35 % kcal)	
Product (Manufacturer)	**CHO (%)**	**Product (Manufacturer)**	**CHO (%)**
Nutren 1.5 (Clintec)	45.0	Glucerna (Ross)	33.3
Replete (Clintec)	45.0	Pulmocare (Ross)	28.2
Replete with Fiber (Clintec)	45.0	NutriVent (Clintec)	27.0
TwoCal HN (Ross)	43.2		
Nepro (Ross)	43.0		
Deliver 2.0 (Mead Johnson)	40.0		
Glytrol (Clintec)	40.0		
Nutren 2.0 (Clintec)	39.0		
Respalor (Mead Johnson)	39.0		
Crucial (Clintec)	36.0		
DiabetiSource (Sandoz)	36.0		

*Product information verified by manufacturers 12/94.

TABLE 13–14 Pediatric Formula Product Comparison*

	Kindercal (Mead Johnson)		Neocate One + (SHS North America)		Nutren JR (Clintec)		Nutren JR with Fiber (Clintec)	
	Source	**per 1000 kcal**	**Source**	**per 1000 kcal**	**Source**	**per 1000 kcal**	**Source**	**per 1000 kcal**
Carbohydrate	Maltodextrin, sucrose	135 g	Maltodextrin, sucrose	46 g	Maltodextrin, sucrose	127.5 g	Maltodextrin, sucrose	127.5 g
Protein	Sodium caseinate	34 g	100% free amino acids	25 g	Intact casein and whey	30 g	Intact casein and whey	30 g
Fat	MCT oil, corn oil, high-oleic sunflower oil	44 g	Fractionated coconut oil, canola oil, high-oleic safflower oil	35 g	Soybean oil, MCT oil, canola oil, lecithin	42 g	Soybean oil, MCT oil, canola oil, lecithin	42 g
Fiber	Soy polysaccharide	6.3 g			—	—	Soy polysaccharide	6 g
Osmolality mOsm/kg H_2O	310		835		350		350	
Caloric density (kcal/ml)	1.06		1.0		1.0		1.0	

BCAA = branched-chain amino acid, MCT = medium-chain triglyceride.
*Product information verified by manufacturers 12/94.

TABLE 13–13   Diabetic Enteral Formula Product Comparison*

	DiabetiSource (Sandoz)	Glucerna (Ross)	Glytrol (Clintec)
Kcal/ml	1.0	1.0	1.0
g Protein/1000 kcal	50	41.8	45.2
% kcal	20	16.7	18
Source	Calcium caseinate, beef	Sodium and calcium caseinates	Calcium and potassium caseinates
g Carbohydrate/1000 kcal	90	93.7	100
% kcal	36	33.3	40
Source	Maltodextrin, fructose, vegetables, fruits	Glucose polymers, soy polysaccharide, fructose	Maltodextrin, modified corn starch, fructose
g Fiber (TDF)/1000 kcal	4.4	14.4	15.2
Source	Vegetables, fruits	Soy polysaccharide	Soy polysaccharide
g Fat/1000 kcal	48.8	55.7	47.6
% kcal	44	50	42
Source	High-oleic sunflower oil, canola, beef	High-oleic safflower oil, unhydrogenated soy oil	Canola oil, high-oleic safflower oil, MCT
Omega-6:Omega-3	2.4:1	17.6:1	3.5:1
Osmolality (mOsm/kg)	360	375	380
ml to meet 100% RDA	1500	1422	1400
NPC:N	100:1	125:1	110:1

TDF = total dietary fiber NPC:N = nonprotein calorie: nitrogen (g) ratio.
*Information obtained from manufacturers and product literature 12/94.

Pediasure (Ross Laboratories)		Pediasure with Fiber (Ross Laboratories)		Peptamen Junior (Clintec)		Vivonex Pediatric (Sandoz Nutrition)	
Source	per 1000 kcal	Source	per 1000 kcal	Source	per 1000 kcal	Source	per 1000 kcal
Hydrolyzed cornstarch, sucrose	109.7 g	Hydrolyzed cornstarch	113.5 g	Maltodextrin, starch	137.5 g	Maltodextrin, modified starch	130 g
Sodium caseinate, low-lactose whey	30 g	Sodium caseinate, low-lactose whey	30 g	Enzymatically hydrolyzed whey, protein	30 g	Free amino acids, 21.6% BCAA, 19.9% glutamine, 6.2% arginine	24 g
High-oleic safflower oil, soy oil, MCT oil	49.7 g	High-oleic safflower oil, MCT oil	49.7 g	MCT oil, soy oil, canola oil, lecithin	38.5 g	MCT oil, soybean oil	24 g
		Soy polysaccharide	5 g				
335		345		260 unflavored 360 flavored		360	
1.0		1.0		1.0		0.8	

cause of excess CO_2 production and heightened ventilatory demand.[111] Decreasing or discontinuing feeding on a short-term basis is an option for critically ill patients with difficulty weaning from the ventilator. For more stable patients, decreasing carbohydrate calories while increasing fat calories should theoretically result in a decreased respiratory quotient and improved gas exchange[112]; however, clinical trials of adequate sample size demonstrating a clear benefit are lacking.[47] Three formulas are currently marketed for use during respiratory failure, although several other products exist with moderate to low carbohydrate content (Table 13–11 and 13–12).

Diabetes Formulas

Noncritically ill patients with diabetes mellitus who need chronic tube feeding require enteral formulas that approximate the American Diabetes Association guidelines for micronutrient intake: 0.8 g/kg of protein (approximately 15 percent of calories), 30 percent fat (one third saturated, one third polyunsaturated, one third monounsaturated), and 55 to 60 percent carbohydrate (primarily complex). High fiber intake is also recommended. For hospitalized patients requiring tube feeding on a more acute basis, limiting carbohydrate intake to less than 50 percent of total calories and the use of formulas with oligosaccharides or polysaccharides rather than simple sugars may facilitate glycemic control.[113-115] If no malabsorption is present, intact protein sources should be used because amino acids may delay gastric emptying. In patients with gastroparesis, concern exists with very high-fat formulas, because fat also prolongs gastric emptying, although it may be beneficial from the standpoint of glucose management. One way to circumvent this problem is to use intraduodenal or jejunal feeding, bypassing the stomach. High-fat formulas with large amounts of polyunsaturated, omega-6 fatty acids should probably be avoided because of the immunocompromising effects described earlier. Complex carbohydrates and fiber offer theoretical benefits to diabetic patients. Alteration of intestinal transit and delay of carbohydrate absorption represent several proposed mechanisms for this. A number of formulas designed for patients with abnormal glucose tolerance are available at this time (Table 13–13).

Pediatric Formulas

In the past, the only choices for tube feeding substrate for children were infant formulas or products designed to meet adult nutrient requirements. Neither of these alternatives conformed to recommended ranges of nutrients proposed by the American Academy of Pediatrics. The recent marketing of products designed for use with pediatric patients (Table 13–14) provides the first step towards developing products better suited for this age category. General characteristics of the pediatric formulas include lower electrolyte levels, lower renal solute load, a better calcium to phosphorus ratio, and improved iron, vitamin D, and taurine concentrations, all of which more closely approximate intake recommendations for children. Such alterations in product composition bring the expectation that improvements in growth and development and clinical outcome will be derived from the use of specialized enteral pediatric solutions. However, efficacy trials are currently pending.

Several polymeric pediatric formulas of standard caloric density are currently available. Two polymeric products are also supplemented with soy fiber. The newest products in this category are hydrolyzed formulas designed for use with pediatric patients who have impaired GI function. The protein source in two of the products is free amino acids, and the other is peptide based. The hydrolyzed products contain moderate levels of fat (24 to 38.5g/1000 Kcal).

Modules

There are patients for whom commercial nutritional products may not be optimal. These patients may benefit from modular feeding systems. Modular formulas may supply a single nutrient or a combination of nutrients and consist primarily of intact macronutrient sources (Table 13–1). There are no complete enteral feeding micronutrient modules available at this time, so clinicians must rely on liquid enteral or parenteral preparations for these nutrients.

Allowing for the tailoring of formulas to meet unique nutritional requirements, modules can be used to alter the caloric or protein density of a base formula or used as a supplement to enhance an oral diet. Another application is the ability to design a new tube-feeding recipe. De novo production permits custom compounding of a formula to meet patients' unique needs and is useful in patients with highly specialized nutritional requirements. Figure 13–4 illustrates a sample modular tube-feeding recipe designed specifically for burn patients. However, the complexity of calculating and ordering a specific nutrient composition and in-

NUTRITION DEPARTMENT
RECIPE CARD

NO.: **RTF #4**
DIET: **Modular Tube Feeding with Glutamine**
EQUIPMENT: Waring blender, gram scale graduated cylinders, 2000 ml
DATE: 6/85: Revised 1/94, 5/94
COST: ___

INGREDIENTS	ML				METHOD
	1000	2000	3000	4000	
Sterile Water	750 ml	1500 ml	2250 ml	3000 ml	1. Measure Sterile Water and pour into Waring Blender.
Centrum Liquid	30 ml	60 ml	90 ml	120 ml	2. Measure Centrum Liquid using graduated cylinder.
Selenium/Copper Mixture	2 ml	4 ml	6 ml	8 ml	3. Add Selenium/Copper Mixture.
Aquasol A	0.1 ml	0.2 ml	0.3 ml	0.4 ml	4. Add Vitamin A preparation. Mix ingredients in blender on low speed for 1 minute.
MaxEPA	6 ml	13 ml	19 ml	25 ml	5. Measure MaxEPA using graduated cylinder and add to blender.
Microlipid	10 ml	20 ml	30 ml	40 ml	6. Shake Microlipid preparation very well. Open and measure using a pipette. Date leftover Microlipid. Discard within 3 days.
Promix RDP	46 g	92 g	138 g	184 g	7. Weigh Promix RDP. Add to liquids in blender.
Polycose	165 g	330 g	495 g	660 g	8. Weigh Polycose. Add to liquids in blender.
Arginine HCL	5 g	10 g	15 g	20 g	9. Weigh Arginine HCL. Add to liquids in blender.
Histidine	1 g	2 g	3 g	4 g	10. Weigh Histidine. Add to liquids in blender.
Cysteine	1 g	2 g	3 g	4 g	11. Weigh Cysteine. Add to liquids in blender.
Glutamine	12 g	24 g	36 g	48 g	12. Weigh Glutamine. Add to liquids in blender.
					13. Add ingredients 4-12 to the Water/Vitamin/Mineral mixture. Mix all ingredients in blender on low for 2 more minutes. Label each container. Deliver to Nursing Unit. Refrigerate immediately.

FIGURE 13–4   Sample modular tube feeding recipe.

creased cost of labor may prevent some facilities from using de novo formulas. De novo formulations also carry the potential risk of microbial contamination from excessive handling of formulas and potential physical incompatibilities with insoluble components.

CONCLUSION

The evolution of defined formula diets as a nutritional intervention tool has been dramatic. Insights into the prophylactic and therapeutic benefits of enteral nutrition support on metabolism have prompted the development and proliferation of a broad range of simple as well as sophisticated enteral formulas. However, there is no consensus on what constitutes the optimal mixture of nutrients. A single ideal combination is unlikely, because the definition of optimal must vary relative to the objectives of the care plan. The objectives of enteral nutrition support differ greatly among patient populations and include promotion of growth and development, support of recovery, nutrient repletion of the malnourished, and compensation for a metabolic aberration.

Because of the recent proliferation of commercially available enteral products, critical evaluation is necessary in choosing products for patients and formularies. Formula selection, relying on commercially available products marketed largely based on theory, still requires considerable scientific validation by comprehensive trials that demonstrate improved outcome under clinical conditions.[47,48,52,116] In the meantime, the increasing number of enteral formulas on the market requires great scrutiny in evaluating their intended use and alleged efficacy.

REFERENCES

1. Bell SJ, Pasulka PS, Blackburn GL: Enteral formulas. In Skipper A (ed): Dietitian's Handbook of Enteral and Parenteral Nutrition. Gaithersburg, MD: Aspen Publishers, 1989:279–292.
2. MacBurney MM, Russell C, Young LS: Formulas. In Rombeau JL, Caldwell MD (eds): Clinical Nutrition: Enteral Tube Feeding, 2nd edition. Philadelphia: WB Saunders, 1990:149–173.
3. Ideno KT: Enteral Nutrition. In Gottschlich MM, Matarese LE, Shronts EP (eds): Nutrition Support Dietetics Core Curriculum, 2nd edition. Silver Spring, MD: American Society for Parenteral and Enteral Nutrition, 1993:71–104.
4. Prosky L, Asp N, Furda I et al: Determination of total dietary fiber in foods and food products: a collaborative study. J Assoc Off Anal Chem 1985;68:677–679.
5. Scheppach W, Burghardt W, Bartram P et al: Addition of dietary fiber to liquid formula diets: the pros and cons. J Parenter Enter Nutr 1990;14(2):204–209.
6. Evans MA, Shronts EP: Intestinal fuels: glutamine, short-chain fatty acids, and dietary fiber. J Am Diet Assoc 1992;92(10):1239–1246, 1249.
7. Frankenfield DC, Beyer PL: Soy-polysaccharide fiber: effect on diarrhea in tube-fed head-injured patients. Am J Clin Nutr 1989;50(3):533–538.
8. Palacio JC, Rombeau JL: Dietary fiber: a brief review and potential application to enteral nutrition. Nutr Clin Prac 1990;5:99–106.
9. Slavin JL, Nelson NL, McNamara EA et al: Bowel function of healthy men consuming liquid diets with and without dietary fiber. J Parenter Enter Nutr 1985;9:317–321.
10. Silk DBA: Fiber and enteral nutrition. Gut 1989;30:246–264.
11. Shorey RL, Day PL, Willis RA et al: Effects of soybean polysaccharide on plasma lipids. J Am Diet Assoc 1985;85:1461–1465.
12. Lo GS, Goldberg AP, Lim A et al: Soy fiber improves lipid and carbohydrate metabolism in primary hyperlipidemic subjects. Atherosclerosis 1986;62:239–244.
13. Krey SH, Lockett GM: Enteral nutrition: a comprehensive overview. In Krey SH, Murray RL (eds): Dynamics of Nutrition Support: Assessment, Implementation, Evaluation. Norwalk, CT: Appleton-Century-Crofts, 1986;279–327.
14. Gottschlich MM: Selection of optimal lipid sources in enteral and parenteral nutrition. Nutr Clin Prac 1992; 7:152–165.
15. Wolfe BM, Ney DM: Lipid metabolism in parenteral nutrition. In Rombeau JL, Caldwell MD (eds): Clinical Nutrition: Parenteral Nutrition. Philadelphia: WB Saunders, 1986;72–99.
16. Mascioli EA, Bistrian BR, Babayan VK et al: Medium chain triglycerides and structured lipids as unique nonglucose energy sources in hyperalimentation. Lipids 1987;22(6):421–423.
17. Babayan VK: Medium-chain triglycerides and structured lipids. Lipids 1987;22(6):417–420.
18. Bell SJ, Mascioli EA, Bistrian BR et al: Alternative lipid sources for enteral and parenteral nutrition: long- and medium-chain triglycerides, structured triglycerides and fish oils. J Am Diet Assoc 1991;91(1):74–78.
19. Haw MP, Bell SJ, Blackburn GL: Potential of parenteral and enteral nutrition in inflammation and immune dysfunction: a new challenge for dietitians. J Am Diet Assoc 1991;91(6):701–709.
20. Wan JM, Teo TC, Babayan VK et al: Invited comment: lipids and the development of immune dysfunction and infection. J Parenter Enter Nutr 1988;12(6): 45S–52S.
21. Sardesai VM: The essential fatty acids. Nutr Clin Prac 1992;7:179–186.
22. Cerra FB, Alden PA, Negro F et al: Sepsis and exogenous lipid modulation. J Parenter Enter Nutr 1988;12(6):635–685.
23. Kinsella JE, Lokesh B: Dietary lipids, eicosanoids and the immune system. Crit Care Med 1990;18(2): S94–S113.
24. Mayes PA: Lipids of physiologic significance. In Murray RK, Granner DK, Mayes PA et al (eds): Harper's Biochemistry, 22nd edition. Norwalk, CT: Appleton & Lange, 1990:134–145.
25. Sucher KP: Medium-chain triglycerides: a review of their use in clinical nutrition. Nutr Clin Prac 1986; 1(3):146–150.
26. Cotter R, D'Alleinne C: Medium-chain triglycerides: a preclinical perspective. In Kinney JM, Borum PR (eds): Perspectives in Clinical Nutrition. Baltimore: Urban and Schwarzenberg, Inc., 1989:393–404.

27. Friedel D, Levine GM: Effect of short-chain fatty acids on colonic function and structure. J Parenter Enter Nutr 1992;16(1):1–4.

28. Koruda MJ, Rolandelli RH, Bliss DZ et al: Parenteral nutrition supplemented with short-chain fatty acids: effect on the small bowel mucosa in normal rats. Am J Clin Nutr 1990;51:685–689.

29. Lynch JW, Miles JM, Bailey JW: Effects of the short-chain triglyceride triacetin on intestinal mucosa and metabolic substrates in rats. J Parenter Enter Nutr 1994;18:208–213.

30. Gollaher CJ, Fechner K, Karlstad M et al: The effect of increasing levels of fish oil containing structured triglycerides on protein metabolism in parenterally fed rats stressed by burn plus endotoxin. J Parenter Enter Nutr 1993;17(3):247–253.

31. Wardlaw GM, Insel PM: Proteins. In Wardlaw GM, Insel PM (eds): Perspectives in Nutrition, 2nd edition. St. Louis: Mosby-Year Book, Inc., 1993:138–171.

32. Oser BL: Method for integrating essential amino acid content in the nutritional evaluation of protein. J Am Diet Assoc 1951;27:396–402.

33. Bell SJ, Bistrian BR, Ainsley BM et al: A chemical score to evaluate the protein quality of commercial parenteral and enteral formulas: emphasis on formulas for patients with liver failure. J Am Diet Assoc 1991;91:586–589.

34. Bell SJ, Bistrian BR, Wade JE et al: Modular enteral diets: cost and nutritional value comparisons. J Am Diet Assoc 1987;87:1526–1530.

35. Dubin S, McKee K, Battish S: Essential amino acid reference profile affects the evaluation of enteral feeding products. J Am Diet Assoc 1994;94:884–887.

36. Silk DBA, Fairclough PD, Clark ML et al: Use of peptide rather than free amino acid nitrogen source in chemically defined elemental diets. J Parenter Enter Nutr 1980;4(6):548–553.

37. Craft IL, Geddes D, Hyde CW et al: Absorption and malabsorption of glycine and glycine peptides in man. Gut 1968;9:425–437.

38. Adibi S, Phillips E: Evidence for greater absorption of amino acid from peptide than from free form in human intestine. Clin Res 1968;16:446.

39. Feller A, Rudman D, Caindec N et al: Clinical trial of Peptamen liquid elemental diet in geriatric patients. In Kinney JM, Borum PR (eds): Perspectives in Clinical Nutrition. Baltimore: Urban and Schwartzenberg, Inc., 1989:339–348.

40. Brinson RR, Hanumanthu SK, Pitts WM: A reappraisal of the peptide-based enteral formulas: clinical applications. Nutr Clin Prac 1989;4(6):211–217.

41. Mowatt-Larssen CA, Brown RO, Wojtysiak SL et al: Comparison of tolerance and nutritional outcome between a peptide and a standard enteral formula in critically ill, hypoalbuminemic patients. J Parenter Enter Nutr 1992;16:20–24.

42. Deitch EA, Xu D, Qi L et al: Elemental diet-induced immune suppression is caused by both bacterial and dietary factors. J Parenter Enter Nutr 1993;17:332–336.

43. Serizawa H, Miura S, Tashiro H et al: Alteration of mucosal immunity after long-term ingestion of an elemental diet in rats. J Parenter Enter Nutr 1994;18:141–147.

44. Blackburn GL, Moldawer LL, Usui S et al: Branched chain amino acid administration and metabolism during starvation, injury and infection. Surgery 1979;86:307–315.

45. Horst D, Grace ND, Conn HO et al: Comparison of dietary protein with an oral branched-chain amino acid supplement in chronic portal-systemic encephalopathy: a randomized, controlled trial. Hepatology 1984;4(2):279–287.

46. McGhee A, Henderson JM, Millikan WJ et al: Comparison of the effects of Hepatic-Aid and a casein modular diet on encephalopathy, plasma amino acids and nitrogen balance in cirrhotic patients. Ann Surg 1983;197(3):288–293.

47. ASPEN Board of Directors: Guidelines for the use of parenteral and enteral nutrition in adult and pediatric patients. J Parenter Enter Nutr 1993;17:1SA–52SA.

48. Talbot JM: Guidelines for the scientific review of enteral food products for special medical purposes. J Parenter Enter Nutr 1991;15:99S–174S.

49. Brennan MF, Cerra F, Daly JM et al: Report of a research workshop: branched-chain amino acids in stress and injury. J Parenter Enter Nutr 1986;10:446–452.

50. Eriksson LS, Persson A, Wahren J: Branched-chain amino acids in the treatment of chronic hepatic encephalopathy. Gut 1982;23:801–806.

51. Christie ML, Sack DM, Pomposelli J et al: Enriched branched-chain amino acid formula versus a casein-based supplement in the treatment of cirrhosis. J Parenter Enter Nutr 1985;9:671–678.

52. Heyland DK, Cook DJ, Guyatt GH: Does the formulation of enteral feeding products influence infectious morbidity and mortality rates in the critically ill patient? A critical review of the evidence. Crit Care Med 1994;22:1192–1202.

53. Naylor CD, O'Rourke K, Detsky AS et al: Parenteral nutrition with branched-chain amino acids in hepatic encephalopathy: a meta-analysis. Gastroenterology 1989;97:1033–1042.

54. Lacey JM, Wilmore DW: Is glutamine a conditionally essential amino acid? Nutr Rev 1990;48(8):297–309.

55. Souba W, Smith RJ, Wilmore DW: Glutamine metabolism by the intestinal tract. J Parenter Enter Nutr 1985;9(5):608–617.

56. van der Hulst RR, van Kreel BK, von Meyenfeldt MF et al: Glutamine and the preservation of gut integrity. Lancet 1993;341:1363–1365.

57. Swails WS, Bell SJ, Borlase BC et al: Glutamine content of whole proteins: implications for enteral formulas. Nutr Clin Prac 1992;7(2):77–80.

58. Smith RJ, Wilmore DW: Glutamine nutrition and requirements. J Parenter Enter Nutr 1990;14(4):94S–99S.

59. Ziegler TR, Benfell K, Smith RJ et al: Sfety and metabolic effects of L-glutamine administration in humans. J Parenter Enter Nutr 1990;14(4):137S–146S.

60. Fischer JE, Chance WT: Total parenteral nutrition, glutamine and tumor growth. J Parenter Enter Nutr 1990;14(4):86S–89S.

61. Klimberg VS, Nwokedi E, Hutchins LF et al: Glutamine facilitates chemotherapy while reducing toxicity. J Parenter Enter 1992;16(6):83S–87S.

62. Austgen TR, Dudrick PS, Sitren H et al: The effects of glutamine-enriched total parenteral nutrition on tumor growth and host tissues. Ann Surg 1992;215(2):107–113.

63. Klimberg VS, Souba WW, Salloum RM et al: Glutamine-enriched diets support muscle glutamine metabolism without stimulating tumor growth. J Surg Res 1990;48:319–323.

64. Seifter E, Rettura G, Barbul A et al: Arginine: an essential amino acid for injured rats. Surgery 1978;84:224–230.

65. Levenson SM, Seifter E: Influence of supplemental arginine and vitamin A on wound healing, the thy-

mus and resistance to infection following injury. In Winters RW, Greene HL (eds): Nutritional Support of the Seriously Ill Patient. New York: Academic Press 1983;53–62.

66. Merimee TJ, Lillicrap DA, Rabinowitz D: Effect of arginine on serum levels of human growth hormone. Lancet 1965;2:668–670.

67. Mulloy AL, Kari FW, Visek WJ: Dietary arginine, insulin secretion, glucose tolerance and liver lipids during repletion of protein-depleted rats. Horm Metab Res 1982;14:471–475.

68. Daly JM, Reynolds J, Thom A et al: Immune and metabolic effects of arginine in the surgical patient. Ann Surg 1988;208(4):512–522.

69. Kirk SJ, Barbul A: Role of arginine in trauma, sepsis and immunity. J Parenter Enter Nutr 1990;14(5):226S–229S.

70. Chyun JH, Griminger P: Improvement of nitrogen retention by arginine and glycine supplementation and its relation to collagen synthesis in traumatized mature and aged rats. J Nutr 1984;114:1697–1704.

71. Bohles H, Segerer H, Fekl W: Improved nitrogen retention during L-carnitine-supplemented total parenteral nutrition. J Parenter Enter Nutr 1984;8(1):9–13.

72. Gottschlich MM, Jenkins M, Warden GD et al: Differential effects of three dietary regimens on selected outcome variables in burn patients. J Parenter Enter Nutr 1990;14:225–236.

73. Hayes KC, Sturman JA: Taurine in metabolism. Annu Rev Nutr 1981;1:401–425.

74. Hayes KC, Pronczuk A, Addesa AE et al: Taurine modulates platelet aggregation in cats and humans. Am J Clin Nutr 1989;49:1211–1216.

75. Thomas EL, Grisham MB, Melton DF et al: Evidence for a role of taurine in the in vitro oxidative toxicity of neutrophils toward erythrocytes. J Biol Chem 1985;260:3321–3329.

76. Chesney RW: New functions for an old molecule. Pediatr Res 1987;22:755–759.

77. Paauw JD, Davis AT: Taurine concentrations in serum of critically injured patients and age- and sex-matched healthy control subjects. Am J Clin Nutr 1990;52:657–660.

78. Desai TK, Maliakkal J, Kinzie JL et al: Taurine deficiency after intensive chemotherapy and/or radiation. Am J Clin Nutr 1992;55:708–711.

79. Martensson J, Larsson J, Nordstrom H: Amino acid metabolism during the anabolic phase of severely burned patients: with special reference to sulfur amino acids. Eur J Clin Invest 1987;17:130–135.

80. Martensson J, Larsson J, Schildt BO: Metabolic effects of amino acid solutions in severely burned patients: with emphasis on sulfur amino acid metabolism and protein breakdown. J Trauma 1985;25:427–432.

81. Borum P: Carnitine. Ann Rev Nutr 1983;3:233–259.

82. Adjei AA, Takamine F, Yokoyama H et al: The effects of oral RNA and intraperitoneal nucleoside-nucleotide administration on methicillin-resistant staphylococcus aureus infection in mice. J Parenter Enter Nutr 1993;17(2):148–152.

83. Rudolph FB, Kulkarni AD, Fanslow WC et al: Role of RNA as a dietary source of pyrimidines and purines in immune function. J Parenter Enter Nutr 1990;6:45–52.

84. Kulkarni AD, Fanslow WC, Rudolph FB et al: Effect of dietary nucleotides on response to bacterial infections. J Parenter Enter Nutr 1986;10:169–171.

85. Carver JD, Pimental BP, Cox WI et al: Dietary nucleotide effects upon immune function in infants. Pediatrics 1991;88:359–363.

86. Vauy R, Stringel G, Thomas R et al: Effect of dietary nucleosides on growth and maturation of the developing gut in the rat. J Pediatr Gastroenterol Nutr 1990;10:497–503.

87. Nunez MC, Ayudarte MV, Morales D et al: Effect of dietary nucleotides on intestinal repair in rats with experimental chronic diarrhea. J Parenter Enter Nutr 1990;14:598–604.

88. Iijima S, Tsujinake T, Kido Y et al: Intravenous administration of nucleosides and a nucleotide mixture diminishes intestinal mucosal atrophy induced by total parenteral nutrition. J Parenter Enter Nutr 1993;17(3):265–270.

89. Gottschlich MM, Warden GD, Michel M et al: Diarrhea in tube-fed burn patients: incidence, etiology, nutritional impact and prevention. J Parenter Enter Nutr 1988;12:338–345.

90. Keohane PP, Attrill H, Love M et al: Relation between osmolality of diet and gastrointestinal side effects in enteral nutrition. Br Med J 1984;288:678–680.

91. Zarling EJ, Parmar JR, Mobarhan S et al: Effect of enteral formula infusion rate, osmolality, and chemical composition upon clinical tolerance and carbohydrate absorption in normal subjects. J Parenter Enter Nutr 1986;10:588–590.

92. Pesola GR, Hogg JE, Eissa N et al: Hypertonic nasogastric tube feedings: do they cause diarrhea? Crit Care Med 1990;18:1378–1382.

93. Davenport HW: Gastric motility. In Davenport HW (ed): Physiology of the Digestive Tract, 4th edition. Chicago: Year Book Medical Publishers, 1977;41–57.

94. Heymsfield SB: Enteral solutions: is there a solution? Nutr Clin Prac 1995;10:4–7.

95. Mueller C, Nestle M: Regulation of medical foods: toward a rational policy. Nutr Clin Prac 1995;10:8–15.

96. Shronts EP, Havala T: Enteral nutrition: formulas. In Teasley-Strausburg KT, Cerra FB (eds): A Compendium of Products with Guidelines for Usage. Cincinnati: Harvey Whitney Publishers, 1992:147–186.

97. Littman A, Hammond JB: Diarrhea in adults caused by deficiency in intestinal disaccharidases. Gastroenterology 1965;48:237–249.

98. Hopkins B: Critical reading of nutrition literature: tools for evaluating specialized formulas. Diet Nutr Supp News 1990;12(3):7–8.

99. Cerra FB, Lehmann S, Konstantinides N et al: Improvement in immune function in ICU patients by enteral nutrition supplemented with arginine, RNA, and menhaden oil is independent of nitrogen balance. Nutrition 1991;7(3):193–199.

100. Daly JM, Lieberman MD, Goldfine J et al: Enteral nutrition with supplemental arginine, RNA, and omega-3 fatty acids in patients after operation: immunologic, metabolic and clinical outcome. Surgery 1992;112(1):56–67.

101. Chandra RK, Whang S, Au B: Enriched feeding formula and immune responses and outcome after *Listeria monocytogenes* challenge in mice. Nutrition 1992;8(6)426–429.

102. Cerra FB, Lehmann S, Konstantinides N et al: Effects of enteral nutrient on in vitro tests of immune function in ICU patients: a preliminary report. Nutrition 1990;6(1)(suppl):84–87.

103. Chlebowski RT, Beall G, Grosvernor M et al: Long-term effects of early nutritional support with new enterotropic peptide-based formula vs standard enteral formula in HIV-infected patients: randomized, prospective trial. Nutrition 1993;9(6):507–512.

104. Brown RO, Hunt H, Mowatt-Larssen CA et al: Comparison of specialized and standardized enteral for-

mulas in trauma patients. Pharmacotherapy 1994;14(3):314–320.

105. Moore FA, Moore EE, Kudsk KA et al: Clinical benefits of an immune-enhancing diet for early postinjury enteral feeding. J Trauma 1994;37(4):607–615.

106. Zapata-Sirvent RL, Hansbrough JF, Ohara MM et al: Bacterial translocation in burned mice after administration of various diets including fiber and glutamine-enriched formulas. Crit Care Med 1994;22(4):690–696.

107. Fischer JE, Baldessarini RJ: Pathogenesis and therapy of hepatic coma. In Popper H, Schaffner F (eds): Progress in Liver Disease, vol V. New York: Grune & Stratton, 1976:363–397.

108. Abel RM, Beck CH, Abbott WM et al: Improved survival from acute renal failure after treatment with intravenous essential L-amino acids and glucose. Results from a prospective, double blind study. N Engl J Med 1973;288:695–699.

109. Feinstein Ei, Blumenkrantz MJ, Healy M et al: Clinical and metabolic responses to parenteral nutrition in acute renal failure. A controlled double-blind study. Medicine 1981;60:124–137.

110. Mirtallo JM, Schneider PJ, Mavko K et al: A comparison of essential and general amino acid infusions in the nutritional support of patients with compromised renal function. J Parenter Enter Nutr 1982;6(2):109–113.

111. Askanazi J, Rosenbaum SH, Hyman AI et al: Respiratory changes induced by the large glucose loads of total parenteral nutrition. JAMA 1980;243:1444–1447.

112. Rothkopf MM, Stanislaus G, Haverstick L et al: Nutritional support in respiratory failure. Nutr Clin Prac 1989;4:166–172.

113. American Diabetes Association: Nutritional recommendations and principles for individuals with diabetes mellitus. Diabetes Care 1987;10:126–132.

114. Charney PJ: Diabetes mellitus. In Gottschlich MM, Matarese LE, Shronts EP (eds): Nutrition Support Dietetics Core Curriculum, 2nd edition. Siver Spring, MD: American Society for Parenteral and Enteral Nutrition, 1993:377–388.

115. Peters AL, Davidson MB: Effects of various enteral feeding products on postprandial blood glucose response in patients with type I diabetes. J Parenter Enter Nutr 1992;16:69–74.

116. Matarese LE: Rationale and efficacy of specialized enteral nutriton. Nutr Clin Prac 1994;9:58–64.

14

Delivery Systems and Administration of Enteral Nutrition

PEGGI GUENTER
SUSAN JONES
MARGOT ROBERTS SWEED
MARTHA ERICSON

Modern improvements in the administration and delivery of enteral nutrition began with Fallis and Barron,[1] who developed fine polyethylene tubes for nasogastric and nasojejunal access, and Pareira and colleagues,[2] who used nasoenteric tube feedings to nourish more than 200 patients. Further technical advances included the development of the enteral feeding pump by Barron[3] and Stephens' and Randall's[4] clinical use of the elemental diet.

The current resurgence of interest in enteral nutrition is partly due to technologic advances, such as the small-bore, flexible tubes constructed of nonreactive materials (polyurethane and silicone rubber), volumetric infusion pumps, and portable and automatic flush pumps, and to the new emphasis on enteral nutrition's efficacy. The new feeding tubes have decreased the incidence of side-effects such as rhinitis, pharyngitis, and atelectasis associated with the larger, stiffer tubes.[5] The newer pumps allow uniform nutrient delivery, increased patient mobility, automatic flushing and thus decreased tube clogging, and a variety of safety features. This chapter discusses the rationale,

indications, methods of delivery, transitional feeding regimens, and monitoring for patients who are receiving enteral nutrition along with the currently available delivery systems.

RATIONALE FOR PRESCRIBING

The rationale for prescribing enteral nutrition rather than parenteral nutrition is based on the following: (1) maintaining gut structure and function, (2) enhancing use of nutrients, (3) safety of administration, and (4) reduced cost.[6]

Both theoretic and scientific evidence confirm that enteral feeding maintains gut structure and function better than parenteral alimentation. Recent studies in humans have demonstrated reductions in septic complications using enteral nutrition compared with parenteral nutrition therapy.[7,8]

Increased safety is a major reason to use enteral feeding. Enteral nutrition avoids the complications of pneumothorax, hydrothorax, arterial puncture, catheter embolus, and sepsis that are associated with central venous catheterization. Although not without its own risks (Chapters 33 and 34), enteral nutrition may be safer than parenteral feeding.[9]

Enteral nutrition is less expensive than total parenteral nutrition (TPN). The major difference in expense is due to formula costs. The average daily cost of TPN is $75 to $350 compared with $18 to $30 for an equivalent amount of enteral formula.[10]

Enteral nutrition does not require the extensive sterile techniques needed for parenteral feedings. In addition, the minimal daily requirements of vitamins and micronutrients are established for enteral feedings, but the parenteral requirements are not as well defined.[11]

PATIENT SELECTION

Patient selection for enteral nutrition can be based on the algorithm in Figure 14–1. Many well-nourished patients have adverse changes in their nutrition status after surgical stress or illness and may need nutritional support.[12] Before initiating nutritional therapy, one must first obtain baseline nutritional data by taking a thorough medical history and dietary review and by performing a complete physical examination (Chapter 10). To establish the need for supplemental feedings, the nutritional assessment and dietary review should demonstrate that the patient's volitional intake is insufficient for his or her nutrient needs. Furthermore, the therapeutic objectives of nutritional support must be clearly identified as either nutritional maintenance or repletion. Stressed or critically ill patients often do not tolerate high caloric intakes, and the nutritional goal is to maintain the nutritional status and prevent further deficits. The repletion of nutritional deficits is undertaken once the acute stress or critical illness is corrected. It usually takes 4 to 5 days to reach the nutritional goal with enteral feeding.[13,14]

Most evidence indicates that enteral nutrition provides satisfactory nutritional therapy. Some patients needing high-caloric nutritional repletion may need supplementary intravenous (IV) feedings to reach their nutritional goals. Peripheral parenteral nutrition is one method by which additional calories can be administered. Although the benefits of this method have not been documented with prospective randomized trials, Young and Hill[15] have published a nonrandomized study that compared combined enteral and peripheral parenteral nutrition with TPN. Their data showed that combination therapy may be as effective as parenteral nutrition alone in decreasing postoperative morbidity and achieving nitrogen and potassium balances.

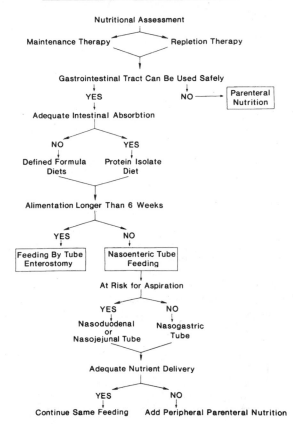

DECISION MAKING FOR NASOENTERIC FEEDING

FIGURE 14–1 Patient selection for nasoenteric feeding.

Once volitional oral intake is shown to be inadequate and it is determined that the patient's nutrient needs are either maintenance or repletion, the route for delivery is selected. Clinical evaluation of the gastrointestinal (GI) tract will determine if it can be used safely and effectively. Safe use of the GI tract is determined by the absence of obstruction, ileus, severe diarrhea, and massive intestinal hemorrhage. Even if the GI tract is not wholly "intact," a defined formula diet may be absorbed with as little as 40 cm of normal small bowel if the ileocecal valve is present.[16] Freeman and coworkers[17] cite the need for at least 100 cm of functioning jejunum or 150 cm of ileum and emphasize the importance of the colon and an intact ileocecal valve for absorption.

INDICATIONS

The indications for nasoenteric tube feedings are listed in Table 14–1. Patients with

TABLE 14–1 Indications for Nasoenteric Tube Feeding

Neurologic and Psychiatric
Cerebrovascular accidents
Neoplasms
Trauma
Inflammation
Demyelinating diseases
Severe depression
Anorexia nervosa
Failure to thrive

Oropharyngeal and Esophageal
Neoplasms
Inflammation
Trauma

Gastrointestinal
Pancreatitis
Inflammatory bowel disease
Short-bowel syndrome
Neonatal intestinal disease
Malabsorption
Preoperative bowel preparation
Fistulas

Miscellaneous
Burns
Chemotherapy
Radiation therapy
Acquired immunodeficiency syndrome
Organ transplantation

neurologic or psychological disorders that prevent satisfactory oral intake and patients with oropharyngeal or esophageal disorders who cannot eat may benefit from nasoenteric feedings. Patients with burns, certain GI diseases, and short gut, and those undergoing chemotherapy or radiotherapy are additional candidates for this type of feeding. Patients with acquired immunodeficiency syndrome (AIDS) who do not have the strength or ability to consume enough to meet their high nutritional requirements are also candidates for enteral nutrition (Chapter 21). Nasoenteric tube feedings can be used in the transition from TPN to combined parenteral and enteral nutrition to volitional oral intake. This feeding progression decreases the time the patient is at risk for complications of parenteral nutrition.

Nasoenteric feedings provide adjunctive nutritional therapy for selected patients with GI fistulas. When fistulas occur in the esophagus, duodenum, or proximal jejunum, placing the nasoenteric tube beyond the fistulous tract and using a liquid diet distal to the fistula may be feasible. One study revealed that 65 percent of

37 heterogenous GI fistulas closed during treatment with an elemental diet,[18] and these findings have been confirmed by other studies.[19] In the presence of a duodenal fistula, defined formula diets administered nasoenterally into the jejunum are efficacious.[20]

Nasoenteric tube feeding is contraindicated in patients with complete gastric or intestinal obstruction. When incomplete obstruction is present, nasoenteric feeding is controversial. Some investigators support the use of a defined formula diet in a patient with incomplete obstruction of the small intestine. These defined formulas were shown to decrease the nausea, vomiting, and bloating normally seen with enteral feeding in such a patient.[21] The clinician should use nasoenteric tube feeding only when the clinical status of the patient's GI tract is fully appreciated. This requirement avoids the possibility of feeding a patient who is completely obstructed but has been misdiagnosed as having a partial obstruction.

When the stomach fails to empty properly, as might occur postoperatively, the risks of nausea, vomiting, and acute gastric dilatation may be reduced by feeding directly into the small intestine.[22] This method may require operative, radiographic, or endoscopic placement of the feeding tube in the small intestine (Chapters 11, 12, and 15). Moss and Friedman advocate an esophagogastric drainage-duodenal feeding tube, which permits esophageal and gastric aspiration during duodenal feedings.[23,24] Moss and others believe that full nutrition can be safely achieved during the immediate postoperative period with this type of tube.

Studies in humans have documented that immediate postoperative feeding leads to positive nitrogen balance and improved wound healing.[25] Enteral nutrition should be performed cautiously in patients with ileus, and careful clinical attention is required because of the increased risk for complications. Those patients with ileus secondary to fluid and electrolyte imbalances, narcotics, infection, sepsis, or trauma are best treated by relieving the underlying condition and feeding through the parenteral route. Nasoenteric tube feeding can be started once the ileus has resolved. When the precipitating factors of small and large bowel ileus cannot be relieved, avoid nasoenteric feedings.

In certain circumstances, the patient's primary illness may be best treated by bowel rest. For example, avoid nasogastric enteral feedings if pancreatic or biliary stimulation is undesirable. In these patients, parenteral nutrition may be the preferred method of therapy. Bowel rest may also be preferred in patients with acute GI hemorrhage or very active inflammatory bowel disease (IBD).

Attempt to anticipate how long the patient will require enteral nutritional therapy. If long-term (greater than 4 weeks) alimentation is needed, the patient's primary disease process and tube preference will influence the type of enteral access. Esophagostomies, gastrostomies, and jejunostomies may be performed when feasible in patients who require long-term enteral feedings. However, nasoenteric tube feedings have been employed for long-term alimentation in the hospital and at home with great success.[26-28]

NASOENTERIC FEEDING TUBES

History

Devices used for artificial alimentation or forced feeding were first described in the Greco-Roman period. The "modern" experience with these devices began with Aquapendente, a monk, who used a tube of silver for nasogastric feeding in 1617. Van HelMont produced flexible leather catheters in 1646; however, a discussion of their use does not appear in the literature.[2,29] The major work related to nasoenteric tube feeding in the 18th century was by John Hunter, who reported successful tube feeding in two patients.[30,31] Nasogastric tubes for feeding purposes were not described in the American literature until 1879.[32] Rankin described the placement of a tube for feeding by the oral and, later, the nasal route in an uncooperative patient in 1882.[33] Use of soft rubber tubes for gavage feeding of pediatric patients was first described in the last half of the 19th century.[34]

The Levin tube had been the most commonly employed nasogastric tube for feeding and is still an appropriate tube for gastric decompression.[35] However, a number of mechanical complications have been reported with the long-term use of this tube for nasoenteric feeding.[36,37] These potential complications and the discomfort to the patient from the tube's size and stiffness make it currently undesirable for feeding.

In the 1950s alternatives to the Levin tube became available when polyethylene tubes were developed. Royce and coworkers[38] and Wagner and coworkers[39] advocated polyethylene tubes for pediatric patients. In 1952 Kunz[40]

suggested that polyethylene tubes could be modified with a paraffin coating to reduce complications from tube stiffness. Concurrently, Fallis and Barron[1] suggested passing polyethylene tubes into the stomach or jejunum using a mercury-filled balloon as a weight to assist with the procedure. However, the mercury-filled balloon was tied in place with surgical catgut, which did not remain intact in the GI tract.

A few years later, Wagner and associates[41] introduced a tube formed from a polyvinyl-type plastic, which was more pliable than polyethylene tubes. In the late 1960s a silicone-elastomer nasoenteric tube with a mercury-filled balloon weight was used by Keoshian and Nelsen.[42] Dobbie and Hoffmeister[43] introduced a tube, the Dobhoff, in 1976 made of polyvinylchloride but with many features that the present-day tubes employ. In the 1970s polyurethane and silicone were being considered and investigated as possibly better materials for tube development.

Today, the soft, small-bore, polyurethane or silicone-elastomer nasoenteric tube, with or without a weighted bolus, is the tube of choice for short-term feeding.

Polyurethane and Silicone Tubes

Polyurethane, which does not stiffen, biodegrade, or discolor in vivo, has become the material of choice for nasoenteral tubes. Polyurethane allows for thinner wall construction for equal strength, increased flow area, and better ability to aspirate gastric contents compared with silicone. It also has an acceptable patient comfort level.[44,45] These tubes have several advantages over the large-bore, stiff polyvinylchoride or Levin tubes. General characteristics of the tubes are outlined in Table 14–2, and comparison of composition is outlined in Table 14–3. Oropharyngeal and esophageal irritation on intubation are minimized with the silicone or polyurethane tube. The small-bore, soft tubes with silicone or tungsten weights can be passed into the stomach more easily, especially in an endotracheally intubated patient. It is still unclear if the weighted tubes facilitate small bowel intubation.[45,46] Smaller-sized tubes may decrease the risk of aspiration because of reduced lower esophageal sphincter compromise and thus decreased reflux of gastric contents. In addition, the softer tube usually does not hinder the patient's ability to swallow.[47]

Polyurethane or silicone-elastomer tubes are usually externally lubricated and may come

TABLE 14–2   Nasoenteric Feeding Tube Characteristics

Characteristic	Comments
Weighted tubes	No advantage in transpyloric passage. Easier intubation with cuffed endotracheal tubes. Controversial whether weights assist in maintaining proper tube tip position.
Tube length	36-inch tube for gastric intubation. 43-inch tube for gastric or intestinal intubation.
Stylet	Stylet stiffens tube for easier passage. Stylet may perforate viscera during placement, especially if force is used. If reinserted in situ can cause perforation.
Self-lubrication	Easier removal of stylet after placement. Easier placement for patient.
Shape and size of tip	
Smooth vs bolus	Smooth tip easier to pass than bolus tip.
Pill or bullet tip vs eyelets or openings in tip	Pill or bullet shape may decrease chance of clogging vs eyelets in tip.
Adaptors	
Incompatible with intravenous tubing	Prevent parenteral administration of enteral formula.
Double/triple ports	Easier administration of medications, modules, fluids, etc.

Adapted with permission from Monturo CA: Enteral access device selection. Nutr Clin Pract 1990;5:207–213.

TABLE 14–3   Nasoenteric Feeding Tube Composition

	Polyvinyl Chloride	Silicone	Urethane
Ease of insertion	Too stiff for comfort	Too soft	Adequate
Ability to aspirate gastric contents	Excellent	Poor to fair	Good
Patient comfort	Very poor	Excellent	Good
Durability/strength	Strong but brittle	Breaks easily	Excellent/strong

Adapted with permission from Monturo CA: Enteral access device selection. Nutr Clin Pract 1990;5:207–213.

with stylets that can be inserted to stiffen the tubes and facilitate their passage. Removal of the stylet after passage is made easier when the interior lumen has also been lubricated.[47,48] Numerous polyurethane and some silicone-elastomer nasoenteric tubes are available in several sizes and lengths (Table 14–4).

Rigid Tubes or Tubes with Rigid Guides

Among the tubes currently available are those with stiff outer tubes for facilitating insertion; these are later removed or left external to the nares, leaving an inner silicone tube in place. The Moss-brand tube is a large rigid tube that decompresses the stomach while allowing feeding through a silicone duodenal feeding tube. This tube has three lumens, a radiographic tip, and a balloon that can be inflated and positioned at the esophagogastric junction. This tube is usually inserted at surgery and removed within 48 hours. The aspiration lumen must be connected to continuous suction to ensure appropriate decompression of the stomach.[25]

The Argyle-brand Duo-Tube has an outer tube of polyvinylchloride for insertion and an inner tube of silicone for feeding. After the polyvinylchloride tube is inserted, the clinician expels the silicone inner tube in the stomach by squeezing a bulb attached to the outer tube.[47]

An enteral tube with a pH sensor, which may help monitor and confirm tube placement, has recently been introduced (Zinetics-brand Accusite pH Enteral Feeding System). This tube helps to reduce the need for radiographic documentation of feeding tube placement.[49-51] The tube has compared favorably with pH tape in determining if the feeding tube is in the stomach or small bowel, and it did not appear that histamine blockers affected its accuracy.[50] However, it remains unclear how reliable pH readings are, since there is room for error, especially in critically ill patients.[52-54]

TABLE 14–4 Nasoenteral Feeding Tubes

Manufacturer/ Tube	Material	Weight	Eyelet Placement	Length (in)	French Size	Features
Clintec						
Clintec Tube	Polyurethane	No weight	Side	20	6	Stylet
	Polyurethane	No weight	Side	37	12	No stylet
	Polyurethane	No weight	Side	37	12	Catheter tip adaptor
	Polyurethane	Tungsten, 3 g	Side	36	8	Stylet
	Polyurethane	Tungsten, 3 g	Side	43	8	Stylet
	Polyurethane	Tungsten, 7 g	Side	43	8	Stylet
	Polyurethane	Tungsten, 7 g	Side	43	8	No stylet
	Polyurethane	Tungsten, 5 g	Side	43	10	Stylet
	Polyurethane	Tungsten, 7 g	Side	43	10	Stylet
	Polyurethane	Tungsten, 5 g	Side	43	12	No stylet
	Polyurethane	Tungsten, 5 g	Side	43	12	Stylet
	Polyurethane	Tungsten, 7 g	Side	43	12	Stylet All hydromer coated, dual port
Cook, Inc.						
Frederick Miller	Polyvinylchloride	Stainless steel, ? Weight	Side	47	8	Luer-lock end guidewire
McLean-Ring	Polyurethane	Stainless steel, ? Weight	Side and tip	51	9.5	Teflon-coated stainless steel guidewire
Corpak Medsystems						
Vitra-Lita NG	Polyurethane	No weight	Outlet Port 3 times girth of tube	36	5	No stylet
	Polyurethane	No weight	Outlet Port 3 times girth of tube	22	6	With or without stylet
	Polyurethane	No weight	Outlet Port 3 times girth of tube	36	6	With or without stylet
	Polyurethane	No weight	Outlet Port 3 times girth of tube	22	8	Stylet
	Polyurethane	No weight	Outlet Port 3 times girth of tube	36	8	With or without stylet
	Polyurethane	No weight	Outlet Port 3 times girth of tube	43	8	With or without stylet
	Polyurethane	No weight	Outlet Port 3 times girth of tube	36	10	With or without stylet
	Polyurethane	No weight	Outlet Port 3 times girth of tube	43	10	Stylet
	Polyurethane	No weight	Outlet Port 3 times girth of tube	36	12	Stylet
	Polyurethane	No weight	Outlet Port 3 times girth of tube	43	12	No stylet
Corflo-Ultra NG	Polyurethane	7 g	Outlet Port 3 times girth of tube	43	8	Stylet
	Polyurethane	7 g	Outlet Port 3 times girth of tube	43	10	(Stylet stiffer for use with fluoroscopy or endoscopy)
	Polyurethane	7 g	Outlet Port 3 times girth of tube	43	12	(Stylet stiffer for use with fluoroscopy or endoscopy)

Table continued on following page

TABLE 14–4   Nasoenteral Feeding Tubes   *Continued*

Manufacturer/ Tube	Material	Weight	Eyelet Placement	Length (in)	French Size	Features
	Polyurethane	3-g pill bolus	Outlet Port 3 times girth of tube	43	8	(Stylet stiffer for use with fluoroscopy or endoscopy)
	Polyurethane	3-g pill bolus	Outlet Port 3 times girth of tube	43	10	(Stylet stiffer for use with fluoroscopy or endoscopy)
	Polyurethane	3-g smooth tip	Outlet Port 3 times girth of tube	36	6	Stylet
	Polyurethane	3-g smooth tip	Outlet Port 3 times girth of tube	36	8	Stylet
	Polyurethane	3-g smooth tip	Outlet Port 3 times girth of tube	43	8	With or without stylet
	Polyurethane	3-g smooth tip	Outlet Port 3 times girth of tube	36	10	With or without stylet
	Polyurethane	3-g smooth tip	Outlet Port 3 times girth of tube	43	10	With or without stylet
	Polyurethane	3-g smooth tip	Outlet Port 3 times girth of tube	36	12	With or without stylet
	Polyurethane	3-g smooth tip	Outlet Port 3 times girth of tube	43	12	With or without stylet
Corflo-Controller NG	Polyurethane	7 g	Staggered side	43	8	Stylet
	Polyurethane	7 g	Staggered side	43	10	Catheter-tip adaptor
	Polyurethane	7 g	Staggered side	43	12	Catheter-tip adaptor
	Polyurethane	3-g pill bolus	Staggered side	43	8	Stylet
	Polyurethane	3-g pill bolus	Staggered side	43	10	Stylet
	Polyurethane	3-g pill bolus	Staggered side	55	10	Stylet
	Polyurethane	3-g smooth bolus	Staggered side	43	8	Stylet
	Polyurethane	3-g smooth bolus	Staggered side	43	10	Stylet
	Polyurethane	3-g smooth bolus	Staggered side	55	10	Stylet
Silk Lite	Polyurethane	No weight	Staggered side	43	12	No stylet
Davol						
Davol tube	Polyvinylchloride	No weight	Side	15	5	No stylet
	Polyvinylchloride	No weight	Side	36	5	No stylet
	Polyvinylchloride	No weight	Side	15	8	No stylet
	Polyvinylchloride	No weight	Side	42	8	No stylet
Entra Care						
Ultraflo	Polyurethane	No weight	Side and tip	36	12	No stylet, all have dual
	Polyurethane	No weight	Side and tip	36	14	No stylet, all have dual
	Polyurethane	Tungsten, 3 g	Side	36	8	Stylet
	Polyurethane	Tungsten, 3 g	Side	43	8	Stylet
	Polyurethane	Tungsten, 3 g	Side	43	8	No stylet
	Polyurethane	Tungsten, 7 g	Side	43	8	Stylet
	Polyurethane	Tungsten, 5 g	Side	43	10	Stylet

TABLE 14–4   Nasoenteral Feeding Tubes   *Continued*

Manufacturer/ Tube	Material	Weight	Eyelet Placement	Length (in)	French Size	Features
	Polyurethane	Tungsten, 5 g	Side	36	12	Stylet
	Polyurethane	Tungsten, 5 g	Side	43	12	Stylet
Ethox Easy Glide	Polyurethane	Tungsten, 4 g	Side	43	8	Stylet
	Polyurethane	Tungsten, 4 g	Side	43	10	Stylet
	Polyurethane	Tungsten, 4 g	Side	43	12	Stylet
Gesco Nutri-Cath	Silicone	No weight	Side and end	15	5, 6.5, 8	Stylet, Luer-lock hub, graduated at 2 cm intervals
	Silicone	No weight	Side and end	24	5, 6.5, 8	Stylet, Luer-lock hub, graduated at 2 cm intervals
IVAC Keofeed II	Polyurethane	3 g	Side	43	8	With or without stylet
	Polyurethane	5 g	Side	43	8	With or without stylet
	Polyurethane	3 g	Side	36	8	With or without stylet
	Polyurethane	3 g	Side	43	12	With or without stylet
Kendall Superior Graduated Pediatric Tubes	Polyvinylchloride	No weight	Side	15	5	Stylet
	Polyvinylchloride	No weight	Side	15	8	Luer-tip adaptor
Moss	Silicone	No weight	Side	44	18	Triple-lumen, decompression while feeding, spring guidewire
Ross Flexiflo	Polyurethane	Tungsten, 3 g	Side and end	45	8	Stylet
	Polyurethane	Tungsten, 3 g	Side and end	45	10	Twin Y-ports
	Polyurethane	Tungsten, 3 g	Side and end	36	8	Twin Y-ports
	Polyurethane	Tungsten, 3 g	Side and end	45	12	Twin Y-ports
	Polyurethane	Tungsten, 3 g	Side and end	45	8	No stylet
	Polyurethane	Tungsten, 3 g	Side and end	36	12	No stylet
	Polyurethane	Tungsten, 3 g	Side and end	36	14	No stylet
	Polyurethane	Tungsten, 3 g	Side and end	36	16	No stylet
Flexiflo "Over the Guidewire"	Polyurethane	Tungsten, 3 g	End	60	10	Twin Y-ports with guidewire
Rusch Entube (3)	Polyurethane	Tungsten, 3.3 g	Open end Outlet Port	45	8	Stylet, triple port connector, can use with luer-lock or slip tip
	Polyurethane	Tungsten, 6.5 g	Open end Outlet Port	45	8	Stylet, triple port connector, can use with luer-lock or slip tip
	Polyurethane	Tungsten, 4.5 g	Open end Outlet Port	45	10	Stylet, triple port connector, can use with luer-lock or slip tip
	Polyurethane	Tungsten, 5.0 g	Open end Outlet Port	45	12	Stylet, triple port connector, can use with luer-lock or slip tip

Table continued on following page

TABLE 14–4   Nasoenteral Feeding Tubes   *Continued*

Manufacturer/ Tube	Material	Weight	Eyelet Placement	Length (in)	French Size	Features
	Polyurethane	Tungsten, 6.5 g	Open end Outlet Port	45	10	Stylet, triple port connector, can use with luer-lock or slip tip
	Polyurethane	Tungsten, 3.3 g	Open end Outlet Port	45	8	No stylet
Entube	Polyurethane	Tungsten, 3.3 g	Side	36	8	Stylet, twin port Y-connector
	Polyurethane	Tungsten, 3.3 g	Side	45	8	Stylet, twin port Y-connector
	Polyurethane	Tungsten, 5.0 g	Side	45	8	Stylet, twin port Y-connector
	Polyurethane	Tungsten, 4.5 g	Side	36	10	Stylet, twin port Y-connector
	Polyurethane	Tungsten, 4.5 g	Side	45	10	Stylet, twin port Y-connector
	Polyurethane	Tungsten, 5.0 g	Side	36	12	Stylet, twin port Y-connector
	Polyurethane	Tungsten, 5.0 g	Side	45	12	Stylet, twin port Y-connector
Entube Plus	Polyurethane	Bolus, 6.5 g	Side	45	8	No stylet
	Polyurethane	Bolus, 6.5 g	Side	55	8	To be placed by nurses in long term care areas
	Polyurethane	Bolus, 6.5 g	Side	45	10	To be placed by nurses in long term care areas
	Polyurethane	Bolus, 6.5 g	Side	45	12	To be placed by nurses in long term care areas
Entube Pediatric Tubes	Polyurethane	Tungsten, 1.5 g	Side	20	6	No stylet
	Polyurethane	Tungsten, 1.5 g	Side	30	6	Twin port Y-connector
	Polyurethane	No weight	Side	20	6	Twin port Y-connector
	Polyurethane	No weight	Side	30	6	No stylet
Enfuse	Polyurethane	Tungsten, 4 g	Side	45	14	Twin port Y
	Polyurethane	No weight	Side	36	12	Stylet
	Polyurethane	No weight	Side	36	14	Stylet
Sherwood Endo-Tube	Polyurethane	Stainless steel, 7 g	Side and end	60	12	Guidewire for fluoroscopy or endoscopic placement
Dobbhoff, Naso-jejunal feeding and gastric decompression	Polyurethane	Tungsten, 3.5 g	Side and end	67	9	Twin Y-ports, jej. dual lumen
					16	Overall guidewire, spiral design reduces kinking
Dobbhoff	Polyurethane	Tungsten, 7 g	Side	55	8	Stylet, rigid outlet
	Polyurethane	Tungsten, 7 g	Side	43	8	With/without stylet
	Polyurethane	Tungsten, 5 g	Side	43	8	Stylet, rigid outlet
	Polyurethane	Tungsten, 7 g	Side	43	10	Stylet, rigid outlet
	Polyurethane	Tungsten, 7 g	Side	43	12	Stylet, rigid outlet
Entriflex	Polyurethane	Tungsten, 3 g	Side	36	8	Hydromer lubricant, dual port option, with or without stylet
	Polyurethane	Tungsten, 3 g	Side	43	8	Hydromer lubricant, dual port option, with or without stylet

TABLE 14–4 Nasoenteral Feeding Tubes *Continued*

Manufacturer/ Tube	Material	Weight	Eyelet Placement	Length (in)	French Size	Features
	Polyurethane	Tungsten, 5 g	Side	43	10	Hydromer lubricant, dual port option, with or without stylet
	Polyurethane	Tungsten, 5 g	Side	36	12	Hydromer lubricant, dual port option, with or without stylet
	Polyurethane	Tungsten, 5 g	Side	43	12	Hydromer lubricant, dual port option, with or without stylet
	Polyurethane	Tungsten, 3.5 g	Side	43	12	No stylet
Argyle/Quest Duo-Tube	Silicone (inner)/ Polyvinylchloride (outer)	Silicone	Side	40	6 inner 15 outer	No stylet
	Silicone (inner)/ Polyvinylchloride (outer)	Silicone	Side	40	8 inner 16 outer	No stylet
	Silicone (inner)/ Polyvinylchloride (outer)	Tungsten	Side	40	8 inner 17 outer	No stylet
Wilson-Cook Nasal Jejunal	Polyvinylchloride	No weight	Side and end	95	8 and 10	Guidewire for endoscopic placement
Zinetics	Polyurethane	No weight	Side	36	6	Single use only, use pH monitor to help aid in tube placement, pH sensor in distal tip
	Polyurethane	Tungsten	Side	43	8 and 10	Single use only, use pH monitor to help aid in tube placement, pH sensor in distal tip

Ideal Tube Characteristics

The ideal nasoenteric feeding tube should be made of pliable, nonstiffening, nonleaching material. It should be the appropriate length for the feeding site, have enough strength to tolerate a pump pressure to 50 psi, and have the correct intraluminal diameter for delivery of formulas with varied viscosities. French sizes describe the outer diameter, not the inner lumen. The adaptor should not be compatible with intravenous tubing, and the tube should have Y-connector access to facilitate irrigation and medication delivery (Fig. 14–2). The distal tip should be smooth and self-lubricated for ease of passage. The inside of the tube should be lubricated as well to facilitate removal of the stylet, if used.

Insertion Techniques

Various procedures are described in the literature to accomplish nasoenteric tube placement while attempting to minimize complications. Although there continues to be conflicting evidence over whether postpyloric feedings may prevent problems associated with reflux of enteral formula and aspiration, it is safe to say that the goal for most enteral tube intubations is the small bowel, preferably distal to the ligament of Treitz (Fig. 14–3).

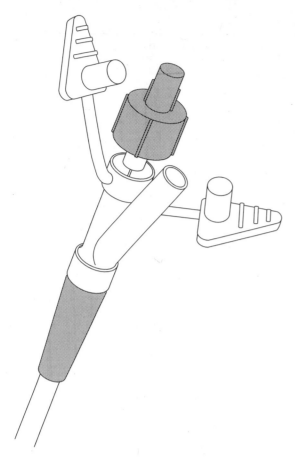

FIGURE 14–2 Nasoenteric feeding tube Y-site end to facilitate irrigation and medication delivery. (Courtesy Corpak Medsystems, Wheeling, IL.)

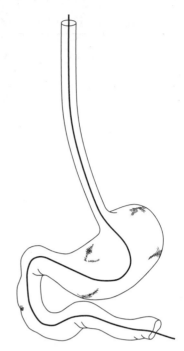

FIGURE 14–3 Optimal position of nasoenteric tube for patients at increased risk for aspiration.

The technique for nasogastric and nasojejunal placement at the bedside is essentially the same. The lubricated tip is passed through the most patent nostril into the nasopharynx and swallowed if the patient is able and the tip of the tube is positioned into the stomach. Many tubes are now packaged with a flexible wire stylet in place to aid with insertion (Table 14–5).

The use of metoclopramide, 10 to 20 mg IV, before the tube is placed has met with varying success.[55-59] Whatley and associates[58] have shown that metoclopramide can aid transpyloric placement if administered before feeding-tube placement but not after tube placement; however, the study size was limited. Kittinger and others looked at 70 patients and found no difference in those who received metoclopramide before intubation and those who did not; however, a subgroup of diabetic patients had a significantly better success rate with the drug. They concluded that metoclopramide may be helpful,

especially in diabetic patients, if administered before tube placement but not after.[55]

Use of erythromycin may also be beneficial when trying to place a feeding tube into the small intestine. A clinical study is currently underway to investigate this issue further.[60,61]

After the tube is passed into the stomach, turn the patient to the right side so that the stomach's peristaltic motion can propel the weighted tube tip through the pylorus into the duodenum. If the tube has not passed spontaneously into the duodenum after 8 to 24 hours, it probably will not.[62]

Other methods of insertion have recently become more widely used. Tubes placed endoscopically and fluoroscopically into the small bowel have proved very successful. These techniques for placement save time and money and allow patients to receive their nutritional requirements in a safer and more timely fashion[63-67] (Chapter 12). Zaloga has also described a method of placing feeding tubes into the small bowel that does not require fluoroscopy or endoscopy and has had a 92 percent success rate. This method requires placing the feeding tube into the patient, removing and bending the stylet, replacing it back into the feeding tube, and then guiding it through the pylorus.[68,69]

When placing any nasoenteric tube for feeding, verify the distal tip. Insufflation of air into

TABLE 14–5 Procedure for Inserting Nasoenteric Tubes

1. Provide privacy.
2. Explain procedure and its purpose.
3. Place patient in sitting position with neck flexed slightly and head of bed elevated to 45 degrees.
4. Estimate distance for placement into the stomach by measuring the length from the tip of the nose to the earlobe and then from the earlobe to the xiphoid process. Add 50 cm to this length. Observe markings on shaft of tube for guidance.
5. Lubricate stylet and insert into feeding tube.
6. Inspect nares and determine optimal patency by having the patient breathe through one nostril while the other is occluded temporarily. Lubricate chosen nostril with water-soluble lubricant.
7. Lubricate the end of the tube or activate the self-lubricant with water and pass it posteriorly. If the patient is alert and cooperative, ask him or her to swallow water to facilitate tube passage.
8. Once the tube is beyond the nasopharynx, allow the patient to rest.
9. Have the patient flex the neck and swallow while the tube is advanced.
10. If the patient begins to cough, withdraw the tube into the nasopharynx and then reattempt passage.
11. Confirm passage into stomach by aspiration of gastric contents first and then obtain abdominal x-ray film.
12. Secure tube to bridge of nose or upper lip with nonallergenic tape or tube attachment device.
13. Once tube placement is confirmed, remove stylet. Do not try to reinsert stylet after removal.

the tube is not sufficient to verify the position in the stomach because auscultation over the stomach can register sound transmitted through a tube that has been inadvertently passed into either mainstem bronchus.[70] Many of these tubes are small enough to pass through the glottis and trachea without markedly interfering with phonation or respiration. Enteral solutions delivered through a tube misplaced into the bronchial tree can cause severe pneumonitis and death. The simplest means of initially confirming proper tube placement in the GI tract is by the aspiration of GI contents. Because small-bore, soft tubes may collapse with negative pressure, a 30 ml or larger syringe, which is recommended by most manufacturers, may not be successful for aspiration of enteric contents. There is continued debate over whether aspiration of enteric contents is a totally reliable test to confirm tube placement.[52-54,71]

If intestinal contents cannot be aspirated through the tube, radiographic confirmation of the tube tip location is the most dependable method for determining tube placement before starting enteral feedings. Because feeding tubes are radiopaque, a simple plain film of the abdomen is usually adequate. If the exact location of the tube is still in doubt, a small amount of contrast material can be injected through the tube.

Techniques for Securing Nasoenteric Feeding Tubes

Maintaining nasoenteric tubes can be a major problem. Skin irritation from the tape is common, and loosening of the tape with accidental removal of the tube occurs frequently even in oriented, cooperative patients.[72] Removal of the tube by confused or uncooperative patients is an even greater dilemma. Various taping methods and holding devices have been developed to address these problems. Except in diaphoretic patients, adhesive or hypoallergenic tape can be safe and effective if applied appropriately.[73]

A nasal tube attachment device is available from the Hollister company. It adheres to the nose and uses an adjustable clip to hold the feeding tube in place. Securing a feeding tube in patients with facial burns can be even more of a challenge. Solem[74] describes a method of securing a tube with plain twilled tape that is tied behind the patient's head. This method is simple and well accepted by patients.

Complications of Nasoenteric Feeding Tube Placement

Small-bore nasoenteral feeding tubes are used frequently in the acute care setting and still present less of a risk for complications than central parenteral access, but their placement does not come without risks.

Recent technologic advances to nasoenteral feeding tubes such as less rigid stylets, fewer side eyelets in styleted tubes, improved radiopaque quality, and self-lubrication, have aided in successful placement. However, complications still occur for various reasons. The number of misplaced tubes over the past 20 years is due to increased use of small-bore nasoenteral feeding tubes in the growing acutely ill population and of health care practitioners' awareness, concern, and documentation. This incidence of complications is documented as 7.6 percent by Ghahremani and Gould.[53] The frequency of nasoenteric feeding tube placement into the trachea has been reported to vary from 0.3 percent to 15 percent in bedside insertions. Table 14–6 lists possible complications and actions to prevent them.

Extra care is needed for intubated patients in the intensive care unit (ICU). Other significant risk factors for problems with tube insertion include advanced age, neurologic impairment, history of tube placement difficulties, and anatomic abnormalities of the maxillofacial area or GI tract. Serious and fatal pneumothoraces as well as fatal intracranial placement has been reported.[75-80] A comprehensive list of these complications can be found in a recent review by Boyes and Kruse.[81]

DELIVERY METHODS AND SITES

After deciding to use a nasoenteric tube for feeding, the clinician must decide whether to feed into the stomach or small bowel (Fig. 14–4). The patient's disease often determines the optimal location for tube placement and method of formula delivery. Either intermittent or continuous feeding may be infused into the stomach. Continuous feeding should be given when the tube is placed in the duodenum or jejunum.

A survey of nutritional support services revealed that 83 percent of enteral nutrition is delivered continuously, whereas only 17 percent is given by the intermittent or bolus method.[82] In the same study, 76 percent of feedings were delivered into the stomach and 24 percent into the small bowel. It was concluded that most feedings are given into the stomach and are administered continuously. In a similar survey of home care patients, no significant difference in the method of administration was observed. Most respondents indicated that more than half their patients used the intermittent delivery method.[83]

Feeding into the Stomach

The advantages of feeding into the stomach include ease of tube placement, physiologic similarity to normal GI function, and the option of continuous or intermittent formula delivery. Numerous factors are considered when choosing between continuous and intermittent feedings into the stomach.

TABLE 14–6 Complications of Nasoenteric Feeding Tube Placement

Complications	Preventive Measures
Cranial	
Intracranial placement	Caution with maxillofacial trauma or basilar skull fracture
	Use oral route
	Use endoscopic technique
Nasal/Laryngeal/Pharyngeal	
Epistaxis, nasopharyngeal erosions, pharyngitis	Caution with placement
	Discontinue procedure if resistance encountered
Otitis media	Use smallest tube possible
Sinusitis	Use polyurethane or silicone tube
Vocal cord paralysis	Obtain permanent access if tube feeding needed long term
Esophageal	
Esophageal perforation	Caution with placement, discontinue placement if resistance
Esophagitis	encountered
Esophageal varices rupture	Caution with guidewires
	Use smaller, softer tube
Tracheal/Pulmonary	
Intratracheal/bronchial placement	Radiographic confirmation before feedings
Pneumothorax, bronchopleural fistula, hemorrhage	Discontinue procedure if resistance met
	Avoid replacing stylet once tube in place
Gastrointestinal	
Gastrointestinal perforation	Discontinue procedure if resistance met
	Avoid replacing stylet once tube in place

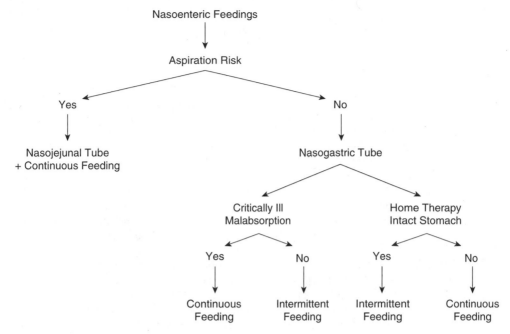

FIGURE 14–4 Decision making for route and method of nasoenteric feedings.

Feeding Continuously into the Stomach

Efficacy. Continuous feedings have demonstrated a decreased risk of gastric distention and aspiration.[5,84,85] In critically ill patients, continuous feedings have been shown to produce fewer metabolic abnormalities, such as increases in postprandial glucose, oxygen consumption, and carbon dioxide production than those produced with intermittently infused nutrients.[86] Because intermittent feedings require energy for storage, research has demonstrated that continuous feedings have less dietary-induced thermogenesis.[87-90] Maintenance energy requirements may then be less during continuous enteral feedings than during intermittent ones. This conflicts with a small study done with 18 adult head and neck patients where Campbell and associates[91] compared 24-hour continuous feedings with 16-hour nocturnal cyclic feedings and found a higher oxygen consumption and nitrogen balance in the continuously fed group. The nocturnally fed group showed more energy efficiency but yielded a poorer nitrogen balance.

Shulman[92] demonstrated an increased intestinal mucosal and protein mass with intermittent feeding compared with 24-hour continuous feeding. Twelve-hour nocturnal feeding was compared with continuous enteral feeding in a larger animal study. Westfall and Heitkemper[93] demonstrated no statistical differences in weight gain, plasma glucose, and glucagon levels with feeding schedules. The 12-hour enteral feeding schedule did, however, significantly influence plasma insulin and corticosterone levels.

Complications. Studies indicate that continuous intragastric feedings are better tolerated than intermittent feedings.[5,84,85] Ciocon,[94] in a study of 60 elderly patients, found higher rates of diarrhea in the intermittent group than in the continuously fed group. There were no significant differences between calories recommended and delivered. In an earlier study, Kocan and Hickisch[95] investigated 34 adult patients in neurologic ICUs, and found no significant differences in stool consistency, number of stools per day, aspiration, or caloric intake between patients receiving continuous feeding and those receiving intermittent feeding.

Gastric feeding and aspiration continues to be examined. Reports include low rates of aspiration in critically ill, adult ventilated patients receiving continuous or intermittent enteral feeding.[56,96] Cogan and Weintraub,[97] in a study of 109 nursing home patients with gastrostomies, found no difference in aspiration rates with continuous versus intermittent enteral feeding.

Continuous feeding associated with pneumonia was examined in a smaller study of 24 ventilated patients. Patients were fed either continuously or for 12 hours nocturnally. Fifty-four percent of the patients who persistently had a gastric pH of more than 3.5 developed pneumonia. This was based only on one gastric aspirate per day.[98] Gastroesophageal reflux has been shown to be higher in critically ill ventilated patients being fed through a nasogastric tube.[99] Gastroesophageal reflux and relaxation of lower esophageal sphincter pressure has been shown to be dramatic after rapid bolus feeding.[100] Saxe[101] measured lower esophageal sphincter (LES) tone in 16 head-injured patients and found that a Glasgow Coma Score below 12 was consistent with a decreased LES tone, which should preclude any gastric feeding.

Intermittent Feeding into the Stomach

Although continuous feeding is frequently the preferred delivery method in the hospitalized patient, intermittent feeding is selected for the home care patient whenever possible. The goal is to return the patient to the normal activities of daily living. As long as the tube is placed in the stomach, a schedule of intermittent feedings, three to six times each day, can usually be developed to accommodate any lifestyle. Today many insurance providers will not reimburse for a feeding pump and continuous intragastric feeding.

One prospective, randomized study in 40 adult patients compared two regimens for converting from continuous to intermittent feedings in patients with feeding gastrostomies. Half the patients were randomized to abruptly changing from continuous to gradually increasing intermittent feedings until reaching their nutritional goals. IV fluids were given to maintain hydration status. The second half of the group received an overlapping regimen, receiving continuous feedings at a decreasing rate while intermittent feedings were progressively increased. Patients receiving the overlapping regimen had a shorter hospitalization, maintained nutritional goals for a greater portion of their hospital stay, used fewer days of IV fluids, and had less diarrheal episodes than the discontinuous regimen-managed patients.[102]

In pediatrics, one method of conversion from continuous to intermittent feedings has been to give the same absolute volume that the infant would receive in a 3-hour period over successively shorter periods. For example, if 30 ml/hour is being delivered continuously, the first step would be to give 45 ml/2 hours and then discontinue the infusion for 1 hour. If this is tolerated for 24 hours, then the following day,

the infusion would be increased to 90 ml/hour, then off for 2 hours, and then repeated.[103]

Feeding into the Small Bowel

The method for feeding into the small intestine is less controversial than feeding into the stomach. Research has demonstrated that the small intestine tolerates intermittent feedings and sudden rate changes poorly, so continuous delivery of nutrients is necessary.[5,9,43,104-106]

Two important unanswered questions remain regarding enteral feeding into the small intestine. First, is nutrient use adequate when feedings are delivered into the small intestine rather than the stomach? Second, are there fewer complications when feeding into the small bowel rather than the stomach?

Efficacy. Use of continuously administered nutrients into the small intestine, compared with the stomach, has been studied in both animals and humans. In an animal model that compared continuous gastric and jejunal feeding, significantly greater weight gain and fewer GI side-effects occurred with gastric feedings.[107] These investigators later studied feedings into the duodenum in the same animal model and found that it may be preferable to either gastric or jejunal sites. Duodenal feedings provided equivalent nutrient use to the stomach without the associated gastroesophageal reflux and aspiration.[108]

In a study of adult humans, serum albumin and transferrin levels improved in a group who received cycled or interrupted enteral nutrition when compared with a group who received continuous enteral nutrition.[109] Infants receiving intermittent nasogastric feedings were compared with a group receiving continuous nasoduodenal feedings; no significant differences in either caloric intake or growth rate were reported.[110] Another infant study comparing nasogastric to transpyloric feedings demonstrated no nutritional benefit from transpyloric feedings.[111] In a study of 38 critically ill patients, nasogastric feedings were compared to nasojejunal. Jejunally fed patients achieved higher percentages of caloric requirements, had a greater rise in prealbumin concentrations, and had less pneumonia than the intragastrically fed group.[112] To date, however, not enough evidence exists in the critical care setting to suggest that one site is safer or more efficient than another.[113] Bypassing the stomach does not effectively reduce the risk of aspiration. Full implications of nutrient delivery to the small bowel, possibly altering the secretions of the upper gut, are unknown.[113]

Complications. The association of aspiration with different sites has been studied. An extensive review of the empiric evidence on aspiration in patients with severe neurogenic oropharyngeal dysphagia did not support the preferential use of either long-term gastric or jejunal feeding.[114] A retrospective study of nursing home patients with feeding jejunostomies found a 16 percent aspiration rate and concluded that use of jejunostomy feeds offers only limited protection against aspiration.[97] In another study of 33 hospitalized patients fed with small-bore nasoenteric tubes, equal aspiration rates were found in two groups of patients, those fed beyond the second portion of the duodenum and those fed intragastrically.[115]

A potential disadvantage of feeding into the duodenum is accidental tube dislodgement. Even tubes with weighted ends can reflux into the stomach because of coughing or vomiting. Although the morbidity associated with unsuspected positional change from nasoduodenal to nasogastric feeding would seem to be minimal, there does appear to be an increased risk of aspiration.[116] This risk is greater in patients with altered gastric motility.

Conclusion

A patient's disease often determines the optimal location for tube placement and continuous or intermittent formula delivery. Numerous studies support continuous feeding into the stomach to produce fewer metabolic abnormalities, decreased risk of gastric distension, and decreased oxygen consumption. No difference in aspiration rates has been found between continuous and intermittent methods of feeding. Decreased LES tone has been demonstrated in more severely head-injured patients, which may preclude intragastric feed-

ing in this population. Rapid bolus administration of formula is not recommended for any patient. Higher rates of diarrhea have been associated with intermittent feedings in hospitalized patients. For those patients receiving intragastric feedings at home, intermittent administration may be better incorporated into their lifestyle.

When nutrient delivery is through the small bowel, feedings must always be delivered continuously. In the critically ill, there is evidence that patients receive a higher percentage of caloric requirements if fed jejunally. Equal aspiration rates have been found in dysphagic patients with permanent gastric and jejunal access as well as in hospitalized patients with small-bore nasoenteric tubes placed either in the stomach or duodenum. The use of feeding jejunostomies in nursing home patients has demonstrated only limited protection against aspiration. In cases of known gastric hypomotility, small-bowel feeding is recommended.

Further controlled prospective randomized trials in different types of patients are needed to identify the optimal feeding site and delivery method.

Starter Regimens

Starter regimens are methods of initiating enteral nutrition based on formula concentration and rate of delivery. Reports recommend that starter regimens be used with isotonic or hypertonic formulas rather than hypotonic feedings.[7,117] Patients started on very dilute (one quarter strength) of an isotonic feeding at slow rates unnecessarily receive very little nutrient intake. Table 14–7 describes a starter regimen that optimizes nutrient intake and minimizes complications. Included are recommendations for monitoring residuals. Acceptable residual volume is lower with gastrostomy

TABLE 14–7   Starter Regimen and Progression Based on Delivery

	Method	
	Intermittent	**Continuous**
Initial regimen	120 ml isotonic formula every 4 hours followed by 30-ml water flush.	30–40 ml/hour of isotonic formula
Rate and method of advancement	Check residuals before next feeding. Residuals acceptable up to half of previously administered volume.	Check residuals every 4 hours. Hold for ≥2 hours worth of rate up to maximum of 150 ml. Hold feeds for maximum of 100 ml in permanent gastrostomy feedings.

tubes because of the higher tip placement in the stomach.[118,119]

Standard Order Form

A standard order sheet is helpful to initiate and maintain nasoenteric tube feeding (Table 14–8). This standardization is especially relevant in institutions where physicians with varied experience are responsible for writing orders. In addition, this checklist helps clinicians to avoid omitting important details. An enteral feeding protocol should be established and followed to ensure that specified nutritional goals are met.

TRANSITIONAL FEEDING

Transitional feeding is defined as the gradual progression from one mode of nutritional therapy to another while maintaining nutrient requirements. Transitional feedings, for the purposes of this discussion, occur when patients are being "weaned" from enteral nutrition to oral feeding. The transition from enteral to oral feeding must be coordinated with the patient's ability and desire to eat by mouth.[120] Frequently, the patient is the best judge of when oral feedings will be tolerated.

Little scientific evidence exists to support the current methods of transitional feeding. Guidelines for transitional feeding that meet the patient's nutritional goals are listed in Figure 14–5. Transitional feedings should be started slowly. An oral intake of greater than 50 percent of normal nutrient requirements is the end point used to progress to the next feeding step. Methods and suggestions to enhance the transition from enteral feedings to oral diet include the following: (1) use cyclic feedings at night to encourage an increased oral intake during the day, (2) use intermittent feedings that do not interfere with meals, (3) select an oral diet that will be most easily ingested, digested, and absorbed, (4) use appetite stimulants as appropriate, (5) have patient select food preferences when possible and include between-meal snacks or supplements, and (6) have families or friends bring in favorite foods from home.

When choosing a transitional feeding plan, the type of formula or diet is important. Certain diseases dictate specific characteristics in the transitional feeding program. Careful observation of dietary tolerance, calorie counts, and standard metabolic monitoring are required during transitional feeding. Successful transitional feeding requires a team approach and good communication with the patient.

MONITORING

Patients who receive nasoenteric feedings require the same careful monitoring as those

---

TABLE 14–8   Enteral Feeding Standard Orders

Feeding tube and location of tip _____

Check items to be completed:

_____   1. Obtain chest x-ray film after placement to confirm position.

_____   2. Before feeding, confirm placement of tube by aspiration of gastric contents.

_____   3. Elevate head of bed 30 degrees when feeding into stomach.

_____   4. Name of formula _____

        a. Intermittent: Give _____ ml over 30 minutes every _____ hours at _____ strength.

        b. Continuous: Give _____ ml per hour for _____ hours at _____ strength.

_____   5. Check for residual every _____ hours with gastric feedings. Return residual to stomach. Hold feedings for 1 hour if residual is greater than _____ ml and recheck in 1 hour.

_____   6. Routinely flush tube with _____ ml of _____ every _____ hours for hydration.

_____   7. Weigh patient every Monday and Thursday and record on chart.

_____   8. Record intake and output daily. Chart volume of formula separately from water or other oral intake for each shift.

_____   9. Record number, volume, and consistency of bowel movements.

_____ 10. Change administration tubing and feeding bag daily.

_____ 11. Obtain complete blood count, complete serum chemistry profile, and prealbumin weekly.

_____ 12. Obtain basic chemistry profile every Monday and Thursday.

_____ 13. Begin 24-hour urine collection for urea nitrogen and creatinine at 7 AM on _____

_____ 14. Notify physician for nausea, vomiting, severe diarrhea, or shortness of breath.

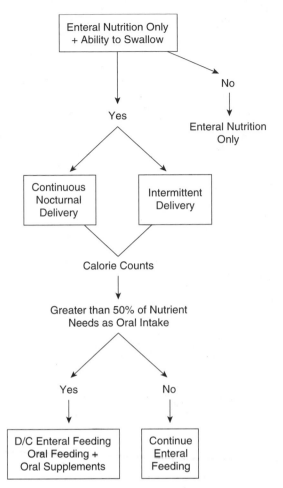

FIGURE 14–5 Transitional feeding from enteral to oral nutrition.

who receive parenteral nutrition. Monitoring is best accomplished by employing protocols, standard orders, and follow-up study of patients by a nutrition support service. Careful attention to the patient's metabolic status and fluid and electrolyte balance is necessary to avoid complications. Complications associated with nasoenteric feeding are briefly outlined in Table 14–9[121] and discussed in Chapter 27.

DELIVERY SYSTEMS: FEEDING CONTAINERS

History

Feeding containers have received little description in the literature. The pig's bladder was one of the first types of containers for administering enteral feeding. Syringelike receptacles followed, but the material from which they were made was not identified.[2] Ceramicware

was widely employed for administering feedings to infants in the late 18th and early 19th centuries.[122] However, no record exists that these devices were adapted for use as feeding tubes. With the discovery of glass, syringelike devices, including the Murphy drip bottle and Asepto syringe, were commonly employed to deliver feedings until the early 1970s. Even metal enema pails were modified to deliver enteral formulas.

When tube-feeding formulas were simply blenderized foods mixed together in the hospital kitchen, they needed to be measured by the nurses and administered by gravity boluses through syringes or funnels attached to rubber tubing. Administration of these viscous, blenderized formulas required that nurses be present throughout the feeding. With the availability of less viscous, commercially prepared feeding formulas, which could pass through IV tubing, the formulas needed to be transferred into recycled glass bottles. During the 1960s and 1970s, bottles that held IV fluids were washed and reused for administering the tube-feeding formula. When empty plastic bags designed for IV administration of fluids became available, they were also used for tube feeding.[104] Tubing used for the IV administration of fluids also provided a screw or roller clamp for controlling the rate of flow. As a consequence, tube feedings could also be administered with more control and less nursing personnel time. The IV tubing also was compatible with the pumps needed for IV administration of fluids.

Present Status

Feeding containers are currently designed with or without preattached tubing. A potential hazard associated with the use of IV containers and tubing is the accidental delivery of an enteral formula intravenously.[123] The introduction of opaque IV fat emulsions has increased the risk of this complication because the emulsions resemble many enteral formulas. Kaminski has suggested that adding food coloring to the enteral formula may decrease the risk of its being delivered intravenously.[123] Manufacturers have taken another approach by labeling the tubing that is connected to the nasoenteric tube. Although this is helpful, a potential hazard is that the lettering on the tubing is difficult to read at night with minimal light. The optimal situation appears to be for the tubing attached to feeding bags and feeding tubes to be designed so that it is not compatible with IV systems. Currently the Association for the Advancement of Med-

TABLE 14–9 Common Complications Associated with Nasoenteric Feeding

Complications	Possible Causes
Gastrointestinal	
Nausea or vomiting	Anxiety
	Large gastric residuals
	Malodorous formula
	Medications
	Tube placement
	Improper patient position
	Cold feedings
	Rapid infusion rate
Aspiration	Improper tube placement
	Improper patient position
Diarrhea	Rapid infusion rate
	Hyperosmolar feedings or medications
	Lactose intolerance
	Antibiotic therapy
	Hypoalbuminemia
	Formula bacterial contamination
	Low-residue formula
Constipation	Low-residue formula
	Dehydration
	Inactivity
	Medications
Metabolic	
Dehydration	Fever or infection
	Inadequate fluid intake
	Excessive fluid losses
Elevated serum electrolytes	Excessive electrolytes in formula
	Inadequate fluid intake
	Excessive fluid losses
Depressed serum electrolytes	Excessive water administration or retention
	Inadequate electrolytes in formula
Hyperglycemia	Metabolic stress
	History of diabetes
	Excessive glucose administration
Mechanical	
Occluded or clogged	Excessive formula residue in feeding tube
	Administration of medications through tube
Nasal irritation or erosion	Improper taping of tube
Tube displacement	Patient coughing or vomiting

Adapted from Bernard M, Forlaw L: Complications and their prevention. In Rombeau JL, Caldwell MD (eds): Enteral and Tube Feeding, vol. 1. Philadelphia: WB Saunders, 1984.

ical Instrumentation is developing a standard for enteral feeding set connections to prevent such a complication.

An alternative developed to alleviate confusion of enteral with IV solutions has been to package commercial tube formulas in single-serving glass bottles with screw-off caps. To administer the solution to a patient, the top must be removed from the bottle and replaced with a screw-on cap with a drip chamber and attached tubing. When the cap is screwed on tightly, the bottle is inverted and the formula is ready to be fed to the patient; the tubing con-

nectors will fit only the feeding tubes. Several types of ready-to-feed bottled formulas are packaged with this adaptation.[124]

Currently, the polyvinylchloride bags, plastic irrigating containers, and semirigid containers are available in 500-, 1000-, 1200-, and 1500-ml sizes. Most of these containers are made with preattached tubing and are filled from the top. One of the benefits of containers designed specifically for enteral feedings is that the large filling ports allow easy transfer of solution into the containers, an advantage not available with IV feeding containers modified for tube feeding. Nonrigid vinyl or vinyl-compound containers (although calibrated with measurement scales in easy-to-read markings) tend to collapse as fluid volume diminishes, thus making it difficult to estimate the volume of feeding delivered. For pump-fed patients, this problem can be avoided because most enteral pumps have an accumulated volume display mechanism. This enables the clinician to better quantify tube formula volume delivered. Semirigid containers do not have this problem, but the calibration marks on these containers are difficult to read if they are not colored.

Powdered formulas that require reconstitution as well as those packaged in unit dose containers must be transferred into enteral feeding containers for administration. Most tube feedings are packaged as clean formulas, and opening them for transfer increases the potential for bacterial contamination. Because bacterial contamination can cause diarrhea in tube-fed patients, the clinician must be aware of this potential problem when solutions are transferred from containers, after reconstitution, or after dilution into containers.[125-132] In response to this problem of contamination, sterile enteral formulas in ready-to-hang "closed" systems were introduced in the mid-1980s.[133] Many prepackaged enteral formula container systems are available from manufacturers in several different sizes and formulas. These are safe and acceptable for patients being fed either continuously or intermittently. According to recent clinical evaluations, these nonvented, closed-delivery containers may be safely infused for as long as 48 hours and are associated with a reduction in both labor and bacterial contamination.[133,134] A spiking set penetrates the sealed bag, carton, or rigid container, thereby delivering the formula to the patient directly. This system eliminates the need for a separate feeding bag.

Manufacturers commonly provide prepackaged feedings in 1-L containers. These save nursing time by eliminating refilling and save storage space previously needed for feeding containers. Patients receive significantly more of the prescribed diet with this type of system.[134-136] The disadvantages of the prefilled system are that formula selection is limited and waste may increase with frequent changes in rate, concentration, or types of formulas prescribed for the patient. Manufacturers have now made available some prepackaged half-strength formulas as well as smaller-volume containers to help eliminate waste.

Ideal Container Design

An enteral feeding container should be easy to fill, close, and hang. It should also be safe, leakproof, and have easy-to-read calibrations and directions for use. Feeding containers should match patient and institutional needs. The container should have an adaptable tubing port that can fit various feeding tube ends; it also must be compatible with the enteral pump in use. Enteral feeding containers should be made from nonleaching material, should be disposable or easy to clean, and should require minimal storage space. Most of the containers currently available are listed in Table 14–10.

ENTERAL FEEDING PUMPS

History

A "stomach pump" for continuous delivery of enteral formulas was first proposed in the late 19th century; however, the first pump designed specifically for use with enteral tube formulas was developed by Dr. James Barron in the 1950s.[137] Tube feedings were generally accomplished by gravity-administered boluses. Pumps for enteral feedings did not come into general use until the early 1970s. As hyperosmolar nutrient solutions became acceptable for feeding patients with compromised GI tracts, the preferred method for administration was continuous slow-drip infusion. Pumps originally designed for IV infusions were employed because of the difficulty in controlling drip rates with screw or roller clamps on IV tubing.[43] Control of enteral infusions with IV pumps has been reported frequently.[11,84,85,138,139] Continuous pump-controlled tube feedings were found to be beneficial in delivering large volumes of liquid formulas with great reliability.[140]

Purpose of Pumps

Pumps ensure a constant rate of flow and reduce the amount of gastric pooling of solution, which are important considerations in lessening the possibility of formula aspiration.[141] With pump-controlled feeding, it has been observed that less time is required for reaching the total volume goal for most patients, with subjectively less abdominal discomfort than with bolus feeding.[84] The use of a pump for controlling enteral infusions has also reduced the incidence of osmotic diarrhea resulting from rapid administration of hypertonic nutrient solutions.[138] This advantage permits a more

TABLE 14–10   Enteral Containers

Manufacturer/ Container	Capacity	Filling	Tubing	Pump/ Gravity	Other Features
Clintec					
Enteral Feeding	1300 ml	Wide mouth	Available	Both	Optional preattached gravity set available with proximal spike; leak resistant cap; marked "not for IV use"
Entri-pack System	1000 ml	Prefilled	Available	Both	Non-air-dependent system; double barrier port; graduated vinyl transparent pouch; color coded
Corpak					
Polar Bag	500, 1200, 2000 ml	Top large mouth port	Available	Both	EVA/Nylon plastic safety lock cap; anti-IV feature designed for freezing; gastric pressure relief system
EntraCare					
Ultraflo Disposables	500, 1000, 1500 ml	Top fill	Attached 8-foot tubing	Pump	Built-in pouch on 1500-ml bags; pump set with spike available for prefilled bags; vinyl
IVAC					
Keofeed II	500, 1500 ml	Top fill	Available	Both	Separate pump set with spike available
Mead Johnson					
Nutritionals Delivery System	500, 1500 ml	Top fill	Attached	Both	Spike tubing set available; vinyl
Plastic Enteral	1000 ml	Top fill	Available	Both	Made of plastic
Ross Labs					
Flexiflo Top Fill Bag	500, 1000 ml	Top fill	Available	Both	Available with 1000-ml flush bag attached
Flexiflo Toptainer	1000 ml	Top fill, 58-mm wide	Available	Both	Two-way graduations allow volume readings when upright or on table
Flexiflo Easy-Feed Bag	1000 ml	Top, rigid neck	Available	Both	Vinyl
Flexitainer	500, 1000 ml	Top fill, 40-mm wide	Not available	Both	
Ready-To-Hang Container	1060 ml	Prefilled	Not available	Both	Semirigid; 24-hour hang time
	240 ml	Prefilled	Not available	Both	Glass bottle
Sandoz					
Compat Enteral Delivery Sets	1000 ml	Top fill	Attached	Pump	Rigid wide mouth; angled funnel neck; attached screw cap
Compat Semi-rigid Containers	500, 1000 ml	Top fill	Attached	Both	Sure-grip design; oversized top fill opening 58 mm; vented screw cap; dual hangers
Sherwood					
Kangaroo Gravity Sets	1000 ml	Top; large mouth port	Available	Gravity	Roller clamp for accurate delivery; sterile and nonsterile available with spike port; temperature control pouch
Kangaroo Easy Cap Closure Bag	1200 ml	Top; large mouth port	Available	Gravity	Graduated in 50-ml increments to 400 ml and in 100 ml increments to 1200 ml; spike port available

rapid advancement of enteral feeding regimens.

IV pumps are a limited resource in most hospitals, and IV infusions retain a higher priority over pump-controlled enteral feedings because of the need for more precise regulation. A plausible solution to the unavailability and expense of parenteral pumps is the development of less expensive pumps for enteral feeding.

The trend is toward manufacturing pumps that require special tubing sets for each type of enteral pump rather than pumps that accept universal tubing. This system increases cost; however, if the extension tubing and the feedings tubes are designed differently for IV tubing, the possibility of accidental IV delivery of enteral formula will be decreased and the special sets for enteral pumps will actually be advantageous.

Another advantage of some of the enteral pumps is an alarm system. The most common systems are the empty-occlusion alarms and the low-battery alarms. Enteral pumps with batteries promote mobility for patients who are ambulatory, and empty-occlusion alarms alert nurses or patients when the formula flow has stopped because of an empty container, an occluded delivery system, or a clogged feeding tube. The alarm system need not be as sophisticated as that of a parenteral pump; thus expense is decreased. More sophisticated alarms include rate change, which indicates any inadvertent manipulation of the tube-feeding rate to avoid overfeeding or underfeeding,[142] and a "set out" feature that indicates that the administration set was not loaded correctly.

Present Status

More reports are appearing in the literature that describe objective evaluations of enteral feeding pumps. In one report, enteral pumps proved efficacious for some patients who were having GI side-effects from gravity-controlled enteral feedings; such patients would have otherwise required parenteral nutrition.[143] The same study found a saving of 30 minutes of nursing time per patient per day with enteral pumps.

With the increase in small-bore feeding tubes and fiber-containing formulas, a study reported that 58 percent of 91 hospitals surveyed had mechanical problems with these tubes that included obstruction or clogging. This report and others suggested that an enteral pump be used.[144,145] The recent introduction of an automatic water flush enteral feeding pump system (Quantum Pump, Ross Laboratories) was aimed at decreasing the frequency of clogged feeding tubes. The pumps are designed to deliver both enteral formula and hourly automatic water flushes during enteral feeding. Manufacturer clinical trials of this pump demonstrated significant reduction in tube clogging compared with typical tube care of manual flushing.[146] The introduction of this pump has led to unique use in clinical practice. One such practice is to add powdered protein module to the water-flush portion of the feeding bag system.[147] Some institutions have incorporated the automatic flush into nursing protocols to decrease nursing time and tube-clogging rates and to take care of patients with severe fluid restrictions.

Various reasonably priced enteral pumps are currently available to serve the needs of hospitalized and at-home patients (Table 14–11). The ideal feeding pump should be portable and inexpensive and should deliver formula accurately (Table 14–12). Areas to investigate when selecting the optimal feeding pump include flow rate, volume-delivered mechanism, alarm system, battery or power source, pressure, service, and maintenance cost.[148,149]

Enteral nutrition pumps are now available for greater mobility and easier transport to allow for increased patient freedom, particularly with the shift of enteral delivery to the home setting and an increase in pediatric at-home patients. Smaller, lighter pumps for this purpose are now marketed. Some individuals who desire greater mobility are using very small parenteral pumps for enteral delivery. The cost of IV portable pumps for enteral delivery is commonly three times the cost of enteral pumps, and the pump tubing set can cost four to five times the enteral set. Justification for this additional expense is often required by third-party payors.[150]

Industry standards require that enteral pump delivery of tube feedings be within 10 percent of the selected flow rate. In a recent study of enteral delivery systems, 15 pumps were evaluated in the delivery of three different formulas, one with the addition of a protein module. The study concluded that there is varying flow rate accuracy of enteral systems depending on the selection of pump and the formula delivered. We recommend frequent monitoring of the volume delivery so that

TABLE 14–11   Enteral Pumps

Manufacturer/ Pump	Flow Rate Increments	Alarms	Power Source	Pressure (psi)	Weight (lb)	Other Features
Clintec Flo-Gard 2100	1–300 ml	Battery low, device, flow, volume to be infused	Electric, 5-hour battery	15	7	Keep tube open; one handed loading, control lock
Clintec 2200	1–295 ml	Battery low, occlusion/empty, dose complete, free flow, rate change	Electric, 8-hour battery	25	5.6	Nonvolatile cap holder adjustable volume control
Corpak Corflo 300	1–300 ml 1-ml increments; dose limit up to 9999 ml	Dose limit, check flow, free flow, hold battery low	Electric, 15-minute recharge	12	4	Compact, 24-hour memory
EntraCare Rate Saver (1, 2, 3)	1–300 ml	(1) Audio/visual, flow hold, dose/volume. complete, battery, system error (2) Set out (3) Door alarm	Electric, 7 hour battery	< 15	5	
Mead Johnson Nutritionals Plus	1–300 ml	Flow rate, free flow, dose/volume delivered, hold, error, low battery, set out	Electric, 8-hour battery	15	5	
Ross Flexiflo Quantum	1–300 ml in 1-ml increments	Empty, dose complete, low battery	Electric, 8-hour battery	15	7.2	Automatic 25-ml water hourly flush
Flexiflo Companion	5–300 ml in 1-ml increments	Empty, reset occlusion, low battery	Electric, 8-hour battery	24	4	Portable, pressure sensor
Flexiflo III	1–300 ml in 1-ml increments	Empty, no flow occlusion, low battery, open door, dose complete	Electric, 8-hour battery	23	7.5	
Sandoz Compat	1–50 ml in 1-ml increments 50–245 ml in 5-ml increments	Occlusion/empty, free flow, dose complete, rate change, hold	Electric, 2-hour battery	15	5.6	Cap holder accumulated volume display
Compat with dose limit	1–295 ml Dose limit 1–9995 in 5-ml increments	Occlusion/empty, free flow, dose complete, rate change, hold	Electric, 2-hour battery	15	5.6	Cap holder accumulated volume display
Compat with dose and memory	1–295 ml Dose limit 1–9995 in 5-ml increments	Occlusion/empty, free flow dose complete, rate change, hold	Electric, 8-hour battery	15	5.7	Cap holder accumulated volume display
Sherwood Kangaroo PET	1–75 ml in 1-ml increments 75-400 ml in 5-ml increments	No set, hold, low battery flow, dose complete, system error	Electric, 14-hour battery	15	2.85	Portable, three-way carrying case
Kangaroo 224	5–30 ml in 5-ml increments	No set, hold, low battery flow error, system error	Electric, recharge 15-minute	12	3.5	Large, easy to read displays
Kangaroo 324	In 1-ml increments 50–300 ml in 5-ml increments	No set, hold, low battery flow, dose complete, system error	Electric recharge 15-minute	12	3.5	Volume total

TABLE 14–12 Characteristics of Ideal Enteral Feeding Pumps

Electrically safe
Simple to use
Clear instructions on pump
Battery lasts minimum of 8 hours
Alarm system
Inexpensive
Volume-infused mechanism
Portable
Quiet
Intravenous pole attachment
Automatic water flush

adjustments can be made and nutritional goals met. Concern exists regarding administration of powdered modules to ready-to-feed formulas, since the study showed significant reduction in prescribed flow rates.[151]

Technical concepts that one must understand to evaluate enteral feeding pumps more effectively are included in the following definitions. A *volumetric* pump is one calibrated to infuse a specific volume of fluid at a specific rate (ml/hour) as opposed to a *nonvolumetric* pump, which is calibrated to infuse at a drop rate (drops/minute). *Peristaltic* is a term that refers to the controlling mechanism.

Some enteral pumps have a rotary peristaltic mechanism for delivery. The basic mechanical principle common to these pumps is a set of rollers attached to a rotating disk that alternately squeezes and releases a portion of the tubing to move fluid. Flow rate and fluid motion are determined by the speed of the rotor device and the diameter of pump chamber tubing.

Another term to become familiar with is *maximum output pressure:* the maximum amount of pressure in pounds per square inch (psi) that a pump will produce. The normal operating pressure depends on the restriction to flow and is determined primarily by feeding tube size and flexibility, and feeding formula viscosity. Some pumps will reach higher pressures, and such pressures could separate connections, affect accuracy, deliver a large bolus, or rupture the feeding tube.[152]

SUMMARY

A renewed interest in nasoenteric tube feeding has occurred because of the improvements in dietary formulas and equipment for nutrient delivery. These feedings are preferred over other routes of nutrient administration in certain situations. Enteral feedings are more physiologic, as efficacious, and less costly than parenteral feedings.

The dictum "when the gut works, and can be used safely, use it" is still a good clinical rule. Many cachectic patients can be maintained or repleted with nasoenteric tube feedings. Most severely malnourished patients in the average general hospital can probably be managed with nasoenteric tube feeding or enteric feeding plus peripheral parenteral nutrition. In those patients who require central venous nutrition, nasoenteric tube feedings can be selected to bridge the gap between parenteral feeding and volitional oral intake.

Prospective, randomized, controlled studies are needed to compare the efficacy of gastric with duodenal feedings and continuous with intermittent techniques. Intermittent feedings are satisfactory for isotonic nasogastric tube feedings in alert, awake patients. Continuous infusion delivered with pumps is necessary when feeding directly into the small intestine.

Further research is needed to determine the best preventive measures for common problems that occur with nasoenteric tube feedings. Starter regimens provide initial nutrition while minimizing delivery-related complications. Use transitional feeding regimens to administer adequate nutrition while moving from one mode of therapy to another. A standard protocol ensures adequate delivery of nutrients and achieves the specified nutritional goals safely.

Equipment for the safe and effective delivery of enteral feedings is commercially available. Tubes, holding devices, containers, and pumps are specifically designed for enteral feeding. Such products have made tube feeding more comfortable and safer for the patient and more reliable and effective for the clinician. Proper selection and use of enteral delivery systems greatly contribute to tube feeding's overall success and accuracy. Interaction between nutritional support teams and industry will continue to enhance the development of high-quality enteral delivery systems.

REFERENCES

1. Fallis LS, Barron J: Gastric and jejunal alimentation with fine polyethylene tubes. Arch Surg 1952;65: 373–381.
2. Pareira MD, Conrad EJ, Hicks W et al: Therapeutic nutrition with tube feeding. JAMA 1954;156:810–816.
3. Barron J: Tube feeding of postoperative patients. Surg Clin North Am 1959;39:1481–1491.

4. Stephens RV, Randall HT: Use of a concentrated, balanced, liquid elemental diet for nutritional management of catabolic states. Ann Surg 1969;170: 642–667.

5. Orr G, Wade J, Bothe A et al: Alternatives to total parenteral nutrition in the critically ill patient. Crit Care Med 1980;8:29–34,.

6. ASPEN Board of Directors: Guidelines for the use of parenteral and enteral nutrition in adult and pediatric patients. J Parenter Enter Nutr 1993;17S:1SA–52SA.

7. Kudsk KA, Croce MA, Fabian TC et al: Enteral versus parenteral feeding: effects on septic morbidity after blunt and penetrating abdominal trauma. Ann Surg 1992;215: 503–513.

8. Moore FA, Feliciano DV, Andrassy RJ et al: Early enteral feeding, compared with parenteral, reduces postoperative septic complications: the results of a meta-analysis. Ann Surg 1992;216:172–183.

9. Rombeau JL, Barot LR: Enteral nutrition therapy. Surg Clin North Am 1981;61:605–620.

10. Steinberg EP, Anderson GF: Implication's of Medicare's prospective payment system for specialized nutrition services. Nutr Clin Pract 1986;1:12–28.

11. Heymsfield SB, Bethel RA, Ansley JD et al: Enteral hyperalimentation: an alternative to central venous hyperalimentation. Ann Intern Med 1979;90: 63–71.

12. Blackburn GL, Bistrian BR, Maini BS et al: Nutritional and metabolic assessment of the hospitalized patient. J Parenter Enter Nutr 1977;1:11–22.

13. Bethel RA, Jansen RD, Heymsfield SB et al: Nasogastric hyperalimentation through a polyethylene catheter: an alternative to central venous hyperalimentation. Am J Clin Nutr 1979;32:1112–1120.

14. Gougeon FW: Enteral hyperalimentation: a new apparatus of administration. Surgery 1976;79:697–701.

15. Young GA, Hill GL: A controlled study of protein-sparing after excision of the rectum. Ann Surg 1980;192: 183–191.

16. Winitz M, Seedman DA, Graff J: Studies in metabolic nutrition employing chemically defined diets. I. Extended feeding of normal human adult males. Am J Clin Nutr 1970;23:525–545.

17. Freeman HJ, Kim YS, Sleisenger MH: Protein digestion and absorption in man: normal mechanisms and protein-energy malnutrition. Am J Med 1979;67: 1020–1036.

18. Rocchio MA, Chung-Ja MC, Haas KF et al: Use of chemically defined diets in the management of patients with acute inflammatory bowel disease. Am J Surg 1974;127:469–475.

19. Voitk AJ, Eschave V, Brown RA et al: Elemental diet in the treatment of fistula of the alimentary tract. Surg Gynecol Obstet 1973;137:68–72.

20. Smith DW, Lee RM: Nutritional management in duodenal fistulas. Surg Gynecol Obstet 1956;103:666.

21. Feldtman RW, Andrassy RJ: Meeting exceptional nutrition needs. II. Elemental enteral alimentation. Postgrad Med 1978;643:65–74.

22. Page CP, Carlton PK, Andrassy RJ et al: Safe cost-effective postoperative nutrition: defined formula diet via needle-catheter jejunostomy. Am J Surg 1979; 133:939–945.

23. Moss G, Friedman RC: Abdominal decompression: increased efficiency by esophageal aspiration utilizing a new nasogastric tube. Am J Surg 1977;133: 225–228.

24. Moss G: Postoperative decompression and feeding. Surg Gynecol Obstet 1977;122:550–554.

25. Moss G: Early enteral feeding after abdominal surgery. In Deitel M (ed): Nutrition in Clinical Surgery. Baltimore: Williams & Wilkins, 1980.

26. Greene HL, Helinek GL, Folk CC et al: Nasogastric tube feeding at home: a method for adjunctive nutritional support of malnourished patients. Am J Clin Nutr 1981;34:1131–1138.

27. Metz G, Dilawari J, Kellock TD: Simple technique for nasoenteric feeding. Lancet 1978;2:454.

28. Newmark SR, Simpson S, Beskitt MP et al: Home tube feeding for long-term nutritional support. J Parenter Enter Nutr 1981;5:76–79.

29. Pareira MD: Therapeutic Nutrition with Tube Feeding. Springfield, IL: Charles C Thomas, 1959.

30. Hunter J: Proposals for recovering persons apparently drowned. Phil Trans Royal Soc London 1776;66 (Part 2).

31. Hunter J: A case of paralysis of the muscle deglutition cured by an artificial mode of conveying food and medicines into the stomach. In The Works of John Hunter, vol. 3. London: Longman, Rees, Orme, Greene and Longman, 1937.

32. Gallagher TJ: On the different methods of artificial alimentation. NY Med J 1879;30:141–149.

33. Rankin DN: Three cases of nasal alimentation. Arch Laryngol 1882;3:355–358.

34. Holt LE: Gavage (forced feeding) in the treatment of acute diseases of infancy and childhood. Med Rec 1894;45:534–551.

35. Levin AL: A new gastroduodenal catheter. JAMA 1921;76:1007.

36. Strohl EL, Holinger PH, Diffenbaugh WG: Nasogastric intubation: indications, complications, safeguards, and alternate procedures. Am Surg 1958;24:721.

37. Hafner CD, Wylie JH Jr, Brush B.E: Complications of gastrointestinal intubation. Arch Surg 1961;83: 147–160.

38. Royce S, Tepper C, Watson W et al: Indwelling polyethylene nasogastric tube for feeding premature infants. Pediatrics 1951;8:79–81.

39. Wagner EA, Jones SV, Koch CA et al: Polyethylene tube feeding in premature infants. J Pediatr 1952;41: 79–83.

40. Kunz HW: Paraffin-tipped polyethylene tubing for feeding of premature babies, infants and children. J Pediatr 1952;41:84–85.

41. Wagner EA, Koch CA, Jones DV: An improved indwelling tube for feeding premature infants. J Pediatr 1954;45: 200–201.

42. Keoshian LA, Nelsen TS: A new design for a feeding tube. Plast Reconstr Surg 1969;44:508–509.

43. Dobbie RP, Hoffmeister JA: Continuous pump-tube enteric hyperalimentation. Surg Gynecol Obstet 1976;143:273–276.

44. Monturo CA: Enteral access device selection. Nutr Clin Pract 1990;5:207–213.

45. Silk DBA, Rees RG, Keohane PP et al: Clinical efficacy and design changes of "fine bore" nasogastric feeding tubes: a seven year experience involving 809 intubations in 403 patients. J Parenter Enter Nutr 1987;11:378–383.

46. Lord LM, Weiser-Maimone A, Pulhamus M et al: Comparison of weighted versus unweighted tubes for efficacy of transpyloric intubation. J Parenter Enter Nutr 1993;17:271–273.

47. Matarese LE: Enteral alimentation: equipment. III. Nutr Supp Serv 1982;2:48–49.

48. Fagerman K, Lysen LK: Enteral feeding tubes: a comparison and history. Nutr Supp Serv 1987;7:11–14.

49. Cort D, Eisenberg P, Methany N et al: Prospective comparison of a combination nasogastric tube-pH microelectrode to aspiration method of pH determination in intensive care unit patients. Gastroenterology 1988;94:A79.

50. Heiselman DE, Vidovich RR, Milkovich B et al: Nasointestinal tube placement with a pH sensor feeding tube. J Parenter Enter Nutr 1993;17:562–565.

51. Strong RM, Gribbon R, Durling S et al: Enteral tube feedings utilizing a pH sensor enteral feeding tube. Nutr Supp Serv 1988;8:11–25.

52. Methany N: Measures to test placement of nasogastric and nasointestinal feeding tubes: a review. Nurs Res 1988;37:324–329.

53. Ghahremani GG, Gould RJ: Nasoenteric feeding tubes: radiographic detection of complications. Dig Dis Sci 1986;31:574–585.

54. Caswell CS: Confirmation of feeding tube placement. Nutr Supp Serv 1987;8:7–8.

55. Kittinger JW, Sandler RS, Heizer WD: Efficacy of metoclopramide as an adjunct to duodenal placement of small-bore feeding tubes: a randomized placebo-controlled double-blind study. J Parenter Enter Nutr 1987;11:33–37.

56. Marian M, Rappaport W, Cunningham D et al: The failure of conventional methods to promote spontaneous transpyloric feeding tube passage and the safety of intragastric feeding in the critically ill ventilated patient. Surg Gynecol Obstet 1993;176: 475–479.

57. Seifert CF, Cuddy PG, Pemberton B et al: A randomized trial of metoclopramide's effects on the transpyloric intubation of weighted feeding tubes. Nutr Supp Serv 1987;7:11–13.

58. Whatley K, Turner WW, Dey M et al: When does metoclopramide facilitate transpyloric intubation? J Parenter Enter Nutr 1984;8:679–681.

59. Kalfarentzos F, Alivizatos V, Panagopoulos K et al: Nasoenteral intubation with the use of metoclopramide. Nutr Supp Serv 1987;7:33–34.

60. Keshavarzian A, Isaac RM: Erythromycin accelerates gastric emptying of indigestible solids and transpyloric migration of the tip of an enteral feeding tube in fasting and fed states. Am J Gastroenterol 1993;88: 193–197.

61. Cacciatore AM, Battey CH, Griffith DP et al: Bedside small intestinal feeding tube placement using intravenous erythromycin in critically ill adult patients. Proceedings of the American Society for Parenteral and Enteral Nutrition, 19th Clinical Congress. Miami, FL: 1995;593.

62. Whatley K, Turner W, Dey M et al: Transpyloric passage of feeding tubes. Nutr Supp Serv 1983;3:18–21.

63. Grant JP, Curtas MS, Kelvin FM: Fluoroscopic placement of nasojejunal feeding tubes with immediate feeding using a nonelemental diet. J Parenter Enter Nutr 1983;7:299–303.

64. Guice KS, Thompson JC: Endoscopic placement of a weighted tip feeding tube in complex surgical patients. Surg Gynecol Obstet 1987;164:272–273.

65. Gutierrez ED, Balfe D: Fluoroscopically guided nasoenteric feeding tube placement: results of a 1-year study. Radiology 1991;178:759–762.

66. Stark SP, Sharpe JN, Larson GM: Endoscopically placed nasoenteral feeding tubes: indications and techniques. Am Surg 1991;57:203–205.

67. Kuipers RJ, van Mourik-van Steyn G, Rijsberman W et al: Direct endoscopic placement of naso-enteral feeding tubes (letter). Endoscopy 1994;26:371.

68. Zaloga GP: Bedside method for placing small bowel feeding tubes in critically ill patients. Chest 1991; 100:1643–1645.

69. Grabenkort WR: Manual placement of small bowel feeding tubes at the bedside: a beginners experience of 53 patients. Proceedings of the American Society for Parenteral and Enteral Nutrition, 18th Clinical Congress. San Antonio, TX: 1994;604.

70. Methany N, McSweeney M, Wehrle MA et al: Effectiveness of ausculatory method in predicting feeding tube location. Nurs Res 1990;39:262–267.

71. Methany N, Reed L, Berglund B et al: Visual characteristics of aspirates from feeding tubes as a method for predicting tube location. Nurs Res 1994;43:282–287.

72. Meer JA: Inadvertent dislodgement of nasoenteral feeding tubes: incidence and prevention. J Parenter Enter Nutr 1987;11:187–189.

73. Cartwright M: Tube feeding by nasal gavage. RN 1959;122:55–61.

74. Solem LD: Enteral elemental nutrition in burn patients. Cont Surg 1986;28:36–40.

75. Bouzarth WF: Intracranial nasogastric tube insertion. J Trauma 1978;18:818–819.

76. Valentine RJ, Turner WW: Pleural complications of nasoenteric feeding tubes. J Parenter Enter Nutr 1985;9:605–607.

77. Olbrantz KR, Gelfand D, Choplin R et al: Pneumothorax complicating enteral feeding tube placement. J Parenter Enter Nutr 1985;9:210–211.

78. Bohnker BK, Artman LE, Hoskins WJ: Narrow bore nasogastric feeding tube complications. Nutr Clin Pract 1987;2:203–209.

79. Aronchick JM, Epstein DM, Gefter WB et al: Pneumothorax as a complication of placement of a nasoenteric tube. JAMA 1984;252:3287–3288.

80. Balogh GJ, Adler SJ, VanderWonde J et al: Pneumothorax as a complication of feeding tube placement. Am J Radiol 1983;141:1275–1277.

81. Boyes RJ, Kruse JA: Nasogastric and nasoenteral intubation. Crit Care Clin 1992;4:865–878.

82. Martin D, Jastram CW: Enteral nutrition. II. Nutr Supp Serv 1987;7:8–10.

83. Reitz MV, Mattfeldt-Beman M, Ridley CM: Current practices in home nutritional support. Nutr Supp Serv 1988;8:8–11.

84. Hiebert JM, Brown A, Anderson RG et al: Comparison of continuous vs. intermittent tube feedings in adult burn patients. J Parenter Enter Nutr 1981;5: 73–75.

85. Parker P, Stroop S, Green HA: A controlled comparison of continuous versus intermittent enteral feeding in the treatment of infants with intestinal disease. J Pediatr 1981;99:360–364.

86. Brandstetter R, Zakkay Y, Gutherz P et al: Effect of nasogastric feedings on arterial oxygen tension in patients with symptomatic chronic obstructive pulmonary disease. Heart Lung 1988;17:170–172.

87. Grant J, Denne S: Effect of intermittent versus continuous enteral feeding on energy expenditure in premature infants. J Pediatr 1991;118:928–932.

88. Heymsfield SB, Casper K, Grossman GD: Bioenergetic and metabolic response to continuous vs. intermittent nasoenteric feeding. Metabolism 1987;36: 570–575.

89. Heymsfield SB, Hill JO, Evert M et al: Energy expenditure during continuous intragastric infusion of fuel. Am J Clin Nutr 1987;45:526–533.

90. Nacht CA, Schutz Y, Vernet O et al: Continuous versus single bolus enteral nutrition: comparison of energy

metabolism in humans. Am J Physiol 1986;251: E524–E529.

91. Campbell I, Morton R, MacDonald I et al: A comparison of the effects of intermittent and continuous nasogastric feeding on the oxygen consumption and nitrogen balance of patients after major head and neck surgery. Am J Clin Nutr 1983;38: 870–878.

92. Shulman RJ, Redel CA, Stathos TH: Bolus versus continuous feedings stimulate small-intestinal growth and development in the newborn pig. J Pediatr Gastro Nutr 1994;18:350–354.

93. Westfall UE, Heitkemper MM: Systemic responses to different enteral feeding schedules in rats. Nurs Res 1992;41:144–150.

94. Ciocon J, Galindo-Ciocon D, Thiessen C et al: Comparison of intermittent versus continuous tube feeding among the elderly. J Parenter Enter Nutr 1992; 16:525–528.

95. Kocan MJ, Hickisch SM: A comparison of continuous and intermittent enteral nutrition in NICU patients. J Neurosci Nurs 1986;18:333–337.

96. Medley F, Stechmiller J, Field A: Complications of enteral nutrition in hospitalized patients with artificial airways. Clin Nurs Res 1993;2:212–223.

97. Cogen R, Weintraub J: Aspiration pneumonia in nursing home patients fed via gastrostomy tubes. Am J Gastroenterol 1989;84:1509–1512.

98. Jacobs S, Chang RWS, Lee B et al: Continuous enteral feeding: a major cause of pneumonia among ventilated intensive care unit patients. J Parenter Enter Nutr 1990;14:353–356.

99. Ibanez J, Penafiel A, Raurich J et al: Gastroesophageal reflux in intubated patients receiving enteral nutrition: effect of supine and semirecumbent positions. J Parenter Enter Nutr 1992;16:419–422.

100. Coben RM, Weintraub A, DiMarino AJ et al: Gastroesophageal reflux during gastrostomy feeding. Gastroenterology 1994;106:13–18.

101. Saxe JM, Ledgerwood AM, Lucas, CE et al: Lower esophageal sphincter dysfunction precludes safe gastric feeding after head injury. J Trauma 1994;37: 581–586.

102. Powers T, Cowan GS, Deckard M et al: Prospective randomized evaluation of two regimens for converting from continuous to intermittent feedings in patients with feeding gastrostomies. J Parenter Enter Nutr 1991;15:405–407.

103. Cochran W: Conversion from continuous to intermittent feedings (letter). J Parenter Enter Nutr 1992;16: 495.

104. Page CP, Ryan JA, Haff RC: Continual catheter administration of an elemental diet. Surg Gynecol Obstet 1976;142:184–188.

105. Dobbie RP, Butterick OD Jr: Continuous pump-tube enteric hyperalimentation: use in esophageal disease. J Parenter Enter Nutr 1977;1:100–104.

106. Evans D, DiSipio M, Barot L et al: Comparison of gastric and jejunal tube feedings. J Parenter Enter Nutr 1980;4:79.

107. Curet-Scot M, Shermata DW: A comparison of intragastric and intrajejunal feedings in neonatal piglets. J Pediatr Surg 1986;21:552–555.

108. Curet-Scot MJ, Mellar JL, Shermata DW: Transduodenal feedings: a superior route of enteral nutrition. J Pediatr Surg 1987;22:516–518.

109. Pinchofsky-Devin GD, Kaminski MV: Visceral protein increase associated with interrupted versus continuous enteral hyperalimentation. J Parenter Enter Nutr 1985;9:474–476.

110. Laing IA, Lang MA, Callaghan O et al: Nasogastric compared with nasoduodenal feeding in low birth weight infants. Arch Dis Child 1986;161:138–141.

111. McDonald PD, Skeoch CH, Carse H et al: Randomised trial of continuous nasogastric, bolus nasogastric and transpyloric feeding in infants of birth weight under 1400 g. Arch Dis Child 1992;67: 429–431.

112. Montecalvo MA, Steger KA, Farber HW et al: Nutritional outcome and pneumonia in critical care patients randomized to gastric versus jejunal tube feedings. Crit Care Med 1992;20:1377–1385.

113. Heyland KK, Cook DJ, Guyatt GH: Enteral nutrition in the critically ill patient: a critical review of the evidence. Intensive Care Med 1993;19:435–442.

114. Lazarus BA, Murphy JB, Culpepper L: Aspiration associated with long-term gastric versus jejunal feeding: a critical analysis of the literature. Arch Phys Med Rehabil 1990;71:46–53.

115. Strong RM, Condon SC, Solinger MR et al: Equal aspiration rates from postpylorus and intragastric-placed small-bore nasoenteric feeding tubes: a randomized, prospective study. J Parenter Enter Nutr 1992;16:59–63.

116. Methany N, Eisenberg P, Spies M: Monitoring patients with nasally placed feeding tubes. Heart Lung 1985; 14:285–286.

117. Keohane P, Attrill H, Love M et al: Relation between osmolality of diet and gastrointestinal side effects in enteral nutrition. Br Med J 1984;288:678–680.

118. Methany N: Minimizing respiratory complications of nasoenteric tube feedings: state of the science. Heart Lung 1993;22:213–223.

119. McClave S, Snider H, Lowen C et al: Use of residual volume as a marker for enteral feeding intolerance: prospective blinded comparison with physical examination and radiographic findings. J Parenter Enter Nutr 1992;16:99–105.

120. Zibrida JM, Carlson SJ: Transitional feeding. In Gottschlich MM, Matarese LE, Shronts EP (eds): Nutrition Support Dietitians Core Curriculum, 2nd edition. Silver Spring, MD: American Society for Parenteral and Enteral Nutrition, 1993.

121. Bernard M, Forlaw L: Complications and their prevention. In Rombeau JL, Caldwell MD (eds): Enteral and Tube Feeding, vol. 1. Philadelphia: W.B. Saunders, 1984.

122. Morse JL: Recollections and reflections on forty-five years of artificial infant feeding. J Pediatr 1935;7: 303–324.

123. Kaminski MV: Enteral hyperalimentation. Surg Gynecol Obstet 1976;143:12–16.

124. Chernoff R (ed): ASPEN Product Resource Manual, 2nd edition. Washington, DC: American Society for Parenteral and Enteral Nutrition, 1982.

125. White WT III, Acuff TE Jr, Sykes TR et al: Bacterial contamination of enteral nutrient solution: a preliminary report. J Parenter Enter Nutr 1979;3(6):459–461.

126. Beyer P, Parrish-Zepeda A, Furtado D: A prospective survey of contamination of enteral feeding solutions in the clinical setting. In Proceedings of the Ross Laboratories Workshop on Contamination of Enteral Products During Clinical Usage. Columbus, OH: Ross Laboratories, 1983.

127. Groshel D: Infection control considerations in enteral feeding. Nutr Supp Serv 1983;3:48–49.

128. Hostetler C, Lipman T, Geraghty M et al: Bacterial safety of reconstituted continuous drip tube feeding. J Parenter Enter Nutr 1982;6:232–235.

129. Kotilainen H, Gantz N: Contamination of enteral feedings and evaluation of environmental and procedural sources. In Proceedings of the Ross Laboratories Workshop on Contamination of Enteral Products During Clinical Usage. Columbus, OH: Ross Laboratories, 1983.

130. Schreiner R, Eitzen H, Gfell M et al: Environmental contamination of continuous drip feedings. Pediatrics 1979;63:232–237.

131. Schroeder P, Fisher D, Volz M et al: Microbial contamination of enteral feeding solutions in a community hospital. J Parenter Enter Nutr 1983;7:364–368.

132. Crocker KS, Krey SH, Markovic M: Microbial growth in clinically used enteral delivery systems. Am J Infect Control 1986;14:250–256.

133. Wagner DR, Elmore MF, Knoll DM: Evaluation of "closed" vs. "open" systems for the delivery of peptide-based enteral diets. J Parenter Enter Nutr 1994; 18:453–457.

134. Rees RGP, Ryan J, Attrill HA: Clinical evaluation of two-liter delivery system: a controlled trial. J Parenter Enter Nutr 1988;12:274–277.

135. Vaughan LA, Manore M, Winston DH: Bacterial safety of a closed-administration system for enteral nutrition solutions. J Am Diet Assoc 1988;88:35.

136. Pemberton LB, Lyman B, Covinsky J: An evaluation of a closed enteral feeding system. Nutr Supp Serv 1985;5:36–42.

137. Champlin L: Enteral nutrition. Med Prod Sales 1982;13:1,8,28–30,32,35.

138. Freeman JB, Fairfull-Smith RJ: Improved nitrogen equilibrium with constant infusion pumps in enteral feeding. J Parenter Enter Nutr 1979;3:27.

139. Kien CL: Employment of a mobile ambulatory infusion system for continuous ambulatory tube feeding. J Parenter Enter Nutr 1981;5:526–527.

140. Butterworth CE, Weinsier RL: Malnutrition in hospitalized patients: assessment and treatment. In Goodhart RS, Shils ME (eds): Modern Nutrition in Health and Disease, 6th edition. Philadelphia: Lea & Febiger, 1980.

141. Gauderer MWL, Olsen MM, Stellato TA et al: Feeding gastrostomy button: experience and recommendations. J Pediatr Surg 1988;23:24–28.

142. Ward J: Evaluation of enteral feeding pumps for pediatric use. J Pediatr Nurs 1986;1:133–136.

143. Jones BJM, Payne S, Silk DBA: Indications for pump-assisted enteral feeding. Lancet 1980;1:1057–1058.

144. Petrosino BM, Christian BJ, Wolf J et al: Implications of selected problems with nasoenteral tube feedings. Crit Care Nurs Q 1989;12:1–18.

145. Andrassy R: Controversies in enteral nutrition. Nutr Supp Serv 1985;5:25–30.

146. Ross Laboratories Medical Department: The effect of hourly flushing on tube clogging using the Flexiflo Quantum Pump. BC 94-2: March 1992.

147. Jones SA, Guenter PA, Roberts MR et al: A practical alternative to frequent bolus protein module administration: utilizing the new technology of automatic flush pumps. Proceedings of American Society for Parenteral and Enteral Nutrition, 18th Clinical Congress. San Antonio, TX: 1994:604.

148. Imbrosciano S, Kovach M: Selecting the optimal enteral feeding pump. Nutr Supp Serv 1986;6:15–16.

149. Lehman S: Advances in parenteral and enteral pumps. Nutr Supp Serv 1988;8:13–14.

150. Young RJ, Murray ND: Adapting intravenous pumps for enteral feeding. Mat Child Nurs 1991;16:212–216.

151. Dietscher JE, Foulks CJ, Waits M: Accuracy of enteral pumps: in vitro performance. J Parenter Enter Nutr 1994;18:359–361.

152. Pipp T: Enteral feeding pumps. Nutr Supp Serv 1986;6:12–18.

15

Enteral Nutrition in the Surgical Patient

ROLANDO H. ROLANDELLI
MICHAEL A. BUCKMIRE

Enteral nutrition should be considered in every patient undergoing major surgery. Patients with illnesses treated by surgical intervention often develop malnutrition, which in turn predisposes patients to postoperative complications. Ideally, to avoid these postoperative complications, proper nutritional assessment and intervention should be done preoperatively. In some patients, however, this is not possible, since surgery cannot be delayed because of life-threatening conditions, and nutritional intervention is then deferred to the postoperative period.

It is more difficult to attain an adequate nutritional status in surgical patients than in nonsurgical patients. Surgical procedures, as well as the perioperative measures required in surgical patients, may interfere with digestion, absorption, or metabolism of nutrients and the ability to establish an access to the alimentary tract for tube feedings.

This chapter will provide the reader with general guidelines regarding the nutritional management of surgical patients and brief discussions regarding certain nutritional issues in special conditions. The special conditions include surgery on specific anatomic regions including head and neck, esophagus, stomach, small intestine, colon and rectum, thorax, and

the musculoskeletal system. Some surgical conditions, such as pancreatic and liver disease or short-bowel syndrome, are sufficiently distinctive that they are addressed in separate chapters (Chapters 23 to 25).

MALNUTRITION IN THE SURGICAL PATIENT

For many years it has been recognized that patients requiring surgery are often malnourished. Early in this century, Studley studied the impact of preoperative malnutrition on the outcome of antiulcer surgery (partial gastrectomy) in 50 consecutive patients.[1] Overall mortality for the study group was 15 percent. When the patients were stratified according to preoperative weight loss, those patients who lost more than 20 percent of their body weight preoperatively were found to have a mortality of 33 percent, compared with a mortality of 3.5 percent in those who lost less than 20 percent of their weight. This study is particularly interesting because it deals with a major surgical procedure (partial gastrectomy) performed for benign disease (peptic ulcer) during a time when medical practitioners lacked the efficacious pharmacotherapy for peptic ulcers and the technology and perioperative support, such as antibiotics, monitoring devices, safe anesthetic agents, and blood banks, that became available throughout the past 50 years.

There are numerous means by which patients requiring surgery may develop malnutrition (Table 15–1). Patients afflicted by some forms of cancer may reduce their intake due to reduced appetite. This has been shown in some experimental studies in rats to be caused by circulating cytokines such as tumor necrosis factor (TNF) or cachectin.[2] However, there are those who feel that TNF is not the sole cause of cachexia.[3] Surgical pathologic conditions may create a mechanical obstruction in the upper alimentary tract, such as esophageal and gastric carcinomas. Other pathologic conditions, such as esophageal dysmotility syndromes or peptic ulcer disease, may leave the patient with an inability to advance food through the alimentary tract. Some surgical conditions may raise the metabolic rate and the consumption of nutrients, leading to acute muscle wasting and weight loss. Typical examples of these types of conditions are burns, infectious processes, and inflammatory bowel disease (IBD).

Another means of malnutrition in surgical patients is the loss of nutrients and body secretions in patients with enteric fistulas. Regardless of the etiology, the pathophysiology of surgical disease tends to predispose patients to malnutrition. To compound matters, the stress alone of the surgical procedure may worsen malnutrition by also increasing the metabolic rate. For these reasons, and because of its correlation with postoperative complications, malnutrition is of paramount concern to the surgeon.

In a 1955 article, Rhoads and Alexander discussed the relationship between nutrition and complications in surgical patients.[4] They described six specific complications secondary to hypoproteinemia. These "dangers of hypoproteinemia" included vomiting after gastroenterostomy, delayed gastrointestinal (GI) motility, wound rupture due to poor fibroplasia, delayed callus formation, increased predisposition to hemorrhagic shock, and decreased resistance to infection. Their study included 102 surgical patients divided into a control group and a hypoproteinemic study group. They defined hypoproteinemia as patients having a serum protein level less than 6.3 g/dL. They found that the incidence of infectious complications in the postoperative period, such as wounds and urinary tract and respiratory tract infections, correlated significantly with hypoproteinemia. This

TABLE 15–1   Causes of Malnutrition in Surgical Patients

Decreased Intake of Nutrients
Cancer
Decreased mental status

Obstruction of the Alimentary Tract
Esophagogastric pathologic state, benign or
    malignant
Small- and large-bowel obstruction

Increased Use of Nutrients
Multiple trauma, burns
Infection

Increased Nutrient Losses
Enterocutaneous fistulas
Short-bowel syndrome

article illustrated the detrimental effect malnutrition can have on the incidence of postoperative complications.

In 1969, Daly reported the effect of protein malnutrition on the healing of colonic anastomoses, as measured by bursting strength.[5] He induced protein-calorie malnutrition in rats by feeding the rats a protein-free diet from 1 to 6 weeks. Then he performed a transection and anastomosis of the descending colon, followed by measurement of bursting pressures of the anastomoses. Rats with weight loss ranging from 2 to 26 percent showed a linear decrease in bursting strength. This study reaffirmed the deleterious effect of protein malnutrition on wound healing; in this case, specifically on colonic wound healing.

The availability of techniques of nutritional support in the late 1970s triggered new studies assessing the impact of malnutrition in the surgical patient. Bistrian and Blackburn investigated the prevalence of malnutrition in an urban general hospital.[6] They used anthropometric and laboratory measurements (such as a weight:height ratio, triceps skin fold, arm-muscle circumference, serum albumin, and hematocrit) to assess nutritional status by comparing the patient's measurements to established standards. Their data show that surgical patients were much more likely to have severe protein depletion vs medical patients due to the catabolic nature of surgical illnesses. They also found that the prevalence of malnutrition in both medical and surgical patients was high and that nutritional status did not improve in most of these patients throughout their hospitalization.[7]

Mullen and Buzby, at the University of Pennsylvania, performed a series of studies during the 1980s to assess more effectively the link between nutritional status and clinical outcome.[8-11] These studies led to the development of the prognostic nutritional index (PNI), a tool to assess the risk of surgical complications based on parameters that reflect preoperative malnutrition. In one of their studies, the population consisted of 64 consecutive elective surgical patients at a Veterans Hospital. They assessed each patient using a total of 16 parameters of nutritional and immunologic state. They found that 35 percent of the group had at least three abnormal nutritional and immunologic measurements. In addition, they found that three of the measurements prospectively identified a subgroup of patients in whom there was a substantial increase in operative morbidity and mortality. These three measurements were the patient's preoperative serum albumin level, serum transferrin level, and delayed hypersensitivity reactivity.[9] Based on this data, they constructed the prognostic nutritional index and applied it to another group of surgical patients. The formula was:

$$PNI\ (\%\ risk) = 158 - 16.6(ALB) - 0.78(TSF) - 0.2(TFN) - 5.8(DH)$$

where PNI was the percentage risk of postoperative complications in an individual patient, ALB was the serum albumin level (g/dL), TSF was the triceps skinfold (mm), TFN was the serum transferrin level (mg/dL), and DH was the maximum cutaneous delayed hypersensitivity reactivity to any of three recall antigens. The patients were stratified into three groups based on the particular patient's PNI. Low risk was a PNI less than 40 percent, intermediate risk was a PNI between 40 and 50 percent and high risk was a PNI more than 50 percent. They found that a PNI of more than 40 percent predicted sepsis with a sensitivity of 86 percent and predicted death with a sensitivity of 93 percent.[8] The possibility of performing a nutritional assessment based on objective parameters was very effective in creating more awareness by various health care workers of the prevalence of malnutrition in surgical patients. However, other investigators have not been able to obtain the same predictive value with the PNI.

Other studies have stressed the importance of a thorough nutritional assessment by clinical means. They argue that a clinical assessment is just as effective as, if not more so, the anthropometric, biochemical, and cell-mediated immunity methods mentioned above.[12] These authors based their nutritional assessments on data collected from a carefully performed history of the patient and a physical examination. The parameters included in their history were weight loss, edema, anorexia, vomiting, diarrhea, decreased or unusual food intake, and chronic illness. Their physical examination emphasized jaundice, cheilosis, glossitis, loss of subcutaneous fat, muscle wasting, and edema. They found that the clinical assessment of the patient's nutritional status was reproducible and was related to clinical morbidity (as measured by incidence of infection, use of antibiotics, and length of hospitalization).

Whether nutritional evaluation is done by "objective" parameters or by a subjective global assessment is not as important as evaluating patients early in the course of the illness. In the current health environment this evaluation is often done in the outpatient setting. Whenever possible, nutritional support should be instituted even in the ambulatory setting before the patient is admitted for surgery.

POSTOPERATIVE RECOVERY AND NUTRITIONAL STATUS

Two physiologic processes crucial to the outcome of surgery are wound healing and resistance to infection (Table 15–2). Wounds that do not heal can result in anastomotic dehiscence, evisceration, or incisional hernias. Increased susceptibility to infection can not only impair proper wound healing but also can lead to pneumonia, enteritis, and urinary tract infections. Another process essential for recovery is adaptation to the change imposed by surgery. If a surgical procedure is performed on the lower extremities, the patient will have to retrain muscles to be able to walk. If the surgery involves an extensive resection of small bowel,

TABLE 15–2 Adverse Effects of Malnutrition on Surgical Outcome

---

Impaired Wound Healing
Dehiscence of surgical incisions
Dehiscence of anatomoses

Decreased Resistance to Infection
Postoperative pneumonia
Postoperative wound infections
Postoperative urinary tract infections

Inability to Adapt to Changes Imposed by Surgery
Insufficient adaptation following resections
Failure to thrive
Decubitus ulcers

---

the remainder of the alimentary tract must compensate for the reduction in absorptive surface to enable the body to assimilate sufficient nutrients. These three phenomena (wound healing, resistance to infection, and rehabilitation) evolve synchronously in the postoperative period, and the outcome of one has a profound influence on the outcome of the others. However, for the purpose of this discussion, each one will be discussed separately.

Wound Healing

Healing of wounds follows a well-characterized sequence of events (Fig. 15–1). Wounds elicit bleeding, which is controlled by constriction of blood vessels and formation of blood clots. Then, an inflammatory process ensues, with release of various substances from all three types of blood cells (i.e., erythrocytes, leukocytes, and platelets). These substances can be enzymes (myeloperoxidase), cytokines (interleukins), or peptide growth factors (EGF, PDGF, etc.). Collagen in the area of wounding is degraded by a group of enzymes collectively known as collagenases. During this phase wounds are weakest and rely on suture materials to maintain coaptation of tissues. The next phase is known as fibroplasia. Under the influence of various growth factors (epidermal, fibroblast, insulinlike, platelet-derived, and transforming growth factors), matrix and epithelial cells replicate and collagen is synthe-

sized and deposited in the wound.[13-15] The last phase is remodelling of the wound, during which the wound contracts while collagen synthesis and degradation take place.

The degree of involvement of each of these processes and their susceptibility to other influences varies among tissues and organs. For instance, the inflammatory response in a colonic anastomosis is much more intense than in a vascular anastomosis. Conversely, hemostasis is more involved in the healing of a vascular anastomosis than in the healing of an intestinal anastomosis. Theoretically, the degree of collagen lysis should be more intense in intestinal wounds because of the presence of bacterial collagenases. Because collagen metabolism takes place in the submucosa, relining the GI wound with epithelium is crucial to isolate collagen from luminal collagenases produced by bacteria. This makes epithelial cell proliferation extremely important for the healing of a GI anastomosis. Nutrition is also believed to play a role in cell proliferation.[16] Luminal nutrients indirectly influence cell proliferation through enterohormones, blood flow, peristalsis, and mechanical stimuli.

Wound healing has been studied mostly in experimental animals because of the need for invasive methods to assess mechanical strength or chemical composition of wounds. In the 1930s and 1940s, Rhoads and Ravdin reported that hypoproteinemia had a deleterious effect on wound healing.[17,18] In a study done in

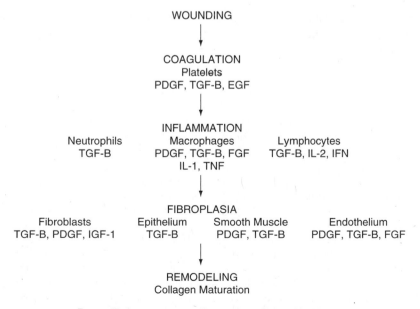

FIGURE 15–1   Sequence of events in wound healing.

the late 1940s, Localio and colleagues showed that tissue protein depletion was related to wound disruption in humans. They concluded that the depletion of tissue protein concentration was an important factor in the etiology of wound disruption in humans.[19] This study reinforced the significance of nutrition in wound healing.

In several studies from New Zealand, the effect of nutritional intervention on wound healing was assessed by implanting a Gore-tex tube in the arms of patients.[20-22] The tube acted as a matrix for healing and was analyzed for the amount of hydroxyproline present in the healing tissue. In one study, the wound healing response was assessed on 66 patients with differing degrees of malnutrition. They found that there was a definite abnormality in malnourished surgical patients' wound healing response.[20] In another study by Windsor, 90 malnourished patients underwent a course of nutritional supplementation and had a Gore-tex tube surgically placed and then excised from the arm.[23] Their results show that the preoperative food intake has a greater effect on the wound healing response than absolute losses of protein and fat from body stores. Windsor concluded that maintaining adequate food intake up until surgery is significant in preventing impairment of the wound healing response. Along these lines, Haydock also reported that the wound healing response is markedly improved by preoperative nutritional supplementation vs postoperative nutritional supplementation.[21]

Specific vitamins and minerals are important in the biochemistry of wound healing, and deficiencies can lead to an alteration of this process (Table 15–3). Deficiency of protein prolongs the inflammatory phase of wound healing and impairs fibroplasia. Specific amino acids have also been shown to have an effect. Specifically, arginine plays an important role in wound repair. Its specific mechanism of action involves the hypothalamic-pituitary axis where arginine acts as a growth hormone secretagogue.[24] Barbul showed significantly minimized immediate postoperative weight loss, increased wound breaking strength and collagen accumulation, and increased thymic weight when arginine was added to the diet. Other amino acids, such as methionine and cystine, may contribute to wound healing. It appears that individual replacement of these amino acids cannot reverse wound healing deficits in hypoproteinemic animals.[25,26] They may, however, play a role as cofactors in the enzyme systems necessary for collagen synthesis. Their specific roles must be further defined.[27]

There is little information on the role of carbohydrates and fats on wound healing. However, carbohydrates, specifically glucose, are needed as an energy source for white blood cells. Adequate leukocyte functioning is necessary during the inflammatory phase of wound repair. Fats are essential to produce cell membranes for new cells. Through these mechanisms, inadequate intake of carbohydrates and fats can have a negative effect on wound healing.[27]

Collagen metabolism is an exceedingly complex enzymatic process crucial to wound repair. A number of specific minerals are important in collagen metabolism.[27] These minerals are cofactors for specific enzymatic steps in collagen synthesis. Iron, manganese, copper, magnesium, and calcium all play a role in collagen metabolism. Specifically, zinc deficiency has been shown to reduce the rate of epithelialization, reduce the rate of gain of wound strength, and decrease collagen strength.[27]

Vitamin C is also necessary for collagen synthesis. Deficiency of vitamin C does not allow proper hydroxylation to take place, which eventually leads to unsatisfactory polymerization of collagen.[28] Clinically, this produces a process of impaired wound healing known as scurvy. Administration of vitamin C quickly reverses the healing process to normal. Vitamin A seems to be able to counteract the inhibitory effects of steroids on wound healing. Also, some of the B vitamins contribute to the wound-healing process.[27] In these ways, nutrition can affect the process of wound repair, which can increase the morbidity of patients undergoing surgical procedures.

TABLE 15–3   Nutrient Deficiencies and Wound Healing

Nutrients	Role in Wound Healing
Calories	Fuel for collagen turnover
Fats	Cell membrane component
Carbohydrates	Fuel for fibroblasts
Protein	Prolongs inflammation
Arginine	Nitric oxide precursor
Glutamine	Fuel for white blood cells
Methionine	Cofactor metalloproteinases
Cysteine	Cross-linking of collagen
Ascorbic acid	Cross-linking of collagen
Zinc	Epithelization
Retinoids	Reverse steroid-induced impairment

Resistance to Infection

A patient's nutritional status also influences the body's ability to resist an infection. Most surgeries, particularly GI procedures, involve some contamination with bacteria. This contamination can be minimal, as in a patient well prepared for elective surgery, or can be enormous, as in a patient with a perforated abdominal viscus. In the latter situation, although surgery is crucial for survival, the body's ability to resist infection is essential to achieve a successful outcome from surgery.

The deleterious effect of malnutrition on the immune system is so consistent that immune parameters are commonly used to assess a patient's nutritional status, such as in the calculation of the PNI mentioned above. Malnourished surgical patients can have any of the following abnormalities: reduced delayed cutaneous hypersensitivity response, decreased number of T-lymphocytes and CD4 + cells, reduced bactericidal capacity of neutrophils, lower IgA antibody titer and depressed complement system. Many of these patients also have vitamin and trace element deficiencies that affect their immune system.[29]

A number of specific micronutrient and vitamin deficiencies impair immunity (Table 15–4). Patients with zinc deficiency have T-lymphocyte and neutrophil abnormalities.[30] Macrophages are also affected by zinc deficiency. Copper deficiency has been associated with an increased incidence of infection. In laboratory animals, the mechanism of impaired immunity in copper-deficiency has been shown to be depressed reticuloendothelial system functioning and reduced microbial activity of granulocytes.[29] There are very few studies on iodine deficiency and immunity. However, because the iodide molecule is linked with the

amount of thyroid hormone in the body, the immunity of hypothyroid patients can give some information on iodine deficiency and immunity. It has been shown that neutrophils' bactericidal capacity is decreased in hypothyroid patients.[31] Animals fed a diet deficient in selenium and vitamin E showed depressed humoral immunity and increased severity and frequency of enteric infections. Selenium-deficient animals have been shown to have decreased microbicidal activity in vitro secondary to decreased peroxidase activity. Iron deficiency has also been studied, but results are controversial.[29] Note that an excessive amount of micronutrients may be deleterious to the immune system as well.

Of the vitamins, vitamin A deficiency is the one that most clearly alters immunity. Vitamin A deficiency reduces the weight of the thymus, decreases lymphocyte proliferation, and increases bacterial binding in respiratory cells. Deficiencies of other vitamins, namely, the B vitamins and vitamins C and E, have all been shown to impair immunity.[29] As with micronutrients, excessive amounts of vitamins can reduce immune system efficiency.

Postoperative Adaptation

Depending on the magnitude of the surgical procedure, the body is often required to implement some mechanisms of adaptation. Resection of one of a paired organ (e.g., lung or kidney) creates a higher workload for the remaining organ. Resection of part, or the whole, of an unpaired organ (e.g., stomach or colon) requires other organs to adapt and compensate for such loss. Processes of adaptation usually involve cellular hyperplasia and hypertrophy with a subsequent increase in function. The increased cellular proliferation is associated with an increase in energy consumption and an increased demand for nutrients used in cellular architecture and function. A perfect example of this process is the adaptation of the alimentary tract to an extensive bowel resection (Chapter 23). In many patients, the combination of the underlying illness, the surgical procedures, and immobilization produce atrophy of skeletal muscles. Muscle atrophy then leads to deconditioning of body functions. This is particularly noticeable in the elderly undergoing orthopedic surgery (see below).

In summary, surgery increases the patient's need for nutrients for proper wound healing. If the underlying illness has already eroded nutritional status, the patient can have a diminished

TABLE 15–4 Nutrient Deficiencies and Infection

Nutrients	Role in Infection
Zinc	T-lymphocyte and PMN function
Copper	RES and PMN bactericidal function
Iodine	PMN bactericidal function
Vitamin E	Humoral immunity
Selenium	PMN bactericidal function
Retinoids	Lymphocyte proliferation

RES = reticuloendothelial system; PMN = polymorphonuclear leukocytes.

resistance to infection and increased possibility of wound complications. Even when a patient survives an operation without complications, full recovery depends on adaptation and rehabilitation, which also depend on nutrient availability.

PREOPERATIVE ENTERAL NUTRITION

Because preoperative malnutrition can lead to postoperative complications, it is reasonable to expect that preoperative nutritional repletion may reduce the incidence of complications. Several studies have been conducted in which parenteral nutrition was used as the means of nutritional repletion. Retrospective studies suggested a positive effect when parenteral nutrition was used in the preoperative period. In the 1980s, Muller, from Germany, performed the first prospective randomized study using preoperative total parenteral nutrition (TPN) in patients undergoing surgery for upper GI malignancies.[32] The study showed a reduction in postoperative morbidity and mortality in patients who received preoperative TPN. However, many questions were raised regarding this study's experimental design. For instance, no nutritional screening was done on the patients, and well-nourished patients had improved clinical outcome when they received TPN. Buzby then conducted a large multicentric study in the Veterans Administration. In this study, the patients were screened for malnutrition and only malnourished patients were included. When the patients were stratified according to degree of malnutrition, only the severely malnourished patients showed an improved outcome. The moderately malnourished patients showed no benefit of receiving preoperative TPN, and, more important, the mildly malnourished patients had a worse outcome when they received TPN.[33]

The benefits of nutritional repletion through TPN can be overshadowed by the side-effects of resting the bowel. Preoperative enteral nutrition can produce not only nutritional repletion, but can also maintain gut integrity. Only one study has been published where enteral nutrition was used in the preoperative period in a randomized fashion.[34] Two groups of patients were studied: 67 patients received a 10-day course of preoperative enteral nutrition, and 43 patients served as controls. The disease processes were equally distributed between the two groups as GI, oral, and breast cancers, and benign diseases. The study group received intragastric feedings with a carbohydrate-based

diet containing a protein hydrolysate. Nutritional and immunologic parameters were improved in the fed group, although in seven patients tube feedings were discontinued due to intolerance or complications. The rate of wound infection was 10.45 percent in the fed group and 37.2 percent in the control group, with a postoperative hospital stay of 10 ± 2.8 and 13 ± 3.4 days, respectively. The mortality was 6 percent in the fed group and 11.7 percent in the control group. This study, albeit the only one in the literature, strongly supports the use of enteral nutrition in the preoperative period.

Several factors limit the use of enteral nutrition in the preoperative period (Fig. 15–2). The main one is lack of access to the GI tract. Nasoenteric tubes are uncomfortable and unappealing to most patients, particularly to ambulatory patients. In some patients, a tube enterostomy (e.g., gastrostomy) can be risky due to esophageal obstruction or undesirable if stomach exposure is needed at surgery, such as in patients undergoing esophogastrectomy with a gastric pull-up. Last, reimbursement by insurance companies is becoming a problem. Most third-party payors will not accept hospitalization for preoperative nutritional repletion. Nutritional repletion in the outpatient environment is definitely possible but not easy to arrange at most institutions.

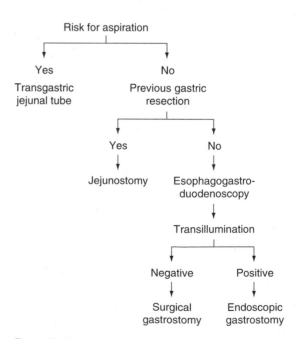

FIGURE 15–2 Decision making regarding enteral access in the surgical patient.

POSTOPERATIVE ENTERAL NUTRITION

The main limiting factor in the use of postoperative enteral nutrition is the common occurrence of ileus. Ileus is paralysis of the GI tract associated with surgery, trauma, infection, metabolic abnormalites, or other pathophysiology of surgical illness. The degree of ileus seems to correlate with the severity of the pathologic state or the magnitude of the surgery. Intra-abdominal and retroperitoneal surgery produce more ileus than surgery on other territories. Postoperative ileus is due to sympathetic discharge in the splanchnic plexus. One other peculiar feature of postoperative ileus is that the degree of paralysis varies along the different segments of the GI tract. Following a substantial abdominal surgery, the stomach usually does not empty properly for 3 to 4 days. The colon may lack motility for 2 to 3 days. The duodenum, jejunum, and ileum, however, recover a few hours after surgery. Therefore, a patient can be enterally fed in the postoperative period as long as the stomach is decompressed and a fiber-free diet is infused into the small intestine. Although there are no data to suggest that bowel rest favors intestinal healing, most surgeons would be reluctant to initiate early jejunal feedings in a patient with a fresh anastomosis in the small bowel. However, it has been shown that immediate postoperative enteral nutrition is feasible and improves the wound-healing response.[35] Also, experimental data on animals suggest that luminal nutrients favor intestinal healing.[36,37]

Since the advent of TPN, the avoidance of enteral nutrition, or bowel rest, was thought to be inconsequential. In fact, bowel rest has been advocated as a therapy for patients with intestinal diseases such as Crohn's disease and ulcerative colitis. However, prospective randomized trials have shown that bowel rest has no added benefit at follow-up examination of 1 year compared with parenteral nutrition in Crohn's disease.[38] In experimental animals, some groups feel that mucosal atrophy with impairment of the mucosal barrier, caused by bowel rest, produces bacterial translocation and endotoxemia.[39] Others feel that mucosal atrophy may have little to do with bacterial translocation.[40,41] The loss of mucosal trophism associated with bowel rest is multifactorial. Some of the factors believed to mediate the trophism induced by enteral nutrition are the provision of epithelial fuels (i.e., glutamine and n-butyrate), the secretion of enterohormones (gastrin, enteroglucagon, peptide YY), biliary and pancreatic secretions, and the workload induced by transport of nutrients.

The human intestine does not seem to have as drastic a response to bowel rest as seen in animals. In animals mucosal atrophy can be seen with simple microscopy, but an electron microscope is needed to detect changes in humans.[42,43] Functional changes do occur in both animals and humans, such as increased permeability to lactulose.[44,45] These observations have led to the hypothesis that the gut is the motor of multiple system organ failure. Patients at increased risk of multiorgan failure are those with significant trauma or burn wounds. Because of these reasons, many studies have been conducted in patients with trauma and burn wounds.

Moore and Moore at the University of Colorado in Denver conducted a study in patients requiring a laparotomy for abdominal trauma.[46] Patients entered into the study were randomized to receive either parenteral nutrition or enteral nutrition with an elemental diet in the immediate postoperative period. The group that received enteral nutrition had a significant reduction in the incidence of major septic complications, such as pneumonia. This study has been reproduced by others, including Kudsk, who included patients with a greater degree of trauma.[47]

ENTERAL NUTRITION IN SPECIAL CONDITIONS

Head and Neck Surgery

Malignancies of the head and neck are often curable with multimodality antineoplastic treatment (i.e., radical surgery, chemotherapy, and radiotherapy). The most common location of these malignancies are the floor of the mouth, tongue, mandible, hypopharynx, and larynx. The success of multimodality therapies usually carries with it significant sequelae, such as dysgeusia, inadequate or excessive salivary secretion, chewing and swallowing disorders, and poor airway protection, which almost unavoidably reduce oral intake and produce malnutrition. It is estimated that greater than 80 percent of patients with head and neck cancer have a significant weight loss during multimodality treatment.[48]

In a study done at Tufts University, 67 consecutive patients with head and neck carcinoma were evaluated for the relationship between nutritional status and treatment-related morbidity, disease recurrence, and survival at 2 years.[49]

They used the presence or absence of the cutaneous delayed hypersensitivity response as a measure of nutritional status. Malnourished patients, as indicated by poor cell-mediated immunity, were at higher risk for treatment complications, recurrence, and death within 2 years after therapy.

A more comprehensive study was carried out by Bassett and Dobie on 50 patients with newly diagnosed head and neck cancer.[50] Their nutritional assessment consisted of anthropometric measurements, skin tests, laboratory values of proteins, and a questionnaire. The overall nutritional score was then computed and categorized as good, fair, or poor as outlined by Copeland and coworkers.[51] Their study found that 40 percent of their population had poor nutrition preoperatively, which concurred with the 39 percent of patients with nutritional impairment found in a previous study by Brookes and Clifford.[52] Bassett and Dobie found that the predominant nutritional impairment was protein-calorie deficiency (marasmus), although there were some elements of visceral protein depletion present as well. They also found that the best predictor of impaired nutritional status was the patient's description of his or her recent diet. Those patients who reported being able to eat a general diet had a good score on the nutritional assessment. Patients whose preoperative diet was reduced to soft or liquid foods had a fair or poor score on the nutritional assessment, with 72 percent accuracy. These data emphasize the importance of a diet history in patients with head and neck malignancies as a good predictor of malnutrition and of increased risk for complications.

Gardine and associates studied a group of 109 patients with squamous cell carcinoma of the oral cavity, larynx, or pharynx over a 5-year period to determine what influenced the need for prolonged postoperative nutritional supplementation.[53] They found that over one third (37.6 percent) of the patients required enteral supplementation for a prolonged period (longer than 1 month). The factors that significantly predicted the need for prolonged nutritional supplementation were preoperative weight loss, stage IV cancers, primary pharyngeal tumors, and the use of combined surgery and radiotherapy. A comparison of three types of enteral access showed that nasogastric feedings were appropriate for short-term use, but for long-term access, a gastrostomy was best for tube feedings. Esophagostomy as a means of access for tube feedings was associated with the most complications. Typical complications in patients with head and neck cancers were aspiration, carotid artery hemorrhage, abscess formation, and skin ulceration or excoriation. Social rehabilitation was also hindered by the use of nasogastric tube feedings, delaying patients' return to work and limiting their social interaction.[53] Because more than half these patients (58 percent) will require enteral supplementation for more than 1 month postoperatively, Gardine recommends gastrostomy tube placement in patients undergoing surgery for head and neck cancer who have two or more of the identified risk factors.

The inability to eat normally, almost always combined with the inability to speak and facial deformities, not only produces malnutrition but also becomes a major source of frustration for the patient and the family. In addition, eating can become a burden when it is laborious, painful, and gruesome to an observer. Ideally, these patients should be counseled by a swallowing therapist and a nutritional support team before initiation of antineoplastic therapies. By reviewing with the patient the expected results of treatment and alternative methods of feeding, much of the anxiety that commonly develops in patients who suddenly realize they cannot carry on basic physiologic processes any longer will be alleviated.

In anticipation of all these problems, a feeding enterostomy can be placed before any treatment. Many patients undergo surgery that may preclude, or make difficult, the placement of feeding enterostomy, endoscopically or even surgically when endotracheal intubation is risky. The unfortunate outcome of these patients is that they remain with the nasogastric tube placed at surgery for a prolonged time. Emphasize the reversibility of a feeding enterostomy to patients, enterostomal therapists, and head and neck surgeons. We have been very satisfied with the use of low-profile gastrostomy devices ("buttons") in this patient population. Regarding oral enteral feeding, retraining for oral alimentation should be done by introducing foods that offer enough consistency for these patients to become accustomed to the sensation of food again and at the same time avoid bronchoaspiration. Typical examples are watermelon and cantaloupe.

Many of these patients depend on opiates for pain control and consequently become constipated. We therefore prefer a fiber-supplemented formula and provide extra free water to lessen the likelihood of this side-effect of opiate usage. In those patients with persistent constipation we recommend a lactulose elixir, 5 to 20 ml through the gastrostomy tube.

The nutritional support team should bear in mind that these patients are not only prone to recurrences of the same cancer but also to development of new cancers, which are typically bronchogenic. Therefore, these patients should have routine laboratory tests for nutrient deficiencies; any indication of tumor activity, such as anemia or abnormal liver function tests, should alert the medical team to suspect cancer. A list of some complications of head and neck cancer is presented in Table 15–5.

Esophageal Surgery

Patients with esophageal pathologic states typically present with painful swallowing, or dysphagia. This can be due to mechanical or functional obstruction. The most common causes of mechanical obstruction are cancer, diverticuli, hiatal hernia, esophagitis, and strictures. Functional obstructions are due to achalasia, diffuse esophageal spasm (DES), and motility disorders secondary to cerebrovascular accidents. Some of these conditions are amenable to surgical treatment. These include resections or bypasses for cancer and myotomies for achalasia. After resections the continuity of the GI tract is reestablished by "pulling up" the stomach to the cervical esophagus or interposing colon or jejunum. All these are major surgical procedures with creation of tenuous anastomoses in severely malnourished patients. Therefore, it is not surprising that many of the studies investigating the use of preoperative nutritional support include a high proportion of patients undergoing esophageal surgery.

The nutritional support of patients with esophageal cancer was reviewed in an article by Burt and Brennan.[54] They listed several potential etiologies for the cachexia commonly seen in esophageal cancer patients. Theories included cachexia caused by anorexia secondary to hypothalamic dysfunction, taste and smell abnormalities, learned food aversions, complications of antineoplastic therapy, increased energy expenditure, and tumor-host competition for substrates. They concluded that host-tumor competition and increased energy expenditure (especially of carbohydrates) were the most likely etiologies contributing to the weight loss, debilitation, and progressive hypophagia seen in these patients.[54] Through their review of the extensive literature, they were able to come to some general findings common to esophageal cancer patients. First,

TABLE 15–5 Complications in Patients with Head and Neck Malignancies

Related to Surgery
Poor chewing
Poor occlusion of the oral cavity
Poor airway protection
Laborious swallowing

Related to Radiotherapy
Dysgeusia
Xerostomia
Salivary hypersecretion

Related to Chemotherapy
Anorexia/nausea/vomiting
Diarrhea

Related to Primary Tumor
Skin ulceration or excoriation
Cellulitis/abscess formation
Carotid artery hemorrhage

Systemic Complications
Metastatic disease
Synchronous or metachronous cancer (e.g., lung)

retrospective studies on these patients show that malnutrition is detrimental and probably affects ultimate clinical outcome. Second, the available biologic evidence indicates that nutritional support benefits this group of patients. Finally, there appears to be a trend toward decreased operative mortality in the studies of patients with esophageal carcinoma, but these trials suffer from having small numbers of patients in each study.[54]

Planning of postoperative nutritional support is just as important as preoperative nutritional support. Many surgeons performing esophageal surgery are overly optimistic regarding the patients' ability to resume oral alimentation postoperatively. The resumption of oral alimentation is often seen as an indicator of surgical success in these patients. This is entirely appropriate, but the surgeon should be aware that it may not happen immediately postoperatively. We feel strongly that all these patients should have a feeding jejunostomy constructed at the time of esophagectomy. Having access to the jejunum allows early feedings and provides nutrition during the management of complications (such as anastomotic leaks). It is much more practical not to delay discharge because of poor oral intake but to deliver sufficient nutrition through a tube enterostomy and plan on the transition to oral alimentation in the ambulatory setting.

As opposed to patients with head and neck malignancies who usually receive a gastros-

TABLE 15–6   Comparison of Gastrostomies and Jejunostomies for Long-Term Feedings

	Gastrostomies	Jejunostomies
Placement	Endoscopic, x-ray, surgical	Only surgical
Laparotomy	Small (when needed)	Full
Bore size	Large	Small
Medications	Well tolerated	Poorly tolerated
Clogging	Uncommon	Very common
Accidental removal	Uncommon	Very common
Exchanges	Easy, elective	Difficult, emergencies

tomy for feedings secondary to their esophageal pathologic state, most patients with a gastric pathologic state require a feeding jejunostomy. Although a jejunostomy is a very effective route for nutrient delivery in the immediate postoperative period, when it is used for long-term feedings it is associated with many more complications than gastrostomies. Table 15–6 compares gastrostomies and jejunostomies as an access to the gastrointestinal tract for long-term feedings.

Gastric Surgery

Gastric surgery today is done mostly to treat patients with cancer. Ulcer surgery has been greatly diminished with the advent of effective medication and by a better understanding of the pathophysiology involved with peptic ulcer disease. A few rare conditions requiring gastric surgery are gastric volvulus and benign tumors. For the most part, three types of procedures are performed on the stomach, excluding gastrostomies: resections (total and subtotal gastrectomies, gastroplasties, and antrectomies), bypass procedures (gastrojejunostomy), and pyloroplasties and vagotomies. After resection of the distal stomach, the GI tract can be reconstructed by connecting the proximal stomach to the duodenum (Billroth I reconstruction) or by closing the duodenal stump and connecting the proximal stomach to the jejunum (Billroth II). Gastric surgery can also result in some serious complications in the early postoperative period, such as anastomotic dehiscence or dehiscence of the duodenal stump following Billroth II reconstructions.

Gastrectomies can produce a wide variety of GI dysfunction grouped under the name of *postgastrectomy syndromes* (Table 15–7). The most common of these is dumping syndrome, which can occur with gastrectomies, gastrojejunostomies, and pyloroplasties. This syndrome is characterized by upper abdominal pain, distention, and sometimes nausea and vomiting. Signs include weakness, sweating, blushing, dizziness, palpitations, and hypotension. They usually occur 20 to 90 minutes after hyperosmolar foods are ingested. These symptoms are caused by the discharge of GI hormones such as serotonin and histamine. Copious diarrhea will relieve these symptoms postprandially.

Patients with postgastrectomy syndromes have been found to develop several nutritional deficiencies as well as significant weight loss. Total gastrectomy can cause up to a 25 to 30 percent decrease in weight. These patients have a functional lactase deficiency because rapid intestinal transit prevents the hydrolysis of lactose.[55] These patients also have high output of bile acids. This causes decreased transit time in the colon, which can produce significant diarrhea.[56]

Another nutrient deficiency commonly seen in patients with gastrectomies is hypocalcemia, which becomes critical in postmenopausal women. Some studies estimate that up to 30 percent of gastric surgery patients have osteoporosis to some degree.[57,58] These patients have an increased tendency to fracture bones.[59] Resection of the distal stomach is associated with poor vitamin B_{12} absorption due to the lack of intrinsic factor. Iron deficiency is also common after gastric surgery.[60] Specifically, gastrojejunostomies bypass the duodenum and variable lengths of jejunum, and this

TABLE 15–7   Postgastrectomy Syndromes

Nutrient Intolerance
Dumping syndrome
Poor emptying of gastric remnant
Lactose intolerance

Nutrient Deficiencies
Osteoporosis (hypocalcemia)
Megaloblastic anemia (vitamin B_{12})
Microcytic anemia (iron deficiency)

can result in iron malabsorption. A major cause is believed to be the lack of gastric acid, which reduces the release of iron bound to protein.[61] Other syndromes include afferent and efferent loop obstructions, gastroparesis, and gastroplegia.

Patients suffering from acute complications of gastric surgery (anastomotic deficiencies or stump leaks) or from postgastrectomy syndromes often require reparative surgery. Another group of patients requiring reparative surgery for gastric complications are patients undergoing surgery for morbid obesity. Reoperation on the stomach can be extremely difficult and often results in a prolonged postoperative recovery. We have found it very useful to perform enterostomies at surgery for continued gastric decompression and jejunal feedings. Various types of tubes for these enterostomies are commercially available. These tubes may be necessary for a short period (a few weeks) or for a significantly longer period (for months to years). An example of such a case is

the patient with gastrojejunostomies performed for decompression of malignant duodenal obstructions.

Transgastric access to the jejunum for simultaneous gastric decompression and jejunal feedings can be established surgically, endoscopically, or radiologically. We have found that surgically placed transgastric tubes are the most effective for this purpose (Fig. 15–3). One advantage is that the internal diameter of the lumen of the jejunal tubes is usually larger in the tubes commercially available for surgical placement. Another advantage is the permanence of the distal tube in the small bowel. When these tubes are placed surgically, access to the stomach is made near the bottom of the stomach, close to the greater curvature, which allows a direct passage of the tube across the pylorus. The placement of jejunal tubes through percutaneous endoscopic gastrostomies, misnomered as percutaneous endoscopic jejunostomies (PEJ), is not as simple as the surgical placement. The main difference

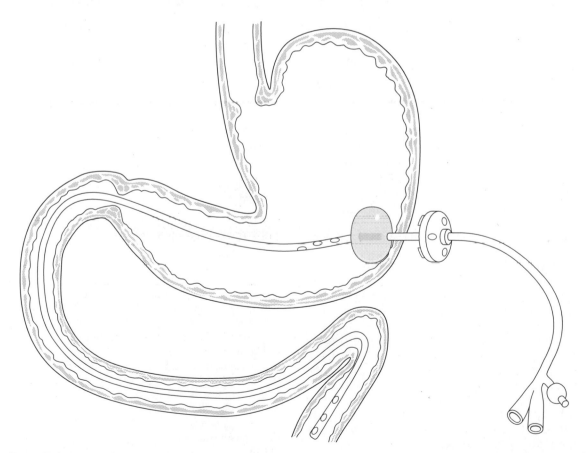

FIGURE 15–3   Transgastric jejunal tube. This dual lumen tube is placed surgically and allows for jejunal feedings while providing gastric decompression.

between these two techniques is the access to the stomach. Although the access chosen at surgery is low, toward the greater curvature, the access used in the endoscopic technique is limited to the midbody of the stomach above the transverse colon. Having such access often directs the jejunal tube either superiorly or laterally, creating a loop in the gastric lumen away from the pylorus. Even when the pylorus is successfully traversed by the tube, it tends to migrate back into the stomach. With the radiologic technique, this approach has a success rate midway between the surgical and endoscopic techniques.

Intestinal Surgery

The most common pathologies of small intestine that require surgical intervention are obstruction, ischemic necrosis due to strangulation, or inflammatory conditions such as Crohn's disease. Segments of intestine can be used as conduits to carry bile (bilioenteric bypass), pancreatic juice (pancreatojejunostomy), or urine (Bricker). Once the segment to be used as a conduit is harvested, it may be reconnected to the bowel as a Roux-Y enteroenterostomy, or remain excluded from the intestine while the remainder of the intestine is reconnected.

Patients afflicted with Crohn's disease or those who develop ischemic bowel undergo excisions of variable lengths of small intestine. Excision of the small bowel can produce malabsorption depending on the extent and the site of resection. Resection of the ileum can produce malabsorption of fats, fat-soluble vitamins, and vitamin B_{12}. The mean length of intestine necessary for proper absorption is 12 feet. When more than 70 to 80 percent of the small intestine is resected, the patient develops a short-bowel syndrome and usually requires parenteral nutrition to survive. There are, however, rare reports of patients who have been able to survive and maintain their nutritional status even after significant small-bowel resection.[62]

A very common dilemma following surgery of the small intestine is when to initiate enteral nutrition because of fear of leakage from the suture line. The parameters used to assess recovery of GI function following abdominal surgery range from bowel sounds to passage of flatus and stool. These parameters, however, do not indicate function of the small intestine but rather function of the large intestine. As mentioned earlier, the large intestine takes longer to

recover function, usually 3 or 4 days, compared with a few hours for the small intestine.

A significant difficulty in the postoperative management of patients undergoing surgery on the small bowel, versus the stomach or large bowel, is our ability to decompress the lumen of the small bowel and reduce the intraluminal contents. Following gastric surgery, a nasogastric tube or a gastrostomy tube can effectively decompress the stomach of fluid and gas. Following colonic surgery, a surgeon may chose to create a colostomy proximal to the anastomosis to divert the fecal stream away from the suture line. Even without a colostomy, the postoperative colonic ileus usually precludes the propulsion of luminal contents, which protects the newly created anastomosis from excessive pressures. The small bowel, however, cannot be decompressed by simple means. Therefore, even though the bowel is deprived of luminal nutrients, bile, pancreatic, and intestinal secretions will continue to be produced and come in contact with the anastomosis. Despite the fact that decompression of small-bowel anastomoses is not possible, the incidence of leakage of small-bowel anastomoses is much less than seen in large-bowel anastomoses.[63,64] The risk of anastomotic breakdown is almost limited to very-well-defined situations (Table 15–8). Other risk factors are technical, such as a bowel anastomosis performed at tension, excessive dissection of the margins of bowel with ischemia or hematoma formation, and closure of the abdomen with excessive tension on the abdominal walls. Whenever one or more of these risk factors is present, it is wise to wait until observing objective signs of total bowel function, such as passage of flatus or stool. On the con-

TABLE 15–8   Factors that Predispose to Anastomotic Leakage and Preclude Early Enteral Nutrition

Intrinsic Disease of the Intestine
Crohn's disease
Radiation enteritis
Dilatation from prolonged obstruction
Ischemic bowel

Intraperitoneal Conditions
Peritonitis (diffuse or localized)
Multiple bowel anastomoses
Urinary and biliary diversion

Systemic Conditions
Immunosuppression
Shock
Sepsis

trary, in patients who undergo a routine bowel resection with normal bowel and no risk factors (e.g., injury secondary to a simple laceration due to a stabbing without shock or peritonitis), there is no reason to withhold enteral nutrition. In fact, many patients sustaining penetrating trauma to the abdomen do so in the postprandial period. We have seen at surgery that not only is the lumen filled with nutrients, but the lymphatic vessels seem to be noticeably loaded with fat being absorbed.

The most common limiting factor in providing enteral nutrition after intestinal surgery is lack of access to the small intestine combined with gastric ileus. In patients undergoing laparotomy for abdominal trauma, the placement of needle catheter jejunostomies has become well established.[46] This is particularly useful in the patient with other traumatic injuries such as head and chest trauma and long bone and pelvic fractures. In patients with lesser injuries or those undergoing elective surgeries, the benefit of having an access to the jejunum for feedings may be outweighed by the complications associated with placement of a jejunostomy tube or catheter. These complications are mainly leakage and obstruction. For these patients, a dual lumen nasoduodenal, or nasojejunal, tube with a gastric port for decompression is a more desirable option. In the past, these tubes were very rigid and limited to tubes of large-bore size that most patients did not tolerate. Fortunately, many different kinds are now commercially available. We have found that an 18 F Silastic dual-lumen tube with some palpable markings below the gastric openings works well in most patients.

The type of formula to be administered into the jejunum varies with the indication and the particular conditions of the GI tract. For early jejunal feedings after abdominal trauma, elemental diets are used until the colon has recovered function. Once the patient is passing flatus or stool, any polymeric, isotonic diet with or without fiber can be administered. In patients with intrinsic bowel disease, such as Crohn's disease or radiation enteritis, peptide-based diets are preferred. Transport of dipeptides and tripeptides across the intestinal mucosa is favored over the transport of free amino acids in both normal and diseased intestine. The process of fat absorption is the first one that suffers when intestinal function is compromised. Therefore, diets for patients with intrinsic intestinal disease should be low in total fat, at least initially. When the intestinal mucosa is diseased or atrophic the tip of the villi becomes blunted. Absorption of log-chain triglycerides takes place at the tip of the villi through a complex process of packaging into chylomicrons and transport through the lymphatics. Medium-chain triglycerides (MCTs) can be absorbed anywhere along the villus/crypt epithelium and then are transported into the portal circulation, just as are amino acids and monosaccharides. For all the above reasons, diets containing short peptides and MCTs are favored in patients with intestinal disease or bowel atrophy from prolonged bowel rest.[62]

Colorectal Surgery

Colonic surgery may be directed to one segment, such as the right colon, the left colon, or the rectum, or to the entire organ. Excision of the rectum and anus results in the need for a permanent colostomy. When the entire colon is excised, in addition to the rectum and anus, stool is evacuated through an ileostomy. In some selected patients, such as those with ulcerative colitis or familial polyposis, the entire colon is excised, as well as the rectal mucosal lining, but the muscle layer of the rectum and the anal sphincters is preserved. Instead of creating a permanent ileostomy, the terminal ileum is folded over and connected in the shape of a pouch with an outlet through the anus. This operation is named ileal-pouch anal anastomosis, or pull-through procedure.

Although the colon has important functions in health, excision of the colon does not produce any permanent nutritional sequelae. However, excision of either a segment of the colon, or the entire organ, can change the pattern of bowel movements. This change may only be transient in the early postoperative period and quickly become compensated for by the remainder of the colon, or it may become permanent. For instance, patients who undergo subtotal colectomy and ileoproctostomy may never regain a normal frequency and consistency of stools. As a permanent new pattern these patients will pass three to five loose stools per day. A colonic anastomosis is quite frequently performed in colonic resections, depending on the extent of colon resected. Malnutrition has been shown to have an adverse effect on colonic healing.[5] The significance of this is that anastomotic leaks are a major source of morbidity and mortality in patients who have undergone colonic surgery.[65]

Of all possible segmental excisions, sigmoid resections are most common. These resections are done not only for cancer but often for complicated diverticular disease. Sigmoid resections do not appear to alter the pattern of bowel movements. Right hemicolectomies involve excision of the cecum, ascending colon, and a short segment of terminal ileum, thereby eliminating the ileocecal valve. In the right colon "antiperistaltic" waves generate retrograde flow of colonic contents back to the cecum to allow for stasis and bacterial fermentation.[66] Both a faster transit time and increased colonic secretion may ensue following right hemicolectomy due to the loss of the ileocecal valve, the loss of the pacemakers in the right colon, and the increased offer of bile salts to the transverse colon. In most patients, the colon can rapidly adapt to these changes, and the bowel pattern is maintained at preoperative levels. However, a small group of patients will develop chronic diarrhea following right hemicolectomy. To reduce the incidence and severity of diarrhea, several dietary measures can be implemented in the immediate postoperative period.

A significant number of patients undergoing colonic surgery are elderly. Age and malnutrition produce chronic constipation, which in turn predisposes to volvulus and complications of diverticular disease. In these patients an access to the GI tract for feedings should be established in conjunction with the colonic procedure.

If the surgery does not involve resection of the colon, then the patient will continue with chronic constipation. These patients need a fiber-supplemented tube feeding formula and extra free water to maintain proper intestinal elimination. In some patients with constipation resistant to psyllium seeds or soy polysaccharide, we have added a daily dose of lactulose. If the colonic procedure involves creating an ileostomy, then dehydration becomes a larger problem. Elderly patients seem to have greater loses of fluid through an ileostomy. A low-residue diet and additional free water should be used.

Anorectal Pathology

Some patients present with severe wounds in the perineal area such as deep decubitus ulcers, Fournier's gangrene of the perineum, or multiple fistula due to Crohn's disease. Constant soiling of these wounds with stool makes management very difficult. In these situations, the best option is to create a diverting colostomy. However, most of these patients are too weak, too old, and too ill to undergo

surgery. Another option is to diminish stool output by dietary and pharmacologic interventions and, in essence, create a medical colostomy. To do that, an access to the GI tract is needed. It can be in the form of a nasoenteric tube or a percutaneous endoscopically placed gastrostomy (PEG) depending on the projected need for tube feedings. A low-residue diet is then infused in a continuous manner to avoid the development of diarrhea.

Orthopedic Surgery

It is important in orthopedic surgery, as in any other surgery, that patients are properly assessed for nutritional status. It is particularly significant in the elderly population. These patients often present with malnutrition. Although the surgical management of orthopedic problems is relatively simple and straightforward, these patients are at great risk of complications and death due to underlying malnutrition. A paper by Smith[67] examined nutrition and its relationship to orthopedic infections.

In a study by Bastow and coworkers,[68] 744 elderly women admitted during an 18-month period with a fracture of the neck of the femur were assessed for nutritional status. The patients were classified into three groups based on their arm circumference and triceps skinfold thickness compared with the mean and standard deviation of home and hospitalized patients. Patients who were classified into groups with nutritional deficits were randomly allocated into either an enteral supplementary feeding group or a control group without supplementary nutrition postoperatively. Bastow's study found that supplementary feedings improved not only anthropometric and plasma protein measurements but also clinical outcome. These differences were especially noted in the group that was most severely malnourished. Specifically, rehabilitation time and hospital stay were shortened. Although this study found a difference in mortality as well, the difference was not statistically significant.[68]

Thoracic Surgery

Thoracic surgery, for the purposes of this discussion, will exclude esophageal surgery, since that was covered in a separate section. As with other types of surgery, nutrition plays an important role in thoracic surgery. Illnesses, such as bronchogenic carcinoma, requiring thoracic surgery are frequently associated with malnutrition because of anorexia and occasionally obstruction. In addition, these patients' postoperative course can be slow with prolonged mechanical ventilation. As with all critically ill postoperative patients, caloric needs are increased by tissue damage, blood, tissue and plasma loss, fever, plasma exudation into surrounding tissues, and clearance of the products of damaged tissues. It is therefore essential to identify the patients at risk of malnutrition. Similar screening measurements can be used to assess the nutritional status of these patients. In general, most thoracic surgeons would like to correct malnutrition before performing the needed operation. However, if that is not possible, some surgeons will place enteral access at surgery.[69]

SUMMARY

Enteral nutrition is now an integral part of the preoperative and postoperative management of surgical patients. Ideally, enteral nutrition should be initiated early in the preoperative period, but this is not always possible in many surgical patients. Surgical patients should undergo nutritional screening and assessment by objective or subjective means. Malnutrition affects surgical outcome by impairing wound healing, predisposing to infection, and interfering with postoperative adaptation and rehabilitation. Surgery performed on the alimentary tract is more likely to render the patient unable to assimilate sufficient nutrients through an oral diet. Therefore, consider placing a tube enterostomy in all patients undergoing major surgery on the alimentary tract. Patients with head and neck malignancies are treated with multimodality antineoplastic therapies that interfere with normal alimentation. These patients benefit from institution of enteral nutrition before initiation of antineoplastic therapy. Enteral nutrition can also accelerate the recovery of elderly malnourished patients undergoing orthopedic procedures. Many patients operated on for thoracic conditions require postoperative enteral nutrition while recovering their ventilatory function. Enteral nutrition is a crucial component in the success of combating surgical illnesses.

REFERENCES

1. Studley HO: Percentage of weight loss: a basic indicator of surgical risk in patients with chronic peptic ulcer. JAMA 1936;106:458–460.
2. Fantino M, Wieteska L: Evidence for a direct central anorectic effect of tumor-necrosis-factor-alpha in the rat. Physiol Behav 1993;53(3):477–483.
3. Grunfeld C, Wilking H, Neese R et al: Persistence of the hypertriglyceridemic effect of tumor necrosis factor despite development of tachyphylaxis to its anorectic/cachectic effects in rats. Cancer Res 1989;49(10):2554–2560.
4. Rhoads JE, Alexander CE: Nutritional problems of surgical patients. Ann NY Acad Sci 1955;63:268–275.
5. Daly JM, Vars HM, Dudrick SJ: Correlation of protein depletion with colonic anastomotic strength in rats. Surg Forum 1970;21:77–78.
6. Bistrian BR, Blackburn GL, Hallowell E et al: Protein status of general surgical patients. JAMA 1974;230(6):858–860.
7. Bistrian BR, Blackburn GL, Vitale J et al: Prevalence of malnutrition in general medical patients. JAMA 1976;235(15):1567–1570.
8. Dempsey DT, Mullen JL, Buzby GP: The link between nutritional status and clinical outcome: can nutritional intervention modify it? Am J Clin Nutr 1988;47:352–356.
9. Mullen JL, Buzby GP, Waldman MT et al: Prediction of operative morbidity and mortality by preoperative nutritional assessment. Surg Forum 1979;30:80–82.
10. Mullen JL, Buzby GP, Matthews DC et al: Reduction of operative morbidity and mortality by combined preoperative and postoperative nutritional support. Ann Surg 1980;192(5):604–613.
11. Mullen JL, Gertner MH, Buzby GP et al: Implications of malnutrition in the surgical patient. Arch Surg 1979;114:121–125.
12. Baker FP, Detsky AS, Wesson DE et al: Nutritional assessment: a comparison of clinical judgment and objective measurements. N Engl J Med 1982;306:969–972.
13. Aaronson SA, Rubin JS, Finch PW et al: Growth factor-regulated pathways in epithelial cell proliferation. Am Rev Respir Dis 1990;142(6 pt 2):S7–S10.
14. Murphy PG, Loitz BJ, Frank CB et al: Influence of exogenous growth factors on the synthesis and secretion of collagen types I and III by explants of normal and healing rabbit ligaments. Biochem Cell Biol 1994;72(9-10):403–409.
15. Kondo H, Matsuda R, Yonezawa Y: Platelet-derived growth factor in combination with collagen promotes the migration of human skin fibroblasts into a denuded area of a cell monolayer. Exp Cell Res 1992;202(1):45–51.
16. Goodlad RA, Wright NA: Peptides and epithelial growth regulation. Experientia 1987;43(7):780–784.
17. Thompson WD, Ravdin IS, Frank IL: Effect of hypoproteinemia on wound disruption. Arch Surg 1938;36:500–508.
18. Rhoads JE, Fliegelman MT, Panzer LM: The mechanism of delayed wound healing in the presence of hypoproteinemia. JAMA 1942;118:21.
19. Localio SA, Chassin JL, Hinton JW: Tissue protein depletion—a factor in wound disruption. Surg Gynecol Obstet 1948;86:107–113.
20. Haydock DA, Hill GL: Impaired wound healing in surgical patients with varying degrees of malnutrition. J Parenter Enter Nutr 1986;10:550–554.
21. Haydock DA, Hill GL: Improved wound healing response in surgical patients receiving intravenous nutrition. Br J Surg 1987;74(4):320–323.
22. Haydock DA, Flint MH, Hyde KF et al: The efficacy of subcutaneous goretex implants in monitoring wound healing response in experimental protein deficiency. Connect Tissue Res 1988;17(3):159–169.
23. Windsor JA, Knight GS, Hill GL: Wound healing response in surgical patients: recent food intake is more

important than nutritional status. Br J Surg 1988;75(2): 135–137.

24. Barbul A, Rettura G, Levenson SM et al: Wound healing and thymotropic effects of arginine: a pituitary mechanism of action. Am J Clin Nutr 1983;37: 786–794.

25. Caldwell FT, Rosenberg IK, Rosenberg BF et al: Effect of single amino acid supplementation upon the gain of tensile strength of wounds in protein-depleted rats. Surg Gynecol Obstet 1964;119:823–830.

26. Irvin TT: The effect of methionine on colonic wound healing in malnourished rats. Br J Surg 1976;63: 237–240.

27. Ruberg RL: Role of nutrition in wound healing. Surg Clin North Am 1984;64(4):705–714.

28. Berg RA, Stienmann B, Rennard SI et al: Ascorbate deficiency results in decreased collagen production: underhydroxylation of proline leads to increased intracellular degradation. Arch Biochem Biophys 1983;226 (2):681–686.

29. Chandra RK: Micronutrients and immune factors: an overview. Ann NY Acad Sci 1990;587:9–16.

30. Good RA, Lorenz E: Nutrition and cellular immunity. Int J Immunopharmacol 1992;14(3):361–366.

31. Farid NR, Woodford G, Au B et al: Polymorphonuclear leucocyte function in hypothyroidism. Hormone Res 1976;7(4-5):247–253.

32. Muller JM, Brenner U, Dienst C et al: Preoperative parenteral feeding in patients with gastrointestinal carcinoma. Lancet 1982;1:68–71.

33. Veterans Affairs Total Parenteral Nutrition Cooperative Study Group: Perioperative total parenteral nutrition in surgical patients. N Engl J Med 1991;325:525–532.

34. Shukla HS, Rao RR, Banu N et al: Enteral hyperalimentation in malnourished surgical patients. Ind J Med Res 1984;80:339–346.

35. Schroeder D, Gillanders L, Mahr K et al: Effects of immediate postoperative enteral nutrition on body composition, muscle function, and wound healing. J Parenter Enter Nutr 1991;15(4):376–383.

36. Rolandelli RH, Saul SH, Settle RG et al: Comparison of parenteral nutrition and enteral feeding with pectin in experimental colitis in the rat. Am J Clin Nutr 1988;47 (4):715–721.

37. Rolandelli RH, Koruda MJ, Settle RG et al: Effects of intraluminal infusion of short-chain fatty acids on the healing of colonic anastomosis in the rat. Surgery 1986;100(2):198–204.

38. Greenberg GR, Fleming CR, Jeejeehboy KN et al: Controlled trial of bowel rest and nutritional support in the management of Crohn's disease. Gut 1988;29(10): 1309–1315.

39. Bark T, Katouli M, Svenberg T et al: Food deprivation increases bacterial translocation after non-lethal hemorrhage in rats. Euro J Surg 1995;161(2):67–71.

40. Barber AE, Jones WG II, Minei JP et al: Bacterial overgrowth and intestinal atrophy in the etiology of gut barrier failure in the rat. Am J Surg 1991;161(2): 300–304.

41. Frankel W, Zhang W, Singh A et al: Fiber: effect on bacterial translocation and intestinal mucin content. World J Surg 1995;19(1):144–148.

42. Guedon C, Schmitz J, Lerebours E et al: Decreased brush border hydrolase activities without gross morphologic changes in human intestinal mucosa after prolonged total parenteral nutrition of adults. Gastroenterology 1986;90(2):373–378.

43. Buchman AL, Moukarzel AA, Ament ME et al: Effects of total parenteral nutrition on intestinal morphology and function in humans. Transplant Proc 1994;26(3):1457.

44. Ziegler TR, Smith RJ, O'Dwyer ST et al: Increased intestinal permeability associated with infection in burn patients. Arch Surg 1988;123:1313–1318.

45. Epstein MD, Tchervenkov JI, Alexander JW et al: Increased gut permeability following burn trauma. Arch Surg 1991;126:198–200.

46. Moore FA, Moore EE, Jones TN et al: TEN versus TPN following major abdominal trauma—reduced septic morbidity. J Trauma 1989;29(7):916–922.

47. Kudsk KA, Croce MA, Fabian TC et al: Enteral versus parenteral feeding. Effects on septic morbidity after blunt and penetrating abdominal trauma. Ann Surg 1992;215(5):503–511.

48. Chencharick JD, Mossman KL: Nutritional consequences of the radiotherapy of head and neck cancer. Cancer 1983;51(5):811–815.

49. Lopez MJ, Robinson P, Madden T et al: Nutritional support and prognosis in patients with head and neck cancer. J Surg Oncol 1994;55:33–36.

50. Bassett MR, Dobie RA: Patterns of nutritional deficiency in head and neck cancer. Neck Surg 1983;91:119–125.

51. Copeland EM III, Daly JM, Dudrick SJ: Nutritional concepts in the treatment of head and neck malignancies. Head Neck Surg 1979;1(4):350–365.

52. Brookes GB, Clifford P: Nutritional status and general immune competence in patients with head and neck cancer. J Roy Soc Med 1981;74(2):132–139.

53. Gardine RL, Kokal WA, Beatty JD et al: Predicting the need for prolonged enteral supplementation in the patient with head and neck cancer. Am J Surg 1988; 156(1):63–65.

54. Burt ME, Brennan MR: Nutritional support of the patient with esophageal cancer. Semin Oncol 1984;11 (2):127–135.

55. McKelvey STD: Gastric incontinence with post-vagotomy diarrhea. Br J Surg 1970;57:741–747.

56. Allan JG, Gerskowitch VP, Russel RI: The role of bile acids in the pathogenesis of postvagotomy diarrhea. Br J Surg 1974;61:516–518.

57. Eddy RL: Metabolic bone disease after gastrectomy. Am J Med 1971;50:442–449.

58. Deller DJ, Witts LJ: Changes in the blood after partial gastrectomy with special reference to vitamin B12. Q J Med 1962;3:71–88.

59. Nilsson BE, Westlin NE: The fracture incidence after gastrectomy. Acta Chir Scand 1971;137:533–534.

60. Clark CG: Medical complications of gastric surgery for peptic ulcer. Compr Ther 1981;7:26–32.

61. Wheldon EJ, Venables CW, Johnston IDA: The relationship of anemia to gastric secretion more than 15 years after vagotomy and gastroenterostomy. Br J Surg 1975;62:356–359.

62. Rodriquez DJ, Clevenger FW: Successful enteral refeeding after massive small bowel resection. West J Med 1993;159:192–194.

63. Wise L, McAlister W, Stein T et al: Studies on the healing of anastomoses of small and large intestines. Surg Gynecol Obstet 1975;141(2):190–194.

64. Hesp FL, Hendriks T, Lubbers EJ et al: Wound healing in the intestinal wall. Effects of infection on experimental ileal and colonic anastomoses. Dis Colon Rectum 1984;27(7):462–467.

65. Irvin TT, Hunt TK: Reappraisal of the healing process of anastomosis of the colon. Surg Gynecol Obstet 1974;138:741–746.

66. Ritchie JA, Truelove SC, Ardan GM et al: Propulsion and retropulsion of normal colonic contents. Am J Dig Dis 1971;16(8):697–704.

67. Smith TK: Nutrition: its relationship to orthopedic infections. Orthop Clin North Am 1991;22(3):373–377.

68. Bastow MD, Rawlings J, Allison SP: Benefits of supplementary tube feeding after fractured neck of femur: a randomised controlled trial. Br Med J 1983;287: 1589–1592.
69. Azarow KS, Molloy M, Seyfer AE et al: Preoperative evaluation and general preparation for chest wall operations. Surg Clin North Am 1989;69:899–910.

BIBLIOGRAPHY

Alexander JW: Nutrition and translocation. J Parenteral Enter Nutr 1990;14(5):170S–174S.

Barbul A, Purtill WA: Nutrition in wound healing. Clin Dermatol 1994;12:133–140.

Bates CJ: Fat-soluble vitamins. Vitamin A. Lancet 1995; 345(8941):31–35.

Beigler DF, Bach BR: Nutritional issues (letters to the editor). Clin Orthop 1982;165:300–301.

Beisel WR: Vitamins and the immune system. Ann NY Acad Sci 1990;587:5–8.

Brookes GB: Nutritional status—a prognostic indicator in head and neck cancer. Otolaryngol Head Neck Surg 1985;93:69–74.

Buzby GP: Perioperative nutritional support. J Parenter Enter Nutr 1990;14(5):197S–199S.

Cannon PR, Wissler RW, Woolridge RL et al: The relationship of protein deficiency to surgical infection. Ann Surg 1944;120:514–525.

Detsky AS, Mendelson RA, Baker JP et al: The choice to treat all, some, or no patients undergoing gastrointestinal surgery with nutritional support: a decision analysis approach. J Parenter Enter Nutr 1984;8(3):245–253.

Ellis LM, Copeland EM, Souba WW: Perioperative nutritional support. Surg Clin North Am 1991;71(3):493–507.

Finkelmeier A: Difficult problems in post-operative management. Thoracic surgical operations. Crit Care Q 1986;9(3):59–70.

Fortunato L, Ridge JA: Surgical palliation of head and neck cancer. Curr Prob Cancer 1995;153–165.

Gottschlich MM, Jenkins M, Warden GD et al: Differential effects of three enteral dietary regimens on selected outcome variables in burn patients. J Parenter Enter Nutr 1990;14(3):225–236.

Iovinelli G, Marsili I, Varrassi G: Nutrition support and total laryngectomy. J Parenter Enter Nutr 1993;17(5): 445–448.

Irvin TT, Hunt TK: Effect of malnutrition on colonic healing. Ann Surg 1974;180(5):765–772.

Localio SA, Morgan ME, Hinton JW: The biological chemistry of wound healing. The effect of methionine on the healing of wounds in protein-depleted animals. Surg Gynecol Obstet 1848;86:582–589.

Moore FA, Moore EE, Kudsk KA et al: Clinical benefits of an immune-enhancing diet for early postinjury enteral feeding. J Trauma 1994;37(4):607–615.

Moore EE, Jones TN: Benefits of immediate jejunostomy feeding after major abdominal trauma—a prospective, randomized study. J Trauma 1986;26(10):874–881.

Moore FA, Feliciano DV, Andrassy RJ: Early enteral feeding, compared with parenteral, reduces postoperative septic complications. Ann Surg 1992;216(2):172–183.

Neumann CG, Lawlor GJ, Stiehm ER et al: Immunologic responses in malnourished children. Am J Clin Nutr 1975:89–104.

Perez-Tamayo R, Ihnen M: The effect of methionine in experimental wound healing. A morphologic study. Am J Pathol 1953;29:233–249.

Pessa ME, Bland KI, Copeland EM: Growth factors and determinants of wound repair. J Surg Res 1987;42(2): 207–217.

Rumore MA: Vitamin A as an immunomodulating agent. Clin Pharmacy 1993;12:506–514.

Saito H, Trocki O, Alexander W et al: The effect of route of nutrient administration on the nutritional state, catabolic hormone secretion, and gut mucosal integrity after burn injury. J Parenter Enter Nutr 1987;11(1):1–7.

Sherman AR: Zinc, copper, and iron nutrition and immunity. J Nutr 1991;122(3S):604–609.

Shizgal HM: Nutrition and immune function. 15–29.

Trockl O, Mochizuki H, Dominioni L et al: Intact protein versus free amino acids in the nutritional support of thermally injured animals. J Parenter Enter Nutr 1986; 10(2):139–145.

16

Enteral Nutrition and the Neurologic Diseases

DONALD F. KIRBY
MARK H. DELEGGE

The spectrum of neurologic diseases can be quite far ranging and requires different decisions regarding nutritional ramifications. The acute brain-injured patient may be well nourished before injury, but hypermetabolism may rapidly erode nutritional stores, especially protein, culminating in a nitrogen death.[1] Other neurologic diseases may alter the patient's ability to initiate the complex swallowing reflex, resulting in gradual nutritional deterioration to a starvation state or death from repeated episodes of aspiration pneumonia. Because patients with neurologic diseases comprise 15 percent of acute care hospital inpatients, over 30 percent of rehabilitation center inpatients, and 50 percent of nursing home patients, their early, effective nutritional management may help improve outcome and reduce medical costs. This chapter discusses the rationale, indications, and special physiologic challenges presented by patients with neurologic diseases.

BACKGROUND

The acuteness of the need to feed patients with neurologic diseases aggressively seems to have lagged behind other areas in medicine. As early as 1947 rapid nutritional deterioration after craniotomy was noted by Drew and colleagues.[2] However, the hypermetabolism asso-

ciated with brain injury was not documented until 1975.[3] There were also few attempts at early feeding until the 1980s, when Rapp and coworkers showed that total parenteral nutrition (TPN) was not only safe but also associated with higher patient survival than attempts at intragastric feeding.[4] This was in contrast to previous beliefs that TPN, with its high fluid volumes and hyperosmolar solutions, would be deleterious to brain-injured patients due to possible progression of cerebral edema.[5] Problems with intragastric feeding due to delayed gastric emptying compounded the issue of early enteral feeding for many patients who required a decision either to start TPN or to starve the patient until adequate gastrointestinal (GI) function returned. Current practice has changed dramatically over the past decade so that aggressive early enteral or parenteral nutrition is a major consideration in the management of brain-injured patients.

ACUTE BRAIN INJURY

Trauma is the fourth leading cause of death in the United States in people under the age of 30.[6] Acute head injury accounts for approximately one fourth of all trauma deaths. These numbers have been increasing coincident with the rise in automobile-related injuries and an explosive increase in firearm-related injuries. The economic impact of this very special disease state involves not only the loss of productive work years in an often very young population, but also the direct cost of the care of these patients. Dramatic improvements in our intensive care capabilities have resulted in a reevaluation of many aspects of care and the acknowledgment that aggressive nutritional therapy plays an important role in the overall management of brain-injured patients.

Head injury is the result of extreme mechanical forces being transmitted to brain tissue. The rigid skull has a very sharp and irregular inner surface that often lacerates and bruises the brain after direct impact. Acute head trauma can be broadly categorized into concussion, contusion, skull fracture, epidural hematoma, subdural hematoma, subarachnoid hemorrhage, and intracerebral hemorrhage. Severely head-injured patients are usually treated in an intensive care unit (ICU), where immediate management focuses on stabilizing vital signs, reducing intracerebral pressure (ICP), and preventing further injury. Resultant cerebral edema and elevated intracerebral pressures can have a devastating effect on cardiorespiratory function and overall neurologic recovery.

Cerebral edema is believed to be the key factor leading to increased ICP pressure. Vasogenic edema results from damage to capillary endothelium with resultant leakage of protein-rich material into interstitial spaces and a rise in osmolality.[7] Free fluid follows into these highly osmotic areas and leads to the development of cerebral edema. Limited compartmental space within the fixed skull allows a substantial rise in intracranial pressure and compromise of local blood flow. Concurrent vasospasm may also accompany head injury, further compromising local blood flow.

Acute Management

Assessment of neurologic function is performed using the Glasgow Coma Scale (Table 16–1). This scale can often predict the severity of head injury and aid in assessing the patient's overall probable outcome. Further evaluation of extraocular movements, corneal and gag reflexes, and swallowing function will allow determination of brain stem injury. Direct intracerebral pressure monitoring permits rapid intervention to help prevent secondary brain injury related to high ICP.

Stabilization of respiratory and cardiovascular function is imperative. Facial injuries often impair attempts at maintaining a patent airway. Gag and cough reflexes are decreased, thus placing the patient at risk for aspiration of body secretions and blood. Mechanical ventilation is generally required, and hyperventilation can be employed to reduce the effect of CO_2 on intracranial pressure by an autoregulatory effect on cerebral blood flow.[8] Arterial blood pressure monitoring and Swan-Ganz catheter measurements of cardiac output and intravascular volume status may be required to prevent further cerebral hypoxia and secondary brain

TABLE 16–1   Glasgow Coma Scale

Eyes	Open	Spontaneously	4
		To verbal command	3
		To pain	2
		No response	1
Best motor response	To verbal	Obeys	6
	To pain	Localizes	5
		Flex—withdraw	4
		Flex—abnormal (decorticate)	3
		Extends-abnormal (decerebrate)	2
		No response	1
Best verbal response		Oriented and converses	5
		Disoriented and converses	4
		Inappropriate words	3
		Incomprehensible	2
		No response	1
		TOTAL	3–15*

* A score between 3–8 denotes a severe head injury.
From Bivins FA, Fath JJ: The patient with acute neurologic injury or disease. In Rombeau JL, Caldwell MD (eds): Clinical Nutrition: Enteral and Tube Feeding, 2nd edition. Philadelphia: WB Saunders, 1990.

damage associated with hypovolemia and hypotension.

Evaluation of intake and output allows assessment of adequate renal function and intravascular volume. Foley catheterization is required to monitor urine production directly and to avoid the devastating complications of either diabetes insipidus or the syndrome of inappropriate antidiuretic hormone (ADH) production. Dehydration and the use of osmotic diuretics, such as mannitol, are a standard approach in reducing intravascular volume in an attempt to reduce the effects of increased cerebral pressures.

Corticosteroids have been used in an attempt to stabilize vascular membranes. However, the evidence supporting their use in the acute brain-injured patient is controversial, and steroids may also increase infectious complications.[9,10]

Pentobarbital coma is used to reduce cerebral metabolism. It is considered a last resort to control the effects of cerebral edema. Some studies have shown a reduction in ICP with the use of a pentobarbital coma.[11] Overall total metabolic demands and resting energy expenditure are also reduced.[12]

Impaired physical activity requires specialized attention. Patients often require frequent repositioning to prevent skin breakdown and to mobilize secretions. Elevation of the head of the bed, use of a rotating bed, placement of antiembolic or pneumatic compression devices on the lower extremities, and implementation of range of motion exercises are critical components in preventing complications associated with immobility.

Acutely head-injured patients also have specialized nutritional needs. Data indicate that these patients often exhibit a marked increase in energy expenditure, increased protein catabolism, and weight loss.[13] Fluid accumulation and rapid volume shifts can make appropriate nutritional assessment difficult. Alterations in gut activity may make enteral nutrition difficult. Aggressive nutritional therapy and its impact on head-injured patients' outcomes remain a widely investigated topic.

Nutrition Assessment

Although a complete discussion of nutrition assessment is provided in Chapter 10, several important issues deserve mention in this population. Predicting a critically ill patient's nutritional needs is not a precise exercise; no single test is able to predict a patient's nutritional sta-

tus under all conditions. The acutely brain-injured patient is often unable to give a weight or diet history, making these data almost impossible to obtain. Fortunately, these patients are usually adequately nourished before their head injury. For those patients in whom a diet and weight history is imperative, such as a patient who appears malnourished or who has been hospitalized and inadequately fed for a prolonged time, this information may be available from family members or previous caregivers.

The complicated physiologic response associated with brain injury makes even the simplest determination of calorie and protein needs difficult, since the brain-injured patient is hypermetabolic.[14] This hypermetabolic response is sustained throughout the patient's injury. Interestingly, an inverse relationship exists between a patient's Glasgow Coma Scale and measured resting energy expenditure (MREE), implying that the severity of brain injury may affect the body's metabolic response.[15] Thus, overall caloric assessment is very important in guiding either parenteral or enteral therapy. The most commonly used formula for caloric determination is the Harris-Benedict equation, which was developed in the early 1900s as an estimate of calorie needs.[16] The Harris-Benedict equation has been shown to underestimate energy expenditure in up to 67 percent of critically ill patients.[17] Resting energy expenditure (REE) can also be measured by indirect calorimetry.[18] True caloric expenditure is calculated by multiplying the REE by an activity factor to arrive at a true resting energy expenditure. Makk and coworkers compared predictive resting energy formulas with indirect calorimetry in traumatic brain-injured patients and found that only 56 percent of the time could the predictive formulas estimate the measured values within ± 25 percent.[19] In addition, daily caloric needs were based on measured resting energy levels and allowed for a stable protein synthesis rate in a group of traumatic brain-injured patients. It was hypothesized that if caloric needs had been based on predictive values, protein synthesis would have been hampered.[19]

Estimation of nitrogen losses plays an important role in determining a patient's protein needs. Urinary nitrogen excretion in the critically ill is believed to result from mobilization of amino acids from muscle to meet increased protein demands. Studies in trauma patients have noted both an increase in protein synthesis and a much larger increase in protein catabolism.[20] Nitrogen losses of up to 30 g/day have been documented in acutely brain-injured patients. No studies have demonstrated a direct correlation between the severity of head injury and the amount of urinary nitrogen losses. However, the amount of nitrogen loss does correlate with serum levels of epinephrine, norepinephrine, and glucagon, all hormones associated with hypermetabolism.[21] More important, immobility may potentiate nitrogen losses. Steroid administration appears to have no significant impact on the degree of nitrogen loss.[22]

Plasma amino acid patterns have been studied in brain-injured patients. Large fluxes in alanine and glutamine were noted, demonstrating skeletal muscle protein release.[23] Branched-chain amino acid (BCAA) (leucine, isoleucine, valine) levels fell and phenylalanine levels rose, as seen in other traumatized patients.[24] The significance of these amino acid profile changes remains controversial.

Attempts at correcting nitrogen balance have had mixed results. High levels of nitrogen intake can reverse nitrogen losses. However, high nitrogen excretion is not reversed by increasing caloric intake alone.[25] Supplementation of BCAAs may retard nitrogen losses; their effect on patient outcome has not been studied.[24]

Biochemical markers of nutritional assessment have proved disappointing. Albumin is the most frequently abused marker of nutrition. Albumin production can be affected by multiple causes, especially interleukin-1 (IL-1) production, which downregulates albumin synthesis to produce acute-phase reactants preferentially in response to stressful stimuli.[26] Serum transferrin and prealbumin are also affected by the protein synthesis rate of the liver.

Global opinions about nutritional status of critically ill patients are not accurate. Only with a detailed review of the history and physical examination, current laboratory data, evaluation of calorie and protein needs, and a combination of available nutritional assessment parameters can the clinician obtain an overall assessment of the patient's nutritional status.

Nutrition Therapy in Acute Head Injury

Determining the appropriate route for nutrition support involves a number of important considerations. When the head injury is associated with other abdominal trauma, the use of the GI tract may be compromised. However, placement of a jejunostomy catheter during laparotomy is becoming more common and allows early enteral feeding, which may limit the progression to multiple organ failure.[27-31] For isolated head trauma, facial injuries and neck stability are important factors in guiding decisions regarding blind passage of oroenteric or nasoenteric tubes and endoscopic or radiologic options for enteral access. If it is unsafe to use the gut, then parenteral nutrition may be useful until safe enteral access can be achieved.

Enteral Nutrition

Enteral nutrition should be used as early as possible in the brain-injured patient's hospital course. Although it is often easier to use parenteral nutrition due to the simplicity of central venous access, many potential complications are associated with parenteral nutrition. After emergent surgery, trauma patients randomized to enteral nutrition had a significant reduction in both the complication rate and overall cost of therapy compared with parenteral nutrition. There were no differences in measured nutritional parameters.[28,31] It is important to provide fuel substrates to the intestinal absorptive surface to stimulate gut immune function and to prevent deterioration of intestinal integrity with resultant bacterial translocation and its potential for promoting sepsis.[32,33]

Feeding through the GI tract requires not only an appropriate access, but a functional GI tract. Gastric function is often abnormal in the critically ill patient. This may be secondary to cytokine influence and GI hypoxia.[34] Gastric function is also altered after severe head injury. Delayed gastric emptying has been noted in the acutely head-injured patient population to a degree similar to patients receiving a surgical vagotomy.[35] Clinically, intolerance to gastric feedings has been reported in up to 50 percent of brain-injured patients, resulting in reduced caloric delivery and a significant incidence of aspiration pneumonia.[36,37] This gastroparesis resulted in early studies reporting improved nutritional parameters with parenteral nutrition compared with enteral nutrition because of the prolonged period required to feed a patient successfully intragastrically.

More recently, interest has focused on postpyloric feeding in the critically ill patient. Critically ill patients randomized to jejunal feeding compared with gastric feedings received a greater number of calories and had improved nutritional parameters. Gastric-fed patients often had their tube feedings held because of high gastric residuals.[38] Recent prospective trials using jejunal tube (J-tube) feeding allowed full caloric delivery in approximately 4 days in a series of severely head-injured patients.[39,40]

Another potential benefit of jejunal feeding is the reduction in GI aspiration and its significant morbidity. Early studies evaluating aspiration pneumonia and enteral feeding did not clearly differentiate between orotracheal or GI aspiration.[41] Obviously, J-tube feeding would not be expected to affect the incidence of orotracheal aspiration. Improperly positioned small-bowel feeding tubes would also not be expected to reduce the risk of GI reflux and resultant GI aspiration. Recently, a prospective study placed methylene blue in all the enteral formulas instilled via a J-tube. Intermittent gastric decompression and orotracheal suctioning was performed monitoring for the presence of methylene blue and thus tube feeding reflux. In all patients whose small-bowel feeding tube was placed in the distal duodenum or in the proximal jejunum, there was no evidence of tube feeding reflux.[42] Thus, it appears that jejunal feeding may allow a more beneficial delivery of calories and protect against tube feeding reflux and aspiration in an at-risk brain-injured patient.

Techniques for Enteral Access

As previously mentioned, in acute brain-injured patients who receive their injury from trauma or accidents, a feeding jejunostomy may be most appropriate, especially if the initial surgical intervention includes a laparotomy.[27-31] In patients with isolated brain injury who have had stabilization of any cervical fractures, radiologic or endoscopic approaches are useful. However, the radiation exposure may not be negligible, especially if multiple tubes are placed, and thus this risk of fluoroscopically guided feeding tubes should be carefully weighed in pediatric populations.[43] Tube placement should be in the distal duodenum or jejunum, preferably using a dual-lumen system that allows for early identification of duodenogastric reflux. This should help limit tube-feeding-related aspiration and provides for gastric decompression if the patient requires mechanical ventilation.[39,40,44]

Oroenteric and Nasoenteric Tubes

Orogastric tubes are used if trauma to the facial area proscribes nasal tube passage. These tubes are tolerated only in patients with an absent gag reflex or depressed levels of consciousness. Use of this route is almost unique to the head-injured population.

A nasoenteric tube (NET) is one that passes through the nasal passage into or beyond the stomach. In general, these are short-term feeding devices because they may cause local nasal irritation, epistaxis, and sinusitis if used long term. Nasoduodenal and nasojejunal feeding tubes are generally smaller than nasogastric tubes; they cause less discomfort but have a higher risk of tube clogging. Although NETs can be passed at the bedside, poor positioning often requires either fluoroscopic or endoscopic guidance.[45] Combination nasogastric/jejunal tubes are available to allow concurrent jejunal tube feeding and gastric decompression.[46] These tubes have a unique over-the-guidewire endoscopic placement technique that has resulted in a 95 percent successful placement rate in under 15 minutes at our center. The major problem limiting nasogastric feeding is the risk of pulmonary aspiration from gastroesophageal reflux of tube feeding with or without delay in gastric emptying, which occurs in a high percentage of acutely head-injured patients. Elevation of the head of the bed has been shown to be useful in reducing, but not eliminating, reflux episodes.[47,48] Unfortunately, in this population these patients must often be kept flat, and the importance of a nasogastric tube or some form of gastric depression cannot be minimized, since most of these acutely ill patients are initially dependent on mechanical ventilation.

Percutaneous Gastrostomy or Gastrojejunostomy

Percutaneously placed gastric tubes and gastrojejunostomy tubes may be inserted either endoscopically (PEG and PEG/J) at the bedside or fluoroscopically in brain-injured patients who may require long-term enteral access. A PEG tube allows direct access to the stomach for feeding or decompression. A PEG/J tube system provides both gastric and jejunal access. A jejunal tube (J-tube) is threaded through the gastric tube (G-tube) into the small bowel. This system allows concurrent feeding into the small bowel through the J-tube and decompression of the stomach through the G-tube. Prospective studies have reported a complication rate of < 5 percent with PEG tube placement in the acutely brain-injured patient in an intensive care setting.[40,42] If the patient recovers, this type of access can be removed endoscopically or percutaneously depending on the type of tube initially placed.

Surgical Options

If it is not placed directly after the initial injury, surgical tube placement continues to remain an option. If endoscopic or fluoroscopic attempts are proscribed or unsuccessful, surgeons at our center often place a gastrojejunostomy apparatus similar to our endoscopic PEG/J tube. This allows gastric suction, jejunal feeding, and easy endoscopic or percutaneous removal, depending on the type of tube, with rapid wound closure. Nasogastric tube use with a standard surgical jejunostomy is also an option and used at many trauma centers. Local expertise and a team approach to enteral access is most beneficial to provide the patient with effective, early enteral nutrition.

Parenteral Nutrition

The absence of a functioning GI tract is an indication for TPN. Central venous access is required to deliver a hyperosmolar solution adequately. The mechanics of providing TPN will not be reviewed here, but once-held fears concerning TPN in the head-injured population appear unfounded.[4] As previously mentioned, a new emphasis on the early enteral feeding of critically ill patients has emerged in the last decade, placing TPN in a more supportive role if one of the following is a factor: enteral therapy is unsafe, enteral access is unobtainable, or TPN may serve as a bridge until full caloric needs are met by the enteral route.

Complications with TPN are well recognized, and the risk of hypophosphatemia, hyperphosphatemia, hypomagnesemia, hypermagnesemia, hypokalemia, hyperkalemia, and hyperglycemia may be increased by the fluid and electrolyte abnormalities commonly seen in the brain-injured patient. Hyperglycemia is a stress response to trauma; increased counterregulatory hormone and cytokine levels are believed to be the etiology.[49] It is most common within the first 24 hours after head injury and correlates to its degree. It may complicate the overall outcome by further damaging brain cells.[50,51] Glucose infused at greater than 7 mg/kg/minute is not oxidized and is synthesized into fat, an energy-consuming process. Severe hepatic steatosis may be a resultant consequence. Thus, aggressive monitoring of serum glucose levels must be performed with the institution of TPN therapy.

The component mixture of TPN should include amino acids, fats, and carbohydrates. The use of a fat-poor TPN solution in critically ill patients may result in negative nitrogen balance even if enough nonprotein calories are provided.[52]

Early animal investigations suggested that the administration of a hyperosmolar solution, such as TPN, to severely brain-injured patients could increase cerebral edema.[53] It was postulated that serum hyperosmolarity from infusion of TPN would initially promote water movement from normal brain tissue to blood. This normal brain tissue would thus be at risk for subsequent rapid water infusion from adjacent areas of injured, edematous brain tissue. However, a recent randomized study of severely brain-injured patients to either TPN or enteral nutrition noted no differences between the groups in measured mean intracranial pressure.[54] Serum glucose levels were carefully monitored and aggressively maintained below 200 mg/dl.

The use of TPN in the brain-injured patient remains an important component of nutritional therapy. Careful monitoring of this invasive therapy and conversion to enteral nutrition at the earliest opportunity are vital to its appropriate use.

Nutritional Goals in Acute Head Injury

As previously reviewed, it may be difficult to assess caloric needs accurately. One standard approach has been to provide 1.4 to 1.5 times the calories estimated by the REE.[55] However, differences in patient movement and other factors may produce large errors by these estimates. The use of metabolic carts may be more accurate and can be performed on subsequent or even sequential days to permit day-to-day adjustments in the nutritional prescription based on the patient's actual clinical course.

In this population, setting a goal to achieve positive nitrogen balance may be unrealistic. Because of this group's hypermetabolism, protein synthesis, turnover, and excretion are all increased. Aggressive nutrition support must be careful not to cause hyperglycemia, which can have many adverse effects. The lack of correlation between caloric intake and nitrogen excretion in severe head injury has been well documented.[56] Many centers will aim for protein intake between 1.5 to 2.2 g/kg/day to attempt to spare protein excretion or even achieve positive protein balance in some patients.[56]

Monitoring should stress maintenance of glycemic control, appropriate volume administration, and careful evaluation of renal function. More research is needed to assist the clinician in determining optimal caloric determination, composition of the nutrient formula, and patient outcome.

Nutritional Outcome in Acute Head Injury

Evaluating the nutritional impact on any disease state is difficult because of the multitude of factors potentially affecting the overall outcome. However, there have been some important studies detailing the importance of adequate nutrition in the severely brain-injured patient. Early prospective studies comparing parenteral nutrition to enteral nutrition in the brain-injured patients demonstrated a greater delivery of calories in the parenteral group, probably secondary to ineffective enteral access techniques. When better fed, these same parenteral patients had fewer deaths and a greater improvement in their Glasgow Coma Scale score than did the poorer-fed enteral patients.[4,57] These studies have not been repeated with today's more aggressive and successful enteral access devices and feeding techniques. Another retrospective study has also demonstrated a direct correlation between calorie deficit and overall outcome.[58] Aggressive, comprehensive management of the severely head-injured patient is critical to overall survival and outcome. Improvement in ICUs and patient care has resulted in improved survival. Nutritional therapy is well recognized as an essential component of this multidisciplinary management. More outcome data are needed in this rapidly changing field.

CHRONIC NEUROLOGIC DISEASES

Many neurologic diseases can affect a patient's ability to feed independently. Depressed levels of consciousness are associated with a decreased ability to protect the airway from episodes of gastroesophageal reflux, vomiting, and even oropharyngeal secretions. Morbidity and mortality from aspiration pneumonia can be significant in this population. Some diseases may disturb the neural or muscular coordination required for successful swallowing, while others may alter gastric or intestinal motility. A review of the signs and symptoms of these disorders can lead to a better understanding of rehabilitation techniques, when possible, and alternative access routes when function is unlikely to return or expected to be significantly delayed.

Dysphagia

Careful evaluation of the swallowing reflex is important in guiding decisions regarding eating orally or using a variety of techniques involving enteral access. A careful history is key to dividing dysphagia into two broad groups: esophageal dysphagia and oropharyngeal (or transfer) dysphagia.[59,60]

Esophageal dysphagia refers to difficulty with a food bolus after successful passage from pharynx to esophagus. There may be intermittent mechanical obstruction to solid food, which suggests an esophageal ring or web or progressive difficulty with solids and then liquids. The latter scenario suggests more intrinsic disease of the esophagus, which may be from a peptic stricture or carcinoma. When a patient describes difficulty with either solids or liquids, even water, it is usually due to a primary neuromuscular or motility disorder. Examples of these disorders include the following: diffuse esophageal spasm, achalasia, and scleroderma. There are other causes of esophageal dysphagia; however, a complete discussion is beyond the scope and intent of this chapter.[60]

Oropharyngeal dysphagia is difficulty swallowing due to a lesion above or proximal to the esophagus. The patient complains of difficulty moving a food bolus into the pharynx and esophagus to initiate the involuntary swallowing reflex. Swallowing is a combination of integrated neural and muscular actions coordinated in the brain stem. Any process that alters the afferent or efferent nerves (the fifth, seventh, ninth, and twelfth cranial nerves) or the brain stem swallowing center can cause oropharyngeal dysphagia. The patient may describe nasal regurgitation, dysarthria, nasal speech from muscular weakness, or coughing during swallowing. Liquids present more difficulty with this disorder than with esophageal dysphagia, in which liquids pass easily until the patient is almost totally obstructed. Table 16–2 lists the diseases associated with oropharyngeal dysphagia, concentrating on neurologic mechanisms.

Dysphagia Evaluation

Table 16–3 lists the tests useful in diagnosing the etiology of the dysphagia. If the diagnosis is obvious, as with a cerebrovascular accident (CVA), then the key issues are how severe is the swallowing deficit and if there is pulmonary aspiration. In this instance, the most important test becomes the modified barium swallow using videofluoroscopy, which is often done by a radiologist and speech therapist.[61] This technique closely examines the initial swallowing mechanisms that lead to a

TABLE 16–2   Conditions Causing Oropharyngeal Dysphagia

Neuromuscular Diseases
Central nervous system (CNS)
   Cerebral vascular accident (brain stem or
      pseudobulbar palsy)
   Cerebral palsy
   Parkinson's disease
   Wilson's disease
   Multiple sclerosis
   Amyotrophic lateral sclerosis
   Brain stem tumors
   Tabes dorsalis
   Miscellaneous congenital and degenerative
      disorders of CNS
   Tardive dyskinesia (usually irreversible and
      drug related—phenothiazines and
      metoclopramide)
   Dystonia (usually reversible and drug related—
      antihistamines and nitrazepam)
Peripheral nervous system
   Bulbar poliomyelitis
   Peripheral neuropathies (diphtheria, botulism,
      rabies, diabetes mellitus)
Motor end plate
   Myasthenia gravis
Muscle
   Muscular dystrophies
   Primary myositis
   Metabolic myopathy (thyrotoxicosis, myxedema,
      steroid myopathy)
   Dermatomyositis
   Amyloidosis
   Systemic lupus erythematosis

Abnormal Upper Esophageal Sphincter (UES)
Relaxation
Incomplete relaxation (cricopharyngeal achalasia):
   CNS lymphoma, oculopharyngeal muscular
   dystrophy
Decreased cricopharyngeal compliance:
   Hypopharyngeal (Zenker's diverticulum),
   cricopharyngeal bar
Delayed UES relaxation: familial dysautonomia
   (Riley-Day syndrome)

Local Structural Lesions
Inflammatory (pharyngitis, abscess, tuberculosis,
   syphilis)
Neoplastic
Congenital webs
Plummer-Vinson syndrome
Extrinsic compression (thyromegaly, cervical spine
   hyperostosis, lymphadenopathy)
Primary head and neck tumors
Surgical resection of the oropharynx
Xerostomia (drugs, autoimmune diseases, radiation
   therapy)

Adapted from Castell DO, Donner MW: Evaluation of dysphagia: a careful history is crucial. Dysphagia 1987;2:68. With permission.

TABLE 16–3   Diagnostic Tools in Dysphagia Evaluation

Careful history
Physical examination (especially neurologic
   examination)
Barium swallow
Modified barium swallow (videofluoroscopy)
Esophageal manometry
Esophageal pH monitoring
Endoscopic evaluation (hypopharynx or
   esophageal)

liquid or solid bolus passing into the upper esophagus and also evaluates the risk of aspiration. Aspiration is the entry of material below the true vocal cords. Identification of aspiration is important because many dysphagic patients may have silent episodes of aspiration without external signs of food or liquid entering the pulmonary tree.[62] If liquids present an aspiration risk, then different food consistencies are also examined to see if any consistency of food is safe. Some patients will be able to swallow more viscous or solid materials safely, and this will have further importance when trying to rehabilitate patients.[63,64] Aspiration risk-reduction diets have been developed and help maximize patient intake while minimizing risk.[65]

Gastrointestinal Motility

Disorders of GI motility can involve primarily the stomach, as in gastroparesis, or be more pervasive and affect any or all areas of the GI tract. Acutely brain-injured patients may exhibit more difficulty with gastroparesis, usually short term, while more chronic patients may have underlying disorders that affect them on a more global basis.

Gastroparesis

Gastroparesis results from impaired contractile capacity of the stomach, which leads to defective gastric emptying. There are many causes of gastroparesis, which can be categorized as primary and secondary GI disorders.[66] Primary disorders include idiopathic forms of gastroparesis where there is no evidence of systemic disease. These disorders comprise one third of the cases and will not be discussed further. Neurologic patients may exhibit secondary disorders with which there is an underlying abnormality in either the smooth muscle or the enteric nervous system or both. The resulting disorder may clinically manifest as gastroparesis or with diffuse defects in GI motility, which occurs more often.

Acutely, gastric antral and duodenal contractions in rabbits are inhibited with increased intracranial pressure.[67] In man, tolerance to gastric feeding is less than 50 percent in acutely brain-injured patients.[68-72] As has been reported with intracranial lesions, the etiology may be from a similar mechanism where elevated intracranial pressure stimulates and compresses the emetic center of the floor of the fourth ventricle.[73] In addition, patients with high spinal cord transections (above T5) may experience delayed gastric emptying.[74]

The actual impact of delayed gastric function or gastroparesis in neurologic diseases is unknown and may be underdiagnosed. Gastric hypomotility has been noted in Duchenne's muscular dystrophy and appears to be a defect in the smooth muscle. These patients usually have bloating, acute gastric dilatation, or intestinal pseudo-obstruction, which can be fatal; therefore, any of these signs or symptoms may warrant an evaluation for gastroparesis.[75-78] Table 16–4 lists neurologic diseases associated with GI motility disorders, and Table 16–5 lists the drugs that can inhibit gastric motility.

Gastrointestinal Motility Evaluation and Treatment

Evaluation of gastroparesis should first exclude an ulcerative, inflammatory or neoplastic process of the stomach and duodenum. This can be accomplished by upper GI endoscopy but may also require an upper GI barium study, which examines the small bowel to exclude a partial obstruction. Also to be considered are

TABLE 16–5   Drugs that Inhibit Gastrointestinal Motility

Anticholinergics
Apomorphine
β-agonists
Bromocriptine
Clonidine (α_2-adrenergic agonists)
Levodopa (and related antiparkinsonian medications)
Opioids
Progesterone
Tricyclic antidepressants

medications and metabolic conditions, especially hypercalcemia.

The gold standard for quantitative evaluation of gastric emptying is radioscintigraphic measurement. This method permits labeling of solid or liquid phases of gastric emptying and allows for measurement of transfer of the radiolabeled phases to different regions of the stomach. It is important to make sure that normal values for a given laboratory are available, since there is variability in the meals and individual protocols used.

Other methods to investigate gastroparesis such as gastric impedance, ultrasonography, and applied potential tomography are available only at a few centers. For evaluating more diffuse disorders of GI motility, manometric evaluation of the stomach and small bowel is becoming more widely available. More in-depth discussion of this area is beyond the scope of this chapter.

Currently available medications that can improve gastric emptying include metoclopramide, cisapride, and erythromycin. Domperidone may be approved for use in the United States soon, and opiate antagonists, cholecystokinin (CCK) antagonists, and gonadotropin-releasing hormone (GnRH) are currently under investigation.[79] The use of these drugs in the acutely brain-injured patient has not been well studied, and some concerns exist about the use of metoclopramide, since it crosses the blood-brain barrier and is associated with many neurologic side-effects. The other listed medications have rare CNS side-effects and deserve further investigation in this population.

Enteral Feeding Considerations for Chronic Neurologic Patients

What follows are the enteral nutrition issues for more chronic neurologic diseases.

TABLE 16–4   Neurologic Diseases Associated with Gastrointestinal Motility Disorders

Diabetic neuropathy and diabetic gastroparesis
    syndrome
Idiopathic orthostatic hypotension
Intracranial lesions
Intrinsic myopathies and neuropathies
    Dystrophia myotonica
    Familial gut myopathies and neuropathies
    Progressive muscular dystrophy
Labyrinthine vertigo
Migraine headaches
Shy-Drager syndrome
Traumatic lesions of the spinal cord (above T5)

1. What is the patient's level of consciousness?
2. Can the patient protect the airway from episodes of gastroesophageal reflux?
3. What is the patient's ability to swallow liquids, thickened liquids, and soft and solid foods?
4. Is the patient at high risk for aspirating oropharyngeal secretions?
5. Will the need for enteral access be short term or long term?
6. Is there a difference between gastric and jejunal feeding in this population?

Level of Consciousness

The ethics of providing prolonged nutrition support for patients in a persistent vegetative state will not be debated here.[80-82] Many patients with depressed levels of consciousness tolerate intragastric feedings well. However, if patients are fed by nasoenteric tubes, the protective barriers to gastroesophageal reflux are compromised.[83] Recent studies show that elevation of the head of the bed has been found to show a marked decrease, but not elimination, of reflux episodes in patients receiving mechanical ventilation.[47,48] Feeding gastrostomies preserve the natural anatomic barriers. However, Park and colleagues compared NET tubes with PEGs in patients with persistent neurologic dysphagia and found no significant difference in episodes of aspiration.[84] The PEG patients received more of their prescribed tube feeding; however, they concluded that for patients who were tolerating NET feedings well, it was not necessary to switch to PEG feedings. Monitoring of patients with depressed consciousness should include examining for abdominal distention, checking for high gastric residuals when they are fed intragastrically, and maintaining elevation of the head of the bed when clinically possible.

Gastroesophageal Reflux

Patients who exhibit multiple episodes of aspiration pneumonia should have gastroesophageal reflux investigated as an etiology; esophageal manometry, pH monitoring, and radionuclide tests may be helpful in this assessment. A recent study evaluated scintigraphy immediately before and 1 week after percutaneous gastrostomy (PG) placement.[85] Evidence of reflux on either examination led to conversion to percutaneous gastrojejunostomy. They concluded that PG did not induce reflux and that scintigraphy was useful in selecting patients who can safely be fed by PG.

Esophagogastroduodenoscopy (upper GI endoscopy) may show other signs of gastroesophageal reflux, mostly complications such as esophagitis, erosions, ulcers, strictures, Barrett's esophagus, and intrinsic masses. Options for patients with severe gastroesophageal reflux are as follows: medications to improve gastric emptying and increase lower esophageal pressure (e.g., metoclopramide and cisapride), feeding into the small bowel rather than the stomach, or performing surgical procedures to limit reflux. Albanese and coworkers retrospectively compared Nissen fundoplication with gastrostomy tube placement with fluoroscopically guided gastrojejunostomy in neurologically impaired children.[86] The nonoperative approach was found to have fewer major complications requiring reoperation. Long-term comparisons of radiologic or endoscopic placement of small-bowel tubes with standard operative jejunostomies are needed.

Swallowing Function

After adequate evaluation of the patient's swallowing function, a treatment plan can be developed.[62-64,87,88] The prognosis of the underlying disease must also be considered. Some patients with CVAs may recover some or all of their swallowing function; thus, a NET or gastrostomy may provide a temporary bridge until recovery. Some patients may have difficulty only with liquids and may benefit from thickening agents with or without additional enteral access to provide hydration or medications. Many PEG tubes now allow for removal without repeated endoscopy and thereby can provide a type of "temporary" access. Patients who have neurologic diseases in which the decline in swallowing function is progressive should be considered for more permanent enteral access options as appropriate to their global treatment plan.

Aspiration of Oropharyngeal Secretions

Aspiration is an important but often misunderstood complication of enteral feeding. Criteria for aspiration in much of the literature are poorly defined, leading to confusion between aspiration of oropharyngeal secretions and stomach contents including enteral alimentation.[41,89,90] This confusion in the literature is part of the reason that the risk of aspiration pneumonia varies from 2 to 95 percent. Few data are available to judge the actual risk of oropharyngeal aspiration of secretions and subsequent aspiration pneumonia in neurologic diseases. Huxley and associates have demonstrated pharyngeal aspiration in humans using indium 111 chloride in 10 patients with depressed consciousness and 20 controls.[91] They showed that 70 percent of the patients and 45 percent of the controls aspirated pharyngeal secretions. Unfortunately, the relationship between this and the development of aspiration pneumonia is not fully understood, but it may occur when normal pulmonary defense mechanisms are either overwhelmed or impaired and the aspirated bacteria can multiply rapidly.[91] In addition, one case report demonstrated that oral aspiration was the etiology of recurrent pneumonias in an infant being fed with a PEG by using a radionuclide salivagram.[92] Once documented, the only way to eliminate oropharyngeal aspiration totally as a cause of recurrent aspiration pneumonia is to perform a tracheostomy and to close the vocal cords surgically. For patients who still can speak, this may not be an attractive solution.

Short- vs Long-Term Access

In choosing between access options in neurologic patients, the clinician should estimate how long access will be needed. Some conditions are difficult to estimate, such as CVAs or acute brain injury. For less than 30 days, nasoenteric options are generally preferred unless contraindications or special circumstances obviate this route.[93] For longer periods, gastrostomies or jejunostomies are preferred and may reduce the risk of aspiration. Monitoring of these patients should include careful assessment of actual tube feeding delivered compared with amounts prescribed so that underfeeding does not occur.[84,94] Local expertise will help direct whether radiologic, endoscopic, or surgical options are used.[93]

Gastric vs Jejunal Feeding

Gastric feeding is very common due to its convenience and ease of feeding. Nasogastric tubes or gastrostomies are common in America and are preferred if there is good patient tolerance of intragastric feeding. In neurologic diseases, one of the main indications for a jejunostomy is gastroesophageal reflux disease or other GI problems leading to aspiration of feedings, not oropharyngeal secretions that in turn may lead to recurrent aspiration pneumonia. Other indications for a jejunostomy include gastroparesis, insufficient stomach from previous resection, and postoperative feeding during major surgical procedures.[93] Jejunostomy feeding is very effective in patients with documented feeding aspiration; however, more data are needed

to document the risks and benefits of long-term enteral access through jejunostomy.[93,95] A more in-depth review of jejunostomy feeding is provided elsewhere in this book (Chapter 14).

CONCLUSION

The past decade has seen a dramatic shift in the nutritional care of the patient with neurologic diseases, especially the acutely brain-injured patient. Initial fears of the safety of parenteral nutrition have been allayed and replaced with a new sense of urgency for early enteral feeding. Nutrition support can now begin on the day of admission with parenteral, enteral, or a combination of both therapies until the enteral route can supply all the patient's needs. New enteral access devices have been created for this population and have been shown to allow enteral feeding soon after admission, if surgical jejunostomy has not already been placed during a laparotomy. Repeated tolerance trials to gastric feeding can now be avoided with these newer options so that effective enteral support can be started early.

For more chronic neurologic diseases, many enteral access options are now available and can be individualized to meet the patient's needs. Patients with recurrent aspiration pneumonias should have an evaluation to determine whether oropharyngeal secretions or intragastric contents are the etiology. Therapy can then be directed toward treating the underlying etiology and not simply performing a jejunostomy when it may not benefit the patient.

The diversity of neurologic diseases has hampered some of the research in this area; however, advancements made in the past decade are likely to improve patient care and outcome. Aggressive, early nutrition support in the acutely brain-injured patient can make the rehabilitation process easier if malnutrition is also not a major recovery issue. Patients with more chronic neurologic diseases can have slow but progressive deterioration in the ability to feed independently and swallow safely. More options are available to the patient and clinician to allow the patient more choices in the final months or years. More research is needed to help guide patients and clinicians in the optimal care of patients with these devastating diseases.

REFERENCES

1. Steffee WP: Malnutrition in hospitalized patients. JAMA 1980;244:2630–2635.
2. Drew JH, Koop CE, Grigger RP: A nutritional study of neurosurgical patients. J Neurosurg 1947;4:7–15.

3. Haider W, Lackner F, Schlick W et al: Metabolic changes in the course of severe brain damage. Eur J Int Care Med 1975;1:19–26.

4. Rapp RP, Young AB, Twyman DL et al: The favorable effect of early parenteral feeding on survival in head-injured patients. J Neurosurg 1983;58:906–912.

5. White RJ: Aspects and problems of total parenteral alimentation in the neurosurgery patient. In Manni C, Magalini SI, Scrascia E (eds): Total Parenteral Alimentation. Amsterdam: Excerpta Medica, 1976:208–214.

6. Kalsbeck W, McLaurin R, Harris B et al: The national head and spine injury survey: major findings. J Neurosurg 1980;53:519–531.

7. Ruelen HJ: Vasogenic brain edema. Br J Anaesth 1976; 48:741–752.

8. Ruelen HJ, Graham R, Spatz M et al: Role of pressure gradients and bulk flow in dynamics of vasogenic brain edema. J Neurosurg 1981;8:754–764.

9. Swain K: Management of severe head injury. In Ropper A, Kennedy S, Zervas N (eds): Neurological and Neurosurgical Intensive Care. Baltimore: University Park Press, 1983:131–152.

10. Deutschman CS, Konstantinides FN, Raup S et al: The metabolic and physiologic response to isolated closed-head injury. The effects of steroids on metabolism. Potentiation of protein wasting and abnormalities of substrate utilization. J Neurosurg 1987;66:388–395.

11. Cooper PR, Moody S, Clark WK et al: Dexamethasone and severe head injury: a prospective double-blind study. J Neurosurg 1979;51:307–316.

12. Dempsey DT, Gunter P, Mullen LJ et al: Energy expenditure in acute trauma to the head with and without barbiturate therapy. Surg Gynecol Obstet 1985;150: 128–134.

13. Young B, Ott L, Haack E et al: Effect of total parenteral nutrition upon intracranial pressure in severe head injury. J Neurosurg 1987;67:76–80.

14. Young B, Ott L, Norton J et al: Metabolic and nutritional sequelae in the non-steroid treated head injury patient. Neurosurgery 1985;17:784–791.

15. Clifton GL, Robertson CS, Grossman RG et al: The metabolic response to head injury. J Neurosurg 1986; 60:89–98.

16. Harris JA, Benedict FG: A biometric study of basal metabolism in man, pub. no. 279. Washington DC: Carnegie Institution of Washington, 1919.

17. Robertson CS, Clifton GL, Grossman RG: Oxygen utilization and cardiovascular function in head-injured patients. J Neurosurg 1984;63:714–718.

18. Weir JB de V: New methods for calculating metabolic rate with special reference to protein metabolism. J Physiol 1949;109:1–9.

19. Makk LJK, McClave SJ, Creech PW et al: Clinical application of the metabolic cart to the delivery of parenteral nutrition. Crit Care Med 1987;13:818–829.

20. Sunderland PM, Heilbrun MP: Estimating energy expenditure in traumatic brain injury: comparison of indirect calorimetry with predictive formulas. Neurosurgery 1992;31:246–253.

21. Birkhahn RH, Long CL, Fitkin D et al: Effects of major skeletal trauma on whole body protein. Surgery 1980;88:294–300.

22. Chiolero R, Schultz Y, Lemerchand T et al: Hormonal and metabolic changes following severe head injury and noncranial injury. J Parenter Enter Nutr 1992;13: 5–12.

23. Zagara G, Scaravilli P, Bellucci CM et al: Effect of dexamethasone on nitrogen metabolism in brain-injured patients. J Neurosurg Sci 1987;31:207–212.

24. Young B, Ott L, Yingling B et al: Nutrition and brain injury. J Neurotrauma 1992;9(suppl 1):S375–383.

25. Ott L, Schmidt J, Young B et al: Comparison administration of two standard intravenous amino acid formulas to severely brain-injured patients. Drug Intell Clin Pharm 1988;22:763–768.

26. Sganga G, Siegel JH, Brown G et al: Reprioritization of hepatic plasma release in trauma and sepsis. Arch Surg 1985;120:187–199.

27. Moore EE, Jones TN: Benefits of immediate jejunostomy feeding after major abdominal trauma: a prospective, randomized study. J Trauma 1986;26: 874–880.

28. Adams S, Dellinger EP, Wertz MJ et al: Enteral versus parenteral nutritional support following laparotomy for trauma: a randomized prospective trial. J Trauma 1986;26:883–890.

29. Moore FA, Moore EE, Jones TN et al: TEN versus TPN following major abdominal trauma: reduced septic morbidity. J Trauma 1989;29:916–922.

30. Kudsk KA, Croce MA, Fabian TC et al: Enteral versus parenteral feeding: effects on septic morbidity after blunt and penetrating abdominal trauma. Ann Surg 1992;215:503–511.

31. Moore FA, Feliciano DV, Andrassy RJ et al: Early enteral feeding, compared with parenteral, reduces postoperative septic complications: the results of a meta-analysis. Ann Surg 1992;216:172–183.

32. Alverdy J, Chi HS, Sheldon GF: The effect of parenteral nutrition on gastrointestinal immunity: the importance of enteral stimulation. Ann Surg 1985;202: 681–684.

33. Deitch EA, Winterton J, Li M et al: The gut as a portal of entry for bacteremia: role of protein malnutrition. Ann Surg 1987;205:681–692.

34. Szabo JS, Stonestreet BS, Oh W: Effects of hypoxemia on gastrointestinal blood flow and gastric emptying in the newborn piglet. Pediatr Res 1985;19:466–471.

35. Ott L, Phillips R, McClain CJ et al: Intolerance to enteral feedings in the brain injured patient. J Neurosurg 1988;68:62–66.

36. Clifton GL, Robertson CS, Contant CF: Enteral hyperalimentation in head injury. J Neurosurg 1985;62: 186–193.

37. Norton JA, Ott LG, McClain C et al: Intolerance to enteral feeding in the brain-injured patient. J Neurosurg 1988;68:62–66.

38. Montecalvo MAS, Steger K, Farber HW et al: Nutritional outcome and pneumonia in critical care patients randomized to gastric versus jejunal tube feedings. Crit Care Med 1992;20:1377–1387.

39. Kirby DF, Clifton GL, Turner H et al: Early enteral nutrition after brain injury by percutaneous endoscopic gastrojejunostomy. J Parenter Enter Nutr 1991;15:298–302.

40. Duckworth PF Jr, Kirby DF, McHenry L Jr. et al: Percutaneous endoscopic gastrojejunostomy (PEG/J) made easy: a new over-the-wire technique. Gastrointest Endosc 1994;40:350–353.

41. Cataldi-Betcher EL, Seltzer MH, Slocum BA et al: Complications occurring during enteral nutrition support: a prospective study. J Parenter Enter Nutr 1983;7: 546–552.

42. DeLegge MH, Duckworth PF Jr, McHenry L Jr et al: Percutaneous endoscopic gastrojejunostomy: a dual center safety and efficacy trial. J Parenter Enter Nutr 1995;19:239–243.

43. Pobiel RS, Bisset GS III, Pobiel MS: Nasojejunal feeding tube placement in children: four-year cumulative experience. Radiology 1994;190:127–129.

44. Baskin WN: Advances in enteral nutrition techniques. Am J Gastroenterol 1992;87:1547–1553.

45. Ugo PJ, Mohler PA, Wilson GL: Bedside postpyloric placement of weighted feeding tubes. Nutr Clin Pract 1992;7:284–287.

46. Baskin WN, Johanson JF: A novel approach to enteral nutrition in the ICU. Gastrointest Endosc 1992;38:272. Abstract.

47. Torres A, Serra-Battles J, Ros E et al: Pulmonary aspiration of gastric contents in patients receiving mechanical ventilation: the effect of body position. Ann Intern Med 1992;116:540–543.

48. Ibañez J, Penafiel A, Raurich JM et al: Gastroesophageal reflux in intubated patients receiving enteral nutrition: effect of supine and semirecumbent positions. J Parenter Enter Nutr 1992;16:419–422.

49. Fong Y, Moldawer LL, Shires T et al: The biologic characteristics of cytokines and their implication in surgical injury. Surg Gynecol Obstet 1990;170:363–378.

50. Young B, Ott L, Beard D et al: Relationship between admission hyperglycemia and neurologic outcome of severe brain-injured patients. Ann Surg 1989;210:466–473.

51. Desalles AA, Kontos HA, Becker DP et al: Prognostic significance of ventricular CSF lactic acidosis in severe head injury. J Neurosurg 1986;65:615–624.

52. Long JM, Wilmore DW, Mason AD et al: Effect of carbohydrate and fat intake on nitrogen excretion during total intravenous feeding. Ann Surg 1977;185:417–422.

53. Waters DC, Hoff JT, Black KL: Effect of parenteral nutrition on cold-induced vasogenic edema in cats. J Neurosurg 1986;64:460–465.

54. Young B, Ott L, Haack D et al: Effect of total parenteral nutrition upon intracranial pressure in severe head injury. J Neurosurg 1987;67:76–80.

55. Phillips R, Ott L, Young B et al: Nutritional support and measured energy expenditure of the child and adolescent with head injury. J Neurosurg 1987;67:846–851.

56. Bivins BA, Twyman DL, Young AB: Failure of nonprotein calories to mediate protein conservation in brain-injured patients. J Trauma 1986;26:980–986.

57. Young B, Ott L, Twyman D et al: The effect of nutritional support on outcome from severe head injury. J Neurosurg 1987;67:668–676.

58. Waters DC, Dechert R, Bartlett R: Metabolic studies in head injury patients: a preliminary report. Surgery 1986;100:531–534.

59. Hendrix TR: Art and science of history taking in the patient with difficulty swallowing. Dysphagia 1993;8:69–73.

60. Castell DO, Donner MW: Evaluation of dysphagia: a careful history is crucial. Dysphagia 1987;2:65–71.

61. Logemann JA: Manual for the Videofluorographic Study of Swallowing, 2nd edition. Austin, TX: Pro-Ed, 1993.

62. Horner J, Massey EW: Silent aspiration following stroke. Neurology 1988;38:317–319.

63. Buchholz DW, Bosma JF, Donner MW: Adaptation, compensation, and decompensation of the pharyngeal swallow. Gastrointest Radiol 1985;10:235–239.

64. Logemann JA: Treatment for aspiration related to dysphagia: an overview. Dysphagia 1986;1:34–38.

65. Curran J, Groher ME: Development and dissemination of an aspiration risk reduction diet. Dysphagia 1990;5:6–12.

66. Malagelada J-R, Azpiroz F, Mearin F: Gastrointestinal motor function in health and disease. In Sleisenger MH, Fordtran JS (eds): Gastrointestinal Disease: Pathophysiology/Diagnosis/Management, 5th edition, vol I. Philadelphia: WB Saunders Co, 1993:486–508.

67. Garrick T, Mulvihill S, Buack S et al: Intracerebroventricular pressure inhibits gastric antral and duodenal contractility but not acid secretion in conscious rabbits. Gastroenterology 1988;95:26–31.

68. Clifton GL, Robertson CS, Contant CF: Enteral hyperalimentation in head injury. J Neurosurg 1985;62:186–193.

69. Hunt D, Rowlands B, Allen S: The inadequacy of enteral nutritional support in head injury patients during the early post-injured period. J Parenter Enter Nutr 1985;9:121. Abstract.

70. Twyman D, Young B, Ott L et al: High protein enteral feedings: a means of achieving positive nitrogen balance in head-injured patients. J Parenter Enter Nutr 1985;9:679–684.

71. Norton JA, Ott LG, McClain C et al: Intolerance to enteral feeding in the brain-injured patient. J Neurosurg 1988;68:62–66.

72. Ott L, Young B, Phillips R et al: Altered gastric emptying in the head-injured patient: relationship to feeding tolerance. J Neurosurg 1991;74:738–742.

73. Wood JR, Camilleri M, Low PA et al: Brainstem tumor presenting as an upper gut motility disorder. Gastroenterology 1985;89:1411–1414.

74. Fealey RD, Szurszewski JH, Merritt JC et al: Effects of traumatic spinal cord transection on human upper gastrointestinal motility and gastric emptying. Gastroenterology 1984;87:69–75.

75. Barohn RJ, Levine EJ, Olson JO et al: Gastric hypomotility in Duchenne's muscular dystrophy. N Engl J Med 1988;319:15–18.

76. Crowe GG: Acute dilatation of stomach as a complication of muscular dystrophy. Br Med J 1961;1:1371.

77. Robin GC, de L Falewski G: Acute gastric dilatation in progressive muscular dystrophy. Lancet 1963;2:171–172.

78. Leon SH, Schuffler MD, Kettler M et al: Chronic intestinal pseudoobstruction as a complication of Duchenne's muscular dystrophy. Gastroenterology 1986;90:455–459.

79. Kendall BJ, McCallum RW: Gastroparesis and the current use of prokinetic drugs. The Gastroenterologist 1993;1:107–114.

80. The Multi-Society Task Force on PVS: Medical aspects of the persistent vegetative state. I. N Engl J Med 1994;330:1499–1508.

81. The Multi-Society Task Force on PVS: Medical aspects of the persistent vegetative state. II. N Engl J Med 1994;330:1572–1579.

82. Swisher KN, Miller KB: An ethical and legal analysis of enteral nutrition. In Kirby DF, Dudrick SJ (eds): Practical Handbook of Nutrition in Clinical Practice. Boca Raton, FL: CRC Press, 1994:263–277.

83. Mittal RK, Stewart WR, Schirmer BD: Effect of a catheter in the pharynx on the frequency of transient lower esophageal sphincter relaxations. Gastroenterology 1992;103:1236–1240.

84. Park RHR, Allison MC, Lang J et al: Randomised comparison of percutaneous endoscopic gastrostomy and nasogastric tube feeding in patients with persisting neurological dysphagia. Br Med J 1992;304:1406–1409.

85. Olson DL, Krubsack AJ, Stewart ET: Percutaneous enteral alimentation: gastrostomy versus gastrojejunostomy. Radiology 1993;187:105–108.

86. Albanese CT, Towbin RB, Ulman I et al: Percutaneous gastrojejunostomy versus Nissen fundoplication for enteral feeding of the neurologically impaired child

with gastroesophageal reflux. J Pediatr 1993;123: 371–375.

87. Logemann JA, Kahrilas PJ: Relearning to swallow after stroke—application of maneuvers and indirect biofeedback: a case study. Neurology 1990;40:1136–1138.

88. Horner J, Massey EW, Riski JE et al: Aspiration following stroke: clinical correlates and outcome. Neurology 1988;38:1359–1362.

89. Winterbauer RH, Durning RB, Barron E et al: Aspirated nasogastric feeding solution detected by glucose strips. Ann Intern Med 1986;95:647–668.

90. Lazarus BA, Murphy JB, Culpepper L: Aspiration associated with long-term gastric versus jejunal feeding: a critical analysis of the literature. Arch Phys Med Rehabil 1990;71:46–53.

91. Huxley EJ, Viroslav J, Gray WR et al: Pharyngeal aspiration in normal adults and patients with depressed consciousness. Am J Med 1978;64:564–568.

92. Heyman S: The radionuclide salivagram for detecting the pulmonary aspiration in an infant. Pediatr Radiol 1989;19:208–209.

93. Kirby DF, DeLegge MH, Fleming CR: AGA technical review on the use of enteral nutrition. Gastroenterology. 1995;108:1282–1301.

94. Kiel MK: Enteral tube feeding in a patient with traumatic brain injury. Arch Phys Med Rehabil 1994;75:116–117.

95. Weltz CR, Morris JB, Mullen JL: Surgical jejunostomy in aspiration risk patients. Ann Surg 1992;215:140–145.

17

Enteral Nutrition in the Cancer Patient

LAWRENCE E. HARRISON
YUMAN FONG

Malnutrition in the cancer population has been associated with increased morbidity and mortality and decreased response to therapy. With an estimated 1,252,000 new cancer cases in 1995,[1] the impact of cancer cachexia on patient outcome and health care resources will continue to be significant. It is therefore important to identify those cancer patients who are malnourished in an attempt to reverse or at least stem the progression of malnutrition. The goal of nutritional supplementation is to translate repletion into clinical benefit, decreasing morbidity or mortality and increasing the response rate to treatment. This chapter reviews the etiology of cancer cachexia, summarizes the biologic and clinical effects of enteral nutrition, and defines specific indications for enteral nutrition in the cancer patient population.

CANCER CACHEXIA

Prevalence

Cancer patients are at high risk for malnutrition, and cachexia is often a presenting manifestation of malignancy. As early as 1932, cancer cachexia was noted to be a common syndrome. In an autopsy series of 500 cancer patients, Warren reported that the immediate cause of death was due to inanition in 114 (22

percent), and up to two thirds of these cancer patients exhibited some degree of cachexia.[2] The scope of malnutrition in the cancer patient has been studied in a variety of patient groups. In a large series, 3047 patients who were enrolled in 12 Eastern Cooperative Oncology Group (ECOG) chemotherapy protocols for a variety of tumor types were assessed for weight loss before starting chemotherapy. Survival was significantly shorter in patients who demonstrated weight loss compared with those who had not lost any weight before chemotherapy treatment. Except for patients with pancreatic and gastric cancer, weight loss correlated with decreasing performance status and the frequency of weight loss increased with increased number of involved sites.

In addition to the presence of cancer, the type and stage of malignancy is an important determinant for weight loss (Table 17–1). In the ECOG study, patients with breast cancer, acute nonlymphocytic leukemia, sarcomas, and favorable subtypes of non-Hodgkin's lymphoma had the lowest frequency of weight loss (31 to 40 percent), while those with colon cancer, prostate cancer, lung cancer, and unfavorable non-Hodgkin's lymphoma presented with an intermediate frequency of weight loss (48 to 61 percent). Patients with pancreatic and gastric cancer had the highest frequency of weight loss (83 to

TABLE 17-1 Incidence of Weight Loss and Effect on Survival

| Tumor Type | No. of Patients | Percentage of Weight Loss in Previous 6 Months | | | | Median Survival (Weeks) | |
		0	0–5	5–10	>10	No Weight Loss	Weight Loss
Favorable non-Hodgkin's lymphoma	290	69	14	8	10	—	138*
Breast	289	64	22	8	6	70	45*
Acute nonlymphocytic leukemia	129	61	27	8	4	8	4
Sarcoma	189	60	21	11	7	46	25*
Unfavorable non-Hodgkin's lymphoma	311	52	20	13	15	107	55*
Colon	307	46	26	14	14	43	21*
Prostate	78	44	28	18	10	46	24*
Small-cell lung	436	43	23	20	14	34	27*
Non-small-cell lung	590	39	25	21	15	20	14*
Pancreas	111	17	29	28	26	14	12
Gastric (nonmeasurable)	179	17	21	32	30	41	27*
Gastric (measurable)	138	13	20	29	38	18	16
Total	3,047	46	22	17	15		

*$P < 0.05$. Survival of patients with weight loss vs no weight loss.
Reprinted by permission of the publisher from Dewys WD, Begg C, Lavin PT et al: Prognostic effect of weight loss prior to chemotherapy in cancer patients. Am J Med 1980; 69:491. Copyright 1980 by Excerpta Medica Inc.

87 percent), with about one third having greater than 10 percent weight loss.[3] Other groups report similar data. In a prospective study of 280 cancer patients, malnutrition was mainly related to tumor type and site, with stomach and esophageal cancer patients demonstrating significant malnutrition compared with other groups. As expected, malnutrition became more severe as the disease advanced.[4] In another study of gastrointestinal (GI) cancer, almost half the 365 patients were determined to be malnourished; the incidence of malnutrition was related to site of disease (Fig. 17-1). Stage also predicted weight loss, with over 50 percent of stage III patients manifesting malnutrition.[5]

Assessment of Malnutrition

Malnutrition has been associated with increased postoperative morbidity and mortality, and therefore assessment of perioperative risk should include a nutritional evaluation. Clinical assessment is the simplest method of nutritional evaluation. The usefulness of a good history and physical examination in this regard cannot be overstated.

Prior medical history provides clues to nutritional deficiencies. For example, previous gastrectomy may lead to dumping syndrome, diarrhea, or folate insufficiency, while ileal resection or chronic pancreatitis may be associated with steatorrhea and deficiencies in fat-soluble vitamins. History of alcoholism is associated with protein-calorie malnutrition as well as deficits in niacin and zinc. A history of perioperative chemotherapy or radiation treatment may indicate a malnourished state. A careful review of systems should focus on recent weight loss, weakness, fatigue, and anorexia. GI symptoms such as nausea, vomiting, abdominal pain, diarrhea, melena, and dysphagia may also provide insight in determining the presence and magnitude of malnutrition.

The physical examination should include overall appearance, noting muscle and fat wasting. Although muscle wasting is commonly associated with protein-calorie malnutrition, most patients will not be overtly emaciated and evaluation of muscle atrophy may be more readily appreciated in the hypothenar muscles of the hand and the muscles of facial expression. Other indicators of malnutrition include loss of subcutaneous adipose tissue, peripheral edema, skin lesions, and loss of skin turgor.[6]

Although body weight is the most commonly used anthropometric measurement, its interpretation as a sole indicator of malnutrition should be tempered. Weight depends greatly on the patient's hydrational status and offers no information about the composition of individual body compartments. Many treatments and conditions in the hospitalized cancer patient lead to edema

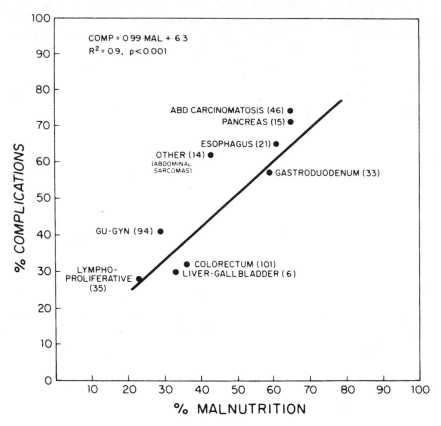

FIGURE 17–1   The relationship between tumor site, extent of malnutrition, and percent complications. (From Meguid MM, Meguid V: Perioperative identification of the surgical patient in need of postoperative supportive nutritional nutrition. Cancer 1985;55:258–262. Copyright © 1985 Wiley-Liss. Reprinted by permission of Wiley-Liss, a division of John Wiley and Sons, Inc.)

and changes in the normal intracellular water:protein ratio and can lead to underestimation of an individual's protein losses.[7] A variety of weight indexes have been developed to standardize weight measurements, including weight:height ratios, percent weight loss, and percent ideal body weight, but these indexes are subject to errors associated with establishing normal or standard values. Serial weight determinations over a sufficient time provide a more reliable indicator of lean body mass (LBM) accrual or loss.[8] Indeed, weight loss has been shown to be an important index of the presence, severity, and progression of malignancy. The importance of weight loss was noted early in the classic study of Studley, who reported that patients who had lost more than 20 percent of their body weight before surgery for peptic ulcer disease had a higher operative mortality.[9]

Skinfold thickness is an anthropometric measurement that may be useful in evaluating fat stores in the cancer patient. Due to ease of measurement and noninvasive nature, body fat assessment by skinfold anthropometrics has been widely used clinically. The skin fold consists of a double layer of skin and subcutaneous fat. Sites of measurement usually include bicep, tricep, subscapular, and suprailiac skinfold thicknesses measured by Lange calipers. A variety of formulas have been proposed to extrapolate subcutaneous fat content to estimate body density and percent body fat. These equations have been derived by multiple regression analysis. One of the most widely used relationships is the regression relationship reported by Durnin and Womersley based on the sum of four skinfolds (triceps, biceps, subscapular, and iliac crest), age, and gender:[10]

$$D = C - m \log_{10}(\Sigma s_i)$$

where D = density, C and m are tabulated linear regression constants, and Σs_i is the sum of the four measured skinfold thicknesses. Body fat can be subsequently calculated from density using Siri's equation:[11]

$$\% \, Fat = (4.95/D - 4.50) \times 100$$

The interpretation of data derived from skinfold measurements is limited in that (1) the technique is only an indirect measurement of body composition, (2) normal values are population specific, (3) observer-to-observer error may be large, and (4) computed tomography (CT) analysis shows that subcutaneous fat distribution is not symmetric.[12]

Another anthropometric indicator of muscle mass is the mid-upper arm muscle circumference (AMC). The mid-upper arm is defined as the midpoint between the olecranon and the acromial process, and the AMC is calculated by subtracting the tricep's skinfold thickness from the arm circumference:

$$AMC = MAC - \pi \, (TSF)$$

where AMC = arm muscle circumference, MAC = midarm circumference, and TSF = triceps skinfold thickness. The AMC is compared with standard tables, and less than 60 percent of standard is consistent with protein depletion. This calculation assumes that the compartment is round, that the skinfold measurement is accurate and consistent around the circumference, and that the humerus is of constant cross-sectional area. None of these assumptions is entirely correct, and interobserver and intraobserver variation may range from 15 to 20 percent.[13,14]

Laboratory measurements aid in the diagnosis and extent of malnutrition. Standard laboratory measurements include albumin, transferrin, prealbumin, and retinol-binding proteins. Albumin is synthesized in the liver with a half-life of approximately 20 days. Normal serum concentration is between 3.5 and 5 mg/dl. Albumin is the main visceral protein, maintaining plasma oncotic pressure and functioning as a carrier for numerous drugs and metabolites. Multiple studies associate increased morbidity and mortality in patients with decreased serum albumin levels.[15,16] The use of albumin as a nutritional index is limited by the fact that (1) albumin levels as an indicator of viseral protein synthesis assume steady-state synthetic rates, which is not the case during acute illness, (2) the long half-life makes it a poor marker to follow acute nutritional changes, (3) reduced serum levels are seen with multiple conditions besides malnutrition, and (4) serum levels are changed by altering hydration status and redistribution. Nevertheless, albumin levels remain the most frequently used index of visceral protein synthesis, since this test is widely available and relatively inexpensive. Serum transferrin has also been used as an indicator of protein malnutrition. Transferrin binds and transports iron in the plasma. The liver is the principle site of synthesis, and the half life of transferrin is 8 to 10 days. Normal serum concentration ranges from 180 to 260 mg/dl. Transferrin levels respond rapidly to nutritional repletion and reflect the severity of protein-calorie malnutrition. Retinol-binding protein (RBP) is a 21 kD α_1-globulin, which is synthesized in the liver, and normal serum concentrations range from 40 to 50 µg/ml. Prealbumin or thyroxine-binding protein (TBP) has a molecular weight of approximately 54 kD, a normal serum concentration of 200 to 300 ug/ml, and circulates in a 1:1 molar ratio with RBP. Because of the short half-lives (10 to 12 hours for RBP and 2 to 3 days for TBP), these proteins reflect rapid changes in hepatic protein synthesis and also provide information about a patient's nutritional state.[14,17]

Protein-calorie malnutrition is often associated with depression of the host's immune response. Several investigators have correlated patient morbidity and mortality with immunologic depression.[18-20] However, it is difficult to quantitate the contribution of malnutrition vs the cancer itself toward impaired immune function. In addition, results can be complicated when patients are receiving steroids or chemotherapy. Although malnutrition impairs both antibody-producing ability and cellular immunity, cellular immunity is affected earlier and more severely. Delayed-type hypersensitivity (DTH) to common skin antigens evaluates the function of the cellular immune system. The common recall antigens used to elicit a DTH response include: (1) purified protein derivatives (PPD), (2) *Candida,* (3) trichophytin, (4) mumps, (5) dinitrochlorobenzene (DNCB), and (6) streptokinase-streptodornase. Antigens are placed intradermally and read at 24 and 48 hours. Induration greater than 5 mm is positive. A patient is considered anergic if induration does not form to *all* antigens.

Another method of evaluating cellular immunity includes in vitro transformation of peripheral lymphocytes with phytohemaglutinin. Although some studies have shown correlation with clinical outcome,[21] the relevance of such in vitro functional testing to the in vivo situation is uncertain.

As an indicator of malnutrition, the humoral response has been less well characterized compared with cell-mediated immunity. Although

TABLE 17-2   Clinical Evaluation of Malnutrition

Degree of Malnutrition	Clinical Findings	Laboratory Findings
None	No weight loss	Normal albumin Normal transferrin Reactive delayed hypersensitivity skin test
Mild	Weight loss < 5%	Albumin < 3.5 Decreased transferrin level
Moderate	5–10% weight loss	Albumin < 3.2 Less than 5 mm reactivity on skin test
Severe	Weight loss > 10% Muscle weakness	Albumin < 2.7 Nonreactive skin test

humoral immunocompetence is influenced by nutritional status, immunoglobulin levels and B-cell function have not been routinely used clinically. Despite a large number of publications advocating such tests of immune competence to evaluate nutritional status, few if any clinicians find such tests to be of significant practical clinical value to justify their use.

All evaluations discussed above have been found to correlate with the level of malnutrition, but most are only relevant in the research setting. The usual health care provider evaluating a cancer patient is unlikely to have mass spectometry or neutron activation available. Nevertheless, most clinicians should and can be effective in evaluating a patient's nutritional status. Some of the best tests for malnutrition are also the most readily available. Table 17-2 shows a useful scale of malnutrition based solely on weight, serum albumin and transferrin, and delayed hypersensitivity skin testing. All cancer patients being evaluated for treatment should have evaluation of nutritional status. All patients with no malnutrition or mild malnutrition should have dietary counseling. Patients with moderate malnutrition should be considered for nutritional supplementation, while patients with severe malnutrition should be referred to a nutritionalist for further evaluation and supplementation.

MECHANISMS OF CANCER CACHEXIA

Host tissue depletion depends on the imbalance between nutrient intake and metabolic demands of the host and tumor. Although diminished food intake is a dominant feature of cancer cachexia, nutrients must also transgress the GI tract into the portal system and ultimately be used systematically to maintain host body mass. Alterations in food intake, absorption, and nutrient use will ultimately lead to cachexia.

Anorexia

Inadequate food intake is a dominant component of cancer cachexia, although the pathogenesis of anorexia is unclear. Many factors have been investigated in an effort to define the mechanism of malignant-associated anorexia. (Table 17-3) The normal physiology of appetite is complex and is regulated by blood nutrient levels, host nutrient resources, liver function, GI capacity and environmental cues such as smell and sight; all of which are processed by the brain.[22] Alterations in one or many of these factors may lead to diminished food intake, resulting in either anorexia (reduced or lack of desire to eat) or early satiety (the desire to eat, but with the ability to eat only reduced amounts of food before feeling full).

Eating is normally a pleasurable and social occasion and is reflected by a sense of well-being. Cancer patients frequently suffer appetite loss as a consequence of their disease and treatment. Based on classic conditioning of animals to associate a conditioned stimulus with an unconditioned stimulus, Berstein reported evidence that learned food aversions to specific foods or tastes develop as a result of the association of food with unpleasant symptoms. Food aversion has been described in tumor-bearing animals and in patients undergoing chemotherapy and radiation therapy.[23-25]

TABLE 17-3   Inadequate Food Intake

Food aversion
Alteration in smell
Alteration in taste
Circulating anorexigenic factor
Tumor obstruction
Surgery
Chemotherapy
Radiation therapy

Alterations in olfactory and gustatory sensation contribute to diminished food intake in cancer patients. Elevated thresholds for sweet and bitter tastes have been correlated with tumor burden.[26] Dewys correlated increased sweet recognition thresholds with decreased appetite and decreased bitter recognition thresholds with a distaste for meat. Elevated threshold for salt has also been reported. Abnormalities in taste may resolve with antitumor therapy and repletion of trace elements such as zinc.[27,28]

Tumor-derived anorexigenic factors have been postulated to play a role in decreased host food intake. Theologides hypothesized that tumors produce peptides that modify host tissue metabolic functions.[29] Support for a circulating mediator emerges from novel models of cancer cachexia. Using a parabiotic MCA sarcoma model, Norton and coworkers demonstrated a decline in food intake and host weight loss in the non-tumor-bearing partner of the parabiotic pair,[30] suggesting the presence of a circulating metabolic mediator. Similar results have been reported when pooled plasma from rats implanted with MCA sarcoma or non-tumor-bearing controls was continuously reinfused into normal rats for 4 days. Rats receiving tumor-bearing serum manifest anorexia, a decrease in total body weight, negative nitrogen balance, and a decrease in gastrocnemius muscle mass compared with rats receiving control serum. In a similar study, infusion of plasma from weight-losing cancer patients into normal F344 rats also caused a decrease in food intake and negative nitrogen balance within 24 hours. These deficits were reversed after animals were crossed over to normal volunteer human serum.[31,32]

Role of Cytokines

In recent years, a class of small protein mediators collectively called cytokines have emerged as putative mediators of the cachectic effects seen in the cancer-bearing state. Initial evidence suggesting that cytokines play a role in cancer cachexia came from studies that reported elevated levels of tumor necrosis factor (TNF)α and interleukin-6 (IL-6) can be detected in the tumor bearing state.[33] Balkwill and colleagues demonstrated that over 50 percent of the cancer patients studied had elevated plasma levels of TNFα.[34] In addition, a variety of studies demonstrated that peripheral blood mononuclear cells from cancer patients spontaneous release significantly more TNFα in

vitro than similar cells from either healthy controls or from patients with benign disease.[35,36] Additional evidence supporting the role of cytokines in cancer cachexia is derived from reports that administration of exogenous cytokines induces metabolic changes seen with cancer cachexia. Fong and associates reported loss of skeletal muscle protein and RNA of rats given escalating doses of IL-1α or TNFα.[37] Oliff and colleagues demonstrated that a CHO cell engineered to produce hTNF, when implanted in nude mice, caused progressive loss of lean body mass and body fat. Similar animals implanted with the CHO xenograft without the TNFα gene inserted failed to demonstrate anorexia or cachexia.[38] A third line of evidence is derived from the work by Sherry and coworkers, who demonstrated that tumor-bearing mice immunized with an anti-TNFα polyclonal antibody delayed both tumor growth and associated anorexia. Similar reductions in tumor growth and anorexia were observed when animals were administered antibody against the IL-1 receptor.[39]

It is evident that increased cytokine production can be seen with the tumor-bearing state and that cytokines can produce many of the changes in host physiology that lead to cachexia. Although the exact roles of these mediators in the pathogenesis of cancer cachexia is incompletely elucidated, it is hoped that future studies will find a role for cytokine-neutralizing agents in the treatment of wasting associated with cancer.

Anatomic Factors

Anatomic factors may play a role in decreased food intake. Patients with head and neck cancers may have diminished oral intake secondary to dysphagia or trismus due to local tumor effects. Patients with esophageal and proximal gastric cancers are also predisposed to partial or complete obstruction. Cancer involving the mid- and lower GI tract may cause a partial or complete obstruction, leading to abdominal discomfort, nausea, and vomiting and thus decreasing food intake.

Once food is ingested, the host must absorb the nutrients, which will be subsequently utilized in biosynthetic pathways. Neoplasms can effect absorption by many ways. Blind-loop syndrome with bacterial overgrowth may lead to malabsorption and vitamin K deficiency. Patients with biliary obstruction may present with steatorrhea. Lymphoma of the small bowel may produce a malabsorptionlike syndrome.

Enterocutaneous fistulas, depending on location, can lead to tremendous loss of nutrient, as well as severe fluid and electrolyte imbalances. Enteroenteric fistulas may cause malnutrition by bypassing large segments of bowel before absorption can occur. In addition, malabsorption may occur due to dismotiliy associated with malignancy.[40]

Treatment of Neoplasms

Treatment of neoplasms contributes to reduced food intake and absorption in the cancer patient. Surgery may delay oral intake for prolonged periods and, when associated with fistula, anastomotic leak, and infection, may last for weeks. Specific anatomic resections are associated with unique nutritional alterations. Gastrectomy may lead to deficiencies in iron, vitamin B_{12}, folate, and a dumping syndrome. Loss of gastric reservoir also leads to smaller meals. Extensive small-bowel resection can produce a short-gut syndrome, while pancreatectomy may result in pancreatic endocrine and exocrine insufficiency.

Radiation therapy may have a significant impact on malnutrition. Head and neck radiation leads to xerostomia, mucositis, dysomia, dysphagia, osteoradionecrosis of the mandible, oral ulcers, trismus, and radiation caries. Intestinal radiation produces early complications such as mucosal edema and ulcers leading to malab-

sorption, diarrhea, nausea, and vomiting. Late complications include fistula, fibrosis, stenosis, obstruction, and perforation. Often symptomatic radiation injury leads to repeat operations, creating a vicious circle contributing to malnutrition.

Chemotherapy also affects the cancer patient's nutritional status. Certain agents have severe GI side-effects (e.g., nausea, vomiting, and enteritis). In addition, generalized weakness contributes to the patient's diminished food intake. Learned food aversion, as mentioned above, has been associated with chemotherapy.

ABNORMALITIES IN HOST METABOLISM

The tumor-bearing state is often associated with abnormalities in energy, protein, carbohydrate, and fat metabolism (Table 17–4 and Fig. 17–2). Although anorexia is a major component of cancer cachexia, restoration of caloric intake does not reverse these alterations. Therefore, additional factors must be involved. Increased nutrient demand by the tumor mass has been suggested as a contributing mechanism, but tumor substrate consumption is rarely significant enough to solely account for host weight loss and metabolic alterations.

Alterations in Energy Expenditure

Attempts have been made to define a hypermetabolic state in the tumor-bearing host to ac-

TABLE 17–4   Metabolic Effects of Malignancy

Metabolic Component	Parameter	Effect	Reference
Energy expenditure			
	Resting energy expenditure	+/–	28-32,40,41,51,129
Protein metabolism			
	Whole body turnover	↑	43-47
	Skeletal synthetic rate	↓	48
	Skeletal catabolic rate	↑	48
	Hepatic synthetic rate	↑	49,52-54
Carbohydrate metabolism			
	Glucose turnover	↑	55,56
	Glucose intolerance	↑	61,62
	Gluconeogenesis	↑	14
	Glucose recycling	↑	13,57-60
	Lactate production	↑	63
	Glucose suppression	↓	56,65-67
Lipid metabolism			
	Fat mobilization	↑	69,71
	Lipoprotein lipase activity	↓	62,72,73
	Fat oxidation	↑	41,74
	Whole body lipolysis	↑	71

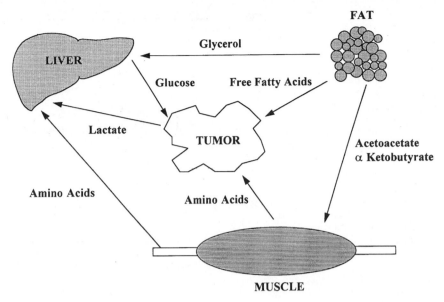

FIGURE 17–2 Intermediary metabolic effects of the tumor-bearing state.

count for the metabolic changes associated with cancer cachexia. Several studies of energy expenditure have been reported with varied results. These inconsistencies are the result of heterogeneous study populations and the sensitivity of resting energy expenditure (REE) measurement to age, gender, body size, and nutritional status. Therefore, although many investigators have reported elevated REE in cancer patients, others have also reported unchanged or decreased REE.[41-43]

Investigators have suggested that the tumor site may predict alterations in REE. Frederix reported that patients with lung cancer had elevated REE, whereas those with gastric and colorectal malignancy were normometabolic.[44] However, Dempsey and colleagues noted that patients with gastric cancer were hypermetabolic, those with esophageal or colorectal were essentially normometabolic, and patients with pancreatic or hepatobiliary cancers were hypometabolic.[45] In contrast to these findings, Hansell and associates reported normal REE in all cancer types.[46] Falconer and colleagues, studying a homogenous population of metastatic pancreatic patients, suggest that the cytokine status might predict extent of abnormality in REE.[47]

Luketich and coworkers measured REE before and after tumor resection in 68 patients. After curative resection, hypometabolic patients increased their REE to normal postoperatively, while those undergoing only palliative surgery increased their REE into the hypermetabolic range (Fig. 17–3). Patients who were normometabolic had no change in their metabolic status, regardless of the type of operation.[48] Similar studies of REE normalization after tumor excision have also been reported.[44,49]

REE is an attractive endpoint, but it has not been demonstrated to correlate or predict which patients will develop cancer cachexia. In patients losing weight, the elevation in REE cannot account for the magnitude of weight loss seen. In summary, there is no agreement on the clinical significance of energy expenditure in cancer patients, and studies looking at serial REE determination, as well as other modalities of evaluating energy state, should be pursued.

Alterations in Protein Metabolism

It has been hypothesized that tumors act as "nitrogen sinks," depleting the host of protein mass, resulting in characteristic alterations in protein metabolism.[50] This tumor avidity for nitrogen accompanies cancer cachexia and involves alterations in whole-body, liver, and skeletal muscle protein metabolism. In general, even though whole-body and hepatic protein synthesis is elevated, muscle protein synthesis is depressed. This pattern is unlike simple starvation, where liver and muscle protein synthetic rates are decreased. These changes have been attributed to a loss of normal host mechanisms designed to conserve body protein in times of stress.[51] Various studies support these

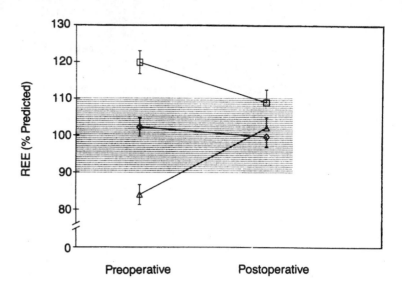

FIGURE 17–3 Resting energy expenditure normalization in response to curative resection in 39 patients with cancer. Shaded area represents normal range; squares, hypermetabolic patients ($P < 0.04$); diamonds, normometabolic patients ($P = 0.034$); and triangle, hypometabolic patients ($P < 0.002$). (From Luketich JD, Mullen JL, Feurer CE et al: Ablation of abnormal energy expenditure by curative tumor resection. Arch Surg 1990;125: 337–341. Copyright 1990, American Medical Association.)

characteristic changes in whole-body, liver, and muscle protein metabolism.

Whole-Body Metabolism

Tumors derive protein at the host's expense, resulting in an increased whole-body protein turnover. With few exceptions, whole-body protein turnover, synthesis, and catabolism have been reported to be elevated in both weight-stable and weight-losing cancer patients. Jeevanandam and coworkers compared whole-body protein kinetics in malnourished cancer patients with malnourished patients with benign disease and with starved healthy controls. They found whole-body protein turnover to be 32 percent and 35 percent higher in the cancer patients than in those with benign disease and starvation, respectively. In addition, the rate of protein synthesis was 35 percent and 54 percent higher in the cancer group than in those with benign disease and healthy starved controls, respectively.[52] Investigators have also reported that extent of disease, dietary manipulation, and nutritional supplementation influence whole-body turnover rates.[53-56]

Skeletal Muscle Metabolism

The tumor-bearing state has been shown to have a pronounced effect on protein metabolism in skeletal muscle. Depression of muscle protein synthetic rates and overall muscle wasting is commonly seen in tumor-bearing animal models and cancer patients. Comparing rectus abdominus muscle biopsied from a heterogenous group of 43 cancer patients with 55 age- and sex-matched controls, Lundholm demonstrated a decreased rate of protein synthesis and increased rate of protein catabolism using in vitro incorporation of ^{14}C leucine.[57] In contrast, Shaw and colleagues determined in vivo fractional synthetic rates (FSR) of muscle in patients with benign disease and weight-stable and weight-losing cancer patients. Although there was no significant difference between the rate of muscle FSR between those with benign disease and weight-stable cancers, there was an increase in FSR in those patients with cancer cachexia.[58]

Hepatic Protein Metabolism

Using both in vitro and in vivo models, Lundholm demonstrated increased liver tissue incorporation of radiolabeled leucine in the MCG101-bearing mouse. In addition, there was a significantly increased RNA and RNA:DNA ratio compared with controls, suggesting increased protein synthesis. Fractions of free and membrane-bound polysomes isolated from liver tissue of tumor-bearing mice combined with cell fractions from control livers incorporated amino acids into nascent peptides at significantly higher rates than did corresponding ribosome fractions from control livers. This provided evidence for an increased translational activity in the liver during tumor-bearing state.[59] Similar results of increased liver FSR have also been reported in both animal[60-62] and cancer patients.[58]

Carbohydrate Metabolism

The literature is replete with evidence documenting alterations of carbohydrate metabolism in the cancer patient. Specifically, these abnormalities include (1) increased hepatic glucose production, (2) decreased skeletal muscle glucose use, (3) increased tumor glucose use with increased lactate production, and (4) increased glucose recycling (Cori cycle). Generally, clinical studies have reported these abnormalities in terms of whole-body, peripheral, and hepatic glucose metabolism. The changes seen are similar to a type II diabetic state but also share elements similar to the stress state.

Whole-Body Metabolism

Increased whole-body turnover (production and use) has been documented in the tumor-bearing state. Both Kolal[63] and Shaw[64] noted increased glucose turnover in cancer patients proportional to extent of disease. Using isotopic methodology, glucose carbon recycling (Cori cycle) has been measured in cancer patients and has been reported as elevated.[20,65-68]

Peripheral Metabolism

Glucose intolerance was one of the earliest recognized metabolic abnormalities in cancer patients. The tumor-bearing state is associated with hyperglycemia and delayed clearance of glucose after an intravenous or oral glucose challenge. In a study of over 600 patients, Glicksman reported that approximately 37 percent of all cancer patients demonstrated abnormal glucose tolerance curves.[69] Yoshikawa and colleagues examined insulin sensitivity in both weight-losing and weight-stable cancer patients compared with normal controls by euglycemic hyperinsulinemic glucose clamp. They reported a significant decrease in clearance and metabolism of glucose in both the weight-stable and weight-losing cancer patients compared with controls. In addition, in six patients, insulin resistance decreased after the tumors were completely resected.[70]

Hepatic Metabolism

Cancer patients, like diabetic patients, have a 25 to 40 percent increase in hepatic glucose production compared with healthy controls. However, unlike diabetics, cancer patients continue to produce increased hepatic glucose in the face of starvation. The mechanism for this increased glucose production has been implicated as either upregulation of gluconeogenic enzyme activity or increased availability of gluconeogenic precursors, such as alanine, lactate, and glycerol.

One such precursor, lactate, may be present in the plasma at increased levels due to tumor production. Elevation in plasma lactate levels have been reported in both tumor-bearing animal models and humans. Richtsmeier measured arterial-venous (A-V) differences across the tumor bed in head and neck cancer patients and demonstrated glucose uptake by the tumor and lactate release into the tumor vein.[71] Recent work with positron emission tomography (PET) scanning in lung cancer patients demonstrated that the tumor had almost a sevenfold increase in glucose uptake compared with the contralateral lung.[72]

The tumor-bearing state is associated with increased lactate production, and the host liver uses this gluconeogenic precursor to supply glucose to both the host and tumor (Cori cycle). This is an energy-wasting process because only two moles of adenosine triphosphate (ATP) are produced by glycolytic degradation of each molecule of glucose, whereas 6 moles of ATP are consumed for the resynthesis of glucose from lactate. The host loses energy through two paths: energy expenditure to synthesize glucose from lactate and loss of available glucose to the tumor itself.

The tumor-bearing state is also associated with reduced suppression of endogenous hepatic glucose production by adequate glucose availability. In healthy volunteers, a 4mg/kg/hour glucose infusion maximally suppresses endogenous glucose production. However, in patients with advanced GI cancers, gluconeogenesis is suppressed only 70 percent. Patients with sarcoma and leukemia demonstrate approximately 30 percent suppression of hepatic glucose production.[64,73-75]

Lipid Metabolism

Although reduced food intake contributes to the depletion of host fat reserves, alterations in lipid metabolism resulting from tumor burden have also been implicated. Alterations reported include increased lipid mobilization, increased free fatty acid (FFA) oxidation, and depressed serum lipid clearance. Animal studies suggest that tumors produce a transmissible fat-mobilizing substance, which increases lipid breakdown and decreases fat synthesis. Investigators have reported normalization of serum FFA after tumors are excised from tumor-bearing animals.[76-78]

Increased fat mobilization has been demonstrated in the cancer patient. Shaw and colleagues studied fatty acid and glycerol kinetics in three populations: weight-losing and weight-stable cancer patients and healthy controls. There was no significant difference between weight-stable cancer patients and healthy controls, but weight-losing cancer patients had increased rates of glycerol and fatty acid turnover. In addition, glucose infusion failed to suppress lipolysis.[79]

Even though the tumor-bearing state is associated with increased lipid mobilization, decreased serum clearance has been noted as well. As a result, hyperlipidemia has been reported to be associated with some tumor types.[47] The hypertriglyceridemia associated with the tumor-bearing state is due in part to suppression of lipoprotein lipase (LPL).[70,80] Synthesized by adipose and muscle parenchymal cells, LPL is responsible for triglyceride clearance from plasma. In the uncomplicated starved state LPL is decreased due to reduced insulin levels. In cancer patients, LPL activity is reduced with no change in insulin levels. Vlassara reported a 35 percent decreased LPL activity in a group of 28 cancer patients with weight loss who had normal or elevated insulin levels. In addition, the degree of reduction correlated with weight loss.[81]

In addition to fat mobilization and depressed triglyceride clearance, evidence supports elevated fat oxidation in the tumor-bearing state. Arbeit and colleagues compared fat oxidation in cancer patients with healthy controls and reported increased fat oxidation rates in patients with metastatic disease.[49] Hansell and colleagues determined the fat oxidation rates in weight-stable and weight-losing cancer patients compared with weight-stable and weight-losing patients with nonmalignant GI. They reported that weight-losing cancer patients had significantly higher fat oxidation rates compared with the other three groups. As in Arbeit's study, patients with metastatic disease had higher rates of fat oxidation compared with those with localized disease.[82] Using glycerol turnover as an estimate of whole-body lipolysis, Eden and associates showed that weight-losing cancer patients had significantly elevated glycerol turnover and oxidation compared with weight-stable cancer patients as well as healthy controls.[83]

ADVANTAGES OF ENTERAL NUTRITION

Nutritional supplementation is an important aspect in the treatment of patients with cancer. Although parenteral nutrition is indicated for patients with nonfunctioning GI tracts, disadvantages of total parenteral nutrition (TPN) include the high cost of parenteral solutions, catheter maintenance, and increased need for absolute sterile technique. In addition, prolonged TPN administration leads to intestinal mucosal atrophy, enterocyte hypoplasia, and decreased intestinal enzyme activity.[84] These changes are associated with a break in the enterocyte barrier, allowing transgression of bacteria and endotoxin into the portal system (bacterial translocation). These observations lead to the hypothesis that the intestinal tract is a source of sepsis in the critically ill patient, and data support that TPN is associated with higher rates of infection in certain patient populations.[85,86]

Therefore, enteral feeding, when possible, is the preferred route of nutrition. Enteral feeds, either by oral supplementation or tube feedings, are less costly, easier to maintain, and more physiologic. Luminal nutrient in the small bowel maintains normal villous architecture and function. Enteral nutrition results in increased total gut weight, mucosal thickness, protein and DNA content, and brush border enzyme activity compared with intravenous nutrition.[87] Enteral feeding has also been reported to decrease infectious complications and sepsis compared with TPN.[85] This is most likely because it maintains the enterocyte barrier and splanchnic immune function.

The human GI tract contains a large collection of bacterial organisms living in symbiosis with the host. The amount and species of bacteria, integrity of the GI barrier, and function of the splanchnic immune cells all contribute to the delicate relationship between bacteria and host. Consequences of illness can affect any or all of these factors, leading to increased translocation of bacteria and compromise of host defenses. Evidence is emerging that the route of feeding may be one factor associated with disease that can affect splanchnic immune function and, specifically, that enteral feedings may help protect the host against potentially harmful changes in bacterial transgression from the GI tract.

Bacterial translocation and its relationship to enteral and parenteral nutrition have been studied extensively in both animals and humans. Factors promoting translocation include (1) bacterial overgrowth, (2) disruption of the intestinal mucosal barrier, and (3) altered host immune status. Disruption of any one of these three may contribute to sepsis and ultimately multisystem organ failure (MSOF) in the cancer patient.

Bacterial overgrowth in the intestine may be associated with oral antibiotic treatment. Postoperative or opiate-induced ileus, intestinal obstruction, and blind loop syndrome all contribute to bacterial overgrowth as well. Jaundice, a common feature in advanced malignancy, is also associated with changes in intestinal microflora and translocation.[88]

Although the enterocyte serves as an absorber of luminal nutrient, it also functions as a barrier to luminal bacteria. There is evidence that the absence of enteral feedings rapidly results in enterocyte atrophy and dysfunction. Once this occurs, the enterocyte barrier is lost, with subsequent translocation of bacteria and endotoxin. Additionally, the GI tract contains a large population of immune cells (lymphocytes and macrophages) that protect the host against potential pathogens from the GI lining when disruption of the intestinal mucosal barrier results in bacterial translocation.

Host immune function is an important determinant in bacterial translocation. Malnutrition by itself is associated with impairment of the immune system. A large proportion of cancer patients present with protein-calorie malnutrition and are therefore at risk for infectious complications. In addition, many of these patients will be treated with chemotherapy, radiation, or surgery, all of which compound the negative effect on host immune function.

Studies have demonstrated that enteral nutrition is superior to TPN in maintaining the host's immunologic function. Fong and coworkers[89] demonstrated that endotoxin administered to human volunteers, maintained on either TPN or enteral nutrition, resulted in an exaggerated counter-regulatory hormone response and hepatic and splanchnic production of TNF in the TPN group (Fig. 17–4). In addition, patients receiving TPN demonstrated increased lactate production and peripheral amino acid release in response to endotoxemia. Importantly, immunologic function has been shown to be improved in postoperative patients receiving enteral nutrition supplemented with arginine.[90]

In summary, enteral feeding is as, if not more, efficient as parenteral alimentation in terms of nutritional repletion. Feeding through the gut is cheaper and easier and helps maintain intestinal enterocyte integrity. This translates into a decreased incidence of bacterial translocation and thus sepsis in a patient population already at high risk for infectious complications.

ENTERAL NUTRITION: METABOLIC EFFICACY

Multiple studies looking at metabolic endpoints have demonstrated that enteral nutrition may reverse many of the detrimental metabolic findings in the cancer patient. In a study designed to compare the metabolic effects of enteral nutrition in malnourished patients with and without cancer, Dresler and associates performed whole-body protein and glucose turnover studies before and after 2 weeks of enteral nutrition. Many similarities were noted between both groups, including (1) decreased protein breakdown, (2) reversal of negative nitrogen balance, and (3) suppressed endogenous glucose turnover. In addition, the cancer patients demonstrated a significant reduction in whole-body protein synthetic rate and elevated lactate and pyruvate production compared with non-tumor-bearing patients.[91]

In a series of reports, malnourished cancer and noncancer patients were studied before and after 2 weeks of enteral nutrition (30 to 40 kcal/kg/day, 165 kcal/g nitrogen through nasogastric tube), and whole-body and peripheral tissue metabolic parameters were reported. Lundholm and colleagues reported that in response to enteral nutrition, the malnourished cancer patients decreased their 3-methylhistidine output, suggesting a decrease in protein breakdown.[92] Nutritional supplementation also resulted in an increased peripheral uptake of glucose, FFAs, and branched-chain amino acids (BCAAs).[93] In addition, Bennegard and colleagues demonstrated an improvement in energy and nitrogen balance after enteral supplementation. They also noted an increase in glucose, pyruvate, lactate, and alanine balance in these patients after the 2-week period. In general, enteral nutrition improved peripheral and whole-body tissue metabolism, but less efficiently than in malnourished noncancer patients.[94]

Edstrom and colleagues studied malnourished patients with and without cancer and evaluated energy balance, glucose turnover, and skeletal muscle metabolism in response to nutrition. Patients were studied before and after 2 weeks of nutritional support. Those patients receiving enteral nutrition demonstrated improved energy balance, increased glucose turnover, and improved protein synthetic capacity in skeletal muscle. However, in this study, there was no difference between the enteral and TPN groups.[95]

Specific enteral nutrients or formulations may offer advantages, which may ultimately translate into improved survival and decreased morbidity. Daly and colleagues studied in a prospective fashion a homogeneous group of bladder cancer patients, comparing high and low BCAA elemen-

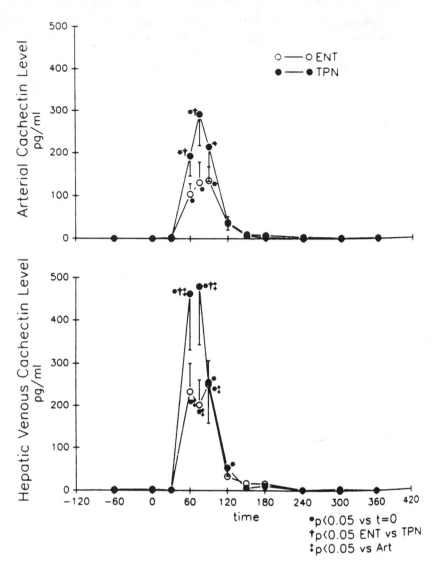

FIGURE 17–4   Cachectin levels in the arterial and hepatic venous blood of volunteers before (t = 0) and after the endotoxin injection. Subjects received either enteral feedings (ENT) or parenteral feedings (TPN) as pretreatment. (From Fong Y, Marano MA, Barber A et al: Total parenteral nutrition and bowel rest modify the metabolic response to endotoxin in humans. Ann Surg 1989;210(4):449–457.)

tal diet formulations with standard dextrose infusions postoperatively. Although the mean caloric intake was significantly higher in the jejunostomy group and the nitrogen balance was significantly less negative in the enterally fed groups, there was no significant difference in length of hospital stay or dietary progression. In addition, a high number of GI complications were noted in the jejunostomy group compared with controls. There was no significant difference between the high and low BCAA groups.[96]

A prospective, randomized study evaluated the impact of enteral nutrition supplemented with arginine, RNA, and omega-3 fatty acids compared with standard enteral tube feeding in patients undergoing surgery for upper GI malignancies. Patients undergoing complete surgical excision were randomized to supplemented or standard feeding regimens. The supplemented group demonstrated improved nitrogen balance and intake. In vitro immunologic studies of lymphocyte mitogenesis were depressed in both groups following surgery but normalized only in the supplemented group by the fifth postoperative day. In a cohort of 77 patients, the authors reported a significant decrease in wound infection rates (11 percent vs 37 percent) in the supplemented group compared with standard. In addition, mean length of hospital stay was significantly shorter (15.8 ± 5.1 days vs 20.2 ± 9.4 days). This is one of the only studies demonstrating a positive outcome in terms of clinical parameters.[90]

There is good evidence that enteral nutrition positively affects the cancer patient in terms of metabolic parameters (Table 17–5). However, at present, few data demonstrate a positive clinical impact for many reasons. Most important, studies demonstrating improvement in survival and morbidity require a large number of patients with significant follow-up time. Few studies are large enough with homogenous populations and sufficient follow-up time to state conclusions about enteral nutrition and its impact on overall survival. Large, prospective, randomized studies are still required before enteral nutrition is instituted globally in cancer patients in an attempt to improve outcome and overall survival.

ENTERAL NUTRITION: SPECIFIC INDICATIONS

Patients with certain types of tumors appear to benefit from enteral nutritional supplementation (Table 17–6).

Head and Neck Cancer

Approximately 40 percent of patients with advanced head and neck cancers will initially present with some form of protein depletion.[97,98] Although malignancy itself contributes to their malnutrition, they often have associated history of chronic alcohol abuse, which places them at an even higher nutritional risk. To compound the problem, treatment of head and neck cancer significantly contributes to the severe malnutrition seen in

TABLE 17–5   Enteral Nutrition: Metabolic Endpoints

Reference	Nutrition	Study Groups	Endpoints
91	Enteral: 14 days	Before vs after treatment	↓ Protein breakdown ↓ Negative NB Suppression of endogenous glucose ↑ Glucose turnover
		Cancer vs noncancer	↓ WB protein synthesis ↑ Lactate/pyruvate production
92 93 94	Enteral: 14 days	Before vs after treatment	↓ 3MH output ↑ Uptake-glucose, FFA, BCAA ↑ NB, energy balance ↑ Glucose, alanine balance → Energy expenditure
		Cancer vs noncancer	→ 3-MH → Tyrosine uptake
130	Enteral/TPN	Cancer vs noncancer	Weight gain: TPN > EN* ↑ Albumin: TPN > EN
95		Before vs after treatment	↑ Glucose turnover ↑ Protein synthetic capacity ↑ Energy balance
96	Enteral: low BCAA Enteral: high BCAA vs IV dextrose	Postoperative Enteral vs IV Low vs high BCAA	↑ Caloric intake Less negative NB → Hospital stay No difference noted
90	Supplemented† vs standard enteral	Postoperative	↑ NB and nitrogen uptake ↓ Wound complication ↓ Length of stay ↑ Immunologic status

3-MH = 3 methyl histidine; NB = nitrogen balance; TPN = total parenteral nutrition; EN = enteral nutrition; BCAA = branch chain amino acids; FFA = free fatty acids.
*Weight gain did not represent synthesis of lean body mass.
†Supplemented—arginine, RNA, omega-3 fatty acids.

TABLE 17–6   Enteral Nutrition: Specific Cancer Populations

Reference	Study Population	Nutrition	Results
99	Head and neck	Preoperative TPN vs EN	No difference in immune parameters, wound complications, or survival
100	Head and neck/radiation	EN vs optimal oral nutrition	↑ caloric intake ↑ weight gain ↑ serum albumin No difference in survival
68	Esophageal	Oral feedings vs TPN vs EN	EN/TPN: ↓ gluconeogenesis ↑ Glucose turnover
102	Esophageal	TPN vs EN	TPN > EN: weight gain earlier positive NB
103	Esophageal	EN: before vs after treatment	+ NB Weight gain ↑ Serum albumin/TIBC ↑ Cellular + humoral immune parameters
96	Bladder cancer	Postoperative Enteral vs IV	↑ Caloric intake Less negative NB → Hospital stay
		Low vs high BCAA	No difference noted

NB = nitrogen balance; TIBC = total iron-binding capacity; BCAA = branched-chain amino acids; EN = enteral nutrition; TPN = total parenteral nutrition.

these patients. Radiation causes salivary gland damage, inducing dysgeusia and xerostomia. The surgical extirpation itself may retard nutritional repletion. Glossectomy, mandibulectomy, and resections of the hard and soft palate may cause difficulties in mastication and deglutition. In addition, these procedures often place the patient at higher risk for aspiration.

Sako and colleagues prospectively randomized 69 patients with head and neck cancer to either preoperative TPN or enteral tube feeding. Nutritional support was given for 14 days. Nitrogen balance was improved in the TPN group, but patients did not demonstrate any differences in terms of immune parameters, wound healing, complications, or survival.[99]

Results of prospective, randomized, enteral nutritional studies in head and neck patients are scarce. In a report of nutritional supplementation in head and neck cancer patients, Daly and coworkers compared nasogastric tube feedings vs optimal oral nutrition during radiation therapy. Caloric intake was higher in the tube-fed group, with significant improvement in body weight and normalization of serum albumin at the completion of radiotherapy. However, there was no significant difference in survival between the two groups.[100]

Head and neck cancer patients are a high-risk group for malnutrition and are perfect candidates for enteral feeding, since the majority of the GI tract is not involved by tumor or affected by treatment. Therefore, these patients may be fed enterally, either by small-bore nasogastric tubes or percutaneously placed gastrostomies or jejunostomies. If anatomy does not allow entry into the GI tract through an endoscopic route, surgical placement of a gastrostomy or jejunostomy tube is a viable option.

Esophageal Cancer

Malnutrition is a common finding in patients with esophageal cancer. The malnutrition associated with esophageal cancer is due in part to mechanical obstruction and anorexia, but tumor-dependent metabolic alterations also contribute to the cachexia syndrome.[101] Therapy associated with esophageal cancer also contributes to worsening nutritional conditions. Radiation may induce esophagitis and subsequent fibrosis and stricture. Chemotherapy causes nausea, vomiting, and anorexia, which further worsen the patient's nutritional status. Surgical treatment may involve esophageal resection, bilateral vagotomy, pyloroplasty, and gastric pullup into the chest. These all interfere with the normal anatomy and invariably result in decreased food intake. In addition, esophageal anastomotic leak, regurgitation, early satiety, decreased gastric emptying, and diarrhea are common complications and sequelae after surgery.

A few studies have attempted to study the effects of enteral nutrition in the esophageal cancer patient. Lim and colleagues treated a small group of esophageal cancer patients with preoperative gastric tube feeding and reported weight gain after approximately 1 week and a positive nitrogen balance after 5 days. After 4 weeks of nutrition, albumin levels increased 7.4 percent. However, the TPN group demonstrated a greater weight gain (although this study did not differentiate whether this reflected protein accrual or just water retention) and early positive nitrogen balance.[102] In another study, Burt and colleagues randomized patients with localized squamous cell carcinoma of the esophagus to three nutritional regimens: oral feeding, jejunal feeding, or TPN. After 2 weeks of therapy, both jejunal feeding and TPN were efficacious in markedly suppressing gluconeogenesis while increasing glucose turnover, pool size, and clearance rate.[68] Haffejee studied 20 patients with esophageal carcinoma. Patients were evaluated for nutritional status and immune status 1 week before and 3 weeks after enteral supplementation. After supplementation, the average weight gain was almost 4 kg, nitrogen balance became positive, and serum albumin and total iron-binding capacity also improved. In addition, both cellular and humoral parameters were improved.[103] Although the cited studies report improved biologic endpoints, they do not demonstrate improved survival or decreased morbidity associated with supplemental nutrition.

Pancreatic Cancer

Pancreatic cancer is associated with a high incidence of malnutrition and weight loss. Numerous etiologies are identified. Mechanical impingement of the tumor can result in gastric outlet obstruction with associated nausea and vomiting, while biliary obstruction can cause fat malabsorption and vitamin K deficiency. Endocrine insufficiency is not usually present. Surgery may contribute to the patient's malnutrition as well. Gastric resection may lead to early satiety and delayed emptying. Reports of pylorus-sparing pancreticoduodenectomy claim to offer patients freedom from dumping syndrome and preserves the stomach's mixing and capacity functions. However, these patients may experience a delay in gastric emptying, in addition to less-encompassing resection. Total pancreatectomy, although eliminating the risk of pancreatic fistula, leaves the patient with both endocrine and exocrine insufficiency, leading to worsening nutritional status.

With these potential mechanical and endocrine problems, it is not surprising that patients with pancreatic cancer often have malnutrition. To date, however, data suggest that perioperative parenteral nutrition may be detrimental[104] and little data exist examining the efficacy of enteral nutrition in this setting. Nevertheless, postoperative enteral nutrition should be considered for patients undergoing pancreatic resection.

Enteral nutrition may be administered through a jejunostomy tube. In addition, nutritional support should include pancreatic enzyme replacement if a total pancreatectomy is performed. In addition, medium-chain triglycerides are more efficiently absorbed in the absence of pancreatic enzymes than long-chain fatty acids. Postoperative diabetes after pancreaticoduodenectomy is uncommon, but close control of blood sugar with insulin is required after total pancreatectomy.

Chemotherapy

Chemotherapeutic agents contribute to host malnutrition by a variety of mechanisms, including nausea and vomiting, mucositis, GI dysfunction, and learned food aversions. These may compound the already malnourished cancer patient, ultimately influencing the outcome after chemotherapy and leading to increased morbidity and mortality. In addition, increased toxicity from chemotherapy is associated with poor nutritional status.[105]

Enteral nutrition studies have demonstrated improvement in biologic endpoints in patients undergoing chemotherapy (Table 17–7). DeVries and colleagues studied 34 patients receiving chemotherapy for acute leukemia and compared tube feeding to ad lib food intake. They reported a decrease in weight loss over 3 weeks with an improvement in serum albumin levels in the tube-fed group compared with controls.[106] In another study, patients receiving fluorouracil (5-FU) were randomized to normal hospital fare ad lib or defined formula diet based on casein hydrosylate as protein source. Rectal biopsies performed after completion of chemotherapy revealed normal histology in all 11 patients fed the elemental diet. This was in

TABLE 17–7   Enteral Nutrition: Chemotherapy Trials

Reference	Study Group	Nutrition	Results
106	Leukemia	EN vs oral	↓ Weight loss ↑ Serum albumin
107	Metastatic GI malignancy	EN vs oral	↑ Caloric intake Rectal biopsy: no histologic change
108	Bone marrow transplant	TPN vs EN	TPN > EN maintaining body cell mass → Hematopoetic recovery → Length of stay No difference in survival
109	Bone marrow transplant	TPN vs PPN + EN	No difference: infection rate, nitrogen balance Decreased diarrhea in PPN/EN
110	Advanced colorectal and non-small-cell lung cancer	Oral vs oral + counseling vs oral + supplementation	No difference: tumor response, toxicity, survival

EN = enteral nutrition; TPN = total parenteral nutrition.

contrast to the control patients, where seven of eight demonstrated signs of mucosal change. In addition, patients on the elemental diet consumed more calories per body weight than did the controls (27.1 vs 20.4 kcal/kg).[107]

Additional information can be culled from the bone marrow transplantation (BMT) literature. BMT requires intensive chemotherapy, resulting in severe adverse nutritional effects. As a result, these patients have received nutritional support as standard of care. In a prospective randomized trial, Szeluga and colleagues randomized 61 patients requiring BMT to either TPN or an individualized enteral feeding program. Although the enteral feeding program was less effective in maintaining body cell mass, there was no difference in rates of hematopoietic recovery, length of hospital stay, or overall survival between the two groups. Furthermore, the average cost for the 28-day study was $2575 for each TPN patient and $1139 for each enteral patient.[108] In a similar study, Mulder and associates randomized 22 consecutive patients to receive either TPN or peripheral intravenous nutrition plus enteral nutrition (PPN/EN). No statistical significance was noted between the TPN and PPN/EN group in terms of hyperglycemia, fever or infection, or nitrogen balance. Interestingly, the enteral group had significantly less diarrhea (31.1 percent vs 54.3 percent) and received better supplementation of calcium, copper, magnesium, and zinc compared with the TPN group.[109] Both studies concluded that enteral support for BMT patients is at least as efficient as TPN.

There is no evidence that enteral nutrition affects overall survival and tumor response. In a prospective randomized trial of 192 previously untreated patients with unresectable non-small-cell lung cancer and colorectal cancer, Evans and colleagues randomized patients to receive either ad lib nutritional intake (control), dietary counseling with a target caloric intake of 1.7 to 1.95 times their basal energy expenditure (standard support), and dietary counseling to the same caloric target but with 25 percent of calories provided as protein and mineral supplementation (augmented support). Caloric intake was increased in both support groups compared with controls. However, they observed no benefit in terms of tumor response, toxicity, or survival duration when comparing ad lib food intake to supplemented or augmented nutritional intervention.[110]

At this time, no strong evidence supports enteral nutrition as effective in patients with advanced disease undergoing chemotherapy. However, there are few studies looking at patients with less advanced tumors. Well-designed prospective randomized trials, studying patients receiving adjuvant or neoadjuvant chemotherapy, are necessary to determine the effects of enteral nutrition on tumor response and overall survival in these patient populations.

Radiation Therapy

In additional to chemotherapy, radiation therapy contributes to the cancer patient's malnourished state. The severity and incidence of malnutrition and weight loss are determined by the body region undergoing radiation, dose, duration, and volume of therapy. Nutritional alterations may result from local therapy to the central nervous system (CNS) (nausea and vomiting), head and neck (mucositis, dysphagia, xerostomia, trismus), thorax (dysphagia, fibrosis, fistula), and abdomen/pelvis (diarrhea, enteritis, malabsorption). Retrospective studies have supported the use of enteral nutrition in patients undergoing radiation, claiming to improve their nutritional state as well as offering a protective effect against acute and chronic radiation changes. However, there are no randomized prospective studies demonstrating improvement in local control or survival with nutritional support.

Experimental evidence supports enteral nutrition as a form of prophylaxis against radiation injury.[111] Bounous reported that elemental nutrition works by suppressing pancreatic and biliary secretions. In addition, he states that it prevents alterations in microvilli, reduces the enterocyte glycocalyx, and suppresses brush border enzymes.[112]

Some of these findings have been reproduced in human trials (Table 17–8). McArdle and colleagues fed 20 patients 3 days before and 4 days during radiotherapy for bladder cancer. All patients underwent cystectomy and ileal conduit. Tube feedings were restarted on the first postoperative day. These patients were compared with treatment-, age-, sex-, and grade-matched historical controls. The authors concluded that the control group had increased diarrhea, nausea, and vomiting both preopera-

tively and postoperatively, and GI function took more time to return to normal. Patients fed the elemental diet remained in positive nitrogen balance during radiation and returned to positive nitrogen balance by postoperative day 4. In addition, histologic examination of biopsy specimens of the terminal ileum in three patients who were not fed the elemental diet demonstrated moderate to severe radiation damage compared with those receiving enteral feedings, who demonstrated normal morphologic findings.[113]

Similar to the data in chemotherapy trials, studies have not shown that nutritional support during radiotherapy improves tumor response or overall survival. In a prospective study, Douglass compared elemental supplementation vs controls in 30 patients undergoing radiotherapy for a variety of locally advanced, nonmetastatic GI malignancies. There was a trend for improved delayed hypersensitivity skin test response in those receiving the supplementation. However, no differences in weight or survival were noted.[114]

Daly and colleagues compared optimal nutrition with tube feeding in 40 patients with advanced head and neck cancers undergoing an average of 8 weeks of radiation therapy. Compared with the orally fed group, the tube-fed group had a higher mean caloric intake, mean protein intake, and less weight loss. The tube-fed patients maintained mid-arm circumference and recovered mean albumin levels after completion of therapy (Fig. 17–5). However, as in other trials, there were no significant differences in tumor response or survival rates.[100]

TABLE 17–8 Enteral Nutrition: Radiation Trials

Reference	Study Group	Nutrition	Results
113	Bladder cancer	EN vs IV dextrose controls	↓ GI symptoms Improved NB Terminal ileum histology: improved radiation changes
114	Locally advanced GI cancers	Elemental supplementation vs controls	Improved DTH No difference in survival
100	Head and neck cancer	EN vs oral	↑ Caloric intake ↑ Protein intake ↓ Weight loss ↑ Recovery of serum albumin No difference in tumor response No difference in survival

DTH = delayed type hypersensitivity; NB = nitrogen balance; EN = enteral nutrition.

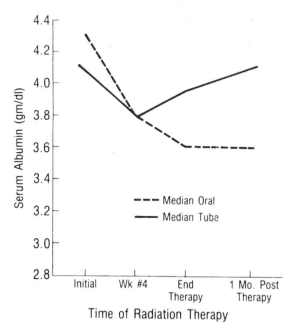

FIGURE 17–5 Median serum albumin levels returned toward normal by the end of radiation therapy in the tube-fed group in contrast to the decline in albumin levels in the orally fed group. (Reprinted by permission of the publisher from Daly JM, Hearne B, Dunaj J et al: Nutritional rehabilitation in patients with advanced head and neck cancer receiving radiation therapy. Am J Surg 1984;148:514–520. Copyright 1984 by Excerpta Medica Inc.)

PHARMACOLOGIC SUPPORT

Anorexia is a major component to cancer cachexia. Although "force feeding" is one approach to overcome nutritional impairment, attempts to improve oral intake should be considered. Control of symptoms such as pain, nausea, constipation, depression, and xerostomia can lead to improved food intake. In addition, certain pharmacologic agents have been shown to improve weight gain in cancer patients.

Patients with advanced cancers will have early satiety based on delayed upper GI motility. In addition, factors such as postoperative ileus and opiate-associated dysmotility contribute to delayed emptying.[115] Metaclopramide, a promotility agent, has been shown to relieve anorexia and early satiety in small trials.[40,116] Although it has been shown to improve gastric emptying and provide symptomatic improvement, it must demonstrate an effect on clinical nutritional endpoints before being used in clinical practice.

Megestrol acetate (Megace), a synthetic progestational agent, has been used for hormonal management of breast cancer. Studies with megestrol acetate noted that the drug produced weight gain and increased appetite and promoted a sense of well-being unrelated to its antitumor effect.[117] In a randomized, double-blind study, 133 cancer patients with anorexia and weight loss were treated with megestrol acetate (800 mg/day) or placebo. Megestrol acetate resulted in significantly improved appetite and food intake while leading to less nausea and vomiting. Although overweight gain was no different, weight gain greater than 10 percent was reported in more patients taking megestrol acetate (16 percent) compared with placebo (2 percent). The only side-effect noted was mild edema.[118] In a multi-institutional, placebo-controlled trial, megestrol acetate was also found to improve weight gain and appetite. Further studies are currently underway.

Corticosteroids are frequently used in cancer patients to improve appetite. In a double-blind crossover study comparing placebo with prednisolone in over 300 cancer patients with advanced disease, 80 percent of the patients experienced improved appetite and a sense of well-being, compared with 50 percent on placebo. However, no increase in caloric intake or body weight resulted.[119] In a randomized, double-blind placebo controlled study, dexamethasone was studied in preterminal gastrointestinal cancer patients and found to improve appetite, but had no effect on weight gain.[120] Although short-term toxicity of steroids is well tolerated, chronic use of steroids would be necessary to achieve clinical improvement. The long-term side-effects and morbidity associated with steroid use outweigh its potential benefit.

Dronabinol (Marinol) is the major active ingredient of marijuana. It is currently approved as a treatment of refractory nausea and vomiting. It has also been noted to stimulate appetite. In a small study, patients with advanced cancers were treated with dronabinol, and although their appetite improved, weight loss continued unabated.[121] In a similar study, dronabinol improved both appetite and reduced the rate of weight loss.[122] Further prospective trials are needed to ascertain this agent's use in clinical practice.

Cryoheptadine is an antiserotonin agent known to stimulate appetite. In a randomized, double-blind, placebo-controlled study, 295 patients with advanced malignancy were treated with cryoheptadine or placebo. Patients receiving the active drug demonstrated a slight improvement in appetite.[123] However, no increase in weight gain was noted. There is currently no role for this medication in the treatment of cancer cachexia.

ETHICS

There is little debate about providing nutritional support for a reversible acute illness. However, controversy exists over initiating and sustaining nutritional support for patients with incurable or end-stage cancer, with little prospect of reversing the underlying disease and regaining nutritional independence. This topic is discussed further in Chapter 35. Patients with cancer may fall anywhere within this spectrum, and patient, family, and physician expectations should be considered in the decision-making process. Two major ethical issues must be addressed. The first relates to the balance of the benefits and burdens of nutritional support and the patient's wishes. The other relates to the allocation of resources, including time, money, personnel, and equipment.

Nutritional support accounts for approximately 1 percent of all health care dollars, which amounted to almost $8 billion in 1992.[124] Health care costs are under great scrutiny at present. Financial burden to both patient and system can be tremendous. Although no patient should be denied nutritional support based on resource issues, rational use of our increasingly limited resources should play a role in the decision-making process.

Through the ages, the act of giving food and drink has been symbolic of caring and compassion. Enteral feeding is believed by some to be a logical continuation of this basic tenet, while others feel that "forced feeding" is an invasive medical intervention, requiring definitive indications and consent. The debate has yet to be resolved, and each case is evaluated by its own merits and circumstances. In terms of legal considerations, almost every court has ruled in favor that nutritional support is a medical intervention that can be refused by either a competent patient or by a surrogate (when there is clear and convincing evidence that the patient would want therapy withdrawn). Excellent reviews and essays on the legal precedent are available.[125-127]

Several principles based on active patient, family, and physician participation can be used to direct the decision process:[128]

1. A patient's expressed wishes, either in the present or through a prior direc-

tive, should be the primary guiding force when tube feeding is a medical option.
2. Although enteral nutrition may prevent dehydration and malnutrition, no data supports its efficacy in providing comfort by alleviating the subjective conditions of thirst or hunger.
3. The decision to use enteral feedings must be made by assessing the benefits and burdens for each case.
4. A therapeutic trial of enteral feeding should be discontinued when the burdens clearly outweigh the benefits.
5. The patient should be the final arbiter in assessing benefits and burdens.

A thoughtful approach is necessary in the initiation and continuation of enteral tube feedings in the cancer patient. Potential benefits must be weighed against burdens, and realistic goals must be evaluated. While the patient is the final arbiter, the family and physician must participate and communicate in the decision making process.

CONCLUSION

Malnutrition is an important element in the cancer syndrome, affecting both the rate of complications and survival in these patients. The exact etiology of cancer cachexia is unclear and probably multifactorial. Putative factors include anorexia, increased energy expenditure, and alterations in intermediate metabolism.

In an attempt to reverse or at least prevent further deterioration of nutritional status, enteral nutrition plays an integral part in the treatment of patients with cancer. Although numerous studies demonstrate that enteral feeding improves biologic and metabolic endpoints in the cancer patient, there is a paucity of prospective data supporting a positive impact on survival. Specific recommendations for enteral nutrition in the cancer patient include the following:

1. All cancer patients should be evaluated for nutritional status.
2. Enteral nutrition should be given priority over TPN, as long as feeding through the gut is not contraindicated.
3. No specific nutritional formulation has yet been proved to have particular efficacy in the cancer patient.
4. Patients who are severely malnourished (more than 10 percent weight loss) may

benefit from preoperative enteral nutrition.

5. Routine use of enteral nutrition is not indicated in patients receiving chemotherapy or radiation treatment. However, severely malnourished patients may require nutritional support to prevent further malnutrition during treatment. Patients receiving bone marrow transplantation may benefit from either enteral nutrition, either by encouraged oral intake or tube feeding.

6. Further studies are needed, with an emphasis on survival and morbidity, to clarify the role of enteral nutrition in the postoperative cancer patient.

REFERENCES

1. Wingo PA, Tong T, Bolden S: Cancer statistics, 1995. CA 1995;45(1):8.
2. Warren S: The immediate causes of death in cancer. Am J Med Sci 1932;184:610.
3. DeWys WD, Begg C, Lavin PT et al: Prognostic effect of weight loss prior to chemotherapy in cancer patients. Am J Med 1980;69:491.
4. Bozzetti F, Migliavacca S, Scotti A et al: Impact of cancer, type, site, stage and treatment on the nutritional status of patients. Ann Surg 1982;196:170.
5. Meguid MM, Meguid V: Preoperative identification of the surgical cancer patient in need of postoperative supportive total parenteral nutrition. Cancer 1985; 55:258.
6. Daly JM, Thom AK: Neoplastic diseases. In Kinney JM, Jeejeebhoy KN, Hill GL et al (eds): Nutrition and Metabolism in Patient Care. Philadelphia: WB Saunders, 1988:567.
7. Hill GL, Beddoe AH: Dimensions of the human body and its compartments. In Kinney JM, Jeejeebhoy KN, Hill GL et al (eds): Nutrition and Metabolism in Patient Care. WB Saunders, 1988:89.
8. Lee J, Kolonel LN, Hinds MW: Relative merits of the weight-corrected-for-height indices. Am J Clin Nutr 1981;34:2521.
9. Studley HO: Percentage of weight loss—a basic indicator of surgical risk in patients with chronic peptic ulcer. JAMA 1936;106:458.
10. Durnin JVGA, Womersley J: Body fat assessed from total body density and its estimation from skinfold thickness: measurements on 481 men and women aged 16 to 72 years. Br J Nutr 1974;32:77.
11. Siri WE: University of California Radiation Publication, No. 3349. 1956.
12. Heymsfield SB, Olafson RP, Kutner MH et al: A radiographic method of quantifying protein-calorie undernutrition. Am J Clin Nutr 1979;32:693.
13. Lukaski HC: Methods for the assessment of human body composition: traditional and new. Am J Clin Nutr 1987;46:537.
14. Torosian MH, Mullen JL: Nutritional assessment. In Kaminski I, Mitchell V (eds): Hyperalimentation: A Guide for Clinicians. New York: Marcel Dekker, 1985: 47.
15. Pettigrew RA, Hill GL: Indicators of surgical risk and clinical judgement. Br J Surg 1986;73:47.
16. Reeds PJ, Laditan AAO: Serum albumin and transferrin in protein-energy malnutrition. Br J Nutr 1976;36:255.
17. Berstein LH, Leukhardt-Fairfield CJ, Pleban W et al: Usefulness of data on albumin and prealbumin concentrations in determining effectiveness of nutritional support. Clin Chem 1989;35(2):271.
18. Smale BF, Mullen JL, Buzby GP et al: The efficacy of nutritional assessment and support in cancer surgery. Cancer 1981;47:2375.
19. Harvey KB, Moldawer, LL, Bistrian BR et al: Biologic measures for the formulation of a hospital prognostic index. Am J Clin Nutr 1981;34:2013.
20. Holroyde CP, Skutches CL, Boden G et al: Glucose metabolism in cachectic patients with colorectal cancer. Cancer Res 1984;44:5910.
21. Saito T, Shimoda K, Shigemitsu Y et al: Complications of infection and immunologic status after surgery for patients with esophageal cancer. J Surg Onc 1994;48:21.
22. Norton JA, Peacock JL, Morrison SD: Cancer cachexia. CRC Crit Rev Oncol Hematol 1987;7:289.
23. Bernstein IL, Bernstein ID: Learned food aversion and cancer anorexia. Cancer Treat Rep 1981;65 (suppl 5):43.
24. Bernstein IL, Sigmundi RA: Tumor anorexia: a learned food aversion. Science 1980;209:416.
25. Smith JC, Blumsack JR: Learned food aversion as a factor in cancer therapy. Cancer Treat Rep 1981;65(suppl 5):37.
26. Abasov IT: Changes of gustatory sensitivity in cancerous patients. Sov Med 1961;25:47.
27. DeWys WD, Walters K: Abnormalities of taste sensation in cancer patients. Cancer 1975;36:1888.
28. DeWys WD: Abnormalities of taste as a remote effect of a neoplasm. Ann NY Acad Sci 1974;230:427.
29. Theologides A: Pathogenesis of cachexia in cancer. Cancer 1972;29(2):484.
30. Norton JA, Moley JF, Green MV et al: Parabiotic transfer of cancer anorexia cachexia in male rats. Cancer Res 1985;45:5547.
31. Illig KA, Maronian N, Peacock JL: Cancer cachexia is transmissible in plasma. J Surg Res 1992;52:353.
32. Pittinger T, Maronian N, Illig K et al: Induction of cachexia in rats by plasma from cancer-bearing patients. SSO 47th Cancer Symposium 1994;138. (Abstract).
33. Gelin J, Moldawer LL, Lonnroth C et al: Appearance of hybridoma growth factor/interleukin-6 in the serum of mice bearing a methylcholanthrene-induced sarcoma. Biochem Biophys Res Commun 1988;157:575.
34. Balkwill F, Osborne R, Burke F et al: Evidence for tumor necrosis factor/cachectin production in cancer. Lancet 1987;2:1229.
35. Aderka D, Fisher S, Levo Y et al: Cachectin/tumor necrosis factor production by cancer patients. Lancet 1985;2:1190.
36. Zembala M, Mytar B, Woloszyn M et al: Monocyte TNF production in gastrointestinal cancer. Lancet 1988;2:1262.
37. Fong Y, Moldawer LL, Marano H et al: Cachectin/TNF or IL-1α induces cachexia with redistribution of body proteins. Am J Physiol 1989;256:R659.
38. Oliff A, Defeno-Jones D, Boyer M et al: Tumors secreting human TNF/cachectin induce cachexia in mice. Cell 1987;50:555.
39. Sherry BA, Gelin J, Fong Y et al: Anticachectin/tumor necrosis factor-α antibodies attenuate development of cachexia in tumor models. FASEB 1989;3:1956.

40. Shivshanker K, Bennet RW, Haynie TP: Tumor-associated gastroparesis: correction with metaclopramide. Amer J Surg 1983;145:221.

41. Burke M, Bryson EI, Kark AE: Dietary intakes, resting metabolic rates, and body composition in benign and malignant gastrointestinal disease. Br Med J 1980;280:211.

42. Hansell DT, Davies JWL, Burns HJG: The relationship between resting energy expenditure and weight loss in benign and malignant disease. Ann Surg 1986; 203(3):240.

43. Macfie J, Burkinshaw L, Oxby C et al: The effect of gastrointestinal malignancy on resting energy expenditure. Br J Surg 1982;69:443.

44. Frederix EWHM, Soeters PB, Wouters EFM et al: Effect of different tumor types on resting energy expenditure. Cancer Res 19??;6138.

45. Dempsey DT, Feurer ID, Knox LS et al: Energy expenditure in malnourished gastrointestinal cancer patients. Cancer 1984;53:1265.

46. Hansell DT, Davies JWL, Burns HJG: The effects on resting energy expenditure of different tumor types. Cancer 1986;58:1739.

47. Falconer JS, Fearon KCH, Plester CE et al: Cytokines, the acute-phase response, and resting energy expenditure in cachectic patients with pancreatic cancer. Ann Surg 1994;219(4):325.

48. Luketich JD, Mullen JL, Feurer ID et al: Ablation of abnormal energy expenditure by curative tumor resection. Arch Surg 1990;125:337.

49. Arbeit JM, Lees DE, Corsey R et al: Resting energy expenditure in controls and cancer patients with localized and diffuse disease. Ann Surg 1984;199(3):292.

50. Kern KA, Norton JA: Cancer cachexia. J Parenter Enter Nutr 1988;12(3):286.

51. Brennan MF: Uncomplicated starvation versus cancer cachexia. Cancer Res 1977;37:2359.

52. Jeevanandam M, Legaspi A, Lowry SF et al: Effect of total parenteral nutrition on whole body protein kinetics in cachectic patients with benign or malignant disease. J Parenter Enter Nutr 1988;12(3):229.

53. Eden E, Ekman L, Bennegard K et al: Whole-body tyrosine flux in relation to energy expenditure in weight-losing cancer patients. Metabolism 1984;33(11):1020.

54. Burt ME, Stein TP, Schwade JG et al: Whole-body protein metabolism in cancer-bearing patients: effect of total parenteral nutrition and associated serum insulin response. Cancer 1984;53(6):1246.

55. Shaw JHF, Wolfe RR: Whole-body protein kinetics in patients with early and advanced gastrointestinal cancer: the response to glucose infusion and total parenteral nutrition. Surgery 1988;103(2):148.

56. Tayek JA, Bistrian BR, Hehir D et al: Improved protein kinetics and albumin synthesis by branched chain amino acid-enriched total parenteral nutrition in cancer cachexia. Cancer 1986;58:147.

57. Emery PW, Edwards RHT, Rennie MJ et al: Protein synthesis in muscle measured in vivo in cachectic patients with cancer. Br Med J 1984;289:584.

58. Shaw JHF, Humberstone DM, Douglas RG et al: Leucine kinetics in patients with benign disease, non-weight-losing cancer, and cancer cachexia: studies at the whole-body and tissue level and the response to nutritional support. Surgery 1991;109(1):37.

59. Lundholm K, Ekman L, Karlberg I et al: Protein synthesis in iver tissue under the influence of a methylcholanthrene-induced sarcoma in mice. Cancer Res 1979;39:4657.

60. Norton JA, Shamberger R, Stein P et al: The influence of tumor-bearing on protein metabolism in the rat. J Surg Res 1981;30:456.

61. Stein TP, Oram-Smith JC, Leskiw MJ et al: Tumor-caused changes in host protein synthesis under different dietary situations. Cancer Res 1976;36:3936.

62. Pain VM, Randall DP, Garlick PJ: Protein synthesis in liver and skeletal muscle of mice bearing an ascites tumor. Cancer Res 1984;44:1054.

63. Kokal WA, McCulloch A, Wright PD et al: Glucose turnover and recycling in colorectal cancer. Ann Surg 1983;198:601.

64. Shaw JHF, Wolfe RR: Glucose and urea kinetics in patients with early and advanced gastrointestinal cancer: the response to glucose infusion, parenteral feeding, and surgical resection. Surgery 1987;101(2):181.

65. Eden E, Edstrom S, Bennegard K et al: Glucose flux in relation to energy expenditure in malnourished patients with and without cancer during periods of fasting and feeding. Cancer Res 1984;44:1718.

66. Lundholm K, Edstrom S, Karlberg I et al: Glucose turnover, gluconeogenesis from glycerol, and estimation of net glucose cycling in cancer patients. Cancer 1982;50:1142.

67. Heber D, Chlebowski RT, Ishibashi DE et al: Abnormalities in glucose and protein metabolism in non cachectic lung cancer patients. Cancer Res 1982;42:4815.

68. Burt ME, Gorschboth CM, Brennan MF: A controlled, prospective, randomized trial evaluating the metabolic effects of enteral and parenteral nutrition in the cancer patient. Cancer 1982;49(6):1092.

69. Glicksman AS, Rawson RW: Diabetes and altered carbohydrate metabolism in patients with cancer. Cancer 1956;9:1127.

70. Yoshikawa T, Noguchi Y, Matsumoto A: Effects of tumor removal and body weight loss on insulin resistance in patients with cancer. Surgery 1994; 116:62.

71. Richtsmeier WJ, Dauchy R, Sauer LA: In vivo nutrient uptake by head and neck cancers. Cancer Res 1987;47:5230.

72. Nolop KB, Rhodes CG, Brudin LH et al: Glucose utilization in vivo by human pulmonary neoplasms. Cancer 1987;60:2682.

73. Shaw JHF, Humberstone DM, Wolfe RR: Energy and protein metabolism in sarcoma patients. Ann Surg 1988;283.

74. Long CL, Spenser JL, Kinney JM et al: Carbohydrate metabolism in normal man and effect of glucose infusion. J Appl Physiol 1971;31:102.

75. Humberstone DM, Shaw JH: Metabolism in hematologic malignancy. Cancer 1988;62:1619.

76. Beck SA, Tisdale MJ: Production of lipolytic and proteolytic factors by a murine tumor-producing cachexia in the host. Cancer Res 1987;47:5919.

77. Kitada S, Hays EF, Mead JF: A lipid mobilizing factor in serum of tumor-bearing mice. Lipids 1980;15:168.

78. Masuno H, Yamasaki N, Okuda H: Purification and characterization of lipolytic factor (toxohormone-L) from cell-free fluid of ascites Sarcoma 180. Cancer Res 1981;41:284.

79. Shaw JHF, Wolfe RR: Fatty acid and glycerol kinetics in septic patients and in patients with gastrointestinal cancer: the response to glucose infusion and parenteral feeding. Ann Surg 1987;205:368.

80. Waterhouse C: Oxidation and metabolic interconversion in malignant cachexia. Cancer Treat Rep 1981;65(suppl 5):61.

81. Vlassara H, Spiegal RJ, Doval DS: Reduced plasma lipoprotein lipase activity in patients with malignancy associated weight loss. Horm Metab Res 1986;18:698.

82. Hansell DT, Davies JWL, Burns HJG et al: The oxidation of body fuel stores in cancer patients. Ann Surg 1986;204(6):637.

83. Eden E, Edstrom S, Bennegard K et al: Glycerol dynamics in weight-losing cancer patients. Surgery 1985;97:176.

84. Rombeau JL, Lew JI: Nutritional-metabolic support of the intestine: implications for the critically ill patient. In Kinney JM, Tucker HN (eds): Organ Metabolism and Nutrition: Ideas for Future Critical Care. New York: Raven Press, 1994:197.

85. Kudsk KA, Croce MA, Fabian TC et al: Enteral versus parenteral feeding: effects on septic morbidity after blunt and penetrating abdominal trauma. Ann Surg 1992;215:503.

86. Sandstrom R, Drott C, Hyltander A et al: The effect of postoperative intravenous feeding (TPN) on outcome following major surgery evaluated in a randomized study. Ann Surg 1993;217:185.

87. Jackson WD, Grand RJ: The human intestinal response to enteral nutrients: a review. J Amer Coll Nutr 1991;10(5):500.

88. Nirgoitis JG, Andrassy RJ: Bacterial translocation. In Borlase BC, Bell SJ, Blackburn GL et al (eds): Enteral Nutrition. Chapman & Hall, 1994:15.

89. Fong Y, Marano MA, Barber A et al: Total parenteral nutrition and bowel rest modify the metabolic response to endotoxin in humans. Ann Surg 1989;210(4):449.

90. Daly JM, Lieberman MD, Glodfine J et al: Enteral nutrition with supplemental arginine, RNA, and omega-3 fatty acids in patients after operation: immunologic, metabolic and clinical outcome. Surgery 1992;112:56.

91. Dresler CM, Jeevanandam M, Brennan MF: Metabolic efficacy of enteral feeding in malnourished cancer and noncancer patients. Metabolism 1987;36(1):82.

92. Lundholm K, Bennegard K, Eden E et al: Efflux of 3-methylhistidine from the leg in cancer patients who experience weight loss. Cancer Res 1982;42:4807.

93. Bennegard K, Lindmark L, Eden E et al: Flux of amino acids across the leg in weight-losing cancer patients. Cancer Res 1984;44:386.

94. Bennegard K, Eden E, Ekman L et al: Metabolic response of whole body and peripheral tissues to eneral nutrition in weight-losing cancer and noncancer patients. Gastroenterology 1983;85:92.

95. Edstrom S, Bennegard K, Eden E et al: Energy and tissue metabolism in patients with cancer during nutritional support. Arch Otolaryngol 1982;108:697.

96. Daly JM, Bonau R, Stofberg P et al: Immediate postoperative jejunostomy feeding: clinical and metabolic results in a prospective trial. Am J Surg 1987;153:198.

97. Bassett MR, Dobie RA: Patterns of nutritional deficiency in head and neck cancer. Otolaryngol Head Neck Surg 1983;91:119.

98. Brooks GB: Nutritional status: a prognostic indicator in head and neck cancer. Otolaryngol Head Neck Surg 1985;93:69.

99. Sako K, Lore JM, Kaufman S et al: Parenteral hyperalimentation in surgical patients with head and neck cancer: a randomized study. J Surg Onc 1981;16:391.

100. Daly JM, Hearne B, Dunaj J et al: Nutritional rehabilitation in patients with advanced head and neck cancer receiving radiation therapy. Amer J Surg 1984;148:514.

101. Burt ME, Brennan MF: Nutritional support of the patient with esophageal cancer. Semin Oncol 1984;11(2):127.

102. Lim STK, Choa RG, Lam KH et al: Total parenteral nutrition versus gastrostomy in the preoperative preparation of patients with carcinoma of the oesophagus. Br J Surg 1981;68:69.

103. Haffajee AA, Angorn IB: Nutritional status and the nonspecific cellular and humoral immune response in esophageal carcinoma. Ann Surg 1979;189(4):475.

104. Brennan MF, Pisters PWT, Posner M et al: A prospective randomized trial of total parenteral nutrition after major pancreatic resection for malignancy. Ann Surg 1994;220(4):436.

105. Kokal WA: The impact of antitumor therapy on nutrition. Cancer 1985;55:273.

106. DeVries EGE, Mulder NH, Houwen B et al: Enteral nutrition by nasogastric tube in adult patients treated with intensive chemotherapy for acute leukemia. Am J Clin Nutr 1982;35:1490.

107. Bounous G, Gentile JM, Hugon J: Elemental diet in the management of the intestinal lesion produced by 5 fluorouracil in man. Can J Surg 1971;14:312.

108. Szeluga DJ, Stuart RK, Brookmeyer R et al: Nutritional support of bone marrow transplant recipients: prospective, randomized clinical trial comparing total parenteral nutrition to an enteral feeding program. Cancer Res 1987;47:3309.

109. Mulder PO, Bouman JG, Gietema JA et al: Hyperalimentation in autologous bone marrow transplantation for solid tumors. Cancer 1989;64:2045.

110. Evans WK, Nixon DW, Daly JM et al: A randomized study of oral nutritional support versus ad lib nutritional intake during chemotherapy for advanced colorectal and non-small-cell lung cancer. J Clin Oncol 1987;5(1):113.

111. McArdle AH, Wittnich C, Freeman CR: Elemental diet as prophylaxis against radiation injury : histologic and ultrastructural studies. Arch Surg 1985;120:1026.

112. Bounous G: The use of elemental diets during cancer therapy. AntiCancer Res 1983;3:299.

113. McArdle AH, Reid EC, Laplante MP et al: Prophylaxis against radiation injury. Arch Surg 1986;121:879.

114. Douglass HO, Milliron S, Nava H: Elemental diet as an adjuvant for patients with locally advanced gastrointestinal cancer receiving radiation therapy: a prospectively randomized study. J Parenter Enter Nutr 1978;2:682.

115. Grosvenor M, Bulcavage L, Chlebowski RT: Symptoms potentially influencing weight loss in a cancer population. Cancer 1989;63:330.

116. Nelson KA, Walsh TD: Metaclopramide in anorexia caused by cancer-associated dyspepsia syndrome (CADS). J Palliat Care 1993;9:14.

117. Aisner J, Tchekmedyian NS, Moody M: High-dose megestrol acetate for the treatment of advanced breast cancer: dose and toxicities. Semin Hematol 1987;24(Suppl 1):48.

118. Loprinzi CL, Ellison NM, Schaid DJ: A controlled trial of megestrol acetate in patients with cancer anorexia/cachexia. Proc Am Soc Clin Onc 1990;9:321.

119. Willox JC, Corr J, Shaw J: Prednisolone as an appetite stimulant in patients with cancer. Br Med J 1984;228:17.

120. Moertel CG, Schutt AJ, Reitemeier RJ: Corticosteroid therapy of preterminal gastrointestinal cancer. Cancer 1974;33:1607.

121. Wadleigh R, Spaulding M, Lembersky B: Dronabinol enhancement of appetite in cancer patients. Proc Am Soc Clin Onc 1990;9:1280.
122. Plasse TF, Gorter RW, Krasnow SH et al: Recent clinical experience with dronabinol. Pharmacol Biochem Behav 1991;40:695.
123. Kardinal CG, Loprinzi CL, Schaid DJ: A controlled trial of cryoheptadine in cancer patients with anorexia and/or cachexia. Cancer 1990;65:2657.
124. Howard L: Home parenteral and enteral nutrition in cancer patients. Cancer 1993;72:3531.
125. Annas GJ: Do feeding tubes have more rights than patients? Hastings Cent Rep 1986;16:26.
126. Paris JL: When burdens of feeding outweigh benefits. Hastings Cent Rep 1986;16:30.
127. King DG, Maillet JO: Position of the American Dietetic Association: issues in feeding the terminally ill adult. J Am Diet Assoc 1987;87:78.
128. Quill TE: Utilization of nasogastric feeding tubes in a group of chronically ill, elderly patients in a community hospital. Arch Intern Med 1989;149:1937.
129. Langstein HN, Norton JA: Mechanisms of cancer cachexia. Hematol Oncol Clin North Am 1991;5(1):103.
130. Nixon DW, Lawson D, Kutner MH et al: Hyperalimentation of the cancer patient with protein-calorie undernutrition. Cancer Res 1981;41:2038.

18

Nutrition and Trauma

Mark J. Koruda
Thomas A. Santora

The majority of critically ill trauma patients are unable to eat voluntarily; therefore, nutrients must be provided by intravenous (IV) or enteral infusion. Since the early 1970s, total parenteral nutrition (TPN) has had an important role in supporting the seriously injured trauma patient; however, enteral nutrition (EN) has recently realized an increasingly important role in the management of this patient population. TPN may maintain the nutritional status of patients who are unable to receive EN, but the absence of nutrients in the gut lumen promotes mucosal atrophy and impaired mucosal barrier functions, which may contribute to hypermetabolism, sepsis, and the multiple organ dysfunction syndrome. The increased enthusiasm for the use of EN in the injured critically ill is due not only to cost savings but to EN's beneficial effects on clinical outcome.

RATIONALE FOR THE USE OF ENTERAL NUTRITION IN CRITICAL ILLNESS

The gastrointestinal (GI) tract is commonly regarded as an organ that is involved solely with the digestion and absorption of nutrients. However, recent investigations have demonstrated that the gut also regulates and processes metabolic substances shuttling through the splanchnic circulation as well as acts as a major component of the host defense system.[1] The gut resists invasion by pathogenic microorganisms by providing secretory IgA antibodies and a translocation barrier consisting of a mucosal component and a submucosal collection of coordinated lymphatic tissue known as the gut-associated lymphatic tissue (GALT). The GALT system provides approximately one lymphocyte for every five enterocytes within the GI tract. Both the epithelial cells of the intestinal mucosa and the lymphocytic cells of the GALT system are being rapidly renewed and thus are markedly affected by nutrient availability, enterohepatic hormones, and intestinal blood flow.

The most important stimulus for mucosal cell proliferation is the direct presence of nutrients in the intestinal lumen.[2] Bowel rest due to starvation or administration of TPN leads to villous atrophy,[3] decreased cellularity, and a reduction in intestinal disaccharidase activities.[4] Some of the effects of nutrients on the GI tract are mediated by enterohormones such as gastrin, bombesine, and enteroglucagon and by nonenteric hormones such as growth hormone and epidermal growth factor.[5]

Many factors affect both the intestinal barrier and the bacterial microflora in critically ill patients (Table 18–1). In the immediate postinjury phase, the intestinal mucosa atrophies due to many factors, including the lack of intraluminal nutrients and a redistribution in the interorgan exchange of metabolic substrates. The intestinal consumption of glutamine increases

TABLE 18–1   Components of the GUT Barrier

Microbial
Contact inhibition
Colonization resistance

Mechanical
Peristalsis
Mucus layer
Epithelial barrier
Junctional complexes
Desquamation

Immunologic
GALT (gut-associated lymphoid tissue)
Reticuloendothelial function

with stress.[6] This demand for glutamine in the intestine may exceed its production from muscle proteolysis, thus resulting in enterocyte fuel deficits if this crucial nutrient is not provided in the gut lumen. The large bowel also suffers a deficit of fuels if fasting is prolonged, and systemic antibiotic administration may exacerbate these colonic deficits by altering the normal intestinal flora responsible for the bacterial fermentation of polysaccharides in the colon. Prolonged fasting in the stressed, critically ill patient can lead to intestinal barrier failure, resulting in increased permeability to bacteria and endotoxins.

In the experimental burn model, gut atrophy and dysfunction is reversed or ameliorated by the administration of early EN.[7] Specific intestinal fuels, such as glutamine, added to the standard enteral diet may further stimulate intestinal trophism. The specific nutritional management of critically ill patients remains controversial; experimental work is underway to determine whether specific intestinal fuels such as glutamine, fiber, or short-chain fatty acids (SCFAs) have beneficial effects for the critically ill.

STUDIES COMPARING ENTERAL AND PARENTERAL NUTRITION

Numerous animal models have investigated the relative benefits of enteral and parenteral nutrition. Enterally fed rats demonstrated improved survival after septic[8-10] and hemorrhagic[11] challenges compared with parenterally fed animals. In animals that sustained femoral fractures, lymphocyte responses returned to normal significantly earlier in animals fed enterally compared with the parenteral group.[12] In a rat model, parenteral nutrition and oral elemental diets promoted bacterial translocation from the gut.[13] Enteral feeding, as compared

with parenteral nutrition, significantly blunted the hypermetabolic response to burn injury.[7]

Several clinical studies have evaluated the efficacy of nutritional support in trauma patients. Border and associates retrospectively examined the effect of enteral feeding on the intensive care unit (ICU) course of 66 victims of multiple blunt trauma.[14] In their study, enteral protein intake was associated with a reduction in septic severity score. Even though patients nourished parenterally received twice the amount of protein that the enterally fed group received, the lack of enteral nutrition resulted in significantly higher septic severity scores.

Although Adams and associates in 1986 demonstrated comparable caloric intakes and nitrogen balance lead to comparable complication rates between 23 enterally fed and 23 parenterally fed trauma patients,[15] recent clinical studies have demonstrated improved outcome with enteral nutrition.[16-19] After burn injury, enteral nutrition was associated with reduced morbidity and mortality[16] and with improved immune function.[17]

Moore and associates demonstrated reduced septic morbidity[18] and improved visceral protein synthesis[19] in patients following major abdominal trauma who received enteral nutrition compared with those managed with TPN. In this study, patients requiring emergent laparotomy for trauma who had an Abdominal Trauma Index (ATI)[20] greater than 15 but less than 40 were randomized to receive either enteral nutrition (Vivonex TEN) or TPN. The ATI, which has been shown to directly correlate with postoperative septic complications,[21] was used to stratify severity of injury in this study. Nutritional support was instituted 12 hours postoperatively in both groups. Despite a slight advantage in protein-caloric intake through the parenteral route, no differences in nitrogen balance were noted between the two groups at postoperative day 5. The overall incidence of septic morbidity was 17 percent in the enterally fed group vs 37 percent in the parenteral group (Table 18–2). The enteral nutrition group had significantly fewer major infections, abdominal abscesses, and pneumonias than the TPN group (3 percent vs 20 percent).

This study has been referred to as the "pivotal clinical trial" that defined the relative benefits of enteral nutrition in the trauma setting. However, a major criticism of this study is that the most severely injured patients—those most prone to infectious complications—were excluded from the analysis.

TABLE 18–2   Septic Complications of Total Enteral Nutrition vs Total Parenteral Nutrition Study Groups

Complications	Group		
	TEN (N = 29)	TPN (N = 30)	*P* Value
Major Infections			
Abdominal abscess	1	2	
	1 (3%)	6 (20%)	0.03
Pneumonia	0	6	
Minor Infections			
Wound	3	1	
Catheter	0	2	
	4 (14%)	5 (17%)	NS
Urinary	0	0	
Miscellaneous	1	0	
Total Patients	5 (17%)	11 (37%)	

Adapted from Moore FA, Moore EE, Jones TN et al: TEN vs. TPN following major abdominal trauma-reduced septic morbidity. J Trauma 1989;29(1):916–923.

Kudsk and associates likewise addressed the issue of enteral vs parenteral nutrition in the trauma patient. This study randomized 98 patients who suffered major abdominal blunt or penetrating trauma with an ATI greater than 15 to either immediate postoperative TPN or enteral nutrition (Vital HN).[22] Unlike the previous report,[18] this study did not exclude the most severely injured patients.

From a nutritional standpoint, there were no significant differences in nitrogen balance between the groups. The enteral group sustained a significantly lower incidence of pneumonia, intra-abdominal abscess, and catheter sepsis (Table 18–3). More important, the most significant differences occurred in the massively injured patients—those requiring more than 20 units of blood—who had an ATI greater than 40 or required reoperation within 72 hours of injury (Fig. 18–1). No significant differences in infection rates were noted in patients with an Injury Severity Score (ISS) of 20 or less or an ATI less than 24. In the group of patients with an ISS greater than 20 or with an ATI greater than 24, the incidence of an infectious complication was six-fold to seven-fold greater in the TPN patients. For patients with an ISS greater than 20 and an ATI greater than 24, TPN was associated with an 11-fold increase in the infection compared with the enterally fed group.

This study also demonstrated that EN produced a greater increase in constitutive proteins and greater decreases in acute-phase proteins after severe trauma when compared with TPN.[24] Previous investigators have drawn an association between the development of sepsis and a decrease in the transport proteins, albu-

TABLE 18–3   Septic Morbidity Associated with Enteral or Parenteral Feeding

Sepsis	Enteral (N = 51)	Parenteral (N = 45)	*P* Value
Pneumonia	11.8%	31%	<0.02
Intra-abdominal abscess	1.9%	13.3%	<0.04
Empyema	1.9%	9%	NS
Line sepsis	1.9%	13.3%	<0.05
Dehiscence	5.9%	8.9%	NS
Abscess (abdominal or empyema)	3.9%	17.8%	<0.03
Pneumonia or abscess	13.7%	37.8%	<0.02
Pneumonia, abscess, or line sepsis	15.7%	40%	NS

Adapted from Kudsk KA, Croce MA, Fabian TC et al: Enteral versus parenteral feeding. Effects on septic morbidity after blunt and penetrating abdominal trauma. J Trauma 1992;215:503–513.

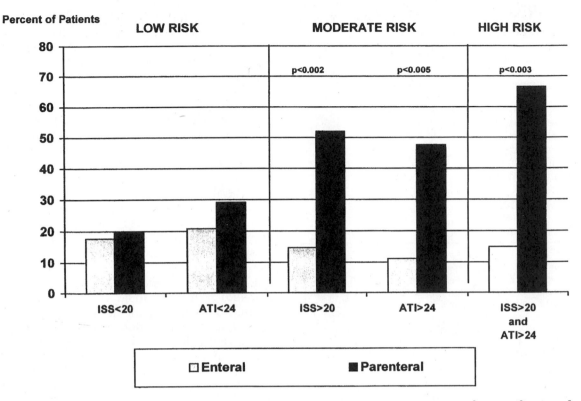

Percent of Patients

FIGURE 18–1 Frequency of infections (pneumonia, intra-abdominal abscess, or empyema) after stratification of patients by severity of injury. (Adapted from Kudsk KA, Croce MA, Fabian TC et al: Enteral versus parenteral feeding. Effects on septic morbidity after blunt and penetrating abdominal trauma. J Trauma 1992;215:503–513.)

min, and transferrin or increased concentrations of acute phase reactants such as α_1-glycoprotein and C reactive protein.[19,25] Although some of the hepatic protein reprioritization appeared to be caused by nutrient route, a more important factor in visceral protein levels is a reduction in septic morbidity associated with enteral feeding.[24]

Moore and others conducted a meta-analysis that combined data from eight prospective-randomized trials that compared the nutritional efficacy of early (within 72 hours) EN and TPN in trauma and other high-risk postoperative general surgical patients.[26] This study of 238 cumulative patients determined that early enteral postoperative nutrition resulted in a significant, two-fold decrease in septic complications compared with those patients administered TPN (Table 18–4). It is worthy of note that in all the studies included in this meta-analysis, the presence of an intestinal anastomosis distal to the site of tube feeding did not preclude the early institution of enteral feeding (i.e., within 24 hours of surgery).

In summary, clinical studies over the past decade have demonstrated that early EN is the preferred route of nutritional support in the trauma patient because it reduces the incidence of septic complications compared with TPN and has beneficial effects on the visceral protein profiles; the exact mechanisms for these effects are not yet clear. Although EN has been shown to maintain intestinal structure and function in various animal models,[27,28] there is no sound clinical evidence that either bacterial translocation or intestinal permeability is improved with enteral nutrition in humans.[29] It is conceivable that TPN itself may promote susceptibility to bacterial infection through immunosuppression or other means; however, there is no direct evidence to support this latter concept either.

"SPECIALIZED" ENTERAL FORMULAS FOR TRAUMA

Perhaps a dozen or more enteral products have been formulated specifically to suit the

TABLE 18–4 Meta-analysis of Postoperative Septic Complications In Patients Fed Enterally or Parenterally

Complication	Enteral (N = 118)	Parenteral (N = 112)
Abdominal abscess	5	7
Pneumonia	6	15
Wound infection	4	3
Bacteremia	2	5
Urinary tract infection	1	3
Catheter sepsis	0	7
Other	6	6
Total events	24	46
No. of patients	19	39
% of patients	16	35*

*$P < 0.05$ for patients: $P < 0.03$ excluding patients with line sepsis.
Adapted from Moore F, Feliciano D, Andrassy R et al: Early enteral feeding, compared with parenteral, reduces postoperative septic complications. Ann Surg 1992;216:173–183.

needs of the trauma or critically ill patient. These diets, in general, have an intermediate to high protein content. Nitrogen is provided as hydrolyzed protein with many containing a significant proportion as short-chain peptides or free amino acids. Specific crystalline amino acids (glutamine, arginine, branched-chain amino acids) have also been supplemented in certain products for their putative end-organ effects.

The proposed advantage for "peptide"-based enteral formulas lies in the greater ease of absorption of the dipeptide and tripeptide protein moieties. Before absorption, intact protein must be hydrolyzed to peptides or free amino acids. The rate-limiting step of protein assimilation lies in the carrier-specific mucosal absorption of individual amino acids. Dipeptides and tripeptides circumvent this rate-limiting step and are directly absorbed by the enterocyte. Although clinical studies have demonstrated increased absorption of dipeptide and tripeptide solutions,[30-32] there remains a lack of data from prospective randomized studies on the suitability and effectiveness of enteral products containing oligopeptides in the trauma setting.[33,34]

Additional attention is currently being focused on the immunostimulatory effects of diets supplemented with the amino acid arginine, omega-3 fatty acids, and ribonucleic acids. Previous prospective randomized clinical studies have demonstrated improved clinical outcome in patients fed an "immune-stimula-tory diet" after burn injury[35] and cancer surgery[36,37] and in ICU patients.[38] Two studies to date have specifically evaluated the relative efficacy of immune-enhancing diets in trauma patients.

In a small, single-center trial 37 trauma patients were randomized to receive a standard diet or a diet supplemented with arginine, β-carotene, and linolenic acid for up to 10 days.[39] Patients who received the specialized formula demonstrated a decreased incidence of infection (3/19 vs 10/18, $P < 0.05$) and improved nitrogen balance. The significant decrease in infectious complications seen with use of the immunoenhancing diet was due to the reduction in incidence of pneumonia (1 vs 7).

Another recent study compared the early use of a standard enteral formula (Vivonex TEN) with an immune-enhancing formula (Immun-aid).[40] In this multicenter, prospective, controlled trial, 98 patients sustaining major torso trauma were randomized to receive early EN with the immune-enhancing diet (study: n = 51) or the standard stress enteral formula (control: n = 48). After 7 days of feeding, the groups had equivalent increases in total protein, albumin, and transferrin concentrations; however, patients receiving the immune-enhancing diet experienced significantly greater increases in total lymphocytes, T-lymphocytes, and T-helper cells. Additionally, these patients had significantly fewer intra-abdominal abscesses (study 0 percent vs control 11 percent, $P = 0.023$) and significantly less multiorgan failure (study 0 percent vs control 11 percent, $P = 0.023$).

The potential to moderate the immune response by nutritional intake shows exciting promise in the management of the high-risk, critically ill trauma patient. Additional clinical trials demonstrating positive patient outcomes are necessary before these specialized enteral formulas can be considered the standard of practice in the management of the trauma patient.

ENTERAL ACCESS

The now-recognized importance of early EN in the trauma patient has made access to the GI tract a high-priority intervention early in the management of this patient population. In the nonoperative trauma patient, nasogastric feeding through small-bore (7 to 10 F) or large-bore (14-18 F) tubes is easy to establish, maintain, and use. Aggressive enteral feeding into the stomach is frequently poorly tolerated in this patient population due to gastric atony, and, in the context of depressed sensorium from associated head injury, places patients at extreme risk for regurgitation and aspiration. Use of weighted tubes to facilitate passage beyond the pylorus may be used in patients with delayed gastric emptying or individuals at high risk for aspiration. Although prudence would indicate feeding patients at risk for aspiration into the duodenum or beyond, transpyloric tube placement does not eliminate the risk of aspiration.[30] Transpyloric feeding does reduce the risk of aspiration in the enterally fed population if the tube is positioned at or beyond the ligament of Treitz. Positioning nasoenteric tubes at or beyond the ligament of Treitz is facilitated by using larger-bore tubes with steerable guidewires; fluoroscopy or endoscopy in experienced hands can hasten proper positioning. Percutaneous endoscopic gastrostomy (PEG) with or without endoscopically placed jejunostomy (PEJ) facilitate removal of tubes from the nose, thus potentially reducing the likelihood of sinusitis resulting from prolonged nasal tube placement. PEG or PEJ is usually reserved for the patient who will require prolonged enteral access.

In the trauma patient who undergoes abdominal exploration for management of injuries, enteral access should be considered if significant injuries are present. In the event of severe injuries that require staged procedures, perform enteral access at the time of definitive management and reconstruction of the GI injuries. Options for enteral access include (1) a nasojejunal tube that is advanced into the stomach by the anesthesiologist and then manually fed into position by the operating surgeon, (2) a combination gastrostomy/transpyloric gastrojejunostomy tube that allows simultaneous gastric decompression and jejunal access for feeding, placed through one gastrotomy and thereby avoiding the potential complications of enterotomy,[41] and (3) a dedicated feeding jejunostomy tube. Several studies have supported the safe and efficacious use of both small-caliber (7 F) needle catheter jejunostomy or larger-bore (16 or 18 F) feeding jejunostomies.[23,33,41-44]

The specific technique of enteral access must be individualized for each patient based on knowledge of the severity of injury, potential for significant postoperative complications, presence of comorbid conditions, and status of preinjury nutritional condition.

ENTERAL NUTRIENT ADMINISTRATION

Administration of EN requires knowledge of a patient's intestinal motility status, the antici-

pated site of nutrient delivery, and preinjury comorbidities that may necessitate specialized nutrient formulation. The most common factor influencing adequate absorption of EN is the status of GI motility in relationship to the site of delivery of EN.

It is well known that abdominal surgery transiently disrupts GI motility in an organized pattern. The small intestine may never lose or rapidly regains normal motility, whereas the stomach may remain atonic for 24 to 72 hours. Dysmotility is most prominent in the colon, where atony may persist for 72 to 96 hours. Thus, in the patient who has undergone abdominal surgery, the most efficacious early EN regimen would be delivered with a low-residual nutrient formulation through jejunal tube placement.

Another important factor in tolerance to early EN administration is the relative tonicity of the nutrient formula. The small bowel can tolerate volume in deference to high tonicity, especially in the early postoperative period when splanchnic blood flow may be altered; conversely, the stomach can tolerate high tonicity but not large volumes. Knowledge of this gut physiology is important when initiating feedings, because early EN has anecdotally been associated with the development of intestinal ischemia.[45] Although no direct cause-and-effect relationship has been established, it is thought increasing lumenal tonicity with EN in an underperfused splanchnic circulation leads to an imbalance in oxygen supply/demand within the enterocyte, resulting in cell death. It is common practice to correct perfusion deficits to normalize splanchnic circulation before initiating EN to minimize this catastrophic complication.

Enteral feedings should be initiated through a gastric tube at full strength regardless of tonicity, at 50 ml/hour, and advanced no faster than 25 ml/hour/8 hours until goal rate is achieved. To minimize the potential for regurgitation and aspiration, the patient is positioned in a 30 degree reverse Trendelenburg position and the gastric tube is aspirated every 4 hours for residual. When enteral feeding is established through intestinal tubes, the initial formulation is delivered at half strength to reduce tonicity, which is especially important in the postoperative patient. The initial rate is 25 ml/hour and is increased no more than 25 ml/hour/8 hours until goal rate is achieved. Once goal rate is achieved, the strength of tube feeding is increased to three quarters and then subsequently to full strength on 8-hour intervals. While administering enteral nutrition, it is prudent to closely follow the abdominal examination for development of pain, tenderness, and distension as well as signs of dysmotility such as reflux of feedings into the proximal GI tract or diarrhea. All the above signs indicate intolerance to the administration of EN, and indicate the need to reduce or eliminate EN.

SUMMARY

In the past 2 decades nutritional support has rapidly become an integral part of the medical care of the critically ill patient. Although parenteral nutrition has been the primary mode of delivering nutrients to this patient population, there has been renewed interest in the use of EN in the management of the critically ill. This interest arises from recognition of the importance of the barrier function of the GI epithelium, the emergence of specialized, immune-enhancing enteral formulas, and innovative techniques and equipment to allow early postoperative feeding.

Even though the benefits of aggressive EN are now known, not every patient undergoing a trauma laparotomy benefits from immediate enteral access and nutrition (Fig. 18–2). Patients who experience mild injury (ATI < 18, ISS < 16) have a low incidence of complica-

tions and are usually expected to resume an oral diet within 4 to 7 days after injury. Extenuating circumstances such as significant head injury (Glasgow Coma Scale ≤ 10), protracted shock, premorbid malnutrition, limited physiologic reserve (such as frequently seen in the elderly), or significant comorbid conditions should prompt consideration of establishment of enteral access at laparotomy with the goal of achieving total EN. In patients who experience postoperative complications, establish enteral access early and institute total EN.

For the moderately injured patient (18 < ATI < 40; 16 < ISS < 40), the possibility of postoperative complications or delayed recovery is such that enteral access should be established at the initial surgery with the intent of initiating early total EN. It is this patient population for whom enteral nutrition has demonstrated clinical benefit.

The massively injured patient (ATI > 40, ISS > 40) is at significant risk for postinjury complications. If feasible, these patients should have gastric or jejunal access or both obtained at laparotomy, either by separate gastrostomy and jejunostomy tubes or by a combination gastrojejunostomy tube. Although the ultimate goal in the nutritional management of these patients is to establish total EN, it is not uncommon for feeding intolerance to occur with

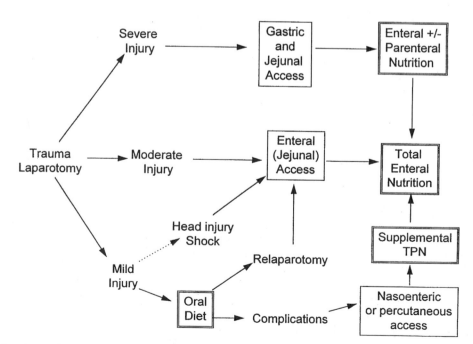

FIGURE 18–2   Algorithm for nutritional support of the trauma patient. (Adapted from Moore FA, Moore EE: Trauma. In Zaloga G (ed): Nutrition in Critical Care. St. Louis: Mosby, 1994:571–586.)

such extensive injuries. Low-dose EN is initiated after resuscitation from surgery and is advanced as tolerated to meet full nutritional goals. Careful monitoring of these patients is necessary to minimize the potential for nutrient-induced abdominal catastrophes. Parenteral supplementation to meet total nutritional goals is prudent until EN intolerance resolves, thus allowing full EN to be accomplished safely.

REFERENCES

1. Udall JN, Walker WA: Mucosal defense mechanisms. In Marsh M (ed): Immunopathology of the Small Intestine. New York: John Wiley & Sons, 1987:3–20.
2. Johnson LR: Regulation of gastrointestinal growth. In Johnson L (ed): Physiology of the Gastrointestinal Tract, 2nd edition. New York: Raven Press, 1987:301–333.
3. Levine GM, Deren JJ, Steiger E: Role of oral intake in maintenance of gut mass and disaccharide activity. Gastroenterology 1974;67:975–982.
4. Raul F, Norieger R, Doffeol M: Modifications of brush border enzyme activities during starvation in the jejunum and ileum of adult rats. Enzyme 1982;28: 328–335.
5. Al-Naffusi AJ, Wright NA: The effect of epidermal growth factor (EGF) on cell proliferation of the gastrointestinal mucosa in rodents. Virchows Arch [Cell Pathol] 1982;40:63–69.
6. Souba WW, Wilmore DW: Postoperative alteration of arteriovenous exchange of amino acids across the gastrointestinal tract. Surgery 1983;94:342–350.
7. Mochizuki H, Trocki O, Domioni L: Mechanism of prevention of postburn hypermetabolism and catabolism by early enteral feeding. Ann Surg 1984;200:297–310.
8. Kudsk KA, Carpenter G, Peterson SR et al: Effect of enteral and parenteral feeding in malnourished rats with hemoglobin-*E. coli* adjuvant peritonitis. J Surg Res 1981;31:105–110.
9. Kudsk KA, Stone JM, Carpenter G et al: Enteral and parenteral feeding influences mortality after hemoglobin *E. coli* peritonitis in normal rats. J Trauma 1983; 23:605–609.
10. Peterson SR, Kudsk KA, Carpenter G et al: Malnutrition and immunocompetence: increased mortality following an infectious challenge during hyperalimentation. J Trauma 1981;21:528.
11. Knowles RCY, Prielipp R, Ward K et al: Peptide-based enteral nutrition is superior to parenteral nutrition and elemental enteral nutrition following hemorrhagic hypotension. J Trauma. In press.
12. Renk CM, Owens DR, Birkhahn RH: Effect of intravenous or oral feeding on immunocompetence in traumatized rats. J Parenter Enter Nutr 1985;4:587.
13. Alverdy JC, Aoys E, Moss GS: Total parenteral nutrition promotes bacterial translocation from the gut. Surgery 1988;104:185–190.
14. Border J, Hassett J, LaDuca J et al: The gut origin septic states in blunt multiple trauma (ISS 40) in the ICU. Ann Surg 1987;206:427–448.
15. Adams S, Dellinger EP, Wertz MJ et al: Enteral versus parenteral nutritional support following laparotomy for trauma: a prospective trial. J Trauma 1986;26: 882–891.
16. Alexander JW, Macmillan BG, Stinnet JD: Beneficial effects of aggressive protein feeding in severely burned children. Surgery 1980;192:505.
17. Antonacci A, Cowles S, Reaves L: The role of nutrition in immunologic function. Infect Surg 1984;3:590.
18. Moore FA, Moore EE, Jones TN et al: TEN versus TPN following major abdominal trauma—reduced septic morbidity. J Trauma 1989;29(1):916–923.
19. Peterson VM, Moore EE, Jones TN et al: Total enteral nutrition versus total parenteral nutrition after major torso injury: attenuation of hepatic protein reprioritization. Surgery 1988;104:199–207.
20. Moore EE, Dunn EL, Jones TN et al: Penetrating abdominal trauma index. J Trauma 1982;21:439–444.
21. Borlase BC, Moore EE, Moore FA: The abdominal trauma index—a critical reassessment and validation. J Trauma 1990;30:1340–1347.
22. Kudsk KA, Croce MA, Fabian TC et al: Enteral versus parenteral feeding. Effects on septic morbidity after blunt and penetrating abdominal trauma. J Trauma 1992;215:503–513.
23. Sagar S, Harland P, Shields R: Early post-operative feeding with elemental diet. Br Med J 1979;1: 293–295.
24. Kudsk KA, Minard G, Wojtysiak SL et al: Visceral protein response to enteral versus parenteral nutrition and sepsis in patients with trauma. Surgery 1994;116: 516–523.
25. Sganga G, Siegel JH, Brown G et al: Reprioritization of hepatic protein release in trauma and sepsis. Arch Surg 1985;120:187–199.
26. Moore F, Feliciano D, Andrassy R et al: Early enteral feeding, compared with parenteral, reduces postoperative septic complications. Ann Surg 1992;216: 173–183.
27. Spaeth G, Berg RD, Specian RD, Deitch EA: Food without fiber promotes bacterial translocation from the gut. Surgery 1990;108:240–247.
28. Alverdy J, Chi HS, Sheldon GF: The effects of parental nutrition on gastrointestinal immunity. The importance of enteral stimulation. Ann Surg 1985;202: 681–684.
29. Moore FA, Moore EE, Poggetti R et al: Gut bacterial translocation via the protal vein: a clinical perspective with major torso trauma. J Trauma 1991;31:629–638.
30. Meredith J, Ditesheim J, Zaloga G: Visceral protein levels in trauma patients are greater with peptide diet than with intact protein diet. J Trauma 1990;30: 825–829.
31. Silk DBA, Fairclough PD, Clark ML et al: Use of a peptide rather than a free amino acid nitrogen source in chemically defined "elemental" diets. J Parenter Enter Nutr 1980;4:548–553.
32. Matthews DM: Memorial lecture: protein absorption—then and now. Gastroenterology 1977;73:1267–1279.
33. Mowatt-Larssen C, Brown R, Wojtysiak S et al: Comparison of tolerance and nutritional outcome between a peptide and a standard enteral formula in critically ill, hypoalbuminemic patients. J Parenter Enter Nutr 1992;16:20–24.
34. Guidelines for the scientific review of enteral food products for special medical purposes. J Parenter Enter Nutr 1991;15:137S.
35. Gottschlich M, Jenkins M, Warden GD et al: Differential effects of three enteral dietary regimens on selected outcome variables in burn patients. J Parenter Enter Nutr 1990;14:225–236.
36. Daly J, Lieberman MD, Goldfine J et al: Enteral nutrition with supplemental arginine, RNA, and omega-3 fatty acids in patients after operation: immunologic, metabolic, and clinical outcome. Surgery 1992;112: 56–67.

37. Daly JM, Weintraub FN, Shou J et al: Enteral nutrition during multimodality therapy in upper gastrointestinal cancer patients. Ann Surg 1995;221:327–338.
38. Bower RH, Cerra FB, Bershadsky B et al: Early enteral administration of a formula (Impact) supplemented with arginine, nucleotides, and fish oil in intensive care unit patients: results of a multicenter, prospective, randomized, clinical trial. Crit Care Med 1995;23: 436–449.
39. Brown RO, Hunt H, Mowatt-Larssen CA et al: Comparison of specialized and standard eneral formulas in trauma patients. Pharmacotherapy 1994;14: 314–320.
40. Moore FA, Moore EE, Kudsk KA et al: Clinical benefits of an immune-enhancing diet for early postinjury enteral feeding. J Trauma 1994;37:607–615.
41. Dent D, Kudsk KA, Minard G et al: Risk of abdominal septic complications after feeding jejunostomy placement in patients undergoing splenectomy for trauma. Am J Surg 1993;166:686–690.
42. Delenay HM, Carenevale NJ, Garvey JW et al: Post-operative nutritional support using needle catheter feeding jejunostomy. Ann Surg 1977;186:165–170.
43. Hoover HC, Ryan JA, Anderson AJ et al: Nutritional benefits of immediate post-operative jejunal feeding of an elemental diet. Am J Surg 1980;139:153–159.
44. Page CP, Ryan JA, Haff RC: Continual catheter administration of an elemental diet. Surg Gynecol Obstet 1976;142:184–188.
45. Kudsk KA, Minard G: Enteral nutrition. In Zaloga G (ed): Nutrition in Critical Care. St. Louis: C.V. Mosby, 1994:331–360.

19

Enteral Nutrition in Burns

CHARLES J. YOWLER
BASIL A. PRUITT, JR.

THE METABOLIC RESPONSE TO BURN INJURY

The metabolic response to burn injury is an exaggerated form of the biphasic posttrauma response originally described by Cuthbertson.[1] Severe burns result in an ebb phase of 24 to 48 hours characterized by decreased to normal resting energy expenditure (REE) and cardiac output. This is followed by a flow phase that peaks between postburn days 6 and 10 and then decreases to normal in a curvilinear fashion over several weeks (Fig. 19–1).

This metabolic response to burn injury is characterized by REEs that are not seen with other illnesses or other major traumatic injuries. REEs of 2 to $2\frac{1}{2}$ times basal metabolic rates were noted in early studies of the metabolic response to burn injury.[2-4] Although current techniques of burn care are associated with more moderate REEs (Fig. 19–2), the hypermetabolism that results from the neuroendocrine, immunologic, and thermoregulatory responses to the burn injury continues to be a significant challenge to the recovery of the burn patient.[5,6]

The opinions or assertions contained herein are the private views of the authors and are not to be construed as official or reflecting the view of the Department of the Army or the Department of Defense.

Neuroendocrine Response

Metabolic rate is primarily controlled by the hypothalamic-pituitary axis. Although thyroid hormone plays a central role in controlling metabolism in the healthy patient, catecholamines appear to be the major mediators of the hypermetabolic response in burn patients.[7] Although mean values for circulating concentrations of triiodothyronine (T_3) and thyroxine (T_4) in burn patients are typically depressed, serum concentrations of free thyroid hormones are generally within normal limits in uncomplicated burn patients. Unstable burn patients, however, have depressed levels of free T_3 and free T_4.[8] These laboratory findings, coupled with the elevated reverse-T_3 present in these unstable burn patients, are consistent with "nonthyroidal illness" or the "euthyroid sick syndrome."[9,10] Consequently, the replacement of T_3 in these critically ill patients does not alter the hypermetabolism of burn patients or the associated morbidity or mortality.[11]

Plasma concentrations of norepinephrine, glucagon, and cortisol are positively correlated with burn size and metabolic rate.[7,12] Infusion of β-agonists in unburned control patients produces metabolic responses similar to those seen with burn injury, while the blockade of β-, but not α-adrenergic receptors blunts many manifestations of the hypermetabolic response including the increases in REE, ventilation, pulse rate, and free fatty acid.[13,14] All these findings

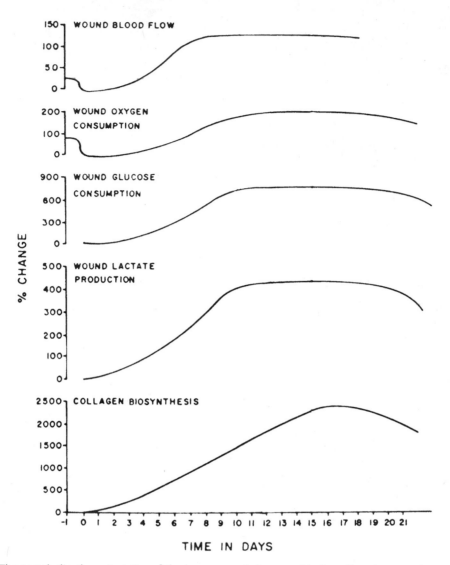

FIGURE 19–1   The metabolic characteristics of the burn wound change with time. Note increase in wound lactate production despite increase in wound oxygen and glucose consumption (Modified from Wilmore DW, Aulick LH: Metabolic changes in burned patients. Surg Clin North Am 1978;58:1173–1187.)

support the central role of catecholamines in regulating the hypermetabolic response to burn injury.

Growth hormone levels are not elevated in burn patients,[15] and in fact the growth hormone response to insulin-induced hypoglycemia, arginine infusion, and nocturnal sleep appears to be blunted. Plasma cortisol concentrations are elevated in proportion to burn size despite normal corticotrophin (ACTH) levels, suggesting that factors other than ACTH contribute to the elevated cortisol levels.[16]

The end result of this hormonal response to the burn injury is an increase in proteolysis, gluconeogenesis, lipolysis, and peripheral insulin resistance. Nutritional regimens must take these changes into account if they are to be effective in countering the negative aspects of this hypermetabolic response.

Immunologic Response

The cytokine response to circulating endotoxin may contribute to the hypermetabolic response to burn injury.[17,18] Endotoxin is thought to be the primary stimulant of tumor necrosis factor (TNF) production by macrophages and lymphocytes. TNF, in turn, appears to be responsible for many of the metabolic changes that occur in catabolic states.

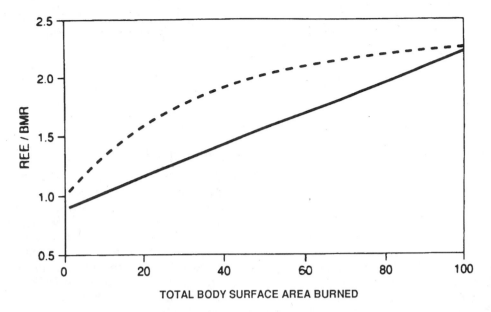

Figure 19–2 The relationship of metabolic rate and burn size has changed over the past 20 years. The previously demonstrated curvilinear relationship of measured resting energy (REE) divided by basal metabolic rate (BMR) (dotted line) is contrasted with the current linear relationship. (Modified from Carlson DE, Cioffi WG, Mason AD et al: Resting energy expenditure in patients with thermal injury. Surg Gynecol Obstet 1992;174:270–276.)

TNF stimulates monocytes and macrophages to produce interleukin (IL)-1, an endogenous pyrogen and proximal mediator of the cytokine cascade. In contrast to TNF, IL-1 concentrations increase in proportion to burn size (Fig. 19–3). As the hypermetabolic response recedes after the third postburn week, IL-1 concentrations decrease in concert with circulating catecholamine levels and a return to positive nitrogen balance.[19]

IL-6, in turn, appears to be the final common mediator elicited by endotoxin, TNF, and IL-1 and is the primary mediator of acute-phase protein production by the hepatocyte. IL-6 levels increase immediately after burn injury but appear to correlate more with the presence of infection than with burn size.[20]

Infusion of endotoxin into unburned animals has resulted in metabolic responses simi-

Figure 19–3 The relationship between plasma cytokines and burn size. IL-1 concentrations increase in proportion to burn size while those of TNF do not. (Modified from Drost AC, Burleson DG, Cioffi WG et al: Plasma cytokines following thermal injury and their relationship with patient mortality, burn size, and time postburn. J Trauma 1993;35:335–339.)

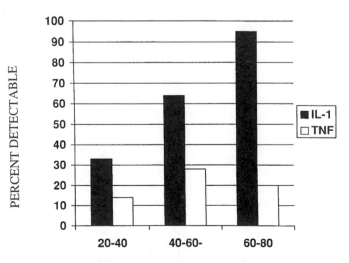

TOTAL BODY SURFACE AREA BURNED

lar to those seen in burned animals.[21] Endotoxemia may occur in burned patients as a result of either bacterial translocation[22] or altered intestinal permeability with absorption of endotoxin directly from the gut.[23,24] Accordingly, immediate postburn enteral feeding has been proposed as a means of preserving enterocyte viability and maintaining gastrointestinal (GI) mucosal integrity to limit both microbial translocation and altered intestinal permeability. Although an initial animal study appeared to confirm that immediate postburn feedings eliminated the hypermetabolic response to burn injury,[25] a subsequent study failed to support this finding.[26] Thus, the exact role of bacterial translocation and altered intestinal permeability in the metabolic response to burn injury and the effect of immediate enteral feedings remain undefined.

Endotoxin may also be absorbed from the wound surface. The importance of burn wound colonization and infection in the metabolic response to burn injury has been confirmed by studies in an animal model in which the degree of hypermetabolism was proportional to the number of bacteria present in the wound.[27,28] The hypermetabolic response in this model could be reduced by topical antimicrobial agents.[29]

Thermoregulatory Response

Initially, it was thought that the hypermetabolic response to burn injury was merely due to increased heat production compensating for increased heat loss through the burn wound. Approximately 0.6 kcal of heat are required to evaporate 1 ml of water. Because thermal injury destroys the water vapor barrier of the skin, evaporative heat loss through the burn wound had been considered by some to be the cause of the hypermetabolic response. However, burn wound coverage with impermeable dressings reduces evaporative water loss but results in only modest REE reduction. Thus, evaporative water loss serves as a convenient route of heat loss but is not the cause of the hypermetabolic response in burn patients.[30]

Central thermoregulation appears to be altered in burn patients with an upward shift of the temperature of comfort and minimum metabolic expenditure.[3] The elevated core and skin temperatures that occur in the initial week following burn injury are the result of the hypermetabolic response, not the cause. Burn patients are "internally warm and not externally cold." However, the metabolic response, while not temperature dependent, is temperature sensitive. Increasing the ambient temperature to 35° C will not eliminate the increase in REE, but failure to maintain a warm environment imposes a cold stress that will increase the metabolic rate and may precipitate cardiovascular collapse in patients who are unable to meet the added physiologic stress.

Substrate Metabolism

Carbohydrate

Glucose is the major metabolic fuel for all cellular components of the healing burn wound. Granulation tissue is relatively hypoxic due to the rapid cell proliferation that occurs in the presence of regenerating capillary beds. This wound environment results in the anaerobic metabolism of glucose to lactate. The lactate produced by the wound is then recycled to glucose by the hepatocyte (Cori cycle). Because of the inefficiency of this anaerobic glycolysis, the increased metabolic demands of the burn wound must be met by increased glucose delivery, which promotes greater uptake.

Blood glucose levels are elevated in burn patients despite the circulating levels of insulin that increase following resuscitation. The increased levels of the anti-insulin hormones (catecholamines, cortisol, glucagon) counter the effects of the elevated insulin levels and are necessary to maintain an adequate rate of gluconeogenesis to meet the patient's energy requirements.

As a result of this altered hormonal state, proteolysis of peripheral muscle is accelerated and amino acids become available for gluconeogenesis. Alanine is the major gluconeogenic amino acid, and measurement of its release from skeletal muscle demonstrates that burn patients increase the rate of peripheral alanine release to approximately three times normal.[31] The magnitude of this peripheral alanine release is proportional to burn size and parallels measured rates of gluconeogenesis and ureagenesis. Hepatic dysfunction secondary to sepsis or preexisting liver disease may interfere with the effective conversion of alanine to glucose and thereby complicate metabolic management.

In summary, the glucose necessary for wound healing and immune function in the burn patient is supplied by the liver from the glucose-lactate-glucose sequence of the Cori cycle and from conversion of amino acids supplied by peripheral muscle breakdown. Glucose supplied by nutritional support will decrease proteolysis and preserve lean body mass. However, burn patients may have difficulty in metabolizing glucose when it is administered at rates greater than 4 to 5 mg/kg/minute.[32] Consequently, additional nutritional support required to meet the calculated caloric requirements of burn patients must be provided by lipids and proteins.

Lipids

Normally, lipid metabolism provides a major portion of the energy used during periods of inadequate glucose availability. Low circulating levels of insulin result in increased lipolysis and ketogenesis, and peripheral tissue converts to the metabolism of glycerol, free fatty acids, and ketone bodies.

However, the neuroendocrine changes that accompany thermal injury significantly alter lipid metabolism.[33] Lipolysis does increase after burn injury in response to elevated circulating levels of catecholamines, and glycerol and free fatty acids are used as fuel by unburned peripheral tissue. Ketogenesis, however, is decreased in burn patients.[34] Because ketone bodies are normally one of the primary alternate energy sources used during periods of starvation, this results in an increased requirement for gluconeogenesis.

Thus, the protein-sparing effect of lipid is limited in the burn patient. Increasing the lipid content of enteral diets above 30 percent of total calories may impair immune function and will not preserve additional lean body mass.

Protein

The burn patient uses amino acids not just for gluconeogenesis but for wound healing and to maintain immune function. Thus, despite the net release of amino acids from unburned tissue, serum concentrations of amino acids are commonly decreased in patients with extensive burns.[35]

The contribution of dietary protein content to immune function has been studied in a group of pediatric patients.[36] A diet in which 16.5 percent of total calories were supplied as protein was compared to one in which the protein content was increased to 23 percent. Although neither group was able to achieve its estimated caloric requirement, the higher protein diet was associated with significant elevations in IgG, transferrin, and complement factor-3. This group also experienced fewer bacteremic days and had a significantly lower mortality rate. Thus, providing adequate protein may be an important factor in maintaining immune function.

In summary, the hypermetabolic response to burn injury is characterized by an increased demand for free amino acids as substrates for gluconeogenesis, collagen formation, and the immune response. The goal of nutritional support is to minimize the proteolysis required to meet this demand by supplying alternate sources of glucose and protein.

GASTROINTESTINAL COMPLICATIONS OF BURN INJURY

The systemic response to burn injury involves the GI tract and may result in complications that interfere with the administration of adequate enteral nutrition. Gastric and intestinal ileus, stress ulceration of the stomach and duodenum (Curling's ulcer), acalculous cholecystitis, acute pancreatitis, nonocclusive ischemic enterocolitis, pseudo-obstruction of the colon, and hepatic dysfunction may all complicate burn injury and limit the effectiveness of enteral nutrition.

Gastric ileus may persist for 24 to 96 hours following burns of more than 20 percent of the body surface area, but small bowel motility is generally adequate to permit transduodenal tube feedings within 24 to 48 hours. Inadequate resuscitation, however, may prolong the duration of the initial ileus, and sepsis occurring later in the hospital course may be associated with profound and prolonged ileus. Burn patients are at increased risk to aspiration secondary to this ileus if the following conditions exist.[37]

1. Altered mentation
2. Enforced supine positioning or prone positioning
3. Absent or decreased cough or gag reflex
4. Presence of an enteric tube

Gastric mucosal erosions have been noted in 86 percent of patients with burn wounds involving more than 35 percent of the body surface. In the absence of acid-reducing therapy,[38,39] progression to frank ulceration has been noted in 22 percent of patients with gastritic changes. Similar changes have been documented in the duodenum.[40] Other studies have shown that gastric acid levels may be markedly elevated following burn injury despite normal gastrin levels.[41] Maintenance of gastric pH above 4.5 by either continuous antacid therapy[42] or histamine$_2$ receptor blockade[43] prevents progression of the mucosal lesions and decreases the incidence of associated bleeding and perforation.

Acute acalculous cholecystitis may occur in critically ill burn patients.[44] Mechanical ventilation, numerous blood transfusions, large doses of narcotics, hypoxia, and shock are associated with an increased risk of acute acalculous cholecystitis.[45] Enteral nutrition promotes gall bladder emptying but does not entirely eliminate the risk of inflammation. Ultrasound evaluation or computed tomography (CT) scanning is indicated to assess gallbladder status in the burn patient with unexplained fever, jaundice, right upper quadrant pain, leukocytosis, abnormalities in liver function tests, or unexplained sepsis. Percutaneous cholecystotomy may facilitate evaluation in the critically ill patient and also prove therapeutic. Emergency cholecystectomy is indicated in the presence of large pericholecystic fluid collections and in the occasional patient who presents with frank peritonitis.

Acute pancreatitis may occur in up to 35 percent of critically ill burn patients.[46] The decrease in visceral perfusion that accompanies thermal injury may result in pancreatic edema and areas of interstitial necrosis and hemorrhage. The associated sludging and inspissation of pancreatic secretions may also contribute to pancreatic injury. Serum amylase levels should be monitored daily in the early postburn period and in the presence of prolonged or recurrent ileus thereafter. Serum lipase levels should be obtained to confirm the diagnosis of pancreatitis in patients with hyperamylasemia. Patients with severe pancreatitis may require parenteral nutrition until the inflammation resolves. The burn patient may then be transitioned to a low-fat enteral diet delivered distal to the ligament of Treitz.

Parenteral nutrition may also be required for nutritional support in patients with small bowel and colonic complications. Nonocclusive intestinal ischemia is being diagnosed more frequently in severely burned patients.[47] This may result in GI hemorrhage or frank bowel necrosis. The lesions of the distal small bowel resemble both endoscopically and histologically those mucosal ulcers noted in the upper GI tract. Segmental ischemic colitis secondary to thrombosis may also occur in the dehydrated patient in whom resuscitation has been inadequate. Pseudo-obstruction of the colon, which occurs with a reported incidence of 1 percent in burn patients,[48] appears to be more common in elderly patients at prolonged bed rest necessitated by multiple skin grafting proce-

dures. Bowel motility in these patients may also be impaired by narcotics administered over prolonged periods for control of pain associated with daily wound care and multiple excision and skin grafting procedures.

ESTIMATION OF NUTRITIONAL REQUIREMENTS

Caloric Requirements

Early formulas devised to estimate the caloric requirements of burn patients have been found to be inaccurate (Table 19–1). The Harris-Benedict equation underestimates caloric requirements without correcting for stress, and studies attempting to determine the stress factor have arrived at values ranging from 1.5 to 2.1. Conversely, the Curreri formula[49] has been shown to overestimate calorie needs.[50,51]

Recent measurements of the metabolic rate of burn patients treated at the United States Army Institute of Surgical Research (USAISR) have been used to derive a nutritional formula based on age, body size, and extent of burn (Table 19–2).[50] Analysis of recently obtained indirect calorimetry data revealed a linear relationship between metabolic rate and burn size in contrast to previous studies, which defined a curvilinear relationship with a plateau of REE at 2 to 2½ times basal metabolic rate when the burn involved 60 percent or more of the body surface (Fig. 19–2). A similar study at the University of Toronto described a linear relationship defined by the percentage of the total body surface area burned, the expected basal energy expenditure (calculated by the Harris-Benedict formula), the body temperature, the number of days after burn, and the thermogenic effect of feeding.[52] Both these studies confirmed that the formulas based on the earlier metabolic studies overestimate the caloric needs of burn patients as currently treated.

The relationship between energy requirements and burn size is fairly consistent for freely breathing patients (Fig. 19–4), but the wide variance of data obtained from mechanically ventilated patients makes estimation of their caloric requirements less accurate (Fig. 19–5). Indirect calorimetry data obtained from mechanically ventilated patients may be inaccurate due to dead space ventilation, air leaks in the ventilatory system, and increased work of breathing due to inadequate sedation. Therefore, caloric requirements in mechanically ventilated burn patients should be initially mea-

TABLE 19–1   Formulas Frequently Used to Estimate Daily Caloric Requirements for Burn Patients (Results in Calories/Day)

Harris-Benedict
Male
$(66 + [13.7 \times W] + [5 \times H] - [6.8 \times A]) \times 2$ (stress factor)
Female
$(655 + [9.6 \times W] + [1.8 \times H] - [4.7 \times A]) \times 2$ (stress factor)

Curreri

Adult		$(25 \times W) + (40 \times \% \text{TBSA burned})$
Junior	(age 0,1)	$(BC \times W) + (15 \times \% \text{TBSA burned})$
	(age 2,3)	$(BC \times W) = (25 \times \% \text{TBSA burned})$
	(age 4–18)	$(BC \times W) + (40 \times \% \text{TBSA burned})$

BC by age for Curreri junior formulae:

A	BC	A	BC	A	BC
0	60	7	48	14	36
1	59	8	47	15	35
2	55	9	46	16	32
3	53	10	45	17	31
4	52	11	44	18	30
5	51	12	40		
6	50	13	38		

Galveston
Children $(1800 \times BSA) + (2200 \times burn[m^2])$

W = weight (kg); H = height (cm); A = age (yr); BSA = body surface area (m²); BC = basal calories.

TABLE 19–2   Calculation of Caloric Needs*

---

1. REE = $(BMR \times [0.89142 + \{0.01335 \times TBS\}]) \times BSA \times 24 \times AF$
2. Calculation of BMR
   Male BMR = $54.337821 - 1.19961 \,(age) + 0.02548 \,(age)^2 - 0.00018 \,(age)^3$
   Female BMR = $54.74942 - 1.54884 \,(age) + 0.0358 \,(age)^2 - 0.00026 \,(age)^3$
3. Calculation of BSA

   $$BSA \,(m^2) = \frac{\sqrt{H + (in) \times wt \,(lb)}}{3131}$$

   $$BSA \,(m^2) = \frac{\sqrt{HT(cm) \times wt \,(kg)}}{3600}$$

4. If preburn weight is in excess of desired body weight (DBW) by more than 25%, use adjusted desired body weight (Adj wt):
   Adj wt = $([actual\ weight - DBW] \times 0.25) + DBW$;
   DBW (male) = 106 lb for first 5 ft and 6 lb for each additional inch;
   DBW (female) = 100 lb for first 5 ft and 5 lb for each additional inch

---

REE = estimated energy requirement; BMR = basal metabolic rate; TBS = Total burn size (ie., for 30% use 30); AF = activity factor (normally 1.25)
*Data from United States Army Institute of Surgical Research.

sured by indirect calorimetry but must then be evaluated in terms of the patient's response to the nutritional support.

Longitudinal studies of REEs in thermally injured patients have found no simple relationship between energy expenditure and wound closure (Fig. 19–6).[53] Although immediate total excision and skin grafting of the entire burn wound eliminate the hypermetabolic response, early burn excision and wound coverage at 48 to 72 hours do not appear to affect metabolic rate.[54,55]

The determination of caloric needs, whether derived from estimates based on formulae or determined by indirect calorimetry, must be corrected for activity. Although it has recently

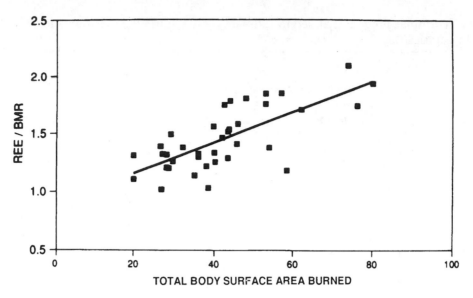

FIGURE 19–4   Resting energy expenditure (REE) as a function of total burn size. Measurements made using a canopy system. (Modified from Carlson DE, Cioffi WG, Mason AD et al: Resting energy expenditure in patients with thermal injury. Surg Gynecol Obstet 1992;174:270–276.)

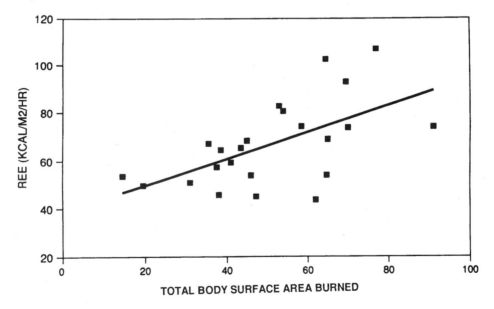

FIGURE 19–5   Resting energy expenditure (REE) vs total burn size in mechanically ventilated patients. (Modified from Carlson DE, Cioffi WG, Mason AD et al: Resting energy expenditure in patients with thermal injury. Surg Gynecol Obstet 1992;174:270–276.)

been reported that bedridden, critically ill patients may require no correction for activity,[56] burn patients are usually involved in extensive physical therapy programs to minimize burn wound complications. Generally, a calorie goal is established that is 20 to 25 percent greater than estimated REE.

Delivery of adequate amounts of carbohydrate and lipid to meet the calorie goal may be complicated by the changes in substrate metabolism and the GI system that have previously been discussed. In general, however, burn patients' calorie requirements may be met by delivery of standard enteral solutions at

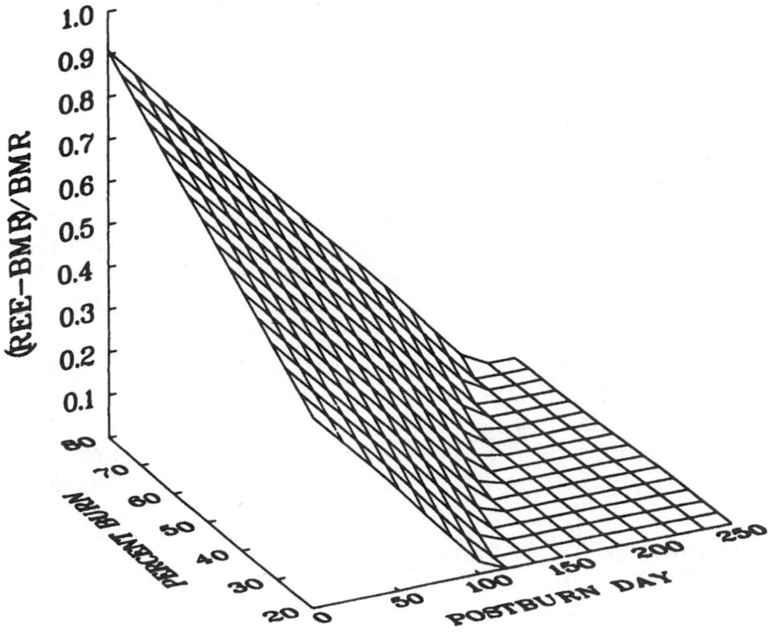

FIGURE 19–6 The metabolic rate expressed as ([REE–BMR]/BMR) increases as burn size increases and decreases with time following injury. (Modified from Milner EA, Cioffi WG, Mason AD et al: A longitudinal study of resting energy expenditure in thermally injured patients. J Trauma 1994; 37:167–170.)

rates tolerated by the GI system. An example of a caloric determination using the USAISR formula is presented in Table 19–3.

Nitrogen Requirements

Enteral solutions with kcal:nitrogen ratios of 150 to 100:1 are optimal to provide sufficient protein and avoid excessive carbohydrate administration. When such solutions are used, a positive calorie balance verified by indirect calorimetry is associated with positive nitrogen balance in the majority of patients.

The determination of nitrogen balance in the burn patient is complicated by protein loss from the open wound. The hypermetabolic starved burn patient may lose 30 g of nitrogen a day, with 20 to 30 percent of the loss occurring in the form of serous exudate from the burn wound.

Waxman and coworkers[57] studied protein loss from the surface of full- and partial-thickness burn wounds. Those investigators found that the average daily protein loss across the burn wound for the first postburn week could be estimated as follows:

$$\text{Protein loss (g)} = 1.2 \times \text{BSA (m}^2) \times \% \text{ burn}$$

These losses decreased by half in the second postburn week:

$$\text{Protein loss (g)} = 0.6 \times \text{BSA (m}^2) \times \% \text{ burn}$$

Nitrogen losses across the burn wound were estimated as:

$$\text{Nitrogen loss (g)} = 0.3 \times \text{BSA} \times \% \text{ burn}$$

TABLE 19–3 Sample Calculation of Caloric Requirement

1. 30-year-old man with 30% TBS burn; ht = 70", wt = 170 lb

2. $\text{BSA (m}^2) = \dfrac{\sqrt{70 \times 170}}{3131} = 1.95 \text{ m}^2$

3. BMR = $54.337821 - 1.19961(30) + 0.02548(30)^2 - 0.00018(30)^3 = 36.42$ kcal

4. REE = (BMR × [0.89142 + {0.01335 × TBS}]) × BSA × 24 × AF
   REE = 36.42 [0.89142 + {0.01335 × 30}]) × 1.95 × 24 × 1.25 = 2752.5 kcal/day

TBS = total burn size; BSA = body surface area; BMR = basal metabolic rate; ht = height; wt = weight; REE = resting energy expenditure; AF = activity factor.

for postburn days 1 to 3 and

$$\text{Nitrogen loss (g)} = 0.1 \times \text{BSA} \times \% \text{ burn}$$

for postburn days 4 to 16. Using the nitrogen balance formula in Table 19–4, daily protein requirements can thus be estimated.

Positive nitrogen balance in burn patients is poorly predicted by serum concentrations of albumin, prealbumin, retinol-binding protein, or transferrin.[58] Changes in the levels of these visceral proteins as nutritional support is implemented also correlate poorly with nitrogen balance. This discrepancy is a manifestation of the protein loss that occurs across the burn wound, along with the variable volumes of fluids infused during the resuscitation period and thereafter.

ADMINISTRATION OF ENTERAL NUTRITION

Delivery of Enteral Solutions

The majority of patients with burn injuries of more than 20 percent of the body surface area will require placement of enteric feeding tubes for nutritional support because of gastric ileus. Enteric feeding tubes must also be used in patients with smaller burns in whom inhalational injury necessitates mechanical ventilation.

At the United States Army Burn Center, enteral feedings are administered through a fluoroscopically placed nasojejunal tube beginning on postburn day 2 or 3. Endoscopic placement past the ligament of Treitz is used when fluoroscopically guided placement fails. Radiologic assessment of tube position is obtained if nasogastric output increases or tracheal secretions become positive for glucose.

The immediate provision of enteral nutrition by intragastric feedings in the burn patient has been reported.[59,60] Proponents of this method believe that the increased integrity of gastric and intestinal mucosa associated with immediate enteral nutrition may prevent complications due to altered intestinal permeability and microbial translocation. However, the risks of aspiration appear to outweigh any proven benefit of immediate intragastric feedings, and delivery of enteral solutions into the jejunum remains the route of choice.

Percutaneous endoscopically placed feeding tubes may be used to provide enteral nutrition in burn patients with associated neurologic or facial injuries. Skin complications at the tube site may occur in patients with abdominal burns, but these are generally minor and respond to aggressive wound and skin care.

The authors initiate enteral nutrition with a half-strength concentration of an isotonic high nitrogen solution at the rate of 25 ml/hour. The patient is closely monitored for abdominal pain, abdominal distention, or increased nasogastric output while the rate is increased by 25 ml/hour every 8 hours until the target rate is achieved. If the patient tolerates target volume, the concentration of the enteral solution is then increased to three fourths strength for 8 hours, after which full-strength solutions are used. If additional protein is required for positive nitrogen balance, protein supplements are added in bolus form every 4 to 6 hours.

Any fluctuation in feeding rates may result in delivery of inadequate calories or nitrogen. Full-volume enteral feedings may be delivered throughout operative procedures with enteral feeding tubes placed distal to the ligament of Treitz. The delivery of enteral nutrition during operative procedures has been shown to reduce caloric deficits and wound infections and does not appear to be associated with an increased risk of aspiration.[61]

Dietary Content

The enteral solution used at the United States Army Burn Center is an isotonic whole-protein solution containing 16.7 percent of calories as protein, 29 percent as fat, and 54 percent as carbohydrate. The delivery of 1400 ml provides 100 percent of the recommended daily allowance (RDA) of vitamins and minerals.

Modular components may be added to this solution to increase the protein or calorie content. Modular protein supplements are occasionally required in patients who remain in negative nitrogen balance despite the delivery of adequate calories. Medium-chain triglycerides are added if necessary to avoid glucose delivery greater than 5 g/kg/minute.

TABLE 19–4   Nitrogen Balance in Burn Patients

Intake = grams protein/6.25
Output = UUN/0.8 + 4 g* + wound factor
Wound factor
    Postburn day 1–3 = 0.3 × (BSA) × (TBS)
    Postburn day 4–16 = 0.1 × (BSA) × (TBS)

*4 g = insensible loss.
UUN = urinary urea nitrogen; TBS = total body surface area burn (%); BSA = body surface area.

Protein

Arginine is not considered an essential amino acid in uninjured humans, but experimental deficiency in the traumatized rat decreases collagen deposition and wound breaking strength.[62] Supplementation of an enteral diet with arginine enhances reparative collagen synthesis, stimulates the release of growth hormone, and appears to promote helper T-cell production.[63,64] A diet in which arginine comprised 2 percent of the total dietary calorie intake improved survival significantly in a guinea pig model of burn injury.[65] However, commercially available enteral solutions are not deficient in arginine, and any recommendation concerning additional arginine supplementation must await further clinical trials.

Similarly, glutamine is believed by many to be an essential amino acid in the critically ill injured patient. Intestinal mucosal cells selectively consume glutamine as a primary fuel, and its deficiency may result in mucosal atrophy and alterations in intestinal permeability. Depressed glutamine levels have been documented in burn patients,[66] but the benefits of supplementation have not yet been established. No metabolic benefits were noted in a guinea pig model of burn injury following glutamine supplementation.[67] At present there is little evidence to support supplementing the nutritional regimen of burn patients with glutamine.

Dietary supplementation with branched-chain amino acids (BCAAs) has also been reported to exert no beneficial effect in a guinea pig model of burn injury.[68] Studies in other critically ill patient groups have similarly failed to demonstrate a role for these amino acids. There is currently no evidence to support supplementation of BCAAs in excess of that found in commercially available products.

Lipids

The addition of fish oil to enteral nutrient solutions has been reported to improve immune functions. Both PGE-1 and PGE-2 produced by the metabolism of the omega-6 fatty acids found in standard vegetable oils have immunosuppressive properties. Metabolism of omega-3 fatty acids found in fish oil produces PGE-3, which is less immunologically active. It has therefore been suggested that postburn immunosuppression may be reduced by replacing the omega-6 fatty acids in the diet with omega-3 fatty acids.[69,70]

However, omega-3 fatty acids may also have deleterious effects in the infected patient.[71] The long-chain, highly polyunsaturated fatty acids in fish oil are prone to autooxidation and may potentially damage cells by forming free radicals. PGE-3 is also less effective in the down-regulation of the tumor necrosis factor response to endotoxin than PGE-1 and PGE-2 and thus may contribute to an exaggerated cytokine response to endotoxin. In one study, mice fed fish oil diets 2 weeks before burn injury and infected with *Pseudomonas* after burning had an increased mortality rate compared with a control group fed a diet rich in vegetable oil.[72] Thus, further research is necessary to identify beneficial effects of omega-3 fatty acids in the burn patient before fish oil can be recommended as a standard supplement.

Vitamins

Most vitamins, particularly A, C, E, and B_6 (pyridoxine), affect immune function, while thiamine, pyridoxine, folic acid, and vitamins C and B_{12} are essential for protein synthesis and wound repair.[63] Although the exact requirements for vitamin supplementation in the burn patient have not been determined, published guidelines have suggested that 500 mg of ascorbic acid (vitamin C), 10,000 units of vitamin A, and a multivitamin tablet should be administered daily.[73] However, the high volumes of enteral solutions delivered to achieve positive calorie balance in burn patients result in delivery of 1.5 to 2 times the recommended daily allowances of vitamins and exceed these recommendations. Therefore, we recommend additional vitamin supplementation only in burn patients with preexisting malnutrition and documented vitamin deficiencies.

Trace Metals

Trace metals play an integral role in wound healing and immune function.[63] Zinc deficiency impairs the use of amino acids for wound healing; copper is essential for maturation of collagen. Selenium-dependent glutathione peroxidase protects the cell from oxidative damage by catalyzing the reduction of hydrogen peroxide.

Commercially available enteral solutions provide adequate concentrations of these and other trace metals without supplementation. Although supplementation with 220 mg of zinc sulfate has been recommended by some,[73] the authors provide zinc supplementation only to those patients with preexisting chronic malnutrition.

Complications of Enteral Delivery

The delivery of adequate enteral nutritional support may be compromised by complications directly attributable to the tube feedings. Daily physical examination of the burn patient should include inspection of the tube to ensure that it has not been displaced and that there is no pressure on the nares or columella. Sinusitis may occur in patients with nasoenteric tubes. The simultaneous presence of a nasotracheal and nasogastric tube has been reported to increase the risk of sinusitis, and prolonged nasotracheal intubation in particular should be avoided. Radiographic studies of the sinuses should be obtained in patients with persistent fevers, and the findings of mucosal thickening or opacification of the sinuses dictate intervention to drain the sinuses. The majority of patients with sinusitis respond to drainage and decongestant use. Antibiotics should be used if cultures reveal bacterial infection.

Abdominal distention may occur as tube feedings are initiated. The majority of burn patients will respond to nasogastric suction and 12 to 24 hours of bowel rest, after which tube feedings may again be gradually advanced as previously described. Initial evaluation, however, must include physical examination, laboratory studies, and radiographs to rule out the presence of an ischemic or perforated viscus, pancreatitis, or sepsis.

Diarrhea commonly occurs following burn injury. In one study of diarrhea in burn patients, the incidence did not appear to correlate with percent body surface area burn, hypoalbuminemia, or osmolality of the enteral solution.[74] The incidence was decreased, however, by initiating tube feedings within 48 hours of burn injury, by vitamin A supplementation, and by reducing fat intake to less than 20 g/day. Continuous rather than intermittent feedings also appear to reduce the incidence of diarrhea.[75]

Evaluation of new-onset diarrhea requires a rectal examination to rule out fecal impaction. Medications should be reviewed to eliminate any sources of an osmolar diarrhea, such as excessive antacid administration. If the diarrhea exceeds 1 L/day, infectious sources should be investigated by laboratory analysis for fecal leukocytes and *Clostridium difficile* toxin. In the absence of infection, antimotility medications or dietary fiber may be added to the enteral solutions to control the diarrhea.

The superior mesenteric artery syndrome may occur in patients with massive burns in whom excessive weight loss occurs.[76,77] Indirect calorimetry may appear to demonstrate positive calorie balances in these patients, and weight loss may be unrecognized due to excision of skin and adipose tissue, amputations, and diuresis. Treatment of this complication requires delivery of enteral solutions at rates that will ensure weight gain using a nasojejunal feeding tube placed past the point of obstruction. Surgical intervention to bypass the obstruction by construction of a duodenojejunostomy or gastrojejunostomy may be required if obstruction persists despite nutritional intervention.

Monitoring Nutritional Support

Reassessment of caloric requirements and nitrogen balance throughout the postburn period is essential to provide optimal nutritional support. Infectious complications, prolonged ventilatory support, and the stress of multiple operative procedures may all contribute to fluctuations in metabolic rate that result in inaccurate initial estimates of calorie and nitrogen requirements and compromise the provision of adequate nutritional support.

All the formulas for predicting calorie requirements become increasingly inaccurate as the interval from burn injury approaches 30 days.[53] Metabolic rate decreases with time after burn but remains elevated throughout hospitalization. REE at hospital discharge is approximately 25 percent above predicted basal metabolic rate, presumably secondary to persistent wound inflammation and remodeling.[53]

Critically ill burn patients commonly require prolonged tube feedings and should be evaluated by indirect calorimetry and nitrogen balance studies weekly. More frequent determinations may be required if the clinical evaluation does not correlate with the initial estimates of calorie and protein requirements. Stable patients may be followed by daily calorie counts and weight measurements as they transition to a regular oral diet. However, the interpretation of daily weight measurements may be complicated by the initial fluid resuscitation and subsequent diuresis as well as the fluids infused during burn wound excision and grafting procedures. A weight gain of more than 0.4 kg/day represents fluid accumulation and does not necessarily correlate with the delivery of adequate calories. Thus, the trend of serial weight measurements must be followed in conjunction with close monitoring of fluid balance and serum sodium concentrations if conclusions concerning nutritional status are to be reliable.

In the past, parenteral nutrition was commonly used to supplement enteral nutrition in burn patients. At the United States Army Burn Center, 13 percent of patients treated between 1987 and 1989 received total or partial parenteral nutrition because of failure to achieve adequate oral intake.[78] Subsequently, Herndon and colleagues found that the mortality rate doubled in burns greater than 50 percent total body surface area if intravenous supplementation was used.[79] Currently, we achieve positive calorie balance by continuing tube feedings throughout operative procedures and by using modular supplements (medium-chain triglycerides, protein supplements) if necessary. TPN is confined to burn patients with GI complications that require bowel rest and in whom return of bowel function is not expected within 3 to 5 days.

NUTRITIONAL ADJUNCTS

One of the most promising areas of current research is the study of pharmacologic agents that may reduce hypermetabolism, promote protein synthesis, speed wound healing, and augment the immune system.

The metabolic effects of pituitary-derived growth hormone in burned patients have been studied since the 1950s. An early study in a series of patients with greater than 50 percent body surface burn injury found that the daily administration of 10 IU of growth hormone reduced mean nitrogen excretion by approximately 25 percent.[80] More recently, basal levels of growth hormone and its second messenger, insulinlike growth factor 1 (IGF-1), have been shown to be depressed following thermal injury.[15] The availability of recombinant human growth hormone (rhGH) and IGF-1 has led to further investigations on the possible usefulness of these two agents as nutritional adjuncts in burn patients.

Growth hormone supplementation has been reported to accelerate skin graft donor site healing in both children[81] and adults.[82] In children with large burns, its use resulted in a significant decrease in time required to close the burn wound. Exogenous growth hormone has also been reported to increase limb and wholebody protein synthesis, suggesting that its use may limit peripheral protein wasting.[83]

The actions of rhGH on protein metabolism may be mediated by IGF-1. In animal models of burn injury, IGF-1 supplementation has been shown to limit postburn hypermetabolism[84] and reduce mucosal atrophy and bacterial translocation.[85] In one human trial, IGF-1 did not have a significant effect on burn patients' REE, even though glucose uptake was promoted and lysine oxidation and overall protein oxidation decreased significantly.[86]

Conversely, rhGH may affect protein metabolism secondary to its effect on glucose metabolism. Administration of rhGH results in peripheral insulin resistance and hyperglycemia, often resulting in a requirement for exogenous insulin administration. Exogenous infusions of insulin and glucose have been shown to stimulate protein synthesis in burn patients. Gore and associates attempted to differentiate between the effects of rhGH and insulin on protein metabolism using a hyperinsulinemic euglycemic clamp technique.[83] Both exogenous growth hormone and insulin appeared to be equally effective in stimulating protein synthesis. However, no further increase in protein synthesis was noted when infusions of glucose and insulin were used in growth hormone–treated patients, suggesting that both rhGH and insulin affect protein kinetics by a common mechanism. Thus, it remains unclear whether rhGH primarily influences protein kinetics through the effects of IGF-1 or the insulin that is concomitantly administered.

At present, rhGH supplementation appears to be efficacious in children with large burns. Sakurai and coworkers have recently reported the results of studies on the effect of long-term (7 days) infusion of insulin on protein metabolism in extensively burned patients ranging in age from 8 to 28. The hyperinsulinemic (plasma insulin ~ 900 µl/ml) euglycemic state was associated with a marked increase in transport of amino acids from the blood, an increase in protein synthesis, and elimination of the pretreatment negative peripheral protein balance. Those investigators also noted that the administration of rhGH during the insulin infusion reduced the rate of glucose uptake by the muscle and significantly decreased the amount of glucose required to maintain euglycemia.[87] Thus, infusions of insulin and glucose may be just as effective as rhGH supplementation, but their use is complicated by the difficulty in maintaining euglycemia. We limit the use of growth hormone (0.2 units/kg/day) in adult burn patients to those with delayed healing of donor sites.

FUTURE DIRECTION

Much of the current research on the metabolic support of the burn patient is centered on manipulation of the metabolic response to burn injury. β-antagonists have been used clinically in attempts to decrease postburn hypermetabolism.[13,14] Decreased heart rates and lower cardiac workloads with an associated decrease in measured metabolic rates have been noted with propranolol. The clinical usefulness of β-adrenergic blockade, however, is severely limited by the associated myocardial depression.

Several β-adrenergic agonists have been recently identified that alter body composition in animals. Cimaterol has been found to decrease fat deposition and increase skeletal muscle accumulation in several animal models.[88,89] The reduction in fat gain appears to result from mobilization of stored triglycerides by stimulation of lipolysis, while the protein gain is associated with elevated lipoprotein lipase activity in muscle. This latter effect increases the metabolism of fatty acids as fuel by skeletal muscle.

Clenbuterol, another β-adrenergic agent, has been found to increase weight gain, muscle mass, and muscle protein content in burned rats.[90,91] Depending on dose, route, and timing of administration, clenbuterol may increase protein synthesis in skeletal muscle[92] or reduce protein degradation rates.[93,94] Both cimaterol and clenbuterol may thus prove to be of therapeutic value in inhibiting or reversing muscle atrophy associated with thermal injury.

In summary, metabolic studies confirm that advances in burn care have resulted in decreased metabolic rates compared with measurements made 2 decades ago. Hormonal manipulations with rhGH, IGF-1 and β-adrenergic agonists may result in further reductions. However, hypermetabolism may be an essential component of the response to burn injury, and if it is pharmacologically reduced it may only impair wound healing and the immune response. Consequently, it is mandatory to meet the patient's elevated energy needs by providing an adequate nutrient supply. The enteral route of nutrient delivery, which can be instituted early and continued perioperatively, preserves GI mucosal integrity and function, maintains muscle mass, and reduces the incidence of infectious complications; it is thus the preferred route of nutritional support in burn patients.

REFERENCES

1. Cuthbertson DP: Observations on the disturbance of metabolism produced by injury to the limbs. Quart J Med 1932;1:233–246.

2. Wilmore DW: Nutrition and metabolism following thermal injury. Clin Plas Surg 1974;1:603–619.

3. Bartlett RH, Allyn PA, Medley T et al: Nutritional therapy based on positive caloric balance in burn patients. Arch Surg 1977;112:974–980.

4. Wilmore DW, Aulick LH: Metabolic changes in burned patients. Surg Clin N Am 1978;58:1173–1187.

5. Waymack JP, Herndon DN: Nutritional support of the burned patient. World J Surg 1992;16:80–86.

6. Goodwin CW: Metabolism and nutrition in the thermally injured patient. Crit Care Clinics 1985;1:97–117.

7. Wilmore DW, Long JM, Mason AD et al: Catecholamines: mediator of the hypermetabolic response to thermal injury. Ann Surg 1974;180:653–668.

8. Becker RA, Wilmore DW, Goodwin CW et al: Free T$_4$, free T$_3$, and reverse T$_3$ in critically ill, thermally injured patients. J Trauma 1980;20:713–721.

9. Vaughan GM, Pruitt BA, Jr: Thyroid function in critical illness and burn injury. Semin Nephrol 1993;13:359–370.

10. Becker RA, Vaughan, GM, Ziegler MG et al: Hypermetabolic low triiodothyronine syndrome of burn injury. Crit Care Med 1982;10:870–875.

11. Becker RA, Vaughan GM, Goodwin CW, Jr et al: Plasma norepinephrine, epinephrine, and thyroid hormone interactions in severely burned patients. Arch Surg 1980;115:439–443.

12. Vaughan GM, Becker RA, Unger RH et al: Nonthyroidal control of metabolism after burn injury: possible role of glucagon. Metabolism 1985;34:637–641.

13. Herndon DN, Barrow RE, Rutan TC et al: Effect of propranolol administration on hemodynamic and metabolic responses of burned pediatric patients. Ann Surg 1988;208:484–492.

14. Baron P, Herndon DN: Chronic propranolol administration safely decreases cardiac work and anxiety in massively burned pediatric patients. Patients Proc Am Burn Assoc 1993;25:87.

15. Jeffries MK, Vance ML: Growth hormone and cortisol secretion in patients with burn injury. J Burn Care Rehabil 1992;13:391–395.

16. Vaughan GM, Becker RA, Allen JP et al: Cortisol and corticotrophin in burned patients. J Trauma 1982;22:263–273.

17. Souba WW: Cytokine control of nutrition and metabolism in critical illness. Current Problems Surg 1994;31:582–595.

18. Youn Y, LaLonde C, Demling R: The role of mediators in the response to thermal injury. World J Surg 1992;16:30–36.

19. Drost AC, Burleson DG, Cioffi WG et al: Plasma cytokines following thermal injury and their relationship with patient mortality, burn size, and time postburn. J Trauma 1993;35:335–339.

20. Drost AC, Burleson DG, Cioffi WG et al: Plasma cytokines after thermal injury and their relationship to infection. Ann Surg 1993;218:74–78.

21. Arita H, Ogle CK, Alexander JW et al: Induction of hypermetabolism in guinea pigs by endotoxin infused through the portal vein. Arch Surg 1988;123:1420–1424.

22. Deitch EA, Berg R: Bacterial translocation from the gut; a mechanism of infection. J Burn Care Rehabil 1987;8:475–482.

23. Levoyer T, Cioffi WG, Pratt L et al: Alterations in intestinal permeability after thermal injury. Arch Surg 1992;127:26–30.

24. Deitch EA: Intestinal permeability is increased in burn patients shortly after injury. Surgery 1990;107:411–416.

25. Mochizuki H, Trocki O, Dominioni L et al: Mechanism of prevention of postburn hypermetabolism and catabolism by early enteral feeding. Ann Surg 1984; 200:297–310.
26. Wood RH, Caldwell FT, Bowser-Wallace BH: The effect of early feeding on postburn hypermetabolism. J Trauma 1988;28:177–183.
27. Aulick LH, McManus AT, Mason AD, Jr et al: Effects of infection on oxygen consumption and core temperature in experimental thermal injury. Ann Surg 1986; 204:48–52.
28. Aulick LH, Wroczyski FA, Coil JA et al: Metabolic and thermoregulatory responses to burn wound colonization. J Trauma 1989;29:478–483.
29. Aulick LH, Hander EH, Wilmore DW et al: The relative significance of thermal and metabolic demands on burn hypermetabolism. J Trauma 1979;19: 559–566.
30. Zawacki BE, Spitzer KW, Mason AD, Jr et al: Does increased evaporative water loss cause hypermetabolism in burned patients? Ann Surg 1970;171: 236–240.
31. Aulick LH, Wilmore DW: Increased peripheral amino acid release following burn injury. Surgery 1979;85: 560–565.
32. Wolfe RR, Durkot MJ, Allsop JR et al: Glucose metabolism in severely burned patients. Metabolism 1979;28: 1031–1039.
33. Wolfe RR, Herndon DN, Peters EJ et al: Regulation of lipolysis in severely burned children. Ann Surg 1987;206:214–221.
34. Abbott WC, Schiller WR, Long CL et al: The effect of major thermal injury on plasma ketone body levels. J Parenter Enteral Nutr 1985;9:153–158.
35. Stinnett JD, Alexander JW, Watanabe C et al: Plasma and skeletal muscle amino acids following severe burn injury in patients and experimental animals. Ann Surg 1982;195:75–89.
36. Alexander JW, MacMillan BG, Stinnett JD et al: Beneficial effects of aggressive protein feeding in severely burned children. Ann Surg 1980;192:505–517.
37. Carlson DE, Jordan BS: Implementing nutritional therapy in the thermally injured patient. Crit Care Nursing Clinics of N Am 1991;3:221–235.
38. Czaja AJ, McAlhany JC, Pruitt BA, Jr: Acute gastroduodenal disease after thermal injury: an endoscopic evaluation of incidence and natural history. N Engl J Med 1974;291:925–929.
39. Czaja AJ, McAlhany JC, Andes WA et al: Acute gastric disease after cutaneous thermal injury. Arch Surg 1975;110:600–605.
40. Czaja AJ, McAlhany JC, Pruitt BA, Jr: Acute duodenitis and duodenal ulceration after burns. JAMA 1975; 232:621–624.
41. Rosenthal A, Czaja AJ, Pruitt BA, Jr: Gastrin levels and gastric acidity in the pathogenesis of acute gastroduodenal disease after burns. Surg Gynecol Obstet 1977;144:232–234.
42. McAlhany TC, Czaja AJ, Pruitt BA, Jr: Antacid control of complications from acute gastroduodenal disease after burns. J Trauma 1976;16:645–648.
43. McElwee HP, Sirinek KR, Levine BA: Cimetidine affords protection equal to antacids in prevention of stress ulceration following thermal injury. Surgery 1979;86:620–626.
44. Munster AM, Goodwin MN, Pruitt BA, Jr: Acalculous cholecystitis in burned patients. Am J Surg 1971;122: 591–593.
45. Babb RR: Acute acalculous cholecystitis. J Clin Gastroenterol 1992;15:238–241.
46. Goodwin CW, Jr, Pruitt BA, Jr: Increased incidence of pancreatitis in thermally injured patients: a prospective study. Proc Am Assoc Surg Trauma 1981.
47. Desai MH, Herndon DN, Rutan RL et al: Ischemic intestinal complications in patients with burns. Surg Gynecol Obstet 1991;172:257–261.
48. Lescher TJ, Teejarden DK, Pruitt BA, Jr: Acute pseudo-obstruction of the colon in thermally injured patients. Dis Colon Rectum 1978;21:618–622.
49. Curreri DW, Richmond D, Marvin J et al: Dietary requirements of patients with major burns. J Am Diet Assoc 1974;65:415–417.
50. Carlson DE, Cioffi WG, Mason AD et al: Resting energy expenditure in patients with thermal injury. Surg Gynecol Obstet 1992;174:270–276.
51. Ireton CS, Turner WW, Hunt JL et al: Evaluation of energy expenditures in burn patients. J Am Diet Assoc 1986;86:331–333.
52. Allard JP, Pichard C, Hoshino E et al: Validation of a new formula for calculating the energy requirements of burn patients. J Parenter Enter Nutr 1990;14: 115–118.
53. Milner EA, Cioffi WG, Mason AD et al: A longitudinal study of resting energy expenditure in thermally injured patients. J Trauma 1994;37:167–170.
54. Rutan TC, Herndon DN, Van Osten T et al: Metabolic rate alterations in early excision and grafting versus conservative treatment. J Trauma 1986;26:140–142.
55. Ireton-Jones CS, Turner WW, Baxter CR: The effect of burn wound excision on measured energy expenditure and urinary nitrogen excretion. J Trauma 1987; 27:217–220.
56. Frankenfield D, Wiles CE, Bagley S et al: Relationships between resting and total energy expenditure in injured and septic patients. Crit Care Med 1994;22: 1796–1804.
57. Waxman K, Rebello T, Pinderski L et al: Evaluation of serum visceral protein loss across burn wounds. J Trauma 1987;27:136–140.
58. Carlson DE, Cioffi WG, Mason AD et al: Evaluation of serum visceral protein levels as indicators of nitrogen balance in thermally injured patients. J Parenter Enter Nutr 1991;15:440–444.
59. McDonald WS, Sharp CW, Deitch EA: Immediate enteral feeding in burn patients is safe and effective. Ann Surg 1991;213:177–183.
60. Hansbrough WB, Hansbrough JF: Success of immediate intragastric feeding of patients with burns. J Burn Care Rehabil 1993;14:512–516.
61. Jenkins ME, Gottschlich MM, Warden GD: Enteral feeding during operative procedures in thermal injuries. J Burn Care Rehab 1994;15:199–205.
62. Nirgiotis JG, Hennessey PJ, Black CT et al: The effects of an arginine-free enteral diet on wound healing and immune function in the post-surgical rat. J Pediatr Surg 1991;26:936–941.
63. Meyer NA, Muller MJ, Herndon DN: Nutrient support of the healing wound. New Horizons 1994;2:202–214.
64. Daly JM, Reynolds J, Thom A et al: Immune and metabolic effects of arginine in the surgical patient. Ann Surg 1988;208:512–523.
65. Saito H, Trocki O, Wang S et al: Metabolic and immune effects of dietary arginine supplementation after burn. Arch Surg 1987;122:784–789.
66. Gottschlich MM, Powers C, Khoury J et al: Incidence and effects of glutamine depletion in burn patients. Proc Am Burn Assoc 1992;24:134.
67. Inoue S, Trocki O, Edwards L et al: Is glutamine beneficial in postburn nutritional support? Curr Surg 1988;45:110–113.

68. Mochizuki H, Trocki O, Dominioni L et al: Effect of a diet rich in branched chain amino acids on severely burned guinea pigs. J Trauma 1986;26:1077–1085.

69. Alexander JW, Gottschlich MM: Nutritional immunomodulaton in burn patients. Crit Care Med 1990;18:S149–S153.

70. Alexander JW, Saito H, Ogle CK et al: The importance of lipid type in the diet after burn injury. Ann Surg 1986;204:1–8.

71. Peck MD: Omega-3 polyunsaturated fatty acids: benefit or harm during sepsis? New Horizons 1994;2:230–236.

72. Peck MD, Alexander JW, Ogle CK et al: The effect of dietary fatty acids on response to Pseudomonas infection in burned mice. J Trauma 1990;30:445–452.

73. Gottschlich MM, Warden GD: Vitamin supplementation in the patient with burns. J Burn Care Rehabil 1990;11:275–279.

74. Gottschlich MM, Warden GD, Michel MA et al: Diarrhea in tube fed burn patients: incidence, etiology, nutritional impact, and prevention. J Parenter Enter Nutr 1988;12:338–344.

75. Heibert JM, Brown A, Anderson RG et al: Comparison of continuous versus intermittent tube feedings in adult burn patients. J Parenter Enter Nutr 1981;5:73–75.

76. Milner EA, Cioffi WG, McManus WF et al: Superior mesenteric artery syndrome in a burn patient. Nutr Clin Prac 1993;8:264–266.

77. Reckler JM, Bruck HM, Munster AM et al: Superior mesenteric artery syndrome as a consequence of burn injury. J Trauma 1972;12:979–985.

78. Becker WK, Pruitt BA, Jr: Parenteral nutrition in the thermally injured patient. Comprehensive Therapy 1991;17:47–53.

79. Herndon DN, Barrow RE, Stein M et al: Increased mortality with intravenous supplemental feeding in severely burned patients. J Burn Care Rehabil 1989;10:309–313.

80. Wilmore DW, Moylan JA, Bristow BF et al: Anabolic effects of human growth and high caloric feedings following thermal injury. Surg Gynecol Obstet 1974;138:875–884.

81. Herndon DN, Barrow RE, Kunkel KR et al: Effects of recombinant growth hormone on donor-site healing in severely burned children. Ann Surg 1990;212:424–431.

82. Sherman SK, Demling RH, LaLonde C et al: Growth hormone enhances re-epithelialization of human split thickness skin graft donor sites. Surg Forum 1989;40:37–39.

83. Gore DC, Honeycutt D, Jahoor F et al: Effect of exogenous growth hormone on whole-body and isolated-limb protein kinetics in burned patients. Arch Surg 1991;126:38–43.

84. Strock LL, Singh H, Abdullah A et al: The effect of insulin-like growth factor I on postburn hypermetabolism. Surgery 1990;108:161–164.

85. Huang KF, Chung DH, Herndon DN: Insulin like growth factor I (IGF-1) reduces gut atrophy and bacterial translocation after severe burn injury. Arch Surg 1993;128:47–54.

86. Cioffi WG, Gore DC, Rue LW et al: Insulin-like growth factor-1 lowers protein oxidation in patients with thermal injury. Ann Surg 1994;220:310–319.

87. Sakurai Y, Aarsland A, Herndon DN et al: Stimulation of muscle protein synthesis by long-term insulin infusion in severely burned patients. Ann Surg 1995;222:283–297.

88. Eadara JK, Dalrymple RH, Delay RL et al: Effects of cimaterol, a beta-adrenergic agonist, on lipid metabolism in rats. Metabolism 1989;38:522–529.

89. Nelson JL, Chalk LL, Warden GD: Anabolic impact of cimaterol in conjunction with enteral nutrition following burn trauma. Trauma 1995;38:237–241.

90. Martineau L, Little RA, Rothwell NJ et al: Clenbuterol, a beta 2-adrenergic agonist, reverses muscle wasting due to scald injury in the rat. Burns 1993;19:26–34.

91. Chance WT, Von Allmen D, Benson D et al: Clenbuterol decreases catabolism and increases hypermetabolism in burned rats. J Trauma 1991;31:365–370.

92. Emery PW, Rothwell NJ, Stock MJ et al: Chronic effects of beta-2 agonists on body composition and protein synthesis in the rat. Biosci Rep 1984;4:83–91.

93. Reeds PJ, Hay SM, Dorwood PM et al: Stimulation of muscle growth by clenbuterol: lack of effect on muscle protein biosynthesis. Br J Nutr 1986;56:249–252.

94. Benson DW, Foley-Nelson T, Chance WT et al: Decreased myofibrillar breakdown following treatment with clenbuterol. J Surg Res 1991;50:1–5.

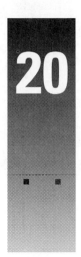

20

Enteral Nutrition in Pediatrics

SUSAN S. BAKER

Children's digestive function and nutritional needs are not the same as adults'. The concept that children are different is particularly important for the design and administration of enteral support for children. Because of growth, nutrient needs are higher on a per kilogram basis than for adults. The digestive process is not completely developed at birth, especially if the birth is premature. Children are never alone as patients. They are part of a family, and often parental and sibling needs must be included in plans for nutrition support. And so, children require a different approach than adults in the design, initiation, and monitoring of nutrition solutions.

GASTROINTESTINAL DEVELOPMENT

Mechanical Function

Sucking is a complex activity involving the cranial nerves and the appreciation of tactile stimulation of facial skin. Partially conscious and partially unconscious, it requires the coordination of sucking, breathing, and swallowing. Swallowing develops before sucking at approximately 11 weeks of gestational age.[1] Mouthing movements, early attempts at sucking, begin by approximately 18 weeks. After 34 to 35 weeks sucking and swallowing rapidly develop.[2] Thus, infants born before 33 or 34 weeks of gestation do not have coordinated sucking activities and cannot rely on sucking for nutrient intake. Rather, they must be fed by

tube. Nonnutritive sucking is sucking activity not associated with the intake of nutrients. Infants offered the opportunity for nonnutritive sucking during tube feeding demonstrate increased oxygenation as measured transcutaneously.[3] Premature infants who are offered the opportunity for nonnutritive sucking gain weight, move more quickly to oral feeding, and leave the hospital earlier than infants not offered nonnutritive sucking.[4-6] The physiologic basis for this observation is unclear. However, offering infants the opportunity to decrease crying may result in decreased activity and energy expenditure.

Gastric emptying may be defined as the time it takes for half the gastric contents to leave the stomach. This time depends on the test meal's volume and composition. Because no standardized method to assess gastric emptying time exists, comparing studies is difficult. Although it is thought that gastric emptying is delayed in the neonate, especially infants born prematurely,[7] no studies have compared adults and neonates using identical liquid meals in volumes normalized for weight.

Motility of the gastrointestinal (GI) tract involves the intraluminal flow of its contents, the motions of the gut wall that cause flow, and the systems that regulate gut wall movement. Motility depends on the integration of neural, smooth muscle, and neural-humoral mechanisms. Few developmental studies have been conducted on humans because of ethical considerations. However, before 30 weeks' gestation, there is little movement of contrast beyond the stomach.[8] By 34 weeks contrast moves into the colon. Duodenal contraction rate increases as a function of gestational age and is associated with an increase in contractions per burst.[9] Both gastric emptying and intestinal motility can be delayed in ill infants and children. Conversely, small enteral feedings result in improved feeding tolerance and earlier progression to full enteral intake compared with a group of infants receiving delayed enteral feedings.[10,11] Thus, the early delivery of some enteral feedings improves GI motility and tolerance to enteral nutrition.

Digestion

The absorption of fat depends on lipases, bile acids, and enterocyte uptake. In premature infants only 65 to 70 percent of ingested fat is absorbed, while in term infants less than 6 months of age 85 percent of ingested fat is absorbed. It is not until approximately 6 months of age that fat absorption, more than 90 percent of ingested fat, approaches that of normal adults.[12] In a series of experiments, Fredrikzon and coworkers[13] demonstrated that duodenal lipase activity is lower in infants than adults and does not increase after a test meal containing a standard per kilogram amount of fat (Fig. 20–1). Hamosh and colleagues[14] found lipase present in gastric aspirates at 26 weeks of gestational age. They proposed that the lingual glands were the source of the lipase and the lipase was important for fat digestion in the neonate. Lipase is present in biopsies of the gastric fundus at 11 weeks' gestational age and reaches adult levels by 3 months of age.[15] Breast-fed infants have the additional advantage of human milk lipase, which aids in the digestion of triglycerides.

Bile acids act to solubilize lipids. Using stable isotope dilution, Watkins and colleagues[12] showed that the bile salt pool and average rate of cholate synthesis is less in normal infants than in normal adults. Infants born prematurely have an even more marked reduction in bile acid pool size[16] compared with term infants (Fig. 20–2).

The digestion of carbohydrates by infants depends on enzymes that hydrolyze starches and disaccharides. The duodenal concentration of amylase is low during infancy.[16] However, infants can digest starch because mammary and salivary amylase and brush border glucoamylase may be involved in the digestion of starch. Further digestion of starches by colonic fermentation into short-chain fatty acids may offer

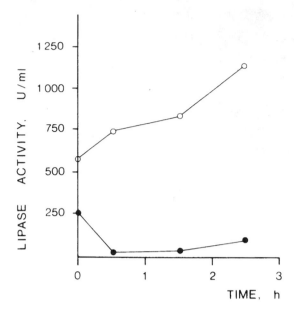

FIGURE 20–1 Lipase activity in duodenal aspirates from infants and adults. (Reproduced with permission from Fredrikzon B, Hernell O, Blackberg L: Lingual lipase. Its role in lipid digestion in infants with low birthweight and/or pancreatic insufficiency. Acta Paediatr Scand Suppl 1982;296:75–80.)

some energy from undigested starches that reach the large bowel.[17] Sucrase, isomaltase, and maltase activities are present at 10 weeks of gestation and reach adult levels by 30 weeks of gestational age.[18] By 28 to 34 weeks of gestation lactase activity is present at approximately one third of the activity found in term infants. Lactase activity peaks at birth and by adulthood is lower than in newborns; nevertheless, infants retain 96 percent of lactose intake and show no clinical sign of intolerance.[19] Monosaccharides such as glucose and galactose are absorbed primarily by a sodium-dependent active transport process that is present as early as the 10th gestational week. In the human newborn the capacity for glucose absorption per unit weight of intestinal tissue is only 50 to 60 percent of the adult level.[20] Fructose, in contrast, is absorbed by sodium-independent facilitated diffusion.

The digestion of protein begins with proteolysis in the stomach. Infants can produce gastric acid, intrinsic factor, and gastrin from approximately 18 weeks of gestational age.[21] However, little protein hydrolysis occurs in their stomach.[22] The pancreas of neonates secretes trypsin at approximately the same level as adults.[23] Chymotrypsin secretion is about 50 to 60 percent of the adult level. Nevertheless, neonates can digest and absorb adequate protein.[24] Premature

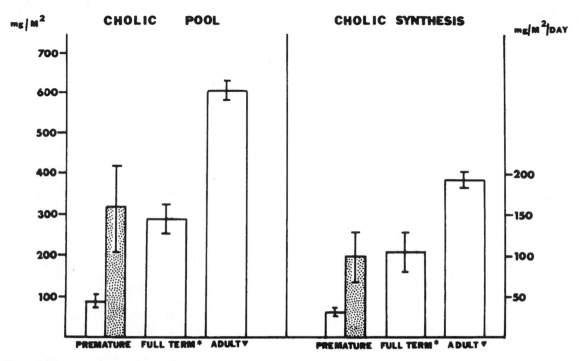

FIGURE 20-2 Comparison of cholic acid pool size and synthetic rates in premature infants, full-term infants, and adults, corrected for body surface area. (Reproduced with permission from Watkins JB, Szczepanik P, Gould JB et al: Bile salt metabolism in the human premature infant. Gastroenterology 1975;69:709.)

infants require higher levels of protein intake, but they have a more limited capacity to digest proteins. Care is essential when supplying excess dietary protein to premature infants, since it may increase their metabolic load and result in uremia, metabolic acidosis, and neurologic disturbances.[25] In addition, undigested proteins may present a source of antigens to the neonate to which allergy can develop.[26]

Barrier Function

The GI tract functions as an important barrier against the passage of viruses, bacteria, and antigenic proteins and acts as an absorptive surface. However, the barrier is not absolute,[27] permitting the passage of some molecules. Under specific conditions[28,29] the barrier may become more permeable. Infants born prematurely demonstrate a higher intestinal permeability than do infants born at term.[30,31] The higher permeability of the GI tract can lead to uptake of potentially harmful infectious agents and antigens.

GROWTH

Growth is extremely rapid in infancy; infants double their birthweight by 6 months of age

and triple it by 12 months of age. Thereafter, growth proceeds at a steady rate of approximately 5 g/day, until the adolescent growth spurt. In addition to this rapid growth, changes occur in body composition.[32] Fuel reserves may be marginal, particularly in prematurely born or sick infants, and the presence of disease may require additional nutrients. During the initial stages of nutrition support in very sick or injured children, growth itself may not be a reasonable goal. However, with time after the acute process, growth becomes important if children are to achieve their full developmental and intellectual potential. Later intellectual achievement may depend on the provision of adequate nutrients in infancy. For some nutrients it is unclear whether the later correction of deficits can completely compensate for earlier lack. An example of this is iron deficiency in infancy and intellectual achievement at age 5 years.[33-35]

ENTERAL NUTRITION SUPPORT

Thus, developmental immaturity and growth are two major factors that must be considered in nutrition support for children. Careful attention to providing nutrients to meet children's additional needs will determine the success of nutrition support.

Before providing enteral nutrients several steps are necessary (Table 20–1). First nutritional needs must be assessed, goals must be set, and a therapeutic plan put in place. Once enteral nutrition begins, careful monitoring and frequent reassessment are needed.

For infants and children a nutritional assessment consists of the anthropometric measurements of weight, height, head circumference, triceps skinfold thickness, and mid-arm muscle circumference (Table 20–2). In addition to the usual anthropometric measures Table 20–2 includes Z-scores, which denote the units of standard deviation from the median. The use of Z-scores permits an observation to be compared with the normal curve. It detects movement toward or away from the median and is more sensitive than percentile changes.[36] In addition, the measurement of hemoglobin, hematocrit, serum proteins, liver function, and renal function tests are helpful.

Nutritional goals may vary with degree of malnutrition, level of metabolic stress, and specific nutrient deficiencies. In general, at least the basal metabolic requirements must be supplied daily. Additional needs can be met by increasing either the concentration of nutrients, the rate at which they are delivered, or the length of time over which they are administered. Specific deficiencies, such as iron, calcium, phosphorus, and zinc, can be corrected by providing the nutrients as supplements.

The therapeutic plan consists of a written set of orders that clearly establishes the nutrient solution, its concentration, and how that concentration is achieved (by adding less water to a powdered or liquid concentrate or by modular nutrients, specifying which modular nutrients and how much of each per unit volume). The therapeutic plan also states the volume of the nutrient solution to be delivered, the rate at which it must be administered, the length of time over which it must be administered, and any additives, such as vitamins, minerals, or trace elements, that must be included.

Reassessment is vital to the successful delivery of enteral nutrition support. It consists of an ongoing evaluation of anthropometrics, biochemistries, delivery of nutrients (did the patient actually receive the volume and concentration of nutrient solutions ordered?), and changes in disease state.

TABLE 20–1   Initiation of Enteral Nutrition

Assess Patient
Anthropomorphics
Biochemistry
Determine if malnourished
Determine level of stress
Determine expected level of GI function
Consider predicted changes in above (planned surgery, chemotherapy, etc)

Set Goals
Deliver at least enough nutrients to supply needs for basal metabolism
Rehabilitate malnutrition
Correct mineral/electrolyte imbalance
Support growth
Initiate catch-up growth
Support through metabolic stress
Account for nutrient needs of disease processes (cystic fibrosis, IBD, etc)
Minimal enteral feeding to support normal GI mucosa
Enteral feeding to potentiate GI development

Design Written Therapeutic Plan
What nutrient solution
Concentration of solution (add modular nutrients?)
Planned rate of advancement
Rate of delivery of solution
Use bolus, continuous administration, cycled administration, or a combination
Site of delivery of nutrition solution (stomach, small bowel)
Determine tools used to monitor each patient

Monitor
Review flow sheets daily
Record amount of solution administered at rate administered
Record fluid composition
Calculate percentage of nutrients from therapeutic plan actually delivered
Record adverse reactions
Record all medications administered enterally

Reassess
Repeat initial assessment
Re-evaluate goals in light of nutritional therapy and changes in metabolic/disease state
Reaffirm goals and therapeutic plan
Modify plan

Indications

The enteral route of nutrition support is preferred unless a specific contraindication such as bowel obstruction exists. The reasons the enteral route is preferred are numerous and have been reviewed recently.[37] Essentially, feeds infused into the GI tract prevent possible atrophy, may induce maturation, may prevent breakdown of the GI barrier, and

TABLE 20-2 Nutritional Assessment

Historic
Recall dietary history
Three-day food diary
Calorie count in hospital

Anthropomorphics
Weight
Height
Weight for height
Body mass index
Head circumference
Mid-arm muscle circumference
Triceps skinfold thickness
Z-Score for each measurement

Biochemical
Electrolytes
Acid-base status
Minerals
Visceral proteins
Renal function
Liver function
Trace elements
Vitamins
Serum triglycerides

---

may directly supply nutrients to enterocytes. The enteral route permits the provision of some nutrients that may be important to the GI tract and are not available in a parenteral form. The GI tract and its vascular system modulates nutrients before they reach the systemic circulation by a passage through the portal circulation. This modulation of nutrients does not occur if nutrients are infused directly into a systemic vein.

In certain situations it may not be possible to supply all necessary nutrients enterally. Nevertheless, as much as possible of the total nutritional needs should be supplied enterally. Gastric and colonic hypomotility may occur in severely injured children, while the small intestine can maintain good motility and absorption. Bowel sounds, produced by the movement of air through the intestines, may not be a good indicator of small bowel function, especially if a nasogastric tube is on constant suction. Instillation of air into the small bowel through a duodenal tube may restore bowel sounds.[38] Sick and injured children who are vomiting, or children with malnutrition or vomiting and reflux may be fed enterally into the small bowel if the stomach is decompressed. Even very small amounts of hypotonic nutrition solutions may benefit the GI tract.[39,40]

Table 20-3 lists criteria for initiating enteral feedings in children with chronic problems,

and Table 20-4 lists some indications for using enteral feedings.

Once enteral nutrition support is identified as the nutrition support of choice, the nutritional formula, concentration, route of delivery, and rate of advancement must be established (Tables 20-5 and 20-6).

Enteral Formulas

The choice for an enteral formula must be individualized, since nutritional requirements, fluid requirements, age, medical condition, gastrointestinal function, food intolerance, and so on must be considered. In general, pediatricians group enteral formulas according to the ages of children for whom they will be used: premature infants, term infants, children aged 1 to 10 years, and children older than 10 years.

Premature Infants

Formulas designed for premature infants have higher calorie, protein, vitamin, and mineral concentrations and lower lactose than term infant formulas. These formulas also contain more medium-chain triglycerides (MCTs).

TABLE 20-3 Indications for Enteral Nutrition Support

Impaired energy consumption	From 50–60% of recommended daily amount despite high-calorie supplements plus total feeding time more than 4–6 hours/day
	plus
Severe and deteriorating wasting	Weight for height >2 standard deviations below the mean plus skinfold thickness below the fifth percentile
	and/or
Depressed linear growth	Fall in height velocity >0.3 standard deviations/year or height velocity <5 cm/year or decrease in height velocity of at least 2 cm from the preceding year during early to mid-puberty

Reproduced with permission from Davis A: Indications and techniques for enteral feeds. In Baker SS, Baker RD, Davis A (eds): Pediatric Enteral Nutrition. New York: Chapman and Hall, 1994:67–94.

TABLE 20–4 Some Indications for Enteral Feedings

Limited Ability to Eat
Neurologic disorders
Acquired immunodeficiency syndrome
Facial trauma
Tumors of face, mouth, or esophagus
Injury of face, mouth, esophagus
Congenital abnormalities of face, mouth, esophagus
Prematurity (less than 34 weeks' gestational age)

Inability to Meet Full Nutrient Needs Orally
Increased metabolic needs
Anorexia, especially from chronic disease
Psychological disorders

Altered Absorption or Metabolism
Chronic diarrhea
Short small bowel
IBD
Glycogen storage disease types I and III
Gastroesophageal reflux
Pseudo-obstruction
Pancreatitis
Amino or organic acidopathies

Adapted from Davis A: Indications and techniques for enteral feeds. In Baker SS, Baker RD, Davis A (eds): Pediatric Enteral Nutrition. New York: Chapman and Hall, 1994:67–94.

Because of concerns over GI immaturity, the formulas designed for premature infants are recommended for infants with weights of approximately 2 to 2.5 kg with normal alkaline phosphatase and serum albumin levels. These specially designed formulas supply adequate nutrients for premature infants when used as the sole nutrient source. The formulas are 24 kcal/oz (0.8 kcal/ml). Breast milk is not adequate as a sole nutrient source for premature infants. Breast milk must be supplemented with calories, protein, vitamins, and minerals, including zinc, calcium, and phosphorus. Human milk fortifiers can be added to human milk (Table 20–7) to achieve adequate enteral nutrition. Nevertheless, premature infants are at risk for rickets and trace element deficiencies.[42,43]

Term Infants

Term infants with normal GI function can be fed human milk or infant formula for the first year of life. If human milk is used as the sole nutrient source, supplementation may be necessary at approximately 6 months of age, when the infant's need for iron outstrips the quantity

TABLE 20–5 Pediatric Enteral Formulas

Clinical Condition	Formula Description
Premature Infant	Premature formula—12% protein, contains MCT oil, carbohydrate, lactose/glucose polymers, calcium, and phosphorus
Term Infant	
Primary or secondary lactose intolerance	Lactose-free cow's milk formula
Primary or secondary lactose intolerance or cow's milk sensitivity	Lactose-free, soy, or hydrolyzed protein formula (sucrose and corn free)
Renal or cardiac disease	Low electrolyte/RSL formula
Steatorrhea associated with bile acid deficiency, ileal resection, or lymphatic anomalies	MCT oil–containing formula
Cow's milk protein and soy protein sensitivity; abnormal nutrient absorption, digestion and transport; intractable diarrhea or protein-calorie malnutrition	Hypoallergenic, hydrolyzed casein, lactose and sucrose free
1–10 Years	
Tube feeding	Complete nutrition in 1100 ml
Oral supplement	Intack protein, 1.0 kcal/ml, glutein free, lactose free, isotonic, appropriate minerals for children
Over 10 Years	
Normal GI function, varying medical conditions	Hypercaloric formula
Fluid restriction	
Abnormal bowel movement	Added fiber
Pulmonary problems/diabetes	High-fat formula
High stress—trauma, sepsis, burns	Hypercaloric, high-protein formula
Lactose intolerance	Lactose-free formula
Compromised GI/pancreatic function	Chemically defined formula
Protein allergy	Elemental formula
Impaired renal function	Low protein, branched-chain amino acid enriched

RSL = renal solute load.

TABLE 20–6   Routes for Delivery of Enteral Nutrition

Site	Advantages	Disadvantages	Complications
Nasogastric	Short term No surgery needed	Vomiting Reflux	Tube dislodgement Possible tactile sensitivity
Passed by mother or child nightly	No visible tube during the day	Difficult for mother/child May irritate nares	May interfere with development of oral motor skills
Indwelling	Infrequently passed	Visible during the day	
Gastrostomy	More stable tube placement Greater patient mobility Does not interfere with development of oral motor skills	Requires invasive procedure May require local skin care	Stomal infections Abdominal leak Tube misplacement
PEG	Easy placement Rapid institution of feedings	Vomiting, reflux not prevented	Tethered colon
Surgery	General anesthesia Longer time to institute feedings	Vomiting, reflux not prevented	Complications of surgery
Jejunal	Bypasses stomach and pylorus Decreased risk of aspiration Decompress stomach while feeding	Continuous feeding	Tube dislodgement Bacterial overgrowth Malabsorption Dumping syndrome
Nasojejunal	No surgery needed	May interfere with development of oral motor skills	
Surgically placed	More stable No visible tube on face	General anesthesia Complications associated with surgery	

PEG = percutaneous gastrostomy.

in human milk. If human milk is used for continuous tube feedings, care must be taken to adjust for nutrient losses caused by fat separation and adherence to the tubing.[44-46] Approximately 20 percent of fat from human milk adheres to the tubing, and those calories must be considered when calculating the enteral feedings. Simply flushing the tubing with water may cause a fat bolus. Adherence of fat to tubing is not a problem with short, intermittent feedings.[47]

Standard infant formulas are available in powder, liquid concentrate, and ready-to-feed forms. In general the powdered forms are the least expensive and the ready-to-feed the most expensive. A proliferation of infant formulas has made it difficult to keep up with each new product. There are, however, major groupings with respect to protein, carbohydrate, fat, and mineral content.

Protein. The most commonly used infant formulas are based on cow's milk protein and can be predominately whey (the liquid portion of milk) or casein (the curd or solid portion). Human milk has proportionately more whey than casein. Soy-based formulas use soy bean protein with the addition of methionine and heat treatment to reduce the activity of trypsin inhibitors and hemagglutinin normally found in soy protein isolates. Since soy-based formulas are also lactose free, they are indicated for infants with cow's milk protein intolerance and lactase deficiency. Hydrolyzed protein formulas are made from cow's milk casein or cow's milk whey protein. The protein is hydrolyzed, or partially hydrolyzed, to polypeptides. Hydrolyzed protein formulas can be used for infants with protein intolerance and pancreatic insufficiency or after gut injury. If food allergy is the basis for the use of a hydrolyzed formula, use only formulas that have been shown clinically to be nonallergenic.[48] Partially hydrolyzed protein formulas may contain polypeptides of sufficient length to cause allergy.[49,50]

TABLE 20–7 Human Milk Fortifiers

Nutrients/dl	Enfamil Human Milk Fortifier (Mead Johnson Laboratories) (liquid)*	Similac Natural Care Milk Fortifier (Ross Laboratories) (packet)†
Energy, kcal	3.5	81.2
Protein, g	0.17	2.2
Source	Whey/sodium caseinate	Nonfat milk and whey
% total calories	20	11
Fat, g	<0.03	4.41
Source	From caseinate	MCT, soy, coconut oils
% total calories	2.5	47
Carbohydrate, g	0.67	8.61
Source	Corn syrup solids, lactose	Lactose, glucose polymers
% total calories	77	42
Vitamins		
E, IU	0.85	3.2
Folic acid, μg	5.8	30.0
D, IU	52	122
Minerals		
Calcium, mg	22	171
Phosphorus, mg	11.2	85
Ca:P ratio	2:1	2:1
Magnesium, mg	NA	10.1
Iron, mg	NA	0.3
Zinc, mg	0.18	1.22
Sodium	1.75	35.0
Potassium	3.9	105.0
Copper, μg	20	203
Renal solute load, mOsm	1.88	14.9
Osmolality, mOsm/kg water	+120	280

*1:1 dilution with breast milk = 22 kcal/oz (0.73 kcal/ml).
†Four packets/50 ml of breast milk = 24 kcal/oz (0.8 kcal/ml).
Data from 1991 product information.

Carbohydrate. Lactose is the main carbohydrate constituent of human milk as well as most cow's milk–based formulas. For lactose intolerance, whether congenital or acquired, a cow's milk–based lactose-free formula is available. Soy-based formulas are lactose free, as are all of the hydrolyzed protein formulas.

Fat. The fat content of infant formulas can vary with the product and the manufacturer. Some fat combinations may be more desirable than others, especially for healthy infants' long-term growth and development. However, for sick or injured infants, the nutritional issues often revolve around the content of MCTs. MCT oil is important in the management of such problems as steatorrhea, chylous ascites, chylothorax, intestinal lymphangiectasia, and ileal resections. Infants receiving formulas containing 86 percent MCT oil must be carefully monitored because they may develop essential fatty acid deficiency with long-term use.[51,52]

Iron. Infant formulas can be purchased with or without iron supplementation. All infant formulas have adequate iron except for the cow's milk–based formulas labeled "low iron formula." Indications for using a low iron formula in infancy are almost nonexistent. Low iron formulas should not be prescribed. Interestingly, the soy formulas and hydrolyzed formulas have adequate iron, as do all the infant formulas manufactured in England and Europe.

Formula Concentrations. The caloric density of infant formulas is 20 kcal/oz (0.67 kcal/ml), the same as human milk. The formulas can be concentrated, either by decreasing the amount of water in which they are diluted or by using modular nutrients. Infant formulas can be safely concentrated to 1.0 kcal/ml by adding less water (JN Udall, personal communication) to concentrated liquid or powdered preparations. Because concentrated infant formulas contain less water than standard formulas, pay careful attention to free water requirements. Inadequate water intake may exceed the kidneys' capacity to concentrate and excrete renal solute (RSL), and the infant may become dehydrated. The RSL consists of nonmetabolizable nutrients, electrolytes, and metabolic products such as urea and can be estimated as follows:

$$RSL\ (mOsm) = (protein\ [g] \times 4) + (Na\ [mEq] + K\ [mEq] + Cl\ [mEq])$$

To estimate the potential renal solute load (PRSL) in formula-fed low birth weight infants, the following formula is used:[53]

$$PRSL\ (mOsm) = \frac{protein\ (g)}{0.175} + \left(Na\ [mEq] + K\ [mEq] + \frac{P(mg)}{Cl\ [mEq] + 31}\right)$$

For infants with increased fluid losses (fever, diarrhea, sweating), in infants with impaired renal concentrating ability, or in those unable to express thirst, dehydration is a risk. Additional free water can be given as a bolus as needed. Caloric supplements, such as fats and carbohydrates, do not increase the RSL. The osmolality of standard infant formulas (90.67 kcal/ml) ranges from 150 to 380 mOsm/kg. The American Academy of Pediatrics recommends that the osmolality of infant formulas be less than 460 mOsm/kg.[54]

Infant formulas can also be concentrated by adding modular nutrients. Modular nutrients can be used to increase the formula's caloric density by adding carbohydrate or fat modules, and to increase the diet's protein content. Modular nutrients can also be used to alter the nutrient composition of diets. Any time nutrient modules are used, the final composition of the diet must be calculated, because a specific nutrient may be diluted or otherwise inadequate in the final diet. For example, the most commonly added nutrient module[55] is a calorie source, such as carbohydrate or fat. If an additional 10 kcal/oz (0.33 kcal/ml) is added to a limited volume of formula, protein, vitamins, and minerals may be inadequate in the final diet. In contrast, adding a noncarbohydrate, nonfat nutrient module may increase the RSL of the final diet.

Children Aged 1 to 10 Years

Enteral nutrition formulas for children are more calorically dense than infant formulas but contain less protein, sodium, potassium, chloride, and magnesium than adult formulas. In addition, they contain more iron, zinc, calcium, phosphorous, and vitamin D.[41] Thus, do not use adult preparations for children without a specific indication. If such an indication exists, the children must be carefully monitored and receive supplements of zinc, iron, calcium, phosphorus, and vitamins. Blenderized diets, either commercially available or prepared in the home, can be used for enteral nutrition support. These feedings generally have a higher osmolality and viscosity than prepared formulas. Home-prepared blenderized diets are cheaper than prepared formulas and may have psychosocial importance for the family. However, home-blenderized diets may have higher bacterial counts, require daily labor, may cause hypernatremic dehydration, and can result in specific nutrient deficiencies if not carefully monitored by a nutritionist.[56,57]

Children Over Age 10 Years

There are many adult formulas available that children over 10 years of age can be fed. The indications are the same as for adults (Chapter 13).

INITIATION OF ENTERAL NUTRITION

Enteral feedings can be initiated in children who are receiving parenteral nutrition with no or little enteral intake for prolonged periods or in children who are on a full diet (Table 20–8). In general, a slow continuous infusion of nutrients is better tolerated as an initial prescription for enteral feeding than bolus feeding. Over time, slow continuous feeds, such as nocturnal feeds, are preferable, no matter what the indication for enteral nutrition support, since continuous feeds are associated with better nutrient absorption and less aspiration[58-62] than bolus feeds.

Transition from Parenteral to Enteral Nutrition

Few controlled studies compare possible feeding schedules. In general, an isotonic, full-strength, lactose-free formula is well tolerated as a first enteral feeding. If the GI tract has not been used for 5 to 7 days, if GI injury has occurred, or if malabsorption or food allergy are present, then choose a hydrolyzed protein–based (elemental) formula. Controversy exists over whether to use a diluted formula. No well-controlled studies exist that demonstrate an advantage to the use of a dilute formula. Greater caloric intake can be achieved when full-strength formula is used, and our experience suggests that a full-strength formula is generally well tolerated. We initiate enteral nutrition with low-volume, full-strength formula. The transition from par-

TABLE 20–8   Guidelines for the Initiation and Advancement of Enteral Feeding

Age	Initial Infusion	Advances	Final Goal
Continuous Feedings			
Preterm	1–2 ml/kg/hour	10–20 ml/kg/day	120–175 ml/kg/day
0–12 months	1–2 ml/kg/hour	1–2 ml/kg/q 2–8 hours	6 ml/kg/hour
1–6 years	1 ml/kg/hour	1 ml/kg/q 2–8 hours	4–6 ml/kg/hour
>7 years	25 ml/hour	25 ml/q 2–8 hours	100–150 ml/hour
Intermittent Feedings			
Preterm (>1200 g)	2–4 ml/kg/feeding	2–4 ml/feeding	120–175 ml/kg/day
0–12 months	10–15 ml/kg/q 2–3 hours (30–60 ml)	10–30 ml/feeding	20–30 ml/kg/q 4–5 hours
1–6 years	5–10 ml/kg/q 2–3 hours (60–90 ml)	30–45 ml/feeding	15–20 ml/kg/q 4–5 hours
>7 years	90–120 ml/q 3–4 hours	60–90 ml/feeding	300–480 ml/kg/q 4–5 hours

Reproduced with permission from Davis A: Transitional and combination feeds. In Baker SS, Baker RD, Davis A (eds): Pediatric Enteral Nutrition. New York: Chapman and Hall, 1994:139–156.

enteral to enteral nutrition is gradual;[63] approximately 1 week is required for an uncomplicated transition from parenteral to enteral nutrition. In some patients with short small bowel or intractable diarrhea, the time to full enteral feeding may be very long.[64]

Once formula tolerance is established at 15 to 50 percent of the desired volume, the formula concentration may be gradually increased. Generally enteral feedings begin at 1 to 2 ml/kg/hour and are advanced (Tables 20–9 and 20–10). As enteral feedings reach 35 to 50 percent of calcu-

TABLE 20–9   Example of Transition from Parenteral to Enteral Nutrition (4-kg Infant)*

Day	Transition[†]	ml/hour	kcal/kg	g protein/kg	Enteral Goal (%)
	PN: 2% amino acid, 2.5% fat, 20% dextrose, 0.93 NP kcal/ml	20	111	2.4	0
1	FS formula = 0.67 kcal/ml	4	16	0.4	16
	PN = 0.93 NP kcal/ml	20	111	2.4	
2	FS formula	8	32	0.7	32
	PN	16	89	1.9	
3	FS formula	12	48	1.1	48
	PN	12	67	1.4	
4	FS formula	16	64	1.4	64
	PN	8	44	1.0	
5	FS formula	20	80	1.8	80
	PN	4	96	0.5	
6	FS formula	24	96	2.2	100
	Discontinue PN				
7	FS formula—concentrate to 24 kcal/oz (0.7 kcal/ml)	24	115	2.6	100

MCT = medium-chain triglycerides; NP = nonprotein; PN = parenteral nutrition; FS = full strength.
*Estimated daily needs:
  Calories 100–120 kcal/kg/day
  Protein 2–3 g/kg/day
  Fluid 100–175 ml/kg/day (17–30 ml/hour)
Selected enteral formula:
  Hydrolyzed protein, 60% MCT, lactose free, elemental
  Formula concentration is full strength (20 kcal/oz [0.67 kcal/ml])
†Formula volume and concentration should not be increased simultaneously.
Reproduced with permission from Davis A: Transitional and combination feeds. In Baker SS, Baker RD, Davis A (eds): Pediatric Enteral Nutrition. New York: Chapman and Hall 1994:139–156.

TABLE 20–10   Transition from Parenteral to Enteral Nutrition (40-kg Adolescent)*

Day	Transition	ml/hour	kcal/kg	g Protein/kg	Enteral Goal (%)
	PN: 3% amino acid, 4% fat, 17.5% dextrose, 1.0 NP kcal/ml	90	54	1.6	0
1	FS formula (30 kcal/oz, 1.0 kcal/ml)	25	15	0.5	25
	PN (1.0 NP kcal/ml)	90	54	1.6	
2	FS formula	50	30	0.9	50
	PN	65	39	1.2	75
3	FS formula	75	45	1.4	75
	PN	40	20	0.7	
4	FS formula	100	60	1.9	100
	Discontinue PN				

FS = full strength; PN = parenteral nutrition; MCT = medium-chain triglycerides; NP = nonprotein.
*Estimated daily needs:
 Calories 50–60 kcal/kg/day
 Protein 1–2 g/kg/day
 Fluid 47–75 ml/kg/day (80–125 ml/hour)
Selected enteral formula:
 Semielemental (350 mOsm/kg), peptides, 35% fat with MCT, lactose free
Reproduced with permission from Davis A: Transitional and combination feeds. In Baker SS, Baker RD, Davis A (eds): Pediatric Enteral Nutrition. New York: Chapman and Hall, 1994:139–156.

lated enteral requirements, parenteral nutrition may be tapered. Tapering parenteral nutrition while advancing enteral feeds prevents rebound hypoglycemia and fluid overload. When enteral feedings are providing 75 to 100 percent of enteral requirements, parenteral nutrition may be discontinued. When parenteral fluids are finally stopped, the enteral infusion must meet the child's full fluid requirement.

Initiation of Enteral Feeding

The initiation of enteral feeding in infants or children with an intact GI tract who have not been receiving parenteral nutrition is similar to the transition from parenteral to enteral nutrition. Generally a polymeric, isotonic, undiluted formula is well tolerated. The feedings can begin as a nocturnal supplement (e.g., in children with failure to thrive) at 1 to 2 ml/kg/hour and after 2 to 4 hours, increasing the rate by 1 to 2 ml/kg/hour until the desired volume is achieved. This process may take more than one night. Alternatively, continuous, 24-hour feedings can begin and the feedings cycled after the full volume is reached.

Transition from Continuous to Intermittent Feedings

Intermittent feedings are administered several times a day, with each feeding lasting for 15 to 45 minutes. Continuous enteral feedings are indicated for transpyloric feeding, for patients with no enteral intake for more than 5 to 7 days, for patients with limited absorption due to bowel resection, GI injury, or malabsorption, and for patients who are at risk for aspiration or who do not tolerate intermittent feedings. Intermittent feedings allow patients to be mobile, simulate oral feeding, and are associated with a more natural hunger-satiety cycle than continuous feeding.[65] However, compared with continuous feeding, diarrhea, cramping, dumping syndrome, delayed gastric emptying, and aspiration are more likely with bolus feeding. Better nutrient absorption occurs with continuous feeding.[61] Overlapping continuous with intermittent feedings is economically and nutritionally more efficient than suddenly discontinuing continuous feeds, since hospital stays, use of intravenous fluids, and complications can be reduced. Optimum infusion rates for intermittent feedings are not greater than 30 ml/minute.[66]

Continuous to Cycled Feedings

Cycled feeding refers to the administration of enteral tube feedings by continuous drip infusion for less than 24 hours. Usually uninterrupted infusions are 8 to 18 hours long, depending on individual patient requirements and tolerance (Tables 20–11 and 20–12). Cy-

TABLE 20–11   Transition/Combination of Continuous Enteral Feeding to Intermittent and Cycled Enteral Feeding (4-kg Infant)*

Day	Formula	ml/hour	Hours Infused	kcal/kg	g Protein/kg
Continuous to Intermittent					
	0.7 kcal/ml formula	24	24	115	2.6
8	0.7 kcal/ml formula	40	q 2	96	2.1
9	0.7 kcal/ml formula	60	q 3	96	2.1
10	0.7 kcal/ml formula	80	q 4	96	2.1
Continuous to Cycled					
	0.7 kcal/ml formula	24	24	115	2.6
8	0.7 kcal/ml formula	28	20	112	2.5
9	0.7 kcal/ml formula	32	18	115	2.6
10	0.7 kcal/ml formula	36	16	115	2.6
11	0.7 kcal/ml formula	40	14	112	2.5
	0.7 kcal/ml formula	24	24	115	2.6
Continuous to Cycled (C) and Intermittent (I)					
8	C-formula[†]	28	17	95	2.1
	I-formula	28	3 feedings	17	0.4
9	C-formula	32	14	90	2.0
	I-formula	38	3 feedings	23	0.5
10	C-formula	36	12	86	1.9
	I-formula	48	3 feedings	29	0.6
11	C-formula	40	10	80	1.8
	I-formula	60	3 feedings	36	0.8

*Estimated daily needs:
  Calories 100–120 kcal/kg/day
  Protein 2–3 g protein/kg/day
  Fluid 100–175 ml/kg/day
[†]Formula concentration is 0.7 kcal/ml.
Reproduced with permission from Davis A: Transitional and combination feeds. In Baker SS, Baker RD, Davis A (eds): Pediatric Enteral Nutrition. New York: Chapman and Hall, 1994:139–156.

TABLE 20–12   Transition of Continuous Enteral Feeding to Cycled/Intermittent Enteral Feeding (40-kg Adolescent)*

Day	Transition to Cycled Feeds	ml/hour	Hours Infused	kcal/kg	g Protein/kg
	1.0 kcal/ml semielemental formula	100	24	60	1.9
8	1.5 kcal/ml polymeric[†] formula	100	16	60	2.2
9	1.5 kcal/ml polymeric formula	125	12	56	2
10	1.5 kcal/ml polymeric[††] formula	150	10	56	2

*Estimated daily needs:
  Calories 40–60 kcal/kg/day
  Protein 1–2 g/kg/day
  Fluid 47–75 ml/kg/day
Enteral formula selection:
  From semielemental (1.0 kcal/ml) to polymeric, lactose-free formula (1.5 kcal/ml) with 77% free water, higher calorie for volume tolerance
[†]Formula volume and concentration not increased simultaneously.
[††]Day 10 of cycled tube feeding provides 1155 ml of free water; if tube feeding is the only intake source, an additional 725 ml of water/day is needed.
Reproduced with permission from Davis A: Transitional and combination feeds. In Baker SS, Baker RD, Davis A (eds): Pediatric Enteral Nutrition. New York: Chapman and Hall, 1994:139–156.

cled feedings are delivered with a pump and are usually administered overnight to enable the infant or child to feed orally during the day. Cycled feedings are associated with less abdominal discomfort than intermittent feedings and are better absorbed.[61] Although infants tolerate up to 6 ml/kg/hour over 24 hours, they can tolerate approximately 10 to 12 ml/kg/hour cycled over 8 to 12 hours. Children receiving 3 to 5 ml/kg/hour over 24 hours can progress to a cycled infusion of 120 to 150 ml/hour. When maximal volume is reached, as assessed by patient tolerance, the caloric density of the formula can be increased (1 to 2 kcal/ml). This method is often used in patients with cystic fibrosis, tracheoesophageal fistula, bronchopulmonary dysplasia, and inflammatory bowel disease (IBD). If children receive nocturnal cycled feeds, the head of the bed should be elevated; if reflux is present, bethanecol, metoclopramide, or cisapride may be useful.

Enteral to Oral Feedings

The goal of all nutrition in pediatrics is to supply nutrients for optimal growth and development while supporting developmentally appropriate eating behavior. Often the development of the normal eating process is interrupted and delayed.[67] Development of mouth sensitivity with distinct oral defensive behaviors and lack of the hunger-satiety cycle due to around-the-clock feedings can make the transition from tube to oral feeding long and difficult. If children are deprived of appropriate oral stimulation during critical development phases, feeding difficulties will arise.[68] Initiating oral feedings in children who have been fed by tube can evoke a resistant or fearful response, such as gagging, choking, or vomiting.[69] Thus, feeding programs for infants must include a speech therapist or occupational therapist to ensure that a vital oral component is in place at the time tube feedings are started. This will help both the infant and family with oral stimulation and simulation of oral feeding behaviors.[70]

The presence of medical complications is a critical factor influencing the time to full transition to oral feeding; the process may vary from days to years. Table 20–13 lists important evaluations that must be in place before initiating a transition to oral feeding.

To begin oral feeding, normalize feedings to approximate meals and snacks. Connect the tube feeding with the process of eating. Introduce the sensation of hunger followed by feeding to alleviate that sensation. This is a gradual process during which behavioral problems may be prominent. The abrupt discontinuation of tube feeding to stimulate oral intake is rarely successful. Careful monitoring of fluids, anthropomorphics, and vitamin and mineral intake as well as motor skill is vital for the transition to full oral feeding.[71]

Monitoring of Enteral Feeds

To manage infants and children receiving enteral feeding, food tolerance and metabolic, mechanical, GI, nutritional, and growth parameters must be carefully and frequently assessed.

Table 20–14 outlines parameters useful to monitor children receiving enteral nutrition support. Tolerance to enteral feeding is followed by noting the presence or absence of vomiting, diarrhea, and abdominal distention. Gastric residuals are not routinely checked un-

TABLE 20–13 Evaluation Before Transition to Oral Feeding

Factor	Status
Original indication for enteral nutrition	Not improved—do not attempt to transition to oral feedings; try to resolve initial problem first
	Improved or resolved—begin transition
Quality of oral motor skills	Determine level of skills: Can child suck, chew? Can child make a bolus? Can child initiate coordinated swallowing? Can child swallow without aspirating? If skills not adequate, do not begin transition; first resolve skill problem if possible.
Parent readiness	Parents agree with transition
	Parent taught skills
	Support for parents—process can be long and frustrating and will fail if parents do not have adequate support
	Support for behavioral problems—common and include food aversion, negative or disruptive behaviors during feeding, refusal to self-feed, power struggles

TABLE 20–14   Suggestions for Monitoring Children and Infants Receiving Enteral Nutrition Support

Parameter	Initial Week	Hospitalization	Outpatient Follow Up
Growth			
Calories, protein, vitamins, minerals	Daily	Weekly	Monthly
Weight for age	Daily	Daily	Monthly
Height for age	Initially	Weekly	Monthly
Weight for height	Initially	Weekly	Monthly
Head circumference	Initially	Weekly	Monthly
Triceps skinfold	Initially	2–4 weeks	1–3 months
Mid-arm muscle circumference	Initially	2–4 weeks	1–3 months
Gastrointestinal			
Gastric residuals	2 hourly	PRN	PRN
Vomiting	Daily	Daily	Daily
Stools			
Frequency/consistency	Daily	Daily	PRN
Reducing substances/pH	Initially	PRN	PRN
Ova/parasites	PRN	PRN	PRN
Mechanical			
Tube position	Initially	8 hourly	8 hourly
Nose care	8 hourly	8 hourly	8 hourly
Ostomy care	PRN	PRN	PRN
Metabolic			
Fluid intake/output	Daily	Daily	Daily
Urine specific gravity	Daily	Weekly	PRN
Electrolytes	Daily until stable	Weekly	Monthly if stable
Glucose	Daily until stable	Weekly	Monthly if stable
BUN/creatinine	Initially	Weekly	Monthly if stable
Visceral proteins	Initially	2–4 weeks	Monthly if stable
Liver function studies	Initially	PRN	PRN
Minerals	Initially, then daily	Weekly	Monthly if stable
Vitamins, trace elements	PRN	PRN	PRN–yearly
Hematology	Initially	PRN	1–3 months
Iron, TIBC, reticulocyte count	Initially	PRN	1–3 months

BUN = blood urea nitrogen; TIBC = total iron binding capacity.
Adapted with permission from Davis A: Indications and techniques for enteral feeds. In Baker SS, Baker RD, Davis A (eds): *Pediatric Enteral Nutrition*. New York: Chapman and Hall, 1994:67–94.

less the patient is at risk for aspiration. A single high gastric residual (> 1.5 to 2 times the hourly rate of formula administration) alone is not enough reason to discontinue enteral feeding. Medications instilled through the feeding tube that decrease gastric motility, such as paralytic agents and morphine, or use of a high osmolar formula may alter GI motility. Decreasing the infusion rate by half for a few hours may resolve the problem with high gastric residuals. If not, transpyloric feeds or metoclopramide or cisapride can be considered.

For children receiving long-term enteral feeding, careful monitoring of growth is essential, since the goal for enteral feeding therapy is to promote normal growth and development. Mechanical complications, such as occluded tubes and malposition of tubes, generally require replacing the apparatus with a new one.

Complications

Table 20–15 lists potential complications of tube feedings and management suggestions. These complications are similar to those occurring in adults and are reviewed in depth elsewhere.[41]

Infections

Careful attention to cleanliness of the gastrostomy tube site promotes healthy tissue. Dirty occlusive dressings with formula leakage promote bacterial growth and increase the risk of infection. Bacterial growth can be limited by using commercially prepared products or confining the time home blenderized diets and breast milk infusions are in the delivery system to 4 hours.[72,73] Delivery systems should be changed every 24 hours and not reused.

TABLE 20-15 Possible Complications of Tube Feeding

Problem	Management Suggestion
Mechanical	
Tubes	
Improper size	Change tube to appropriate size
Improper placement	Change placement
Aspiration	Elevate head of bed 30–45 degrees, confirm tube placement, use continuous feeding rather than bolus, consider antireflux medication
Occlusion	Flush before and after intermittent feedings and every 8 hours with continuous feedings, thoroughly mix powder additives, use only liquid preparations of medications, crush medications well if using pills
Medications	Use liquid whenever possible, assess physical compatibility of drug/formula, avoid mixing formulas with liquid medications with pH < 5.0
Metabolic	
Overhydration, malnutrition, refeeding	Monitor input and output, include all other fluid intake (oral, IV)
Dehydration	Evaluate osmolality of formula, provide more fluids
Diarrhea	Culture stools, stools for *Clostridium difficile* toxin titer, evaluate osmolality of all medications, ?medications as GI stimulants, evaluate osmolality of formula, stools for pH, and reducing substances, give additional fluids
Hyperglycemia	Slow or stop feeding, monitor blood sugar, reduce carbohydrates, give insulin if diabetic
Hyperkalemia	Change formula, give potassium binders, give insulin and glucose, correct acidosis
Hyperphosphatemia	Change formula, use phosphate binder, give calcium supplement
Hypokalemia	Give potassium, monitor electrolytes, evaluate adequacy of formula
Hypophosphatemia	Give phosphorus, evaluate formula
Hyponatremia	Evaluate fluid balance, if overhydrated restrict fluids, evaluate adequacy of formula
Fatty acid deficiency	Change formula, add modular fat, add 5 ml safflower oil
Abnormal liver function tests	Determine etiology, evaluate formula in light of liver status
Rapid/excessive weight gain	Evaluate electrolytes, evaluate fluid balance, decrease amount or concentration of formula
Azotemia	Decrease protein
Congestive heart failure	Decrease sodium, slow rate, give diuretics
Inappropriate weight gain	Evaluate macronutrient and micronutrient intake, monitor daily input and output, correct deficiencies
Gastrointestinal	
Diarrhea	
Mucosal atrophy	Use isotonic or dilute hypertonic formula, start at a slow rate and increase gradually
Medications (changes motility, flora, increases osmolality when given with feedings)	Change time medication is given, type, or prescribe an antidiarrheal agent, check sorbital content of medication
Hyperosmolar solution	Dilute to isotonicity and slowly increase concentration
Rapid delivery	Slow rate and gradually increase
Bacterial contamination	Use aseptic preparation techniques and limit time the formula hangs in bag
Intolerance of formula component	Use formula without intolerant component (e.g., if lactose intolerant, use lactose-free formula)

MCT = medium-chain triglyceride.
Adapted with permission from Davis A: Indications and techniques for enteral feeds. In Baker SS, Baker RD, Davis A (eds): Pediatric Enteral Nutrition. New York: Chapman and Hall, 1994:67–94.

Table continued on following page

TABLE 20–15   Possible Complications of Tube Feedings *Continued*

Problem	Management Suggestion
Malabsorption	Use elemental or semielemental formula, MCT oil
Gastric residuals	
High osmolality	Dilute to isotonicity and slowly increase concentration
High fat content	Consider changing formula to one having < 30–40% total calories from fat
Intermittent feedings	Consider continuous feeding
Medications that slow peristalsis	If unable to stop medication, consider addition of medications that stimulate peristalsis
Gastroparesis	Small bowel feedings
Gastric residuals on initiating feedings	Advance slowly
Nausea and vomiting	
Rate too fast	Slow rate
High osmolality	Dilute formula to isotonicity, then gradually increase
Mechanical problems	Check tube placement
Delayed gastric emptying	Consider metoclopramide, patient position, transpyloric feeds, continuous infusion, isotonic formula
Medications given with feeding	Consider changing time of medication, check contents of medications
Obstruction	Stop feeding
Patient positioning	Elevate head of bed
Delayed gastric emptying	Consider medication, reposition patient, transpyloric feeds, continuous infusion, isotonic formula
Constipation	
Inadquate fluids	Monitor fluid balance, increase fluids by increasing the rate and decreasing the formula
Inadequate fiber	Consider formula with fiber or fiber supplement
Inactivity	Encourage activity
Obstruction	Stop feedings
Fecal impaction	Disimpact, consider stool softeners
Developmental	
Prevent delayed feeding skills development	Nonnutritive sucking, offer small amounts of food from spoon, fluids from cup, develop an association between oral activity and satiety
Food refusal	Consult an occupational or speech therapist

Mechanical

Mechanical complications are similar to those occurring in adult patients receiving enteral feedings. Nasogastric or enteric tubes can cause erosion of the nares or esophagus. GI perforation can occur with the use of stiff tubes or improper placement of those with a removable stylet. These problems can be lessened by careful attention to tube position, choosing a small soft tube, and using trained personnel to introduce tubes with stylets. In addition, nasoduodenal or jejunal tubes can be placed under fluoroscopic guidance. The incidence of tube occlusion can be lessened by infusing only liquid preparations of all nutrients and medications through feeding tubes and thorough flush-

ing of the tubes. Often tubes can simply lie within a gastric fold, and a gentle water flush with repositioning of the patient will resolve the occlusion. Pancreatic enzymes, cranberry juice, water, carbonated beverages, and papain have been used to declog tubes.[74-79]

Metabolic

Overhydration and underhydration can occur with enteral feedings. Overhydration can occur as the transition is made from parenteral to enteral feedings or if excessive free water flushes are used, especially in small children or infants. Children with renal, cardiac, hepatic, or other diseases who may require fluid restriction are at greater risk for fluid overload than children who do not require fluid restriction.

Dehydration can occur if inadequate fluids are given, if the child has increased losses, such as occur with diarrhea, or if hyperosmolar feedings are given. Dehydration can be prevented by calculating the fluid in the final feeding and ensuring adequate free water is supplied.

Other metabolic complications, such as electrolyte imbalance and hypoglycemia (if feedings are more then 6 to 8 hours apart) can occur. Children receiving long-term enteral feeding can develop calcium, phosphorus, vitamin D, and zinc deficiencies.[80-82]

Gastrointestinal

GI complications include nausea, vomiting, diarrhea, and constipation. Sometimes the smell of the formula may make children nauseous. Flavorings and mixing the formula at a distance so children cannot smell it may be helpful. Vomiting can result because of improper tube placement, slow GI motility, rapid infusion rate, hyperosmolality, and medications. Reflux may occur in infants. It can be treated by positioning the infant so the head of the bed is at a 30- to 40-degree angle, using a slow infusion rate, and possibly using bethanecol, metoclopramide, or cisapride.

Constipation can be a problem for children receiving enteral feeding and can be helped by choosing a formula with fiber, giving adequate fluids, and encouraging as much physical activity as possible. At times stool softeners are useful.

Diarrhea can also be a problem. Before the enteral feeding itself is assumed to be the cause of the diarrhea, infections, such as pseudomembraneous colitis, or medications that increase GI motility or have a high osmolality, should be considered.[83] The use of a formula with fiber can be helpful. For children with short small bowel, agents that slow GI motility or bind bile salts may be considered.

CONCLUSION

Enteral nutritional support is a powerful medical tool to support children through critical illnesses or to sustain long-term growth and development. However, the delivery of enteral nutrition support in children requires recognition that the GI tract is immature and that children have high requirements for growth.

REFERENCES

1. Prichard JA: Fetal swallowing and amniotic fluid volume. Obstet Gynecol 1966;28:606–610.
2. Golubera EL, Shuleikina KV, Vainshsteinii V: Development of reflex and spontaneous activity of the human fetus in the process of embryogenesis. Obstet Gynecol (USSR) 1959;3:59–62.
3. Treloar DM: The effect of nonnutritive sucking on oxygenation in healthy, crying full-term infants. Appl Nutr Res 1994;7:52–58.
4. Bernbaum JC, Pereira CR, Watkins JB et al: Nonnutritive sucking during gavage feeding enhances growth and maturation in premature infants. Pediatrics 1983;71:41–45.
5. Measel CP, Anderson GC: Nonnutritive sucking during tube feedings: effect on clinical course in premature infants. J Obstet Gynecol Neonatal Nurs 1979;8:265–272.
6. Field T, Ignatoff E, Stringer S et al: Nonnutritive sucking during tube feedings: effects on preterm neonates in an intensive care unit. Pediatrics 1972;70:381–384.
7. Deren JS: Development of structure and function in the fetal and newborn stomach. Am J Clin Nutr 1971;24:144–159.
8. McLain CR: Amniography studies of the gastrointestinal motility of the human fetus. Am J Obstet Gynecol 1965;86:1079–1087.
9. Morris FH, Moore M, Weisbroodt NW et al: Ontogenic development of gastrointestinal motility. IV: duodenal contractions in preterm infants. Pediatrics 1986;78:1106–1113.
10. Slagle TA, Gross SJ: Effect of early low-volume enteral substrate on subsequent feeding tolerance in very low birth weight infants. J Pediatr 1988;113:526–531.
11. Morris FH: Neonatal gastrointestinal motility and enteral feeding. Semin Perinatol 1991;15:478–481.
12. Watkins JB, Ingall D, Szczepanik P et al: Bile-salt metabolism in the newborn. Measurement of pool size and synthesis by stable isotope technic. New Engl J Med 1973;288:431–434.
13. Fredrikzon B, Hernell O, Blackberg L: Lingual lipase. Its role in lipid digestion in infants with low birthweight and/or pancreatic insufficiency. Acta Paediatr Scand Suppl 1982;296:75–80.
14. Hamosh M, Scanlon JW, Ganot D et al: Fat digestion in the newborn. Characterization of lipase in gastric aspirates of premature and term infants. J Clin Invest 1981;67:838–846.
15. Sarles J, Maori H, Verger R: Human gastric lipase: ontogeny and variation in children. Acta Pediatr 1992;81:511–513.
16. Areca S, Rubin A, Murset G: Intestinal glycosidase activities in the human embryo, fetus and newborn. Pediatrics 1965;36:944–954.
17. Bond JK, Levitt MD: Fate of soluble carbohydrate in the colon of rats and man. J Clin Invest 1976;57:1158–1162.
18. Grand RJ, Watkins JB, Torti FM: Development of the human gastrointestinal tract. A review. Gastroenterology 1976;70:790–810.
19. Kein CL, Sumners JE, Stetina JS et al: A method for assessing carbohydrate energy absorption and its application to premature infants. Am J Clin Nutr 1982;36:910–915.
20. Mobashaleh M, Montgomery RK, Biller JA et al: Development of carbohydrate absorption in the fetus and neonate. Pediatrics 1985;75(suppl):160–165.
21. Kelly EJ, Brownlee KG: When is the fetus first capable of gastric acid, intrinsic factor and gastrin secretion. Biol Neonate 1993;63:153–156.

22. Berfenstam R, Jagenburg R, Mellander O: Protein hydrolysis in the stomach of premature and full term infants. Acta Pediatr 1955;44:348–341.

23. Lebenthal E, Lee PC: Development of functional response in human exocrine pancreas. Pediatrics 1980;66:556–561.

24. Hirata Y, Matsur P, Kobubu H: Digestion and absorption of milk proteins in infants' intestine. Kobe J Med Sci 1965;11:103–106.

25. Lebenthal E, Lee PC, Heitlinger LA: Impact of development of the gastrointestinal tract on infant feeding. J Pediatr 1983;102:1–5.

26. Raiha NCR: Nutritional proteins in milk and the protein requirement of normal infants. Pediatrics 1985;75(suppl):136–142.

27. Fordtran JS, Rector FC, Ewton MF et al: Permeability characteristics of the human small intestine. J Clin Invest 1965;44:1935–1944.

28. Jackson D, Walker-Smith JA, Phillips AD: Macromolecular absorption by histologically normal and abnormal small intestinal mucosa in childhood: an in vitro study using organ culture. J Pediatr Gastroenterol Nutr 1983;2:235–247.

29. Ziegler TR, Smith RJ, O'Dwyer ST et al: Increased intestinal permeability associated with infection in burn patients. Arch Surg 1988;123:1313–1319.

30. Weaver LT, Laker MF, Nelson R: Intestinal permeability in the newborn. Arch Dis Child 1984;59:236–241.

31. Beach RC, Menzies IS, Clayden GS et al: Gasrointestinal permeability changes inthe preterm neonate. Arch Dis Child 1982;57:141–145.

32. Widdowson EM: Growth and body composition in childhood. In Brunser O, Carrazza FR, Gracey M et al (eds): Clinical Nutrition of the Young Child. New York: Raven Press, 1991:1–14.

33. Pollitt E, Leibel R: Iron deficiency and behavior. J Pediatr 1976;88:372–381.

34. Walter R, De Andraca I, Chadud P et al: Iron deficiency anemia: adverse effects on infant psychomotor development. Pediatrics 1989;84:7–17.

35. Lozoff B, Jimenez E, Wolf AW: Long term developmental outcome of infants with iron deficiency. New Engl J Med 1991;325:687–694.

36. Dibley MJ, Staehling N, Nieburg P et al: Interpretation of Z score anthropometric indicators derived from the International Growth Reference. Am J Clin Nutr 1987;20:503–510.

37. Seidman EG: Gastrointestinal benefits of enteral feeds. In Baker SS, Baker RD, Davis A (eds): Pediatric Enteral Nutrition. New York: Chapman and Hall, 1994:46–67.

38. Jenkins M, Gottschlich M, Alexander JW et al: Effect of immediate enteral feeding on the hypermetabolic response following severe burn injury. J Parenter Enter Nutr 1989;13(suppl 1):12S–15S.

39. Berseth CL: Effect of early feeding on the maturation of the preterm infant's small intestine. J Pediatr 1992;120:947–953.

40. Slagle TA, Gross SJ: Effect of early low-volume enteral substrate on subsequent feeding tolerance in very low birth weight infants. J Pediatr 1988;113:526–531.

41. Davis A: Indications and techniques for enteral feeds. In Baker SS, Baker RD, Davis A: Pediatric Enteral Nutrition. New York: Chapman and Hall, 1994:67–94.

42. Kulkarni PB, Hall RT, Rhodes PG et al: Rickets in very-low-birthweight infants. J Pediatr 1980;96:249–253.

43. Hambridge K: Zinc deficiency in the premature infant. Pediatr Rev 1985;6:209–215.

44. Stocks RJ, Davies DP, Allen F et al: Loss of breast milk nutrients during tube feeding. Arch Dis Child 1985;60:164–167.

45. Lavine M, Clark RM: The effect of short term refrigeration and addition of breast milk fortifier on the delivery of lipids during tube feeding. J Pediatr Gastroenterol Nutr 1989;8:496–500.

46. Narayanan I, Singh B, Harvey D: Fat loss during feedings of human milk. Arch Dis Child 1984;59:745–748.

47. Geer FR, McCormick A, Laker J: Changes in fat concentration of human milk during delivery by intermittent bolus and continuous mechanical pump infusion. J Pediatr 1984;105;745–749.

48. American Academy of Pediatrics Committee on Nutrition: Hypoallergenic infant formulas. Pediatrics 1989;83:1068–1069.

49. Eastham EJ, Lichauco T, Grady MI et al: Antigenicity of infant formulas: role of immature intestine on protein permeability. J Pediatr 1978;93:561–564.

50. Crawford LV, Grogan FT: Allergenicity of cow's milk protein. II: studies with serum-agar precipitation technique. Pediatrics 1961;28:362–366.

51. Kaufman SS, Murray ND, Wood RP et al: Nutritional support for the infant with extrahepatic biliary atresia. J Pediatr 1987;110:679–681.

52. Kaufman SS, Scrivner DJ, Murray ND et al: Influence of portagen and pregestamil on essential fatty acid status in infantile liver disease. Pediatrics 1992;89:151–154.

53. Ziegler EE, Ruy JE: Renal solute load and diet in growing premature infants. J Pediatr 1976;89:609–615.

54. American Academy of Pediatrics Committee on Nutrition: Commentary on breast feeding and infant formulas, including proposed standards for formulas. Pediatrics 1979;63:52–54.

55. Davis A, Baker SS: The use of modular nutrients in pediatrics. J Parenter Enter Nutr 1995 (In press).

56. Listernick R, Sidransky E: Hypernatremic dehydration in children with severe psychomotor retardation. Clin Pediatr 1985;24:440–445.

57. Chernoff R, Block AS: Liquid feedings: considerations and alternatives. J Am Diet Assoc 1977;70:4–6.

58. Leider A, Sullivan L, Mullen MA: Intermittent tube feeding: pros and cons. Nutr Supp Serv 1984;4:59–61.

59. Lavine JE, Hattner RS, Heyman MB: Dumping in infancy diagnosed by radionuclide gastric emptying technique. J Pediatr Gastroenterol Nutr 1988;7:614–617.

60. Parathyras AJ, Kassak LA: Tolerance, nutritional adequacy, and cost-effectiveness in continuous drip versus bolus and/or intermittent feeding techniques. Nutr Supp Serv 1983;3(5):56–62.

61. Parker P, Stroop S, Greene H: A controlled comparison of continuous versus intermittent feeding in the treatment of infants with intestinal disease. J Pediatr 1981;99:360–364.

62. Coben RM, Weintraub A, DiMarino AJ et al: Gastroesophageal reflux during gastrostomy feeding. Gastroenterology 1994;106:13–18.

63. Davis A: Transitional and combination feeds. In Baker SS, Baker RD, Davis A (eds): Pediatric Enteral Nutrition. New York: Chapman and Hall, 1994:139–156.

64. Kurkchubasche AG, Rowe MI, Smith SD: Adaptation in short-bowel syndrome: reassessing old limits. J Pediatr Surg 1993;28:1069–1071.

65. Leider Z, Sullivan L, Mullen MA: Intermittent tube feeding: pros and cons. Nutr Supp Serv 1984;4:59.

66. Heitkemper ME, Martin DC, Hansen BC et al: Rate and volume of intermittent enteral feeding. J Parenter Enter Nutr 1981;5:125.

67. Satter EM: The feeding relationship. J Am Dietet Assoc 1986;86:352–356.

68. Illingwith RS, Lister J: The critical or sensitive period with special reference to certain feeding problems in infants and children. J Pediatr 1964;65(6):839–842.

69. Harris NB: Oral motor management of the high risk neonate. Phys Occup Ther Pediatr 1986;6:231–235.

70. Tuchman DN: Oralpharyngeal and esophageal complications of enteral tube feeding. In Baker SS, Baker RD, Davis A (eds): Pediatric Enteral Nutrition. New York: Chapman and Hall, 1994:179–191.

71. Byzyk S: Factors associated with the transition to oral feeding in infants fed by nasogastric tubes. Am J Occup Ther 1990;44:1070–1072.

72. White WE, Acuff TE, Sykes TR et al: Bacterial contamination of enteral solution: a preliminary report. J Parenter Enter Nutr 1979;3:459–461.

73. Hostetler C, Lipman T, Gearaghty M et al: Bacterial safety of reconstituted continuous drip tube feedings. J Parenter Enter Nutr 1983;3:232–375.

74. Macuard SP, Stegall KL, Trogdon S et al: Clearing obstructed feeding tubes. J Parenter Enter Nutr 1989; 13:81.

75. Haynes-Johnson V: Tube feeding complications: causes, prevention, and therapy. Nutr Supp Serv 1986; 6:17.

76. Cataldi-Betcher EL, Seltzer MH, Slocum BA et al: Complications occurring during enteral nutrition support. A prospective study. J Parenter Enter Nutr 1983;7:546.

77. Marcuard SP, Perkins AM: Clogging of feeding tubes. J Parenter Enter Nutr 1988;12:403.

78. Nicholson LJ: Declogging small-bore feeding tubes. J Parenter Enter Nutr 1987;11:594.

79. Marcuard SP, Stegall KS: Unclogging feeding tubes with pancreatic enzyme. J Parenter Enter Nutr 1990;14:198.

80. Brammer EM: Shortcomings of current formula for long-term enteral feeding in pediatrics. Nutr Clin Pract 1990;5:160.

81. Bowen PE, Mobarhan S, Henderson S et al: Hypocarotenemia in patients fed enterally with commercial diets. J Parenter Enter Nutr 1988;12:484–489.

82. Kenny F, Sriram K, Hammond JB et al: Clinical zinc deficiency during adequate enteral nutrition. J Am Coll Nutr 1989;8:83–86.

83. Edes TE, Walk B, Austin JL: Diarrhea in tube-fed patients: feeding formula not necessarily the cause. Am J Med 1990;88:91–93.

21

Enteral Nutrition in HIV Infection

LEE M. OBERMAN
DONALD P. KOTLER

Protein energy malnutrition frequently develops in individuals infected with the human immunodeficiency virus (HIV). The Centers for Disease Control (CDC) recognize malnutrition as an acquired immunodeficiency syndrome (AIDS)-defining disease complication.[1] As physicians become more adept at treating patients with AIDS-related complications, and as their overall survival is prolonged, appreciation of malnutrition as a serious problem in AIDS patients in the United States has increased. Its prominence in the developing world has long been recognized and is exemplified by the syndrome of "Slim's disease" in Africa.[2]

The nutritional consequences of HIV infection have been the focus of much study over the past 10 years, but knowledge deficits persist. The development of malnutrition may affect clinical outcome. The Multicenter AIDS Cohort Study (MACS) showed malnutrition to be an independent predictor of mortality in persons with marked CD4+ lymphocyte depletion.[3] Other studies indicate that malnutrition in AIDS increases morbidity and diminishes quality of life, as it does in other diseases.[4-6] Some authors have suggested that malnutrition may intensify the severity of immune dysfunction. Similarly, malnutrition may hasten disease progression, reduce the tolerance of or response to other treatments, and increase the need for hospitalization or chronic custodial care. In this context, not only the HIV-positive patient but the entire health care system may

be burdened by the development of malnutrition. However, these potential consequences have not been proved, so that the role of malnutrition in the context of HIV infection remains uncertain.

This chapter will review the effects of HIV infection and AIDS on nutritional status, both of macronutrients and micronutrients. The pathogenesis of malnutrition will be discussed, with particular emphasis on small-intestine disease and nutrient malabsorption. The effects of nutritional support will be reviewed, with an emphasis on studies using oral supplements, appetite stimulants, and nonvolitional enteral feeding. In addition, other AIDS-related nutritional issues including the ethics of feeding, clinical decision making, and adjunctive nutritional recommendations will be discussed.

EFFECTS OF HIV INFECTION AND AIDS ON NUTRITIONAL STATUS

Macronutrients

Many studies have documented the effects of HIV infection on body composition. Several groups studied hospitalized AIDS patients and found a high prevalence of significant weight loss (>10 percent of premorbid weight).[7] Clinical disease progression and the development of opportunistic infections often were found to follow or coincide with noticeable weight loss. A cross-sectional study analyzed the composition of weight lost by AIDS patients.[8] Body cell mass, fat content, and body water volumes, both intracellular and extracellular, were measured and the results compared with studies in controls. Body cell mass, as reflected by total body potassium content, was markedly reduced in men with AIDS, whereas body fat content was similar to homosexual male controls. The loss in weight was less profound than the loss in body cell mass. Intracellular water volume depletion directly correlated with the losses of body cell mass, whereas relative extracellular water volumes were increased.

Other forms of malnutrition such as kwashiorkor[9] and sepsis[10] also manifest with increases in extracellular water volumes. The increase in extracellular water content, along with the relative lack of fat depletion, diminished the measured change in weight. Thus, the malnutrition seen in patients with AIDS may be even more severe than the given weight loss would suggest. In addition, a normal weight does not necessarily equate with adequate nutritional status. The composition of weight loss in the AIDS patients studied suggested a stressed rather than a starved condition. The loss of body cell mass evinces a protein-wasting state, which was corroborated in a follow-up study showing depletion of total body nitrogen content.[11] Other studies have revealed visceral protein depletion by analysis of serum proteins.[5,6,8] Further analyses of body composition, by Ott and colleagues, confirm the depletion of body cell mass in HIV-infected patients, including subjects relatively early in their disease course.[12] In contradistinction, some AIDS patients have normal body composition studies, implying that the condition of immune deficiency alone does not determine the existence or degree of malnutrition.

The composition of weight loss in men and women appears to differ. The cross-sectional study cited above[8] revealed that HIV-infected women had greater losses of body fat than body cell mass, similar to findings in people with eating disorders, such as anorexia nervosa. These findings were confirmed in a study by Thea and coworkers of HIV-infected Africans[13] and in two other studies from the United States.[14,15] The explanation for the gender-specific differences is uncertain.

To examine the consequences of malnutrition in AIDS, the relationship between body cell mass depletion and death in patients not receiving nutritional support was examined.[4] There was a progressive fall in normalized body cell mass as patients neared death, with an extrapolated body cell mass at death of about 50 percent of normal. Extrapolated body weight was about one third below ideal. Historical studies of lethal starvation, such as in Leningrad and in the Warsaw Ghetto in World War II, also inferred this value of two thirds of ideal body weight as the point at which the risk of dying rose substantially. The results imply that the timing of death from wasting in AIDS patients is related to the degree of body cell mass depletion rather than the specific cause of the wasting process. Other measures of malnutrition also are associated with increased mortality in AIDS patients.[3-6]

Longitudinal studies of nutritional status conducted in clinically stable AIDS outpatients were performed to determine if progressive wasting is a constant phenomenon in AIDS patients.[16] Body cell mass was preserved over a 6-week follow up in the patients studied. Food consumption in the AIDS patients was similar to that in healthy homosexual and heterosexual controls. Stable AIDS patients have demonstrated normal food consumption in other studies as well.[17,18] These studies demonstrated mild to moderate malabsorption of sugars and fats. Unexpectedly, resting energy expenditure (REE) was less than that of the controls, which could compensate for the excess enteric energy losses. Because progressive wasting is not invariably seen in AIDS, its occurrence must correspond to the presence of specific disease complications.

MaCallum and coworkers performed longitudinal follow up of nutritional status in their patients by using weight charts.[19] Weight loss was found to be episodic, with frequent reversal, either spontaneously or in response to treatment of a specific disease complication. Systemic infections commonly produced acute weight loss, while intestinal diseases more often manifested with subacute, progressive wasting. Failure to reverse weight loss predicted a terminal course. Such findings underscore the thesis that wasting accompanies disease complications and is not an intrinsic characteristic of AIDS per se.

Micronutrients

Micronutrient deficiencies occur in HIV-infected individuals, often relatively early in the disease course. A comparison of the development and progression of macronutrient and micronutrient deficits remains unpublished. The most commonly recognized micronutrient to be deficient is vitamin B_{12}. Several studies have shown a prevalence of subnormal vitamin B_{12} concentrations in up to one third of patients. One study showed absent intrinsic factor secretion in some patients, while several have documented abnormal Schilling tests including part 2 (vitamin B_{12} complexes to intrinsic factor), implying abnormalities in ileal absorption. Serum levels of other water-soluble vitamins also have been reported to be low, despite apparent normal intake.[20] Of note is pyridoxine (vitamin B_6),[20,21] whose content parallels immune function in several experimental models.[22] Pyridoxine deficiency adversely affects lymphocyte responsiveness to mitogens and natural killer cell function, independent of CD4 cell number. It has been suggested that monitoring serial vitamin B concentrations may help identify subjects at increased risk for opportunistic infection. Vitamin B_6 deficiency in the general population has been associated with anorexia and decreased food intake. Deficiencies of fat-soluble vitamins also occur, especially in patients with fat malabsorption. Vitamin A deficiency, like vitamin B_6 deficiency, produces anorexia and decreased food intake. Decreased serum zinc and selenium concentrations have been reported.[23,24] Zinc deficiency is relevant to nutritional status, since its deficiency has been linked with a decrease in both taste and olfaction[25] and, consequently, decreased appetite and food intake. Studies have shown that serum zinc levels correlate with progression to AIDS in HIV-infected subjects,[26] but a cause-and-effect relationship has not been demonstrated. Selenium deficiency has been associated with cardiomyopathy,[27] and decreased selenium contents were found in cardiac muscle from autopsied AIDS patients in one study.[28] Various reports have documented subnormal serum concentrations of copper, magnesium, calcium, and potassium as well.

The implications of these micronutrient deficiencies are unclear. It is risky to base therapy on serum levels of zinc and selenium, since serum concentrations may fall as a result of the acute-phase response and may indicate extravascular sequestration rather than deficiency. On the other hand, a recent study did identify neuropsychological changes associated with low serum vitamin B_{12} concentrations and normalization as a result of specific supplementation.[29]

Studies in HIV-infected subjects have revealed glutathione depletion,[30] believed to reflect increased antioxidant requirements. The finding of increased rate of HIV replication in cells undergoing oxidative stress and the inhibition of this HIV replication by N-acetyl-L-cys-

teine suggest a possible association between a specific nutritional deficiency and disease progression.[31] Important studies continue to evaluate the clinical significance of these micronutrient deficits, and, likewise, the clinical significance of micronutrient replacement therapy.

PATHOGENESIS OF MALNUTRITION DURING DISEASE PROGRESSION

In-depth analysis of nutritional needs and nutritional alterations during the progression of HIV infection has yet to be performed. The general consensus is that nutritional needs vary with disease status. In essence, the progression of HIV disease can be categorized into three basic stages: early, intermediate, and late. HIV seropositivity alone, without clinical or immunologic evidence of immune deficiency, represents early disease. Few nutritional studies have been performed in patients at this stage of disease. Laboratory evidence without clinical evidence of immune deficiency or any AIDS-specific symptoms represents the intermediate stage of disease. This phase is associated with nutritional alterations, although progressive wasting is rare. Studies have shown mild-to-moderate depletion of body cell mass,[12] mild elevations in REE,[32,33] and serologic evidence of a chronic, systemic inflammatory disorder.[34,35] The specific causes of these metabolic abnormalities are uncertain but are felt to be epiphenomena of HIV replication and the anti-HIV immune response. It is also possible that the metabolic abnormalities occur in response to other overt or occult infections.[36] Cell marker studies of peripheral blood lymphocytes[37] and studies in cytokine expression in lymphoid tissues[38,39] both showed evidence of immune activation. Patients with AIDS or undergoing disease progression to AIDS are in the late stage of HIV disease. Nutritional deficiencies may be severe and progressive at this stage.

PATHOGENIC MECHANISMS

Nutritional deficiencies in any disease develop from alterations in food intake, nutrient absorption, or intermediary metabolism. Intake, absorption, and metabolism are highly regulated and interrelated, so that any disease may affect all three simultaneously.

Alterations in Food Intake

Oral, pharyngeal, or esophageal pathology (Fig. 21–1); medications; and psychosocial and

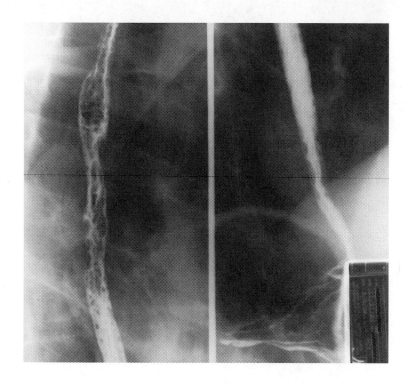

FIGURE 21–1 Barium esophogram demonstrating characteristic diffuse involvement of the esophagus by *Candida albicans.*

economic factors may act alone or together to reduce food intake. Diagnosis can be based on an algorithmic approach (Fig. 21–2). In addition, food intake may be reduced in response to intestinal malabsorption[40] or systemic disease.[41] Cytokines mediate the anorexia of systemic infection,[42] while the precise mediators of changes in appetitive behavior related to malabsorption are unknown. Regardless of the primary cause of disease, decreased food intake may contribute to wasting. As a corollary, effective therapy should produce a return of appetite. This point was clearly demonstrated in a longitudinal study of HIV-infected and AIDS patients with and without systemic infection.[43] Increased REE was demonstrated in all HIV groups, and results were comparable in AIDS patients with and without infection. Short-term weight loss was documented in the AIDS patients with infections and correlated with decreased food intake rather than increased energy expenditure. Although other studies have demonstrated higher metabolic rates in patients with active infections,[44] the confounding effects of disease on appetite are important and should be considered in the design of nutritional strategies.

Malabsorption

Chronic diarrhea is a very common complaint of HIV-infected individuals, occurring in about 60 percent of patients at some point in their disease course in the United States and approaching 100 percent in patients in developing countries.[45] Abnormalities in absorption also have been noted repeatedly, which range from occult to clinically severe. Efficient evaluation and diagnosis in such cases can often be obtained with use of diagnostic algorithm (Fig. 21–3). An opportunistic infection can be demonstrated in most patients with severe malabsorption (Fig. 21–4).[46] In the absence of opportunistic infections, small intestinal structure and function may be normal.[46,47] In our experience, chronic, severe malabsorption is limited mainly to patients with severe immune depletion (CD4+ <100 cells/mm^3). These findings imply that small intestine damage results from a disease complication and is not an intrinsic characteristic of AIDS and that absorptive function should suffice to preserve homeostasis in patients lacking small intestine injury. Given that infections such as cryptosporidiosis are often acquired through ingestion of contaminated water,[48] such infections may account for a substantial percent of cases of malnutrition associated with HIV in countries without effective public health measures.

Protozoa including *Cryptosporidium* spp, *Isospora* spp, and *Microsporidia* spp are the most common organisms found on clinical evaluation of small intestinal disease.[49] *My-*

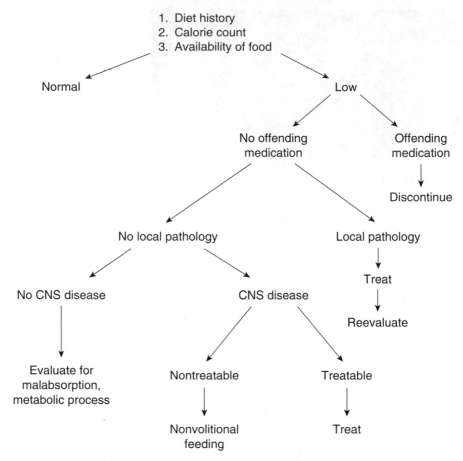

FIGURE 21–2   Clinical evaluation of food intake.

cobacteria spp such as *Mycobacterium avium-intracellulare* complex (MAC), also may cause an enteropathy characterized by marked fat malabsorption associated with evidence of systemic infection.[50] Increasing evidence reveals that bacteria that adhere to the mucosa of the ileum and the colon contribute to malabsorption.[51] Some studies have shown the frequent presence of exotic enteric viruses, although clinical-pathologic correlations have not been performed.[52] The possible presence of other organisms remains to be studies. In a recent series, 15 to 25 percent of comprehensive evaluations for intestinal malabsorption revealed no pathogenic organisms.

Different classes of pathogens have been noted to produce differing patterns of intestinal injury. Intracellular pathogens, such as cryptosporidiosis, microsporidiosis, and isosporiasis, lead to excess losses of enterocytes and hyperplastic villus atrophy. Malabsorption may result from infiltration of the lamina propria, submucosa, and intestinal lymphatics with macrophages containing mycobacteria, which produces a physical barrier to the transport of nutrients and leads to an exudative enteropathy. Bacterial adherence is associated with cytoskeletal alterations and epithelial cell cytotoxicity, especially in the ileum.[53] Some cryptosporidial infections also are localized in the ileum.[54] Some authors have suggested that small intestinal alterations may reflect the response to a T-cell-mediated reaction, including, possibly, the response to infection with HIV itself.[55]

Malabsorption secondary to intracellular pathogens develops as a result of chronic, excess loss of epithelial cells. Normally, homeostasis is maintained through the coordinated regulation of cell proliferation and loss.[56] The typical turnover rate for a villus epithelial cell is about 72 hours, during which time functional maturation occurs, followed by senescence. Specific maturational events occur independently.[57,58] For example, the specific activities of the brush border disaccharidases, maltase

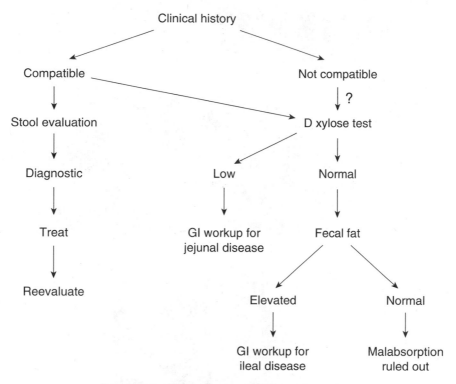

FIGURE 21–3 Clinical evaluation of malabsorption.

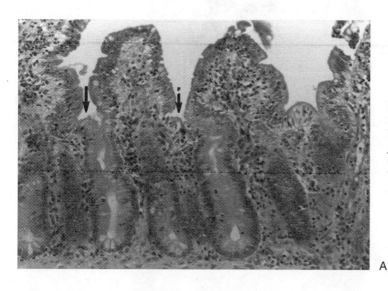

A

FIGURE 21–4 Infections that promote nutrient malabsorption. *A,* Partial villus atrophy and crypt hyperplasia in a jejunal biopsy from a patient with microsporidiosis (H&E 250X). The crypt villus junction is shown by the arrows. *Illustration continued on following page*

and sucrase, are similar in the upper and lower villus, while the specific activities of lactase and the enzymes of fatty acid esterification are absent in the lower villus and reach peak activity in the upper villus, implying that the latter enzymes require more time to be expressed.[59,60] For this reason lactase and fatty acid esterifying enzyme activities are more vulnerable to alterations in epithelial cell turnover.

Many physiologic and pathologic stimuli affect the rates of cellular production and loss.[56] Increased enterocyte losses lead to a compensatory crypt hyperplasia in an attempt to maintain a normal villus architecture. However, enterocytes may not achieve functional maturation secondary to increased migration rates. As predicted, functional deficits in lactose and fat absorption are more common and of greater

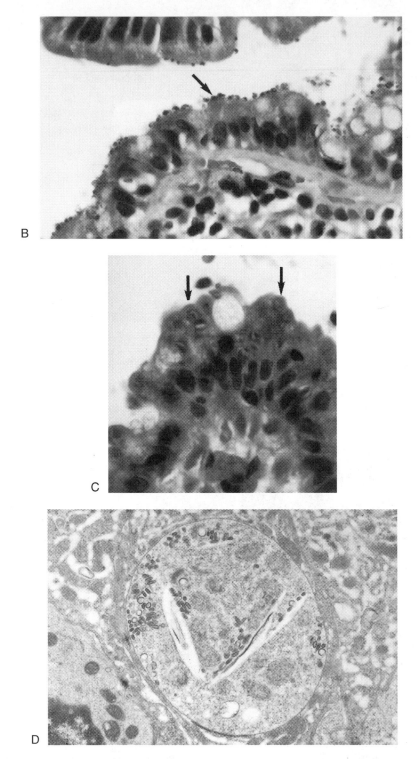

Figure 21–4   *Continued B* through *D   B,* Cryptosporidia involving jejunal enterocytes. Note their location at the luminal membrane (arrow). Most of the organisms actually are intracellular (H&E 400X). *C,* Microsporidia appearing as supranuclear inclusions (arrows) in cells located at the villus tip in the jejunum (H&E 400X). *D,* Transmission electron micrograph of a developing plasmodium (meront) of *Enterocytozoon bieneusi* (15,000X). (Electron micrographs courtesy of Jan M. Orenstein, MD, PhD, George Washington University School of Medicine.)

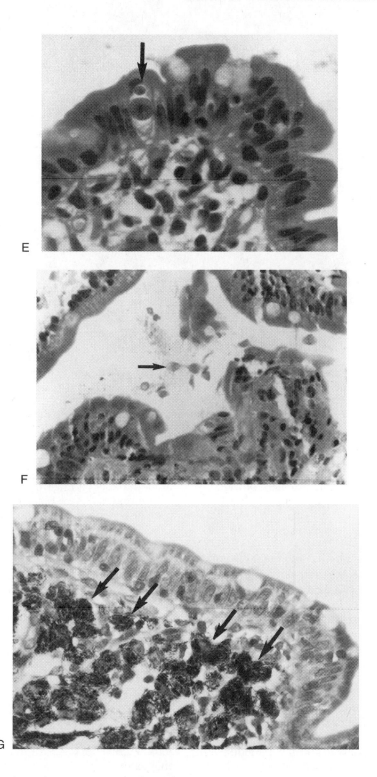

FIGURE 21–4 *Continued E* through *G E,* Macrogametocyte of *Isospora belli* (arrow) located in a jejunal villus epithelial cell (H&E 400X). *F,* Trophozoites of *Giardia lamblia* (arrow) located in the intervillus space (H&E 250X). *G, Mycobacterium avium intracellulare* infection of the small intestine. Acid-fast staining reveals clusters of bacilli (arrows) in macrophages in the lamina propria (Ziehl Nielson 400X).

Illustration continued on following page

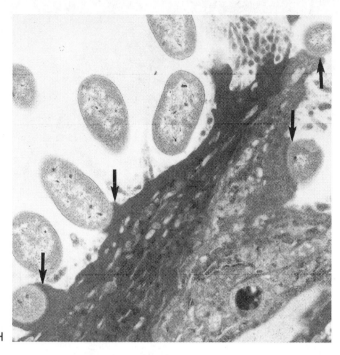

Figure 21–4 *Continued H,* Transmission electron micrograph of bacilli adhering to the luminal membrane of ileal enterocytes and producing an "attaching and effacing" lesion (arrows). The apical cytoplasm of the cell on the left is becoming dark and amorphous, reflecting cell death, while the increased density immediately beneath the attachment site in the cell on the right represents and earlier stage in the cytolytic process (22,500X).

clinical consequence than are deficits in starch and sucrose absorption in diseases producing hyperplastic villus atrophy. Histopathologic examination reveals partial villus atrophy and crypt hyperplasia in such cases, similar to findings in tropical sprue.[46,47,61]

Evaluation of small intestine function in AIDS patients, using D xylose absorption as a measure of mucosal integrity, revealed a bimodal distribution of results, with both normal and grossly abnormal values.[47,49] Partial villus atrophy and crypt hyperplasia were typical in AIDS patients with microsporidiosis and cryptosporidiosis but not in the majority of patients lacking identifiable enteric pathogens.[47,62,63] Transmission electron microscopy revealed full preservation of small intestine ultrastructure in many of the patients without enteric pathogens.[47] Likewise, decreased specific activities of sucrase, lactase, and maltase were typical of biopsies from AIDS patients with cryptosporidiosis and microsporidiosis, while enzyme-specific activities were normal in most patients without enteric pathogens. Lactase:sucrase and lactase:maltase ratios were lower in patients with parasitic infections than in those without such infections, implying a disproportionate loss of lactase, as explained above. However, not

every case of small intestine injury results from an identifiable organism.

The role of HIV in producing intestinal injury and dysfunction, including malabsorption, remains to be elucidated, although Ulrich and colleagues noted decreased activities of mucosal enzymes in HIV-infected individuals, which increased after therapy with zidovudine (AZT) (Retrovir). Altered local concentrations of cytokines and other proinflammatory mediators may play an as-yet-to-be determined role.

Interference of solute transport distal to the epithelial cell also may lead to malabsorption. MAC infections are known to produce malabsorption, particularly of fats. Exudative enteropathy occurs secondary to lymphatic blockade by infected macrophages. The pathophysiologic process resembles that seen in Whipple's disease,[64] which similarly is linked with a chronic bacterial infection of macrophages in the intestinal mucosa and elsewhere (Chapter 33).

Intraluminal bacterial overgrowth has been suggested as a pathogenic factor in malabsorption.[65] Intraluminal bacterial colony counts have been quantitated, with divergent results.[65,66] Although elevations in colony counts to the degree seen in scleroderma and other such motility disorders are not seen in AIDS patients, some bacterial overgrowth may occur secondary to the presence of hypochlorhydria.[67,68] Of note, these studies measured only the intraluminal colony counts and may fail to reflect the numbers of bacteria adherent to the epithelial surface. Adherent bacteria may increase independently of intraluminal bacterial colonies; adherence may reflect impaired local immune defenses, whereas intraluminal bacterial counts are largely regulated by peristalsis. There is little evidence for impaired peristalsis in AIDS patients.[69,70]

Ileal Dysfunction

Several lines of evidence suggest that ileal dysfunction occurs in HIV-infected and AIDS patients. As noted above, there is a high prevalence of subnormal serum vitamin B_{12} concentrations,[20,29,71,72] which were linked in some cases with ileal B_{12} malabsorption.[72] Ileal dysfunction is further suggested by separate studies documenting abnormal bile salt breath tests[73] and decreased whole body retention of a synthetic bile salt (SeHCAT).[66,74] Ileal dysfunction may occur as an isolated phenomenon or in association with diffuse intestinal disease and other signs of malabsorption. The spectrum of enteric pathogens responsible for ileal dysfunction has yet to be elucidated in full.

Clinically, bile salt malabsorption affects the net absorption of water, ions, and fat. Intraluminal bile salts may act as secretagogues in the colon, inducing active chloride secretion in the right colon through cyclic adenosine monophosphate (AMP)–mediate pathways.[75] The likelihood that fat malabsorption will occur is determined by the quantitative defect in bile salt absorption, as it is in cases of ileal resection related to inflammatory bowel disease (IBD).[76] The liver will compensate for lesser degrees of bile salt malabsorption, thereby permitting normal micelle formation and fatty acid solubilization, through compensatory increases in bile salt synthesis. Greater degrees of bile salt malabsorption will lead to reduced intraluminal bile salt concentrations in the small intestine, with attendant fat malabsorption.

Metabolic Alterations

Metabolic alterations occur in HIV infection and may or may not be associated with hypermetabolism. Systemic infections cause derangements of intermediary metabolism and produce protein wasting, even in the presence of adequate nutrient intake. *Pneumocystis carinii* pneumonia (PCP), among the most common initial infections in HIV-seropositive patients, produces fevers, hypermetabolism, and marked and progressive weight loss. Mycobacterial infections are classically hypermetabolic infections. Systemic fungal diseases are similar to mycobacteria in both their clinical presentation and in their metabolic effects. Cytomegalovirus (CMV) produces a disseminated disease in AIDS patients, typically presenting as retinitis or colitis, and also is hypermetabolic.

HIV-infected men, and probably HIV-infected women, may become hypogonadal at some point during the disease course.[77] Although hypogonadism primarily affects a man's sexual function, the decreased testosterone level may also promote protein wasting, because testosterone is an anabolic hormone as well as an androgen.

Fasting hypertriglyceridemia is another metabolic alteration associated with AIDS, and its presence has been associated with elevated levels of circulating α-interferon.[78,79] This association appears to relate a metabolic alteration directly to immune activation. Increased de novo fatty acid synthesis and esterification into triglycerides as well as decreased clearance of circulating triglycerides both contribute to hypertriglyceridemia.[80,81] Hypertriglyceridemia was not associated with progressive wasting in one study, and its implications are unclear.[79] In contrast, Zangerle showed that weight loss in HIV infection is associated with immune activation, although the specific mechanism was not defined in that study.[82]

NUTRITIONAL SUPPORT

General Issues

The importance of designing effective and cost-efficient nutritional support therapies for HIV-infected patients is obvious, given the large number of HIV-infected people and the extent of their malnutrition. The rationale for providing nutritional support to AIDS patients is based on the suppositions that nutritional status can be enhanced and that such enhancements provide clear advantages for the patient. Limited studies do support the first supposition, that nutritional support enhances nutritional status. The second supposition, although anecdotally clear, remains largely unstudied. Improvement in immune functions and other antimicrobial resistance, in "quality of life," in physical and mental performance, and in longevity, as well as avoidance of costs of supportive, custodial care, all are possible advantages of adequate nutritional support. No study has demonstrated reversibility of cell-mediated immune deficiency in AIDS through nutritional repletion. On the other hand, cell-mediated immune deficiencies due to uncomplicated malnutrition are reversed by nutritional repletion. The lack of reversibility in AIDS likely is due to the HIV-associated CD4 cell loss. Although other aspects of host defense independent of CD4 could be improved by nutritional therapies, no such reports have yet been published.

The indications for nutritional support for HIV-infected patients are the same as for nutritional support in other chronic diseases. They include progressive wasting producing objective evidence of morbidity and little likelihood of self-correction, occurring in a patient with the potential for a prolonged comfortable life. The circumstances for *not* providing nutritional support, e.g. for wasting associated with advanced HIV dementia and little hope for recovery, are far more complex. Is it "right" to insert a percutaneous endoscopic gastrostomy (PEG) in such a patient? Is it "right" not to do so? Such conundrums exist in all of medicine and are not limited to AIDS. The patient's role, the doctor's role, the family's role, and society's role all must be taken into account when decisions are made. The broad discussion in Chapter 35, "Ethics and the Terminally Ill," raises many of the issues involved in such complex decisions.

Several approaches to nutritional support have been tried in AIDS patients. The most straightforward involves treating the underlying disease complication responsible for malnutrition. A longitudinal study of patients with CMV colitis demonstrated the impact of successfully treating underlying disease complications.[83] Progressive wasting in such patients was demonstrated before the availability of effective therapy, whereas patients treated with the antiviral agent ganciclovir regained body weight, body cell mass, and body fat without the addition of formal nutritional support. The antiviral agent AZT also promoted weight gain in some HIV-infected patients, again without formal nutritional support.[84] Thus, effective disease treatment can reverse wasting. As a corollary, nutritional supplementation may be futile in the presence of untreated, serious disease complications.

Enteral and Parenteral Therapies

Nutritional therapy falls into two broad categories. The first is intended to promote nutritional repletion chiefly by providing a balanced diet, whereas the second employs supraphysiologic or pharmacologic doses of specific micronutrients to affect the underlying disease process. More studies have focused on nutritional repletion than on nutritional pharmacology.

Food-based strategies of nutritional support often achieve best results by creating a diet composed of the individual's own food preferences. The intended dietary intake is between 25 and 35 kcal/kg body weight. If intake is not hindered by active disease complications, many people can adjust their intake and achieve caloric balance, so that weight gain[85] or maintenance is possible. Several publications offer practical guidelines to food-based nutritional therapy.[86]

Oral Enteral Supplements

Although food supplements are often advised, supporting data demonstrating their usefulness are limited.[87] The list of commercial nutritional formulae, which differ widely in composition and palatability, continues to grow. Standard polymeric diets have a nutrient composition similar to food-based diets. Their advantage is simply ease of preparation and administration. Some formulae are low in residue; others are modified in being lactose free or in containing high contents of medium-chain triglycerides (MCTs) rather than long-chain triglycerides in the event of malabsorption; others are semielemental or elemental in the event of severe malabsorption; others also contain enhanced quantities of specific nutrients to serve a pharmacologic role.

Each type of diet might have a role in the AIDS patient, depending on the clinical circumstances. However, few studies have compared different oral enteral formulae. Chapter 13, "Defined Formula Diets," covers extensively the indications for the various formulae, including a section on the rationale for the use of MCTs. Chlebowski and colleagues studied a novel enterotropic peptide-based enteral formula, which contained a patented polypeptide and a mixture of carbohydrates and lipids, including MCTs, plus β-carotene, omega-3 fatty acids, selected vitamins (B_6, B_{12}, C, E), minerals (iron, zinc, and selenium), and soluble fiber in HIV-infected individuals and found evidence of benefit compared with a standard polymeric diet.[88] Although the weight gained was small and no objective improvement in immune function was detected, hospitalizations in the experimental group appeared to fall. If corroborated in other studies, the results could provide strong evidence of a benefit of nutritional support beyond its effects upon body composition.

Pediatric HIV-infected patients also may benefit from enteral elementation. Extremely ill infants with AIDS and multiple medical problems were provided an intensive oral regimen of a standard formula and exhibited a clinically significant gain in weight.[89]

Appetite Stimulants

The appetite stimulants megestrol acetate (Megace) and dronabinol (Marinol) have been shown to promote weight gain, with an increase in over 6 percent in body weight after 12 weeks of therapy at 800 mg/day.[90,91] Appetite stimulation is most beneficial in the absence of local pathologic lesions affecting chewing and swallowing, malabsorption syndromes, and in patients without active systemic infections. Since megestrol acetate is a progestational agent, it may interfere with gonadotropin secretion and effects. Women may become amenorrheic or develop other menstrual irregularities. There is a high incidence of impotence in men treated with megestrol acetate, probably due to suppression of gonadotropin release. A suppressant effect on serum testosterone concentration can be shown, which could explain the proclivity of megestrol acetate to promote weight gain through increases in body fat content.[92] Dronabinol (delta-9-tetrahydrocannabinol, THC) is a principal psychoactive substance present in *Cannabis sativa* (marijuana). Additional benefits include the drug's antiemetic effect and its purported ability to improve mood. Dronabinol's effect on the composition of weight gained, that is, fat vs lean mass, has yet to be studied. Side-effects commonly encountered with dronabinol therapy are predominantly those of the central nervous system and include drowsiness, anxiety, poor concentration, impairment of coordination, and confusion. In addition, tachycardia, palpitations, and vasodilation have been reported. Cyproheptadine (Periactin) has received little formal study. It was found to have a mild stimulatory effect on food intake in one study.[93] Cyproheptadine may cause sedation but has few other side-effects. Additional clinical trials in adults are needed to show if cyproheptadine truly has a positive effect on appetite.

Nonvolitional Feeding

When supplements and appetite stimulants fail to moderate wasting, aggressive nutritional support regimens may be required for improvement. Several studies have evaluated nonvolitional feeding regimens. The effect of total parenteral nutrition (TPN) on body composition was assessed in AIDS patients with diverse gastrointestinal (GI) and systemic diseases.[94] The clinical efficacy of TPN was largely determined by the underlying clinical problem.

In patients with eating disorders or malabsorption syndromes, repletion of body cell mass was noted. On the other hand, progressive depletion of body cell mass occurred despite TPN in patients with systemic infections, while body fat accumulation occurred. Presumably, the differing pathogenic mechanisms for malnutrition produced the divergent results. The former set of patients experience caloric deprivation but do not necessarily have derangements in intermediary metabolism. The latter patients have a disorder of metabolic regulation leading directly to protein wasting and may not sustain an anabolic response (i.e., nitrogen retention), even with sufficient calories. The potential for TPN to prolong survival in patients with refractory malabsorption and progressive wasting is intuitive, although survival in AIDS patients receiving TPN for longer than one year is uncommon.* The complication of catheter sepsis in TPN patients is frequently encountered, with gram-positive cocci most typically isolated.[95]

A formal assessment of the effect of TPN on survival will be difficult to perform in AIDS patients as in other diseases, for several reasons. These reasons include difficulties with the use of nutritional placebos and limitations in using death as an endpoint in an intervention study because other potentially important factors may not be controllable. No published studies have compared the effect of TPN with other nutritional therapies. The relative efficacies of TPN and oral intake of a semielemental diet in AIDS patients with severe malabsorption are currently being compared.

In AIDS patients with primary eating disorders and no objective evidence of severe malabsorption or systemic infection, enteral nutrition might be expected to replete body cell mass. This was shown in a prospective case series using a formula diet administered through a PEG for 2 months.[96] In addition to increases in body cell mass, body fat content, serum albumin concentration, and serum iron-binding capacity, the last a reflection of transferrin, also increased. Thus, the enteral

---

*Kotler DP, personal observations.

feeding regimen repleted both somatic and visceral protein compartments. Of note, repletion succeeded despite the persistence of systemic infection in several patients. In this study, total lymphocyte counts in peripheral blood increased significantly during the period of nutritional support, associated with an increase in the number of T-suppressor cells (CD8 +), although no changes were noted in the number of helper CD4 + lymphocytes. Functional improvement, including subjective improvements in cognitive function, was appreciated in those patients receiving nutritional support. The results of this study suggest that nutritional repletion produces benefits beyond simply repleting body mass, although prospective controlled studies that include careful analyses of such clinical outcomes are needed. Nutritional therapies have been shown to promote weight gain in several other trials, including studies using gastrostomy feeding.[97]

The thrust of these studies is that nutritional support may be beneficial in properly selected patients. These studies also underline the multifactorial nature of malnutrition in AIDS and the notion that clinical application will require tailored therapeutic approaches based on specific pathogenic mechanisms. The published studies of nutritional support in HIV-positive patients do not definitively indicate its usefulness, nor do they provide enough information to allow patients or primary care health providers to make rational choices. Further studies must clarify the most appropriate form of nutritional support in specific clinical settings, preferably using comparative trials in well-defined patient populations and analyzing clinically relevant outcomes in addition to specific nutritional endpoints. Pharmacoeconomic considerations also must be taken into account in data analysis.

Other Nutritional Therapies

Ongoing trials are testing various anabolic agents for the long-term treatment of wasting. Recombinant growth hormone has been shown in short-term studies (7 days to 3 months) to produce positive nitrogen balance[98] and repletion of fat-free mass.[99] Cytokine inhibitors, such as pentoxyfylline (Trental) and thalidomide, also have been proposed to treat malnutrition associated with HIV infection. One study analyzed the potential of omega-3 fatty acids to modify cytokine responses and

metabolic derangements, but no treatment effects were found.

CLINICAL DECISION MAKING

The indications for nutritional support in an AIDS patient are the same as in any other patient (i.e., significant body cell mass depletion, negative caloric balance, no overwhelming or untreatable disease complications, and the potential for prolonged comfortable survival). Criteria for choosing specific therapies also should be similar to those employed in other chronic diseases. As in other diseases, a prudent course is to use nutritional interventions on a progressive basis starting with the least intrusive measures, unless the clinical situation dictates otherwise. Initially, oral, pharyngeal, or esophageal conditions that impair food intake should be diagnosed and treated and spontaneous food intake should be stimulated as possible. Several compendia of dietary recommendations for HIV-positive patients have been published.[86] The selection of oral enteral supplements has been discussed above.

If caloric intake is sufficient but improvement is slow, anabolic agents might be useful to optimize retention of fat-free mass, although definitive studies have not been published. If intake remains inadequate, appetite stimulants can be employed. If the patient is unable to maintain an adequate intake by oral means, the enteral route should be used for alimentation, unless contraindicated by obstruction, malabsorption, or other factors. The choice of feeding tube, transnasal vs transabdominal, should be based on the expected duration of therapy (Fig. 21–5) and on the risks of recurrent sinus infections, aspiration pneumonia, and nasal cartilage erosion associated with long-term nasogastric tube placement (Chapter 14). However, patients and caregivers are often reluctant to accept any feeding tubes.

If parenteral nutrition becomes necessary, partial parenteral nutrition through a peripheral IV may be used for short periods (< 2 weeks) in patients likely to resume normal intake; TPN is needed in patients with irreversible gut failure. Gut failure includes severe, intractable malabsorption, frequent and persistent vomiting, or another intestinal condition precluding adequate absorption. The choice of tube used is often based on personal preferences. For patients with aesthetic concerns a subcutaneous reservoir, which is accessed by a removable needle, may be preferred, rather than an external

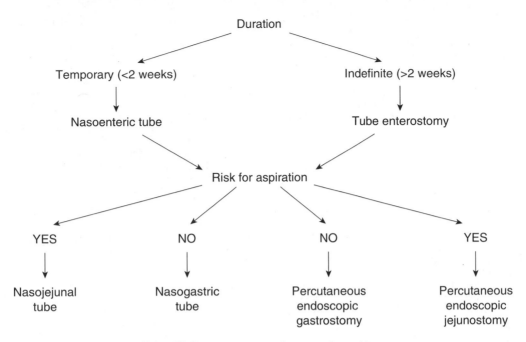

FIGURE 21–5 Decision tree for enteral nutrition.

catheter. Success has been achieved using peripherally inserted central venous catheters for TPN (PICC line). As stated above, untreated, active infections are significant obstacles to nutritional repletion, so nutritional support should be employed in conjunction with an aggressive overall diagnostic and treatment plan.

The current state of knowledge does not allow specific recommendations for micronutrient intakes to be made. There is evidence suggesting that overall requirements for many of the water-soluble vitamins is increased as a result of disease activity, to a level between three to five times normal. Many clinicians recommend intake of one or two multivitamins in addition to a balance diet. Ongoing and planned studies will help define the needs and benefits of other micronutrients, especially antioxidants, on nutritional status.

CONCLUSION

Proper nutritional management can have a positive impact on the clinical course of HIV-infected patients. Further information is required to assign nutrition its proper priority in the clinical management of HIV-infected individuals. The respective roles of macronutrients and micronutrients remain unclear. Occult malabsorption especially, and intestinal dysfunction in general, play a role in nutritional status that must be clarified. Metabolic alterations, including hypogo-

nadism, which can be easily treated, and hypermetabolism, which may be cytokine driven, may play important roles in the pathogenesis of malnutrition associated with HIV infection. These subjects require further study. The role of nutritional supplements in altering the progression of HIV infection and in limiting the severity of the clinical immune deficiency is poorly understood. The overall impact of malnutrition and of nutritional support on clinical outcomes in addition to nutritional status must be studied. Whether the development of progressive malnutrition can be prevented by early intervention with nutritional therapies remains to be answered.

Acknowledgments

We are indebted to Richard N. Pierson, Jr., Jack Wang, and the staff of the Body Composition Unit and to Anita R. Tierney, MPH, for continuing contributions to the research program on nutrition in AIDS.

REFERENCES

1. Revision of the CDC surveillance case definition for acquired immunodeficiency syndrome. MMWR 1987; 36:3–15.
2. Serwadda D, Mugerwa RD, Sewankambo NK et al: Slim disease: a new disease in Uganda and its association with HTLV-III infection. Lancet 1985;2:849–852.
3. Palenicek JG, He D, Graham NMH et al: Weight loss as a predictor of survival after AIDS among HIV-infected

gay men enrolled in the MACS. (Abstract). Proc Int Conf AIDS 1993;1:77.

4. Kotler DP, Tierney AR, Wang J et al: The magnitude of body cell mass depletion determines the timing of death from wasting in AIDS. Am J Clin Nutr 1989;50: 444–447.

5. Chlebowski RT, Grosvenor MB, Bernhard NH et al: Nutritional status, gastrointestinal dysfunction, and survival in patients with AIDS. Am J Gastroenterol 1989; 84:1288–1293.

6. Guenter P, Muurahainen N, Simons G et al: Relationships among nutritional status, disease progression, and survival in HIV infection. J AIDS 1993;6:1130–1138.

7. Greene JB: Clinical approach to weight loss in the patients with HIV infection. Gastroenterol Clin N Am 1988;17:573–586.

8. Kotler DP, Wang J, Pierson RN: Studies of body composition in patients with the acquired immunodeficiency syndrome. Am J Clin Nutr 1985;42:1255–1265.

9. Barac-Nieto M, Spurr GB, Lotero H et al: Body composition in chronic undernutrition. Am J Clin Nutr 1978; 31:23–40.

10. Long CL, Schaffel N, Geiger JW et al: Metabolic response to injury and illness: estimation of energy and protein needs from indirect calorimetry and nitrogen balance. J Parenter Enteral Nutr 1979;3:452–456.

11. Kotler DP, Tierney AR, Dilmanian FA et al: Correlation between total body potassium and total body nitrogen in patients with acquired immunodeficiency syndrome. Clin Res 1991;39:649A.

12. Ott M, Lambke B, Fischer H et al: Early changes of body composition in human immunodeficiency virus-infected patients: tetrapolar body impedance analysis indicates significant malnutrition. Am J Clin Nutr 1993;57:15–19.

13. Keusch G, Thea D, Ngoy N et al: Body composition by bioelectric-impedance analysis in HIV+ and – adults in Kinshasa, Zaire. Proc Int Conf AIDS 1992;2:B231.

14. Kosok A, Muurahainen N, Simons G et al: Demographic correlations of malnutrition in HIV disease. Abstract. Tenth International Conference on AIDS. 1994;2:225.

15. Kotler DP, Babameto G, Burastero S et al: Application of a single frequency bioimpedance analysis for the study of body composition in HIV-infected individuals. Abstract. Clin Res 1994;42:279.

16. Kotler DP, Tierney AR, Brenner SK et al: Preservation of short-term energy balance in clinically stable patients with AIDS. Am J Clin Nutr 1990;57:7–13.

17. Trujillo EB, Borlase BC, Bell SJ et al: Assessment of nutritional status, nutrient intake, and nutrition support in AIDS patients. JAMA 1992;92:477–478.

18. Sharkey SJ, Sharkey KA, Sutherland LR et al: Nutritional status and food intake in human immunodeficiency syndrome. J Acquired Immune Defic Syndr 1992;5:1091–1098.

19. Maccallan DC, Noble C, Baldwin C et al: Prospective analysis of patterns of weight change in stage IV human immunodeficiency virus infection. Am J Clin Nutr 1993;58:417–424.

20. Beach RS, Mantero-Atienza E, Shor-Posner G et al: Specific nutrient abnormalities in asymptomatic HIV infection. AIDS 1992;6:701–708.

21. Baum MK, Mantero-Atienza E, Shor-Posner G et al: Association of Vitamin B6 status with parameters of immune function in early HIV-1 infection. J Acquired Immune Defic Syndr 1991;4:1122–1132.

22. Robson LC, Schwarz RM, Perkins WD: The effects of Vitamin B_6 deficiency on the lymphoid system and immune responses. In Tryfiates CP (ed): Vitamin B_6 Me-

tabolism and Role in Growth. Westport, CT: Food and Nutrition Press, 1980:205–222.

23. Falutz J, Tsoukas C, Gold P: Zinc as a cofactor in human immunodeficiency virus-induced immunosuppression. JAMA 1988;259:2850–2851.

24. Dworkin BM, Rosenthal WS, Wormser GW et al: Selenium deficiency in the acquired immunodeficiency syndrome. J Parenter Enter Nutr 1986;10:405–407.

25. Henkin RI, Bradley DF: Regulation of taste acuity threshold by thiols and metal ions. Proc Natl Acad Sci (USA) 1969;62:30–37.

26. Graha NMH, Sorenson D, Odaka N et al: Relationship of serum copper and zinc to HIV-1 seropositivity and progression to AIDS. J Acquir Immune Defic Syndr 1991;4:976–980.

27. Johnson RA, Baker SS, Fallon JT et al: An occidental case of cardiomyopathy and selenium deficiency. N Engl J Med 1981;304:1210–1212.

28. Dworkin BM, Antonecchia PP, Smith F et al: Reduced cardiac selenium content in the acquired immunodeficiency syndrome. J Parenter Enter Nutr 1989;13: 644–647.

29. Beach RS, Morgan R, Wilkie F et al: Plasma cobalamin levels as a potential cofactor in studies of HIV-1 related cognitive changes. Arch Neurol 1992;49:501–506.

30. Staal FWT, Ela SW, Roederer M et al: Glutathione deficiency and human immunodeficiency virus infection. Lancet 1992;339:909–912.

31. Roederer M, Staal FJT, Raju PA et al: Cytokine-stimulated human immunodeficiency virus replication is inhibited by N-acetyl-L-cysteine. Proc Natl Acad Sci (USA) 1990;87:4884–4888.

32. Hommes MJT, Romijn JA, Endert E et al: Resting energy expenditure and substrate oxidation in human immunodeficiency virus (HIV)-infected asymptomatic men: HIV affects host metabolism in the early asymptomatic stage. Am J Clin Nutr 1991;54:311–315.

33. Hommes MJT, Romijn JA, Godfried MH et al: Increased resting energy expenditure in human immunodeficiency virus-infected men. Metabolism 1990;39: 1186–1190.

34. Grieco MH, Reddy MM, Kothari HB et al: Elevated B₂ — microglobulin and lysozyme levels in patients with acquired immune deficiency syndrome. Clin Immunol Immunopathol 1984;32:174–178.

35. Eyster ME, Goedert JJ, Poon M-C et al: Acid-labile interferon: a possible preclinical marker for the acquired immunodeficiency syndrome in hemophilia. N Engl J Med 1983;309:583–587.

36. Lange M, Klein E, Kornfield H et al: Cytomegalovirus isolation from healthy homosexual men. JAMA 1984; 252:1908–1910.

37. Giorgi JV, Detels R: T-cell subset alterations in HIV-infected homosexual men. NIAID Multicenter AIDS Cohort Study. Clin Immunol Immunopathol 1989;52:10–18.

38. Reka S, Garro ML, Kotler DP: Variation in the expression of HIV, RNA and cytokine mRNA in rectal mucosa during the progression of HIV infection. Lymphokine Cytokine Res 1994;13:391–398.

39. Reka S, Garro ML, Kotler DP: Evaluation of cytokine expression in lymph nodes of HIV-infected individuals by RNA in situ hybridization. Abstract. Ninth International Conference on AIDS. 1993;1:171.

40. Sclafani A, Koopmans HS, Vasselli J et al: Effects of intestinal bypass surgery on appetite, food intake, and body weight in obese and lean rats. Am J Physiol 1978;234:E389–E398.

41. Fong Y, Moldower LL, Marono M et al: Cachectin/TNF or IL-1 alpha induces cachexia with redistribution of body proteins. Am J Physiol 1989;256:R659–R665.

42. Moldawer LL, Anderrson C, Gelin J et al: Regulation of food intake and hepatic protein synthesis by recombinant-derived cytokines. Am J Physiol 1988;254: G450–G456.

43. Grunfeld C, Pang M, Shimizu L et al: Resting energy expenditure, caloric intake, and short-term weight change in human immunodeficiency virus infection and AIDS. Am J Clin Nutr 1992;55:455–460.

44. Melchior J-C, Salmon D, Rigaud D et al: Resting energy expenditure is increased in stable, malnourished HIV-infected patients. Am J Clin Nutr 1991;53: 437–441.

45. Piot P, Quinn T, Taelman H et al: Acquired immunodeficiency syndrome in a heterosexual population in Zaire. Lancet 1984;2:65–79.

46. Kotler DP, Francisco A, Clayton F et al: Small intestinal injury and parasitic disease in the acquired immunodeficiency syndrome (AIDS). Ann Intern Med 1990; 113:444–449.

47. Kotler DP, Reka S, Chow K et al: Effects of enteric parasitoses and HIV infection upon small intestinal structure and function in patients with AIDS. J Clin Gastro 1993;16:10–15.

48. Hayes EB, Malte TD, O'Brien TR et al: Large community outbreak of cryptosporidiosis due to contamination of a filtered public water supply. N Engl J Med 1989;320:1372–1376.

49. Kotler DP, Orenstein JM: Prevalence of intestinal microsporidiosis in HIV-infected individuals referred for gastroenterological evaluation. Am J Gastroenterol 1994;89:1998–2002.

50. Roth RI, Owen RL, Keren DF et al: Intestinal infection with *Mycobacterium avium* in acquired immunodeficiency syndrome (AIDS): histological and clinical comparison with Whipple's disease. Dig Dis Sci 1985; 30:497–500.

51. Kotler DP, Orenstein JM: Diarrhea and malabsorption due to enterocyte-adherent bacterial infection in a patient with AIDS. Ann Intern Med 1993;119:127–128.

52. Grohmann GS, Glass RI, Pereira HG et al: Enteric viruses and diarrhea in HIV-infected patients. N Engl J Med 1993;329:14–20.

53. Kotler DP, Giang TT, Thiim M et al: Chronic bacterial enteropathy in patients with AIDS. J Infect Dis 1995; 171:552–558.

54. Clayton FC, Heller TH, Reka S et al: Variation in the distribution of cryptosporidiosis in AIDS. J Clin Pathol 1994;102:420–425.

55. Hodges JR, Wright R: Normal immune responses in the gut and liver. Clin Sci 1982;63:339–347.

56. Johnson LR: Regulation of gastrointestinal mucosal growth. Physiol Rev 1988;68:456–469.

57. Holt PR, Tierney AR, Kotler DP: Delayed enzyme expression: a defect of aging rat gut. Gastroenterology 1986;89:1026–1034.

58. Nordstron C, Dahlqvist A, Josefsson L: Quantitative determination of enzymes in different parts of the villi and crypts of rat small intestine: comparison of alkaline phosphatase, disaccharidases and dipeptidases. Cytochemistry 968;15:713–721.

59. Boyle JT, Celano P, Koldovsky O: Demonstration of a difference in expression of maximal lactase and sucrase activity along the villus in the adult rat jejunum. Gastroenterology 1980;79:503–507.

60. Shiau YF, Kotler DP, Levine GM: Can normal small bowel morphology be equated with normal function? Gastroenterology 1979;76:1246A.

61. Schenk EA, Samloff IM, Klipstein FA: Morphologic characteristics of jejunal biopsies in celiac disease and in tropical sprue. Am J Pathol 1965;47:765–772.

62. Cummins AG, LaBrooy JT, Stanley DP et al: Quantitative histological study of enteropathy associated with HIV infection. Gut 1990;31:317–321.

63. Ullrich R, Zeitz M, Heise M et al: Small intestinal structure and function in patients infected with human immunodeficiency virus (HIV): evidence for HIV-induced enteropathy. Ann Intern Med 1989;111:15–21.

64. Roth RI, Owen RL, Keren DF et al: Intestinal infection with *Mycobacterium avium* in acquired immunodeficiency syndrome (AIDS): histological and clinical comparison with Whipple's disease. Dig Dis Sci 1985; 30:497–502.

65. Budhraja M, Levandoglu H, Kocka F et al: Duodenal mucosal T cell population and bacterial culture in acquired immunodeficiency syndrome. Am J Gastroenterol 1987;82:427–433.

66. Sciaretta G, Bonazzi L, Monti M et al: Bile acid malabsorption in AIDS-associated chronic diarrhea: a prospective 1-year study. Am J Gastroenterol 1994;89:379–381.

67. Wolfe MM, Soll A: The physiology of gastric acid secretion. N Engl J Med 1988;319:1707–1712.

68. Lake-Bakaar G, Quadros E, Beidas S et al: Gastric secretory failure in patients with the acquired immunodeficiency syndrome (AIDS). Ann Intern Med 1988; 109:502–504.

69. Griffin GE, Miller A, Batman P et al: Damage to jejunal autonomic nerves in HIV infection. AIDS 1988;2: 379–382.

70. Batman P, Miller ARO, Sedgwick PM et al: Autonomic denervation in jejunal mucosa of homosexual men infected with HIV. AIDS 1991;5:1247–1252.

71. Coodley GO, Coodley MK, Nelson HD et al: Micronutrient concentrations in the HIV wasting syndrome. AIDS 1993;7:1595–1600.

72. Harriman GR, Smith PD, McDonald KH et al: Vitamin B_{12} malabsorption in patients with the acquired immunodeficiency syndrome. Arch Intern Med 1989; 149:2039–2041.

73. Kotler DP, Haroutiounian G, Greenberg R et al: Increased bile salt deconjugation in AIDS. Abstract. Gastroenterology 1985;88:1455.

74. Sciarretta G, Vicini G, Fagioli G et al: Use of 23-Selena-25-homosholyltaurine to detect bile acid malabsorption in patients with ileal dysfunction or diarrhea. Gastroenterology 1986;91:1–9.

75. Hofmann AF: The syndrome of ileal disease and the broken enterohepatic circulation: cholerrheic enteropathy. Gastroenterology 1967;52:752–757.

76. Hofmann AF, Poley JR: Role of bile acid malabsorption in the pathogenesis of diarrhea and steatorrhea in patients with ileal resection. Gastroenterology 1967;52: 752–757.

77. Coodley GO, Loveless MO, Nelson HD et al: Endocrine function in the HIV wasting syndrome. J Acquired Immune Defic Syndr 1994;7:46–51.

78. Grunfeld C, Kotler DP, Hamadeh R et al: Hypertriglyceridemia in the acquired immunodeficiency syndrome. Am J Med 1989;86:27–31.

79. Grunfeld C, Kotler DP, Shigenga JK et al: Circulating interferon alpha levels and hypertriglyceridemia in the acquired immunodeficiency syndrome. Am J Med 1991;90:154–162.

80. Grunfeld C, Pang M, Doerrler W et al: Lipids, lipoproteins, triglyceride clearance and cytokines in human immunodeficiency virus infection and the acquired immunodeficiency syndrome. J Clin Endocrinol Metab 1992;74:1045–1052.

81. Hellerstein MK, Grunfeld C, Wu K et al: Increased de novo hepatic lipogenesis in human immunodeficiency virus infection. J Clin Endo Metab 1993;7:559–565.

82. Zangerle R, Reibnegger G, Wachter H et al: Weight loss in HIV infection is associated with immune activation. AIDS 1993;7:175–181.

83. Kotler DP, Tierney AR, Altilio D et al: Body mass repletion during ganciclovir therapy of cytomegalovirus infections in patients with the acquired immunodeficiency syndrome. Arch Intern Med 1989;149:901–905.

84. Fischl MA, Richman DD, Grieco MH et al: The efficacy of azidothymidine (AZT) in the treatment of patients with AIDS and AIDS-related complex. N Engl J Med 1987;317:185–191.

85. Burger B, Ollenschlager G, Schrappe M et al: Nutritional behavior of malnourished HIV-infected patients and intensified oral nutritional intervention. Nutrition 1993;9:43–44.

86. Newman CF: Practical dietary recommendations in HIV infection. In Kotler DP (ed): Gastrointestinal and Nutritional Consequences of AIDS. New York: Raven Press, 1991:247–277.

87. Burger B, Olenschlager G, Schrappe M et al: Nutrition behavior of malnourished HIV-infected patients and intensified oral nutritional intervention. Nutrition 1993;9:43–44.

88. Chlebowski RT, Beall G, Grosvenor M et al: Long-term effects of early nutritional support with new enterotropic peptide-based formula vs. standard enteral formula in HIV-infected patients: randomized prospective trial. Nutrition 1993;9:507–512.

89. Fennoy I, Leung J: Refeeding and subsequent growth in the child with AIDS. Nutr Clin Prac 1990;5:54–58.

90. Von Roenn JH, Armstrong D, Kotler D et al: A placebo-controlled trial of megestrol acetate in patients with AIDS-related anorexia and cachexia. Ann Intern Med 1994;121:400–408.

91. Gorter R, Seefried M, Volberding P: Dronabinol effects on weight in patients with HIV infection. AIDS 1992; 6:127.

92. Engelson ES, Tierney AR, Pi-Sunyer FX et al: Effects of megestrol acetate therapy upon body composition and serum testosterone in patients with AIDS. Clin Res 1994;42:281A.

93. Summerbell CD, Youle M, McDonald V et al: Megestrol acetate vs cyproheptadine in the treatment of weight loss associated with HIV infection. Intl J STD AIDS 1992;3:278–280.

94. Kotler DP, Tierney AR, Wang J et al: Effect of home total parenteral nutrition upon body composition in AIDS. J Parenter Enter Nutr 1990;14:454–458.

95. Raviglione MO, Battan R, Pablos-Mendez A et al: Infections associated with Hickman catheters in patients with acquired immunodeficiency syndrome. Am J Med 1989;86:780–786.

96. Kotler DP, Tierney AR, Ferraro R et al: Effect of enteral feeding upon body cell mass in AIDS. Am J Clin Nutr 1991;53:149–154.

97. Cappell MS, Godil A: A multicenter case controlled study of percutaneous endoscopic gastrostomy in HIV seropositive patients. Am J Gastroenterol 1993;88: 2059–2066.

98. Mulligan K, Grunfeld C, Hellerstein MK et al: Anabolic effects of recombinant human growth hormone in patients with wasting associated with human immunodeficiency virus infection. J Clin Endocrinol Metab 1993;77:956–962.

99. Schembelan M, LaMarca A, Mulligan K et al: Growth hormone therapy of AIDS wasting. Abstract. Proc Int Conf AIDS 1994;2:35.

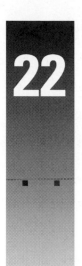

Enteral Nutrition in the Elderly

EDWARD SALTZMAN
JOEL B. MASON

The elderly, defined as persons over 65 years of age, are a rapidly growing segment of the population with unique nutritional needs. These unique characteristics and demographic trends make nutritional support of this group an increasing challenge. Persons over the age of 65 now comprise 12 percent of the U.S. population and are predicted to increase to 22 percent by the year 2030.[1,2] Similar predictions have been made in Canada,[3] and even greater numbers are predicted in Europe.[4] In absolute numbers, the size of the elderly population in the United States has increased by 50 percent in the last 20 years[2] and is now over 25 million.[5] In particular, the elderly over age 85 are the fastest expanding of all age groups,[1,6] as evidenced by a 41 percent increase in the U.S. over-85 population between 1970 and 1981.[7]

Despite considerable increases in longevity, the elderly experience substantially more disease than younger groups.[7] The elderly are hospitalized more frequently and for longer durations.[1,7] Eighty-five percent of the elderly have one or more chronic illnesses, and 30 percent have three or more.[1] The high prevalence of illness contributes to increased risk for primary and secondary malnutrition in the elderly.[8] It has been estimated that 85 percent of the non-institutionalized elderly suffer from at least one condition that could be improved by proper nutrition.[9] Although the elderly comprise 12 percent of the population, it is estimated that at least 30 percent of health care dollars are spent on this age group.[1,3] Nutrition screening and intervention in selected settings has therefore been recently proposed as an appropriate, cost-effective measure.[10]

In community-dwelling elderly, maintenance of independence and function is vital. Proper nutrition contributes to maintenance of functional status, whereas nutritional deficits have been linked to declines in mobility and independence.[11] Malnutrition among community-dwelling elderly may also predispose these individuals to acute illness and hospitalization.[12] There is an estimated 5 to 10 percent prevalence of protein-calorie malnutrition (PCM) among community-dwelling elderly.[13] However, in many cases, PCM in ambulatory patients remains unrecognized by clinicians.[14,15] Physicians also often fail to recognize functional deficits[16] that may reflect underlying malnutrition.

As the elderly population grows, so does the number of institutionalized elderly. Only 1 percent of those under the age of 74 reside in institutions, but the number is substantially increased to 22 percent of those over 85 years.[1] In a recent review of malnutrition in nursing homes, Abbasi and Rudman[17] noted alarmingly high rates (30 to 50 percent) of PCM in nursing home patients, which were associated with increased rates of mortality. The authors provide convincing evidence that much of the malnutrition is preventable or reversible (Table 22–1).

Nutritional status in acute illness is a determinant of morbidity, length of hospital stay, and mortality.[18-21] Although malnutrition may predispose younger patients to similar negative outcomes, the risk is increased in the elderly due to baseline loss of reserves, likelihood of preadmission nutritional deficiencies, and difficulties in repletion.[21,22]

Some wasting and nutrient deficiencies will result from disease and will not be preventable or reversible. Numerous studies, however, have demonstrated that malnutrition is neither integral to aging nor is it unavoidable in illness. Nutritional intervention has resulted in improvements in quality of life and in indexes of nutritional status in the community-dwelling, the chronically institutionalized, and the acutely ill elderly.[17,22-27] It is now clear that better attempts must be made to prevent and treat malnutrition in the elderly.

This chapter addresses the nutritional assessment, requirements, and delivery of enteral nutrition in the elderly. It is inappropriate to discuss the elderly as a homogeneous group because the diversity in age, presence or absence of illnesses, and level of function are all features that dictate a stratified approach. Accordingly, when possible we have tried to differentiate the needs and strategies that reflect the unique characteristics of these subgroups of the elderly.

ASSESSMENT OF NUTRITIONAL STATUS

A thorough assessment of nutritional status in the elderly includes historical data, physical examination, anthropometric measurements, and biochemical tests. Functional assessment adds information about strength, mobility, and ability to perform activities necessary for daily living. Functional assessment is also often more sensitive than other methods in detecting nutritional deficits[27,28] and in predicting outcome.[21,29]

TABLE 22–1   Modifiable Causes of Malnutrition in the Nursing Home

Cause	Method of Identification	Corrective Action
Staff unawareness	Lack of documentation in chart by MD, RN, or RD	Staff education
Inappropriate use of restricted diets	Patient receiving a restricted diet no longer indicated	Replace by ad lib diet
Use of drugs that impair desire or ability to eat	Review of medications	Discontinue or replace offending drug
Unmet need for eating assistance or self-help eating devices	Observation and calorie count	Provide assistance or devices
Suboptimal technique of eating assistance	Observation	Retrain the nursing aide
Suboptimal dining environment	Observation	Improve the environment
Prescription of maintenance instead of repletion dietary intakes (oral or enteral)	< 1.5 × RDA of calories and protein prescribed	Increase prescription to 1.5 × RDA calories and protein
Inadequate nutritional support during intercurrent illness	Weight or albumin decline during illness; inadequate nutrition support	Project MD will consult on each patient during intercurrent illness
Unrecognized febrile illness	Daily temperatures reveal elevations	Identify and treat infections
Unmet need for modified diet	Clinical review	Prescribe indicated modified diet
Inadequate management of tube-feeding complications	Prescribed tube-feeding volume not being administered or absorbed	Correct management of complication
Poor dental status	Oral examination	Prompt dental care
Unmet need for dysphagia work-up	Clinical signs suggest dysphagia; work-up not requested	Consult speech pathology for swallowing evaluation
Suboptimal treatment of dysphagia	Recommendations of speech pathology not being followed	Speech pathologist retrains nursing staff

Adapted from Abbasi AA, Rudman DR: Undernutrition in the nursing home: prevalence, consequences, causes and prevention. Nutr Rev 1994;52:113. © International Life Sciences Institute. Reprinted with permission.

Unfortunately, only limited reference standards for many assessment parameters are currently available for elderly populations. The third National Health and Nutrition Examination Survey (NHANES III) incorporated data from persons up to the age of 94, with subdivision of age by 10-year increments.[30] As these data become available, they will provide much needed normative standards for many parameters of nutrition status in the elderly.

The diversity of the elderly population has made the development of a comprehensive screening or assessment tool difficult. Perhaps the best effort to date toward this goal is The Nutrition Screening Initiative, which is a multiagency collaboration designed to improve nutritional status in the U.S. elderly.[31] Screening is performed using a two-stage approach. The Level I screen is a simple questionnaire that can be completed by the patient or a surrogate and directs the patient to appropriate professionals (Fig. 22–1). The Level II screen is more complex and relies on historical, anthropometric, biochemical, and functional data. These screening devices include many of the assessment parameters discussed below and can be recommended as valuable tools for identifying the elderly patient at risk for malnutrition. The Nutrition Interventions Manual for Professionals Caring for Older Americans,[31] also developed by the Nutrition Screening Initiative, is an excellent compendium of detailed approaches to nutritional assessment and intervention and contains examples of the Level I and Level II screens.

History

As in all age groups, the diet history is essential. Accurate dietary assessment in the elderly may be hampered by cognitive deficits, and, like other age groups, the elderly are prone to underreporting.[32] Many patients may follow restricted diets, such as those low in sodium, fat, or lactose. These diets can impair nutrient intake by reducing palatability or variety.

Important components of the history include ability to obtain, prepare, and consume nutritionally sound foods.[11,22] Oral health must be evaluated. Dental disease is common in the elderly, including approximately 40 percent of the elderly who are endentulous.[33] Poor dentition can result in changes in food choices and quantity. Alterations associated with aging in the senses of taste and smell may contribute to decreased food intake.[34] Schiffman and Warwick[26] have demonstrated that enhancing food flavors increases food intake and nutritional status in elderly institutionalized patients. Altered bowel habits, especially constipation, also contribute to food intake and choices. The elderly experience decreased sensation of thirst in response to dehydration and osmotic stimuli;[35,36] thus it cannot be assumed that even those with free access to fluids will remain appropriately hydrated.

Disturbances of mood and affect are common in the elderly,[37] particularly following the death of a spouse, and can dramatically influence appetite and food intake. Alterations in cognition not only predispose the elderly to malnutrition, but also can result from protein-calorie malnutrition, dehydration, and deficiencies of thiamine, vitamin B_{12}, and folate.[38,39]

Living arrangements and the environment in which meals are taken may influence the quantity and composition of food intake.[40] Socioeconomic and educational factors may result in inadequate or suboptimal nutrient intake.[41] Improvements in nutritional status have been made by delivery of supplements to housebound elderly,[27] and programs for home-delivery or congregate meals are available in many areas.[42]

Drug-nutrient interactions occur in all age groups, but the elderly are at especially increased risk because they generally take more medications. Impairments in renal or hepatic metabolism and excretion, hypoalbuminemia,[43] and changes in body composition may affect drug volume of distribution and concentration. Detailed reviews of drug-nutrient interactions are available in this volume (Chapter 31) and elsewhere.[44-46]

Physical Examination

Physical manifestations of nutritional deficiency in the elderly may be atypical.[47] The elderly may not present with classic signs of PCM, micronutrient deficiency, or dehydration due to age-related alterations in skin and hair, mucous membranes, and losses in muscle mass. Similarly, neurologic or cognitive impairment may mask deficiency states, including deficiencies of thiamine, vitamin B_6, and vitamin B_{12}. Because the prevalence of marginal vitamin B_{12} status is common (see the section on Micronutrients, below) and can result in impaired cognition, alterations in cognition should never be ascribed merely to "normal aging." The immobile patient must be examined for the presence of decubitus ulcers, which may signify deficiencies of energy, protein, or

Level I Screen

Body Weight

Measure height to the nearest inch and weight to the nearest pound. Record the values below and mark them on the Body Mass Index (BMI) scale to the right. Then use a straight edge (ruler) to connect the two points and circle the spot where this straight line crosses the center line (body mass index). Record the number below.

Healthy older adults should have a BMI between 22 and 27.

Height (in):_____
Weight (lbs):_____
Body Mass Index:_____
(number from center column)

Check any boxes that are true for the individual:

☐ Has lost or gained 10 pounds (or more) in the past 6 months.

☐ Body mass index <22

☐ Body mass index >27

For the remaining sections, please ask the individual which of the statements (if any) is true for him or her and place a check by each that applies.

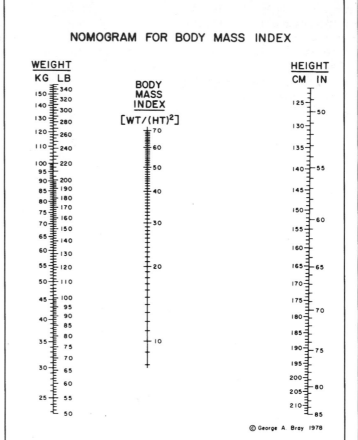

Eating Habits

☐ Does not have enough food to eat each day

☐ Usually eats alone

☐ Does not eat anything on one or more days each month

☐ Has poor appetite

☐ Is on a special diet

☐ Eats vegetables two or fewer times daily

☐ Eats milk or milk products once or not at all daily

☐ Eats fruit or drinks fruit juice once or not at all daily

☐ Eats breads, cereals, pasta, rice, or other grains five or fewer times daily

☐ Has difficulty chewing or swallowing

☐ Has more than one alcoholic drink per day (if woman); more than two drinks per day (if man)

☐ Has pain in mouth, teeth, or gums

FIGURE 22–1 Nutrition screening initiative level I screen. (Reprinted with permission by the Nutrition Screening Initiative, a project of the American Academy of Family Physicians, the American Dietetic Association, and the National Council on the Aging, Inc., and funded in part by a grant from Ross Products Division, Abbott Laboratories.)

A physician should be contacted if the individual has gained or lost 10 pounds unexpectedly or without intending to during the past 6 months. A physician should also be notified if the individual's body mass index is above 27 or below 22.

Living Environment

- ☐ Lives on an income of less than $6000 per year (per individual in the household)

- ☐ Lives alone

- ☐ Is housebound

- ☐ Is concerned about home security

- ☐ Lives in a home with inadequate heating or cooling

- ☐ Does not have a stove and/or refrigerator

- ☐ Is unable or prefers not to spend money on food (<$25-30 per person spent on food each week)

Functional Status

Usually or always needs assistance with (check each that apply):

- ☐ Bathing

- ☐ Dressing

- ☐ Grooming

- ☐ Toileting

- ☐ Eating

- ☐ Walking or moving about

- ☐ Traveling (outside the home)

- ☐ Preparing food

- ☐ Shopping for food or other necessities

If you have checked one or more statements on this screen, the individual you have interviewed may be at risk for poor nutritional status. Please refer this individual to the appropriate health care or social service professional in your area. For example, a dietitian should be contacted for problems with selecting, preparing, or eating a healthy diet, or a dentist if the individual experiences pain or difficulty when chewing or swallowing. Those individuals whose income, lifestyle, or functional status may endanger their nutritional and overall health should be referred to available community services: home-delivered meals, congregate meal programs, transportation services, counseling services (alcohol abuse, depression, bereavement, etc.), home health care agencies, day care programs, etc.

Please repeat this screen at least once each year--sooner if the individual has a major change in his or her health, income, immediate family (e.g., spouse dies), or functional status.

These materials developed by the Nutrition Screening Initiative.

FIGURE 22–1 *Continued* Nutrition screening initiative level I screen (page 2).

vitamin C.[48] Physical strength and gait should be assessed and are discussed in the section on functional assessment below.

Anthropometric Measurements

To understand the role of anthropometric measurements in assessment of the elderly, the effect of aging on body composition must first be briefly discussed. Aging is associated with the loss of lean body mass (LBM) and a concomitant gain in fat mass. In a longitudinal study using the total body potassium tech-nique, Flynn and colleagues[49] found that LBM decreases by an average of 0.45 kg/year after age 60. Loss of LBM occurs disproportionately more from skeletal muscle than from viscera.[50] Because a gain in body fat accompanies the loss of LBM, total body weight may not change despite underlying changes in body composi-tion. Gains in fat mass may also be accompa-nied by shifts in the distribution of fat from subcutaneous to intramuscular depots[50-52] re-sulting in a phenomenon called "marbling" of muscle.[53] Figure 22–2 illustrates these changes in body composition.

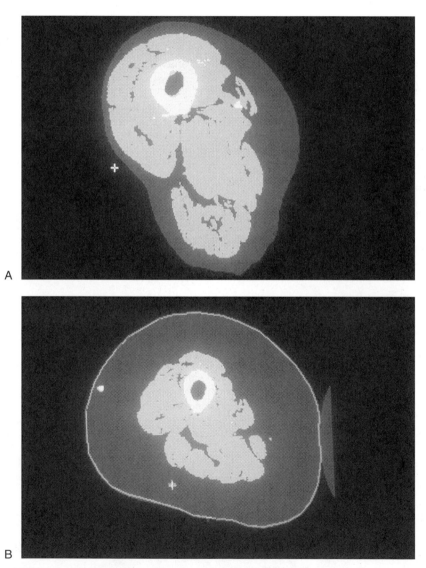

FIGURE 22–2   Mid-thigh CT image of women aged 63 (*A*) and 93 years (*B*) depicting age-associated changes in lean and fat mass. (Courtesy of Dr. Miriam Nelson, Jean Mayer USDA Human Nutrition Research Center on Aging at Tufts University, Boston, MA.)

Functionally, the loss of LBM is associated with impairments of many physiologic functions, including pulmonary function,[54] depressed immunity and hematopoiesis,[24,55,56] and losses of strength and independence.[11,57] The etiology and teleology of these changes in body composition with aging are subjects of considerable debate and research effort. Possible causes include the "normal" aging process, catabolic effects of chronic or acute illness, deconditioning or disuse, changes in hormone or cytokine levels or action, and malnutrition.

Stature declines with age due to losses in vertebral bone, intervertebral disks, and the resultant kyphosis.[58-60] Accurate measurement of height is difficult in those who are unable to stand erect or who are bedbound.[51] If a surrogate measurement for height is required, an effective method is calculation of stature from knee height.[61-63] Stature can be calculated from knee height by a nomogram (Fig. 22–3) or by the equations of Chumlea:[61]

$$\text{Stature for men (cm)} = (2.02 \times \text{knee height}) - (0.04 \times \text{age}) + 64.19$$

$$\text{Stature for women (cm)} = (1.83 \times \text{knee height}) - (0.24 \times \text{age}) + 84.88$$

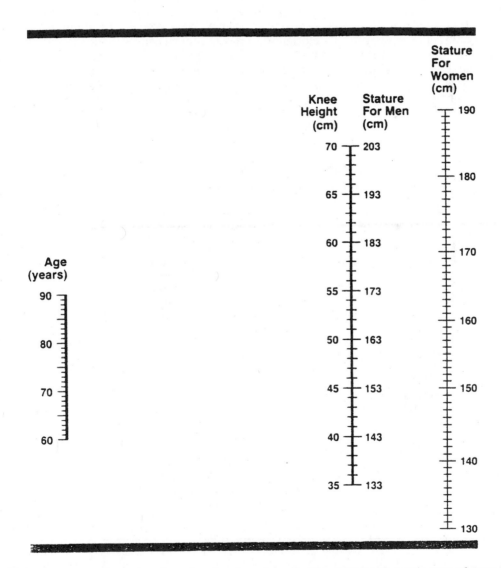

Figure 22–3 Nomogram for estimation of stature from knee height. (Used with permission of Ross Products Division, Abbott Laboratories, Columbus, OH, from Chumlee WC: Nutritional Assessment of the Elderly Through Anthropometry, 1988.)

Other surrogate measures of height include armspan[61,64-66] and recumbent length.[67]

Anthropometric measurements are useful for comparing values obtained in an individual patient to normative standards or for repeated measures in the same individual over time. Because of the quantitative and qualitative changes in body composition and stature with aging, anthropometric reference standards derived from younger subjects cannot be assumed to be accurate in the elderly. It is also unclear if standards derived from a particular age range within the elderly are applicable to other age ranges. Of the available surveys of normative anthropometric data in the elderly, none is without flaws.[39,51,68] Masters and coworkers[69] established weight for height norms for healthy whites up to age 94. However, these data were not related to mortality data and were derived from individuals born from 1865 to 1895, which reflects little overlap with the "oldest old" of today.[51] Frisancho[70] compiled weight standards for height, gender, and age up to 74 years using NHANES I and II

data. Use of these standards is limited because all ages over 55 years were grouped together. Andres[71] used weight for height data from the Build Study 1979,[72] and related this to mortality data to determine "desirable weights" up to age 69 by 10-year increments. The Andres standards[71] (Table 22–2) are similar to those of Frisancho,[70] adding confidence in the accuracy of estimating desirable weight from these tables.[68]

Andres[71] also demonstrated that when weight for height is expressed as the body mass index (BMI) (weight in kg/height in m^2), modest increases in BMI with aging are advantageous for survival. In the Build Study 1979,[72] the optimal BMI at age 69 was approximately 27 kg/m^2. Nevertheless, it is worthwhile noting that at least one recent study as well as the most recent Dietary Guidelines for Americans are more stringent in setting desirable upper limits for BMI.[30,72a] No provisions for increased BMI with aging are included in the latter documents, suggesting that a modest weight gain with aging is undesirable. This controversy ne-

TABLE 22–2 Comparison of the Weight-for-Height Tables from Actuarial Data: Non-Age-Corrected Metropolitan Life Insurance Company and Age-Specific Gerontology Research Center Recommendations*†

Height (ft and in)	Metropolitan 1983 Weights (25–59 yr)		Gerontology Research Center Age-Specific Weight Range for Men and Women				
	Men	Women	20–29 yr	30–39 yr	40–49 yr	50–59 yr	60–69 yr
4 10		100–131	84–111	92–119	99–127	107–135	115–142
4 11		101–134	87–115	95–123	103–131	111–139	119–147
5 0		103–137	90–119	98–127	106–135	114–143	123–152
5 1	123–145	105–140	93–123	101–131	110–140	118–148	127–157
5 2	125–148	108–144	96–127	105–136	113–144	122–153	131–163
5 3	127–151	111–148	99–131	108–140	117–149	126–158	135–168
5 4	129–155	114–152	102–135	112–145	121–154	130–163	140–173
5 5	131–159	117–156	106–140	115–149	125–159	134–168	144–179
5 6	133–163	120–160	109–144	119–154	129–164	138–174	148–184
5 7	135–167	123–164	112–148	122–159	133–169	143–179	153–190
5 8	137–171	126–167	116–153	126–163	137–174	147–184	158–196
5 9	139–175	129–170	119–157	130–168	141–179	151–190	162–201
5 10	141–179	132–173	122–162	134–173	145–184	156–195	167–207
5 11	144–183	135–176	126–167	137–178	149–190	160–201	172–213
6 0	147–187		129–171	141–183	153–195	165–207	177–219
6 1	150–192		133–176	145–188	157–200	169–213	182–225
6 2	153–197		137–181	149–194	162–206	174–219	187–232
6 3	157–202		141–186	153–199	166–212	179–225	192–238
6 4			144–191	157–205	171–218	184–231	197–244

*Adapted from Andres R: Mortality and obesity: the rationale for age–specific height–weight tables. In Andres R, Bierman E, Hazzard W (eds): Principles of Geriatric Medicine. New York: McGraw-Hill, 1985:311–318. Reproduced with permission of The McGraw-Hill Companies. From Mason JB, Russell RM: Parenteral nutrition in the elderly. In Rombeau JL, Caldwell MD (eds): Clinical Nutrition: Parenteral Nutrition, 2nd edition. Philadelphia: WB Saunders, 1993.
†Values are for height without shoes and weight without clothes.

cessitates further research to better define the range of ideal weights or BMI in the elderly.

Anthropometric measures other than weight or weight for height include determination of skin folds and circumferences of torso and extremities. Uses and limitations of these measures are discussed in depth elsewhere.[51,52] Briefly, use of these measurements in the elderly at present is limited by the lack of standards derived from elderly populations that relate anthropometric measures to body composition, variability associated with levels of hydration, age-associated changes in skin integrity, and the need for examiner training and consistency.

Biochemical Indexes

Serum albumin has traditionally been used as an indicator of visceral protein nutriture. Albumin concentration is determined by nutritional as well as many nonnutritional factors. Although hypoalbuminemia may suggest protein-calorie malnutrition in this age group, alterations in level of hydration, changes in albumin synthesis and distribution within body compartments seen during illness,[73] and alterations in liver and kidney function also affect albumin concentrations.[68] Albumin concentration may decline slightly with aging, ranging from a 3 to 8 percent loss per decade after age 70.[74-77] Given this minimal age-related decline, hypoalbuminemia should never be ascribed to aging and warrants a thorough evaluation of nutritional and nonnutritional causes. Despite its limitations as an indicator of visceral protein status, albumin concentration has been shown to be an important independent predictor of morbidity, length of hospitalization, disposition after discharge, and mortality.[29,77-82]

Clinically significant declines in hemoglobin or hematocrit should not be attributed to aging alone.[83,84] Like hypoalbuminemia, anemia in the elderly should stimulate consideration of nutritional and nonnutritional causes.

Functional Assessment

Assessment of function in the elderly aids in the detection of physical and cognitive deficits that can result from malnutrition or may render the patient susceptible to malnutrition.[85] Assessment is accomplished by direct observation or reported by the patient or a surrogate. The functions to be assessed can be simple, such as handgrip strength, or can reflect more complex integration, such as the activities of daily living. Many indexes for functional assessment are available, ranging from those for evaluating the severely demented patient to those for the active community-dwelling elderly.[86] Common to most functional assessment tools, however, is evaluation of the skills needed to procure, prepare, and consume food.

Loss of strength and muscle mass is associated with functional declines, impaired mobility, and impaired independence.[87-89] Handgrip strength has been shown to correlate with body protein depletion[90] and respiratory strength.[54,91] During repletion of malnourished patients, handgrip strength improves along with other indexes of strength and can precede measurable protein accretion.[90,91] The ease with which handgrip strength can be measured, along with its sensitivity to nutritional repletion, make this simple functional test extremely valuable in the elderly.

Handgrip dynamometry is best used to determine strength changes over time in an individual elderly patient. Two attempts have been made to establish normative standards for handgrip strength in the elderly[92,93] that would allow comparison of individual values to population norms. Bassey and associates[92] collected normative data using a strain-gauged dynamometer in 920 men and women over the age of 65. Handgrip strength was negatively associated with age and illness and was positively associated with indexes of overall physical activity and of handgrip use (Fig. 22–4).

Handgrip strength was then followed longitudinally in 620 of the original subjects, who displayed greater decreases in strength after 4 years than would have been predicted (with aging) by the original cross-sectional data. In a study by Webb and colleagues,[93] a mechanical dynamometer was used, making direct comparison with Bassey and coworkers[92] difficult. Unresolved issues highlighted by these studies suggest that before handgrip dynamometry measurements in individuals can be applied to population norms, further data are needed.

NUTRIENT REQUIREMENTS

Energy and Macronutrients

Energy

In general, energy goals in the elderly have been traditionally set for either maintenance or for repletion. However, as both life expectancy and the prevalence of obesity increase, the goal of weight loss in the elderly may become more common. In NHANES III, the prevalence of

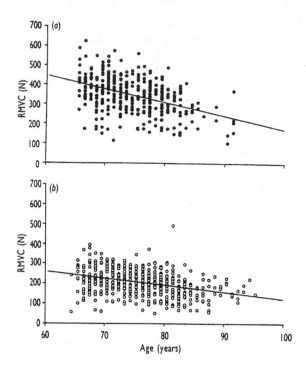

FIGURE 22–4   Maximum handgrip strength with aging in men (top) and women (bottom). (Adapted from Bassey EJ, Harries UJ: Normal values for handgrip strength in 920 men and women aged over 65 years, and longitudinal changes in 620 survivors. Clin Sci 1993;84:331.)

overweight in the 60 to 74 age group was 41 percent, increased from the 32 percent found in NHANES II.[30] Although the prevalence of overweight decreased with age after age 59, 22 percent in the over-80 group were categorized as overweight.[30] However, as discussed earlier, controversy exists regarding the criteria used to define overweight in the elderly.

As in all ages, energy requirements represent the sum of resting energy expenditure (REE), the thermic effect of food, and the energy cost of arousal and activity. REE declines with age, primarily due to decreases in LBM.[94,95] The elderly are, in general, less active than those younger and thus expend less energy on activity. The energy cost of some activities may be greater in the elderly than in those younger,[96,97] but there is no evidence to date to suggest that the energy cost of activity in the elderly is uniformly different.

Estimating energy needs in the elderly is accomplished by prediction equations or by direct measurement. Few prediction equations for estimating REE have been derived from elderly populations.[98-104] Most equations

in clinical use were derived from populations that included small numbers of elderly subjects,[99] and almost all equations were derived from measurements in persons under the age of 80, making their use in the "oldest old" questionable.[102] In addition, the paucity of data derived from elderly populations is compounded by the wide variation in the resting metabolic rate among the elderly,[101] which makes prediction of individual energy expenditure from group norms difficult. Some equations may improve accuracy in predicting REE but include factors that may be cumbersome for routine clinical assessment, such as inventories of physical activity and skinfold measurements.[100] No equations to our knowledge are as easily calculated and have prospectively predicted REE in the elderly as accurately as those of the World Health Organization (WHO).[100,103] For ages over 60 years the WHO equations are:

$$\text{Men: REE} = 8.8W + 1128H - 1071$$

$$\text{Women: REE} = 9.2W + 637H - 302$$

where REE is expressed as kilocalories per day, W is weight in kilograms, and H is height in meters. Use of WHO equations[103] derived from age, sex, and weight, but not height, modify estimated REE by approximately 5 percent. These equations serve as the basis for the current U.S. Recommended Daily Allowances (RDAs) for energy.[104] Because accurate height is often difficult to obtain in the elderly, these equations can be used with only a minor loss of accuracy in predicting REE:[68]

$$\text{Men: REE} = 13.5W + 487$$

$$\text{Women: REE} = 10.5W + 596$$

An advantage of the WHO equations is that REE can be calculated without reference to height. Disadvantages include the need to use different equations for other adult age ranges. The Harris-Benedict equations, although commonly used, have been demonstrated to be inaccurate in multiple situations,[105-107] including malnourished nursing home patients.[106]

Equations predicting resting energy requirements necessitate the use of appropriate stress and activity factors. No evidence suggests that these factors differ in the elderly from those applied to younger patients. In the many studies evaluating the degrees of hypermetabolism or hypometabolism in disease states (Chapter 18), the elderly are not routinely distinguished from other age groups.

The doubly labeled water (DLW) method measures total energy expenditure over days to weeks, eliminates the need for estimating stress or activity factors, and has been employed to estimate the energy needs of the healthy free-living elderly.[108] In a recent review of DLW studies to date, Roberts[108] proposes that the current RDA[104] underestimates energy needs of elderly adults and suggests that an increased activity factor should be employed. This is not to suggest that elderly adults should eat more but that current predictions of needs may underestimate actual energy intakes needed to maintain weight in the free-living elderly. DLW has been used to determine energy expenditure in chronically ill patients to a limited extent, but unfortunately DLW cannot be used in acutely ill patients due to methodologic limitations.

Measurement of REE by indirect calorimetry eludes pitfalls associated with prediction equations, and it has been suggested that REE in the elderly be assessed by this method.[105] The clinical application of indirect calorimetry has been reviewed in depth by McClave and Snider.[109] However, no known studies actually demonstrate a benefit from routine use in an elderly population.

The importance of accurately assessing energy needs in the elderly is illustrated by a recent report of controlled underfeeding and overfeeding in weight-stable young and elderly men.[110] After 3 weeks of underfeeding or overfeeding, elderly men were less able than young men to return to previous or compensatory levels of spontaneous energy intake. This suggests that environmental influences may play an increasingly important role in energy regulation with aging. DeCastro[111] also suggests that with aging, food intake is more influenced by external factors and less influenced by internal factors such as hunger. These findings have significant implications because intake is externally controlled for many disabled or institutionalized elderly.

Protein

Studies of protein metabolism in aging provide a conflicting picture, and protein needs in healthy elderly adults have been difficult to determine due to methodologic problems and inconsistencies between studies.[108,112] Given the conflicting evidence for protein requirements in the elderly, it seems prudent to follow the current RDA[104] for adults of 0.8g/kg of body

weight in the healthy elderly. Because the ratio of LBM to fat mass decreases with aging, more protein per kilogram LBM is provided to the elderly by the adult RDA.

Although the issue of protein requirements in the healthy elderly is unresolved despite considerable research effort, studies in the elderly addressing protein needs induced by illness are relatively scarce. Clark and coworkers[113] followed seven chronically ill elderly women with intercurrent acute complications for 6 months while determining nutrient intakes, nitrogen balance, and other anthropometric and biochemical parameters. They found that average protein needs to maintain nitrogen (N) balance were 0.8g/kg of "desired body weight." Tube-fed nursing home patients with pressure ulcers have been reported to have increased needs for protein (1.4 vs 0.9 g/kg of actual body weight for patients without ulcers) and energy.[114] In acutely ill elderly patients, optimal protein delivery also remains unresolved. When Clevenger and associates[115] delivered 2 g/kg of protein to acutely ill young and elderly patients, elderly patients were less likely to achieve N balance and had increased rates of azotemia compared with younger patients.

In studies investigating protein requirements, the level of energy delivered has varied considerably. Since energy intake influences N balance,[108] the optimal protein:energy ratio is important. Shizgal[116] evaluated the effects of different levels of energy delivery on body composition of 325 well-nourished and malnourished patients of different ages, all of whom were receiving parenteral nutrition. In malnourished patients of all ages, improvements in body cell mass (BCM) were positively related to total energy intake. As age increased, more energy was required for BCM accretion. Further prospective trials of enteral feeding in the elderly are needed to determine if the optimal protein:energy ratio is altered with aging, which would have implications for clinical practice.

Energy and Protein Prescriptions

We recommend using a factorial approach for energy based on REE, to be calculated by the WHO equations[104] or measured by indirect calorimetry, with the addition of stress and activity factors. Until more definitive studies are available, protein delivery in the chronically and acutely ill elderly must be dictated by clinical judgement and functional and biochemical parameters of nutrition status. Protein delivery should be guided by 0.8 g/kg of body weight and multiplied by appropriate factors. In response to acute illness, energy and protein requirements generally increase in parallel,[68] although protein requirements increase to a proportionally greater degree in many circumstances.

Growth Hormone

Although not a macronutrient, human growth hormone (hGH) has been investigated as an agent for arresting or reversing the age-associated losses of LBM as well as bone mass.[117-120] Of concern are reports of side-effects, such as hyperglycemia, fluid retention, carpal tunnel syndrome, and possibilities of cancer promotion or stimulation.[121-123] Questions still remain about appropriate patient selection, dose, and long-term effects.[123-125] Because of these unresolved issues the routine use of hGH in elderly patients cannot be recommended at this time.

Fluid

The capacity of the kidney to adapt to perturbation of fluid and electrolyte status is impaired with aging.[68] Responses to sodium depletion or sodium excess may be blunted, as is the ability to concentrate or dilute the urine in response to changing states of hydration. These changes in renal adaptive capacity predispose the elderly to both dehydration and volume overload and therefore dictate a more gradual approach to changes in fluid delivery. Dehydration in the elderly leads to multiple problems, including hypotension, lethargy, and depressed levels of consciousness.[67] Factors contributing to dehydration include fluid restriction, confusion, impaired thirst,[36] medications, lack of ready access to fluid, and immobility.[67] Given the reduced volume of formula required to meet the decreasing energy needs of the elderly, patients receiving tube feeding may need additional fluid to maintain adequate hydration.

Micronutrients

Because many enteral formulas are designed to meet the RDA for micronutrients/2000 kcal of energy, intakes below this level may result in inadequate micronutrient intakes. Thus, a diet reduced in energy may need to be micronutrient-rich or supplemented to meet RDAs. Requirements for several micronutrients change sufficiently with aging to warrant specific discussion here.

Vitamin A

Although in general the elderly are more prone to nutrient deficiency, vitamin A is an exception. The elderly have a lower threshold and greater risk for vitamin A toxicity for several reasons. These include the common use of vitamin A supplements, the apparent increase of vitamin A stores in liver and plasma with aging, and decreased plasma clearance of vitamin A in the elderly.[126-128] Chronic renal insufficiency, common in the elderly, can lead to increased plasma levels of vitamin A resulting from diminished renal degradation of retinol-binding protein (RBP).[129-132] This presents significant risk to those receiving chronic hemodialysis.[68] In the hyperlipoproteinemias associated with severely elevated chylomicrons and very low density lipoproteins, elevations of retinol and retinyl esters have been noted.[133] Given the increased risk of hypervitaminosis A in the elderly, the following guidelines are recommended. The RDA for vitamin A is recommended for healthy elderly patients, a large portion of which should be from β-carotene-containing foods.[5] For those elderly patients with serum creatinine > 2mg/dl or a glomerular filtration rate less than 25 ml/minute, and particularly those receiving chronic hemodialysis, half the RDA is recommended.[68]

Vitamin D and Calcium

Vitamin D deficiency causes osteomalacia, and it has been estimated that 30 to 40 percent of those elderly with hip fractures have inadequate vitamin D nutriture.[134] The reasons for impaired vitamin D status in the elderly are multiple. A main dietary source in the United States is milk, consumption of which may be limited due to the increased frequency of lactose intolerance in the elderly. In addition to dietary insufficiency, the skin of the elderly is less able to synthesize previtamin D.[135] Compounding this is decreased exposure to sunlight, an important factor in the institutionalized elderly.[136] Sunlight exposure through plate glass windows or Plexiglass does not stimulate skin synthesis of vitamin D.[134] Furthermore, the seasonal variations in sunlight found in temperate climates are associated with wintertime vitamin D insufficiency and lead to bone loss.[137] Chronic use of sunscreen, common in the elderly residing in warmer climates, can result in diminished or deficient levels of 25-OH-D.[138] As a result of these factors, vitamin D nutriture in the elderly is commonly compromised. Calcium intake may also be compromised in the elderly due to lactose intolerance, and impaired renal responsiveness to 1,25-OH-D[139] may hinder calcium absorption.

To prevent the development or worsening of metabolic bone disease, all elderly, especially the housebound or institutionalized, should receive the RDA of 5 μg (200 IU) of vitamin D daily as food or supplement.[101] Some elderly may require an additional 5 μg to maintain normal vitamin D status. Although the optimal intake of calcium for bone maintenance is debated, the diet should contain 1500 mg of calcium per day.[139a] Calcium intake more than 2400 mg/day can result in renal disease.[140]

Vitamin B$_6$

Evidence now suggests that there is a high prevalence of marginal vitamin B$_6$ status in the elderly. Vitamin B$_6$ requirements for the elderly may be greater than previously thought and appear to be approximately 20 percent greater than those for younger adults.[127,141] Assessing vitamin B$_6$ status by use of plasma levels is problematic, as many acute and chronic diseases have been associated with decreased levels of vitamin B$_6$ (or B$_6$ as pyridoxal phosphate [PLP]).[142-145] Also plasma levels are not accurate biochemical indicators of muscle levels of vitamin B$_6$ (the main repository of vitamin B$_6$ stores in humans) in vitamin B$_6$-depleted subjects.[146] The clinical significance of depressed vitamin B$_6$ levels in the ill elderly is not clear at this time. Until vitamin B$_6$ needs in the diverse elderly population are better defined, vitamin B$_6$ intake of 2 mg pyridoxine/day, as defined by the current RDA,[101] is recommended.

Vitamin B$_{12}$

Plasma vitamin B$_{12}$ levels may decline in the elderly as a whole, and marginal or frank vitamin B$_{12}$ deficiency in the elderly is not uncommon.[147-149] Sensitive biochemical markers of vitamin B$_{12}$ deficiency have been used to demonstrate that cellular depletion can occur despite normal blood concentrations of the vitamin. Serum methylmalonic acid (MMA) concentration appears to be the most sensitive indicator of vitamin B$_{12}$ deficiency[150-152] and is becoming widely available. Studies employing MMA and other markers have revealed that plasma levels of vitamin B$_{12}$ previously thought to be within a low-normal range (150 to 400 pg/ml) can be associated with neuropsychiatric or hematologic manifestations of B$_{12}$ deficiency.[152,153] Present estimates suggest 7 to 10 percent of the elderly with "low-normal" plasma vitamin B$_{12}$ levels may actually be functionally deficient. Recog-

nition of vitamin B$_{12}$ deficiency is further complicated, since biochemical and neuropsychiatric manifestations of vitamin B$_{12}$ deficiency may occur in the absence of the hematologic signs.[152]

Diminished levels of vitamin B$_{12}$ have been found in the subset of the elderly with atrophic gastritis (AG), which comprises approximately 20 percent of 60-year-olds and almost 40 percent of 80-year-olds.[154] In AG, digestion of food-bound vitamin B$_{12}$ is impaired due to decreases in gastric acid and pepsin, and ingested vitamin B$_{12}$ may be consumed by increased numbers of small bowel bacteria.[127,155] Free (crystalline or non-food-bound) vitamin B$_{12}$, as found in oral supplements, appears to be adequately absorbed by those with AG[127,156] unless defects in intrinsic factor production exist. Use of drugs that inhibit gastric acid secretion may result in decreased food-bound vitamin B$_{12}$ absorption.[157] The inhibitory effects on vitamin B$_{12}$ absorption of some drugs can be overcome by increasing intake of vitamin B$_{12}$-containing foods, but the long-term nutritional significance of newer drugs such as omeprazole is unknown. Particular attention to the vitamin B$_{12}$ status of elderly patients taking these drugs is warranted.

Any patient who is, or is suspected to be, vitamin B$_{12}$ deficient should receive a course of parenteral vitamin B$_{12}$ to replete stores. When the etiology of the vitamin B$_{12}$ deficiency is ascertained, appropriate maintenance therapy can be initiated. Even in disease states associated with decreased vitamin B$_{12}$ absorption, oral supplements in appropriate doses (1 mg/day[156]) usually maintain vitamin B$_{12}$ stores.

B Vitamins and Homocysteine

The importance of diminished vitamin B$_{12}$ status in the elderly is underscored by the role that vitamin B$_{12}$, along with folate and vitamin B$_6$, play in the pathogenesis of homocysteinemia. Modest elevations of this amino acid have been related to coronary artery disease[158,159] as well as other types of occlusive vascular disease.[160,161] Selhub and coworkers[162] evaluated the elderly component of the original Framingham Heart Study[163] cohort and concluded that the majority of hyperhomocysteinemia could be ascribed to inadequate intake of these vitamins. Homocysteine levels can be normalized in many instances with vitamin repletion or supplementation,[145,164] but there is not yet a clinical trial that convincingly demonstrates that correction of homocysteine results in improvement of occlusive vascular disease.

NUTRIENT SUPPLEMENTATION IN THE ELDERLY

Given the high prevalence of PCM in the elderly, early and persistent intervention to provide adequate energy and protein is likely to be beneficial. Guidelines for supplementation should always be guided by nutritional and clinical goals. The use of nutritional supplements in institutionalized patients may not always be based on sound nutritional assessment,[165] and indiscriminant supplementation may be wasteful and lead to nutrient excess.

Despite growing epidemiologic evidence that intake of particular nutrients or foods is associated with longevity or reduced incidence of disease, few controlled prospective clinical trials are available to support routine supplementation of the healthy elderly. Chandra[166] demonstrated that a daily multivitamin may reduce rates or complications of infections in an elderly free-living population; this important observation has yet to be reproduced. There is little scientific basis for recommending supplementation in amounts greater than the RDA for micronutrients at present.

CONCLUSION

The rapid growth of the elderly population, and their disproportionately great reliance on the health care system, will necessitate considerable attention to their nutritional needs. Assessment of nutritional status demands a multifactorial and flexible approach. Loss of lean mass and bone are not immutable side-effects of aging, and nutritional support can help to preserve the function and health of the elderly.

REFERENCES

1. Katz MS, Gerety MB, Lichenstein MJ: Gerontology and geriatric medicine. In Stein JH (ed): Internal Medicine. St. Louis: Mosby, 1994:2825.
2. Jahnigen DW: The geriatric patient. In Matzen RN, Lang RS, Mosby S (eds): Clinical Preventative Medicine. St. Louis: Mosby, 1993:659.
3. Chandra RJ, Imbach A, Moore C et al: Nutrition of the elderly. Can Med Assoc J 1991;145(11):1475.
4. Dall JLC: The greying of Europe. Br Med J 1994; 309:1282.
5. Ausman LM, Russell RM: Nutrition in the elderly. In Shils ME, Olson JA, Shike M (eds): Modern Nutrition in Health and Disease, 8th edition, Vol I. Philadelphia: Lea & Febiger, 1994:770.
6. Karkeck JM: Nutrition support for the elderly. Nutr Clin Prac 1993;8(5):211.
7. Public Health Service, Centers for Disease Control, National Center for Health Statistics: Health United States 1993 Chartbook. DHHS Pub. No. (PHS) 94-1232-1. Hyattsville: US Department of Health and Human Services, 1994.
8. Rolandelli RH, Ullrich JR: Nutritional support in the frail elderly surgical patient. Surg Clin North Am 1994;74(1):79.
9. U.S. Senate Committee on Education and Labour. Cited by: American Academy of Family Physicians, The American Dietetic Association, National Council on the Aging, Inc: Incorporating Nutrition Screening and Interventions into Medical Practice: A Monograph for Physicians. Washington: Nutrition Screening Initiative, 1994.
10. Carey M, Gillespie S: Position of the American Dietetic Association: cost-effectiveness of medical nutrition therapy. J Am Diet Assoc 1995;95(1):88.
11. Galanos AN, Pieper CF, Cornoni-Huntley JC et al: Nutrition and function: is there a relationship between body mass index and the functional capabilities of community-dwelling elderly? J Am Geriatr Soc 1994;42:368.
12. Mowé M, Bøhmer T, Kindt E: Reduced nutritional status in an elderly population (> 70 y) is probable before disease and possibly contributes to the development of disease. Am J Clin Nutr 1994;59:317.
13. Fiatorone M: Nutrition in the geriatric patient. Hosp Pract 1990;September 30:38.
14. Morley JE: Why do physicians fail to recognize and treat malnutrition in older persons? J Am Geriatr Soc 1991;39:1139.
15. Manson A, Shea S: Malnutrition in elderly ambulatory medical patients. Am J Publ Health 1991;81(9):1195.
16. Calkins DR, Rubenstein LV, Cleary PD et al: Failure of physicians to recognize functional disability in ambulatory patients. Ann Intern Med 1991;114:451.
17. Abbasi AA, Rudman DR: Undernutrition in the nursing home: prevalence, consequences, causes and prevention. Nutr Rev 1994;52(4):113.
18. Constans T, Basq Y, Bréchot J-F et al: Protein-energy malnutrition in elderly medical patients. J Am Geriatr Soc 1992;40:263.
19. Robinson G, Goldstein M, Levine GM: Impact of nutritional status on DRG length of stay. J Parenter Enter Nutr 1987;11(1):49.
20. Windsor JA, Hill GL: Risk factors for postoperative pneumonia: the importance of protein depletion. Ann Surg 1988;208(2):209.
21. Phillips P: Grip strength, mental performance and nutritional status as indicators of mortality risk among female geriatric patients. Age Ageing 1986;15:53.
22. ASPEN Board of Directors: Geriatric conditions. J Parenter Enter Nutr 1993;17(4):24SA.
23. Kaminski MV, Nasr NJ, Freed BA et al: The efficacy of nutritional support in the elderly. J Am Coll Nutr 1982;1:35.
24. Lipschitz DA, Mitchell CO: The correctability of the nutritional, immune, and hematopoietic manifestations of protein calorie malnutrition in the elderly. J Am Coll Nutr 1982;1:17.
25. Winograd CH, Brown EM: Aggressive oral feeding in hospitalized patients. Am J Clin Nutr 1990;52:967.
26. Schiffman SS, Warwick ZS: Effect of flavor enhancement of foods for the elderly on nutritional status: food intake, biochemical indices, and anthropometric measures. Physiol Behav 1993;53(2):395.
27. Gray-Donald K, Payette H, Boutier V et al: Evaluation of the dietary intake of homebound elderly and the feasibility of dietary supplementation. J Am Coll Nutr 1994;13(3):277.
28. Kalfarentzos F, Spiliotis J, Velimezis G et al: Comparison of forearm muscle dynamometry with nutritional

prognostic index, as a preoperative indicator in cancer patients. J Parenter Enter Nutr 1989;13(1):34.

29. Corti MC, Guralnik JM, Salive ME et al: Serum albumin level and physical disability as predictors of mortality in older persons. JAMA 1994;272(13):1036.

30. Kuczmarski RJ, Flegal KM, Campbell SM et al: Increasing prevalence of overweight among US adults: The National Health and Nutrition Examination Surveys, 1960 to 1991. JAMA 1994;272(3):205.

31. American Academy of Family Physicians, The American Dietetic Association, National Council on the Aging: nutrition interventions manual for professionals caring for older Americans: executive summary. Washington: Nutrition Screening Initiative, 1992.

32. Johnson RK, Goran MI, Poehlman ET: Correlates of over- and underreporting of energy intake in healthy older men and women. Am J Clin Nutr 1994;59:1286.

33. DePaola DP, Faine MP, Vogel RI: Nutrition in relation to dental medicine. In Shils ME, Olson JA, Shike M (eds): Modern Nutrition in Health and Disease, 8th edition, Vol II. Philadelphia: Lea & Febiger, 1994:1007.

34. Rolls BJ: Aging and appetite. Nutr Rev 1992;50(12):422.

35. Phillips PA, Johnston CI, Gray L: Disturbed fluid and electrolyte homeostasis following dehydration in elderly people. Age Ageing 1993;22:26.

36. Phillips PA, Bretherton M, Johnston CI et al: Reduced thirst in healthy elderly men. Am J Physiol 1991;261:R166.

37. Blazer D, Williams CD: Epidemiology of dysphoria and depression in an elderly population. Am J Psychiatry 1980;137(4):439.

38. Gray GE: Nutrition and dementia. J Am Diet Assoc 1989;89:1795.

39. Fischer J, Johnson MA: Low body weight and weight loss in the aged. J Am Diet Assoc 1990;90:1697.

40. Davis MA, Murphy SP, Neuhaus JM: Living arrangements and eating behaviors of older adults in the United States. J Gerontol 1988;43(3):S96.

41. Ryan VC, Bower ME: Relationship of socioeconomic status and living arrangements to nutritional intake of the older person. J Am Diet Assoc 1989;89:1805.

42. Read M, Schenkler ED: Nutrition and the continuum of health care in older adults. In Schlenker ED (ed): Nutrition in Aging. St. Louis: Mosby, 1993:313.

43. Larson EB: Albumin levels and mortality in healthy elderly persons: commentary. ACP Journal Club 1992; Nov/Dec:91.

44. Roe DA: Diet, nutrition, and drug reactions. In Shils ME, Olson JA, Shike M (eds): Modern Nutrition in Health and Disease, 8th edition, Vol II. Philadelphia: Lea & Febiger, 1994:1399.

45. Cook MC, Taren DL: Nutritional implications of medication use and misuse in elderly. J Florida MA 1990;77(6):606.

46. Sacks GS, Brown RO: Drug-nutrient interactions in patients receiving nutritional support. Drug Ther 1994;March:35.

47. Gupta KL, Dworkin B, Gambert SR: Common nutritional disorders in the elderly: atypical manifestations. Geriatrics 1988;43(Feb):87.

48. Allman RM: Pressure ulcers among the elderly. N Engl J Med 1989;320:850.

49. Flynn MA, Nolph GB, Baker AS et al: Total body potassium in aging humans: a longitudinal study. Am J Clin Nutr 1989;50:713.

50. Borkan GA, Hults DE, Gerzof SG et al: Age changes in body composition revealed by computed tomography. J Gerontol 1983;38(6):673.

51. Chumlea WC, Guo SS, Kuczmarski RJ et al: Bioelectric and anthropometric assessments and reference data in the elderly. J Nutr 1993;123:449.

52. Roubenoff R, Rosenberg IH: Anthropometry in clinical situation. World Health Organization Technical Report. In press.

53. Fiatarone MA, Marks EC, Ryan ND et al: High-intensity strength training in nonagenarians. JAMA 1990;263:3029.

54. Enright PL, Kronmal RA, Manolio TA et al: Respiratory muscle strength in the elderly: correlates and reference values. Am J Respir Crit Care Med 1994; 149:430.

55. Roubenoff R, Kehayias JJ: The meaning and measurement of lean body mass. Nutr Rev 1991;49(6): 163.

56. Torún B, Chew F: Protein-energy malnutrition. In Shils ME, Olson JA, Shike M (eds): Modern Nutrition in Health and Disease, 8th edition, Vol II. Philadelphia: Lea & Febiger, 1994:950.

57. Evans WJ, Campbell WW: Sarcopenia and age-related changes in body composition and functional capacity. J Nutr 1993;123:465.

58. Hertzog K, Garn S, Hempy H III: Partitioning the effects of secular trend and aging on stature on adult stature. Am J Phys Anthropol 1969;31:11.

59. Nappa H, Anderson M, Bengtsson C et al: Longitudinal studies of anthropometric data and body composition: the population study of women in Götenburg, Sweden. Am J Clin Nutr 1980;33:155.

60. Miall W, Ashcroft M, Lovell H et al: A longitudinal study of the decline with age in two Welsh communities. Hum Biol 1967;33:155.

61. Chumlea WC, Roche AF, Steinbaugh ML: Anthropometric approaches to the nutritional assessment of the elderly. In Munro HN, Danford DE (eds): Nutrition, Aging, and the Elderly. New York: Plenum Press, 1989:335.

62. Roubenoff R, Wilson PWF: Advantage of knee height over height as an index of stature in expression of body composition in adults. Am J Clin Nutr 1993;57: 609.

63. Prothro JW, Rosenbloom CA: Physical measurements in an elderly black population: knee height as the dominant indicator of stature. J Gerontol 1993;48(1): M15.

64. Mitchell CO, Lipschitz DA: Arm length measurement as an alternative to height in nutritional assessment of the elderly. J Parenter Enter Nutr 1982;6(3):226.

65. Kwok T, Whitelaw MN: The use of armspan in nutritional assessment of the elderly. J Am Geriatr Soc 1991;39:492.

66. Van Hoeyweghen RJ, De Leeuw IH, Vandewoude MFJ: Creatinine arm index as alternative for creatinine height index. Am J Clin Nutr 1992;56:611.

67. Chernoff R, Lipschitz D: Enteral feeding and the geriatric patient. In Rombeau JL, Caldwell MD (eds): Clinical Nutrition: Enteral and Tube Feeding, 2nd edition. Philadelphia: WB Saunders, 1990:386.

68. Mason JB, Russell RM: Parenteral nutrition in the elderly. In Rombeau JL, Caldwell MD (eds): Clinical Nutrition: Parenteral Nutrition, 2nd edition. Philadelphia: WB Saunders, 1993:737.

69. Master AM, Lasser RP, Beckman G: Tables of average weight and height of Americans aged 65 to 94 years. JAMA 1960;172:658.

70. Frisancho AR: New norms of upper limb fat and muscle areas for assessment of nutritional status. Am J Clin Nutr 1981;34:2540.

71. Andres R, Elahi D, Tobin JD et al: Impact of age on weight goals. Ann Intern Med 1985;103(6):1030.

72. Build Study 1979. Chicago: Society of Actuaries and Association of Life Insurance Medical Directors of America, 1980.

72a. Dietary Guidelines for Americans. U.S. Department of Health and Human Services and U.S. Department of Agriculture, 1995.

73. Gray GE, Meguid MM: The myth of serum albumin as a measure of nutritional status. Gastroenterology 1990;99:1845.

74. Cooper JK, Gardner C: Effect of aging on serum albumin. J Am Geriatr Soc 1989;37:1039.

75. Mitchell CO, Lipschitz DA: The effect of age and sex on the routinely used measurements to assess the nutritional status of hospitalized patients. Am J Clin Nutr 1982;36:340.

76. Campion EW, deLabry LO, Glynn RJ: The effect of age on serum albumin in healthy males: report from the normative aging study. J Gerontol 1988;43(1):M18.

77. Salive ME, Cornoni-Huntley J, Phillips CL et al: Serum albumin in older persons: relationship with age and health status. J Clin Epidemiol 1992;45(3):213.

78. Ferguson RP, O'Connor P, Crabtree B et al: Serum albumin and prealbumin as predictors of clinical outcomes of hospitalized elderly nursing home residents. J Am Geriatr Soc 1993;41:545.

79. Klonoff-Cohen H, Barrett-Connor EL, Edelstein SL: Albumin levels as a healthy predictor of mortality in the healthy elderly. J Clin Epidemiol 1992;45(3):207.

80. McEllistrum MC, Collins JC, Powers JS: Admission serum albumin level as a predictor of outcome among geriatric patients. South Med J 1993;86(12):1360.

81. Herrmann FR, Safran C, Levkoff SE et al: Serum albumin level on admission as a predictor of death, length of stay, and readmission. Arch Intern Med 1992;152:125.

82. Agarwal N, Acevedo F, Leighton LS et al: Predictive ability of various nutritional variables for mortality in elderly people. Am J Clin Nutr 1988;48:1173.

83. Resnik NM: Geriatric medicine. In Isselbacker KJ (ed): Harrison's Principles of Internal Medicine. New York: McGraw-Hill, 1994:30.

84. Zauber NP, Zauber AG: Hematologic data of healthy very old people. JAMA 1987;257(16):2181.

85. Solomons NW, Allen LH: The functional assessment of nutritional status: principles, practice and potential. Nutr Rev 1983;41(2):33.

86. Applegate WB, Blass JP, Williams TF: Instruments for the functional assessment of older patients. N Engl J Med 1990;322(17):1207.

87. Fiatarone MA, Evans WJ: Exercise in oldest old. Top Geriatr Rehabil 1990;5(2):63.

88. Fiatarone MA, Evans WJ: The etiology and reversibility of muscle dysfunction in the aged. J Gerontol 1993;48:77.

89. Ensrud KE, Nevitt MC, Yunis C et al: Correlates of impaired function in older women. J Am Geriatr Soc 1994;42:481.

90. Hill GL: Body composition research: implications for the practice of clinical nutrition. J Parenter Enter Nutr 1992;16(3):197.

91. Stokes M, Hill GL: Peripheral parenteral nutrition: a preliminary report on its efficacy and safety. J Parenter Enter Nutr 1993;17(2):145.

92. Bassey EJ, Harries UJ: Normal values for handgrip strength in 920 men and women aged over 65 years, and longitudinal changes over 4 years in 620 survivors. Clin Sci 1993;84:331.

93. Webb AR, Newman LA, Taylor M et al: Hand grip dynamometry as a predictor of postoperative complications: reappraisal using age standardized grip strengths. J Parenter Enter Nutr 1989;13(1):30.

94. Vaughan L, Zurlo F, Ravussin E: Aging and energy expenditure. Am J Clin Nutr 1991;53:821.

95. Fukagawa NK, Bandini LG, Young JB: Effect of age on body composition and resting metabolic rate. Am J Physiol 1990;25:E233.

96. Didier JP, Mourey F, Brondel L et al: The energetic cost of some daily activities: a comparison in a young and old population. Age Ageing 1993;22:90.

97. Voorrips LE, van Acker TMJ, Deurenberg P et al: Energy expenditure at rest and during standardized activities: a comparison between elderly and middle-aged women. Am J Clin Nutr 1993;58:15.

98. Mifflin MD, St Jeor ST, Hill LA et al: A new predictive equation for resting energy expenditure in healthy individuals. Am J Clin Nutr 1990;51:241.

99. Arcerio PJ, Goran MI, Gardner AM et al: A practical equation to predict resting metabolic rate in older females. J Am Geriatr Soc 1993;41:389.

100. Arcerio PJ, Goran MI, Gardner AW et al: A practical equation to predict resting metabolic rate in older men. Metabolism 1993;42(8):950.

101. Fredrix EWHM, Soeters PB, Deerenberg IM et al: Resting and sleeping energy expenditure in the elderly. Eur J Clin Nutr 1990;44:741.

102. Bell S: Current summaries: a practical equation to predict resting metabolic rate in older men. J Parenter Enter Nutr 1994;18(2):193.

103. FAO/WHO/ONU: Energy and Protein Requirements. Technical report series 724. Geneva: World Health Organization, 1985.

104. National Research Council: Recommended Dietary Allowances, 10th edition. Washington: National Academy Press, 1989.

105. Foster GD, Knox LS, Dempsey DT et al: Caloric requirements in total parenteral nutrition. J Am Coll Nutr 1987;6(3):231.

106. Hoffman P, Richardson S, Giacoppe J et al: Failure of the Harris-Benedict equation to predict energy expenditure in undernourished nursing home residents. FASEB J 1995;9:A438.

107. Roza AM, Shizgal HM: The Harris Benedict equation reevaluated: resting energy requirements and the body cell mass. Am J Clin Nutr 1984;40:168.

108. Roberts SB: Energy requirements of older individuals. Eur J Clin Nutr. In press.

109. McClave SA, Snider HL: Use of indirect calorimetry in clinical nutrition. Nutr Clin Prac 1992;7(5):207.

110. Roberts SB, Fuss P, Heyman MB et al: Control of food intake in older men. JAMA 1994;272(20):1601.

111. DeCastro JM: Age-related changes in spontaneous food intake and hunger in humans. Appetite 1993;21:255.

112. Young VR: Macronutrient needs in the elderly. Nutr Rev 1992;50(12):454.

113. Clark NG, Rappaport JI, DiScala C et al: Nutritional support of the chronically ill elderly female at risk for elective or urgent surgery. J Am Coll Nutr 1988;7(1):17.

114. Breslow RA, Hallfrisch J, Goldberg AP: Malnutrition in tubefed nursing home patients with pressure sores. J Parenter Enter Nutr 1991;15(6):663.

115. Clevenger FW, Rodriguez DJ, Demarest GB et al: Protein and energy tolerance by stressed geriatric patients. J Surg Res 1992;52:135.

116. Shizgal HM, Martin MF, Gimmon Z: The effect of age on the calorie requirement of malnourished individuals. Am J Clin Nutr 1992;55:783.

117. Rudman D, Feller AG, Nagraj HS et al: Effects of human growth hormone in men over 60 years old. N Engl J Med 1990;323(1):1.

118. Rudman D, Feller AG, Cohn L et al: Effects of human growth hormone on body composition in elderly men. Horm Res 1991;36(suppl 1):73.

119. Borst SE, Millard WJ, Lowenthal DT: Growth hormone, exercise, and aging: the future of therapy for the frail elderly. J Am Geriatr Soc 1994;42(5):528.

120. Holloway L, Butterfield G, Hintz RL et al: Effects of recombinant human growth hormone on metabolic indices, body composition, and bone turnover in healthy elderly women. J Clin Endocrinol Metab 1994;79(2):470.

121. Lehmann S, Cerra FB: Growth hormone and nutritional support: adverse metabolic effects. Nutr Clin Prac 1992;7:27.

122. Cohn L, Feller AG, Draper MW et al: Carpal tunnel syndrome and gynaecomastia during growth hormone treatment of elderly men with low circulating IGF-1 concentrations. Clin Endocrinol 1993;39:417.

123. Rudman D, Shetty KR: Unanswered questions concerning the treatment of hyposomatotropism and hypogonadism in elderly men. J Am Geriatr Soc 1994;42(5):522.

124. Inzucchi SE, Robbins RJ: Clinical review 61: effects of growth hormone on human bone biology. J Clin Endocrinol Metab 1994;79(3):691.

125. Ross RJM: Growth hormone replacement in adults: what dose? Clin Endocrinol 1993;39:401.

126. Krasinski SD, Russell RM, Otradovec CL et al: Relationship of vitamin A and vitamin E intake to fasting plasma retinol, retinol-binding protein retinyl esters, carotene, α-tocopherol, and cholesterol among elderly people and young adults: increased plasma retinyl esters among vitamin A-supplement users. Am J Clin Nutr 1989;49:112.

127. Russell RM, Suter PM: Vitamin requirements of elderly people: an update. Am J Clin Nutr 1993;58:4.

128. Krasinski SD, Cohn JS, Schaefer EJ et al: Postprandial retinyl ester response is greater in older subjects compared with younger subjects: evidence for delayed plasma clearance of intestinal lipoproteins. J Clin Invest 1990;85:883.

129. Cano N, Di Costanzo-Dufetel J, Calaf R et al: Prealbumin-retinol-binding-protein-retinol complex in hemodialysis patients. Am J Clin Nutr 1988;47:664.

130. Stewart WK, Fleming LW: Plasma retinol and retinol binding protein concentrations in patients on maintenance haemodialysis with and without vitamin A supplements. Nephron 1982;30:15.

131. Muth I: Implications of hypervitaminosis A in chronic renal failure. J Renal Nutr 1991;1(1):2.

132. Hendriks HFJ, Verhoofstad WAMM, Brouwer A et al: Perisinusoidal fat-storing cells are the main vitamin A storage sites in rat liver. Exp Cell Res 1985;160:138.

133. Ellis JK, Russell RM, Makrauer FL et al: Increased risk for vitamin A toxicity in severe hypertriglyceridemia. Ann Intern Med 1986;105:877.

134. Holick MF: Vitamin D—new horizons for the 21st century. McCollum Award Lecture, 1994. Am J Clin Nutr 1994;60:619.

135. MacLaughlin J, Holick MF: Aging decreases the capacity of human skin to produce vitamin D_3. J Clin Invest 1985;76:1536.

136. Webb AR, Pilbeam C, Hanafin et al: An evaluation of the relative contributions of exposure to sunlight and of diet to the circulating concentrations of 25-hydroxyvitamin D in an elderly nursing home population in Boston. Am J Clin Nutr 1990;51:1075.

137. Dawson-Hughes B, Dallal GE, Krall EA et al: Effect of vitamin D supplementation on wintertime and overall bone loss in healthy postmenopausal women. Ann Intern Med 1991;115(7):505.

138. Matsuoka LY, Wortsman J, Hanifan N et al: Chronic sunscreen use decreases circulating concentrations of 25-hydroxyvitamin D. Arch Dermatol 1988;124:1802.

139. Gallagher JC, Riggs BL, Eisman J et al: Intestinal calcium absorption and serum vitamin D metabolites in normal subjects and osteoporotic patients: effect of age and dietary calcium. J Clin Invest 1979;64:729.

139a. Optimal calcium intake. NIH Consensus Statement 1994;12(4):1–31.

140. Allen LH, Wood RJ: Calcium and phosphorus. In Shils ME, Olson JA, Shike M (eds): Modern Nutrition in Health and Disease, 8th edition, Vol I. Philadelphia: Lea & Febiger, 1994:144.

141. Ribaya-Mercado JD, Russell RM, Sahyoun et al: Vitamin B-6 requirements of elderly men and women. J Nutr 1991;121:1062.

142. Leklem JE: Vitamin B_6. In Shils ME, Olson JA, Shike M (eds): Modern Nutrition in Health and Disease, 8th edition, Vol I. Philadelphia: Lea & Febiger, 1994:383.

143. Dellaripa PF, Selhub J, Nadeau MR et al: Dissociation between plasma pyridoxal-5'-PO_4 (PLP) and evidence of PLP deficiency in chronic inflammation. FASEB J 1995;9:A153.

144. Roubenoff R, Roubenoff RA, Selhub J et al: Abnormal vitamin B_6 status in rheumatoid cachexia. Arth Rheum 1995;38(1):105.

145. Saltzman E, Mason JB, Jacques PF et al: B vitamin supplementation lowers homocysteine levels in heart disease. Clin Res 1994;42(2):172A.

146. Coburn SP, Ziegler PJ, Costill DL et al: Response of vitamin B-6 content of muscle to changes in vitamin B-6 intake in men. Am J Clin Nutr 1991;53:1436.

147. Elsborg L, Lund V, Bastrup-Madsen P: Serum vitamin B_{12} levels in the aged. Acta Med Scand 1976;200:309.

148. Lindenbaum J, Rosenberg IH, Wilson PWF et al: Prevalence of cobalamin deficiency in the Framingham elderly population. Am J Clin Nutr 1994;60:2.

149. Allen LH, Casterline J: Vitamin B_{12} deficiency in elderly individuals: diagnosis and requirements. Am J Clin Nutr 1994;60:12.

150. Allen RH, Stabler SP, Savage DG et al: Diagnosis of cobalamin deficiency. I: usefulness of serum methylmalonic acid and total homocysteine concentrations. Am J Hematol 1990;34:90.

151. Joosten E, Pelemans W, Devos P et al: Cobalamin absorption and serum homocysteine and methylmalonic acid in elderly subjects with low serum cobalamin. Eur J Haematol 1993;51:25.

152. Lindebaum J, Savage DG, Stabler SP et al: Diagnosis of cobalamin deficiency. II. Relative sensitivities of serum cobalamin, methylmalonic acid, and total homocysteine concentrations. Am J Hematol 1990;34:99.

153. Lindebaum J, Healton EB, Savage DG et al: Neuropsychiatric disorders caused by cobalamin deficiency in the absence of anemia or macrocytosis. N Engl J Med 1988;318:1720.

154. Krasinski SD, Russell RM, Samloff M et al: Fundic atrophic gastritis in an elderly population: effect on hemoglobin and several serum nutritional indicators. J Am Geriatr Soc 1986;34:800.

155. Logan RF, Elwis A, Forrest MJ et al: Mechanisms of vitamin B_{12} deficiency in elderly patients. Age Ageing 1989;18:4.

156. Hathcock JN, Troendle GJ: Oral cobalamin for treatment of pernicious anemia? JAMA 1991;265(1):96.

157. Saltzman JR, Kemp JA, Golner BB et al: Effect of hypochlorhydria due to omeprazole treatment or atrophic gastritis on protein-bound vitamin B_{12} absorption. J Am Coll Nutr 1994;13(6):584.

158. Clarke R, Daly L, Robinson K et al: Hyperhomocysteinemia: an independent risk factor for vascular disease. N Engl J Med 1991;324(17):1149.

159. Stampfer MJ, Malinow MR, Willett WC et al: A prospective study of plasma homocyst(e)ine and risk of myocardial infarction in US physicians. JAMA 1992;268(7):877.

160. Kang SS, Wong PWK, Malinow MR: Hyperhomocyst(e)inemia as a risk factor for occlusive vascular disease. Ann Rev Nutr 1992;12:279.

161. Wenzler EM, Rademakers AJJM, Bjoers GHJ et al: Hyperhomocysteinemia in retinal artery and retinal vein occlusion. Am J Ophthalmol 1993;115:162.

162. Selhub J, Jacques PF, Wilson PWF et al: Vitamin status and intake as primary determinants of homocysteinemia in an elderly population. JAMA 1993; 270(22):2693.

163. Dawber TR, Moore FE, Mann GV et al: Coronary heart disease in the Framingham Study. Am J Public Health 1957;47(suppl):4.

164. Ubbink JB, Vermaak WJH, Van der Merwe A et al: Vitamin requirements for the treatment of hyperhomocysteinemia in humans. J Nutr 1994;124:1927.

165. Johnson LE, Dooley PA, Gleick JB: Oral nutritional supplement use in elderly nursing home patients. J Am Geriatr Soc 1993;41:947.

166. Chandra RK: Effect of vitamin and trace-element supplementation on immune responses and infection in elderly patients. Lancet 1992;340:1124.

23

Enteral Nutrition in Inflammatory Bowel Disease

MIQUEL A. GASSULL
FERNANDO FERNÁNDEZ-BAÑARES
EDUARD CABRÉ
MARIA ESTEVE-COMAS

Inflammatory bowel disease (IBD) includes a complex group of clinical situations that until now have been grouped into two main clinical entities—ulcerative colitis (UC) and Crohn's disease (CD), also know as granulomatous enteritis.[1] Both have as common features the presence of chronic inflammation of the gastrointestinal (GI) tract with various degrees of severity, but the inflammatory response pattern differs. In UC, inflammation is confined to mucosa and submucosa, whereas in CD it involves the whole thickness of the intestinal wall from mucosa to serosa. The two entities also differ in the location and extension of the inflamed areas; in UC the disease is confined to the colon, whereas CD potentially involves the whole GI tract, including the anal and perianal regions. A further important difference is that in UC proctocolectomy is a curative procedure, whereas the surgical resection of the inflamed areas is not curative in CD, because the disease is likely to recur at any level of the GI tract.

Diarrhea, with or without blood, is the predominant symptom in both entities, which may be accompanied by other digestive and systemic manifestations. The onset of both diseases may be acute or subacute. The length of the inflamed bowel does not correlate with the severity of the symptoms, and it is possible to observe acute severe symptoms in patients with a short segment of inflamed bowel while other patients with extensive disease and important weight loss show only symptoms of mild inflammation.

On the other hand, CD has different clinical presentations and evolutive forms, from acute to indolent, in relation to the predominant variant of the disease (inflammatory, stenosing, or fistulizing). The diagnosis is made by a set of clinical, endoscopic, and histologic characteristics. A group of patients (up to 15 percent) with findings of either disease confined to the large bowel are classified as having indeterminate colitis.[1] The established standard treatment consists of steroids or 5-aminosalicylic acid (5-ASA) drugs (sulfasalazine, mesalazine, olsalazine). Occasionally, when resistance or dependence to steroids appears, alternative immunosuppressive drugs (azathioprine or its derivative 6-mercaptopurine and cyclosporine) are used.

The incidence of UC and CD varies around the world from 2 to 10, and 1 to 6 new cases per 100,000 inhabitants per year, respectively.

The prevalence varies from 35 to 100, and 10 to 100 cases per 100,000 inhabitants for UC and CD, respectively.[2] Of unknown etiology, both entities share a trend of family aggregation, but no definite pattern of the major histocompatibility complex has been consistently associated with either disease. A racial and ethnic predominance is observed, with the incidence of both diseases being higher in whites and Jewish populations; there is also a slightly higher prevalence in females than in males.[3] In UC patients the number of smokers is lower than expected, whereas the opposite is observed in CD.[4,5] An anomalous or exaggerated immune response to intestinal, bacterial, alimentary antigens or autoantigens, or a normal response to a persistent stimulus, is thought to be involved in the pathogenesis of these diseases.[6,7] These would trigger the release of inflammatory mediators (e.g., cytokines and eicosanoids), which would cause the clinical and histologic manifestations of the disease.[8-10]

In summary, both diseases have various patterns of clinical presentation and evolution, patient response to medical treatment, and patient outcome. This, together with a failure to recognize etiologic agents or clear genetic traits, suggests that UC and CD represent a spectrum of diseases with different etiologies and common clinical features.

MALNUTRITION IN INFLAMMATORY BOWEL DISEASE

Protein-energy malnutrition (PEM), a common finding in most diseases of the digestive system both in hospitalized[11] and outpatients,[12] is also common in UC and CD.[12-17] Changes in the status of micronutrients have also been described in IBD.[18-27] Some are involved in important metabolic pathways such as lipid peroxidation, protein degradation, and cellular death. These nutritional derangements may play a role in the pathobiologic mechanisms of inflammation and may consequently influence the patient's outcome. Therefore, the role of nutritional support in UC and CD may theoretically become more than administering energy and nitrogen, since providing certain nutrients may exert an adjuvant action in IBD treatment.

Protein-Energy Nutritional Status

The prevalence of PEM in adults with IBD varies in the literature from 20 to 85 percent.[11-17] This wide range may be explained by the fact that the different series published use different methods to assess nutritional status in a clinical setting, from anthropometry and biologic nutritional markers to more sophisticated methods of body composition assessment. Besides, these reports seldom differentiate between UC and CD and between inpatients and outpatients. The result is often a mixture containing data of patients with mild to severe inflammatory disease activity, different clinical evolution (from recurrent acute bouts to chronic indolent illness), and disease involving the small or the large intestine or both. A careful prospective study[17] that assessed the nutritional status in IBD patients at hospital admission by objective anthropometric and biologic parameters[11] found PEM to be as high as 85 percent. Some of these patients receiving the usual medical treatment and eating the prescribed hospital diet became more malnourished while in the hospital.[17]

Vitamin, Mineral and Trace-Element Status

Derangement of micronutrient status has been described in IBD as in other GI and liver diseases,[28,29] but reports assessing the status of a wide range of vitamins, minerals, and trace elements in the same subjects are scarce. This is important when one considers the possible role of micronutrient deficits in the pathogenesis of the inflammatory process. Further problems, such as the absence of reference values obtained from the same area where the study is carried out, together with the fact that the assays are performed in different types of samples (serum, plasma, whole blood, urine, tissues), with different methodologies, add more burden to the interpretation of results. In evaluation of the micronutrient status in IBD, as in all disease states, the concept of subclinical or biochemical deficiency may be of relevance,[30] because clinically evident vitamin or trace element deficits (except for folate and iron) very seldom occur. Such subclinical deficiencies may be important in the metabolic pathways of inflammation and tissue injury.[31]

Most studies on vitamin status in patients with IBD report data on a single vitamin. In this way, deficient status of vitamins A,[21,22] K,[23] D,[24,25] and C[26] have been reported. Only a few studies[18,27] have simultaneously studied a wide range of fat- and water-soluble vitamins in the same group of patients compared with a group of healthy individuals living in the same geographic area. The findings suggest that there is a wide variety of vitamin deficiencies in patients with IBD. In one of these studies,[18] the intestinal area involved (ileal/ileocecal vs extensive colitis) was taken into account when the results were analyzed. Blood levels of biotin, folate, β-carotene, and vitamins A, C, and B₁ were found to be significantly lower in patients with both ileal/ileocecal and extensive colonic disease than in healthy subjects. In addition, low levels of riboflavin were observed in patients with acute colonic disease, and, as expected, low values of vitamin B_{12} were found when the ileal or ileocecal areas were involved. No patient showed clinical evidence of vitamin deficiency, but the percentage of patients at risk of developing hypovitaminosis (plasma levels of a given vitamin below the 15th percentile of healthy controls) was greater than 40 percent for vitamin A, β-carotene, folate, biotin, vitamin C, and vitamin B₁ both in patients with acute colitis and patients with small bowel disease. Only a weak correlation was found between vitamin values and the protein-energy nutritional status.

In IBD, iron deficiency secondary to blood loss and hypomagnesemia has been reported.[32,33] Zinc and selenium status has often been low in IBD.[22,34-45] There are few reports on copper status in IBD.[40,45] Deficiencies in other trace elements, such as chromium, manganese, or molybdenum, have not been demonstrated in these patients,[46] although they may occur in long-term parenteral nutrition.[47]

Zinc status has been evaluated in relation to changes in taste[34] and growth failure.[39] Zinc deficiency was more prevalent in the early days of total parenteral nutrition (TPN). In active CD, low zinc levels have been observed in plasma, urine, and hair[34,40] in relation to disease activity and plasma albumin levels. In UC, plasma zinc is also low[40] but is not related to serum albumin levels and inflammatory activity. An interesting finding is that in UC plasma zinc positively correlated with low vitamin A values. This is probably due to the negative impact of zinc deficiency on the hepatic synthesis of retinol-binding protein[48] and may be a contributing factor in maintaining low plasma vitamin A levels in UC.

The assessment of total-body zinc status in acute attacks of IBD has met with some difficulties. Alternatives to serum zinc levels, such as plasma zinc-dependent enzyme activities (e.g., alkaline phosphatase),[49] hair or urinary zinc,[50] or leukocyte zinc contents[44] have been used to detect true zinc deficiency. These tech-

niques are of limited use because they are not always available. Moreover, plasma alkaline phosphatase is of little help in detecting zinc deficiency in IBD, since increases in the values of this enzyme, mostly unrelated to zinc status, are frequently observed in these patients.[51]

Thus, are serum zinc levels of any use in the assessment of zinc status in IBD? Studies have shown that between 60 to 70 percent of circulating zinc is loosely bound to albumin, considered exchangeable, and delivered to metabolically active tissues.[50] In fact, serum zinc concentration correlates well with ileal mucosal zinc levels in patients with and without CD.[52] In addition, studies on serum zinc kinetics in patients with CD have shown low serum levels in relation to an accelerated total body clearance of zinc from the circulation. In turn, zinc clearance positively correlates with the severity of the disease.[53] Thus, these arguments allow us to hypothesize that serum zinc levels could be useful in the assessment of the metabolically active zinc status in IBD, but this remains to be proved.

Pathophysiology of Malnutrition in Inflammatory Bowel Disease

IBD is a peculiar pathophysiologic model of multiple possible etiologies for the development of malnutrition. Both UC and CD have, in general terms, distinct clinical presentations and evolution. When inappropriately treated, patients invariably become malnourished. The clinician who is aware of this fact can avoid adding the consequences of malnutrition to the sometimes severe complications of both diseases. Patients with severe UC usually have an acute disease, passing a large number of bloody loose stools per day, as opposed to most CD patients, who often have an insidious course, passing loose, usually bloodless stools. Patients with UC tend to seek medical advice quite early, within a few days, whereas CD patients may wait for months. Patients with severe UC thus come to the hospital in a fairly good nutritional state, which will, however, rapidly deteriorate if nutritional support is not supplied, even when the appropriate medical treatment is administered. Conversely, CD patients used to be admitted with substantial losses of body weight, subcutaneous fat, and, in some cases, skeletal muscle mass. CD also may have different clinical presentations and evolutive forms, in relation to the predominant variety of the disease (inflammatory, stenosing, or fistulizing), making the medical and nutritional management of these patients more difficult.

As mentioned, the etiology of PEM in IBD is multifactorial and involves various mechanisms related mainly to the disease itself (inflammation, ulceration, stenosis, fistulas) together with some therapeutic maneuvers (e.g., dietary restrictions or fasting, steroids). The possible causes leading to malnutrition in these patients are shown in Table 23–1. However, all these causes act through four basic mechanisms:

1. Decreased nutrient intake
2. Nutrient malabsorption
3. Increased intestinal protein loss
4. Increased metabolism

Low nutrient intake is common in patients with acute IBD, in whom anorexia, nausea, and even vomiting may occur. Increases in cytokines, such as interleukin-1 and tumor necrosis factor (TNF), may account for anorexia in these patients.[54,55] In CD, recurrent episodes of intestinal obstruction appear in about 34 percent of patients during the course of the disease, whereas upper GI involvement (esophagus, stomach, and duodenum) is observed in up to 30 percent of patients.[56,57] Treatments with sulfasalazine, 5-ASA, or metronidazole may produce gastric upset.[58,59] In addition, metronidazole therapy and zinc deficiency may alter taste perception.[34] All these factors may account for reduced food intake in these patients.

The idea that the presence of food in the intestinal lumen may aggravate diarrhea leads the patients themselves, or even their doctors, to restrict dietary intake. Moreover, the concept that foods may act as antigens to the intestinal mucosa, triggering or perpetuating the anomalous or exaggerated immune response responsible for the clinical and histologic manifestations of IBD, has made bowel rest (i.e., no oral intake), together with steroids and intravenous fluids, the cornerstone of treatment of acute UC and CD. Such an approach leads to malnutrition. As much as 44 percent of the theoretical food ingestion in the hospital was uneaten because of the combined effect of therapeutic fasting and anorexia in hospitalized IBD patients.[60]

Severe malabsorption occurs in CD when it involves large areas of the small intestine or when extensive surgical resection has been carried out, resulting in a short bowel. Less severe degrees of malabsorption can occur because of terminal ileum involvement or bacter-

Table 23–1 Possible Etiologic Mechanisms of Malnutrition in Inflammatory Bowel Disease

Related to the Disease Itself
Decreased food intake
- Anorexia, vomiting
- Dietary restrictions because of diarrhea
- Intestinal obstruction
- Altered taste perception (zinc deficiency, metronidazole therapy)

Increased intestinal loss of nutrients
- Altered intestinal mucosa permeability (inflammation)
- Mucosal ulcerations
- Difficult lymphatic drainage

Onset and evolution
- Acute: rapidly developing malnutrition
- Insidious: slowly established severe malnutrition

Disease location and pattern
- Colon: nutrient losses, increased requirements
- Small intestine extensive disease or resection: malabsorption
- Small intestine/colon—inflammatory:
  Increased nutrient losses
  Increased requirement
- Small intestine—stenosing:
  Bacterial overgrowth
- Small intestine/colon—fistulizing:
  Increased nutrient losses
  Increased requirements

Septic complications: increased requirements

Related to Therapy/Iatrogenic
Dietary restrictions because of diarrhea
"Therapeutic" fasting
Drug-induced gastric upset
Steroids

ial overgrowth.[61,62] Terminal ileum involvement or ileocecal resection is associated with bile salt malabsorption and diarrhea, leading to a diminished bile acid pool, abnormal micelle formation, and malabsorption of fat and fat-soluble vitamins.[62] However, this does not explain the low vitamin A and E levels found in both CD and UC patients,[18,21,22] as gross malabsorption is rare in the former and is not expected to occur in the latter. Ileal CD or resection may produce vitamin B_{12} malabsorption. In addition, intestinal strictures or resection of the ileocecal valve result in bacterial overgrowth, which occurs in 30 percent of patients with CD,[20] with overconsumption of vitamin B_{12} and derangement of carbohydrate, protein, and bile salt absorption.[61] Changes in the biotin-forming intestinal bacterial flora induced by diarrhea, fasting, or antibiotics might explain biotin subclinical deficiency in IBD.[18] Drugs such as cholestyramine, used to treat diarrhea in extensive ileal disease or resection, induce malabsorption by binding bile salts, fat, fat-soluble vitamins, and calcium. Also, folate deficiency is a well-recognized side-effect of sulfasalazine therapy.[19]

The inflamed and ulcerated intestinal mucosa may be an additional factor for the development of malnutrition in IBD.[63] Protein losses are directly related to the degree of severity of mucosal inflammation, and their quantification is an index of disease activity.[64] Also, changes in the intercellular epithelial tight junctions of the inflamed mucosa[65] and, in CD, altered lymphatic drainage[66] and bacterial overgrowth,[61] may contribute to a negative nitrogen balance in these patients. The increased intestinal losses of carrier proteins, such as prealbumin or retinol-binding protein, may contribute to the low plasma vitamin A levels found in both CD and UC patients.[18,21,22]

Increased energy and nitrogen requirements may contribute to the development of PEM in IBD because of the existence of inflammation, fever, and metabolic stress.[67-70] In such situations, energy and nitrogen supplies should be provided above the calculated requirements. In UC, it was observed that resting energy expenditure (REE) was 19 percent higher than predicted for healthy adults using the Harris-Benedict equation.[67] Other studies have shown that energy expenditure is increased only in those patients whose body weight is lower than 90 percent of normal.[68,69] More recently, the measurement of total energy expenditure has provided conflicting results by showing modest increases[71] or no changes[72] in different studies. These variations may be explained by the different methods of measurement and by whether REE or total energy expenditure is assessed. In addition, most series do not state the disease activity of the patients studied and do not differentiate between UC and CD.

A further question is whether to increase nitrogen supply to these patients because of an enhanced protein breakdown. In a clinical study of medically treated hospitalized patients with active IBD who were eating the prescribed ward diet, significant loss of muscle protein (as assessed by serial measurements of mid-arm muscle circumference) during admission was observed, compared with a group of active patients nutritionally supported with enteral nutrition.[17] In adults with active IBD it was shown that protein synthesis and breakdown increased in parallel to disease activity.[73] In children with IBD, both protein synthesis and degradation were increased in active disease, but protein degradation was always higher than synthesis, even when disease was inactive.[74] A further argument is that inflammation favors protein degradation by the action of inflammatory mediators (cytokines, eicosanoids),[75] causing negative nitrogen balance.[76] It remains unclear if an increased nitrogen supply is needed in patients with active IBD, and this may be particularly relevant to children and adolescents with IBD and their adult height.

Consequences of Malnutrition in Inflammatory Bowel Disease

Despite the lack of objective demonstration, PEM is thought to have a number of primary consequences, as well as to modify the course and the therapeutic response of the underlying disease (Table 23–2). The clinician's impression, however, is that the malnourished CD patient with fistulizing disease must be nourished to overcome severe complications, while surgeons prefer to proceed with colectomy in a fairly well-nourished UC patient.

In children with IBD, PEM is considered an important contributing factor to growth failure and delayed sexual maturation, which are seen in 20 to 30 percent of these patients,[77-79] especially in those with CD. In fact, growth failure is considered to be the most frequent extraintestinal complication of CD in child-

TABLE 23–2   Consequences of Protein-Energy Malnutrition in Inflammatory Bowel Disease

Primarily Related to PEM
Immunosuppression (increased susceptibility to infection)
Impairment in tissue repair (poor wound healing)
Intestinal villous atrophy (malabsorption, PEM self-perpetuation)
Derangement of gut mucosal barrier (increased uptake of bacterial products and other macromolecules)
Growth failure and delayed sexual maturation
Deficient binding of drugs to plasma proteins
Increased surgical risk
Increased mortality

Modulation of IBD Course
Immunosuppression
Impaired defense against free-radical damage
Changes in PUFA and eicosanoid synthesis
Increased mucosal dysplasia (folate deficiency)

PUFA = polyunsaturated fatty acids; PEM = protein-energy malnutrition; IBD = inflammatory bowel disease.

hood. In a recent study analyzing the records of 48 adults diagnosed with IBD during childhood, 31 percent of the subjects had permanent adult growth deficiency; this was more prominent in those diagnosed with CD.[80] Another retrospective study reviewing 100 children with CD found that 50 percent of children below the third height percentile at diagnosis failed to reach the third percentile for adult height.[81] Because growth deficit may become a permanent feature in adulthood, its improvement is a major therapeutic objective when IBD is diagnosed in childhood and adolescence. Growth failure in these patients has been attributed to nutritional, hormonal, and disease-related factors. The finding that growth resumes when children receive nutritional rehabilitation[82,83] supports the idea that malnutrition is a major factor for this complication.

A point worth mentioning is the possibility that malnutrition may influence the evolution of IBD itself. In this sense, a number of pathophysiologic consequences of both macronutrient and micronutrient deficiencies on immune response and tissue repair should be discussed. Malnutrition is a major cause of secondary immunodeficiency, both cellular and humoral. This is not only due to the lack of energy and protein substrates in immune cells but to deficiencies of a variety of specific nutrients. These include nucleotides,[84] glutamine,[85] arginine,[86] biotin,[87] and zinc.[88,89] On the other hand, a deficit of antioxidant micronutrients, such as vitamins E, C, β-carotene, zinc, manganese, and selenium, decreases the host's defense against free-radical-induced damage.[90,91] Likewise, copper and zinc are necessary for polyunsaturated fatty acid (PUFA) biosynthesis, and a high copper:zinc ratio may impair arachidonate and eicosanoid synthesis.[92]

Gut immune response and regional host defense also may be influenced by malnutrition. PEM is closely associated with gut mucosal atrophy and may affect the integrity of the GI mucosal barrier, leading to bacterial translocation and increased macromolecule uptake eliciting a chronic immune challenge.[93]

The reparative tissue processes after inflammation may also be impaired by protein-energy deficiency. In addition, vitamin C is an essential cofactor for collagen synthesis.[94] Moreover, zinc is a cofactor for collagenase and is a potent inhibitor of prolyl hydroxylase, an enzyme that plays a key role in collagen synthesis.[95,96] Moreover, deficit of some micronutrients such as folate has been associated with

abnormal nucleic acid synthesis and development of dysplasia in UC.[97]

Some of the above-mentioned phenomena could be viewed as immunosuppressive and might improve inflammation. In contrast, others may promote the self-perpetuation of the inflammatory process in IBD. The true significance of nutritional deficiencies on the pathophysiology of IBD is far from being fully understood.

ENTERAL NUTRITION AS NUTRITIONAL SUPPORT IN INFLAMMATORY BOWEL DISEASE

Artificial nutrition was introduced as an adjuvant therapy to steroids in IBD because of the high prevalence of PEM in severe acute attacks, long-standing moderate bouts of the disease, and especially when fistulas complicated the clinical course of CD. TPN was the first way to provide artificial nutritional support to IBD patients. As in other disease states, this was partly due to historical reasons, since TPN was introduced earlier than total enteral nutrition (TEN) in clinical practice. In addition, TPN maintained the bowel at rest, which was believed crucial in the management of active IBD. Now, however, the concept of "therapeutic bowel rest" in IBD is questioned. Its theoretical advantages were to decrease bowel movements and to drastically reduce the bulk of intraluminal alimentary antigens to the intestinal mucosa.[98] However, complete bowel rest also had disadvantages, because the presence of nutrients in the gut lumen is the most important trophic factor for the intestinal mucosa. Villous hypoplasia, documented in patients with protracted fasting and in those treated with TPN,[99] is a self-perpetuating factor for PEM and may limit tolerance to conventional food after TPN. In the last decade, the concept that "complete bowel rest" is unnecessary for the management of IBD has gained acceptance, since no differences in clinical outcome could be demonstrated between patients managed with or without this therapeutic maneuver.[100-102]

TEN is a safer alternative to TPN for artificial nutritional support. Early attempts of TEN in IBD patients used predigested, chemically defined elemental diets that provided nitrogen in the form of free L-amino acids. The rationale for using such diets was based on the lower antigenicity of free amino acids compared with whole protein. In addition, amino acids, not requiring digestion, were thought to be well absorbed in the upper segments of the small bowel. This was considered to result in some degree of bowel rest. In addition, elemental diets contained only small amounts of fat, often in the form of medium-chain triglycerides, which required relatively little luminal lipolysis and micellar solubilization before absorption. Based on results of physiologic studies showing better nitrogen absorption from dipeptides or tripeptides that form isonitrogenous free amino acid mixtures,[103] the amino acid source of some elemental diets was replaced by peptide mixtures of varying chain length. However, in recent years, whole-protein enteral diets have proved nutritionally effective and well tolerated by most patients with IBD.[16,17]

Enteral nutrition may be administered as supplemental feedings or as the major source of nutrition. In the first case, sip feeding can be used. However, when TEN is envisaged (especially in patients with severe or extensive disease), enteral diets should be infused through a proper feeding tube and at a constant rate throughout the day with the aid of a peristaltic pump.[104] In extreme cases, when nutritional requirements cannot be met by enteral tube feeding, TPN should be used.

Absolute contraindications to TEN in IBD include massive hemorrhage, bowel perforation, complete intestinal obstruction, toxic megacolon, and the presence of mid-jejunal fistulas in which nutrients cannot be infused distal to their origin.[104]

Ulcerative Colitis

Artificial nutritional support (TEN or TPN) is advisable as an adjunct to steroid therapy in UC patients who are moderately or poorly malnourished. It is also indicated in those patients with severe attacks (mainly if surgery is planned). In these patients, PEM may develop within a short time and may increase surgical risk.

The possibility of using TEN in severe UC was opened by the results of two controlled trials performed in steroid-treated patients, comparing TPN plus bowel rest and oral diet. TPN plus bowel rest did not influence clinical outcome in terms of achievement of clinical remission and need for surgery in these patients.[101,105] However, long-term outcome, specifically surgery-related complications, was not fully evaluated.

The question of which type of artificial nutrition is better as adjuvant therapy to steroids in severe UC has been recently examined in a prospective controlled trial of isocaloric and isonitrogenous TPN vs TEN.[106] Clinical remission was achieved in 54 and 50 percent of patients in TEN and TPN groups, respectively, with a similar number of patients requiring surgery. However, postoperative infections and nutritional support–related complications were significantly more frequent in the TPN group than in the TEN patients. Nutritional assessment showed a greater increase in serum albumin levels in the TEN group than in the TPN group. These results suggest that TEN should be the preferred modality of artificial nutrition in severe UC, unless the above-mentioned contraindications for enteral feeding are present.

However, is a conventional oral diet nutritionally enough in severe UC? Only in one trial comparing TPN vs hospital diet was total-body nitrogen evaluated before and after treatment in a subset of matched patients in each group. A significant decrease in total-body nitrogen was found in patients receiving an oral diet but not in those receiving TPN.[105] On the other hand, data from retrospective nonrandomized studies suggest that TEN, but not hospital diet, is able to prevent nutritional derangement in patients with acute attacks of UC.[16,17] Moreover, TEN is an easy way to secure an adequate nutrient intake in these patients, who often must be encouraged to eat. Randomized clinical trials comparing TEN vs oral diet are needed to answer this query.

Crohn's Disease

Patients with CD often have complications that require, in addition to drugs, specific dietary restrictions, such as low-fiber or low-fat diets, which often result in suboptimal energy intake.[107] In such cases, enteral or parenteral nutrition is the only way to ensure a correct energy supply. As in UC, TPN plus bowel rest makes little difference on clinical outcome in CD, irrespective of its location, even when complications such as fistula or inflammatory mass are present.[102] On the other hand, artificial nutrition often must be administered for longer periods in CD than in UC, and it is well known that the rate of TPN-related complications and deleterious effects on intestinal mucosa increase in parallel with the time a patient receives parenteral feeding. All these arguments have prompted the use of the enteral instead of the parenteral route in CD. The interest in the enteral route has also been related to its simplicity and its lower cost compared with TPN.

Home enteral tube feeding is feasible in difficult cases. Percutaneous endoscopic gastrostomy has facilitated this approach. A combination of daily oral diet and nocturnal tube feeding can also be nutritionally effective. Patients with multiple intestinal resections and short-bowel syndrome may require combined TPN and TEN to meet nutritional requirements and promote intestinal adaptation. Except in certain situations, whole-protein-based diets are recommended because they are well tolerated and allow higher nitrogen supply than amino acid– or peptide-based diets.[104] This occurs because of the osmolar strength of free amino acids and peptides is greater than that of isonitrogenous amounts of whole protein, thus increasing the risk of diarrhea.

ENTERAL NUTRITION AS PRIMARY THERAPY IN INFLAMMATORY BOWEL DISEASE

No study has assessed the role of artificial support as the only therapeutic measure in UC. However, studies evaluating the effect of TEN or TPN as adjunct therapy to steroids do not suggest that artificial nutrition either increases the number of patients achieving remission or accelerates the therapeutic response.[101,105,106] On the other hand, severe UC usually follows a more acute course than CD, with emergency surgery being required more often in the former. In this setting, rapidly acting therapeutic measures are necessary, which is not expected to be the case for enteral nutrition. All these circumstances make questionable the performance of controlled trials on the primary effect of TEN in UC.

In contrast to UC, some studies have suggested that enteral nutrition may be effective in inducing clinical remission in acute exacerbations of CD. However, after more than 10 years of investigation on the effect of TEN as primary treatment of active CD, no clear conclusions about this therapy exist.

Amino acid–based diets were initially introduced as primary treatment of active CD because of their low allergenicity, since whole protein was thought to act as a dietary antigen in the gut. It was also argued that these diets would favor bowel rest. After the first randomized clinical trial in 1984,[108] two other trials showed that amino acid–based diets were as effective as steroid therapy in achieving short-term remission in active CD.[109,110] After these early reports, further studies using not only amino acid– but peptide- or whole-protein-based diets yield controversial results.[111-129] In a large trial comparing a peptide-based tube-fed diet with steroids, Lochs and associates found that the diet was less effective than a combination of methylprednisolone and sulfasalazine in treating active CD.[114] However, the finding that 44 percent of patients did not respond to an enteral diet is surprising, since it is a figure considerably higher than those found in other small-sized trials.[112,117,122,124] On the other hand, some authors have claimed that whole-protein diets were worse than amino acid–based diets,[118] whereas others found that they were as good as steroids.[116]

In an attempt to clarify the role of enteral nutrition as primary therapy of Crohn's disease, a meta-analysis of the randomized clinical trials has recently been performed.[130] Nine randomized trials comparing enteral nutrition with steroids and seven comparing elemental (amino acid based) with nonelemental diets were selected, and their results were analyzed on an intention-to-treat basis. This study indicates that steroids are better than enteral nutrition in inducing remission in active CD (the 95 percent confidence interval of the pooled odds ratio for all types of enteral diets compared with steroid therapy ranged from 0.23 to 0.53). As a whole, the probability of achieving remission was 65 percent lower with TEN than with steroids. These results were consistent for all trials combined, for the best four studies (as assessed by a quality score) combined, after excluding trials using sip feeding, and when noncompliant patients were withdrawn. However, subgroup analysis according to the type of diet showed that this trend was markedly definite when peptide-based diets were administered, but it was inconclusive for amino acid– or whole-protein-based diets.[130]

In light of these results, is there a therapeutic role for enteral nutrition in inducing clinical remission in active Crohn's disease? In the above-mentioned meta-analysis, the overall remission rate after total enteral nutrition was about 60 percent, a figure higher than those reported responses to placebo in CD (20 to 30 percent).[131,132] Although such comparison must be taken with caution, it supports the idea that enteral nutrition has some therapeutic effect in active CD. A placebo-controlled trial of enteral nutrition in active CD would appropriately answer this question. Because this approach is at present doubtfully ethical, the primary therapeutic role of enteral nutrition in CD will be difficult to establish.

The time elapsed until remission is achieved is important data and is reported only in four studies.[114,116,117,122] In three of them it was similar for enteral diets and steroids.[116,117,122] In the remaining study,[114] time until remission was significantly longer in the enteral group, but the datum was obtained pooling together responders and nonresponders.

It would be interesting to investigate the possibility that enteral nutrition was particularly advantageous in some subset of patients (in terms of extent, evolutive type, or location of disease). Unfortunately, such assessment is difficult to perform with the published data. Also, the influence of the differences in diet composition, other than the nitrogen source, on the primary therapeutic effect of enteral nutrition in CD must be evaluated.

THE FUTURE

It is now well established that there is a close relationship between the composition of dietary lipids, immune function, and inflammatory response.[133-137] This may be due to changes in the fatty acid composition and function of cell membranes (including those of the immune cells),[138,139] the modulation of eicosanoid synthesis,[140,141] and the production of other inflammatory mediators.[142,143] The modulation of eicosanoid synthesis by administering long-chain n3-PUFA (fish oil) as a diet supplement has been used in some trials in IBD patients, yielding controversial results. Although some studies suggest that fish oil induces a clinical, sigmoidoscopic, and histologic improvement of active UC,[144-147] others have not found any therapeutic effect.[148-150] Active CD did not improve with fish oil supplementation in one study.[148] However, the design and methodology of some of these trials have been recently criticized.[151] The effect of TEN or TPN using n3-PUFA-enriched diets has not been evaluated in IBD.

The possibility that clinical remission achieved with enteral diets in CD might be related to the administration of both the type and amount of fat has been suggested.[152] This hypothesis is based on the observation that those diets with larger amounts of linoleic acid were associated with a poorer outcome. In contrast, the outcome of patients receiving insufficient substrate for n6-PUFA-derived eicosanoid synthesis, either as low-fat diets or as diets with normal amounts of fat but containing large proportions of monounsaturated fatty acids (i.e., oleic acid), was more favorable. This hypothesis must be verified in controlled studies.

On the basis that butyrate is a major energy-yielding substrate to colonocytes[153] and that in UC there is both a decreased fecal concentration[154] and a deficient colonocyte use of this short-chain fatty acid (SCFA),[155,156] treatment with butyrate enemas has been used in active distal UC.[157-159] Results suggest that this approach may be useful in some UC patients unresponsive to standard therapy. Larger clinical studies are needed to evaluate butyrate enemas as a new therapy in UC. To our knowledge, a controlled investigation on the effect of either oral supplementation with SCFA substrate (i.e., fiber) or butyrate-enriched TEN/TPN in these patients has yet to be performed.

L-arginine is a semiessential amino acid with possible immunostimulating effects.[86] It is also the precursor of nitric oxide, which has been suggested to promote mucosal injury in IBD.[160] Experimental studies have shown that L-arginine administration has different effects depending on the different models of intestinal inflammation used. Thus, it may prevent intestinal damage in a model of necrotizing enterocolitis[161] but may increase colonic lesions in a model of trinitrobenzenesulfonic acid–induced colitis.[162] All these data raise the need of further studies to assess which would be the amount of L-arginine suitable for IBD patients.

A number of animal studies suggest an important role for using various intestinal growth factors in states of gut mucosal injury and inflammation. Epidermal growth factor administration has been useful after methotrexate-induced small-intestinal mucosal damage and in experimental colitis.[163-165] The effect of this and other trophic factors, such as polyamines, glutamine, and nucleotides, remains to be evaluated in IBD. Finally, because oxidative stress may play a major role in the pathogenesis of tissue injury in IBD,[90] should the amounts of antioxidant micronutrients be increased in enteral diets for patients with IBD?

In summary, enteral nutrition has been demonstrated to be the preferred modality of artificial nutrition in patients with IBD, since it is safer, cheaper, and at least as nutritionally effective as TPN. Furthermore, some published data suggest that enteral nutrition may play a role as primary treatment in CD. However, solid data still have not been obtained confirming this possibility. Future work should aim to ascertain the actual performance of diets now in the market and the improvements that could be achieved by adding other nutrients with possible specific pathobiologic roles in IBD.

REFERENCES

1. Kirsner JB, Shorer RG: Recent developments in 'non-specific' inflammatory bowel disease. N Engl J Med 1982;306:775.
2. Stenson WF, McDermot RP: Inflammatory bowel disease. In Yamada T (ed): Textbook of Gastroenterology, Vol 2. Philadelphia: JB Lippincott Co. 1991:1589.
3. Yang H, Rotter JI: Genetics of inflammatory bowel disease. In Targan SR, Shanahan F (eds): Inflammatory Bowel Disease. From Bench to Bedside. Baltimore: Williams & Wilkins, 1994:32.
4. Calkins BM: A meta-analysis of the role of smoking and its relationship to inflammatory bowel disease. Dig Dis Sci 1989;34:1841.
5. Osborne MJ, Stansby GP: Cigarette smoking and its relationship to inflammatory bowel disease: a review. J Royal Soc Med 1992;85:214.
6. Podolsky DK: Inflammatory bowel disease (Part I). N Engl J Med 1991;325:928.
7. Shanahan F, Targan SR: Mechanisms of tissue injury in inflammatory bowel disease. In Targan SR, Shanahan F (eds): Inflammatory Bowel Disease. From Bench to Bedside. Baltimore: Williams & Wilkins, 1994:78.
8. Fiocchi C: Immunology of inflammatory bowel disease. Curr Opin Gastroenterol 1991;7:654.
9. Fiocchi C: Cytokines. In Targan SR, Shanahan F (eds): Inflammatory Bowel Disease. From Bench to Bedside. Baltimore: Williams & Wilkins, 1994:106.
10. Wallace JL: Eiscosanoids. In Targan SR, Shanahan F (eds): Inflammatory Bowel Disease. From Bench to Bedside. Baltimore: Williams & Wilkins, 1994:123.
11. Gassull MA, Cabré E, Vilar LI et al: Protein-energy malnutrition: an integral approach and a simple new classification. Hum Nutr Clin Nutr 1984;38C:419.
12. Gee MI, Grace MGA, Wensel RH et al: Protein-energy malnutrition in gastroenterology out-patients: increased risk in Crohn's disease. J Am Dietet Assoc 1985;85:1466.
13. Harries A, Jones L, Heatley RV et al: Malnutrition in inflammatory bowel disease: an anthropometric study. Hum Nutr Clin Nutr 1982;36C:307.
14. Heatley RV: Nutritional implications of inflammatory bowel disease. Scand J Gastroenterol 1984;19:995.
15. Rosenberg IH, Bengoa JM, Sitrin MD: Nutritional aspects of inflammatory bowel disease. Ann Rev Nutr 1985;5:463.
16. Abad A, Cabré E, Giné JJ et al: Total enteral nutrition in inflammatory bowel disease. J Clin Nutr Gastroenterol 1986;1:1.
17. Gassull MA, Abad A, Cabré E et al: Enteral nutrition in inflammatory bowel disease. Gut 1986;27(suppl 1):76.
18. Fernandez-Bañares F, Abad-Lacruz A, Xiol X et al: Vitamin status in patients with inflammatory bowel disease. Am J Gastroenterol 1989;84:744.
19. Hoffbrand AV, Steward JS, Booth CC et al: Folate deficiency in Crohn's disease: incidence, pathogenesis and treatment. Br Med J 1968;2:71.
20. Farivar S, Fromm H, Schindler D et al: Tests of bile acid and vitamin B12 metabolism in ileal Crohn's disease. Am J Clin Pathol 1980;73:69.
21. Imes S, Pinchbeck B, Dinwoodie A et al: Vitamin A status in 137 patients with Crohn's disease. Digestion 1987;37:166.
22. Schoelmerich MS, Becher MS, Hoppe-Seyler P et al: Zinc and vitamin A deficiency in patients with Crohn's disease is correlated with activity but not with localization or extent of the disease. Hepatogastroenterology 1985;32:34.
23. Krasiski SD, Russell RM, Furie BC et al: The prevalence of vitamin K deficiency in chronic gastrointestinal disorders. Am J Clin Nutr 1985;41:639.
24. Driscoll RH, Meredith SC, Sitrin M et al: Vitamin D deficiency and bone disease in patients with Crohn's disease. Gastroenterology 1982;83:1252.
25. Harris AD, Brown R, Heatley RV et al: Vitamin D status in Crohn's disease: association with nutrition and disease activity. Gut 1985;26:1197.
26. Imes S, Dinwoodie A, Walker K et al: Vitamin C status in 137 out-patients with Crohn's disease: effect of diet counseling. J Clin Gastroenterol 1986;8:443.
27. Kuroki F, Iida M, Tominaga M et al: Multiple vitamin status in Crohn's disease. Correlation with disease activity. Dig Dis Sci 1993;38:1614.
28. Leevy CM, Cardi L, Frank O et al: Incidence and significance of hypovitaminosis in randomly selected municipal hospital population. Am J Clin Nutr 1965;17:259.
29. Lemoine A, Le Devehat C, Codacchioni JL et al: Vitamin B1, B2, B6 and C status in hospital inpatients. Am J Clin Nutr 1980;33:2595.
30. Pietzrik K: Concept of borderline vitamin deficiency. Int J Vitam Nutr Res 1985;27:61.
31. Gassull MA, Fernandez-Bañares F, Esteve-Comas M: Nutrition in inflammatory bowel disease. In Payne-James J, Grimble G, Silk D (eds): Artificial Nutrition in Clinical Practice. London: Edward Arnold Publishers, 1994:443.
32. Barr M, Delava S, Zetterstrom R: Studies of the anaemia in ulcerative colitis with special reference to iron metabolism. Acta Pediatr 1975;44:62.
33. Valentin N, Nielsen OV, Olesen KH: Muscle cell electrolytes in ulcerative colitis and Crohn's disease. Digestion 1975;13:284.
34. Penny WJ, Mayberry OV, Agget PJ et al: Relationship between trace elements sugar consumption, and taste in Crohn's disease. Gut 1983;24:288.
35. McClain C, Soutor C, Zieve L: Zinc deficiency: a complication of Crohn's disease. Gastroenterology 1980;78:272.
36. Solomons NW, Rosenberg IH, Sandstead H et al: Zinc deficiency in Crohn's disease. Digestion 1977;16:87.
37. Fleming CR, Huizenga KA, McCall JT et al: Zinc nutrition in Crohn's disease. Dig Dis Sci 1981;26:865.
38. Valberg LS, Flanagan PR, Kertesz A et al: Zinc absorption in inflammatory bowel disease. Dig Dis Sci 1986;31:724.
39. Nishi Y, Lifshitz F, Bayne MA et al: Zinc status and its relation to growth retardation in children with chronic inflammatory bowel disease. Am J Clin Nutr 1980;33:2613.
40. Fernandez-Bañares F, Mingorance MD, Esteve M et al: Serum zinc, copper, and selenium levels in inflammatory bowel disease: effect of total enteral nutrition on trace element status. Am J Gastroenterol 1990;85:1584.
41. Porchen R, Fisher CH, Purrmann J et al: Urinary excretion and plasma concentration of trace elements in Crohn's disease: zinc and selenium deficiency is not compensated by treatment with an elemental diet. Gastroenterology 1989;96:A396.
42. Jacobson S, Plantin LO: Concentration of selenium in plasma and erythrocytes during total parenteral nutrition in Crohn's disease. Gut 1985;36:50.
43. Loechke K, Köning A, Heaberlin ST et al: Low blood selenium concentration in Crohn's disease (letter). Ann Intern Med 1987;106:908.

44. Hinks LJ, Inwards KD, Lloyd B et al: Reduced concentrations of selenium in mild Crohn's disease. J Clin Pathol 1988;41:198.

45. Ringstad J, Kildebo S, Thomassen Y: Serum selenium, copper and zinc concentrations in Crohn's disease and ulcerative colitis. Scand J Gastroenterol 1993; 28:605.

46. Fernández-Bañares F, Mingorance MD, Cabré E et al: Serum mineral and trace element levels in hospitalized patients with inflammatory bowel disease. Clin Nutr 1988;7(suppl):86.

47. Goldschmid S, Graham M: Trace-element deficiencies in inflammatory bowel disease. Gastroenterol Clin North Am 1989;18:579.

48. Smith JE, Brown ED, Smith JD: The effect of zinc deficiency on the metabolism of retinol-binding in the rat. J Lab Clin Med 1974;84:692.

49. Hendricks KM, Walker WA: Zinc deficiency in inflammatory bowel disease. Nutr Rev 1988;46:401.

50. Solomons NW: On the assessment of zinc and copper nutriture in man. Am J Clin Nutr 1979;32:856.

51. Dew MJ, Thompson H, Allan RN: The spectrum of hepatic dysfunction on inflammatory bowel disease. Q J Med 1979;48:113.

52. Clarkson JP, Elmes ME: Correlation of plasma zinc and ileal enterocyte zinc in man. Ann Nutr Metab 1987;31:259.

53. Nakamura T, Higashi A, Takano S et al: Zinc clearance correlates with clinical severity of Crohn's disease. A kinetic study. Dig Dis Sci 1988;33:1520.

54. Hellerstein MK, Meydani SN, Meydani N et al: Interleukin 1 induced anorexia in the rat. Influence of prostaglandins. J Clin Invest 1989;84:228.

55. Bodnar RJ, Pasternak GW, Mann PE et al: Mediation of anorexia by human recombinant tumour necrosis factor through a peripheral action in the rat. Cancer Res 1989;49:6280.

56. Danesh BJZ, Park RHR, Upadhyay R et al: How useful are upper gastrointestinal biopsies with Crohn's disease? Gut 1988;29:A703.

57. Farmer RG, Hawk WA, Turnbull RB: Clinical patterns in Crohn's disease: a statistical study of 615 cases. Gastroenterology 1975;68:627.

58. Singleton JW, Law DH, Kelley ML et al: National Cooperative Crohn's Disease Study: adverse reactions to drugs. Gastroenterology 1979;77:870.

59. Riley SA, Mani V, Goodman MJ et al: Comparison of delayed-release 5-aminosalicylic acid (mesalazine) and sulfasalazine as maintenance treatment for patients with ulcerative colitis. Gastroenterology 1988; 94:1383.

60. Gassull MA, Cabré E, Vilar LI et al: Nival de ingesta hospitalaria y su posible papel en el desarrollo de malnutrición calórico-proteica en pacientes gastroenterológicos hospitalizados. Med Clin (Barc) 1985; 85:85.

61. King CE, Toskes PP: Small intestine bacterial overgrowth. Gastroenterology 1979;76:1035.

62. Hoffmann AF, Poley JR: Role of bile acid malabsorption in the pathogenesis of diarrhoea and steatorrhoea. Gastroenterology 1972;62:918.

63. Seinfield JL, Davidson JD, Gordon RS Jr et al: The mechanisms of hypoproteinemia in patients with regional enteritis and ulcerative colitis. Am J Med 1960;29:405.

64. Crama-Bohbouth G, Peña AS, Biemond J et al: Are activity indexes helpful in assessing active intestinal inflammation in Crohn's disease? Gut 1989;30:1236.

65. Bjarnason I, O'Morain C, Levi AJ et al: Absorption of 5-chromium-labelled ethylendiamine tetra-acetate in

inflammatory bowel disease. Gastroenterology 1983; 85:318.

66. Kovi J, Duong HD, Hoand CT: Ultrastructure of intestinal lymphatics in Crohn's disease. Am J Clin Pathol 1981;76:385.

67. Klein S, Meyers S, O'Sullivan P et al: The metabolic impact of active ulcerative colitis: energy expenditure and nitrogen balance. J Clin Gastroenterol 1988; 10:34.

68. Barot LR, Rombeau JL, Feurer ID et al: Caloric requirements in patients with inflammatory bowel disease. Ann Surg 1982;195:214.

69. Barot LR, Rombeau JL, Steinberg JJ et al: Energy expenditure in patients with inflammatory bowel disease. Arch Surg 1981;116:460.

70. Rigaud D, Alberto LA, Sobhani I et al: Increased resting energy expenditure during flare-ups in Crohn's disease. Gastroenterol Clin Biol 1993;17:932.

71. Kushner RF, Schoeller DA: Resting and total energy expenditure in patients with inflammatory bowel disease. Am J Clin Nutr 1991;53:161.

72. Stokes MA, Hill GL: Total energy expenditure in patients with Crohn's disease. Measurement by the combined body scan technique. J Parenter Enter Nutr 1993;17:3.

73. Powel-Tuck J, Garlick P, Lennard-Jones JE et al: Rates of whole-protein synthesis and breakdown increase with the severity of the disease. Gut 1984;25:460.

74. Thomas AG, Miller V, Taylor F et al: Whole-body protein turnover in childhood Crohn's disease. Gut 1992;33:675.

75. Baracos V, Rodemann HP, Dinarello CA et al: Stimulation of muscle protein degradation and prostaglandin release by leukocytic pyrogen (interleukin 1). A mechanism for the increased degradation of muscle protein during fever. N Engl J Med 1983; 308:553.

76. Hartig W, Matkowtiz R, Faust H: Post-aggression metabolism: hormonal and metabolic aspects. J Clin Nutr Gastroenterol 1986;1:255.

77. Kirshner BS, Voinchet O, Rosenberg IH: Growth retardation in inflammatory bowel disease. Gastroenterology 1978;75:504.

78. Burbige EJ, Huang SH, Bayles TM: Clinical manifestations of Crohn's disease in children and adolescents. Pediatrics 1975;75:866.

79. McCafferty TD, Nasr K, Lawrence AH et al: Severe growth retardation in children with inflammatory bowel disease. J Pediatr 1970;45:386.

80. Markowitz J, Grancher K, Rosa J et al: Growth failure in pediatric inflammatory bowel disease. J Pediatr Gastroenterol Nutr 1993;16:373.

81. Griffiths AM, Nguyen P, Smith C et al: Growth and clinical course of children with Crohn's disease. Gut 1993;34:939.

82. Kirschner BS, Klich JR, Kalman SS et al: Reversal of growth retardation in Crohn's disease with therapy emphasizing oral nutritional restitution. Gastroenterology 1981;80:10.

83. Morin CL, Roulet M, Roy CC et al: Continuous elemental enteral alimentation in children with Crohn's disease and growth failure. Gastroenterology 1980; 79:1205.

84. Pizzini RP, Kumar S, Kulkarni AD et al: Dietary nucleotides reverse malnutrition and starvation-induced immunosuppression. Arch Surg 1990;125:86.

85. Newsholme E, Parry-Billings M: Properties of glutamin release from muscle and its importance for the immune system. J Parenter Enter Nutr 1990;14 (suppl):63S.

86. Barbul A: Arginine and immune function. Nutrition 1990;6:53.

87. Obake N, Urabe K, Fujita K et al: Biotin effects in Crohn's disease. Dig Dis Sci 1988;33:1495.

88. Kruse-Jarres JD: The significance of zinc for humoral and cellular immunity. J Trace Elem Electrolytes Health Dis 1989;3:1.

89. Chandra RK, McBean LD: Zinc and immunity. Nutrition 1994;10:79.

90. Grisham MB, Granger DN: Neutrophil-mediated mucosal injury. Role of reactive oxygen metabolites. Dig Dis Sci 1988;33(suppl):6S.

91. Blake DR, Allen RE, Lunee G: Free radicals in biological systems: a review orientated to inflammatory processes. Br Med Bull 1987;43:371.

92. Cunnane SC: Differential regulation of essential fatty acid metabolism to the prostaglandins: possible basis for the interaction of zinc and copper in biological systems. Prog Lipid Res 1982;21:73.

93. Alexander JW: Nutrition and translocation. J Parenter Enter Nutr 1990;14(suppl):170S.

94. Barnes MJ: Function of ascorbic acid in collagen metabolism. Ann NY Acad Sci 1975;258:264.

95. Seltzer JL, Jeffrey JJ, Eisen AZ: Evidence for mammalian collagenases as zinc ion metalloenzymes. Biochim Biophys Acta 1977;485:179.

96. Anttinen H, Puistola U, Pihlajaniemi T et al: Differences between proline and lysine hydroxylations in their inhibition by zinc or by ascorbate deficiency during collagen synthesis in various cell types. Biochim Biophys Acta 1981;674:336.

97. Lashner BA, Heidenreich PA, Su GL et al: Effect of folate supplementation on the incidence of dysplasia and cancer in chronic ulcerative colitis. A case-control study. Gastroenterology 1989;97:255.

98. Rhodes J, Rose J: Does food affect acute inflammatory bowel disease? The role of parenteral nutrition, elemental and exclusion diets. Gut 1986;27:471.

99. Dowling RH: Small bowel adaptation and its regulation. Scand J Gastroenterol 1982;17(suppl 74):53.

100. Lochs H, Meryn S, Marosi L et al: Has bowel rest a beneficial effect in the treatment of Crohn's disease? Clin Nutr 1983;2:61.

101. McIntyre PB, Powell-Tuck J, Wood SR et al: Controlled trial of bowel rest in the treatment of severe acute colitis. Gut 1986;27:481.

102. Greenberg GR, Fleming CR, Jeejeebhoy KN et al: Controlled trial of bowel rest and nutritional support in the management of Crohn's disease. Gut 1988;29:1309.

103. Silk DBA: Physiology of protein absorption. Res Clin Forums 1979;1:29.

104. Cabré E, Gassull MA: Enteral tube-feeding in digestive tract diseases: a pathophysiological challenge. J Clin Nutr Gastroenterol 1986;1:97.

105. Dickinson RJ, Ashton MG, Axon ATR et al: Controlled trial of intravenous hyperalimentation and total bowel rest as an adjunct to the routine therapy of acute colitis. Gastroenterology 1980;79:1199.

106. González-Huix F, Fernández-Bañares F, Esteve-Comas M et al: Enteral versus parenteral nutrition as adjunct therapy in acute ulcerative colitis. Am J Gastroenterol 1993;88:227.

107. Fernández-Bañares F, Gassull MA: Role of dietary management and artificial nutritional support in the treatment of inflammatory bowel disease. In Gassull MA, Obrador A, Chantar C (eds): Management of Inflammatory Bowel Disease. Barcelona: Prous Editores, 1994:299.

108. O'Moráin C, Segal AW, Levi AJ: Elemental diet as primary treatment of acute Crohn's disease: a controlled study. Br Med J 1984;288:1859.

109. Seidman EG, Bouthillier L, Weber AM et al: Elemental diet versus prednisone as primary treatment of Crohn's disease (abstract). Gastroenterology 1986;90:A1625.

110. Saverymuttu S, Hodgson HJF, Chadwick VS: Controlled trial comparing prednisolone with an elemental diet plus non-absorbable antibiotics in active Crohn's disease. Gut 1985;26:994.

111. Gorard A, Hunt JB, Payne-James JJ et al: Initial response and subsequent course of Crohn's disease treated with elemental diet or prednisolone. Gut 1993;34:1198.

112. Sanderson IR, Udeen S, Davies PSW et al: Remission induced by an elemental diet in small bowel Crohn's disease. Arch Dis Child 1987;61:123.

113. Malchow H, Steinhartdt HJ, Lorenz-Meyer H et al: Feasibility and effectiveness of a defined-formula diet regimen in treating active Crohn's disease. European Cooperative Crohn's disease study III. Scand J Gastroenterol 1990;25:235.

114. Lochs H, Steinhardt HJ, Klaus-Wentz B et al: Comparison of enteral nutrition and drug treatment in active Crohn's disease. Results of the Europen Cooperative Crohn's disease study IV. Gastroenterology 1991;101:881.

115. Lindor KD, Fleming CR, Burnes JU et al: A randomized prospective trial comparing a defined formula diet, corticosteroids, and a defined formula diet plus corticosteroids in active Crohn's disease. Mayo Clin Proc 1992;67:328.

116. González-Huix F, de Leon R, Fernández-Bañares F et al: Polymeric enteral diets as primary treatment of active Crohn's disease. A prospective steroid controlled trial. Gut 1993;34:778.

117. Seidman E, Griffiths A, Jones A et al: (Canadian Collaborative Pediatric Crohn's disease study group). Semi-elemental diet vs prednisone in pediatric Crohn's disease (abstract). Gastroenterology 1993;104:A778.

118. Giaffer MH, North G, Holdsworth CD: Controlled trial of polymeric versus elemental diet in treatment of active Crohn's disease. Lancet 1990;335:816.

119. Rigaud D, Cosnes J, Le Quintrec Y et al: Controlled trial comparing two types of enteral nutrition in treatment of active Crohn's disease: elemental vs polymeric diet. Gut 1991;32:1492.

120. Park RHR, Galloway A, Danesh BJZ et al: Double-blind controlled trial of elemental and polymeric diets as primary therapy in Crohn's disease. Eur J Gastroenterol Hepatol 1991;3:483.

121. Raouf AH, Hildrey V, Daniel J et al: Enteral feeding as sole treatment for Crohn's disease: controlled trial of whole protein vs amino acid based feed and a case study of dietary challenge. Gut 1991;32:702.

122. Middleton SJ, Riordan AM, Hunter JO: Comparison of elemental and peptide-based diets in the treatment of acute Crohn's disease (abstract). Ital J Gastroenterol 1991;23:609.

123. Mansfield JC, Giaffer MH, Holdsworth CD: Amino-acid versus oligopeptide based enteral feeds in active Crohn's disease (abstract). Gut 1992;33(suppl 2):S3.

124. Royall D, Jeejeebhoy KN, Baker JP et al: Comparison of amino acid vs peptide based enteral diets in active Crohn's disease: clinical and nutritional outcome. Gut 1994;35:783.

125. Alun Jones V: Comparison of total parenteral nutrition and elemental diet in induction of remission of Crohn's disease. Long-term maintenance of remissions by personalized food exclusion diets. Dig Dis Sci 1987;32(suppl):100S.

126. Larsen PM, Rasmussen D, Ronn B et al: Elemental diet: a therapeutic approach in chronic inflammatory bowel disease. J Intern Med 1989;225:325.

127. Okada M, Yao T, Yamamoto T et al: Controlled trial comparing an elemental diet with prednisolone in the treatment of active Crohn's disease. Hepato-Gastroenterology 1990;37:72.

128. Rigaud D, Cerf M, Melchior JC et al: Nutritional assistance (NA) and acute attacks of Crohn's disease (CD): efficacy of total parenteral nutrition (TPN) as compared with elemental (EEN) and polymeric (PEN) enteral nutrition (abstract). Gastroenterology 1989;96: A416.

129. Engelman JL, Black L, Murphy GM et al: Comparison of a semi elemental diet (Peptamen) with prednisolone in the primary treatment of active ileal Crohn's disease (abstract). Gastroenterology 1993; 104:A697.

130. Fernández-Bañares F, Cabré E, Esteve M et al: How effective is enteral nutrition in inducing clinical remission in active Crohn's disease? A meta-analysis of the randomized clinical trials. J Parenter Enter Nutr 1995;19:356.

131. Summers RW, Switz DM, Sessions JT Jr et al: National cooperative Crohn's disease study: results of drug treatment. Gastroenterology 1979;77:847.

132. Singleton JW, Hanauer SB, Gitnick GL et al: Mesalamine capsules for the treatment of active Crohn's disease: results of a 16-week trial. Gastroenterology 1993;104:1293.

133. Kinsella JE, Lokesh B, Broughton S et al: Potential effects of the modulation of inflammatory and immune cells: an overview. Nutrition 1990;6:24.

134. Morrow WJW, Homsy J, Swanson CA et al: Dietary fat influences the expression of autoimmune disease in MLR 1pr/1pr mice. Immunology 1986;89:439.

135. Schreiner GF, Flye W, Brunt E et al: Essential fatty acid depletion of renal allografts and prevention of rejection. Science 1988;240:1032.

136. Denko CW: Modification of adjuvant inflammation in rats deficient in essential fatty acids. Agents Actions 1976;65:636.

137. Lohoues MJ, Russo P, Gurbindo C et al: Essential fatty acid deficiency improves the course of experimental colitis in the rat: possible role of dietary immunomodulation. Gastroenterology 1992;102:A655.

138. Kinsella JE: Lipids, membrane receptors, and enzymes: effects of dietary fatty acids. J Parenter Enter Nutr 1990;14(suppl):200S.

139. Hartl WH, Wolfe RR: The phospholipid/arachidonic acid second messenger system: its possible role in physiology and pathophysiology of metabolism. J Parenter Enter Nutr 1990;14:416.

140. Strasser T, Fischer S, Weber PC: Leukotriene B5 is formed in human neutrophils after dietary supplementation with eicosapentaenoic acid. Proc Natl Acad Sci USA 1985;82:1540.

141. Lee TH, Hoover RL, Williams JD et al: Effect of dietary enrichment with eicosapentaenoic and docosahexaenoic acids on in vitro neutrophil and monocyte leukotriene generation and neutrophil function. N Engl J Med 1985;312:1217.

142. Endres S, Ghorbani R, Kelley VE et al: The effect of dietary supplementation with n-3 polyunsaturated fatty acids on the synthesis of interleukin-1 and tumour necrosis factor by mononuclear cells. N Engl J Med 1989;320:265.

143. Endres S: Messengers and mediators: interactions among lipids, eicosanoids and cytokines. Am J Clin Nutr 1993;57(suppl):798S.

144. Tobin A, Suzuki Y, O'Morain CO: Controlled double blind cross over study of eicosapentaenoic acid (EPA) in chronic ulcerative colitis (UC). Gastroenterology 1990;98:A207.

145. Hillier K, Jewell R, Dorrell L et al: Incorporation of fatty acids from fish oil and olive oil into colonic mucosal lipids and effects upon eicosanoid synthesis in inflammatory bowel disease. Gut 1991;32: 1151.

146. Stenson WF, Cort D, Rodgers J et al: Dietary supplementation with fish oil in ulcerative colitis. Ann Intern Med 1992;116:609.

147. Aslan A, Triadafilopoulos G: Fish oil fatty acid supplementation in active ulcerative colitis: a double-blind, placebo-controlled, crossover study. Am J Gastroenterol 1992;87:432.

148. Lorenz R, Weber PC, Szimnau P et al: Supplementation with n-3 fatty acids from fish oil in chronic inflammatory bowel disease—a randomized, placebo-controlled, double-blind cross-over trial. J Intern Med 1989;225(suppl 1):225.

149. Hawthorne AB, Daneshmend TK, Hawkey CJ et al: Treatment of ulcerative colitis with fish oil supplementation: a prospective 12 month randomized controlled trial. Gut 1992;33:922.

150. Greenfield SM, Green AT, Teare JP et al: A randomized controlled study of evening primrose oil and fish oil in ulcerative colitis. Aliment Pharmacol & Ther 1993;7:159.

151. Esteve M, Gassull MA: Is there a role for omega-3 fatty acids in the treatment of IBD? In Gebos K, Rutgeerts P, Vantrappen G (eds): Update in Inflammatory Bowel Disease. Leuven: Katholieke Universiteit Leuven, 1992:121.

152. Fernández-Bañares F, Cabré E, González-Huix F et al: Enteral nutrition as primary therapy in Crohn's disease. Gut 1994;35(suppl 1):S55.

153. Reilly KJ, Rombeau JL: Metabolism and potential clinical applications of short-chain fatty acids. Clin Nutr 1993;12(suppl 1):S97.

154. Vernia P, Gnaedinger A, Hauck W et al: Organic anions and the diarrhoea of inflammatory bowel disease. Dig Dis Sci 1988;33:1353.

155. Roediger WEW: The colonic epithelium in ulcerative colitis: an energy-deficiency disease? Lancet 1980; 2:712.

156. Chapman MAS, Grahn MF, Boyle MA et al: Butyrate oxidation is impaired in the colonic mucosa of sufferers of quiescent ulcerative colitis. Gut 1994;35: 73.

157. Breuer RI, Buto SK, Christ ML et al: Rectal irrigation with short-chain fatty acids for distal ulcerative colitis. Preliminary report. Dig Dis Sci 1991;36:185.

158. Scheppach W, Sommer H, Kirchner T et al: Effect of butyrate enemas on the colonic mucosa in distal ulcerative colitis. Gastroenterology 1992;103:51.

159. Senagore AJ, MacKeigan JM, Scheider M et al: Short-chain fatty acid enemas: a cost-effective alternative in the treatment of nonspecific proctosigmoiditis. Dis Colon Rectum 1992;35:923.

160. Boughton-Smith NK, Evans SM, Hawkey CJ et al: Nitric oxide synthase activity in ulcerative colitis and Crohn's disease. Lancet 1993;342:338.

161. Di Lorenzo M, Bass J, Krantis A: Treatment of experimental necrotizing enterocolitis wiht L-arginine. Gastroenterology 1994;106:A604.

162. Neilly PJD, Anderson NH, Kirk SJ et al: Nitric oxide synthase inhibition blocks the pro-inflammatory action of arginine in experimental colitis. Proceedings of the Falk Symposium No. 76, Estoril-Cascais, Portugal, 1994.

163. Petschow BW, Carter DL, Hutton GD: Influence of orally administered epidermal growth factor on normal and damaged intestinal mucosa in rats. J Pediatr Gastroenterol Nutr 1993;17:49.

164. Luck MS, Bass P: Effect of epidermal growth factor on experimental colitis in the rat. J Pharmacol Exp Ther 1993;264:984.

165. Procaccino F, Reinshagen M, Hoffmann P et al: Protective effects of epidermal growth factor in an experimental model of colitis in rats. Gastroenterology 1994;107:12.

24

Enteral Nutrition and Liver Failure

FREDERICK D. WATANABE
ELAINE A. KAHAKU
ACHILLES A. DEMETRIOU

The liver is an integral organ for the synthesis and metabolism of most nutrients. The clinician must have a basic understanding of its vital functioning to prescribe nutritional treatment for liver dysfunction. This chapter reviews (1) normal nutrient metabolism, (2) the pathogenesis of liver disease, and (3) the nature of liver failure as it relates to nutritional therapy.

NORMAL NUTRIENT METABOLISM

The liver has a primary role in the synthesis and metabolism of nutrients. It is the center for glucose metabolism and storage. As in other cells, glucose brought into hepatocytes by facilitated diffusion is promptly phosphorylated to glucose 6-phosphate. The phosphorylated molecule is unable to pass back through the cell membrane; instead it is either used by the mitochondia to produce energy or is stored in the form of glycogen. Hepatocytes can store a larger amount of glycogen than most cells, although this represents a minor amount of energy reserve relative to the body's energy needs. Also unique to hepatocytes is the presence of glucose 6-phosphatase. This vital enzyme allows the dephosphorylation of glucose 6-phosphate to glucose, which can then be freely transported though the hepatocyte cell membrane to the bloodstream for delivery to the rest of the body.

Amino acid processing also depends largely on the liver. The major plasma proteins are albumin, globins, and fibrinogen; all but half the circulating globins are synthesized by the liver. The liver also degrades these proteins into their amino acid constituents for release into the circulation. Hence, the liver makes possible the steady availability of amino acids for protein synthesis in the body by using the plasma protein pool for amino acid storage. The liver's second major contribution to amino acid processing is its ability to deaminate amino acids so that their carbon chain can be used to synthesize glycogen and in the Krebs cycle. Although muscle can also catabolize branched-chain amino acids (BCAAs) to glutamine and keto acids, the liver is the sole organ able to process the aromatic amino acids (AAAs) for this purpose.

The liver is the primary organ for the detoxification of ammonia produced by deamination. Two scavenging mechanisms exist in the liver. Over 90 percent of the hepatocytes can synthesize urea—a small, water-soluble molecule subsequently excreted by the kidney. All hepatocytes, except those surrounding the central veins, can carry out ureagenesis. The majority of ammonia is detoxified through the urea cycle; however, a significant amount of ammonia escapes ureagenesis.[1] Additionally, deamination of amino acids by hepatocytes

417

produces more ammonia than is cleared by ureagenesis.

The removal of unprocessed and liver-derived ammonia is performed by hepatocytes surrounding the central vein.[1] These hepatocytes use a second system of ammonia salvaging, resulting in glutamine formation. These perivenular hepatocytes are positioned optimally as the "back-up" system for ammonia removal since they are the last hepatocytes encountered by the blood flow before blood exits the liver. Additionally, this glutamine salvage pathway has a much higher affinity for ammonia than the urea cycle. In vitro perfusion and isolated hepatocyte studies demonstrate a large reserve capacity for ammonia detoxification by these cells.[1] Glutamine is subsequently recycled into the normal amino acid pool; thus glutamine synthesis, although a method of plasma ammonia clearance, is unable to remove nitrogen waste products from patients.

The liver plays a primary role in lipid metabolism. The liver synthesizes apoproteins and phospholipids, regulates and synthesizes cholesterol, degrades fatty acids into smaller carbon fragments used for energy production, and desaturates fatty acids. Fats are metabolized in the gastrointestinal (GI) tract to triglycerides. Triglycerides combine with apoproteins and phospholipids to form chylomicrons, which travel through the lymphatics to the systemic circulation. Chylomicrons are cleared from the circulation by the adipose tissue—the repository for triglycerides—and by the liver. The adipose tissue removes the triglycerides from the chylomicron, leaving behind a lipoprotein remnant, low-density lipoprotein (LDL). LDL is in turn cleared by the liver by receptor-mediated endocytosis where it is catabolized to amino acids and cholesterol. The breakdown of LDL is an important regulatory mechanism because cholesterol downregulates endogenous cholesterol synthesis by the liver.

Hepatocyte mitochondria are a major site for free fatty acid (FFA) oxidation and ketogenesis. FFAs are released as a result of triglyceride catabolism in the adipose tissue or the hepatocyte itself. Subsequent cleavage of two-carbon fragments from the FFA chain result in acetyl coenzyme A (acetyl Co-A) formation. A fraction of the acetyl Co-A produced is directly oxidized to form adenosine triphosphate (ATP); the majority is condensed to acetoacetic acid. Acetoacetic acid and its oxidation product β-hydroxybutyric acid diffuse freely across the hepatocyte membrane where they are taken to other cells for conversion back to acetyl Co-A and use in energy generation.

The liver helps process vitamins and trace minerals. The formation and secretion of bile salts is essential for proper intestinal absorption of vitamins A, D, E, and K. Micelle formation and absorption of long- and short-chain fatty acids (LCFAs and SCFAs) is also a bile-salt-dependent process. The first hydroxylation step in vitamin D activation occurs in the liver, thereby influencing calcium homeostasis in the body. Additionally, trace metal metabolism—such as iron and copper—requires normal hepatocellular function.

Based on the preceding brief summary of the multiple synthetic, regulating, and detoxifying functions of the liver and its key role in metabolism, it is not surprising that liver failure often results in massive metabolic, physiologic, and nutritional derangement.

LIVER FAILURE

Definition

Attempts have been made to stratify and define the degree of liver dysfunction and quantitate its physiologic impact. The terminology describing liver dysfunction is confusing and continues to evolve as knowledge of the etiology and natural history of liver disease expands.[2] The etiologic factors of liver disease are multiple and varied (Table 24–1). Clinically, patients with liver disease can be stable, partially decompensated, or in overt failure.

Stable disease is seen in patients who are either asymptomatic or have well-compensated chronic disease. Chronic liver disease is generally accepted as liver dysfunction persisting longer than 6 months. Compensated chronic liver disease patients are stable, without exacerbation of the complications of liver disease, and generally are able to function well in society. As liver dysfunction persists, hepatocyte death and scarring take place with eventual development of cirrhosis. It is not known in cirrhotic patients what is the critical, minimal, normal mass needed to maintain adequate liver function and keep a patient well compensated. However, such patients have minimal tolerance to stress due to concomitant disease, prolonged fasting, or complications of liver disease.

Decompensated liver disease describes the inability of the patient who is either acutely ill or has chronic liver disease to maintain normal homeostasis. Sufficient decompensation re-

TABLE 24–1 Etiology of Liver Disease

Viral Hepatitis
Hepatitis A, B, C, D, E
Hepatitis Non-A, Non-B, Non-C (indeterminate)
Hepatitis due to herpes simplex, cytomegalovirus, Epstein-Barr virus, adenovirus, giant-cell hepatitis, echovirus

Drugs
Nonsteroidal anti-inflammatory drugs
  Acetaminophen, salicylates, piroxicam, pirprofen, ibuprofen, indomethcin, naproxen, diclofenac
Neuropsychiatric
  Valproic acid, diphenylhydantoin, iproclozide, prochloroperazine, imipramine, desipramine, amitriptyline
Antibiotics
  Tetracycline, sulfasalazine, isoniazid (with or without rifampicin), ketoconozole, 2'3'-dideoxyinosine (ddl), nitrofurantoin, sulfonamides
Anesthetics
  Halothane, enflurance, dimethylformamide (veterinary)
Herbal medicines
Hormonal drugs
  Propylthiouracil, flutamide
Hallucinogenic drugs
  Cocaine, phencyclidine
Cardiovascular drugs
  Lisinopril, methyldopa, hydralazine
Miscellaneous
  Nicotinic acid, disulfiram, cyproteron

Toxins
Mushrooms: *Amanita phalloides,* verna and virosa; *Lepiota* species
Hydrocarbons: Carbon tetrachloride, tichloroethylene, 2-nitropropane chloroform, monochlorobenzene
Aflatoxin
Yellow phosphorous

Miscellaneous Conditions
Wilson's disease
Acute fatty liver of pregnancy
Reye's syndrome
Hypoxic liver cell necrosis
Hyperthermia
Budd-Chiari syndrome
Veno-occlusive disease of the liver
Autoimmune hepatitis
Massive malignant infiltration of the liver
Partial hepatectomy
Liver transplantation
Galactosemia
Hereditary fructose intolerance
Tyrosinemia

sults in acute hepatic failure (AHF). AHF is specifically defined by liver dysfunction resulting in prothrombin time prolongation and coagulation factor V level less than half normal.[3] Implied is the elevation of serum liver transaminase levels and presence of cholestasis with elevated bilirubin. The presence of marked coagulopathy distinguishes the AHF patient from stable patients with liver disease; AHF patients have a less favorable prognosis.[2]

Liver failure ensues as hepatic function deteriorates; as a result, cognitive and neurologic encephalopathic changes appear. The development of encephalopathy bodes poorly for the AHF patient. The degree of encephalopathy varies from mild sedation to frank coma. Attempts to categorize encephalopathic AHF patients based on prognosis led to the development of two nomenclature systems. The first system was introduced by Trey and Davidson,[4] who were the first to define the term *fulminant hepatic failure* (FHF) (Table 24–2). This definition specified the development of encephalopathy within 8 weeks from the onset of liver dis-

TABLE 24–2   Nomenclature of Liver Failure

	Acute Hepatic Failure	Fulminant Hepatic Failure	Subfulminant Hepatic Failure	Hyperacute Liver Failure	Acute Liver Failure	Subacute Liver Failure	Late Onset Liver Failure
Encephalopathy	No	Yes	Yes	Yes	Yes	Yes	Yes
Time from onset of jaundice to encephalopathy	None	< 8 weeks or < 2 weeks	2–12 weeks	0–7 days	8–28 days	5–12 weeks	2–6 months
Cerebral edema	No	Frequent	Rare	Frequent	Frequent	Rare	Rare
Ascites	None	Rare	Frequent	Rare	Rare	Frequent	Frequent
Prognosis	Good	Poor to fair	Poor	Fair	Poor	Poor	Poor

ease and also stipulated the absence of preexisting liver disease. This definition soon proved to be too rigid because patients with chronic liver disease also developed acute, massive liver insufficiency. Furthermore, the natural history of disease identified patients with extremely rapid development of encephalopathy and others with gradually developing encephalopathy. Thus Bernuau and associates[3] proposed a refined definition that further divided patients based on how rapidly encephalopathy developed. The term FHF is used when encephalopathy develops within 2 weeks of the onset of jaundice; the term *subfulminant hepatic failure* (SFHF) describes patients in whom encephalopathy develops 2 to 12 weeks after jaundice appears. Bernuau also eliminated the stipulation that liver dysfunction appear in the absence of preexisting liver disease. This variation of the Trey and Davidson FHF definition is presently widely used.

Gimson and associates[5] further expanded the Trey and Davidson definition by proposing a category called *late onset hepatic failure* (LOHF). This describes patients in whom encephalopathy develops 2 to 6 months after the initial onset of liver dysfunction. These patients represent a group of individuals most likely to have chronic liver disease as opposed to the episodic nature of liver disease in FHF.

A second nomenclature has been proposed by O'Grady and colleagues[6] based on their experience with FHF. Using the descriptive term *liver failure*, O'Grady uses 1 week, 1 month, 3 months, and 6 months to define hyperacute, acute, subacute, and late onset failure, respectively. When adjusted for time-course of encephalopathic changes, the two classification systems seem to arrive at similar conclusions regarding outcome.[2] The O'Grady classification, however, found that patients with hyperacute liver failure had a better outcome than those in the acute liver failure subgroup.[6] This

finding remains insufficiently explained. For the purpose of this discussion, we will use the Bernuau variation of the Trey and Davidson nomenclature system.

Clinical Presentation

FHF afflicts over 2000 individuals annually; up to 10 times this number have chronic liver disease.[7] The presentation of FHF—whether in an individual without prior liver disease or in the patient with a cirrhotic liver from long-standing liver disease—is a rapidly debilitating process requiring admission into the intensive care unit (ICU).[8] Despite advances in medical care, mortality ranges from 70 to 90 percent.[8-12] Introduction of orthotopic liver transplantation (OLTx) has greatly improved survival,[13] but a large number of patients with FHF are unable to receive a transplant either because an organ is unavailable or because complications preclude transplantation.[7]

Metabolic disturbances are common in patients with FHF. Catabolic metabolism is the rule, with negative nitrogen balance and increased caloric demands well documented.[7,14-18] Hyponatremia, hypokalemia, hypocalciuria, hypophosphatemia, and hypomagnesemia develop.[8] Hypoglycemia from loss of glycogen stores—both actual and functional loss from reduced liver mass—is frequently encountered. A reduction in plasma zinc levels is also seen and felt to be clinically significant; however, its true relationship to hepatic encephalopathy is unclear.[19-22]

The severity of illness and rapidity of clinical deterioration preclude the routine use of enteral nutrition in FHF patients. Among the functional abnormalities observed in FHF patients, ileus is a well-recognized and frequent complication. Furthermore, present management of patients with hepatic encephalopathy seeks to reduce the amount of ammonia in the bloodstream. Coliforms in the GI tract produce ammonia through intraluminal urea lysis, which passively diffuses into the bloodstream. Normally this is quickly cleared from the portal blood by the liver; in patients with FHF this becomes a significant, persistent ammonia source. Therapy therefore includes administration of antibiotics to reduce bacterial activity in the GI tract and lactulose to reduce the absorption of ammonia in the colon.[7-12] Ileus and need for gut decontamination often make enteral feeding impractical.

When patients with subacute and late onset hepatic failure deteriorate, they also exhibit the aforementioned metabolic disturbances. However, because of their protracted illness before they developed encephalopathy, nutritional intervention is an important component of their management. The increased incidence of milder—stage I and II—encephalopathy with protracted clinical course and lack of ileus allows for use of enteral nutrition. Similarly, individuals with stable chronic liver disease may also benefit from nutritional supplementation and support.

The presentation of the patient with long-standing liver disease is highly variable and depends on the etiology of the underlying disease, the rate of its progression, and the development of complications. In general, patients with decompensated chronic liver disease have significant fibrosis and cirrhosis. As a result, development of portal hypertension, cholestasis, and hepatic encephalopathy are frequently seen complications during the late stages of the disease.

Portal vein pressure is normally low. The portal vein is unique in not having valves to prevent retrograde blood flow. Thus as the liver becomes cirrhotic and vascular resistance through the liver rises, the increase in portal vein pressure is transmitted to other collateral venous drainage systems. As a result, initially, collateral veins are able to accommodate the increased pressure and subsequent increase in blood flow. However, as portal pressure continues to rise, anatomically susceptible regions of venous drainage expand in caliber, forming varices. Over time, the vessel walls become unable to tolerate the high luminal pressure and rupture. Profuse bleeding can then ensue, resulting in shock and death. Regions particularly prone to development of varices include the venous plexus located at the esophagogastric junction as well as the luminal veins along the intestinal tract and colon. The resultant nitrogen load in the GI tract subsequently results in an increase in serum ammonia and can precipitate hepatic encephalopathy. Portal hypertension also leads to increased congestion within the GI tract. Relative venous stasis with increased vascular pressure inhibits nutrient and bile acid absorption. This also directly impairs intrinsic enterocyte functions, exacerbating the problem. Damage to the mucosal tight junctions also increases the risk of bacterial translocation from the gut and subsequent development of sepsis.

Shunting and diversion of blood flow through collateral veins effectively decreases the liver's functional mass. Ammonia and toxins freely pass into the general systemic circulation. Translocated bacteria remain unfiltered by Kupffer's cells in the liver, making the development of sepsis more likely. Glucose regulation and storage, amino acid metabolism, and lipid metabolism are all impaired.

Associated with the development of cirrhosis and portal hypertension is the accumulation of serous fluid in the peritoneum. The mechanism of ascites formation is not fully understood; it has been shown that there is inappropriate retention of sodium and water by the kidneys despite the patient's being in a hyperdynamic, hypervolemic state.[23] Currently it is believed that in portal hypertension, there is initial accommodation of the retarded blood flow by the splanchnic venous plexus. As hypertension persists and increases, this accommodation is maximized with spillover into the systemic venous circulation, resulting in excessive peripheral vasodilatation. The resultant decrease in systemic vascular resistance invokes a cascade of regulatory hormonal factors, leading to renal sodium and volume retention and subsequent extravasation of this extra fluid into the peritoneal cavity.

Ascites formation can be rapid and unrelenting. Increased intraperitoneal fluid content has been known to compromise diaphragmatic motion and respiration, compress the stomach and intestines, and become a physical burden for the patient when ambulating. Decompression—paracentesis—is performed by inserting a sterile needle into the abdomen and withdrawing the ascitic fluid. Several liters of fluid can be removed in this fashion; unfortunately, this procedure may have to be performed very frequently. Aside from the physical risk of needle insertion (viscus perforation, bleeding), paracentesis also causes large fluid shifts between the intravascular and extravascular spaces. Large amounts of electrolytes and protein accompany the ascitic fluid, necessitating

25 percent albumin intravenous (IV) infusion following these procedures. Infection of the ascitic fluid may result in spontaneous bacterial peritonitis (SBP). The usual causative agents are enteric; the increased risk of bacterial translocation from the gut in portal hypertension places patients with ascites in a precarious position. Modern antibiotic management has decreased the mortality from this complication, although SBP remains troublesome in the cirrhotic, relatively immunocompromised patient.

Development of cholestasis can either be a primary event in liver disease, as in primary sclerosing cholangitis and biliary atresia, or it may be secondary to liver inflammation, fibrosis, and cirrhosis. Lack of bile flow is clinically recognized by the development of hyperbilirubinemia; however, the mechanism of cholestasis is not always understood. Bile acids are cholesterol-derived salts formed by hepatocytes and excreted through the bile cannuliculi into the bile duct. Joining pancreatic digestive secretions on entering the duodenum, bile salts function as detergents, forming micelles required for intestinal absorption of LCFAs as well as other fat-soluble compounds such as vitamins A, D, E, and K. Reducing the secretion of bile salts or obstructing the flow of bile decreases the intestinal absorption of fats. Absorption is significantly impaired in up to half of all cirrhotic patients, resulting in steatorrhea.[18] However, malabsorption of essential fatty acids and fat-soluble vitamins can occur without overt symptoms. Bile acids are also inherently hepatotoxic. Impaired flow out of the hepatocyte results in accumulation of these potent detergents with subsequent disruption of cellular membranes and hepatocellular necrosis. Hence the process of cholestasis is a self-perpetuating insult on the liver, leading to more hepatocellular damage, fibrosis, and worsening cholestasis.

As previously mentioned, development of encephalopathy is a late clinical finding suggesting severe end-stage liver disease. For the medical management of patients with severe liver disease, it is important to recognize and avoid exacerbating factors that can induce hepatic encephalopathy. Controversy still exists regarding the pathogenesis of hepatic encephalopathy.[8,24,25] Interestingly, "hepatic encephalopathy" encompasses two distinct processes. In the patient with acute disease, encephalopathy is characterized by increased brain edema and increased intracranial pressure with decreased cerebral blood perfusion. The patient with chronic liver disease develops encephalopathy without cerebral edema; intracranial

pressure and perfusion pressure are usually normal. This latter presentation is referred to as portal-systemic encephalopathy (PSE), since the critical clinical event appears to be shunting of blood directly into the systemic circulation, thereby bypassing the liver. PSE may develop slowly from increasing collateralization or acutely with the medical or surgical placement of a decompressive shunt for treatment of bleeding due to portal hypertension.

The role of ammonia and protein degradation in hepatic encephalopathy was first recognized at the turn of the century when dogs with Eck fistulas developed encephalopathy on meat feeding.[24] Hyperammonemia was later associated with the development of both forms of encephalopathy,[8,24,25] while reduction in ammonia was often associated with improved mental status.[8,24,25] Ammonia has been demonstrated to accumulate in the neurons of experimental animals, interfering with both inhibitory and excitatory synaptic functions.[24] Ammonia accumulation also has been associated with impaired cerebral energy metabolism,[26] blood-brain barrier alteration,[24] and alterations in extraneuronal parenchymal elements, especially astrocytes.[24]

Alternatively, a number of other studies indicate that ammonia is not the only important factor in the development of encephalopathy. Ammonia levels alone do not predict either the development or severity of hepatic encephalopathy.[24,25] A particular arterial ammonia level may be found in both a comatose and a fully alert patient. Additionally, threshold levels do not exist that correlate with severity or have prognostic significance. Other factors that have been implicated in the pathogenesis of hepatic encephalopathy include the composition of amino acids in the brain and the specific role of tryptophan.

Transport of amino acids across the blood-brain barrier is a carrier-mediated, gradient-dependent process. During liver failure, the serum amino acid profile changes as the concentration of AAAs—especially phenylalanine, methionine, tyrosine, tryptophan, aspartate, and glutamate—rises relative to the BCAAs, resulting in preferential transport of AAAs into the brain. AAAs are themselves neurotransmitter precursors; development of encephalopathy therefore could be due to inappropriate synaptic activity, competitive inhibition by AAAs, or subsequently synthesized neurotransmitters.[24,25]

The AAA tryptophan has been specifically implicated in the development of hepatic encephalopathy.[24] Tryptophan is a precursor of the neurotransmitter serotonin (5HT), which is in turn associated with sleep and psychiatric disorders. Animal studies using direct infusion of tryptophan demonstrated increased 5HT synthesis and turnover;[27] human autopsy studies demonstrate increased levels of monoamine oxidase,[28] increased levels of 5HT metabolites,[29] and increased 5HT receptor density.[24] Collectively, experimental data suggest that accumulation of 5HT metabolites or a net paradoxic decrease in synaptic 5HT can result in the sleep disturbance and psychiatric changes associated with hepatic encephalopathy.[24]

Other theories have been put forth attempting to explain the pathophysiology of hepatic encephalopathy, including altered cerebral energy metabolism, glutamine synthesis, and endogenous g-aminobutyric acid analog synthesis.[24,25] None to date has been shown to explain reliably and completely the pathogenesis of hepatic encephalopathy. Nevertheless, hyperammonemia is believed to be an integral part of hepatic encephalopathy; its management has relied on reducing ammonia by lowering protein intake and thus simultaneously reducing amino acid ingestion.

NUTRITIONAL ASSESSMENT IN LIVER DISEASE

The role of nutritional support in patients with varying degrees of liver failure is to prevent or treat malnutrition. It is clear that liver failure is accompanied by significant metabolic derangement; in addition, with increasing severity of failure, it becomes very difficult to assess the patient's nutritional status properly and provide balanced nutritional supplementation. However, proper nutritional management appears to improve patient survival and reduce the incidence of complications. Furthermore, specific use of nutrients is an essential and integral part of the management of patients with liver failure in general and of those with hepatic encephalopathy and ascites in particular.

Determining the nutritional status of a patient with severe liver disease is difficult. Most currently used clinical signs and nutritional markers for standard nutritional assessment are affected by the degree of liver failure, and it is difficult to determine whether a specific abnormality is a result of malnutrition or liver failure. For example, assessing weight gain or loss is made difficult by changes in the volume of ascites and tissue edema. Anthropomorphic measurements are also affected by the presence of tissue edema. Delayed-type hypersensitivity skin testing may demonstrate anergy due to immunosuppression secondary to liver failure and decreased liver synthetic function rather than to malnutrition. Similarly, serum albumin, prealbumin, retinol-binding protein, and transferrin levels as well as levels of other serum protein markers may be depressed due to poor liver synthetic function rather than to malnutrition. Bone marrow suppression can also develop as part of the liver failure syndrome, thus making the use of total lymphocyte count monitoring for nutritional assessment difficult. For the same reasons, determining the efficacy of a specific nutritional intervention in patients with liver failure is also difficult.

In patients with chronic liver disease, close follow-up study and serial examination of a patient are required to understand the pattern of disease (improvement vs deterioration) and nutritional status in the context of dietary habits, socioeconomic environment, coexisting diseases, active use of alcohol, and physical examination findings. Serial weight measurements in conjunction with abdominal girth and tension determinations and anthropomorphic determinations will usually provide insight into a patient's nutritional status. In patients with stable compensated chronic liver failure, intimate clinical knowledge of the patient allows some degree of nutritional assessment. Serologic and other laboratory markers are used in the same manner. The issue of nutritional assessment becomes more challenging when patients have acute exacerbation and fluctuations in the level of liver failure, making nutritional assessment very difficult. In patients with FHF, nutritional assessment is usually not a problem because these patients do not have chronic disease with ascites and other stigmata, and they were usually in good nutritional status before the onset of their illness.

As mentioned previously, cholestasis impairs absorption of fat-soluble vitamins, making serum levels of vitamins A and E nonspecific but useful indicators of fat malabsorption in the absence of steatorrhea. Although important in assessing compliance to therapy, the measurement of 25-OH vitamin D reflects the liver's synthetic properties more than nutritional status. Vitamin K is the other fat-soluble vitamin of importance; indirect measurement of vitamin K activity is usually made by determining the prothrombin time. However, since liver-related abnormalities of the coagulation cascade also prolong the prothrombin time, the use of this measurement for nutritional evaluation is limited.

MALNUTRITION IN LIVER DISEASE

Despite the described difficulties in assessing patients with severe liver disease, a number of studies attempted to determine the incidence and degree of malnutrition in patients with liver disease. As expected, patients with alcoholic cirrhosis have the highest incidence of malnutrition. Mendenhal and colleagues[30] found the prevalence of malnutrition to reach 72.2 percent in severely ill patients with alcoholic liver disease. The incidence of malnutrition in patients with nonalcoholic liver disease (chronic cirrhosis) is 10 to 70 percent.[14,31]

Numerous risk factors exist for the development of malnutrition in patients with liver disease. As alluded to above, alcoholic liver disease, because of its chronicity and other socioeconomic factors, is associated with a high incidence of malnutrition. In addition, biliary disorders result in malabsorption of fats and fat-soluble vitamins. PSC is frequently accompanied by inflammatory bowel disease, with the latter contributing to water, electrolyte, and blood loss and exacerbation of malabsorption. Congenital inborn errors of metabolism may affect carbohydrate, amino acid, and lipid metabolism in organs other than the liver, creating multiorgan deficits affecting proper nutrient use.

Liver disease alters the palatability of ingested nutrients, thereby reducing their consumption. Anorexia and nausea occur in up to 87 percent of patients with advanced liver disease.[32] Alterations in taste and satiety also contribute to decreased nutrient intake.[33] The natural tendency to reduce enteral intake may be exacerbated by medical restrictions on diet. Ascites formation is initially treated by restricting salt and liquid intake. Hepatic encephalopathy is managed by restricting protein intake. Both result in diets that place additional constraints on the volume, quality, and palatability of ingested food.

The repetitiveness and severity of complications of liver disease also affect a patient's nutritional status and increase nutritional requirements. Massive blood loss with hospitalization in variceal bleeding, sepsis, and SBP are all likely complications that place increased stress on the patient. Ascites alone increases resting energy expenditure (REE) by approximately 10 percent.[18] Large-volume paracentesis of ascites removes albumin and other proteins contributing to protein malnutrition.

In addition to decreased nutrient absorption and portosystemic blood shunting, the changes occurring in patients with severe liver disease also affect nutrient use. Healthy subjects obtain only 35 percent of their energy from fat sources after an overnight fast.[14-16,31] This is increased to 75 percent in cirrhotics.[14,15] This alteration in fuel use resembles that seen following prolonged starvation and probably results from the development of insulin resistance in these patients.[15] Hence, even if "true" malnutrition cannot be adequately evaluated in a patient, chronic cirrhosis appears to be the physiologic equivalent of starvation.

NUTRITIONAL THERAPEUTIC CONSIDERATIONS IN LIVER FAILURE

The overall goal of nutritional management is to establish adequate protein-calorie intake while respecting the limitations and restrictions imposed by underlying disease therapy and the extent of liver failure. Nutritional education and close follow-up examination are mandatory for these patients. As already discussed, liver disease is a dynamic process with variable presentation, clinical course, and outcome. The need for serial examinations to assess a patient's nutritional status alone necessitates closely following the patient. Further, educating the patient about nutritional goals, the rationale behind therapy, and food choices empowers them to take responsibility for their care, resulting in better compliance.

The energy requirement in liver disease depends highly on the patient's clinical status. Using indirect calorimetry, Owen and coworkers[34] demonstrated that stable, compensated cirrhotic patients had an overall caloric requirement similar to that of healthy controls. This finding has been subsequently confirmed by other investigators.[35-36] However, when caloric expenditure was adjusted for lean body mass using creatinine clearance, cirrhotic patients were found to have a higher REE. Interpreting these findings is difficult, however, since both lean body mass and energy expenditure determinations have inherent variability. Furthermore, the development of ascites and other acute complications (e.g., infection, bleeding) makes individualization of nutritional objectives imperative.

Generally, a caloric intake of 30 to 35 kcal/kg/day should be adequate for a stable adult cirrhotic patient. During periods of increased stress (e.g., after a surgical procedure, gastrointestinal bleeding, infection) the caloric intake should be increased to 40 to 45 kcal/kg/day. In the presence of ascites, an additional upward caloric adjustment of 10 percent is also required. Whatever the starting caloric intake, frequent assessment to establish adequacy of a nutritional supplementation plan is necessary. Caloric intake should be adjusted empirically; caloric loads up to 55 kcal/kg/day may be necessary in malnourished individuals suffering from multiple complications of end-stage liver disease. However, overzealous administration of calories should be avoided to prevent fatty infiltration in the liver.[15]

Perhaps as important as the total caloric requirement are the caloric sources and frequency of meals. Low-fat diets are not necessary in the patient with liver failure. As mentioned earlier, alterations in the sense of taste, abnormal satiety, and nausea decrease the palatability of food. A diet that derives 30 to 40 percent of calories from fat will improve patient compliance by making meals more appetizing. Additional benefits include a more calorie-dense meal, reducing meal volume in the anorectic patient, and ingestion of more fat-soluble vitamins.

Protein requirements in stable adult cirrhotic patients can be met with a total protein load of 0.8 to 1.0 g/kg/day or 40 to 60 g of protein/day for the average adult patient. The presence of stress or preexisting malnutrition may necessitate 1.5 to 2 g/kg/day of protein intake. Generally, protein intake should be accompanied by an appropriate nonprotein calorie load to ensure maximal anabolic use. Intake should begin slowly (20 to 30 g/day) and gradually rise on a daily basis because hepatic encephalopathy can be precipitated or exacerbated even with low protein loads. Development of hepatic encephalopathy should prompt reduction of protein intake. Earlier recommendations suggested dietary abstinence from protein to minimize ammonia production. However, the resultant catabolism of endogenous proteins negates this advantage, and nutritional therapy should now be directed at providing 0.5 to 0.8 mg/kg/day of protein. The actual protein load for a specific patient must be individualized based on patient tolerance.

In addition to the amount of protein administered, the source and amino acid composition of protein products delivered have also been investigated. Vegetable protein diets have received considerable attention in the treatment of patients with hepatic encephalopathy.[37-39] Vegetable proteins are high in fiber and accelerate intestinal transit time. Weber and coworkers[37] found a 160 percent increase in stool output with increased nitrogen content in the bacterial flora of the stool. Unfortunately, a high-vegetable protein regimen is calorically less dense and relatively unpalatable. The difficulty in achieving proper caloric intake and the poor compliance associated with its unpalatability render a vegetable-protein diet impractical.[15,40]

Diets increasing the consumption of BCAAs have been introduced since Fischer and Baldessarini first put forth their theory of false neurotransmitters and their potential role in the pathogenesis of hepatic encephalopathy.[41] This subject has been reviewed numerous times, with the balance of clinical data failing to establish a significant advantage of BCAA preparations over standard amino acid regimens.[15,40,42-45] Munoz[15] reviewed nine clinical trials that examined the impact BCAA formulations had on nitrogen balance vs conventional protein preparations and casein preparations. In two studies, the BCAA group demonstrated a superior improvement in nitrogen balance; however, Marchensini and associates[46] extended their study to 6 months, at which time the control group also demonstrated similar positive changes in nitrogen balance. Six other studies demonstrated equivalent improvement in nitrogen balance between control and experimental groups. This equivalence fails to make a compelling case for the use of BCAA preparations, especially with the significant additional cost incurred relative to conventional amino acid preparations.

BCAA therapy, however, has also been proposed not simply as a nutritional supplement but rather as a therapy for hepatic encephalopathy. Naylor and colleagues[47] performed a meta-analysis on five randomized controlled studies from a total of nine randomized controlled studies found in the literature through December 1987. All the studies administered parenteral BCAA solutions as part of the treatment of patients with acute hepatic encephalopathy. The results demonstrated a significant reversal of hepatic coma; however, the heterogeneity of the study designs makes further interpretation unreliable.

The use of enteral BCAA formulations for the treatment of patients with hepatic encephalopathy was examined by Cerra and coworkers,[48] who studied 22 patients with "refractory" hepatic encephalopathy in a double-blind controlled study. Here, improvement in hepatic encephalopathy and protein use were demonstrated, with the treatment group being able to tolerate twice the nitrogen load of the control group. Unfortunately, there has been no subsequent confirmation of these findings. The present status of BCAA use is limited to specific instances where conventional amino acid preparations are not tolerated and adequate amounts of protein cannot be administered.

A nutritional intervention that should be considered is increasing meal frequency to five or six times per day, including a late-evening snack. This minimizes the fasting period and subsequently spares fat and protein stores as alluded to earlier. Furthermore, patients with significant cholestasis benefit from the smaller boluses of fat delivered with each meal by minimizing bile salt requirements, maximizing the efficiency of fatty acid absorption, and reducing steatorrhea.

Dietary supplementation regimens in cholestatic liver disease are well established for fat-soluble vitamins and controversial for trace metals and minerals. Vitamin A, D, E, and K enteral absorption relies on bile salt micellular formation and fatty acid absorption in the GI tract. Additionally, specific liver-derived binding proteins are required for the proper use of vitamins A and D. Supplementation should be preceded by direct serum measurement of vitamin A and 25-hydroxy vitamin D. Vitamin E is best assessed by calculating the ratio of the serum vitamin E level to the total serum lipid concentration (serum cholesterol, triglycerides, and phospholipids); vitamin K is indirectly assessed by measuring prothrombin time. Initiation of vitamin supplementation is probably not warranted unless vitamin deficiency is documented. Risk factors justifying screening for vitamin deficiency include infancy, cholestasis for longer than 1 year, serum total bilirubin greater than 4 mg/dl, and malnutrition.

An interesting development has been the introduction of the water-soluble form of vitamin E, D-α-tocopheryl-polyethylene glycol-1000 succinate (TPGS). TPGS has been found efficacious in correcting vitamin E deficiency in refractory cases treated with "traditional" oral vitamin E preparations (α-tocopheryl, α-tocopheryl acetate, and α-tocopheryl succinate).[49,50] Additionally, TPGS augments absorption of other fat-soluble substrates when the two are administered concomitantly.[51,52] Further clinical investigations are being carried out to examine the use of TPGS to enhance the efficiency of absorption of other fat-soluble vitamins.

Trace metal and mineral requirements in patients with liver failure have been investigated extensively with major focus on zinc, selenium, chromium, copper, and iron. The latter two are known to be directly hepatoxic in excess quantities; selenium and chromium deficiencies have been described, but the practical clinical implications are questionable and the efficacy of supplementation has not been adequately investigated.[53] Zinc deficiency in liver disease has been well documented.[54-56] Depressed serum zinc levels have been associated with anorexia, altered taste, hepatic encephalopathy, acrodermatitis,[57-59] immune dysfunction,[60] altered protein metabolism, and impaired wound healing. Zinc deficiency is also correlated with the exacerbation of copper and iron overload. Supplementation with either enteral or parenteral zinc has been reported to correct most of the signs and symptoms associated with zinc deficiency; however, general routine zinc supplementation in patients with acute and chronic liver disease awaits proof of efficacy based on controlled, prospective clinical trials.

Salt restriction is a vital component of the diet of patients with ascites. Mobilization of extravascular fluid is usually accomplished by the simultaneous administration of diuretics and the creation of a net negative balance of sodium.[61] Simply lowering sodium to 40 mEq/day improves ascites in up to 20 percent of cirrhotic patients; dietary restriction of sodium is more efficient than diuretic therapy alone in reducing total body sodium stores.[62] In many instances of "resistant" ascites, a careful history will reveal noncompliance with the dietary regimen.

The vehicle delivering enteral nutrition is as important as the nutrients being administered. The only absolute contraindication to enteral feeding in these patients is mechanical obstruction; however, the patient's individual needs must be considered in deciding between enteral and parenteral approaches. Stable cirrhotic patients with no more than mild hepatic encephalopathy are usually able to comply with a dietary regimen of nutritional therapy. However, individuals with either worsening encephalopathy or severe anorexia will require enteral supplementation. Enteral feeding devices include nasoenteric tubes (nasoduodenal and nasojejunal), percutaneous gastrostomy and jejunostomy feeding tubes placed under endoscopic or radiologic guidance, and surgically placed gastrostomy and jejunostomy tubes. A thorough review of these tube-feeding devices, including detailed discussion of complications associated with their use, has been recently published.[63] Nasoenteric devices should be reserved for situations requiring less than 30 days of mechanical intervention. Prolonged placement of nasoenteric tubes can result in nasal mucosal ulceration, sinusitis, otitis media, and gastroesophageal reflux with pulmonary aspiration. The latter is the result of both mechanical stenting of the lower esophageal sphincter (LES) as well as the induction of inappropriate transient relaxation of the LES by pharyngeal stimulation.[63] In the cirrhotic patient with varices there is also the potential risk of esophageal erosive or traumatic bleeding;[64] however, this must be weighed against that of more invasive procedures.

The percutaneous or surgical placement of a gastrostomy or jejunostomy tube should be reserved for individuals requiring feeding support for more than 30 days. Gastric varices and coagulopathy potentially increase the risk for bleeding during tube placement, making portal hypertension a relative contraindication for this procedure. Additionally, the presence of severe ascites must be taken into account. Generally, most patients with liver failure will not need this extent of enteral support; if they do, such a device must be placed carefully. If enteral support is not possible, the patient will require parenteral nutritional support.

CONCLUSION

Enteral nutritional therapy in liver failure is restricted to patients with subacute, late onset, and chronic failure before complete loss of hepatic function. Although patients with hepatic failure are catabolic and probably have some degree of malnutrition, accurate, rational nutritional management is impaired by limitations of our ability to assess the degree of malnutrition. At present, serial examination by a skilled clinician represents the best means of following these patients.

Nutritional therapy in patients with liver failure is limited by lack of clear understanding of the etiology of development of cerebral edema and encephalopathy, and the complexities of the liver. The primary objective remains the reduction of catabolism and replenishment of depleted nutrients. However, the role of nutritional therapy is expanding. Therapy for ascites is based on salt and fluid management. The traditional line drawn between hepatic encephalopathy and the administration of proteins has changed; severe protein restriction is giving way to careful protein administration to maintain nitrogen balance and possibly use of specific amino acid formulations. It is possible that nutritional therapies will become more important in managing the complex physiologic and metabolic derangements seen in patients with liver failure.

REFERENCES

1. Haussinger D: Nitrogen metabolism in the liver: structural and functional organization and physiological relevance. Biochem J 1990;267:281–290.
2. Woolf G: Definitions and etiology. In Demetriou AA (ed): Support of the Acutely Failing Liver. Austin, TX: RG Landes, 1994:5–21.
3. Bernuau J, Rueff B, Benhamou J: Fulminant and subfulminant liver failure: definitions and causes. Semin Liver Dis 1986;6:97–106.
4. Trey C, Davidson C: The management of fulminant hepatic failure. Prog Liver Dis 1970;3:282–298.
5. Gimson AES, O'Grady J, Ede RJ et al: Late onset hepatic failure: clinical, serological and histological features. Hepatology 1986;6:288–294.
6. O'Grady J, Schalm SW, Williams R: Acute liver failure: redefining the syndromes. Lancet 1993;342:273–275.
7. Lee WM: Acute liver failure. N Engl J Med 1993;329: 1862–1868.
8. Watanabe F, Rosenthal P: Medical therapy. In Demetriou AA (ed): Support of the Acutely Failing Liver. Austin, TX: RG Landes, 1994:22–32.
9. Capocaccia L, Angelico M: Fulminant hepatic failure: clinical features, etiology, epidemiology and current management. Dig Dis Sci 1991;36:775–779.
10. Douglas DD, Rakela J: Fulminant hepatitis. In Kaplowitz N (ed): Liver and Biliary Diseases. Baltimore: Williams & Wilkins, 1992:279–288.
11. Fingerote RJ, Bain VG: Fulminant hepatic failure. Am J Gastroenterol 1993;88:1000–1010.
12. O'Grady JG, Portmann B, Williams R: Fulminant hepatic failure. In Schiff L, Schiff ER (eds): Diseases of the Liver, 7th edition. Philadelphia: JB Lippincott, 1993:1077–1090.
13. Hoofnagle JH, Carithers RL, Shapiro C et al: Fulminant hepatic failure: summary of a workshop. Hepatology 1995;21:240–252.
14. McCullough AJ, Tavill AS: Disordered energy and protein metabolism in liver disease. Semin Liver Dis 1991;11:265–277.
15. Munoz SJ: Nutritional therapies in liver disease. Semin Liver Dis 1991;11:278–291.
16. Marsano L, McClain CJ: Nutrition and alcoholic liver disease. J Parenter Enter Nutr 1991;15:337–344.
17. Keohane PP, Attrill H, Grimble G et al: Enteral nutrition in malnourished patients with hepatic cirrhosis and acute encephalopathy. J Parenter Enter Nutr 1983;7: 346–350.
18. Munoz SJ: Difficult management problems in fulminent hepatic failure. Semin Liver Dis 1993;13: 395–413.
19. Reding P, Duchateau J, Bataille C: Oral zinc supplementation improves hepatic encephalopathy. Results of a randomised controlled trial. Lancet 1984;2: 493–495.
20. McClain CJ, Marsano L, Burk RF et al: Trace metals in liver disease. Semin Liver Dis 1991;11:321–339.
21. Riggio O, Ariosto F, Merli M et al: Short-term oral zinc supplementation does not improve chronic hepatic encephalopathy. Results of a double-blind crossover trial. Dig Dis Sci 1991;36:1204–1208.
22. Kimball SR, Chen SJ, Risica R et al: Effects of zinc deficiency on protein synthesis and expression of specific mRNAs in rat liver. Metabolism 1995;44:126–133.

23. Wong F, Blendis L: Pathophysiology of sodium retention and ascites formation in cirrhosis: role of atrial natriuretic factor. Semin Liver Dis 1994;14(1):59–70.

24. Butterworth RF: Hepatic encephalopathy. In Arias IM, Boyer JL, Fausto N et al (eds): The Liver: Biology and Pathobiology, 3rd edition. New York: Raven Press, 1994:1193–1208.

25. Marsano L, McClain C: How to manage both acute and chronic hepatic encephalopathy. J Crit Illness 1993; 8:579–599.

26. Bessman SP, Wang W, Mohan C: Ammonia inhibits insulin stimulation of the Krebs cycle: further insight into mechanism of hepatic coma. Neurochem Res 1991;16:805–811.

27. Ogihara K, Mozai T, Hirai SN: Tryptophan as a cause of hepatic coma. N Engl J Med 1966;275:1255.

28. Bergeron M, Reader TA, Pomier Layrargues B et al: Monoamines and metabolites in autopsied brain tissue from cirrhotic patients with hepatic encephalopathy. Neurochem Res 1989;14:853–859.

29. Raghavendra Rao VL, Giguere JF, Pomier Layrargues G et al: Increased activities of MAO_A and MAO_B in autopsied brain tissue from cirrhotic patients with hepatic encephalopathy. Brain Res 1993;621:349–352.

30. Mendenhall CL, Anderson S, Weesner RE et al: Protein-calorie malnutrition associated with alcoholic hepatitis. Am J Med 1984;76:211–222.

31. Kestell MF, Lee SP: Clinical nutrition in acute and chronic liver disease. Semin Gastrointest Dis 1993;4: 116–126.

32. McCullough AJ, Tavill AS: Disordered energy and protein metabolism in liver disease. Semin Liver Dis 1991;11:277.

33. Deems RO, Friedman MI, Friedman LS et al: Chemosensory function, food preference and appetite in human liver disease. Appetite 1993;20:209–216.

34. Owen OE, Trapp VE, Reichard GA et al: Nature and quantity of fuels consumed in patients with alcoholic cirrhosis. J Clin Invest 1983;72:1821–1832.

35. Jhangiani SS, Agarwal N, Holmes R et al: Energy expenditure in chronic alcoholics with and without liver disease. Am J Clin Nutr 1986;44:323–329.

36. John WJ, Phillips R, Ott L et al: Resting energy expenditure in patients with alcoholic hepatitis. J Parenter Enter Nutr 1989;13:124–127.

37. Weber FL, Minco D, Fresard KM et al: Effects of vegetable diets on nitrogen metabolism in cirrhotic subjects. Gastroenterology 1985;85:538–544.

38. Greenberger NJ, Carley J, Schenker S et al: Effect of vegetable and animal protein diets in chronic hepatic encephalopathy. Dig Dis Sci 1977;22:845–855.

39. Uribe M, Marquez MA, Ramos GG et al: Treatment of chronic portal systemic encephalopathy with vegetable and animal protein diets: a controlled crossover study. Dig Dis Sci 1982;27:1109–1116.

40. Mullen KD, Weber FL: Role of nutrition in hepatic encephalopathy. Semin Liver Dis 1991;11:292–304.

41. Fischer JE, Baldessarini RJ: False neurotransmitters and hepatic failure. Lancet 1971;ii:75.

42. McCullough AJ, Mullen KD, Smanik EJ et al: Nutritional therapy and liver disease. Med Clin North Am 1989;18:619–643.

43. Eriksson LS, Conn HO: Branched-chain amino acids in the management of hepatic encephalopathy: an analysis of variants. Hepatology 1989;10:228–246.

44. Horst D, Grace ND, Conn HO et al: Comparison of dietary protein with an oral, branched-chain enriched amino acid supplement in chronic protal-systemic encephalopathy. Hepatology 1984;4:279–287.

45. Guarnieri GF, Tolgo G, Situlin R: Muscle studies on malnutrition in patients with liver cirrhosis. In Capoccaia

L, Fisher JE (eds): Hepatic Encephalopathy in Chronic Liver Failure. New York: Plenum Press, 1984:193–208.

46. Marchensini G, Dioguardi FS, Bianchi GP et al: Long term oral branched chain amino acid treatment in chronic hepatic encephalopathy. A randomized double blind casein controlled trial. J Hepatol 1990;11: 92–101.

47. Naylor CD, O'Rourke K, Detsky A et al: Parenteral nutrition with branched-chain amino acids in hepatic encephalopathy: a meta-analysis. Gastroenterology 1989; 97:1033–1042.

48. Cerra FB, McMillen M, Angelico R et al: Cirrhosis, encephalopathy and improved results with metabolic support. Surgery 1983;94:612–619.

49. Sokol RJ, Butler-Simon N, Bettis D et al: Tocopheryl polyethylene glycol 1000 succinate (TPGS) therapy for vitamin E deficiency in chronic childhood cholestasis. Gastroenterology 1991;100:A799. Abstract.

50. Sokol RJ, Heubi JE, Butler-Simon N et al: Treatment of vitamin E deficiency during chronic childhood cholestasis with oral D-alpha tocopheryl polyethylene glycol-1000 succinate. Gastroenterology 1987;93:975.

51. Sokol RJ, Johnson KE, Karrer FM et al: Improvement of cyclosporin absorption in children after liver transplantation by means of water-soluble vitamin E. Lancet 1991;96:212.

52. Argao EA, Heubi JE, Hollis BW et al: D-alpha-tocopheryl-polyethylene-glycol-1000 succinate enhances the absorption of vitamin D in chronic cholestatic liver disease of infancy and childhood. Pediatr Res 1992; 31:146.

53. McLain CJ, Marsano L, Burke RF et al: Trace metals in liver disease. Semin Liver Dis 1991;11:321–339.

54. Grungreiff K, Abicht K, Kluge M et al: Clinical studies on zinc in chronic liver diseases. Zeitschrift fur Gastroenterologie 1988;26:409–415.

55. Grungreiff K, Presser HJ, Franke D et al: Correlations between zinc, amino acids and ammonia in liver cirrhosis. Zeitschrift fur Gastroenterologie 1989;27: 731–735.

56. Nabdu SS, Chawla YK, Nath R et al: Serum and urinary zinc in fulminant hepatic failure. J Gastroenterol Hepatol 1989;4:209–213.

57. McLaine CJ, Souter C, Steele N et al: Severe zinc deficiency presenting with acrodermatitis during hyperalimantation: diagnosis, pathogenesis and treatment. J Clin Gastroenterol 1980;2:125–131.

58. McLaine CJ: Trace metal abnormalities in adults during hyperalimentation. J Parenter Enter Nutr 1981;5: 424–429.

59. Ecker RI, Achroeter AL: Acrodermatitis and acquired zinc deficiency. Arch Dermatol 1978;114:937–939.

60. Taniguchi S, Kaneto K, Hamada T: Acquired zinc deficiency associated with alcoholic liver cirrhosis. Inter J Derm 1995;34:651–652.

61. Forns X, Gines A, Gines P et al: Management of ascites and renal failure in cirrhosis. Semin Liver Dis 1994;14: 82–96.

62. Kirby DF, DeLegge MH, Fleming CR: American Gastroenterological Association technical review on tube feeding for enteral nutrition. Gastroenterology 1995; 108:1282–1301.

63. Mittal RK, Stewart WR, Schirmer BD: Effect of a catheter in the pharynx on the frequency of transient lower esophageal sphincter relaxations. Gastroenterology 1992;103:1236–1240.

64. Ritter DM, Rettke SR, Hughes RW Jr et al: Placement of nasogastric tubes and esophageal stethoscopes in patients with documented esophageal varices. Anesth Analg 1988;67(3):283–285.

25

Nutritional Support in Pancreatic Disease

AMY M. KUSSKE
DONNA REBER KATONA
HOWARD A. REBER

PANCREATIC PHYSIOLOGY

Exocrine Pancreas

The pancreas secretes 1 to 2 L/day of an alkaline (pH 8.0 to 8.3) fluid that contains more than 20 different digestive enzymes. The alkaline pancreatic juice helps to neutralize gastric acid in the duodenum and provides the optimal pH for the activity of the pancreatic digestive enzymes, which are synthesized in, stored in, and released from the pancreatic acinar cells. Pancreatic enzymes are proteolytic (e.g., trypsins, chymotrypsin, carboxypeptidases, ribonucleases, deoxyribonucleases, elastase), lipolytic (e.g., lipase, colipase, phospholipase A_2), and amylolytic (e.g., amylase). Although lipase and amylase are secreted in their active forms, the proteolytic enzymes and phospholipase A_2 are secreted as inactive "zymogens." Activation of trypsinogen to trypsin occurs when the zymogen is exposed to the duodenal enzyme enterokinase. Trypsin then converts the other zymogens to their active forms. In the intestine, the proteolytic enzymes digest proteins into peptides, lipase breaks fats into glycerol and fatty acids, phospholipase A_2 catalyzes the conversion of biliary lecithin to lysolecithin, and amylase converts starch to dissaccharides and dextrins.

Regulation of Secretion

Pancreatic secretion is under complex neurohormonal control. Ductal fluid and bicarbonate are secreted chiefly in response to the hormone secretin, which is released from the mucosa of the duodenum and proximal small bowel when acid enters the bowel lumen. Bicarbonate secretion is triggered when the pH of the duodenal lumen falls below 4.5. Acinar enzyme secretion is stimulated both by vagal cholinergic discharge and by the hormone cholecystokinin (CCK). CCK is released from the proximal small bowel by fatty acids, oligopeptides, and some amino acids.

Pancreatic secretion has been divided artificially into cephalic, gastric, and intestinal phases.[1] The *cephalic* phase begins with the sight, smell, and anticipation of food, and is mediated by vagal cholinergic pathways. Although mostly enzymes are secreted, some bicarbonate is also produced.[2] The *gastric* phase begins when food enters the stomach. Gastric distention, as well as the exposure of the stomach mucosa to nutrients (e.g., peptides), causes primarily an enzyme rich pancreatic secretion. This effect is blocked by atropine or truncal vagotomy. The *intestinal* phase begins when the chyme empties into the duodenum. This phase is important for the maintenance of enzyme output as gastric distention diminishes. Gastric acid is also responsible for pancreatic bicarbonate secretion. When the buffering effect of the food is lost, the duodenal pH begins to fall, and secretin is released.[3] Both neural and hormonal mechanisms are responsible for this phase, which involves both stimulatory (e.g., secretin, CCK, gastrin releasing peptide [GRP], bombesin, neurotensin, vasoactive intestinal polypeptide [VIP]), and inhibitory (e.g., pancreatic polypeptide [PP], calcitonin gene related peptide [CGRP], peptide YY [PYY], neuropeptide Y [NPY], somatostatin) effects on the pancreas.[4-7] In addition to these stimulatory and inhibitory effects, there is also evidence for a negative feedback mechanism for pancreatic secretion. The presence of pancreatic proteases and bile within the duodenum appears to inhibit the release of CCK. Thus, pancreaticobiliary diversion from the intestine is characterized by elevated plasma CCK levels and stimulation of pancreatic secretion. This may have some clinical relevance in patients with pain from chronic pancreatitis who are sometimes treated with large amounts of oral pancreatic enzymes in an effort to inhibit pancreatic secretion. There is some evidence that inhibition of secretion in this way relieves the pain.[8-10] In this circumstance, the enzymes are not being given to treat pancreatic insufficiency.

The quantity of pancreatic enzymes that is secreted in response to a meal is almost 90 percent in excess of what is actually needed for normal digestion. Thus, patients develop symptoms of malabsorption only when secretion falls to about 10 percent or less of normal.[11] Pancreatic insufficiency can result from blockage of the main pancreatic duct, which prevents the enzymes from entering the intestine (e.g., pancreatic cancer), from destruction of the pancreatic secretory parenchyma (e.g., chronic pancreatitis), and from surgical procedures that remove the pancreas or result in poor mixing of the gastric chyme with the pancreatic secretions (e.g., partial gastrectomy with gastrojejunostomy).

Pancreatic insufficiency affects fat absorption much more than protein or carbohydrate absorption because protein digestion is aided by gastric pepsin and small bowel brush border enzymes, and carbohydrate digestion is aided by salivary amylase. Moreover, fat malabsorption causes troublesome diarrhea, whereas malabsorption of protein and carbohydrate is generally asymptomatic.[12] On a diet containing 100 g of fat a day, normal subjects excrete 5 to

7 g/day of fat in the feces (i.e., 5 to 7 percent fat malabsorption is normal). A total pancreatectomy causes 70 percent fat malabsorption; partial pancreatic resections may not cause any malabsorption provided that the pancreatic remnant is normal. Vitamin malabsorption is rarely a problem in adults since water soluble B vitamins are absorbed throughout the small intestine, and fat soluble vitamins do not require pancreatic enzymes for absorption. Vitamin B_{12} malabsorption occurs in some patients, but is rarely a significant problem. Therefore, vitamin B_{12} replacement is usually unnecessary.

Among the specialized organs in the body, the pancreas exhibits, along with the liver and small intestine, the highest rate of protein synthesis and turnover. The acinar tissue synthesizes and secretes between 6 g and 20 g of digestive enzymes per day. As a result the pancreas is extremely vulnerable to protein deficiency states.

Endocrine Pancreas

The islets of Langerhans comprise 1 to 2 percent of the pancreatic mass, but they receive about 20 percent of the total pancreatic blood flow. They are dispersed throughout the pancreatic parenchyma, but some of the hormone secreting cells are concentrated in specific areas. The insulin secreting cells are evenly distributed and are usually localized in the core of each islet, where they form 60 to 80 percent of the cells. They are surrounded peripherally by a mantle of other cells that are specialized to secrete glucagon (15 to 20 percent of the islet cells), somatostatin (5 to 10 percent), or PP (15 to 20 percent). The PP cells are found chiefly in the islets of the head of the pancreas. The glucagon cells occur mainly in the body and tail of the gland.

Insulin is synthesized by the B-cells through the precursor proinsulin. Insulin is an anabolic hormone that lowers blood glucose concentration by enhancing glucose uptake by all of the body cells, promoting glycogenesis, and inhibiting gluconeogenesis. It also stimulates lipogenesis, inhibits lipolysis, and enhances protein synthesis. Although the factors that govern insulin secretion are multiple and complex, the most important is an elevation of the blood glucose concentration. The primary sites of action of the hormone are the liver, muscle, and fat cells.

Glucagon is formed in the A-cells of the islets. It increases blood glucose by causing hepatic glycogenolysis and gluconeogenesis.

Thus, the effects of glucagon counterbalance those of insulin. These processes are critical in the maintenance of fasting glucose levels, thereby minimizing glucose fluctuations despite variability in nutrient intake and energy utilization. Glucagon also relaxes and dilates smooth muscle, such as the stomach, duodenum, and sphincter of Oddi. The hormone is released by a low blood glucose concentration, amino acids, catecholamines (e.g., during stress), sympathetic nervous discharge, and CCK. Insulin and hyperglycemia suppress glucagon release.

Somatostatin arises in the D-cells of the islets. Both oral and intravenous nutrients stimulate somatostatin secretion. The hormone inhibits the release of insulin, and in turn, its own release is inhibited by insulin.[13] It may act as an important local paracrine regulator of glucose homeostasis. Somatostatin has a wide spectrum of activities, most of which are inhibitory. These include suppression of the release of gastrin, secretin, VIP, PP, gastric acid, pepsin, pancreatic enzymes, and glucagon. Somatostatin also inhibits intestinal, biliary, and gastric motility.

Pancreatic polypeptide arises in the PP cells. Orally ingested protein, vagal cholinergic stimulation, and hypoglycemia are all potent stimulants for the release of PP. PP itself inhibits pancreatic exocrine secretion.

NUTRITIONAL ABNORMALITIES IN PANCREATIC DISEASES

Acute Pancreatitis

Acute pancreatitis is an inflammatory disorder of the pancreas that may be caused by gallstones that obstruct the pancreatic duct, trauma to the pancreas, acute ethanol intoxication, reactions to certain toxins or drugs, and a variety of other more obscure conditions. Regardless of the etiology, the final common pathway involves autoactivation of pancreatic enzymes, inflammation, and autodigestion of the gland and peripancreatic tissues.[14] The resulting systemic response is similar to that seen in sepsis and burns. A hypermetabolic state characterized by increases in energy expenditure, gluconeogenesis, protein degradation, and urea turnover occurs in these patients.[15] Peripheral insulin resistance results in hyperglycemia. These changes collectively result in an overall catabolic state that makes patients with pancreatitis more susceptible to malnutrition and infection. In severe cases,

hypocalcemia may also occur. Unionized calcium losses are proportional to the amount of third space losses of albumin; ionized calcium losses are a result of deposition of calcium within areas of fat necrosis. Hypomagnesemia may also be present as a result of vomiting, urine losses, and magnesium deposition in areas of fat necrosis.

Chronic Pancreatitis

Chronic pancreatitis is a disease in which both the exocrine and endocrine tissues of the pancreas are gradually replaced by fibrous scar tissue. When 10 percent or less of either tissue remains, the patient may exhibit exocrine insufficiency (malabsorption) and diabetes.[11] The usual cause of chronic pancreatitis is chronic alcoholism, and the disease usually becomes apparent after at least 5 years of alcohol consumption. However, there are other causes such as pancreatic duct obstruction or a congenital predisposition, and in many patients there is no obvious explanation for the disease. Even before large amounts of functional pancreatic tissue are lost, most patients experience abdominal pain, which brings them to a physician for help. They may also have episodes of acute inflammation of their chronically scarred pancreas, which are indistinguishable from attacks of acute pancreatitis and should be treated the same way.

Variable weight loss occurs in 75 percent of the patients with chronic pancreatitis. This is because food usually aggravates the pain, and food intake is voluntarily restricted. Significant weight loss from malabsorption is less common. Even when malabsorption occurs, most patients who are able to eat maintain their weight by eating more.

Significant exocrine insufficiency does not occur until 90 percent of the secretory capacity of the pancreas is lost. This can be the result either of progressive parenchymal destruction or obstruction of the major ducts (e.g., from stones, strictures) which prevents the pancreatic digestive enzymes from reaching the duodenum. In either case, it is a late development. The major consequences are steatorrhea and creatorrhea, excessive loss of fat, and protein in the stools. Carbohydrate digestion is not impaired because amylase is also produced by the salivary glands. The patients may complain of bulky, offensive, fatty, or oily stools.

About two thirds of patients with chronic pancreatitis have abnormal glucose tolerance and half of these have diabetes mellitus.[16] In patients with diabetes, some degree of malabsorption is also present since exocrine and endocrine insufficiency usually develop in parallel. The diabetes is usually easily controlled with insulin, but hypoglycemia may be a problem in alcoholics with irregular eating habits.

Pancreatic Cancer

Pancreatic cancer, which usually occurs in the head of the gland, may cause pancreatic exocrine insufficiency if the tumor obstructs the main pancreatic duct. When duct obstruction occurs in the body or tail of the pancreas from tumors in that area, enough enzymes from the unobstructed portion of the gland still enter the duodenum so that absorption and digestion remain normal.[17] Patients with pancreatic cancer often have lost 10 percent or more of their normal body weight by the time the diagnosis is made. In part, this may be due to the malabsorption that can be present. However, there is some evidence that other factors alter the normal metabolic responses in these patients, and that profound weight loss is due to an unidentified substance(s) produced by the tumor itself. These patients also may suffer significant abdominal and back pain, which decreases their appetite and contributes to the weight loss.

Operations for Pancreatic Diseases

Various operations that are performed to treat pancreatic diseases may alter the normal physiology of digestion and absorption of nutrients. The two most common operations are discussed.

Pancreaticoduodenectomy (Whipple Procedure and Pylorus Preserving Whipple Procedure)

The Whipple procedure is an operation in which the head of the pancreas is resected, along with the distal stomach (antrum), duodenum, proximal jejunum, distal common bile duct, and gallbladder (Fig. 25–1A). It is performed most commonly for patients with tumors in the head of the pancreas, but is also used for patients with severe chronic pancreatitis involving the same area. The operation may be followed by nutritional problems in some patients, but it is hard to predict who will experience difficulty. Two factors explain the symptoms: (1) after a partial gastrectomy, the gastric emptying of both liquids and solids is often more rapid than normal, and food particles that are too large to be digested completely may enter the intestine, and (2) the pancreatic juice and bile now enter the intestine some distance proximal to the point where the food does. Thus, even if the remaining pancreas is normal, and the *amount* of digestive enzymes is adequate for normal absorption, malabsorption may result from inadequate mixing of the gastric chyme with bile and pancreatic juice. In practice, by 1 year after the operation, most patients have stabilized at a new weight which is 5 to 10 percent less than their preoperative one. In some cases, this requires dietary modifications and drug therapy, or both; in others, in spite of the alterations described, no adjustments are required. The pylorus preserving modification of the Whipple resection was developed to avoid these problems (Fig. 25–1B). It was hoped that preservation of the stomach and pylorus would maintain gastric emptying closer to normal, and that fewer patients would develop gastrointestinal symptoms. In the few studies that compare the two operations, there seems to be no significant difference, however.[18]

Lateral Pancreaticojejunostomy (Puestow Procedure)

In patients with painful chronic pancreatitis whose main pancreatic duct is dilated to 7 mm or more in diameter (up to 5 mm is normal), the Puestow operation often is done to relieve pain (Fig. 25–2). Although pancreatic enzymes that were blocked from entering the duodenum before the operation now can empty freely into the jejunum, absorption and digestion are not improved. This is because the enzymes enter the gut away from where the food does, and the two do not mix well. However, patients may gain weight after the operation because they no longer have pain when they eat, so they eat more.

Cystic Fibrosis

Cystic fibrosis (CF) is the most frequent cause of pancreatic insufficiency in children, adolescents, and young adults. It is a common, severe autosomal recessive disorder that occurs primarily in the white population, but is seen also in Asians, blacks, Hispanics, and others. Although it is associated with high morbidity and mortality rates, the median life expectancy of CF patients born in 1990 was estimate to be 40 years, about double what it was in 1975. The disease is caused by a genetic defect in the CF transmembrane conductance

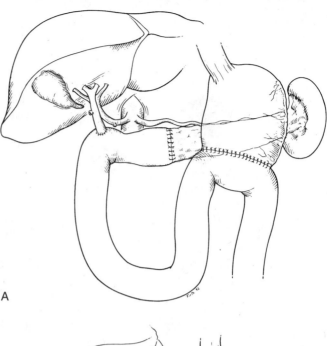

A

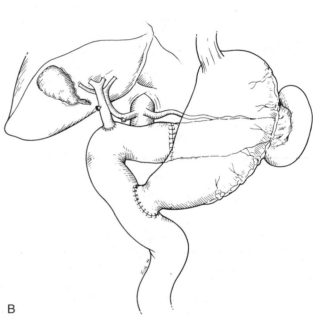

B

FIGURE 25–1   *A,* The Whipple procedure. *B,* The pylorus preserving modification of the Whipple procedure.

regulator (CFTR). The CFTR gene is located on the long arm of chromosome 7, and it is currently estimated that there are over 200 different mutations that can cause CF clinical disease.

While all exocrine glands in the body are affected, symptoms are primarily associated with abnormalities in the lungs and the pancreas. Patients suffer from recurrent pulmonary infections and varying degrees of pancreatic insufficiency, which may cause severe retardation of growth and development. Pancreatic function is abnormal in 90 percent of

patients with CF, and in 85 to 90 percent of them, pancreatic enzyme secretion is decreased or absent. Overall, 85 to 90 percent of CF patients have symptoms from malabsorption and require treatment. This is important to recognize because normal growth and development and sound overall nutritional status greatly increase the ability of these patients to resist and combat pulmonary infections, which are the most common cause of death.[19]

Impaired nutrition in CF patients is usually caused by inadequate treatment of the malabsorptive state rather than by progression of the

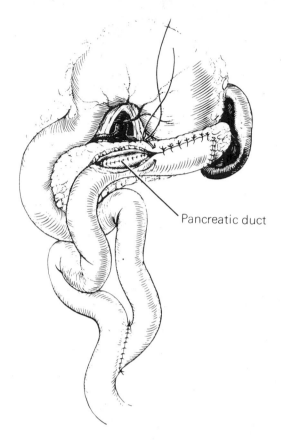

FIGURE 25–2   The Puestow procedure.

disease. These patients are at particular risk be-cause their energy and protein needs are higher than those for healthy children and adults. Factors that further increase the nutri-tional needs of CF patients are the worsening of the lung disease, the presence of infection, increased rate of growth, and increased physi-cal activity. Meeting these increased energy needs is often the greatest challenge for both the patient and the physician.[20]

NUTRITIONAL SUPPORT IN PANCREATIC DISEASES

Acute Pancreatitis

Early studies of nutrition in acute pancreati-tis sought to determine whether total paren-teral nutrition, which avoids secretory stimula-tion of the inflamed pancreas, hastened the resolution of the inflammation. Numerous studies concluded that it does not.[21-23] In fact, during the acute inflammatory phase of the disease, the pancreas is thought to be unre-sponsive to all forms of stimulation. Thus, it is

generally agreed today that parenteral nutrition has no *specific* role in the treatment of this dis-ease. On the other hand, nutritional support (parenteral or enteral) is an important part of the management of patients with acute pan-creatitis, especially those with severe and pro-tracted disease who cannot eat for long peri-ods.[14]

One concern in the provision of enteral nu-trition to these patients involves the fear of stimulating pancreatic secretion, which may aggravate the inflammation. As outlined earlier, pancreatic secretion is stimulated when certain components of protein and fat digestion enter the lumen of the small intestine. Indeed, some patients will experience pain and exacerbation of the disease when they begin to eat again during the period of recovery, and oral intake must be withheld once more.

Rarely pancreatitis itself may be precipitated by very high levels of serum lipids called *hy-perlipidemic pancreatitis.* The mechanism by which the lipids provoke the pancreatic inflam-mation is obscure. Thus, there has been con-cern about whether to provide lipid as part of the parenteral nutrition formulation in these particular patients, as well as to patients with other forms of the disease.

Recommendations. Regardless of etiology, most patients with acute pancreatitis are best managed by withholding oral feeding and pro-viding fluids and electrolytes intravenously. No specific nutritional support is required since most recover quickly and are eating within 4 to 5 days.[23] In those with more serious disease, to-tal parenteral nutrition (TPN) should be started by the end of the first week of hospitalization if it seems clear that oral intake is not going to be possible by that time.[24,25] Careful monitoring of blood glucose levels and appropriate insulin ad-ministration are important, and glucose levels should be maintained in the 200 to 250 mg/dl range. In all patients except those with hyper-lipidemic pancreatitis, intravenous lipids al-most always can be used without concern of aggravating the disease. If the disease persists beyond several weeks, we try to gain access to some route for the provision of enteral nutri-tion (e.g., feeding tube), although this is not al-ways possible. Enteral feeding can either sup-plement the parenteral route, or, if adequate amounts of calories and nutrition can be pro-vided, it can be the sole source of nourishment. However, it is often not possible to supply all of the calories that these patients require during the acute phase of their illness through the en-teral route alone (4000 to 5000 kcal/day). Enteral feeding is important because there is evidence that maintaining the mucosal integrity of the gut by providing luminal nutrients minimizes translocation of bacteria and endotoxin from the bowel lumen into the blood, and may improve the outcome. If patients require surgery to treat the pancreatitis, a feeding jejunostomy should be placed to use for this purpose. As the pancreatic inflammation subsides and the patient improves, oral feedings may resume. There is neither theoretical nor practical support for the feeding of special diets (e.g., low fat) to minimize the chances of recurrent attacks of pancreatitis. Patients should be instructed on a well-balanced, nutritious, and palatable diet.

Several investigators have examined whether specific TPN formulations (e.g., branched chain amino acids, glutamine enrichment) would benefit patients with acute pancreatitis. No clear role has emerged for such an approach.

Chronic Pancreatitis, Pancreatic Cancer, Operations on the Pancreas

Pancreatic Insufficiency

The principles of treatment of the malabsorption that occurs in chronic pancreatitis, pancreatic cancer, or after various pancreatic operations are similar. Pancreatic insufficiency affects fat absorption more than that of protein or carbohydrate because protein digestion is aided by gastric pepsin and carbohydrate digestion is aided by salivary amylase.

Recommendations. The diet should supply 3000 to 6000 kcal/day, emphasizing carbohydrate (400 g or more) and protein (100 to 150 g). Patients with steatorrhea may or may not have diarrhea, and dietary restriction of fat is important mainly to control diarrhea. Patients with diarrhea may be restricted to 50 g of fat/day and the amount increased until diarrhea appears. Permissable fat intake averages 100 g/day distributed equally throughout four meals. Pancreatic enzyme replacement may be accomplished with pancreatic extracts (e.g., Cotazym, Ilozyme, Pancreas MT, Viokase, Ultrase) containing 30,000 to 50,000 units of lipase given with each of four daily meals. If enzymes alone do not improve the malabsorption sufficiently, the problem is probably due to the destruction of lipase by gastric acid. Then an enteric coated enzyme preparation may be substituted or an H_2 receptor blocking agent should be added to the regimen.

It is important to realize that the malabsorption of fat can never be eliminated entirely. Nevertheless the diarrhea should cease and patients should be able to regain weight with the proper combination of diet, enzyme replacement, and (in some cases) acid antisecretory drugs.

If patients have undergone some form of gastric resection as part of their pancreatic operation, five or six smaller meals/day may be better tolerated than the usual three to four meals since stomach capacity is smaller. The enzymes should be given with each meal.

Diabetes Mellitus

In patients with diabetes from chronic pancreatitis, ketoacidosis is rare even if blood glucose levels are quite high. However, even small amounts of subcutaneous insulin may induce a profound hypoglycemia. This is probably because there is also a deficiency of glucagon, which normally corrects hypoglycemia by converting liver glycogen to glucose. Thus the patient must be instructed thoroughly on the dangers of hypoglycemia, its symptoms, and management. Mild elevations in blood sugar do not require treatment, but fasting elevations in excess of 250 mg/dl should be managed with insulin. Frequently only 20 to 30 units a day are required. Rigid control of blood sugar is not advisable, and it is reasonable to maintain the fasting level around 200 mg/dl. Oral agents are almost never successful. In those patients who are not yet diabetic and who are to undergo pancreatic resection, the chance for the development of diabetes is related to the amount of pancreas removed. Most patients with abnormal glucose tolerance before operation will require insulin after a resection of 50 percent or more.

Cystic Fibrosis

The goal of pancreatic enzyme replacement therapy in CF patients is similar to that in the other pancreatic insufficiency states already discussed. However, because of the age of most of these patients, their coexisting pulmonary disease, and the energy requirements associated with growth and development, certain aspects of their management are different and will be discussed in detail.

A number of different pancreatic enzyme preparations, which vary in potency and have different physicochemical characteristics, are available.[26] For infants and children with CF, enteric coated enzyme preparations usually have been used. The enteric coating is pH sensitive and protects the enzymes from the acid environment of the stomach that would otherwise inactivate the lipase. The enteric coating remains intact until the enzymes enter the small intestine where the higher intraluminal pH allows the enzymes to be released together with the chyme, where digestion begins.[27]

For infants with CF, the recommended dose to begin treatment is 500 to 1000 IU lipase per feeding. Adjustments should be made according to the growth rate, stool volume, and frequency. One must be aware that protein deficiency is more common in infants than in adolescents or adults since the protein requirements in infants are three times as great. Soy based formulas and human milk (7 percent kcal from protein) generally provide adequate amounts of protein, as long as enough enzymes are added to the diet. If the volume required to deliver adequate calories and nutrition is too great, infant formulas may be concentrated to maximize caloric intake and minimize volume.[28]

In older children, enzyme dosage should not exceed 3000 units lipase/kg body weight/meal. Higher doses have been associated with the development of colonic strictures, and the development of hyperuricosuria.[28] The amount of enzymes for each meal should be individualized for each patient.[29] In general, the amount required depends on the degree of pancreatic insufficiency, the nutritional status, the quantity of food eaten and its composition, and the type of enzyme replacement used. Enzymes are adjusted until adequate growth and an acceptable pattern of stooling (1 to 2/day) are achieved. A fat balance study to measure fecal fat excretion helps to determine the efficacy of the enzyme replacement therapy. For optimal activity, enzymes should be taken at the beginning of each meal. For infants and young children who are unable to swallow capsules, the capsules can be opened and the enzyme beads mixed with soft foods, such as applesauce or hot cereal, and swallowed. The beads should not be crushed or chewed to retain the benefits of the enteric coating.

Nutritional guidelines for children with CF are based on the recommended dietary allowance (RDA) for DBW based on height and age. In some patients, calorie needs can be as high as 120 to 150 percent RDA, and protein needs as high as 200 percent RDA. Caloric intake is monitored closely and may be adjusted depending on linear growth and weight gain. Routine plotting of a child's height and weight

on growth charts helps to detect suboptimal growth and the need for additional intervention.[29]

The recommended diet for a CF patient is high calorie, high protein, and moderate fat, with emphasis on nutrient dense foods. In the past, fat used to be restricted to help control steatorrhea. However, with improved enzyme preparations, fat is well tolerated in most CF patients and can add extra calories, provide essential fatty acids, and improve the palatability of many foods. Tolerance to high-fat diets varies: some patients experience increased signs of malabsorption when eating high fat foods like pizza or french fries. Patients are instructed to take extra enzymes with the high fat foods to help control steatorrhea and improve digestion. Clinical signs of malabsorption (increase in the number of stools, abdominal cramps, or greasy stools) should be monitored.

Extra calories and protein can easily be added to traditional foods without increasing volume. Adding nutrient dense snacks and choosing higher calorie foods are helpful. Enteral supplementation by mouth is often useful, and is well accepted by CF patients. Examples of fortified beverages include Ensure, Pediasure, and Scandishakes (intact protein formulas) and Pregestimil and Reabilan (elemental formulas). Modular products are also available (e.g., Polycose, Promod, medium-chain triglyceride oil) as powdered and liquid additions to traditional foods. Enzymes are required with the nonelemental formulas and occasionally are needed with the elemental products. The advantages of specialty nutritional supplements include the convenience and nutrient density of these items. The major disadvantage is the high cost.

In CF patients, malabsorption also can lead to micronutrient deficiency.[30] Patients are at risk for fat soluble vitamin and essential fatty acid deficiencies. Vitamin and mineral supplementation is an important part of therapy. The water soluble vitamins are well absorbed in CF and the need can usually be met by diet alone. The fat soluble vitamins (A, D, E, and K) are often poorly absorbed because of fat malabsorption and are routinely supplemented. One to two multivitamins/day are often prescribed as well as additional vitamins based on documented deficiencies. Fat soluble vitamins prescribed in water miscible form are most effective. Yearly monitoring of serum vitamin A and E levels is helpful to avoid unnecessary supplementation. In warm climates with sun exposure, vitamin D supplements are not needed;

they may be required in climates with long winters. Vitamin K is only supplemented when the patient has hemoptysis or bleeding from another source, liver disease, or is on chronic antibiotic therapy.

The need for sodium is increased in CF because excessive sodium is lost in the sweat. Some individuals require salt supplementation during the summer months or during physical exertion and fever. Infants may require extra salt if they are fed solely breast milk or infant formulas. Other minerals (iron, zinc, selenium) are not routinely supplemented; however, their status should be monitored at intervals.

Those patients who present with severe malabsorption, frequent infections, or advanced lung disease may experience progressive nutritional failure. For this group, continuous enteral feeds (via nasogastric, gastric, or jejunal tubes) or even parenteral feeding may be required. Nocturnal feeds of a calorically-dense formula may improve nutritional status and prevent further deterioration. The choice of feeding tube depends on the patient's lifestyle and the physician's experience. All types of tubes have been used successfully. Enzymes should be administered at the beginning of the feed (preferably by mouth), again 4 to 6 hours later, and once more upon waking. Adjustments in dosage may be needed based on the type of formula and the rate of infusion. Supplemental feedings have also been given during the day and delivered as bolus feedings.[31]

Parenteral nutrition may be indicated short term in CF patients with acute complications (e.g., pancreatitis, surgery). Those with short-gut syndrome sometimes require long-term TPN.[32]

REFERENCES

1. Solomon TE: Control of exocrine pancreatic secretion. In Johnson LR (ed): Physiology of the Gastrointestinal Tract, 3rd Edition. New York: Raven Press, 1994.
2. Anagostides A, Chadwick VS, Selden AC et al: Sham feeding in pancreatic secretion. Evidence for direct vagal stimulation of output. Gastroenterology 1984;87:109–114.
3. Annis D, Hallenbeck GA: Effect of excluding pancreatic juice from duodenum on secretory response of pancreas to a meal. Proc Soc Exp Biol Med 1977;383:1951.
4. Adrian TE, Besterman HS, Mallinson CN et al: Inhibition of secretin stimulated pancreatic secretion by pancreatic polypeptide. Gut 1978;20:37.
5. Adrian TE, Savage AP, Sagor GR et al: Effect of Peptide YY on gastric, pancreatic, and biliary function in humans. Gastroenterology 1985;89:494.
6. Hanssen LE, Hanssen KF, Myren J: Inhibition of secretin release and pancreatic bicarbonate secretion by

7. somatostatin infusion in man. Scand J Gastroenterol 1977;12:391.
7. Shapiro H, Ludwig RM: The effect of glucagon on the exocrine pancreas: a review. Am J Gastroenterol 1978;70:274.
8. Slaff J, Jacobson D, Tillman CR et al: Protease-specific suppression of pancreatic exocrine secretion. Gastroenterol 1984;87:44–52.
9. Isaksson G, Ihse I: Pain reduction by an oral pancreatic enzyme preparation in chronic pancreatitis. Dig Dis Sci 1983;28:97–102.
10. Owyang C, Louie DS, Tatum D: Feedback regulation of pancreatic enzyme secretion. Suppression of cholecystokinin release by trypsin. J Clin Invest 1986;77:2043–2047.
11. Sarles H, Pastor J, Pauli AM et al: Determination of pancreatic function. A statistical analysis conducted in normal subjects and in patients with proven chronic pancreatitis (duodenal intubation, glucose tolerance test, determination of fat content in the stools, sweat test). Gastroenterologia 1963;99(3):279–300.
12. Doty JE, Fink AS, Meyer JH: Alterations in digestive function caused by pancreatic disease. Surg Clin North Am 1989;69(3):447–465.
13. Schusdziarra V: Somatostatin—a regulatory modulator connecting nutrient entry and metabolism. Horm Metab Res 1980;12:563.
14. Pisters PWT, Ranson JHC: Nutritional support for acute pancreatitis. Surg Gynecol Obstet 1992;175:275–284.
15. Bouffard YH, Delafosse BX, Annant GJ et al: Energy expenditure during severe acute pancreatitis. J Parenter Enter Nutr 1989;13:26–29.
16. Kalthoff L, Layer P, Clain JE et al: The course of alcoholic and nonalcoholic chronic pancreatitis. Dig Dis Sci 1984;29:953.
17. DiMagno EP, Malagelada JR, Go VLW: The relationships between pancreatic ductal obstruction and pancreatic secretion in man. Mayo Clin Proc 1979;54:157.
18. Fink AS, DeSouza LR, Mayer EA: Long-term evaluation of pylorus preservation during pancreaticoduodenectomy. World J Surg 1988;12:663.
19. Luder E: Nutritional care of patients with cystic fibrosis. Top Clin Nutr 1991;6:39–50.
20. Creveling S, Light M, Gardner P et al: Cystic fibrosis, nutrition and the health care team. Ped Nutr 1994;18:1–14.
21. Goodgame JT, Fischer JE: Parenteral nutrition in the treatment of acute pancreatitis: effect on complications and mortality. Ann Surg 1977;186:651–658.
22. Grant JP, James S, Grabowski V et al: Total parenteral nutrition in pancreatic disease. Ann Surg 1984;200:627–631.
23. Sax HC, Warner BW, Talamini MA et al: Early total parenteral nutrition in acute pancreatitis: lack of beneficial effects. Am J Surg 1987;153:117–124.
24. Sitzman JV, Steinborn PA, Zinner MJ et al: Total parenteral nutrition and alternate energy substrates in treatment of severe acute pancreatitis. Surg Gynecol Obstet 1989;168:311–317.
25. Feller JH, Brown RA, MacLaren Toussant GP et al: Changing methods in the treatment of severe pancreatitis. Am J Surg 1974;127:196–201.
26. George DE, Mangos JA: Nutritional management and pancreatic enzyme therapy in cystic fibrosis patients: state of the art in 1987 and projections into the future. J Pediatr Gastroenterol Nutr 1988;7:S49–S57.
27. Kraisinger M, Hochhaus G, Stecenko A et al: Clinical pharmacology of pancreatic enzymes in patients with cystic fibrosis and in vitro performance of microen-

capsulated formulations. J Clin Pharmacol 1994;34: 158–166.

28. Adams E: Nutrition care in cystic fibrosis: focus on infancy through adolescence. Nutr News 1988;3: 1–6.

29. Ramsey BW, Farrell PM, Pencharz P et al: Nutritional assessment and management in cystic fibrosis: a consensus report. Am J Clin Nutr 1992;55:108–116.

30. Gaskin KJ: Cystic fibrosis: nutritional problems and their management. Semin Pediatr Gastroenterol Nutr 1993;4:9–15.

31. Gaskin KJ: The impact of nutrition in cystic fibrosis: a review. J Pediatr Gastroenterol Nutr 1988;7:S12–S17.

32. Durie PR: Cystic fibrosis: gastrointestinal and hepatic complications and their management. Semin Pediatr Gastroenterol Nutr 1993;4:3–9.

26

Enteral Nutrition in Renal Disease

WILFRED DRUML
WILLIAM E. MITCH

Even though enteral nutrition has become the first line of nutritional support and tube feeding is performed routinely in many institutions, there are remarkably few reports containing systematic investigations of its efficacy in improving nutritional status. The most extensive reviews of artificial nutrition in patients with renal failure have focused mainly on parenteral nutrition, and there are only single references to enteral or tube feeding.[1-4] Even the manufacturers of specialized formulas for enteral nutrition in renal failure rarely have systematic studies of their products.

This scarcity of information about enteral nutrition in renal disease reflects several basic difficulties in approaching the subject. First, the spectrum of disease states associated with renal dysfunction is heterogenous, ranging from stable, advanced chronic renal failure (CRF) to acute renal failure (ARF) occurring in a patient with multiple organ dysfunction, often as part of complex drug regimens in an intensive care unit (ICU). Consequently, the goals of nutritional therapy, the patient's nutritional requirements, and the enteral formulas will differ fundamentally among patients. Second, the patient's degree of renal function impairment and hence ability to excrete nitrogen-containing waste products, electrolytes, and minerals limits the amounts of protein and other constituents that can be given. Third, the metabolic abnormalities associated with renal insufficiency (or the diseases causing renal failure) must be taken into account when an enteral feeding formula is used.[4] These factors make it

difficult if not impossible to design a standard formula for all patients with renal disease. In short, the diverging aims of nutritional therapy have created uncertainties that result in inconsistent or even divergent recommendations for enteral nutritional support.

Based on available information and our experience, we believe that enteral nutrition may become especially important in three groups of patients with renal failure. The first group is the catabolic patient with ARF or CRF requiring dialysis as well as patients being treated by regular hemodialysis therapy (RDT) or peritoneal dialysis therapy (CAPD) who have a superimposed acute illness. In these patients, the optimum nutrient intake should be provided in the enteral formula. The goal of using the formula is to meet the increased nutrient demands arising from the hypercatabolic disease and to prevent the loss of lean body mass. Ancillary goals are to stimulate wound healing and improve immunocompetence. For such patients, electrolyte disorders or the accumulation of fluid and metabolic waste products should be prevented by adjusting the intensity of dialysis.

The second group includes patients with stable CRF who are not being treated by dialysis. Small children with congenital or acquired forms of renal dysfunction or malnourished (mostly elderly) patients with CRF but no evidence of hypercatabolism should be treated differently. In sharp contrast to acutely ill patients treated with dialysis, nutritional support for CRF patients who do not have a catabolic illness is aimed at minimizing uremic toxicity arising from accumulated waste products and retarding the progression of renal insufficiency while delaying the time until dialysis will become necessary. These goals must be done while maintaining lean body mass or stimulating growth.

The third group includes patients treated by hemodialysis or CAPD but without a catabolic illness. When dialysis patients are found to have an inadequate intake of nutrients, malnutrition develops and becomes a major determinant of morbidity (especially infections) and mortality. Dietary supplementation for this group is aimed at the repletion and maintenance of body protein stores. The goals are to improve visceral protein synthesis, stimulate immunocompetence, and improve the quality of life as well as physical well-being.

To establish recommendations for these groups, we will first review the alterations of gastrointestinal (GI) function in patients with renal disease, then define the characteristics of groups of patients and their nutrient requirements, and summarize the techniques and types of nutrient application and enteral formulas that have been used in patients with renal disease. The impact of nutrition on the progression of renal insufficiency, including the use of very-low-protein diets and supplements of essential amino acids or keto acids will not be reviewed. Information on this topic has been covered elsewhere.[5]

GASTROINTESTINAL FUNCTION IN UREMIA

Abnormalities of the structure and function of virtually every segment of the GI tract have been described in patients with renal failure.[6] Many of these reports contain divergent if not contradictory findings. In part, these discrepancies are due to the fact that investigations have been performed in patients with different stages and types of renal insufficiency. Moreover, many abnormalities have been uncovered in animal models of uremia, but animal models may not provide an accurate picture of patients. Regardless, there are alterations in GI function that are clinically relevant to enteral feeding strategies.

Oral Cavity and Esophagus

Stomatitis, gingivitis, parotitis, mucosal ulcerations with bleeding, and an altered sense of taste due to bacterial overgrowth are frequent findings in uremic patients.[6] The metallic taste associated with uremia has been linked to the conversion of urea to ammonia because of urease activity from an excess of bacteria in the GI tract. Esophagitis caused by gastroesophageal reflux, bacterial colonization, or fungal or secondary viral infections can be present in renal failure patients and is even more common after renal transplantation. These factors, plus a decreased appetite, dysgeusia, and psychosocial factors such as loneliness and depression, are all indications for initiating nutritional therapy in uremic patients. Obviously, severe esophagitis can complicate the placement of a feeding tube and may even force the use of a gastrostomy tube.

Stomach

It is believed that untreated CRF patients secrete less acid than healthy subjects both in the basal state and after gastrin stimulation of acid secretion. The lower secretory rate occurs despite high serum gastrin levels. Acid secretion returns to normal after institution of routine hemodialysis therapy and even hypersecretion of acid can develop because of the persistent hypergastrinemia.[7] Gastric mucosal permeability is increased in CRF patients, but this defect is reversed by RDT.[7]

Hemorrhagic gastritis is an important cause of upper GI bleeding in patients with renal failure.[8,9] It is more frequent in CRF patients than in patients treated by RDT but is even more frequent after kidney transplantation. Gastric mucosal alterations range from mucosal edema with scattered petechiae to hemorrhagic infarction, pseudomembrane formation, or frank ulceration. Impaired clotting and platelet function contribute to the bleeding tendency.

Earlier studies suggested there is an increased incidence of peptic ulcers in uremic patients. The conclusions were based largely on the presence of symptoms suggesting peptic ulcer disease, which were reported in 40 to 60 percent of patients. Recent investigations using endoscopic biopsies with histologic verification of ulceration do not support an increased frequency of peptic ulcers in CRF patients.[10]

Gastric emptying is reported to be delayed in patients with CRF but is reversed following institution of RDT.[11,12] In diabetic patients, gastroparesis associated with polyneuropathy can aggravate a defect in gastric motility. With or without diabetes, delayed gastric emptying plus incompetence of the lower esophageal sphincter can result in gastroesophageal reflux.

In such cases, duodenal intubation of the feeding tube will be necessary.

Pancreas

A mild degree of pancreatic insufficiency is present in many patients with end-stage renal disease. Basal bicarbonate secretion appears to be decreased, but both stimulated and peak bicarbonate secretions are usually normal.[13] Measurements of lipase and trypsin secretion in response to cholecystokinin produce variable results, while amylase secretion is consistently decreased. As with many other peptide hormones, blood cholecystokinin levels are increased in patients with end-stage renal failure. Generally, the higher levels are ascribed to decreased degradation of peptides by the damaged kidney, but there probably is also an impairment in the responsiveness of the end-organ to the hormone, since the rate of hormone production should adjust to maintain the blood level in the normal range. Chronic pancreatic insufficiency has been suggested to be an important contributor to the syndrome of wasting of lean body mass found in some patients with end-stage renal disease.[13]

Despite the low amylase secretory levels, the blood amylase concentration can be raised in uremia, predominantly because of a decreased renal clearance.[14] Plasma trypsinogen and lipase concentrations can also be elevated. Regardless, there is no link between these slightly high levels and symptomatic acute pancreatitis.[6,15] It is unclear whether the hypertriglyceridemia, hypercalcemia, and hyperparathyroidism found in most CRF patients predispose them to develop pancreatitis. Fortunately, acute pancreatitis is unusual in CRF or dialysis patients.

Small Intestine

Digestion and absorption of carbohydrates and proteins is normal or only mildly impaired in uremia.[16,17] The many alterations in intestinal function that have been reported are probably of little functional importance, in part because of the enormous capacity of intestinal function. For example, brush border disaccharidases are reported to be decreased in uremic patients, but glucose uptake is decreased, normal, or even increased.[18] Lactase deficiency is not increased in uremia, and the uptake of amino acids or peptides is not grossly affected by uremia even though peptidase activity was reported to be reduced in CRF rats but increased in acutely uremic rats.[19] There may be abnormal amino acid absorption, however, because there is evidence of bacterial overgrowth in the intestines of uremic patients that could affect absorption, plus there is increased intestinal loss of albumin.[20] Mucosal edema or uremic enterocolitis also could stimulate protein-losing enteropathy and contribute to altered absorption and motility.

Uremia is associated with mild fat malabsorption. After a test meal of long-chain triglycerides (LCTs), the expected increase in blood triglyceride levels is retarded and fecal fat excretion is enhanced in RDT patients.[21] Biliary dysfunction, pancreatic insufficiency, changes in intestinal structure and function, and altered intestinal motility have been implicated as potential causes of this problem. Absorption of the essential fatty acid, linoleic acid, was shown to be decreased in rats with experimental uremia while intestinal absorption of medium chain triglycerides (MCTs) was not evaluated.[22]

Malabsorption of calcium is common in renal failure and has been linked to defects in vitamin D metabolism. Loss of kidney mass results in reduced conversion of monohydroxyvitamin D_3 into $1,25\text{-}(OH)_2D_3$ or calcitriol, the active form of vitamin D. Vitamin D appears to be necessary for normal metabolism, replication, and structure of intestinal mucosal cells including crypt mitotic activity and lengthening of crypts and villi.[23]

The intestinal absorption of only a few micronutrients has been systemically evaluated in uremic patients. In experimental uremia, folate absorption is impaired.[24] Iron absorption by normal adults depends on iron stores in the body, and this same relationship is preserved in patients treated by RDT.[25] Nevertheless, some investigators believe that intestinal iron absorption is impaired in dialysis patients, and for this reason, when iron requirements are increased (e.g., with erythropoietin treatment), they suggest that iron should be supplemented parenterally.[26]

Colon

There is an increased incidence of colonic ulcers and pseudomembranous colitis in predialysis CRF patients and in patients following renal transplantation but not in patients treated by hemodialysis.[27] Although unusual, angiodysplasia of the colonic mucosa appears to be an important cause of lower GI bleeding in uremia. Besides bleeding, colonic motility can be impaired and constipation is frequent; in elderly hemodialysis patients, constipation is aggravated by autonomic neuropathy, by drugs impairing intestinal motility, and by phosphate-binding drugs. Still, diarrhea may occur and is most often linked to mucosal inflammation from infection, to ischemic damage to the intestine, or to altered bile-acid metabolism.[28]

Colonic flora probably play a role in nitrogen retention as well as generation of toxic products. In fact, antibiotic therapy improved nitrogen balance in uremic patients.[29,30] However, the bacteria in intestines of CRF patients do not clear more urea than the intestinal flora of healthy subjects, even though the mass of intestinal bacteria is increased in uremia.[6,31] The increased secretion of potassium by the large bowel in uremic patients is a compensatory means of achieving potassium homeostasis as renal potassium excretion declines.[32]

Summary

GI function in uremia can be altered in a variety of ways and could affect enteral nutrition. There are mild digestive and absorptive insufficiencies that are probably of little clinical importance in determining the assimilation of substrates because there is a large functional reserve in intestinal function. Fat malabsorption (and especially LCTs) may be important and should be kept in mind when one chooses whether the enteral formula contains predominantly LCTs or MCTs. Problems that might impair tolerance to enteral nutrition include abdominal cramping, constipation, or diarrhea.

Careful investigations of GI motility in the various causes and degrees of renal failure have not been published, but available information indicates the problems are not excessive in uremic patients. Whether the intestinal mucosa is more prone to injury remains controversial.[33] Despite dramatic results from animal experiments, it remains to be shown whether enteral nutrition can prevent the development of erosions and ulcerations or decrease the frequency of intestinal bleeding.[34]

As reviewed in Chapter 29, the multiple organ dysfunction syndrome is generally associated with edema of the intestinal mucosa, impaired production of mucus, and intestinal enzymes plus altered peristalsis. All these abnormalities can lead to intestinal paralysis, an increase in intestinal permeability, and impaired absorption of nutrients. Acute or chronic renal dysfunction may aggravate or modify these findings; it certainly will not improve them.

METABOLIC ALTERATIONS IN UREMIA

Energy Metabolism

In experimental animals, renal failure is associated with decreased oxygen consumption even when hypothermia and acidosis are corrected.[35] The term "uremic hypometabolism" was coined to describe this phenomenon, and impaired oxidative phosphorylation has been implicated as the cause of reduced oxygen use. In contrast, the oxygen consumption of patients with various forms of renal failure is unchanged[36,37] but energy expenditure is increased in uremic patients who have other illnesses such as sepsis.[36] In the multiple organ failure syndrome, oxygen consumption is significantly higher in patients without impairment of renal function compared with those with acute renal failure (ARF), suggesting that uremia "dampens" the defect.[38] Taken together, these data indicate that in well-controlled uremia (by hemodialysis or hemofiltration), there is little if any change in energy metabolism.

In renal failure, the pattern of substrate oxidation is similar to that in other disease states. The oxidation of fat is increased and carbohydrate oxidation is reduced after an overnight fast.[36] This shift from carbohydrate to fat oxidation may reflect insulin resistance or decreased hepatic glycogen stores.

Protein and Amino Acid Metabolism

A hallmark of ARF and CRF, including uremia treated by hemodialysis or CAPD, is abnormal nitrogen metabolism. Acute renal failure alone even without a superimposed acute illness causes accelerated protein catabolism and sustained negative nitrogen balance resulting in excessive release of amino acids from skeletal muscle.[39-41] There also is defective use of amino acids for protein synthesis in muscle.[41,42] This has led to the conclusion that amino acids are redistributed, flowing from skeletal muscle (because of increased protein degradation and impaired protein synthesis) to the liver, where extraction of amino acids is increased. These changes are associated with increased gluconeogenesis (and ureagenesis) as well as increased synthesis of acute-phase proteins.[41,43] There is also evidence that amino acid transport across muscle and adipocyte cell membranes is impaired in both ARF and CRF. Presumably, abnormal amino acid transport is linked to changes in cellular sodium transport.[44]

The elimination of amino acids given intravenously to uremic patients is abnormal. In fact, the clearance of all α-amino nitrogen plus the clearance of histidine, tryptophan, and to a lesser degree of arginine are all increased, while the clearances of phenylalanine and valine are decreased.[47,48] There is thus an imbalance in amino acid pools in plasma and in the intracellular compartment. In patients with ARF or CRF or in dialysis patients, there are characteristic plasma amino acid patterns.[46,47]

An important catabolic factor in renal failure is insulin resistance. In muscle of rats with ARF, the maximal rate of insulin-stimulated protein synthesis is depressed while protein degradation is increased, even in the presence of insulin.[41] In ARF, there appears to be a common defect in both protein and glucose metabolism because protein catabolism in muscle is highly correlated with the ratio of lactate released to glucose uptake by muscle.[41] In this formulation, inefficient energy metabolism in muscle would stimulate protein breakdown, thereby interrupting the control of protein turnover.

Other endocrine abnormalities have been implicated as causes of the accelerated protein degradation occurring in uremia. For example, secondary hyperparathyroidism may stimulate protein breakdown in muscle.[49] Plasma levels of other "catabolic hormones" (e.g., catecholamines, glucagon, and corticosteroids) are elevated in uremia, and indirect evidence suggests that glucocorticoids stimulate protein catabolism in ARF.[50-52] For example, an inhibitor of steroid receptors reduced the rate of protein degradation in acutely uremic rats.[52]

Acidosis is an important factor causing growth retardation and an increase in muscle protein breakdown in renal failure. Metabolic acidosis was shown to activate the catabolism of protein and the oxidation of branched-chain amino acids in muscle independently of azotemia.[53,54] These responses are mediated by glucocorticoid-dependent pathways.[55,56] The catabolic effects of acidosis, together with the untoward effects of acidosis on lipolysis, insulin resistance, erythropoietin resistance, and hyperparathyroidism, indicate that alkali therapy should be a cornerstone of the treatment of CRF patients.

There is evidence for increased activity of circulating proteases in the plasma of uremic patients. The proteases are released from gran-ulocytes during hemodialysis and may stimulate catabolism of proteins in ARF patients.[57,58] Finally, inflammatory cytokines such as interleukins and tumor necrosis factor (TNF) could be mediators of hypercatabolism in acute disease states.[51]

The failure of different regimens of nutritional support to suppress endogenous protein breakdown and gluconeogenesis from amino acids in catabolic patients with ARF or CRF (with or without a superimposed illness) means that it is virtually impossible to achieve positive nitrogen balance. On the other hand, experimental evidence indicates that with renal failure, neutral or positive nitrogen balance can be achieved. Insulin-like growth factor-1 (IGF-1) accelerates functional recovery from ischemic ARF in the rat and improves nitrogen balance.[59] However, initial clinical experience does not support these positive results.[51]

In metabolically stable, nonacidotic patients with CRF, protein turnover is remarkably stable and nitrogen balance is neutral.[60-63] However, when malnutrition or an intercurrent catabolic stimulus, such as acidosis, trauma, or infection is present, protein breakdown accelerates.[39,64] In such cases, inadequate oral nutrient intake or lack of dietary compliance will cause a loss of lean body mass and overt malnutrition.

In patients treated by hemodialysis, a catabolic effect of renal replacement therapy must be taken into account. The evidence for catabolism is that nitrogen balance is negative on dialysis days by an amount that cannot be attributed solely to the loss of substrates during therapy.[65] Stimulation of protein breakdown occurs, possibly mediated by activation of neutrophils and macrophages, by release of proteases, by activation of the complement system, or by mediators such as TNF and interleukins.[65,66]

Besides stimulation of protein degradation by acidosis and dialysis, there is suppression of protein synthesis and impaired protein and amino acid metabolism in renal failure because of the loss of metabolically active renal tissue. Amino acids that are synthesized and released into the circulation by the kidneys include cysteine, tyrosine, arginine, and serine.[67] A decreased release of these amino acids from the damaged kidneys could contribute to the altered amino acid pools. Moreover, those amino acids usually termed as nonessential (NEAA) may become conditionally indispensable (e.g., tyrosine).[68,69] The kidney is also an important organ for degrading proteins. Small peptides, including hormones, are filtered and catabolized in proximal tubule cells with resulting amino acids recycled into the metabolic pool.[70] Because the kidney accounts for 30 to 70 percent of the total metabolic clearance of peptides, including hormones such as insulin, glucagon, or growth hormone, plasma levels of peptides are elevated in patients with renal failure.[71] As noted earlier, the higher blood levels of hormones suggest impaired responsiveness of the target organ to the hormone but overall, the impact of this change on metabolic processes is uncertain.

Carbohydrate Metabolism

Renal failure is associated with impaired glucose tolerance and insulin resistance.[72,73] Because the plasma insulin level is higher, the fasting blood glucose concentration may be normal despite glucose intolerance. Maximal insulin-stimulated glucose uptake by skeletal muscle is decreased by 50 percent, and glycogen synthesis in muscle is impaired but the insulin concentration causing half-maximal stimulation of glucose uptake is normal, pointing to a postreceptor defect rather than impaired insulin sensitivity as the cause of defective glucose metabolism in uremia.[73] This abnormality, coupled with accelerated hepatic gluconeogenesis from extraction of amino acids, leads to increased production of glucose and urea.[74-76] In contrast to patients with stable CRF or healthy subjects, hepatic gluconeogenesis cannot be suppressed by glucose infusion.[76] Finally, the increased circulating levels of catabolic hormones, hyperparathyroidism, metabolic acidosis, inflammatory cytokines such as interleukins, and TNF can contribute to insulin resistance.[77] As detailed earlier, alterations in glucose and protein metabolism in ARF appear to be interrelated because impaired glucose metabolism in muscle is highly correlated with the accelerated rate of protein catabolism.[41,73] Interestingly, administration of a glucocorticoid receptor antagonist not only improves protein breakdown but also suppresses gluconeogenesis.[78]

Insulin metabolism is grossly abnormal in uremia. Basal insulin secretion is reduced, and the response to glucose infusion is limited.[72] Because the kidney is the main organ of insulin disposal, insulin degradation is decreased.[71] The defect is aggravated because insulin catabolism by the liver is consistently reduced, at least in dogs with ARF.[79] The higher plasma insulin concentration resulting from impaired renal and hepatic degradation reduces the insulin requirements of diabetic subjects. This occurs

gradually in advancing CRF and more rapidly in patients with ARF.[80]

Lipid Metabolism

The most relevant alteration in lipid metabolism in the nonnephrotic patient with renal failure is impaired lipolysis.[81,82] Reduced activities of lipolytic enzymes, including peripheral blood lipoprotein lipase and hepatic triglyceride lipase, have been identified as the major cause of defective lipoprotein catabolism.[83,84] The result is that total triglycerides and the triglyceride content of plasma lipoproteins, especially very low density lipoproteins and low density lipoproteins, are increased while cholesterol is reported to be increased, normal, or even decreased in uremic patients. Cholesterol levels in high density lipoproteins have been found to be consistently low in patients with ARF or CRF or those treated by RDT. Thus, in most nonnephrotic patients in renal failure, the lipoprotein profile corresponds to a type IV hyperlipidemia of the Frederickson classification. Additionally, the protein composition of lipoproteins is abnormal: concentrations of apoproteins A I and A II are decreased, and the ratio of C II (an activator of lipoprotein lipase) and C III (an inhibitor of lipolysis) are increased.[85]

Impaired lipolysis affects the metabolism and hence use of LCTs and MCTs. During an intravenous infusion of artificial fat emulsions, hydrolysis of MCTs and LCTs is equally delayed.[86] Reduced lipolysis coupled with delayed intestinal fat absorption after a fat-rich meal results in a slower and higher rise in plasma triglycerides in dialysis patients compared with healthy subjects.[21] A circulating inhibitor has been implicated as the cause of the impaired lipolysis found in uremia. For example, chronic hemofiltration therapy or high-flux dialysis (using a dialysis membrane that will eliminate middle molecules) ameliorates the abnormal lipid profile.[87] In experimental animals, parathyroidectomy or therapy with a calcium channel blocker prevents the development of lipid abnormalities.[88] The presence of metabolic acidosis can impair lipolysis by inhibiting lipoprotein lipase.[89] Finally, repeated heparin administration to dialysis patients (plus depletion of lipoprotein lipase stores) aggravates hypertriglyceridemia. To achieve a lesser impact on the lipolytic system, some workers recommend substituting low-molecular-weight heparin for conventional heparin in hopes of improving the lipid profile.[90]

In summary, the main feature of abnormal lipid metabolism in the nonnephrotic patient with kidney failure is reduced catabolism rather than increased synthesis of very low density lipoproteins or triglyceride.[91] However, intraperitoneal infusion of massive amounts of acetate, lactate, or glucose stimulates triglyceride synthesis, yielding the higher triglyceride levels found in CAPD patients.[92] Hepatic lipid synthesis in CAPD patients can also be stimulated because of peritoneal protein losses, maintaining a condition mimicking "chronic nephrosis".[92,93] Enhanced synthesis of fatty acids and triglycerides plus increased very low density lipoprotein secretion induced by inflammatory mediators such as TNF also contribute to hyperlipidemia.[94]

Carnitine deficiency does not seem to play a major role in the altered use of triglycerides and free fatty acids, at least in ARF. In contrast to CRF or chronic dialysis patients, plasma carnitine levels are increased in ARF patients because there is increased carnitine release from catabolism of muscle tissues plus increased hepatic carnitine synthesis.[95] Because carnitine deficiency has been linked to the lipid abnormalities of CRF (and particularly hemodialysis patients), a carnitine supplement has been advocated for these patients.[96] Consequently, several enteral diets designed for patients in renal failure are enriched with carnitine.

Electrolytes

Potassium

Uremia frequently is associated with hyperkalemia because of impaired renal excretion and potassium release during accelerated protein catabolism. There also can be altered distribution of potassium between intracellular and extracellular spaces.[97] Decreased cellular potassium uptake can be caused by factors associated with uremia.[44,98,99] These factors decrease potassium tolerance, resulting in a greater increase in serum potassium after a potassium-rich meal.[97] Despite the frequency of hyperkalemia, body stores of potassium are decreased in most patients with CRF including those treated by dialysis. The low potassium stores mainly reflect a decrease in lean body mass because of malnutrition. Consequently, dialysis patients with a poor nutritional state or patients with ARF may also present with a low serum potassium concentration, especially if potassium intake is restricted.[100]

Phosphate

Serum phosphate increases in uremic patients not only because of decreased renal excretion but also because phosphates are released from bone with hyperparathyroidism and during catabolism. Like potassium, body stores of phosphates are decreased in many CRF patients because of a low lean body mass.[101] When receiving nutritional support with a low-electrolyte-composition supplement, hypophosphatemia and hypokalemia will develop in many uremic patients.[61,102] Malnourished patients treated by hemodialysis can even develop overt hypophosphatemia. In subjects with normal kidneys, potassium or phosphate depletion increases the risk of developing ARF and will retard the recovery of renal function following ARF.[103]

Calcium

The majority of uremic patients have a low serum calcium, including both protein-bound and ionized fractions. The major reasons for a low serum calcium are reduced calcium absorption from the GI tract (due to reduced synthesis of $1,25\text{-}(OH)_2$ vitamin D_3), the presence of hyperphosphatemia, skeletal resistance to the calcemic effect of parathyroid hormone, and aluminum toxicity.[104] ARF and CRF are frequently associated with hypocalcemia.[105] Unlike CRF patients, however, plasma levels of $1,25\text{-dihydroxy-vitamin } D_3$ are more variable because both its production and metabolic clearance are reduced in ARF patients.[106]

Hypercalcemia can develop with calcitriol administration or calcium-containing antacids, a high calcium concentration in the dialysis fluid, chronic immobilization, or tertiary hyperparathyroidism. In ARF associated with rhabdomyolysis, a persistent increase in serum calcitriol can cause a "rebound" hypercalcemia during the recovery or diuretic phase of ARF.[107]

Magnesium

A high serum magnesium is common in patients with uremia but rarely causes clinical problems. Symptomatic hypermagnesemia may develop when magnesium hydroxyl gels or magnesium-containing cathartics are used. Hypomagnesemia can occur with GI disorders associated with steatorrhea or prolonged diarrhea.

Micronutrients

Vitamins

Serum levels of water-soluble vitamins are low in dialysis patients mainly because of losses during dialysis.[108] A deficiency of pyridoxine (vitamin B_6) has been linked to abnormal amino acid and lipid metabolism in uremia while depletion of thiamine (vitamin B_1) during continuous hemofiltration has been associated with lactic acidosis.[109]

Regarding fat-soluble vitamins, calcitriol levels are low in patients with CRF because of reduced conversion of vitamin D_3 to its most active form, 1,25-dihydroxy vitamin D_3. Vitamin K deficiency has been reported only in patients receiving certain antibiotics that impair vitamin K production by intestinal bacteria.[110] Plasma vitamin A levels are almost always high in patients with ARF and CRF and in hemodialysis patients because of hepatic release of retinol and retinol-binding protein plus reduced renal catabolism of the transport protein.[111] Although a similar defect may be present for other protein-transporting vitamins/trace elements, the abnormality has only been identified with vitamin A. Plasma and erythrocyte concentrations of vitamin E (α-tocopherol) are decreased, normal, or increased in patients treated by hemodialysis or CAPD; in most patients with ARF, vitamin E levels are low.[112]

Trace Elements

Available reports on trace element metabolism in uremic subjects provide conflicting evidence.[113] The cause and degree of renal disease as well as the type of tissue being studied must all be considered when interpreting reports of abnormalities in trace element metabolism.[114] Geographic location and treatment strategies such as the mineral content of water, the type of therapy and medications, and especially the possibility of contaminated dialysis fluids can profoundly affect trace element balance.[115]

Except for aluminum, the contribution of trace element toxicity or deficiency to symptoms in patients with renal disease has not been established. Decreased levels of zinc in tissues in patients with CRF or in dialysis patients have been linked to uremic symptoms including loss of appetite, an altered sense of taste and smell, and impaired sexual function. Although some of these problems may be alleviated by zinc supplements, a positive response has not been confirmed by others.[116]

Selenium concentrations in plasma and erythrocytes are uniformly decreased in patients in renal failure, and selenium deficiency has been implicated as an important factor in lipid peroxidation and the development of cardiomyopathy and ischemic heart disease, malignancy, or impaired immune function. It is not known whether selenium can help patients with such problems.[117]

Many dialysis patients will develop complications from iron overload because they have had multiple blood transfusions. With the widespread use of erythropoietin to correct anemia, this problem is infrequent, and in fact the daily iron requirement is increased.

Micronutrients are important for the defense mechanisms against oxygen free-radical injury. A reduced antioxidant status has been found in patients with ARF and CRF.[112] In rats with ARF, antioxidant deficiency (determined as low blood levels of vitamin E or selenium) exacerbates ischemic renal injury and increases mortality from ARF.[118] These results suggest a crucial role for reactive-oxygen species causing peroxidation of lipid membrane components resulting in tissue injury.[119]

NUTRIENT REQUIREMENTS IN UREMIA

Energy

Renal failure per se has little impact on oxygen consumption; energy requirements are largely determined by the burden of the illness causing renal failure. In patients with ARF, energy requirements have been grossly overestimated, leading to recommendations for more than 50 kcal/kg of body weight/day (i.e., about 200 percent of the calculated basal energy expenditure [BEE]) in attempts to achieve positive nitrogen balance.[120,121] Fortunately, the adverse effects and dangers of such an exaggerated nutrient intake are now known, and it is agreed that the energy supply for ARF, CRF, or dialysis patients should not exceed the actual energy consumption. Even in patients with hypermetabolic conditions such as sepsis or multiple organ failure, energy requirements rarely exceed 130 percent of the calculated BEE.[36,38]

Unfortunately, a patient's energy requirements are not easily measured so the energy requirement should be calculated using standard formulas such as the BEE of the Harris-Benedict equation. This value is then multiplied by a "stress factor" depending on associated illnesses (Table 26–1). The older practice of adding 1.3 or 1.25 multiples of the BEE should be discarded.

The optimal energy intake for metabolically stable CRF dialysis patients with normal physical activity and no accompanying acute illness is at least 35 kcal/kg/day (i.e., about 40 percent above BEE).[122,123] This intake will be sufficient to achieve neutral nitrogen balance unless there is a catabolic illness. If there is, increasing calories alone will not correct the abnormality.

TABLE 26–1 Estimation of Energy Requirements

Calculation of Basic Energy Expenditure (BEE)
Harris-Benedict equation:
  Males: 66.47 + (13.75 × BW) + (5 × height) − (6.76 × age)
  Females: 655.1 + (9.56 × BW) + (1.85 × height) − (4.67 × age)
The average BEE is approximately 25 kcal/kg of body weight/day

Stress Factors
Correct calculated energy requirement for hypermetabolism:
  Postoperative (no complications) =   1.0
  Long bone fracture   1.15–1.30
  Cancer   1.10–1.30
  Peritonitis/sepsis   1.10–1.30
  Severe infection/multiple trauma   1.20–1.40
  Multiple organ failure syndrome   1.20–1.40
  Burn   1.20–2.00
  (= approximately BEE + % burned body surface area)

Corrected Energy Requirements
(kcal/day) = Bee × stress factor

On the other hand, if calorie intake is restricted, energy expenditure will not adapt, so protein conservation will be impaired and contribute to the development of malnutrition.[123]

Amino Acids and Proteins

Assessment of Protein Catabolism

Because virtually all nitrogen arising from amino acid catabolism following protein degradation is converted to urea, the quantity of protein degraded can be judged clinically by calculating the urea nitrogen appearance rate (UNA). When UNA is multiplied by 6.25, it is converted to protein equivalents. Because muscle contains about 20 percent of protein, multiplying the estimated protein loss by 5 yields an approximation of the loss of muscle mass. Obviously, UNA is not a "true" rate of protein catabolism because it does not take into account the high endogenous rate of protein turnover (3 to 4 g of protein/kg of body weight/day in normal adults).[51]

In patients with renal insufficiency, urea produced is not rapidly excreted but accumulates in body fluids. Because urea is distributed equally throughout the body water (about 60 percent of body weight)[124] changes in urea pool can easily be calculated (Table 26–2). Besides urea nitrogen lost in urine, losses in other body fluids (e.g., GI losses) must be added to calculate UNA accurately. Besides urea nitrogen, nonurea nitrogen must be taken into account. According to Maroni and colleagues, these nonurea nitrogen losses do not vary substantially with the diet and average 0.031 g of nitrogen/kg of body weight/day.[124] If this value is added to UNA, total waste nitrogen production can be estimated, and when nitrogen intake from the diet or parenteral nutrition is known, nitrogen balance can be estimated accurately.

The UNA can also serve as a guide to dietary compliance or to monitor the adequacy of a dietary prescription in metabolically stable subjects with CRF.[124,125] In this calculation, nitrogen output is assumed to be equal to dietary nitrogen intake so that UNA plus the average value of nonurea nitrogen excretion is assumed to be equal to nitrogen intake. For dialysis pa-

TABLE 26–2 Estimating the Extent of Protein Catabolism and Compliance to Nutritional Prescription

UNA (g/day)
  = Urinary urea excretion
  + Change in urea nitrogen pool
  = (UUN × V) + (BUN-2 − BUN-1) 0.006 × BW
  + (BW-2 − BW-1) × BUN-2/100
If there are substantial GI losses, add the urea
  nitrogen in secretions:
  = Volume of secretions × BUN-2
Net protein breakdown (g/day) = UNA × 6.25
Muscle loss (g/day) = UNA × 6.25 × 5
The assumptions are that 6% of weight is water,
  that short-term changes in weight are due to
  changes in body water, that protein is 16%
  nitrogen, and that muscle is 20% protein (see
  text).

UNA = Urea nitrogen appearance; UUN = urea nitrogen concentration in urine in grams of nitrogen/liter; V = urine volume in liters/day; BUN-1 and BUN-2 = BUN in mg/dl on days 1 and 2; BW-1 and BW-2 = body weights in kg on days 1 and 2.

tients, the protein catabolic rate (PCR) can be calculated from urea kinetic modeling.[126] Again, this calculation assumes a steady-state condition between nitrogen intake and output; consequently, do not use these calculations if there is an acute intercurrent disease.

Essential Amino Acids in Uremia

Rose originally proposed that eight amino acids are essential for human nutrition.[127] Histidine is now recognized as essential both in health and disease, a fact that was overlooked because of the large body pools, especially as a component of carnosine.[68] In patients with impaired renal function, other amino acids may become "conditionally indispensable." For example, the normal kidney releases arginine, and an arginine-free diet can cause disturbances in ammonia detoxification, even to the point of hyperammoniemic coma in patients with ARF or CRF.[128,129] Arginine also is important as a component of the L-arginine-nitric oxide pathway, and arginine deficiency is suggested as a cause for several aspects of the uremic syndrome, such as impaired blood pressure control, atherogenesis, vascular smooth muscle cell proliferation, macrophage toxicity, and impaired antibacterial defense.[130,131] Thus, arginine can be regarded as a conditionally essential amino acid in uremia, and an arginine-free diet should not be given to uremic subjects. Similarly, tyrosine formation from phenylalanine is impaired in ARF and CRF because there is reduced activity of the hepatic enzyme that accomplishes this conversion, phenylalanine hydrolase.[69] The decreased renal conversion of phenylalanine to tyrosine indicates that diets for uremic subjects should contain tyrosine. Serine and cysteine are also released from the kidneys and could become conditionally indispensable in patients with renal failure.[67,68]

As a general principle, many so-called nonessential amino acids can exert important physiologic functions but also are necessary for protein synthesis, and "nonessential nitrogen" has been shown to be important for normal growth and protein synthesis.[132,133] Thus, the distinction between essential and nonessential amino acids is no longer justified, and enteral diets containing only essential amino acids should not be used for prolonged periods.

Amino Acid and Protein Requirements

Few studies have attempted to define the optimal intake of protein or amino acids for patients with ARF or CRF or those treated by hemodialysis or CAPD. In noncatabolic patients during the polyuric phase of ARF, a protein intake of 0.97 g/kg of body weight/day was required to achieve a positive nitrogen balance; a similar value (1.03 g/kg of body weight/day) was required in another study, but unfortunately energy intake was not kept constant.[120,134] In the polyuric, recovery phase of ARF, a nitrogen intake of 15 g/day (averaging an amino acid intake of 1.3 g/kg of body weight/day) was superior in improving nitrogen balance compared with an intake of 4.4 g/day (about 0.3 g/kg amino acids), at least in patients with sepsis-induced ARF.[135] A prospective, randomized trial was conducted in 13 ARF patients to compare an intake of 21 g of essential amino acids (EAA) only (averaging 0.25 g/kg of body weight/day) with enough EAA plus nonessential amino acids to equal the urea nitrogen appearance rate of the previous day (the mean intake was 76 g amino acids/day).[136] Not surprisingly, the UNA increased rapidly in the group receiving more nitrogen, but their nitrogen balance tended to improve. Unfortunately, all regimens resulted in negative nitrogen balance. These results emphasize the problems that will occur with a strategy based on "pushing" protein intake to achieve nitrogen balance. We conclude that the optimal intake of protein or amino acids in patients with ARF is influenced more by the nature of the illness causing ARF and the extent of protein catabolism plus the type and frequency of dialysis rather than renal dysfunction per se. In most clinical situations, daily requirements will exceed the minimal requirement of 0.6 g of protein/kg of body weight/day or even the recommended allowance for normal subjects of 0.8 g/kg of body weight/day.

Unless the period of renal insufficiency will be brief, (e.g., in aminoglycoside-induced ARF), and unless there is no accompanying catabolic illness, the intake of protein or amino acids, respectively, should not be below 0.8 g/kg of body weight/day. In patients treated with hemodialysis, peritoneal dialysis, or continuous hemofiltration, protein or amino acid intake should be increased by 0.2 g/kg of body weight/day. In the hypercatabolic patient with ARF treated by continuous hemofiltration, protein needs have been estimated to range from 1.4 to 1.7 g/kg of body weight/day.[127] In similar patients, Kierdorf and colleagues showed that 1.7 g protein/kg of body weight/day was superior to 0.7 g and 1.5 g, respectively, in improving nitrogen balance but nitrogen balance still remained negative.[139] Because more protein and amino acid intake will increase waste products, it is not justified to supply more than 1.5 g of protein/amino acids/kg of body weight/day in critically ill patients even when they are treated by dialysis or hemofiltration.[140,141]

Hypercatabolism and loss of lean body mass cannot be controlled simply by increasing protein or amino acid intake. Besides the evidence from published trials,[134,136] it is clear that accelerated hepatic conversion of amino acids to glucose in an acute illness can be reduced but not eliminated simply by providing more protein or energy.[137] Moreover, the level of UNA should not be confused with a nitrogen requirement, but rather it should serve as an index of nitrogen intake plus the degree of catabolism. A protein or amino acid intake above maximal value of about 1.5 g/kg of body weight/day should not be used because it simply promotes the formation of urea and other nitrogenous waste products.

Any low-protein diet must be carefully monitored when given as enteral feeding to avoid complications and malnutrition. Correction of acidosis to control protein catabolism is crucial in the treatment of patients with CRF because this measure will permit them to use dietary protein optimally.[142]

Protein requirements in hemodialysis patients are not well defined but are thought to be considerably higher than in healthy subjects or stable patients with CRF. At least 1.2 g/kg of body weight/day should be given and even more is needed by patients with overt malnourishment; 1.5 g/kg of body weight/day has been recommended.[65] The protein intake of patients treated by CAPD should be enough to compensate for losses of amino acids and proteins into the peritoneal fluid. In a metabolic balance study of a few, clinically stable CAPD patients, it was shown that 1.4 g protein/kg of body weight/day is superior to 0.98 g protein/kg of body weight/day in achieving a positive nitrogen balance.[143]

Electrolytes

Electrolyte requirements for any patient with renal failure who requires nutritional support are limited, so enteral products specifically designed for uremic patients generally have a low mineral content. If a patient develops an electrolyte deficiency (e.g., phosphate or potassium), these minerals should be added to the supplement.[102,144]

Micronutrients

The requirements for water-soluble vitamins are increased in uremic patients, except for ascorbic acid (vitamin C).[108] It is a precursor of oxalic acid, and vitamin C intake should be kept below 200 mg/day to prevent secondary oxalosis.[145] Regarding fat-soluble vitamins, plasma vitamin A levels are increased in patients with renal failure, so dietary requirements are decreased; the same may be true for vitamin K.[110] Recommendations for vitamin E are conflicting, and there is a need to supplement $1,25\text{-(OH)}_2$ vitamin D_3 in the dialysis patient; there is no evidence that vitamin D should be replaced in patients with ARF. No firm recommendations can be made for supplementing selenium or zinc above the level for normal adults. In fact, most enteral formulations contain the recommended daily allowances of vitamins and trace elements.

Parenteral administration of trace elements to a patient with renal failure carries the risk of inducing toxicity because the major control of trace element homeostasis is a balance between its GI absorption and renal excretion, and both elements would be bypassed by intravenous infusion.

METABOLIC IMPACT OF EXTRACORPOREAL THERAPY

Amino acid elimination during hemodialysis accounts for about 4 g amino acids/hour of dialysis therapy.[146] There is another 4 g of peptide-bound amino acids plus the blood lost in the extracorporeal circuit. These losses contribute to the negative nitrogen balance that occurs during dialysis.[65] Recently, it was shown that reprocessing of the dialyzer by bleaching increases amino acid losses, presumably by modifying membrane properties.[147] During CAPD, losses of free amino acids average about 3 to 4 g/day, and there is an additional loss of 9 g of protein/day (6 g of albumin/day).[148]

For critically ill ARF patients treated by continuous arteriovenous hemofiltration or continuous hemodialysis, the sieving coefficient of amino acids is within the range of 0.8 to 1.0. Thus, amino acid losses can be estimated from the volume of the filtrate and the average plasma amino acid plasma concentration.[149] Usually, the loss amounts to approximately 0.3 g/L or 5 to 10 g of amino acids/day.

Interestingly, the infusion of a supplemental nutritional solution during dialysis does not augment amino acid losses substantially; only about 10 percent of amino acids given are lost in the dialysate/hemofiltrate.[150] Amino acid losses are negligible because the endogenous clearance of amino acids into cells exceeds their clearance by the dialysis procedure by 10 to 100 times.[42] However, an exaggerated protein/amino acid intake may increase dialysis-induced elimination by raising the plasma amino acid concentrations.

Synthetic dialysis membranes that filter small proteins and peptide hormones cause additional losses, but because the plasma half-life of these compounds is short, hormone losses do not cause major physiologic abnormalities. Besides amino acids or peptides and proteins, water-soluble vitamins and carnitine are eliminated during dialysis. Because trace elements have a very large volume of distribution and fat-soluble vitamins are protein bound, there are negligible losses of these elements with dialysis. Finally, in an experimental study of the effects of dialysis, the dialysis membrane was shown to cause muscle protein catabolism related to the degree of biocompatibility of the dialysis membrane.[66] This factor may be clinically important because a recent study using more "biocompatible" dialyzer membranes showed improved survival of ARF patients compared with those treated with "bioincompatible" membranes.[151] Hemodialysis also promotes the generation of oxygen radicals, which contribute to tissue injury, accelerated atherosclerosis, impaired immunocompetence, and protein wasting.[152,153]

NUTRITIONAL STRATEGIES

The decision to initiate nutritional support is influenced by the following:

1. The patient's ability to achieve nutritional requirements by eating. Preterm or small infants, patients with neurologic disabilities or with mechanical obstructions in the upper GI tract, the anorectic elderly, and critically ill patients will require artificial nutritional support.
2. The patient's nutritional status as determined from values of serum albumin and transferrin concentrations, anthropometric measurements, and, most important, clinical judgement. In the presence of an acute illness, or evidence of malnourishment, nutritional intervention should be initiated even if the patient is judged likely to eat.
3. The degree of accompanying catabolism, the type of accompanying complications, or underlying illness. In the presence of excessive protein catabolism, nutritional support should be initiated early.

When should nutritional support be started? The time to initiate nutritional support will be determined by the patient's nutritional status and the degree of catabolism. In general, the greater the extent of malnutrition and the more pronounced the degree of catabolism, the earlier nutritional support should be initiated.

During the acute phase of ARF (within the first 24 to 48 hours after trauma or surgery) nutritional support must be avoided. Infusions of large quantities of amino acids or glucose during this "ebb phase" will not only increase oxygen requirements but also may aggravate tubular damage and the degree of renal functional loss.[154,155]

At what degree of renal dysfunction should the nutritional regimen be modified? Experimental and clinical studies have shown that the metabolic alterations associated with renal failure occur when creatinine clearance falls below 40 ml/minute.[42,156,157] Thus, when serum creatinine is above 3 mg/dl or creatinine clearance is below 40 ml/minute, nutritional regimens should be designed to counteract the metabolic abnormalities of renal failure.

PATIENT CLASSIFICATION

Ideally, a nutritional program should be designed for each patient with renal failure, but because nutritional needs will differ among patients, uniform recommendations and standardization of nutrition protocols are almost impossible. The following recommendations for specific patient groups should serve as guidelines:

1. The noncatabolic patient with ARF and the patient with stable CRF. This group includes patients without excess catabolism (a UNA of less than 5 g of nitrogen above nitrogen intake/day) (Table 26–3). ARF in these patients is usually caused by nephrotoxins (e.g., aminoglycosides, contrast media, or mismatched blood transfusions). Even in stable CRF, the nutritional state is impaired in as many as 40 percent of patients, and

TABLE 26–3   Patient Classification and Substrate Requirements

Patient Classification	Non-catabolic ARF or Stable CRF +/– Malnutrition	Stable RDT/CAPD +/– Malnutrition	ARF, CRF, RDT/CAPD + Superimposed Catabolic Illness Catabolism	
			Moderate	Severe
Excess urea appearance (above nitrogen intake)	0–5 g/day	0–5 g/day	6–12 g/day	> 13 g/day
Route of nutrient administration	Oral/enteral	Oral/enteral	Enteral or parenteral or both	Enteral or parenteral or both
Energy recommendations (kcal/kg/day)	25–35	30–40	25–35	30–40
Protein g/kg/day	0.6–0.8	1.2–1.5	0.8–1.2	1.0–1.5
Nutrients used				
Oral	Food or specific enteral formulas +/– EAA/KA supplement	Enteral formulas Specific/standard	Enteral formulas Specific/standard	Enteral formulas Specific/standard
Enteral				
Parenteral	EAA solution glucose 20–40%	EAA + NEAA solution (adapted or standard) plus 50–70 g/dl glucose and fat emulsion (10–20%)		
	Plus supplements of vitamins, trace elements, and electrolytes as required			

EAA = essential amino acids; NEAA = nonessential amino acids; KA = keto acids of EAA.

there are multiple metabolic abnormalities including abnormal regulation of protein turnover, an enhanced response to catabolic factors, and nutrient deficiencies. Nutritional repletion in these subjects requires a delicate balance between minimizing uremic toxicity by avoiding too much dietary protein to avoid further loss of renal function[5] while promoting positive nitrogen balance.

2. The stable patient treated by hemodialysis/peritoneal dialysis. Evidence of malnutrition has been observed in 20 to 70 percent of patients in this group.[65] Aside from disturbances in protein and energy metabolism, hormonal derangements, metabolic acidosis, infections and superimposed illness, losses of nutrients during dialysis, and the catabolic effect of dialysis per se all contribute to muscle wasting. In these patients, anorexia is very common, and there may be nausea, vomiting, and psychosocial factors such as loneliness and depression. Nutritional status has been identified as an important denominator of morbidity and survival in dialysis patients.[158] These patients should receive 1.2 g/kg/day of protein and 35 kcal/kg/day.

3. The dialysis patient with a superimposed acute illness. The primary goal is to maintain nutrition and correct fluid and electrolyte disorders. The accumulation of waste products is prevented by adjusting the intensity of dialysis. Nutritional therapy should not be aimed at avoiding or reducing dialysis frequency, nor should protein or amino acid intake be raised with the unrealistic goal of forcing nitrogen balance to become positive. In clinical practice, it is useful to distinguish which acutely ill patients are catabolic and evaluate the extent of protein breakdown associated with the underlying disease. This practice relies on repeated measurements of the UNA and can provide guidelines to assess dietary requirements (Table 26–3).

The first category consists of patients with moderate hypercatabolism and a UNA exceeding nitrogen intake by 6 to 12 g of nitrogen/day (Table 26–3). Such patients frequently suffer from complicating infections, peritonitis, or moderate injury and have renal dysfunction. Tube feeding or intravenous nutritional support is generally required, and dialysis/hemofiltration often become necessary to limit waste product accumulation.

In a second group of patients, renal failure is associated with severe trauma, burns, or overwhelming infections. UNA is markedly elevated (more than 12 g of nitrogen above nitrogen intake). Treatment strategies are usually complex and include enteral or parenteral nutrition, hemodialysis or continuous hemofiltration, and blood pressure and ventilatory support. To reduce the impact of catabolism and minimize protein depletion, nutrient administration is generous and dialysis is needed to maintain fluid balance and blood urea nitrogen (BUN) below 100 mg/dl (Table 26–3). Mortality in this group of patients exceeds 60 to 80 percent. It is not renal dysfunction that accounts for the poor prognosis but rather the superimposed hypercatabolism and the severity of underlying illness and complications. Unfortunately, there are no reliable methods for stopping hypercatabolism, and nutritional therapy should be directed at minimizing the loss of protein mass.

NUTRIENT ADMINISTRATION

Enteral nutrition should always be the first line of nutrient administration in artificial nutrition. Among the well-documented advantages (Chapter 23) is the fact that intestinal nutrients are needed to maintain GI functions such as secretion of mucus and IgA, bile flow, and intestinal motility and especially to support the barrier function of the intestinal mucosa. Enteral nutrition helps to preserve the structural integrity of the mucosal layer and prevent the development of ulcerations and translocation of bacteria with a systemic infection.[159] However, in the critically ill patient, it may be impossible to achieve nutrient requirements exclusively by the enteral route, and parenteral nutrition may become necessary.[160] Regardless, even when intestinal motility is severely compromised and nutritional requirements cannot be met enterally, providing small amounts of enteral nutrients regularly (i.e., 100 ml/day several times each day) can help support intestinal function.[161]

Enteral Nutrition

Feeding Tubes

Use only soft-bore feeding tubes to prevent the development of pressure ulcerations in the esophagus. Usually, the tip of the tube is positioned in the stomach, but in patients with impaired gastric emptying and vomiting due to gastroparesis, persistent duodenogastric, or gastroesophageal reflux or for small infants, advance the tip of the tube into the small intestine, preferably into the jejunum. Consider percutaneous endoscopic gastrostomy (PEG) (Chapter 14) if prolonged enteral nutritional support is needed for confused patients or those with neurologic disabilities or mechanical obstruction in the upper GI tract. PEG is contraindicated in patients with peritoneal dialysis because a gastric leak can cause peritonitis.[162,163] With special precautions including a sufficient interval between positioning the feeding tube and beginning peritoneal dialysis to guarantee a stable seal between stomach and abdominal wall, PEG has been used in patients treated by CAPD. In a 155-month experience with PEG in 13 small infants treated by peritoneal dialysis, no major complications were observed.[164] A report of 9 children during 64 months reported only one peritoneal dialysis fluid leak from the PEG exit site.[165] In infants treated by continuous cycling peritoneal dialysis, a gastrotomy button device has been used for long-term feeding.[166]

Enteral Formulas

The difficulty in designing an enteral diet for patients with renal failure lies not only in the broad clinical spectrum of patients with renal dysfunction but with diverse individual requirements. These problems prevent widespread use of a common enteral, nutritional mixture. An enteral diet often is a compromise between supplying nutrients and tailoring the mixture for an individual's requirements and ability to excrete minerals and waste products. There also have been fewer systematic investigations of commercially available diets.[167] Essentially, three types of enteral formulas have been used in uremic patients (Table 26–4).

Elemental Powder Diets Containing Mainly Essential Amino Acids. Low-protein diets supplemented with essential amino acids were designed in the 1960s to provide adequate oral nutrition for patients with advanced CRF, and these have been extended for use as enteral nutrition supplements. These diets contain the eight, classic, essential amino acids plus histidine but are not complete because they must be supplemented with energy substrates, vitamins, and trace elements. Major disadvantages of the

TABLE 26–4 Specialized Enteral Formulas for Nutritional Support in Patients with Renal Failure

	Amin-Aid	Travasorb renal*	Salvipeptide nephro†	Survimed renal‡	Suplena§	Nepro§
Volume (ml)	750	1050	500	1000	500	500
Calories (kcal)	1467	1400	1000	1320	1000	1000
cal/ml	1.96	1.35	2.00	1.32	2.00	2.00
Energy distribution proteins: fat: carbohydrates (%)	4:21:75	7:12:81	8:22:70	6:10:84	6:43:51	14:43:43
kcal/g N	832:1	389:1	313:1	398:1	427:1	179:1
Proteins (g)	14.6	24.0	20.0	20.8	15.0	35
AA:EAA (%)	100	60	23			
NEAA (%)	—	30	20			
Hydrolysate (%)	—	—	23	100		
Full protein (%)	—	—	34	—	100	100
Nitrogen (g)	1.76	3.6	3.2	3.32	2.4	
Carbohydrates (g)	274	284	175	276	128	108
Monosaccharides/ Disaccharides (%)	100	100	3		10	12
Oligosaccharides (%)	—	—	28			
Polysaccharides (%)	—	—	69	88		90
Fat (g)	34.6	18.6	24	15.2	48	47.8
LCT (%)		30	50		100	100
Essential FA (%)		18	31	52	22	
MCT (%)		70	50	30	0	0
Nonprotein (calories/g nitrogen)	800	363	288	3741	54	393
Osmol (mOsm/kg)	1095	590	507	600	635	615
Sodium (mmol/l)	11	—	7.2	15.2	36.1	34.0
Potassium (mmol/l)	—	—	1.5	8	27.0	28.5
Phosphate (mmol/l)	—	16.1	6.13	6.4	11.0	11.0
Vitamins	b	a	a	a	a	a
Minerals	b	b	a	a	a	a

a = 2000 kcal/day meets RDA for most vitamins/trace elements; b = must be added; EAA = essential amino acids; NEAA = nonessential amino acids; FA = fatty acid.
*3 bags + 810 ml = 1050 ml.
†1 × component I + 1 × component II + 350 ml = 500 ml.
‡4 bags + 800 ml = 1000 ml
§Liquid formula, cans a 8 fl oz (= 237.5 ml), supplemented with carnitine, taurine.

available enteral diets are the limited spectrum of nutrients and the high osmolality of the solution plus the problems of mixing a powder. Still, they can be used as a dietary supplement for patients with advanced CRF or for dialysis patients. If total enteral nutrition is necessary, these diets should be replaced by a more complete formula.

After modification, an experimental diet was designed to include six amino acids and four nitrogen-free keto-analogs of essential amino acids. The aim was to provide minimal nitrogen to reduce waste products and retard the progression of renal failure.[168] Even though effective, few clinical situations require the mixture, so it has not become commercially available.[169]

Standard Enteral Formulas for Nonuremic Patients. In patients with renal insufficiency requiring intensive care, standard enteral formulas have been used.[140,170] A disadvantage of these diets is the fixed nutrient composition. In addition, the amount and types of protein are fixed, and there is a high content of electrolytes and especially potassium and phosphate.

Standard pediatric formulas such as Similac PM 60/40 or SMA have been given to uremic infants. Generally, so-called nonessential nutrients and protein or energy supplements are added to avoid growth retardation.[171,172]

Specific Enteral Formulas Adapted to Meet the Metabolic Alterations of Uremia. Two concepts have been followed in designing a specialized enteral diet for patients with renal failure. First, modular diets can circumvent many of the problems arising from an individual's special requests. With these mixtures, the diet can be adapted to a patient's needs by altering the number and types of components and thus could be useful for renal failure patients.[173] The main disadvantages are that the powders must be mixed and there is a risk of contaminating the fluid.

Second, "ready-to-use" liquid diets have been introduced recently, including one preparation designed as a supplement for patients with CRF. This preparation has a lower protein and electrolyte concentration (Table 26–4, Nepro). A second preparation has been adapted for dialysis patients and contains more protein but still has a reduced electrolyte content (Table 26–4, Suplena). Both diets are supplemented with taurine and carnitine and have a high energy content of 1.5 kcal/ml. Originally designed as an oral supplement, these diets can be used in enteral nutrition and for hypercatabolic patients.

Enteral Nutrient Administration

The techniques of enteral nutrition in patients with renal failure are identical to those employed for other patient groups (Chapter 13). Feeding solutions can be administered intermittently or continuously into the stomach or continuously into the jejunum, preferably by pump. If given continuously, the stomach should be aspirated every 2 to 4 hours to check for fluid retention until adequate gastric emptying and intestinal peristalsis are established. This will prevent vomiting and will reduce the risk of bronchopulmonary aspiration. To avoid high-osmolality-induced diarrhea, the formula (especially elemental diets with free amino acids and a high osmolality) should be diluted and the amount and concentration of the solution gradually increased until nutritional requirements are met. This practice usually avoids potentially treatable side-effects such as nausea, vomiting, abdominal distension, and cramping and diarrhea. Gradually increasing the rate of nutrient infusion will help to ensure adequate use while avoiding metabolic derangements in patients with reduced tolerance. In malnourished dialysis patients, nocturnal enteral supplementation by nasogastric feeding tubes has been advocated.[174] The necessity of repeatedly placing a feeding tube, the risk of intrabronchial insertion, or inadvertent removal by a confused patient combine to make this type of nasogastric feeding unadvisable. Instead, a PEG should be used.[166]

It has been suggested that enteral nutrition should be stopped during hemodialysis because splanchnic blood flow might decrease and increase GI symptoms.[1] This has not been a major problem, and if a patient tolerates intradialytic nutrient supply, nutrients can be provided during treatment.

Clinical Experience with Enteral Nutrition in Renal Disease

Most available investigations have focused on the feasibility and tolerance of enteral diets in only a few patients, and data regarding nutritional efficiency are rarely provided. Abras and Walser gave continuous nasogastric feeding to four patients with advanced CRF using an experimental, low-nitrogen diet composed of amino and keto acids and oligosaccharides.[168,169] The subjects were permitted unlimited quantities of other foods, but about 70 percent of the substrates were delivered by feeding tube. Despite the extremely limited nitrogen intake (averaging only 3.3 g of nitrogen/day) nitrogen balance became positive in all subjects, body weight was maintained, and plasma protein concentrations remained stable.

Douglas and colleagues provided nasogastric feeding using conventional diets with 44 g of protein and 2060 kcal while studying malnourished hemodialysis patients.[175] In some, feeding was given overnight for only 8 hours and provided 55 g of protein and 1450 kcal. The feedings were tolerated. Several authors have investigated the use of oral supplements (mostly amino acids) in malnourished patients treated by hemodialysis or CAPD.[176] Note that the amounts of amino acids given in many of these studies hardly compensated for the dialysis losses of amino acid. The benefit of adding a supplement to improve nitrogen retention is controversial.

Gretz and colleagues reported their experience (Table 26–4) with a modular, enteral formula (Salvipeptid Nephro) given to two patients: one was treated by RDT and another had advanced CRF.[144] Nutritional indexes (e.g., plasma proteins) improved. Remarkably, the low phosphate content of the diet required that one of the patients needed a phosphate supplement.

Regarding the "ready-to-use" liquid diets, oral tolerance studies are available. A formula comparable to the product, Suplena (Table 26–4), was tested in 18 patients with CRF during 4 weeks.[177] The patients ate other foods and added the supplement at a rate of 10 kcal/kg of body weight/day and this combination raised energy and protein intake to the recommended level for hemodialysis patients. Blood chemistry values remained stable in all patients, and GI tolerance was good. Nepro, a diet designed for RDT patients, was tested in 19 patients during 21 days as the primary source of nutrition. It was given at 28 or 35 kcal/kg of body weight/day, respectively; tolerance was good while nitrogen balance became positive.[178] The sodium and chloride content was low so patients were given sodium chloride supplement. Several subjects developed hypercalcemia, which has been observed during enteral nutrition with standard diets.

Most published studies on enteral nutrition in patients with renal failure have been performed in pediatric patients. Trapper and colleagues reported on eight infants with end-stage renal failure in whom a Tenckoff and a gastrostomy tube were placed to supplement oral nutrition.[172] Kidney transplantation was performed when body weight exceeded 10 kg, and growth and development were adequate in all survivors. Abitbol and coworkers investigated forced-feeding regimens in 12 children with a creatinine clearance below 70 ml/minute/1.73 m^2. Six patients received supplemental enteral feedings, initially by intermittent (nocturnal) or continuous nasogastric intubation.[171] Three infants could not tolerate nasogastric feedings and had surgical placement of a gastrostomy tube. Again, growth and development in these children was excellent. Dabbagh and associates evaluated the incidence of infections and need for hospitalization during "aggressive" nutrition in 37 pediatric patients treated by CAPD.[179] The frequency of peritonitis decreased, and there was a 55 percent decline in number of hospitalization days during enteral nutritional support. Positive experiences with enteral nutrition in pediatric patients with renal failure have also been reported by other groups.[180-183]

Complications and Monitoring of Enteral Nutrition

Side-effects and complications of nutritional support in patients with renal failure are similar to those observed in other patient groups, except that the tolerance to volume is much more limited, electrolyte derangements can develop rapidly, and excessive protein or amino acid intake results in accumulation of urea (and other waste products). Furthermore, glucose intolerance and decreased fat clearance can cause hyperglycemia and hypertriglyceridemia, respectively. Thus, nutritional therapy in renal failure patients requires a tighter schedule of monitoring to avoid metabolic complications of nutritional intervention (Table 26–5). In critically ill patients with multiple organ dysfunctions and renal failure, it is unclear whether the incidence of GI side-effects of enteral nutrition and especially diarrhea are increased. In small infants, exclusive nutrient supply by tube feeding can result in developmental or eating disorders.[184]

Parenteral Nutrition

For parenteral nutrition in renal disease, there are extensive reviews.[1,2,3,5] Parenteral nutrition should not be viewed as an alternative to enteral feeding but rather as a complementary method of nutritional support.

TABLE 26–5 A Minimal Schedule for Monitoring of Parenteral Nutrition

	Patients	
Variables	**Metabolically Unstable**	**Metabolically Stable**
Blood glucose	1–6 times daily	Daily
Osmolality	Daily	Twice weekly
Electrolytes (Na$^+$, K$^+$, Cl$^+$)	Daily	Daily
Calcium, phosphate, magnesium	Daily	3 times weekly
Creatinine, BUN/BUN rise/day	Daily	Daily
UNA	Daily	Twice weekly
Triglycerides	Daily	Twice weekly
Blood gas analysis/pH	1–6 times daily	Once weekly
Ammonia	2 times weekly	Once weekly
Transaminases + bilirubin	2 times weekly	Once weekly

BUN = blood urea nitrogen; UNA = urea nitrogen appearance.

For many patients, it is not possible to meet nutritional requirements by the enteral route alone.[160] Moreover, ARF often occurs in patients with severe GI dysfunction, such as pancreatitis or in hypercatabolic patients with multiple organ dysfunction, so a supplementary parenteral nutrient supply may become necessary. In selected dialysis patients with overt malnutrition, in whom attempts at oral or enteral nutritional supplements have failed, intradialytic parenteral nutrition may improve nutritional state and reduce morbidity.[185]

CONCLUSION

Enteral nutrition has become the preferred type of artificial nutritional support in patients with renal failure and is a standard of care even in ICUs, in pediatric nephrology, and in malnourished patients treated by RDT or CAPD. Whenever possible, nutrients should be supplied orally or enterally, even if only small amounts of luminal nutrients can be used because they help maintain GI functions and integrity. However, our knowledge of the alterations in GI functions present in patients with renal disease and the impact of enteral nutrients is incomplete; the optimal type and composition of enteral diets remain to be specified. The tremendous heterogeneity of patient groups, the diverging aims of nutritional support, and differences in individual requirements make general recommendations impossible. Modular diets that can be adapted to individual needs present the most promising concept for enteral products. Unfortunately, nutrient administration alone cannot control catabolism in acute disease states.[137] For the future, alternative endocrine or metabolic interventions, such as growth factors,[59,185] must be devised to improve the efficiency of nutritional support.

REFERENCES

1. Compher C, Mullen JL, Barker CF: Nutritional support in renal failure. Surg Clin North Am 1991;71: 597–608.
2. Varella L, Utermohlen V: Nutritional support for the patient with renal failure. Crit Care Nurs Clin North Am 1993;5:79–96.
3. Seidner DL, Matarese LE, Steiger E: Nutritional care of the critcally ill patient with renal failure. Semin Nephrol 1994;14:53–63.
4. Druml W: Nutritional management of acute renal failure. In Mitch WE, Klahr S (eds): Nutrition and the Kidney. Boston: Little, Brown & Co. 1993:314.
5. Mitch WE: Restricted diets and slowing the progression of chronic renal insufficiency. In Mitch WE,

Klahr S (eds): Nutrition and the Kidney. Boston: Little, Brown & Co. 1993:243.
6. Gilbert RJ, Goyal RK: The gastrointestinal system. In Eknoyan G, Knochel JP (eds): The systemic consequences of renal failure. New York: Grune & Stratton, 1984:133.
7. Shapira N, Skillman JJ, Steinman TI: Gastric mucosal permeability and gastric acid secretion before and after hemodialysis in patients with chronic renal failure. Surgery 1978;83:1859–1862.
8. Margolis DM, Saylor JL, Geisse G: Upper gastrointestinal disease in chronic renal failure: appropriate evaluation. Arch Intern Med 1978;138:1214–1217.
9. Zuckerman GR: Upper gastrointestinal bleeding in patients with chronic renal failure. Ann Intern Med 1985;102:588–592.
10. Andriulli A, Malfi B, Rechia S et al: Patients with chronic renal failure are not at risk of developing chronic peptic ulcers. Clin Nephrol 1985;23: 245–248.
11. Wright RA, Clemente R, Wathene R: Gastric emptying in patients with chronic renal failure receiving hemodialysis. Arch Intern Med 1984;144:495–496.
12. McNamee PT, Moore GW, McGeown MC: Gastric emptying in chronic renal failure. Br Med J 1985; 291:310–311.
13. Sachs EF, Hurwitz J, Block HM et al: Pancreatic exocrine hypofunction in the wasting syndrome of end stage renal disease. Am J Gastroenterol 1983;78: 170–174.
14. Araki T, Ueda M, Takeda K et al: Pancreatic type hyperamylasemia in renal insufficiency. Dig Dis Sci 1989;34:1425–1427.
15. Rutzky EA, Robards V, VanDyke A et al: Acute pancreatitis in patients with end stage renal disease without transplantation. Arch Intern Med 1986;146: 1741–1745.
16. Arvanitakis C, Nakos V, Kalekou-Greka H et al: Small intestinal function and structure in patients with chronic renal failure. Clin Nephrol 1985;29:235–243.
17. Haines DJ, Swan CHJ, Green JRG et al: Mucosal peptide hydrolase and brush-border marker enzyme activities in three regions of the small intestine of rats with experimental uraemia. Clin Sci 1990;79: 663–668.
18. Wizemann V, Ludwig D, Kuhl R et al: Digestive-adsorptive function of the intestinal brush border in uremia. Am J Clin Nutr 1978;31:1643–1646.
19. Sterner G, Lindberg T, Denneberg T: In vivo and in vitro absorption of amino acids and dipeptides in small intestine of uremic rats. Nephron 1982;31: 273–276.
20. Johansson SV, Oder-Cederlof I, Plantin LO et al: Albumin metabolism and gastrointestinal loss of protein in chronic renal failure. Acta Med Scand 1977;201: 353–358.
21. Drukker A, Levy E, Bronza N et al: Impaired intestinal fat absorption in chronic renal failure. Nephron 1982;30:154–160.
22. Pahl MV, Barbari A, Vaziri ND: Intestinal absorption of linoleic acid in experimental renal failure. Br J Nur 1991;66:467–477.
23. Goldstein DA, Hurowitz D, Petit S et al: The duodenal mucosa in patients with renal failure: response to 1,25(OH)2D3. Kidney Int 1981;19:324–331.
24. Said HM, Vaziri ND, Kariger RH et al: Intestinal absorption of 5-methylatrahydrofolate in experimental uremia. Acta Vitaminol Enzymol 1984;6:339–342.
25. Hughes RT, Smith T, Hesp R et al: Regulation of iron absorption in iron loaded subjects with end stage re-

nal disease: effects of treatment with recombinant human erythropoietin and reduction of iron stores. Br J Haematol 1992;82:445–454.

26. Domoto DT, Martin KJ: Failure of CAPD patients to respond to an oral iron absorption test. Adv Perit Dial 1992;8:102–104.

27. Dave PB, Romeu J, Antonelli A et al: Gastrointestinal telangiectasias: a source of bleeding in patients receiving hemodialysis. Arch Intern Med 1984;144: 1781–1783.

28. Gordon SJ, Miller LJ, Haeffner LJ et al: Abnormal intestinal bile acid distribution in azotemic man: a possible role in the pathogenesis of uremic diarrhea. Gut 1976;17:58–67.

29. Mitch WE: Effects of intestinal flora on nitrogen metabolism in patients with chronic renal failure. Am J Clin Nutr 1978;31:1594–1600.

30. Mitch WE, Walser M: Effects of oral neomycin and kanamycin in chronic uremic patients. II. Nitrogen balance. Kidney Int 1977;11:123–127.

31. Simenhoff ML, Burke JF, Sankkonen LG et al: Amine metabolism and the small bowel in uremia. Lancet 1976;2:818–822.

32. Hayes CP, McLeod MD, Robinson RR: An extrarenal mechanism for the maintenance of potassium balance in severe chronic renal failure. Trans Assoc Am Physicians 1967;58:207–216.

33. Pahl MV, Erickson RA, Vaziri ND et al: Intestinal morphometry and bile acid-induced mucosal injury in chronic experimental renal failure. J Lab Clin Med 1990;15:572–578.

34. Ephgrave KS, Leiman-Wexler RL, Adair CG: Enteral nutrients prevent stress ulceration and increase intragastric volume. Crit Care Med 1990;18:621–626.

35. Om P, Hohenegger M: Energy metabolism in acute uremic rats. Nephron 1980;25:249–253.

36. Schneeweib B, Graninger W, Stockenhuber F et al: Energy metabolism in acute and chronic renal failure. Am J Clin Nutr 1990;52:596–601.

37. Cotton JR, Woodward T, Carter NW et al: Resting skeletal muscle membrane potential as an index of uremic toxicity. J Clin Invest 1979;63:501–506.

38. Soop M, Forsberg E, Thörne A et al: Energy expenditure in postoperative multiple organ failure with acute renal failure. Clin Nephrol 1989;31:139–143.

39. Mitch WE: Amino acid release from the hindquarter and urea appearance in acute uremia. Am J Physiol 1981;241:E415–E419.

40. Flügel-Link RM, Salusky IB, Jones MR et al: Protein and amino acid metabolism in posterior hemicorpus of acutely uremic rats. Am J Physiol 1983;244: E615–E622.

41. Clark AS, Mitch WE: Muscle protein turnover and glucose uptake in acutely uremic rats. J Clin Invest 1983;72:836–845.

42. Baliga R, George VT, Ray PE: Effects of reduced renal function and dietary protein on muscle protein synthesis. Kidney Int 1991;39:831–835.

43. Lacy WW: Effect of acute uremia on amino acid uptake and urea production by perfused rat liver. Am J Physiol 1969;216:1300–1305.

44. Druml W, Kelly RA, Mitch WE et al: Abnormal cation transport in uremia. J Clin Invest 1988;81: 1197–1203.

45. Maroni BJ, Haesemeyer RW, Kutner MH et al: Kinetics of system A amino acid uptake by muscle: effects of insulin and acute uremia. Am J Physiol 1990;258:F1304–F1310.

46. Fürst P: Amino acid metabolism in uremia. J Am Coll Nutr 1989;8:310–323.

47. Druml W, Bürger U, Leinberger G et al: Elimination of amino acids in acute renal failure. Nephron 1986; 42:62–67.

48. Druml W, Fischer M, Liebisch B et al: Elimination of amino acids in renal failure. Am J Clin Nutr 1994;60:418–423.

49. Garber AJ: Effects of parathyroid hormone on skeletal muscle protein and amino acid metabolism. J Clin Invest 1983;71:1806–1810.

50. Campese VM, Romoff MS, Levitan D et al: Mechanisms of autonomic nervous system dysfunction in uremia. Kidney Int 1981;20:246–253.

51. Wilmore DWL: Catabolic illness: strategies for enhancing recovery. N Engl J Med 1991;325:695–702.

52. Schaefer RM, Teschner M, Eiegel W et al: Reduced protein catabolism by the antiglucocorticoid RU 38 486 in acutely uremic rats. Kidney Int 1989;36(suppl 27):S208–S211.

53. May RC, Kelly RA, Mitch WE: Mechanisms for defects in muscle protein metabolism in rats with chronic uremia: the influence of metabolic acidosis. J Clin Invest 1987;79:1099–1103.

54. Hara Y, May RC, Kelly A et al: Acidosis, not azotemia, stimulates branched-chain amino acid catabolism in uremic rats. Kidney Int 1987;32:808–814.

55. Mitch WE, Medina R, Greiber S et al: Metabolic acidosis stimulates muscle protein degradation by activating the ATP-dependent pathway involving ubiquitin and proteasomes. J Clin Invest 1994;93: 2127–2133.

56. Price SR, England BK, Bailey JL et al: Acidosis and glucocorticoids concomitantly increase ubiquitin and proteasome subunit mRNAs in rat muscle. Am J Physiol 1994;267:C955–C960.

57. Hörl WH, Heidland A: Enhanced proteolytic activity—cause of protein catabolism in acute renal failure. Am J Clin Nutr 1980;33:1423–1427.

58. Horl WH, Gantert C, Auer LA et al: In vitro inhibition of protein catabolism by alpha 2-macroglobulin in plasma from a patient with posttraumatic acute renal failure. Am J Nephrol 1982;2:32–34.

59. Ding H, Kopple JD, Cohen AH et al: Recombinant human insulin-like growth factor-1 accelerates recovery and reduces catabolism in rats with ischemic acute renal failure. J Clin Invest 1993;91: 2281–2287.

60. Berkelhammer CH, Baker JP, Leiter LA et al: Wholebody protein turnover in adult hemodialysis patients measured by 13 C-leucine. Am J Clin Nutr 1987;46: 778–783.

61. Goodship THJ, Mitch WE, Hoerr RA et al: Adaptation to low-protein diets in renal failure: leucine turnover and nitrogen balance. J Am Soc Nephrol 1990;1: 66–75.

62. Masud T, Young VR, Chapman T et al: Adaptive responses to very low protein diets: the first comparison of ketoacids to essential amino acids. Kidney Int 1994;45:1182–1192.

63. Tom K, Young VR, Chapman T et al: Long-term adaptive responses to dietary protein restriction in chronic renal failure. Am J Physiol 1995;268:E668–E677.

64. Li JB, Wassner SJ: Protein synthesis and degradation in skeletal muscle of chronically uremic rats. Kidney Int 1986;29:1136–1143.

65. Bergstrom J: Nutritional requirements of hemodialysis patients. In Mitch WE, Klahr S (eds): Nutrition and the Kidney. Boston: Little, Brown & Co, 1993:263.

66. Gutierrez A, Alvestrand A, Bergström J: Membrane selection and muscle protein catabolism. Kidney Int 1992;42(suppl 38):S86–S90.

67. Mitch WE, Chesney RW: Amino acid metabolism by the kidney. Miner Electrolyte Metab 1983;9:190–202.

68. Laidlaw SA, Kopple JD: Newer concepts of indispensable amino acids. Am J Clin Nutr 1987;46:593–605.

69. Druml W, Roth E, Lenz K et al: Phenylalanine and tyrosine metabolism in renal failure. Kidney Int 1989;36(suppl 27):282–286.

70. Druml W, Lochs H, Roth E et al: Utilization of tyrosine dipeptides and acetyl-tyrosine in normal and uremic humans. Am J Physiol 1991;260:E280–E285.

71. Rabkin R, Kitaji J: Renal metabolism of peptide hormones. Miner Electrolyte Metab 1983;9:212–226.

72. DeFronzo RA, Smit D, Alvestrand A: Insulin action in uremia. Kidney Int 1993;24(suppl 16):S102–S114.

73. May RC, Clark AS, Goheer MA et al: Specific defects in insulin-mediated muscle metabolism in acute uremia. Kidney Int 1985;28:490–497.

74. Frölich J, Hoppe-Seyler G, Schollmeyer P et al: Possible sites of interaction of acute renal failure with amino acid utilization for gluconeogenesis in isolated perfused rat liver. Eur J Clin Invest 1977;7:261–268.

75. Grolich J, Scholmerich J, Hoppe-Seyler G et al: The effect of acute uremia on gluconeogenesis in isolated perfused rat livers. Eur J Clin Invest 1974;4:453–458.

76. Cianciaruso B, Sacca L, Terraciano V et al: Insulin metabolism in acute renal failure. Kidney Int 1987;23(suppl 27):109–112.

77. Weisinger J, Swenson RS, Greene W et al: Comparison of the effects of metabolic acidosis and acute uremia on carbohydrate tolerance. Diabetes 1972;21:1109–1115.

78. Schaefer RM, Riegel W, Stephan E et al: Normalization of enhanced hepatic gluconeogenesis by the antiglucocorticoid RU 384 86 in acutely uremic rats. Eur J Clin Invest 1990;20:35–40.

79. Cianciaruso B, Bellizzi V, Napoli R et al: Hepatic uptake and release of glucose, lactate and amino acids in acutely uremic dogs. Metabolism 1991;40:261–290.

80. Naschitz JE, Barak C, Yeshurun D: Reversible diminished insulin requirement in acute renal failure. Postgrad Med J 1983;59:269–271.

81. Bagdade JD, Casaretto A, Albers J: Effects of chronic uremia, hemodialysis and renal transplantation on plasma lipids and lipoproteins in man. J Lab Clin Med 1976;87:37–48.

82. Druml W, Laggner A, Widhalm K et al: Lipid metabolism in acute renal failure. Kidney Int 1983;24(suppl 16):139–142.

83. Mordasini R, Frey F, Flury W et al: Selective deficiency of hepatic triglyceride lipase in uremic patients. N Engl J Med 1977;297:1362–1366.

84. Druml W, Zechner R, Magometschnigg D et al: Postheparin lipolytic activity in acute renal failure. Clin Nephrol 1985;23:289–293.

85. Attman P, Alaupovic P, Gustafson A: Serum apolipoprotein profile of patients with chronic renal failure. Kidney Int 1987;32:368–375.

86. Druml W, Fischer M, Sertl S et al: Fat elimination in acute renal failure: long chain versus medium chain triglycerides. Am J Clin Nutr 1992;55:468–472.

87. Seres DS, Strain GW, Hashim SA et al: Improvement of plasma lipoprotein profiles during high-flux hemodialysis. JASN 1993;3:1409–1415.

88. Akmal M, Perkins S, Kasim SE et al: Verapamil prevents chronic renal failure-induced abnormalities in lipid metabolism. Am J Kidney Dis 1993;22:158–163.

89. Breier C, Dzien A, Lisch HJ et al: Decreased activity of post-heparin lipoprotein lipase during acidosis. Klin Wochenschr 1984;62:593–594.

90. Schrader J, Stibbe W, Armstrong VW et al: Comparison of low molecular weight heparin to standard heparin in hemodialysis/hemofiltration. Kidney Int 1988;33:890–896.

91. Cattran DC, Fenton SSA, Wilson DR et al: Defective triglyceride removal in lipemia associated with peritoneal dialysis and hemodialysis. Ann Intern Med 1976;85:29–33.

92. Lindholm B, Norbeck HE: Serum lipids and lipoproteins during continuous ambulatory peritoneal dialysis. Acta Med Scand 1986;220:143–151.

93. Kaysen GA: Nephrotic hyperlipidemia: primary abnormalities in both lipoprotein catabolism and synthesis. Miner Electrolyte Metab 1992;18:212–216.

94. Nitzan M: Hepatic lipogenesis in acute uremic syndrome. Nutr Metab 1971;13:292–297.

95. Druml W, Laggner AN, Lenz K et al: Lipid metabolism and lipid utilization in renal insufficiency. Infusionstherapie 1983;10:206–212.

96. Wanner C, Riegel W, Schaefer RM et al: Carnitine and carnitine esters in acute renal failure. Nephrol Dial Transplant 1989;4:951–956.

97. Salem MM, Rosa RM, Batle DC: Extrarenal potassium tolerance in chronic renal failure. Am J Kidney Dis 1991;18:421–440.

98. Kelly RA, O'Hara DS, Mitch WE et al: Endogenous digitalis-like factors in hypertension and chronic renal insufficiency. Kidney Int 1986;30:723–729.

99. Kelly RA, Canessa ML, Steinman TI et al: Hemodialysis and red cell cation transport in uremia: role of membrane free fatty acids. Kidney Int 1989;35:595–603.

100. Mitch WE, Wilcox CS: Disorders of body fluids, sodium and potassium in chronic renal failure. Am J Med 1982;72:536–550.

101. Kurtin P, Kouba J: Profound hypophosphatemia in the course of acute renal failure. Am J Kidney Dis 1987;10:346–349.

102. Kleinberger G, Gabl F, Gabner A et al: Hypophosphatemia during parenteral nutrition in patients with renal failure. Wien Klin Wochenschr 1978;90:169–172.

103. Lumlertgul D, Harris DCH, Burke TJ et al: Detrimental effects of hypophosphatemia on the severity and progression of ischemic acute renal failure. Miner Electrolyte Metab 1986;12:204–209.

104. Ritz E, Matthias S, Seidel A et al: Disturbed calcium metabolism in renal failure pathogenesis and therapeutic strategies. Kidney Int 1992;38(suppl 38):S37–S42.

105. Massry SG, Arieff AI, Coburn JW: Divalent ion metabolism in patients with acute renal failure: studies on the mechanism of hypocalcemia. Kidney Int 1974;5:437–445.

106. Hsu CH, Patel S, Young EW et al: Production and metabolic clearance of calcitriol in acute renal failure. Kidney Int 1988;33:530–535.

107. Akmal M, Bishop JE, Telfer N et al: Hypocalcemia and hypercalcemia in patients with rhabdomyolysis with and without acute renal failure. J Clin Endocrinol Metab 1986;63:137–142.

108. Whitehead VM, Compty CH, Posen GA et al: Homeostasis of folic acid in patients undergoing maintenance hemodialysis. N Engl J Med 1968;279:970–974.

109. Madl CH, Kranz A, Liebisch B et al: Lactic acidosis in thiamine deficiency. Clin Nutr 1993;12:108–111.

110. Robert D, Jorgetti V, Leclercq M et al: Does vitamin K excess induce ectopic calcifications in hemodialysis patients? Clin Nephol 1985;24:300–304.

111. Gerlach TH, Zile MH: Effect of retinoic acid and apo-RBP on serum retinol concentration in acute renal failure. FASEB J 1991;5:86–92.

112. Druml W, Bartens C, Steltzer H et al: Impact of acute renal failure on antioxidant status in multiple organ failure syndrome. JASN 1993;4:314A.

113. Smythe WR, Alfrey AC, Craswell PW et al: Trace element abnormalities in chronic uremia. Ann Intern Med 1992;96:302–310.

114. Thomson NM, Stevens BJ, Humphery TJ et al: Comparison of trace elements in peritoneal dialysis, hemodialysis, and uremia. Kidney Int 1983;23:9–14.

115. Padovese P, Gallieni M, Brancaccio D et al: Trace elements in dialysis fluids and assessment of the exposure of patients on regular hemodialysis, hemofiltration and continuous ambulatory peritoneal dialysis. Nephron 1992;61:442–448.

116. Rodger RSC et al: Zinc deficiency and hyperprolactinemia are not reversible causes of sexual dysfunction in uremia. Nephrol Dial Transplant 1989;4:488.

117. Fischer M, König JS, Elmadfa I et al: Anti-oxidant status in chronic hemodialysis patients: impact of selenium supplementation. JASN 1991;3:364A.

118. Joannidis M, Bonn G, Pfaller W: Lipid peroxydation—an initial event in experimental acute renal failure. Renal Physiol Biochem 1989;12:47–55.

119. Nath KA, Paller MS: Dietary deficiency of antioxidants exacerbates ischemic injury in the rat kidney. Kidney Int 1990;38:1109–1117.

120. Spreiter SC, Myers BD, Swenson RS: Protein-energy requirements in subjects with acute renal failure receiving intermittent hemodialysis. Am J Clin Nutr 1980;33:1433–1437.

121. Mault JR, Bartlett RH, Dechert RE: Starvation: a major contributor to mortality in acute renal failure. Trans Am Soc Artif Intern Organs 1983;29:390–394.

122. Monteon F, Laidlaw S, Shaib J et al: Energy expenditure in patients with chronic renal failure. Kidney Int 1986;30:741–747.

123. Kopple JD, Monteon F, Shaib J: Effect of energy intake on nitrogen metabolism in nondialyzed patients with chronic renal failure. Kidney Int 1988;29:734–742.

124. Maroni BJ, Steinman T, Mitch WE: A method for estimating nitrogen intake of patients with chronic renal failure. Kidney Int 1986;27:58–63.

125. Maroni BJ: Requirements for protein, calories, and fat in the predialysis patient. In Mitch WE, Klahr S (eds): Nutrition and the Kidney. Boston: Little, Brown & Co. 1993:185.

126. Sargent JA, Gotch F, Borak M et al: Urea kinetics: a guide of nutritional management of renal failure. Am J Clin Nutr 1978;31:1696–1702.

127. Rose WC: Amino acid requirements of man. Fed Proc 1949;8:546–552.

128. Motil KJ, Haron WE, Grupe WE: Complications of essential amino acid hyperalimentation in children with acute renal failure. J Parenter Enter Nutr 1980;4:32–35.

129. Grazer RE, Sutton JM, Friedstrom S et al: Hyperammoniemic encephalopathy due to essential amino acid hyperalimentation. Arch Intern Med 1984;144:2278–2279.

130. Moncada S, Palmer RMJ, Higgs EA: Nitric oxide: physiology, pathophysiology, and pharmacology. Pharmacol Rev 1991;43:109–142.

131. Ritz E, Vallance P, Nowicki M: The effect of malnutrition on cardiovascular mortality in dialysis patients: is L-arginine the answer? Nephrol Dial Transplant 1994;9:129–130.

132. Snyderman SE, Holt LE, Dancis J et al: "Unessential" nitrogen: a limiting factor for human growth. J Nutr 1962;78:57–72.

133. Stucki WP, Harper AE: Importance of dispensable amino acids for normal growth of chicks. J Nutr 1961;74:377.

134. Hasik J, Hryniewiecki L, Baczyk K et al: An attempt to evaluate minimum requirements for protein in patients with acute renal failure. Pol Arch Med Wewn 1979;61:29–36.

135. Lopez-Martinez J, Caparros T, Perez-Picouto F: Nutrition parenteral en enfermos septicos con fracaso renal agudo en fase poliurica. Rev Clin Esp 1980;157:171–178.

136. Feinstein EI, Kopple JD, Silberman H et al: Total parenteral nutrition with high or low nitrogen intakes in patients with acute renal failure. Kidney Int 1983;26(suppl 16):S319–S323.

137. Shaw JHF, Wildbore M, Wolfe RR: Whole body protein kinetics in severely septic patients. Ann Surg 1987;205:288–294.

138. Chima CS, Meyer L, Hummell AC et al: Protein catabolic rate in patients with acute renal failure on continuous arteriovenous hemofiltration and total parenteral nutrition. JASN 1993;3:1516–1521.

139. Kierdorf H, Kindler J, Sieberth HG: Nitrogen balance in patients with acute renal failure treated by continuous arteriovenous hemofiltration. Nephrol Dial Transplant 1985;1:72.

140. Reynolds HN, Borg U, Frankenfield D: Full protein alimentation and nitrogen equilibrium in a renal failure patient treated with continuous hemodialfiltration. J Parenter Enter Nutr 1992;16:379–383.

141. Frankenfeld DC, Badellino MM, Reynolds N et al: Amino acid loss and plasma concentration during continuous hemodiafiltration. J Parenter Enter Nutr 1993;17:551–561.

142. Reaich D, Channon SM, Scrimgeous CM et al: Correction of acidosis in humans with CRF decreases protein degradation and amino acid oxidation. Am J Physiol 1993;265:E230–235.

143. Blumenkantz MJ, Kplle JD, Moran JK et al: Metabolic balance studies and dietary protein requirements in patients undergoing continuous ambulatory peritoneal dialysis. Kidney Int 1982;35:849–861.

144. Gretz N, Meisinger E, Kehry I et al: Tube feeding in patients with renal insufficiency: first long term experience with a specialized diet. Klin Ernahr 1986;20:129–135 (In German).

145. Friedman AL, Chesney RW, Gilbert EF et al: Secondary oxalosis as a complication of parenteral alimentation in acute renal failure. Am J Nephrol 1983;3:248–252.

146. Kluthe R, Luttgen FM, Capetianu R et al: Protein requirements in maintenance hemodialysis. Am J Clin Nutr 1978;31:1812–1820.

147. Ikizler TA, Flakoll PJ, Parker RA: Amino acid and albumin losses during dialysis. Kidney Int 1994;46:830–837.

148. Blumenkrantz MJ et al: Protein losses during peritoneal dialysis. Kidney Int 1981;19:593.

149. Davies SP, Reaveley DA, Brown EA et al: Amino acid clearances and daily losses in patients with acute renal failure treated by continuous arteriovenous hemodialysis. Crit Care Med 1991;19:1510–1515.

150. Wolfson M, Jones MR, Kopple JD: Amino acid losses during hemodialysis with infusion of amino acids and glucose. Kidney Int 1982;21:500–506.

151. Hakim RM, Wingard RL, Parker RA: Effect of the dialysis membrane in the treatment of patients with acute renal failure. N Engl J Med 1994;331:1338–1342.

152. Toborek M, Wasik T, Drozdz M et al: Effect of hemodialysis on lipid peroxidation and antioxidant system in patients with chronic hemodialysis. Metabolism 1992;41:1229–1232.

153. Cristol JP et al: Enhancement of reactive oxygen species production and cell surface markers expression due to hemodialysis. Nephrol Dial Transplant 1994;9:389–394.

154. Zager RA, Venkatachalam MA: Potentiation of ischemic renal injury to amino acid infusion. Kidney Int 1983;24:620–625.

155. Moursi M, Rising CL, Zelenock GB et al: Dextrose administration exacerbates acute renal ischemic damage in anesthesized dogs. Arch Surg 1987;122:790–794.

156. Grutzmacher P, Marz W, Peschke B et al: Lipoproteins and apolipo-proteins during the progression of chronic renal disease. Nephron 1988;50:103–111.

157. Grutzmacher P, Radtke HW, Schifferdecker E et al: Early changes in plasma lipid status and glucose tolerance during the course of chronic renal failure. Contr Nephrol 1984;41:332–336.

158. Lowrie EG, Lew NL: Death risk in hemodialysis patients: the predictive value of commonly measured variables and an evaluation of death differences between facilities. Am J Kid Dis 1990;15:458–482.

159. Deitch EA, Winterton J, Berg R: The gut as a portal of entry for bacteremia. Role of protein malnutrition. Ann Surg 1987;681–692.

160. Abernathy GB, Heizer WD, Holcombe BJ et al: Efficacy of tube feeding in supplying energy requirements of hospitalized patients. J Parenter Enter Nutr 1989;13:387–391.

161. Inoue S, Epstein M, Alexander JW et al: Prevention of yeast translocation across the gut by a single enteral feeding after burn injury. J Parenter Enter Nutr 1989;13:565–571.

162. Ponsky JL, Gauderer MWL: Percutaneous endoscopic gastrotomy: indications, limitation, techniques and results. World J Surg 1989;13:165–170.

163. Andrews PA, Webb M: PEG. Br Med J 1992;305:116.

164. O'Regan S, Garel L: Percutaneous gastrojejunostomy for caloric supplementation in children on peritoneal dialysis. Adv Peritoneal Dialysis 1990;6:273–275.

165. Wood EG, Bunchman TE, Khurana R et al: Complications of nasogastric and gastrostomy tube feeding in children with end stage renal disease. Adv Peritoneal Dialysis 1990;6:262–264.

166. Watson AR, Coleman JE, Taylor EA: Gastrotomy buttons for feeding children on continuous cycling peritoneal dialysis. Adv Periton Dial 1992;8:391–395.

167. Talbot JM: Guidelines for the scientific review of enteral food products for special medical purposes. J Parenter Enter Nutr 1991;15(suppl):99S–174S.

168. Abras E, Walser M: Growth of rats fed by a continuous intragastric infusion containing amino acids and keto acids. Am J Clin Nutr 1982;36:154–161.

169. Abras E, Walser M: Nitrogen utilitzation in uremic patients fed by continuous nasogastric infusion. Kidney Int 1982;22:392–397.

170. Schiller HJ, Galvin M, Meguid MM: Acute nutrition managements in insulin-dependent diabetes: presentation of an index case. Nutrition 1993;9:360–364.

171. Abitol CL, Zilleruelo G, Montane B et al: Growth of uremic infants on forced feeding regimens. Pediatr Nephrol 1993;7:173–177.

172. Trapper D, Watkins S, Burns M et al: Comprehensive management of renal failure in infants. Arch Surg 1990;125:1276–1281.

173. Gretz N, Jung M, Scigalla P et al: Tube feeding in patients suffering from renal failure. In Giovanetti S (ed): Nutritional Treatment of Chronic Renal Failure. Boston: Kluwer Academic Publishers, 1989:339.

174. Wolfson M: The cost and bother of intradialytic parenteral nutrition are not justified by available scientific studies. ASAIO J 1993;39:864–867.

175. Douglas E, Lomas L, Prygrodzka F et al: Nutrition and malnutrition in renal patients: the role of nasogastric nutrition. Proc EDTA 1982;11:17–20.

176. Wolfson M: Use of nutritional supplements in dialysis patients. Semin Dialysis 1992;5:285–290.

177. Cockram DB, Moore LW, Acchiardo SR: Response to an oral nutritional supplement for chronic renal failure patients. J Renal Nutr 1994;4:78–85.

178. Ross Products Division, Abbott Laboratories. Clinical report BE51. Use of Nepro specialized liquid nutrition as a sole source of nutrition in hemodialyzed renal patients. 1994, Data on request.

179. Dabbagh S, Fassinger N, Clement K et al: The effect of aggressive nutrition on infection rates in patients maintained on peritoneal dialysis. Adv Peritoneal Dial 1991;7:161–164.

180. Guillot M, Broyer M, Cathelineau L et al: Nutrition enterale a debit constant en nephrologie pediatrique. Arch Fr Pediatr 1980;37:497–505.

181. Brewer ED: Growth of small children managed with chronic peritoneal dialysis and nasogastric tube feedings: 203-month experience in 14 patients. Adv Peritoneal Dial 1990;6:265–268.

182. Strife C, Quinal M, Mears K et al: Improved growth of three uremic children by nocturnal nasogastric feedings. Am J Dis Child 1986;140:438–443.

183. Jones JW, Nevins T, McHugh L et al: Nutrition and growth in pediatric renal transplant recipients. Transplant Proc 1994;26:62–63.

184. Kamen RS: Impaired development of oral-motor functions required for normal oral feeding as a consequence of tube feeding during infancy. Adv Peritoneal Dial 1990;6:276–278.

185. Capelli JP, Kushner H, Camiscioli TC et al: Effect of intradialytic parenteral nutrition on mortality rates in end-stage renal disease care. Am J Kidney Dis 1994;23:808–816.

27

Enteral Nutrition and Diabetes Mellitus

■ ■ ■ ■ ■ ■ ■ ■ ■ ■ ■ ■ ■ ■ ■ ■ ■

M. MOLLY MCMAHON
DANIEL L. HURLEY

Diabetes mellitus is caused by an absolute (insulin-dependent diabetes mellitus, Type I) or a relative (noninsulin-dependent diabetes mellitus, Type II) lack of insulin. Insulin-dependent diabetes mellitus is associated with onset at an early age, tendency toward ketosis, and an absolute dependency on insulin. Noninsulin-dependent diabetes mellitus, by far the more common type, is associated with adult onset, obesity, and insulin resistance. Because of the prevalence of diabetes mellitus and the comorbidity of the disease, most physicians will manage diabetic patients receiving nutritional support. This review will cover the effects of diabetes mellitus, illness, and feeding on carbohydrate metabolism and will discuss diabetic enteropathy and the use of enteral tube feeding in hospitalized diabetic patients.

REGULATION OF CARBOHYDRATE METABOLISM

Normal Physiology

In nondiabetic subjects, the plasma glucose concentration is closely regulated in both the postabsorptive (6 to 14 hours after a meal) and the postprandial period. In the postabsorptive period, plasma glucose is primarily derived from the liver, since cellular glucose release requires the action of glucose-6-phosphatase, an

enzyme present in significant amounts only in the liver and kidney. Endogenous glucose production results both from glycogenolysis (the breakdown of glucose stored as glycogen) and gluconeogenesis (the formation of glucose from precursors).[1,2] Euglycemia is maintained because the rate of hepatic glucose release (glucose production) approximates the rate of glucose uptake (glucose use) by the liver, brain, and peripheral tissues. These rates average approximately 2 mg/kg/minute in the healthy, nondiabetic subject in the postabsorptive period, or approximately 200 g day for the 70-kg subject.

After a meal (or infusion of dextrose), the increase in plasma glucose leads to an increase in plasma insulin level. The postprandial plasma insulin concentration increases from the fasting level of approximately 6 to 10 μU/ml to approximately 40 to 100 μU/ml and then returns to basal levels within 3 to 4 hours after eating. Both hyperglycemia and hyperinsulinemia are key modulators of glucose turnover rates (the rate of glucose release and of glucose uptake). Hyperglycemia suppresses hepatic glucose release by decreasing both glycogenolysis and gluconeogenesis and by activating glycogen synthetase (the enzyme stimulating glycogen synthesis).[3,4] During euglycemic conditions, an increase in the plasma insulin level from 10 μU/ml (average preprandial concentra-

461

tion) to approximately 25 to 30 µU/ml suppresses hepatic glucose release with near-maximal suppression at an insulin concentration of 50 to 60 µU/ml.[5] Both hyperglycemia (due to mass effect) and hyperinsulinemia stimulate glucose uptake.[6,7] Half-maximal increase in glucose uptake occurs at a plasma insulin concentration of approximately 50 to 60 µU/mL with a near-maximal effect observed at insulin concentrations in excess of 200 µU/mL.[5]

The hyperglycemia and hyperinsulinemia of the fed state convert the liver from an organ that produces glucose to one that takes up glucose and stimulates peripheral glucose uptake, thereby preventing the postprandial glucose concentration from exceeding 150 mg/dl. Postprandially, as the plasma glucose and insulin fall, the rates of glucose release and glucose uptake are restored to preprandial levels. The decrease in insulin level permits an increase in hepatic glucose release and a decrease in glucose uptake in insulin-sensitive tissues, namely, liver, muscle, and fat. A lack of suppression of hepatic glucose release in the presence of hyperinsulinemia denotes a resistance to the action of insulin at the liver (i.e., hepatic insulin resistance). A lack of appropriate glucose uptake in the presence of hyperinsulinemia denotes resistance to the action of insulin in peripheral tissues (i.e., peripheral insulin resistance). Both sickness and diabetes mellitus are characterized by insulin resistance.

Effect of Diabetes Mellitus

Patients with diabetes mellitus have preprandial and postprandial hyperglycemia. The hyperglycemia is due to excessive hepatic glucose release and impaired glucose uptake that results from both decreased insulin secretion and action.[8-11]

Effect of Illness

Under conditions of severe stress, patients without an antecedent diagnosis of diabetes mellitus may develop hyperglycemia.[12,13] "Stress diabetes," included under the category of secondary diabetes,[14] is an important cause of hyperglycemia in critically ill patients. Severe stress is accompanied by a marked increase in the plasma concentration of glucagon, epinephrine, and cortisol. These counterregulatory hormones increase hepatic glucose release[15-18] and decrease glucose uptake,[19-21] resulting in hyperglycemia. Animal and human studies have evaluated the role and

interactions of counterregulatory hormones in the pathogenesis of stress-induced hyperglycemia. The hormones were infused individually and together in healthy subjects in doses designed to reproduce the hormonal milieu of stress (Fig. 27–1).[22,23] Although single hormone infusion caused only mild hyperglycemia, com-

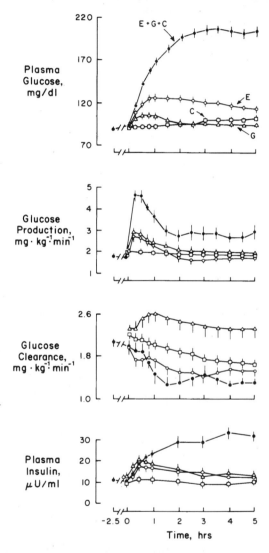

FIGURE 27–1 Effect of combined hormonal infusion (epinephrine [E] plus glucagon [G] plus cortisol [C]) on plasma glucose concentration, glucose production, glucose clearance, and plasma insulin concentration in nondiabetic subjects. The responses are compared with those during the individual infusion of epinephrine, glucagon, and cortisol. (From Shamoon M, Hendler R, Sherwin R: Synergistic interactions among anti-insulin hormones in the pathogenesis of stress hyperglycemia in humans. J Clin Endocrinol Metab 1981;52:1235–1241. © The Endocrine Society.)

bined hormone infusion resulted in plasma glucose levels over 200 mg/dl due to increased hepatic glucose release and decreased glucose uptake.[23] The exaggerated glucose response following a stress-dose counterregulatory hormone infusion in healthy diabetic subjects compared with nondiabetic subjects is one explanation for the deterioration in glucose control in stressed diabetic patients.[24]

Cytokines may have profound effects on carbohydrate metabolism. Interleukin-1 and tumor necrosis factor (TNF) stimulate hepatic glucose output,[25-27] with the former either inhibiting or stimulating insulin secretion depending on the concentration and length of exposure. Interleukin-1 can create a stress hormone profile that can also lead to stress diabetes mellitus.[28]

DIABETES MELLITUS AND THE GASTROINTESTINAL TRACT

Esophageal Dysmotility

Diabetes mellitus can affect the entire gastrointestinal (GI) tract. Retrospective chart reviews report a relatively low prevalence of GI problems in patients with diabetes mellitus.[29,30] However, when patients were questioned during diabetes clinic visits, 76 percent reported the presence of at least one GI symptom.[31] Although abnormal esophageal pressures (particularly lower esophageal sphincter pressure) and esophageal dysmotility are reported to occur in the majority of patients with diabetic gastroparesis, these esophageal disturbances are often asymptomatic.[32-35]

Diabetic Gastroparesis

Symptoms

Gastroparesis diabeticorum is a term that denotes gastric atony and delayed gastric emptying in diabetic patients.[36] It is now clear that the symptoms of diabetic gastroparesis are related to dysmotility not only of the stomach but also of the small bowel.[37,38] In one study, isolated gastric or small bowel dysmotility was detected in approximately one quarter of diabetic patients with nausea, vomiting, and epigastric pain yet manometric abnormalities of both stomach and small bowel were confirmed in three quarters of the patients.[38] It is estimated that as many as one fifth of diabetic patients without GI symptoms have radiographic evidence of gastric retention.[39] Common manifestations of diabetic enteropathy include heartburn, dysphagia, nausea, early satiety, postprandial vomiting (especially partially digested food retained from earlier meals), and epigastric pain. Markedly delayed gastric emptying may make the regulation of blood glucose difficult, and hyperglycemia may further delay gastric emptying. In contrast, hypoglycemia may develop in those who take insulin and fail to absorb ingested food because of delayed gastric emptying.[40-42] Peripheral neuropathy, retinopathy, and nephropathy are frequently found in patients with symptomatic gastroparesis.[29] It is generally believed that autonomic neuropathy is the cause of gastroparesis. However, a study of 84 consecutive diabetic patient referrals for evaluation of GI symptoms reported that, in 95 percent of patients, the severity of documented dysmotility was not associated with the presence of autonomic neuropathy, type of diabetes (type I or type II), duration of diabetes, daily insulin dose, or glycated hemoglobin level.[38]

It is important to diagnose diabetic gastroparesis accurately to avoid attributing the GI symptoms to tube feeding alone or to other factors capable of affecting gut motility. Review of the patient's medication list will help exclude the use of commonly prescribed medications that may delay gastric emptying. These include anticholinergics, antidepressants, α-2 adrenergic agonists, calcium channel blockers, and opiates. Glucose levels should be closely monitored and appropriately managed because gastric emptying can be slowed by hyperglycemia.[43] In addition, knowledge of the tube-feeding formula's fat content is important because fat can also delay gastric emptying. The diagnosis of diabetic gastroparesis should be strongly suspected from the history. Physical examination may reveal gastric dilatation with a succussion splash. Demonstration of a delay in gastric emptying establishes the diagnosis of gastroparesis. Standard barium roentgenographic studies generally demonstrate gastric dilatation and retained solid residue even after a prolonged fast.[37] Follow-up films show a marked delay of emptying, with more than 50 percent of contrast remaining in the stomach after 30 minutes. However, because gastric emptying of liquids may be normal even in the presence of moderately severe symptoms,[44,45] scintigraphic assessment of emptying of solids has become the preferred test.[46,47] Endoscopy can exclude organic causes of gastric atony and delayed emptying.

Guidelines for Therapy

The treatment of diabetic gastroparesis has been recently reviewed.[48-50] The primary goals of therapy are to control blood glucose levels and to relieve GI symptoms. The evaluation of various modalities used to treat gastroparesis is confounded by the intermittent and variable course of symptomatic gastroparesis, the poor correlation between the degree of gastric stasis and severity of symptoms,[31,36,50-53] and the effect of hyperglycemia on gastric emptying.[54-57] These features may help to explain why some patients have objective measures indicating dysmotility but experience no symptomatic relief after treatment.

Treatment of diabetic gastroparesis is necessary when the patient's symptoms are significant and persistent, diabetes control is suboptimal, or nutritional state is compromised. Because gastric emptying is slowed during hyperglycemia (252 to 288 mg/dl) compared with euglycemia (72 to 126 mg/dl)[55] and is reported to be inversely related to the degree of hyperglycemia,[54,56] aggressive control of blood glucose is indicated. Although conventional antiemetic drugs (e.g., prochlorperazine) may provide relief of nausea and vomiting, the anticholinergic properties may adversely affect gastric emptying. Prokinetic agents are the treatment of choice. Metoclopramide, a central and peripheral antidopaminergic agent, releases acetylcholine from the myenteric plexus and facilitates cholinergic transmission in enteric smooth muscle. Metoclopramide crosses the blood-brain barrier and exerts an antiemetic effect. Mild neurologic side-effects (e.g., anxiety, drowsiness, lassitude) occur in up to 20 percent of patients, and dystonic reactions may be seen in 1 percent of patients. In contrast, domperidone, a peripheral dopamine antagonist, lacking cholinergic activity, does not cross the blood-brain barrier and has few neurologic side-effects. Domperidone will soon be clinically available. Cisapride, like metoclopramide, stimulates acetylcholine release from the myenteric plexus but does not have antidopaminergic action. In vitro studies have shown that cisapride acts as a serotonin receptor agonist, increasing GI motility. Erythromycin enhances gut motility by acting as an agonist of the GI peptide motilin. Bethanechol, a cholinomimetic agent, is rarely used due to its lack of efficacy and frequent side-effects.

Metoclopramide,[45,58-61] domperidone,[62,63] cisapride,[61,64] and erythromycin[65] all increase the rate of gastric emptying following a single dose. The magnitude of response appears to be related to both dose[61] and severity of dysmotility.[64] Because the prokinetic effects of metoclopramide,[32,59] domperidone,[62,66] and erythromycin[65] may diminish with time, we recommend their use only during symptomatic gastroparesis. Only one study using a controlled crossover design comparing the results of metoclopramide and cisapride vs placebo has been performed, and no symptomatic relief was found with either drug.[67] Only a few studies using a randomized, double-blind, placebo-controlled crossover design have evaluated symptomatic relief of gastroparesis. Two of the three trials with metoclopramide[60,67,68] and neither of the two studies with cisapride[67,69] showed improvement in symptoms. Many studies using a randomized, double-blind, placebo-controlled parallel design have reported symptomatic improvement with the use of domperidone,[63] metoclopramide,[70] and cisapride.[64,71]

Controversy exists in the literature concerning the drug of first choice.[48-50] We prefer to use metoclopramide initially rather than cisapride. Our preference is based on the lack of significant difference in efficacy between the two agents, the availability of an intravenous preparation of metoclopramide for use during acute exacerbations, and its lesser cost. If side-effects occur or if there is no symptomatic relief with metoclopramide, cisapride should be substituted. Cisapride is well tolerated and may have a more sustained effect with long-term therapy.[64,69,72-74] In patients with acute and severe symptoms of gastroparesis, intravenous erythromycin may be beneficial. Prokinetic agents should be administered in low dose 30 minutes before meals and before the bedtime snack and the dose increased as tolerated. Although data regarding the dosing of prokinetic agents during continuous tube feeding is limited, we suggest drug administration every 6 hours. Only metoclopramide and erythromycin can be intravenously administered. Metoclopramide may also be administered by rectal suppository. Because absorption of tablets may be compromised by gastroparesis, liquid preparations may be more effective in these patients.

Constipation, Diarrhea, and Fecal Incontinence

Constipation, diarrhea, and fecal incontinence may develop with long-standing diabetes mellitus. Constipation is the most common symptom of diabetic enteropathy, and its prevalence increases with the progression of severe neuropathy.[29] Constipation often alternates with diarrhea.[29] Diabetic diarrhea affects approximately 10 percent of all diabetic patients; of these, 40 percent have fecal incontinence, both of which are more likely in the presence of symptomatic neuropathy.[75-79]

If the history suggests steatorrhea, a 48- or 72-hour stool fat collection should be completed. The differential diagnosis of steatorrhea is similar in diabetic and nondiabetic patients. However, celiac sprue,[80] pancreatic insufficiency,[81] and bacterial overgrowth[82] occur more frequently in diabetics than in nondiabetics and can be evaluated by jejunal biopsy, pancreatic function tests, and cultures of jejunal fluid aspirate, respectively. Other causes of diarrhea, such as infection, medications, and bacterial overgrowth, should also be excluded. A stool specimen for leukocytes and *Clostridium difficile* toxin should be obtained in patients recently treated with antibiotics. The medication list should be reviewed for antibiotics, drugs with high sorbitol (poorly absorbed carbohydrate added to certain elixirs for its solvent and sweetener properties), or magnesium content and for drugs with a high osmolality, all of which could increase stool output. The management of diarrhea should include correction of water and electrolyte imbalance and vigorous blood glucose control. If infectious diarrhea has been excluded, loperamide or deodorized tincture of opium can be used to treat the diarrhea. Lomotil is used less frequently long term because of potential anticholinergic side-effects from the atropine content. Although oral clonidine has been shown to reduce the number and volume of stools in patients with diabetic diarrhea,[83] adverse side-effects (e.g., orthostatic hypotension and slowed gastric emptying) limit its use.

Low-volume "diarrhea" may be a clue to fecal incontinence because patients may mistake the passage of frequent, small, but semiformed stool for diarrhea. Fecal incontinence is associated with decreased basal internal anal sphincter pressure (autonomic innervation of smooth muscle) compared with both nondiabetic and diabetic subjects without incontinence.[78] Objective tests of anorectal function include manometry and neurophysiologic evaluation of the pelvic floor. If pelvic function is normal, colonic transit time can be assessed by reliable and noninvasive radiopaque marker studies.

INDICATIONS FOR NUTRITION SUPPORT

Over the short term, the indications for nutritional support and the daily estimate of caloric, protein, and lipid requirements are similar in hospitalized diabetic and nondiabetic patients with comparable medical problems. The percentage of recent (previous 3- to 6-month period) weight loss, the presence of clinical markers of stress, and the anticipated time that the patient will be unable to meet nutritional needs orally all influence the need for nutritional support.[84,85] In general, a recent weight loss of less than 10 percent from usual weight is well tolerated. For the well-nourished and unstressed (afebrile, normal leukocyte count and differential) or mildly stressed patient who is anticipated to be eating in the next 7 to 10 days, provision of dextrose-containing fluid and electrolytes should be sufficient. Those who have recently lost 10 to 20 percent of their usual weight should receive supplemental nutrition if moderately or severely stressed. Prompt nutritional support should generally be provided for severely stressed patients (e.g., after closed-head injury, major burn, multiple trauma, or severe sepsis), since the stress response generally exceeds 7 to 10 days, and to those who have recently lost more than 20 percent of their usual weight.

DESIGN OF NUTRITIONAL PROGRAM

A patient's daily caloric requirement can be estimated by nomograms, such as the Harris-Benedict equation, which is based on the premise that basal caloric needs are related to body cell mass.[86,87] Direct measurement of daily energy requirements by indirect calorimetry is useful in selected situations. For years it was believed that patients requiring nutrition support had elevated energy requirements, especially when stressed by surgery, trauma, or sepsis. Over the last decade numerous studies have shown that the majority of patients have surprisingly normal energy expenditure, usually between 100 and 120 percent of predicted energy expenditure.[88-92] Avoidance of overfeeding is crucial in diabetic patients, since excessive calories can cause hyperglycemia. An indirect calorimetric measurement of energy needs may be helpful in the following types of patients: severely malnourished, volume overloaded if a "dry weight" estimate is uncertain, severely stressed (i.e., following closed-head injury, trauma, or burn because the measured daily caloric requirements often exceed estimated daily caloric requirements), morbidly obese, severely marasmic, or the ventilator-dependent patient experiencing weaning difficulty. It is our practice to deliver approximately 1 g protein/kg body weight to mildly stressed diabetic patients and approximately 1.5 g protein/kg body weight to moderately and severely stressed diabetic patients, assuming normal hepatic and renal function. For obese patients, we provide 1.5 g protein/kg of estimated "ideal" weight, assuming normal hepatic and renal function.

Because peritoneal dialysis (PD) may be used in diabetic patients with renal failure, it is helpful to review certain points. Dextrose in the PD fluid serves as the osmotic gradient for fluid removal. Since high-dextrose-containing PD fluid is frequently employed in fluid-overloaded patients to achieve negative fluid balance, a significant proportion of the dextrose instilled into the peritoneal cavity may be absorbed.[93,94] Using indirect calorimetry and analyzing the dialysis effluent for dextrose concentration, investigators studied the effects of high-dextrose-containing dialysates in five patients with acute renal failure undergoing PD.[95] Despite minimal caloric intake, all five patients had a respiratory quotient in excess of 1 consistent with net lipogenesis due to dextrose absorbed from the peritoneal cavity. Four of the five patients absorbed more than 500 g of dextrose/day from the peritoneal cavity. For diabetic patients on PD who are receiving tube feeding, the caloric content can be appropriately decreased to avoid providing an excess of calories.

GLYCEMIC GOALS

A major goal in the care of the hospitalized diabetic patient is to minimize the extremes of hyperglycemia and hypoglycemia. Desirable glycemic goals are different for healthy diabetic subjects than for stressed, hospitalized diabetic patients. The landmark Diabetes Control and Complications Trial convincingly showed the protective value of near-normal blood glucose control in preventing and delaying diabetic-related complications in healthy patients with insulin-dependent diabetes mellitus.[96] It is likely that the results are applicable to patients with noninsulin-dependent diabetes mellitus. However, for stressed hospitalized diabetic patients a sound aim is to maintain the plasma glucose values between 100 and 200 mg/dl. Once nutritional support is established, more tightly regulated plasma glucoses (i.e., 100 to 150 mg/dl) may be desirable in stable patients.

Hypoglycemia: Clinical Presentation and Treatment

Hypoglycemia can cause adrenergic or neuroglycopenic symptoms. The most common adrenergic symptoms are sweating, palpitations, anxiety, tachycardia, and hunger. Neuroglycopenic symptoms include headache, visual changes, and alterations in behavior. The identification of neuroglycopenia is often difficult in sedated or ventilator-dependent patients. In addition, patients with long-standing diabetes mellitus may lose the ability to recognize warning symptoms of hypoglycemia, that is, hypoglycemic unawareness. Therefore, avoidance or minimization of hypoglycemia is crucial. Although prompt restoration of glucose to normal usually completely reverses symptoms and signs of hypoglycemia, prolonged hypoglycemia can cause irreversible neurologic damage. Thus, a standardized approach to the treatment of hypoglycemia (i.e., plasma glucose ≤ 60 mg/dl) has merit (Table 27–1). If the patient has symptoms suggesting hypoglycemia, the health care provider should provide treatment promptly without waiting to check the blood glucose level. The physician should attempt to identify the factor(s) responsible for hypoglycemia. Potential causes include discontinuation of enteral tube feeding, resolution of severe stress, discontinuation or decreased dose of corticosteroids or sympathomimetic agents, renal dysfunction, acute hepatitis, septic shock, and diabetic gastroparesis. If no explanation is found, the daily dosage of the insulin active at the time of hypoglycemia should be reduced by approximately 10 percent. A more aggressive decrease in dose is needed if the hypoglycemia recurs.

Hyperglycemia: Adverse Effects

Over the short term, hyperglycemia can adversely affect fluid balance and immune function. As with hypoglycemia, the physician should attempt to identify factors responsible for hyperglycemia (Table 27–2). Hyperglycemia can cause an osmotic diuresis.[97] As the filtered load of glucose (glomerular filtration rate times the plasma glucose concentration) rises, it may exceed renal tubular reabsorptive capacity. As a result, glucose remains in the tubular lumen and acts as an osmotic diuretic, increasing the urinary loss of electrolytes and water.

Hyperglycemia can also adversely affect immune function. Abnormalities in granulocyte adherence, chemotaxis, phagocytosis, respiratory burst, and microbicidal function in patients with poorly controlled diabetes mellitus improve with more aggressive glycemic control.[98-104] Complement function is impaired in the presence of hyperglycemia.[105-108] Covalent

TABLE 27–1   Treatment of Hypoglycemia in Hospitalized Patients with Diabetes Mellitus

I. We define hypoglycemia in the hospitalized diabetic patient as a blood glucose level less than or equal to 60 mg/dl.

II. If a patient has symptoms or signs compatible with hypoglycemia, prompt treatment should be administered without waiting to confirm a low glucose value. Patients with documented hypoglycemia who are asymptomatic should also receive prompt treatment.

   A. Oral administration of glucose is preferable if the patient is able to swallow safely. The patient should ingest approximately 15 g of dextrose. An enteral tube can be used to provide dextrose. Examples of 15 g of dextrose include:

   1. 2 sugar packets/cubes
   2. 15 g of glucose tablets/gel
   3. ½ cup (4 oz) of fruit juice

   B. If the patient is not able to take oral feeding safely, is nil per os (NPO) for any reason, or has severe hypoglycemia, the following treatment is indicated:

   1. If intravenous access is available, 50% dextrose solution (D 50%) should be intravenously administered, using an initial dose of ½ ampule or 12.5 g of dextrose.
   2. If there is no intravenous access, 1 mg of glucagon should be administered by subcutaneous or intramuscular injection.

III. Glycemic monitoring following treatment

   A repeat plasma glucose determination should be obtained in 15 minutes. If the glucose value is not greater than 80 mg/dl, the treatment outlined above should be repeated and the glucose value rechecked in 15 minutes. Further treatment (and glucose checks at 15-minute intervals) should be repeated until the glucose is greater than 80 mg/dl.

TABLE 27–2   Potential Causes of Sudden Hyperglycemia

Nutritional program
  Excess calories
  Excess dextrose load (nutrition + crystalloid + peritoneal dialysis)
  Insufficient insulin
Infection/inflammation
  Role of counterregulatory hormones
  Role of cytokines
Medications
  Glucocorticoid
  Phenytoin
  Sympathomimetic infusion
  Cyclosporine
Volume depletion

---

attachment of the third component of complement (C3) to the microbial surface is a critical determinant of phagocytic recognition. This opsonic process is regulated by the internal thiolester bond of C3. Theoretically, attachment of glucose to the opsonic binding site within the C3 thiolester bond diverts this protein from the surface of invading bacteria and generates a dysfunctional complement/glucose complex. In addition, compared with controls the basal levels of cytosolic calcium in polymorphonuclear cells of diabetic patients are increased whereas ATP content and phagocytic ability are decreased. There was a direct correlation between cytosolic calcium concentration and fasting glucose levels. Three months of treatment with oral hypoglycemic agents improve glucose control, ATP content, and phagocytosis, and decrease cytosolic calcium concentration. All of this information suggests that adequate glucose control is required for normal leukocyte function.[109] Although the clinical significance of these findings is unclear, a growing body of clinical evidence indicates that hyperglycemia increases the risk of nosocomial infection in stressed patients.

First, the rate of central catheter–related infections was approximately five times higher in diabetic patients receiving central parenteral nutrition compared with nondiabetic patients receiving the same nutrition.[109a] Second, hyperglycemia (plasma glucose greater than 200 mg/dl) within 3 days before the isolation of *Candida albicans* was the most common risk factor for candida infection in hospitalized patients.[105] Certain unique properties of *C. albicans* promote its virulence in the presence of hyperglycemia. This yeast expresses a surface protein, and expression of the protein increases in a dose-dependent fashion. An abrupt increase in expression was observed as the glucose concentration increased from 180 mg/dl to 360 mg/dl. The surface protein impairs phagocytic recognition and mediates adhesion of the yeast to endothelial surfaces. Third, investigators monitoring perioperative glucose control in 100 diabetic patients undergoing elective surgery and the subsequent development of postoperative infection found that a higher glucose value on postoperative day 1 was associated with subsequent development of infection.[110] It is unlikely that infection would be the cause of the hyperglycemia that early in the postoperative period. A postoperative day 1 glucose greater than 220 mg/dl was associated with a 20 percent incidence of severe infection (bacterial) or pneumonia during the postoperative period in these patients, while the incidence was 0 percent when the blood glucose was less than 220 mg/dl on the first postoperative day.

The final clinical example of hyperglycemia associated with infectious risk is found in a meta-analysis of randomized clinical trials comparing parenteral nutrition to enteral nutrition in critically ill patients.[111] A significant reduction (35 percent vs 16 percent) in infection was reported during tube feeding compared with parenteral nutrition. However, hyperglycemia may have been a contributing variable because the average blood glucose was greater than 220 mg/dl in the parenteral nutrition group and significantly lower at approximately 130 mg/dl in the tube-feeding group.

ENTERAL TUBE FEEDING: USE IN PATIENTS WITH DIABETES MELLITUS

Formula Selection

As discussed in Chapter 13, the enteral route should be used to provide nutrition in malnourished patients with a functioning GI tract. The recent availability of an enteral tube feeding formula that is lower in carbohydrate and higher in fat content than standard formulas prompted studies comparing the glycemic response. Although standard formulas contain approximately 50 percent simple carbohydrate and 30 percent fat, one of the novel formulas contains 18 percent glucose oligosaccharides, 7 percent fructose, 8 percent soluble fiber, and 50 percent fat. The glucose response to these products was studied in ten patients with insulin-dependent diabetes mellitus.[112] Even though an initial report suggested that the glycemic response to the lower carbohydrate product was blunted compared with standard formulas, a follow-up study reported that the glycemic response was quite variable in each patient.[113] The clinical significance of these studies is unclear because the subjects ingested very small amounts of the formula over a few

hours, a very different pattern than that of continuous or gravity tube feeding. The high fat content could impair gastric emptying in patients with gastroparesis. With regard to fiber content, the current American Diabetes Association position statement on nutrition states that although selected soluble fibers can delay glucose absorption from the small intestine, the effect of dietary fiber on glycemic control is probably insignificant.[114] Therefore, the fiber intake recommendations for diabetics are probably the same as for the general hospitalized population. As discussed in Chapter 13, a fiber-containing formula may be advantageous for diabetic patients with diarrhea or constipation. During hospitalization, avoidance of overfeeding is likely more important than is the use of a specific enteral formula. Outcome studies will be necessary to definitively address this subject.

Tube Feeding and Gastroparesis

The selection of gastric vs jejunal feeding was discussed in Chapter 13, and in general the same guidelines apply to patients with diabetes mellitus. A unique situation in diabetic patients is diabetic gastroparesis. These patients may require supplemental or total nutrition support by tube feeding. The majority of these patients will tolerate jejunal tube feeding when isoosmolar feedings are started at a low rate (e.g., 20 ml/hour) and advanced slowly (10 to 20 ml/hour increment every 12 to 24 hours). It is important not to advance the rate too quickly in these patients, since a rapid progression may lead to tube-feeding intolerance. The use of a decompression (or venting) nasogastric tube may provide symptomatic relief in patients with gastroparesis.

Method of Tube-Feeding Administration

The method of nutrient delivery varies with tube location. If gastric feedings have been selected, continuous administration of feeding is preferred for stressed patients. Gravity administration of feeding is desirable in stable patients, since the hormonal profile more closely approximates the hormonal milieu profile following meal ingestion in healthy diabetic subjects. In addition, an infusion pump is not required, which decreases expense and facilitates patient mobility. There may be theoretical advantages of nocturnal tube feeding (i.e., decreased insulin levels during the nutrition-free period in nondiabetic patients), but there are also potential disadvantages. During nocturnal feeding, the caloric provision is both compressed and continuous, causing a sustained, nonphysiologic hyperinsulinemia that may have adverse sequelae. If jejunal feedings have been selected, continuous feeding is preferred because intermittent feeding usually creates dumping symptoms.

Long-Term Tube Feeding

Enteral feeding has been shown to be effective in the long-term nutritional support of diabetic patients with gastroparesis.[115] Long-term tube feeding should be considered in diabetic patients with gastroparesis who, despite adequate medical therapy (antiemetic or prokinetic agents), are hospitalized frequently for symptoms of gastroparesis or who cannot maintain weight or hydration. Before placement of a permanent enteral feeding tube, a trial of nasoenteric feeding is important to confirm that the patient can tolerate at least 30–40 ml/hour of tube feeding. Tubes can be successfully placed either endoscopically[116] or surgically. Patients with significant gastroparesis often require a feeding jejunostomy and a decompression gastrostomy. The initial enthusiasm to convert percutaneous endoscopic gastrostomies to percutaneous jejunostomies has waned as higher rates of tube dysfunction, without elimination of aspiration, have been reported.[117-119]

The presence of disordered motility throughout the GI tract and the unpredictable clinical course of diabetic enteropathy should make physicians wary of surgical intervention. However, the use of gastric decompression may provide symptomatic relief. For nondiabetic patients with pseudo-obstruction and severe and persistent symptoms due to GI stasis despite medical therapy, gastric decompression significantly reduced the number of hospital admissions.[120] This disorder resembles gastroparesis both in symptoms and in manometric findings.

Parenteral Nutrition: Indications for Use in Gastroparesis

Parenteral nutrition should be reserved for those patients who have severe small bowel dysmotility (characterized by low-amplitude contractions less than 15 mm Hg on small bowel manometry) and who have failed a reasonable trial of nasojejunal tube feeding.[50]

PRINCIPLES OF GLYCEMIC MANAGEMENT

The glycemic management of diabetic patients receiving enteral tube feeding is challenging. Oral hypoglycemic agents administered by feeding tube can be used to treat hyperglycemia in medically stable patients with well-controlled noninsulin-dependent diabetes mellitus and normal renal and hepatic function. We do not recommend the use of metformin in this group of patients. A major (although very uncommon) risk of metformin is lactic acidosis, which can occur in patients with hepatic or renal disease or with tissue ischemia. Patients admitted to the hospital on insulin or with consistent fasting glucose values greater than 200 mg/dl will require insulin, and enteral tube-feeding calories generally can be covered with subcutaneously administered insulin. Short-acting (Regular) insulin supplementation is often required in addition to intermediate-acting (NPH or Lente) insulin, and adherence to an insulin algorithm for the subcutaneous administration of regular insulin is important (Tables 27–3 and 27–4). The algorithm should be individualized depending on such variables as type of diabetes (type I vs type II), physiognomy, degree of metabolic

TABLE 27–3   Insulin Preparation Pharmacokinetics (Human)

Preparation	Route	t$_{1/2}$ (Minutes)	Glucose Nadir (Hours)	Effects (Hours)
Rapid onset				
Regular	SC	60	2–6	4–12
	IV	3–6	0.5	3.5
Intermediate acting				
NPH	SC		6–16	12–18
Lente	SC		6–16	12–18
Long acting				
Ultralente	SC		14–24	16–32

SC = subcutaneous; IV = intravenous.

TABLE 27–4 Algorithm for Subcutaneous Administration of Regular Insulin

Plasma Glucose (mg/dl)*	Subcutaneous Insulin Dose (Units)†‡
200–250	2–3
251–300	4–6
301–350	6–9
351–400	9–12

*Notify physician if glucose value < 80 mg/dl or > 200 mg/dl. The algorithm may need to be modified for certain patients.

†Do not use subcutaneous administration of regular insulin more often than every 4 hours.

‡This recommended insulin dose should be doubled if the dose suggested by the algorithm does not result in a decrease in glucose toward goal levels.

stress, and glucocorticoid or sympathomimetic agent use. It is our practice to measure glucose by reflectance meter because the results are rapidly obtained and the need for venipuncture is avoided. However, a strenuous control program involving glucose meter calibration, personnel training, comparison measurements, and monitoring of results needs to be in place to ensure adequacy of glucose results.

Until tube-feeding tolerance has been established, cautious use of intermediate-acting insulin and reliance on short-acting insulin is preferred. This approach should minimize the risk of hypoglycemia that could result from the prolonged action of NPH or Lente insulin following unexpected discontinuation of tube feeding. Once the continuous tube-feeding rate has reached 30 to 40 ml/hour, the use of intermediate-acting insulin (Table 27–3) should be safe. We initially provide one half the patient's preadmission morning insulin dose as intermediate-acting insulin. In general, do not increase the tube-feeding infusion rate until adequate glycemic control has been achieved. As the feeding rate is increased, the intermediate-acting insulin dose often must be increased. Twice-daily administration of subcutaneous intermediate-acting insulin may be necessary if the feedings are continuous. Short-acting insulin should be added to the insulin regimen if glucose goals are not achieved with intermediate-acting insulin alone.

If the feedings are infused by gravity administration, check the glucose level immediately before initiating feeding and no sooner than 4 hours after the end of the prior feeding. As stated earlier, desirable blood glucose goals are 100 to 200 mg/dl during initiation of tube feeding or in stressed patients and 100 to 150 mg/dl in stable patients. It is generally not helpful to check glucose levels during or immediately following the gravity feeding. Although some patients receiving this form of feeding can be managed with intermediate-duration insulin alone, others will need combined treatment with intermediate-acting and short-acting insulin.

A common management error occurs when the physician relies on the Regular insulin algorithm exclusively for insulin management throughout the entire hospitalization. Once the patient is medically stable, the preferred management is to review the amount of Regular insulin required over the preceding 24-hour period and then appropriately adjust the intermediate-acting and short-acting insulin programs. Because of the dramatic results of the Diabetes Control and Complications Trial, more diabetic patients will be managed with multiple-dose insulin therapy (e.g., Ultralente insulin and premeal Regular insulin). In general, the dose of Ultralente insulin (Table 27–3) should initially be continued at the preadmission dose, and dose adjustments should be made in the short-acting insulin. Consultation with an endocrinologist for assistance with glycemic management is appropriate in this select group of patients.

In patients with unsatisfactory glucose control or a changing clinical condition, initiation of an intravenous insulin infusion is indicated; guidelines for its use are provided in Table 27–5. Plasma levels of potassium, phosphorus, and magnesium may decrease following initiation of an intravenous insulin infusion, so these values should be carefully monitored. When adequate glycemic control has been achieved, conversion from intravenous to subcutaneous insulin management is indicated. It is important to continue the intravenous insulin infusion for several hours after the first subcutaneously administered insulin dose to prevent rebound hyperglycemia.

MONITORING FOLLOWING INITIATION OF NUTRITION SUPPORT

Inadequate attention to blood glucose monitoring and insulin/oral hypoglycemic agent administration may lead to the development of significant hyperglycemia and even the hyperosmolar nonketotic syndrome. The potential for fever, leukocytosis, overfeeding, or initiation of corticosteroids, cyclosporine, or sympathomimetic infusion to cause significant hyper-

TABLE 27–5 Insulin Infusion Algorithm: A Suggested Initial Insulin Infusion*

Plasma Glucose (mg/dl)	IV Infusion Rate (ml/hour)	Insulin Infusion Rate (units/hour)
> 400	8	8
351–400	6	6
301–350	4	4
250–300	3	3
200–249	2.5	2.5
150–199	2	2
120–149	1.5	1.5
100–119	1	1
70–99	0	0
< 70	0	0

*Define glucose goals for each patient. In stressed patients, a glucose goal range of 100–200 mg/dl is reasonable. Monitor glucose hourly until the glucose concentrations have stabilized in the patient's goal range for 4 hours. Then decrease the frequency of testing to every 2 hours; once the glucose control remains stable, decrease testing to every four hours.

This infusion is designed for the average 70-kg patient and may require modification for smaller or larger patients. This infusion is not appropriate for treatment of diabetic ketoacidosis. Patients with insulin resistance often require more insulin. Suspect this possibility when a high glucose does not decrease by at least 50 mg/dl/hour. If hyperglycemia persists, increase this algorithm by 50% increments for each glucose range greater than 200 mg/dl. The risk of hypoglycemia may be greater if the insulin infusion is increased for glucose ranges less than 200 mg/dl.

In hyperglycemic patients treated with insulin infusions, plasma potassium, phosphorus, and magnesium may decrease rapidly and should be monitored. Finally, at conversion from intravenous to subcutaneous insulin therapy, continue the intravenous insulin infusion for 2 to 3 hours after administering the first subcutaneous dose.

TABLE 27–6 Guidelines for Frequency of Glucose Testing*

Frequency	Clinical Situations
Daily (morning)	Stable oral hypoglycemic agent program with average glucoses in goal range
Twice daily (0700, 1600)	Once daily or twice daily NPH or Lente program with average glucoses in goal range
Four times daily (0700, 1100, 1600, 2100)	Initiation of tube feeding and during progression to goal feeding rate
	Deterioration in medical status
	Regular insulin algorithm program
	Split/mixed program, such as once-daily NPH (or Lente) and Regular insulin program twice-daily NPH (or Lente) and Regular program
	Ultralente/Regular insulin program
Every hour to every fourth hour	Intravenous insulin infusion

*Refer to text for glucose monitoring guidelines during gravity administration of tube feeding.

glycemia should be considered. The frequency of glucose monitoring should be increased during these situations and the insulin program appropriately modified. Conversely, unanticipated discontinuation of enteral tube feeding may cause hypoglycemia in patients who have received subcutaneous insulin, and blood glucose levels should be closely monitored to see if initiation of a dextrose-containing crystalloid solution is necessary. A decrease in the average glucose values should also be anticipated with resolution of severe stress, deterioration in renal function, decrease in dose of corticosteroids or sympathomimetic agents, or significant weight loss. Anticipation of these effects and careful observation of glucose trends over the preceding few days should allow adjustment of the insulin program and thereby minimize wide fluctuations in glucose control. Guidelines for blood glucose monitoring follow-

ing initiation of tube feeding are provided in Table 27–6.

Careful monitoring of the diabetic patient receiving nutritional support is key to safe use of this form of therapy. Accurate recording of daily weight and fluid balance is essential. After initiation of tube feeding, careful monitoring of the patient's vital signs, hemodynamic data (if applicable), weight, fluid balance, acid-base status, and biochemical parameters is important. Hemodynamic data, fluid balance, creatinine, urea, and sodium should be reviewed to determine the appropriate volume of fluid and nutrition. An osmotic diuresis should be considered in patients with hyperglycemia and increased urine output. In the stressed patient, day-to-day weight changes generally reflect shifts in fluid balance. A daily weight increase in excess of 0.25 kg should be attributed to fluid gain rather than to the accretion of lean tissue.

Base-line biochemical monitoring should include a glycated hemoglobin, complete blood count, glucose, electrolytes, creatinine, urea nitrogen, liver function tests, phosphorus, magnesium, calcium, and albumin. A baseline glycated hemoglobin is useful both to establish recent glucose control and to help determine the appropriate diabetes treatment after hospital dismissal. Hyperglycemia may cause a pseudohyponatremia.[98] Because glucose penetrates cells slowly, an increase in the plasma glucose level raises the plasma osmolality and causes water to move from the cells to the extracellular volume. This lowers the plasma sodium concentration by dilution. In general, every 62 mg/dl increment in the plasma glucose level will draw enough water out of the cells to reduce the plasma sodium concentration 1 mEq/L. Potassium levels should be interpreted in light of the glucose value. Hyperkalemia, if accompanied by hyperglycemia, is often effectively treated by supplemental insulin. Plasma magnesium, zinc, and copper levels should be measured in patients with impaired absorption or increased GI (zinc, copper), or renal (magnesium) output. Although the extent and frequency of biochemical monitoring following initiation of tube feeding should be individualized, at a minimum plasma glucose, electrolytes, and phosphorus levels should be checked until levels are stable.

With an acute increase in plasma insulin (e.g., following refeeding or exogenous insulin administration), renal sodium excretion decreases, which may lead to salt and water retention. The hyperinsulinemia stimulates tubular reabsorption of sodium independent of changes in the filtered load of glucose, glomerular filtration rate, renal blood flow, and plasma aldosterone.[121] The effect of chronic hyperinsulinemia on sodium excretion is not known. Hyperinsulinemia may also decrease the plasma levels of potassium, phosphorus, and magnesium if the supplementation is inadequate.[122] Insulin increases the sodium permeability of skeletal muscle cells, increases cytosolic sodium concentration, and activates Na, K-adenosine triphosphatase.[123] As sodium is then transported from the cell, electronegativity is generated. This promotes the passage of potassium from the extracellular space to the intracellular space, resulting in hypokalemia. Hypokalemia can also be caused by malnutrition or anabolism. Total body potassium is stored almost entirely within lean tissue. Because the amount of lean tissue is decreased in malnutrition, the body stores of potassium may also be decreased. Finally, during the accretion of lean tissue during anabolism, potassium requirements may increase, since 3 mEq of potassium are retained per 1 g of nitrogen.[124] Phosphorus

plays an important role in intermediary metabolism. Glucose- and insulin-stimulated glycolysis enhance cellular uptake and use of phosphorus for the phosphorylation of glycolytic intermediates and for the synthesis of adenosine triphosphate synthesis. Thus, insulin infusion may cause hypophosphatemia. Hyperinsulinemia can increase tissue uptake of magnesium, resulting in hypomagnesemia.

CONCLUSION

In summary, over the short-term hospitalization, the tenets underlying the design of tube-feeding programs for hospitalized patients with diabetes mellitus are similar to those for feeding nondiabetic patients. The finely tuned homeostatic mechanisms regulating carbohydrate metabolism in the healthy subject can be affected by diabetes mellitus, feeding, and stress. An appreciation of the clinical presentation and the management of diabetic enteropathy is important for effective use of enteral tube feeding in this subset of patients. Finally, an understanding of the importance of glycemic control and development of guidelines for glucose management should facilitate safe use of enteral tube feeding in diabetic patients.

REFERENCES

1. Dietz G, Wicklmayr M, Hepp K et al: On gluconeogenesis of human liver: accelerated hepatic glucose formation induced by increased precursor supply. Diabetologia 1976;12:555–561.
2. Wahren J, Felig P, Ahlborg G et al: Glucose metabolism during leg exercise in man. J Clin Invest 1971; 50:2715–2725.
3. Buschiazzo H, Exton J, Park C: Effects of glucose on glycogen synthetase, phosphorylase, and glycogen deposition in the perfused rat liver. Proc Natl Acad Sci USA 1971;65:383–387.
4. Ruderman N, Herrera M: Glucose regulation of hepatic gluconeogenesis. Am J Physiol 1968;214:1346–1351.
5. Rizza R, Mandarino L, Gerich J: Dose-response characteristics for effects of insulin on production and utilization of glucose in man. Am J Physiol 1981;40: E630–E639.
6. Verdonk C, Rizza R, Gerich J: Effects of plasma glucose concentration on glucose utilization and glucose clearance in normal man. Diabetes 1981;30: 535–537.
7. Cherrington A, Williams P, Harris M: Relationship between the plasma glucose level and glucose uptake in the conscious dog. Metab Clin Exp 1978;27: 787–791.
8. Pehling G, Tessari P, Gerich J et al: Abnormal carbohydrate disposition in insulin-dependent diabetes: relative contributions of endogenous glucose production and initial splanchnic uptake and effect of intensive insulin therapy. J Clin Invest 1984;74:985–991.

9. Firth R, Bell P, Marsh H et al: Postprandial hyperglycemia in patients with noninsulin-dependent diabetes mellitus. J Clin Invest 1986;77:1525–1532.

10. McMahon M, Rizza R: The contribution of initial splanchnic glucose clearance and gluconeogenesis to postprandial hyperglycemia in noninsulin-dependent diabetes mellitus. Clin Res 1987;35:899A.

11. Bell P, Firth R, Rizza R: Assessment of insulin action in insulin-dependent diabetes mellitus using [6-^{14}C] glucose, [3-^{3}H] glucose, and [2-^{3}H] glucose. J Clin Invest 1986;78:1479–1486.

12. Batstone G, Aloberti K, Hinks L et al: Metabolic studies in subjects following thermal injury. Intermediary metabolites, hormones, and tissue oxygenation. Burns 1976;2:207–225.

13. Willerson J, Hutcheson D, Leshin S et al: Serum glucagon and insulin levels and their relationship to blood glucose values in patients with acute myocardial infarction and acute coronary insufficiency. Am J Med 1974;57:747–753.

14. Harris M, Cahill G, Bennett P et al: National Diabetes Data Group. Diabetes 1979;28:1039–1057.

15. Exton J: Gluconeogenesis. Metabolism 1972;21:945–989.

16. Exton J, Park C: The role of cyclic AMP in the control of liver metabolism. Adv Enzyme Regul 1968;6:391–407.

17. Long C, Smith O, Fry E: Actions of cortisol and related compounds on carbohydrate and protein metabolism. In Wolstenholm O, Connor M (eds): Metabolic Effects of Adrenal Hormone. London: Churchill, 1960.

18. Shulman G: Glucose disposal during insulinopenia in somatostatin-treated dogs: the roles of glucose and glucagon. J Clin Invest 1978;62:487–492.

19. Hers H: The control of glycogen metabolism in the liver. Ann Rev Biochem 1976;45:167–189.

20. Walaas O, Walaas E: Effect of epinephrine on rat diaphragm. J Biol Chem 1950;187:769–776.

21. Munck A: Studies on the mode of action of glucocorticoids in rats. Biochem/Biophys Acta 1962;57:318–326.

22. Shamoon M, Hendler R, Sherwin R: Synergistic interactions among antiinsulin hormones in the pathogenesis of stress hyperglycemia in humans. J Clin Endocrinol Metab 1981;52:1235–1241.

23. Bessey P, Watters J, Aoki T et al: Combined hormonal infusion stimulates the metabolic response to injury. Ann Surg 1984;200:264–281.

24. Shamoon M, Hendler R, Sherwin R: Altered responsiveness to cortisol, epinephrine, and glucagon in insulin-infused juvenile-onset diabetics. Diabetes 1980;29:284–291.

25. Fukushima R, Saito H, Taniwaka K et al: Different roles of IL-1 and TNF on hemodynamics and interorgan amino acid metabolism in awake dogs. Am J Physiol 1992;262:E275–E281.

26. Flores EA, Istfan N, Pomposelli JJ et al: Effect of interleukin 1 and tumor necrosis factor/cachectin on glucose turnover in the rat. Metabolism 1990;39:738–743.

27. Pomposelli JJ, Flores EA, Bistrian BR: Role of biochemical mediators in clinical nutrition and surgical metabolism. J Parenter Enter Nutr 1988;12:212–218.

28. Besedovsky H, Del Ray A, Sorkin E et al: Immunoregulatory feedback between interleukin-1 and glucocorticoid hormones. Science 1986;233:652–654.

29. Rundles RW: Diabetic neuropathy: general review with report of 125 cases. Medicine 1945;24:111–160.

30. Zitomer BR, Gramm HF, Zozak GP: Gastric neuropathy in diabetes mellitus: clinical and radiologic observations. Metabolism 1968;17:199–211.

31. Feldman M, Schiller LR: Disorders of gastrointestinal motility associated with diabetes mellitus. Ann Intern Med 1983;98:378–384.

32. Loo FD, Dodds WJ, Soergel KH et al: Multipeaked esophageal peristaltic pressure waves in patients with diabetic neuropathy. Gastroenterology 1985;88:485–491.

33. Sundkvist G, Hillarp B, Lilja B et al: Esophageal motor function evaluated by scintigraphy, video-radiography and manometry in diabetic patients. ACTA Radiol 1989;30:17–19.

34. Borgstrom PS, Olsson R, Sundkvist G et al: Pharyngeal and oesophageal function in patients with diabetes mellitus and swallowing complaints. Br J Radiol 1988;61:817–821.

35. Kesharvarzian A, Iber FL, Nasrallah S: Radionuclide esophageal emptying and manometric studies in diabetes mellitus. Am J Gastroenterol 1987; 82(7):625–631.

36. Kassander P: Asymptomatic gastric retention in diabetics (gastroparesis diabeticorum). Ann Intern Med 1958;48:797–812.

37. Camilleri M, Malagelada JR: Abnormal intestinal motility in diabetics with the gastroparesis syndrome. Eur J Clin Invest 1984;14:420–427.

38. Kim CH, Kennedy FP, Camilleri M et al: The relationship between clinical factors and gastrointestinal dysmotility in diabetes mellitus. J Gastrointest Motil 1991;3(4):268–272.

39. DePonti F, Fealey RD, Malagelada JR: Gastrointestinal syndromes due to diabetes mellitus. In Dyck PJ, Thomas PK, Asbury AK et al (eds): Diabetic Neuropathy. Philadelphia: W.B. Saunders, 1987:155.

40. Campbell A, Conway H: Gastric retention and hypoglycemia in diabetes. Scot Med J 1960;5 167–168.

41. Wooten RL, Meriwether TW: Diabetic gastric atony: a clinical study. JAMA 1961;176:1082–1087.

42. Gupta KK, Hedge KP, Lal R: Diabetic gastric neuropathy with acute hypoglycemic attacks. J Indian Med Assoc 1971;57:258–259.

43. MacGregor IL, Gudler R, Watts HP et al: The effect of acute hyperglycemia on gastric emptying in man. Gastroenterology 1976;70:90–196.

44. Campbell IW, Heading RC, Tothill P et al: Gastric emptying in diabetic autonomic neuropathy. Gut 1977;18:462–467.

45. Loo FD, Palmer DW, Soergel KH et al: Gastric emptying in patients with diabetes mellitus. Gastroenterology 1984;86:485–494.

46. von der Ohe MR, Camilleri M: Measurement of small bowel and colonic transit: indications and methods. Mayo Clin Proc 1992; 67:1169-1179.

47. Lartigue S, Bizais Y, Des Varannes SB et al: Inter- and intrasubject variability of solid and liquid gastric emptying parameters: a scintigraphic study in healthy subjects and diabetic patients. Dig Dis Sci 1994;39(1):109–115.

48. Horowitz M, Smout AJPM: Disordered esophageal and gastric motility in diabetes mellitus. In Mazzaferri EL, Bar RS, Kreisberg RA (eds): Advances in Endocrinology & Metabolism, Vol 4. St. Louis: Mosby, 1993:81–114.

49. Drenth JPH, Engels LGJB: Diabetic gastroparesis: a critical reappraisal of new treatment strategies. Drugs 1992;44(4):537–553.

50. Camilleri M: Appraisal of medium- and long-term treatment of gastroparesis and chronic intestinal dysmotility. Am J Gastroenterol 1994;89(10):1769–1774.

51. Horowitz M, Harding PE, Maddox AF et al: Gastric and oesophageal emptying in patients with type II (non-insulin-dependent) diabetes mellitus. Diabetologia 1989;32:151–159.

52. Van dijl PW, Hofma SJ, Van doormaal JJ et al: Low prevalence of symptomatic gastric and esophageal motor dysfunction in diabetes mellitus. Gastroenterology 1989;96:a524.

53. Wright RA, Clemente R, Wathen R: Diabetic gastroparesis: an abnormality of gastric emptying of solids. Am J Med Sci 1985;289:240–242.

54. Horowitz M, Maddox AF, Wishart JM et al: Relationships between oesophageal transit in solid and liquid gastric emptying in diabetes mellitus. Eur J Nucl Med 1991;18:229–234.

55. Fraser R, Horowitz M, Maddox AF et al: Hyperglycemia slows gastric emptying in type I diabetes mellitus. Diabetologia 1990;30:675–680.

56. Kawagishi T, Nishizawa Y, Okuno Y et al: Antroduodenal motility and transpyloric fluid movement in diabetic patients studied using duplex sonography. Gastroenterology 1994;107:403–409.

57. Llebbard GS, Sun WM, Dent J et al: Acute hyperglycemia increases proximal gastric compliance. Gastroenterology 1994;108a.

58. Campbell JW, Heading RC, Tothill P et al: Gastric emptying in diabetic autonomic neuropathy. Gut 1977;18:462–467.

59. Schade RR, Dugas MC, Lhotsky DM et al: Effect of metoclopramide on gastric liquid emptying in patients with diabetic gastroparesis. Dig Dis Sci 1985;30:10–15.

60. Ricci DA, Saltzman MB, Meyer C et al: Effect of metoclopramide in diabetic gastroparesis. J Clin Gastroenterol 1985;7:25–32.

61. McHugh S, Lico S, Diamant NE: Cisapride vs. metoclopramide: an acute study in diabetic gastroparesis. Dig Dis Sci 1992;37:997–1001.

62. Horowitz M, Harding PE, Chatterton BE et al: Acute and chronic effects of domperidone on gastric emptying in diabetic autonomic neuropathy. Dig Dis Sci 1985;30:1–9.

63. Champion MC, Gulenchyn K, O'Leary T et al: Domperidone (Motilium) improves symptoms and solid phase gastric emptying in diabetic gastroparesis. Am J Gastroenterol 1987;82:213.

64. Horowitz M, Maddox A, Harding PE et al: Effect of cisapride on gastric and oesophageal emptying in insulin-dependent diabetes mellitus. Gastrotenterology 1987;92:1899–1907.

65. Janssens J, Peeters TL, Vantrappen G et al: Improvement of gastric emptying in diabetic gastroparesis by erythromycin: preliminary studies. N Engl J Med 1990;322:1028–1031.

66. Coch KL, Stern RM, Stewart WR et al: Gastric emptying and gastric myoelectrical activity in patients with diabetic gastroparesis: effect of long-term domperidone. Am J Gastroenterol 1989;84:69–75.

67. DeCaestecker JS, Ewing DJ, Tothill P et al: Evaluation of oral cisapride and metoclopramide in diabetic autonomic neuropathy: an eight-week double-blind crossover study. Aliment Pharmacol Ther 1989;3:69–81.

68. Snappe WJ, Battle WM, Schwartz SS et al: Metoclopramide to treat gastroparesis due to diabetes mellitus. A double-blind controlled trial. Ann Intern Med 1982;96:444–446.

69. Havelund T, Oster-Jorgensen E, Eshoj O et al: Effect of cisapride on gastroparesis in patients with insulin-dependent diabetes mellitus: a double-blind controlled trial. Acta Med Scand 1987;222:339–343.

70. McCallum RW, Ricci DA, Rakatansky H et al: A multicenter placebo-controlled clinical trial of oral metoclopramide in diabetic gastroparesis. Diabetes Care 1983;6:463–467.

71. Champion MC, Gulenchyn K, Braaten J et al: Cisapride improves symptoms and solid phase gastric emptying in diabetic gastroparesis. Diabetes 1988;37(supp 1):48a.

72. Camilleri M, Brown ML, Malagelada JR: Impaired transit of chyme in chronic intestinal pseudo-obstruction: correction by cisapride. Gastroenterology 1986;91:619–626.

73. Champion MC: Management of idiopathic, diabetic and miscellaneous gastroparesis with cisapride. Scand J Gastroenterol 1989;165:44–53.

74. Horowitz M, Dent J: Disordered gastric emptying: mechanical basis, assessment and treatment. Baillieres Clin Gastroenterol 1991;5:371–407.

75. Ogbonnaya KI, Arem R: Diabetic diarrhea. Pathophysiology, diagnosis, and management. Arch Intern Med 1990;150:262–267.

76. Spengler U, Stellaard F, Ruckdeschel G et al: Small intestinal transit, bacterial growth, and bowel habits in diabetes mellitus. Pancreas 1989;4(1):65–70.

77. Dooley CP, el-Newihi HM, Zeidler A et al: Abnormalities of migrating motor complex in diabetes with autonomic neuropathy and diarrhea. Scand J Gastroenterol 1988;23:217–233.

78. Schiller LR, Santa Ana CA, Schmulen AC et al: Pathogenesis of fecal incontinence in diabetes mellitus: evidence for internal anal sphincter dysfunction. N Engl J Med 1982;307:1666–1671.

79. Marzuk PM: Biofeedback for gastrointestinal disorders: a review of the literature. Ann Intern Med 1985;103:240–244.

80. Thompson MW: Heredity, maternal age, and birth order in etiology of celiac disease. Am J Hum Genet 1951;3:159–166.

81. Frier BM, Saunders JHB, Wormsley KG et al: Exocrine pancreatic function in juvenile-onset diabetes mellitus. Gut 1976;17:685–691.

82. Goldstein F, Wirts CW, Kowlessar OD: Diabetic diarrhea and steatorrhea: microbiologic and clinical observations. Ann Intern Med 1970;72:215–218.

83. Fedorak R, Field M, Chang E: Treatment of diabetic diarrhea with clonidine. Ann Intern Med 1985;102:197–199.

84. Bistrian BR: Nutritional assessment of the hospitalized patient: a practical approach. In Wright RA, Heymsfield S (eds): Nutritional Assessment. Boston: Blackwell Scientific Publications, 1984:183–205.

85. McMahon M, Bistrian BR: The physiology of nutritional assessment and therapy in protein-calorie malnutrition. Disease-a-Month 1990; XXXVI 7:375–417.

86. Harris JA, Benedict FG: A biometric study of basal metabolism in man, pub. no. 279. Washington DC: Carnegie Institute of Washington, 1919.

87. Roza AM, Shizgal HM: The Harris-Benedict equation re-evaluated: resting energy requirements and the body cell mass. Am J Clin Nutr 1984;40:168–182.

88. Quebbeman EJ, Ausman RK, Schneider TC: A re-evaluation of energy expenditure during parenteral nutrition. Ann Surg 1982;195:282–286.

89. Hunter DC, Jaksic J, Lewis D et al: Resting energy expenditure in the critically ill. Crit Care Med 1985;13:173–177.

90. Paauw JD, McCamish MA, Dean RE: Assessment of caloric needs in stressed patients. J Am Coll Nutr 1984;3:51–59.

91. Mann S, Westenskow DR, Houtchens BA: Measured and predicted caloric expenditure in the acutely ill. Crit Care Med 1985;13:173–177.

92. McMahon MM, Farnell MB, Murray MJ: Nutritional support of critically ill patients. Mayo Clin Proc 1993; 68:911–920.

93. Albert A, Takamatsu H, Fonkalsrud E: Absorption of glucose solutions from the peritoneal cavity in rabbits. Arch Surg 1984;119:1247–1251.

94. Schade D, Eaton R, Friedman W et al: Prolonged peritoneal infusion in a diabetic man. Diabetes Care 1980;3:314–317.

95. Manji N, Shikora S, McMahon M et al: Peritoneal dialysis for acute renal failure: overfeeding resulting from dextrose absorbed during dialysis. Crit Care Med 1990;18:29–31.

96. The Diabetes Control and Complications Trial Research Group: The effect of intensive treatment on the development and progression of long-term complications in insulin-dependent diabetes mellitus. N Engl J Med 1993;329:977–986.

97. Rose BD: Hypoosmolal states — hyponatremia. In Rose BD (ed): Clinical Physiology of Acid-Base and Electrolyte Disorders. New York: McGraw-Hill, 1989: 601–638.

98. Bagdade J, Stewart M, Walters E: Impaired granulocyte adherence. A reversible defect in host defense in patients with poorly controlled diabetes. Diabetes 1978;27:677–681.

99. Mowat A, Baum J: Chemotaxis of polymorphonuclear leukocytes from patients with diabetes mellitus. N Engl J Med 1971;284:621–627.

100. Bagdade J, Nielson K, Bulger R: Reversible abnormalities in phagocytic function in poorly controlled diabetic patients. Am J Med Sci 1972;263:451–456.

101. Bagdade J, Koot R, Bulger R: Impaired leukocyte function in patients with poorly controlled diabetes. Diabetes 1974;23:9–15.

102. Nolan C, Beaty H, Bagdade J: Impaired granulocyte bactericidal function in patients with poorly controlled diabetes. Diabetes 1978;127:889–894.

103. Repine J, Clawson C, Goetz F: Bactericidal function of neutrophils from patients with acute bacterial infections and from diabetes. J Infect Dis 1980;142: 869–875.

104. Karnovsky M: The metabolism of leukocytes. Semin Hematol 1968;5:156–165.

105. Hostetter MK: Handicaps to host defense: effects of hyperglycemia on C3 and *Candida albicans*. Diabetes 1990;39:271–275.

106. Gilmore BJ, Retsinas EM, Lorenz JJ et al: An iC3b receptor on *Candida albicans*: Structure, function, and correlates for pathogenicity. J Infect Dis 1988;157: 38–46.

107. Hostetter MK, Krueger RA, Schmeting DJ: The biochemistry of opsonization: central role of the reactive thiolester of the third component of complement. J Infect Dis 1984;150:653–661.

108. Hostetter MK, Lorenz JS, Preus L et al: The iC3b receptor on *Candida albicans:* subcellular localization and modulation of receptor expression by glucose. J Infect Dis 1990;161:761–768.

109. Alexiewicz JM, Kumar D, Smogorzewski M et al: Polymorphonuclear leukocytes in noninsulin dependent diabetes mellitus: abnormalities in metabolism and function. Ann Intern Med 1995;123:919–924.

109a. Overett TK, Bistrian BR, Lowry SF et al: Total parenteral nutrition in patients with insulin-requiring diabetes mellitus. J Am Coll Nutr 1986;5:79–89.

110. Baxter JK, Babineau T, Apovian CM et al: Perioperative glucose control predicts increased nosocomial infection in diabetics. Crit Care Med 1990;18:5705.

111. Moore FA, Feliciano DV, Andrassy RJ et al: Early enteral feeding, compared with parenteral, reduces postoperative septic complications. Ann Surg 1992; 216:172–183.

112. Peters AL, Davidson MB, Isaac RM: Lack of glucose elevation after simulated tube feeding in patients with type I diabetes. Am J Med 1989;87:178–182.

113. Peters AL, Davidson MB: Effects of various enteral feeding products on postprandial blood glucose response in patients with type I diabetes. J Parenter Enter Nutr 1991;16:69–74.

114. American Diabetes Association: Nutrition recommendations and principles for people with diabetes mellitus. Diabetes Care 1995;18:16–19.

115. Jacober SJ, Narayan A, Strodel WE et al: Jejunostomy feeding in the management of gastroparesis diabeticorum. Diabetes Care 1986;9:217–219.

116. Larson DE, Burton DD, Schroeder KW et al: Percutaneous endoscopic gastrostomy: indications, success, complications, and mortality in 314 consecutive patients. Gastroenterology 1987;93:48–52.

117. Kaplan DS, Murthy UK, Linscheer WG: Percutaneous endoscopic jejunostomy: long-term follow-up of 23 patients. Gastrointest Endosc 1989;35:403–406.

118. Wolfsen HC, Kozarek RA, Ball TJ et al: Tube dysfunction following percutaneous endoscopic gastrostomy and jejunostomy. Gastrointest Endosc 1990;36: 261–263.

119. DiSario JA, Foutch PG, Sanowski RA: Poor results with percutaneous endoscopic jejunostomy. Gastrointest Endosc 1990;36:257–260.

120. Pitt HA, Mann LL, Berquist WE et al: Chronic intestinal pseudo-obstruction. Management with total parenteral nutrition and a venting enterostomy. Arch Surg 1985;120:614–618.

121. DeFronzo R, Cooke C, Andres R et al: The effect of insulin on renal handling of sodium, potassium, calcium, and phosphate in man. J Clin Invest 1985;55: 845–855.

122. Knochel JP: Complications of total parenteral nutrition (letter to the editor). Kidney Int 1985; 27: 489–496.

123. Moore RD: Stimulation of NA:H exchange by insulin. Biophys J 1981;33:203–210.

124. Acheson KJ, Flatt JP, Jequier E: Glycogen synthesis versus lipogenesis after a 500 gram carbohydrate meal in man. Metabolism 1982;31:1234–1240.

28

Enteral Nutrition and Respiratory Diseases

Susan K. Pingleton

Nutrition is an important aspect of patient care in any patient with respiratory disease. Malnutrition adversely effects lung function by diminishing respiratory muscle strength, altering ventilatory capacity, and impairing immune function. Repletion of altered nutritional status or refeeding improves altered function and may improve outcome. When spontaneous oral intake is inadequate, enteral feeding is preferred over parenteral feeding in all but those with nonfunctional gastrointestinal (GI) tracts. Unfortunately, as with any therapy, complications of nutritional support exist. Those complications presenting special problems to the patient with respiratory disease are nutritionally related hypercapnia and aspiration of enteral feedings. This article considers the association of respiratory disease and malnutrition, the determinants of appropriate nutritional support in respiratory disease, the use of enteral nutritional support to reverse malnutrition, and the complications associated with enteral feeding. Although patients with a variety of respiratory diagnoses are appropriate targets for this discussion, this chapter will deal largely with patients with chronic pulmonary lung disease (chronic obstructive pulmonary disease [COPD]), because this is the respiratory disease most commonly studied. General principles involved in the nutritional care of the COPD patient can be applied to patients with other respiratory diagnoses.

ADVERSE EFFECTS OF MALNUTRITION

A substantial proportion of patients with chronic obstructive lung disease are malnourished. The incidence depends largely on disease severity as determined several ways. As many as 25 percent of outpatients with COPD may be malnourished, while almost 50 percent of patients admitted to the hospital have evidence of malnutrition.[1,2] Critically ill COPD patients with acute respiratory failure have an incidence of malnutrition of 60 percent.[3] Disease severity can also be assessed by the degree of pulmonary function and gas exchange abnormalities. In patients with chronic hypoxemia as well as normoxemic patients with severe airflow obstruction (forced expiratory volume in 1 second [FeV$_1$] < 35 percent), malnutrition occurs in 50 percent, but 25 percent of patients with moderate airflow obstruction are malnourished.[4]

Poor nutritional status can adversely affect thoracopulmonary function in spontaneously breathing as well as mechanically ventilated patients with respiratory disease by impairing respiratory muscle function, ventilatory drive, and pulmonary defense mechanisms (Table 28–1).[5] The adverse effects of malnutrition occur independently of the presence or absence of primary lung disease. However, malnutrition's adverse effects can be additive in some patients with acute respiratory failure such as those with respiratory failure due to COPD. In COPD, pri-

TABLE 28–1 Adverse Effects of Malnutrition on Thoracopulmonary Function in Patients with Respiratory Disease

---

Decreased respiratory muscle strength
Altered ventilatory drive
Impaired immunologic function

---

mary abnormalities of decreased inspiratory pressure and increased work of breathing are found. Inspiratory muscle weakness as assessed by maximal inspiratory pressure results from both mechanical disadvantage to inspiratory muscles consequent to hyperinflation and generalized muscle weakness.[6,7] In COPD, inspiratory muscle weakness must be severe for hypercapnia to occur. In patients with myopathy, hypercapnia occurs when inspiratory pressures are less than one third.[7] However, hypercapnia is found in a majority of COPD patients when inspiratory pressures are only less than half normal.[8] Thus hypercapnia occurs with much less respiratory muscle weakness when other mechanical abnormalities are present that increase the work of breathing. Thus, malnutrition may further compromise an already compromised lung function. Dyspnea may worsen in the spontaneously breathing COPD patient. Hypercapnic respiratory failure or difficulty in weaning from mechanical ventilation may be more easily precipitated in the malnourished patient with COPD than the normally nourished patient with COPD.

In simple starvation or undernutrition, fat and protein are lost, but the loss of protein is minimized by reducing the need to use it as a source of energy.[9] Nitrogen loss is modified by mobilization of fat, and enhanced fat oxidation is the principal source of energy in the starving individual. Some protein wasting does occur despite the availability of fat as a source of energy, and this becomes markedly accelerated when fat stores are used up. When body weight drops to less than 80 percent of ideal body weight, protein catabolism occurs in the spontaneously breathing COPD patient. In critical illness, protein catabolism occurs to provide energy. With inadequate caloric intake in critically ill patients, energy sources are derived from protein breakdown and gluconeogenesis. Of various protein "pools" available, the muscle protein pool is susceptible to catabolism to provide fuel.[10] Inspiratory and expiratory respiratory muscles, primarily the diaphragm and intercostals, are skeletal muscles and therefore susceptible to this catabolic effect. Because the

diaphragm is the principal respiratory muscle, the following discussion will focus on it, although these considerations are generally valid for all respiratory muscles. Note that little if any data exist directly examining respiratory muscle function and malnutrition in critically ill, mechanically ventilated patients with COPD.

Malnutrition reduces diaphragmatic muscle mass in health and disease.[11,12] In necropsy studies, body weight and diaphragmatic muscle mass were reduced to 70 percent and 60 percent, respectively, of normal in underweight patients dying of a variety of diseases.[12] Animal studies confirm the loss of diaphragmatic strength in prolonged and acute nutritional deprivation.[13,14] Respiratory muscle function is also impaired in poorly nourished humans. When malnourished patients without lung disease were studied, respiratory muscle strength, maximum voluntary ventilation, and vital capacity were reduced 37, 41, and 63 percent, respectively.[15] Respiratory muscle strength in patients without a systemic disease is also decreased. Maximal inspiratory pressures were lower in malnourished postoperative patients compared with normally nourished patients.[16] Similar data have also been recently described in anorexia nervosa patients, a relatively pure model of malnutrition without systemic disease.[17] Transdiaphragmatic pressures elicited by phrenic nerve stimulation were markedly diminished in anorexia patients before institution of enteral nutritional support.

The effect of nutritional status on respiratory muscle function in patients with chronic obstructive lung disease is controversial. In COPD, primary abnormalities of decreased inspiratory pressure and increased work of breathing are found. Inspiratory muscle weakness as assessed by maximal inspiratory pressure results from mechanical disadvantages to inspiratory muscles consequent to hyperinflation and perhaps generalized muscle weakness.[18] Controversy exists over the additive role of denutrition in the etiology of the measured inspiratory muscle weakness. Cystic fibrosis (CF) patients with both hyperinflation and malnutrition were compared with asthmatics with hyperinflation but no malnutrition and anorexia nervosa patients with malnutrition but no hyperinflation as well as control patients with neither.[19] Peak inspiratory pressures in CF with hyperinflation were decreased as were pressures in anorexia nervosa patients. With volume correction, however, the difference in inspiratory strength in the CF group disappeared. These data suggest hyperinflation may be a major cause of diminished respiratory muscle weakness in COPD. In contrast to these data, renutrition studies in COPD as well as CF patients documenting improved muscle strength suggest that malnutrition is an important cause of diminished muscle strength.[20,21]

In addition to diminished muscle mass and hyperinflation, other factors can alter diaphragmatic strength in patients with respiratory disease (Table 28–2). Mineral and electrolyte deficiencies can impair respiratory muscle function. Hypophosphatemia reduces diaphragmatic contractile strength as measured by transdiaphragmatic pressures in mechanically ventilated patients with acute respiratory failure.[22] Hypocalcemia and hypomagnesemia are also associated with decreased diaphragmatic function.[23,24] Improvement in diminished diaphragmatic strength was found in hypomagnesemic patients after institution of magnesium replacement.[22,24]

Malnutrition also affects ventilatory drive.[25] The interaction of nutrition and ventilatory drive appears to be a direct function of the influence of nutrition on metabolic rate.[26] In general, conditions that reduce metabolic rate reduce ventilatory drive. A decrease in metabolic rate occurs with starvation. A parallel fall in metabolic rate and hypoxic ventilatory response has been documented in humans.[26] A 58 percent reduction in the ventilatory response to hypoxia was found in volunteers placed on a balanced 550-kcal/day diet for 10 days. The ventilatory response returned to normal with refeeding. Ventilatory response is also affected by constituents of the diet. After a 7-day protein-free diet, a blunted ventilatory response to carbon dioxide was noted.[27]

Consequences of decreased respiratory strength and decreased ventilatory drive could include decreased cough and thus increased likelihood for atelectasis and subsequent pneumonia in spontaneously breathing patients with any type of respiratory disease. Decreased respiratory muscle strength and drive also can prolong the duration of mechanical ventilation in patients who are otherwise candidates for weaning. Thus potential for adverse outcomes are present in patients who are initially malnourished from their disease as well as in patients with respiratory disease who develop malnutrition due to intercurrent diseases.

Malnutrition alters immune function. Protein-calorie malnutrition is the most frequent cause of acquired immunodeficiency in humans.[28] Polymorphonuclear leukocytes are normal in number but chemotaxis, opsonic function, and phagocytic function usually re-

TABLE 28–2 Nutritional Factors that Decrease Diaphragmatic Strength

Malnutrition
Electrolyte deficiencies
   Hypophosphatemia
   Hypomagnesemia
   Hypocalcemia

main or are mildly depressed while intracellular killing decreases.[29] Thymus, spleen, and lymph nodes become markedly atrophic, and lymphocytes may decrease. Although immunoglobulins remain normal or slightly increased, antibody response may be depressed.[29]

EFFECT OF RENUTRITION ON MALNUTRITION

Nutritional repletion can improve diminished respiratory muscle strength in some patients. A 37 percent increase in maximal inspiratory pressure and a 12 percent increase in body cell mass was found in 21 of 29 hospitalized patients given parenteral nutrition for 2 to 4 weeks.[16] Short-term oral refeeding in malnourished COPD patients can also improve respiratory muscle function, although it appears to depend on the presence of weight gain.[20] When six ambulatory patients with COPD were given oral nutritional repletion for 2 weeks, body weight increased by 6 percent and transdiaphragmatic pressures increased by 41 percent.[20] In contrast, when 8 weeks of nutritional supplementation in 21 malnourished COPD patients produced no change in weight, no change in respiratory muscle function was found.[30] Intensive nocturnal nasoenterally administered nutrition in COPD and CF patients can result in weight gain and improved respiratory muscle and pulmonary function.[31] Renutrition has also been found to improve diaphragmatic contractility in a more "pure" model of malnutrition, that of anorexia nervosa.[17] After 1 month of enteral nutrition (weight gain 15 percent), stimulated diaphragmatic pressure (Pdi) was increased from 16 ± 5 cm H_2O to 23 ± 7 cm H_2O, documenting improved diaphragmatic function with renutrition. With long-term nocturnal enteral feeding, CF patients had improved pulmonary function tests in conjunction with significant weight gain.[21]

The mechanism of improved muscle performance with renutrition is not known with certainty. In animal and human studies chronic hypocaloric dieting produces changes in skeletal muscle that may be important in the genesis of muscle dysfunction. In addition to protein catabolism, these changes include depletion of glycolytic and oxidative enzymes, reduction in high energy phosphate stores, and increases in intracellular calcium. Severe malnutrition depresses muscle glycolytic energy activity, thus reducing the availability of energy from glycolysis during contraction.[32] Succinate dehydrogenase, phosphofructokinase, and hydroxyacyl-COA-dehydrogenase were reduced in skeletal muscle homogenates of malnourished rats.[33] Energy stores are also decreased in severe malnutrition. Creatine phosphate fell in a 2-day fasting rat model, which was associated with a loss of muscle total creatinine.[34] Thus the reserves of energy phosphorus were decreased and the calculated free adenosine diphosphate (ADP) rose, suggesting deficient oxidative phosphorylation. These findings suggest that reduced glycolytic and oxidative enzymes such as phosphofructokinase and succinate dehydrogenase may limit the flux of glycolytic and oxidative pathways. Succinate dehydrogenase activity, when quantified in individual muscle fibers, does not appear to be altered in diaphragmatic muscle in chronic undernutrition.[35] Oxidative muscle activity may depend in part on a particular muscle's fiber type and exercise activity.

The muscle's electrophysiologic properties can also be altered by modifying cell membrane properties to decrease the sodium potassium pump activity, alter ionic permeability, and thus unbalance the intercellular electrolyte composition.[34] These data suggest that alterations in muscle contractile and endurance properties are not simply or solely due to changes in lean tissue. Indeed renutrition studies in hypocaloric dieting and fasting and severe starvation of anorexia nervosa patients document improvement in muscle performance at a time when significant changes in body composition could not be detected.[36] Changes in intracellular electrolytes may be responsible for early improvement in muscle contractile and endurance properties.

NUTRITIONAL SUPPORT

Appropriate nutritional care of the patient with respiratory disease depends on physician assessment of several variables: the presence or absence of malnutrition, assessment of the adequacy of nutritional intake with the patient's current mode of nutrition, determination of the appropriate total energy requirements and substrate mix, and complications associated with nutritional support. The optimum mode of nutrition in any patient is oral, spontaneous intake of appropriate balanced diet. Unfortunately, patients with respiratory disease may require supplementation or even complete nutritional support depending on the severity and intensity of illness. However, the principles of nutritional support are independent of the type of respiratory disease, the mode of nutritional administration, or the severity of respiratory illness. Whether patients require either supplementation or total support, the following discussion will focus on enteral nutrition because the enteral route is preferred whenever nutritional support is indicated.

Energy Needs

Several methods exist for estimating caloric requirements of patients with respiratory disease. Levels of energy expenditure can be estimated, calculated with formulas or nomograms, or determined by using measurements of energy expenditure (Table 28–3). In mechanically ventilated patients with respiratory disease, guidelines of 25 kcal/kg/day have been suggested.[37] Estimates of basal metabolic rate (BMR) through a resting energy expenditure (REE) can be obtained from the Harris-Benedict equation, which relates energy expenditure to sex, weight in kilograms (W), height in centimeters (H), and age in years (A).

$$\text{BMR (Males)} = 66.47 + 13.75 \,(W) + 5.0 \,(H) - 6.76 \,(A)$$

$$\text{BMR (Females)} = 655.1 + 9.56 \,(W) + 4.85 \,(H) - 4.68 \,(A)$$

A stress factor or percentage increase in energy requirements is then added to this determina-

TABLE 28–3 Determination of Daily Energy Expenditure in Patients with Respiratory Disease

Estimation
  25 kcal/kg/day for respiratory failure
Calculation
  Resting energy expenditure
  Harris-Benedict plus stress factor
Measurement
  Indirect calorimetry
  Pulmonary artery catheter measurements

tion based on the severity of the patient's illness. Stress factors are based on estimated metabolic needs over and above resting needs and vary with respect to body temperature, degree of physical activity, or extent of injury.[38] Most critically ill patients with respiratory disease require a stress factor of 1.2. The use of the Harris-Benedict equation in clinical practice is controversial. Caloric needs may be inaccurate with overestimation of caloric requirements.[39] It is, however, a relatively simple method of estimating caloric requirements, especially in critically ill patients.

The most accurate method of determining energy requirements is indirect measurement of actual energy expenditure with a metabolic cart. In this case, caloric requirements can be indirectly determined by measuring the rate of oxygen consumption, each liter representing approximately 4 to 5 kcal. Metabolic carts can be used to measure oxygen consumption in both mechanically ventilated and spontaneously breathing patients, but they are expensive and require technical expertise. Unfortunately the stringent conditions that must be imposed during these study periods are not the ordinary conditions of clinical care. Also, although indirect calorimetry may accurately reflect the energy requirements over the 30- to 60-minute period of measurements, it is difficult to know how to extrapolate this measure to a 24-hour period. Energy expenditure can also be measured using a pulmonary artery catheter by determining the oxygen consumption from the measured thermodilution cardiac output and the oxygen content differences between arterial and mixed venous blood.[40]

Energy requirements in COPD patients follow general guidelines with several caveats. Malnourished, spontaneously breathing COPD patients have increased resting energy requirements, approximately 15 percent above values predicted by Harris-Benedict equations, resulting in far greater expected energy requirement.[41] The relative hypermetabolism is explained by the increased energy needs of the ventilatory muscles.[42] The energy cost of respiratory muscles can be approximated from the severity of lung hyperinflation. Assessment of these points should be kept in the perspective of whether the COPD patient is spontaneously breathing or being mechanically ventilated. Nutritional support in the spontaneously breathing COPD patient should also take into account the limitations that COPD patients have in augmentation of caloric intake, such as early satiety, anorexia, bloating, and fatigue.

When calculating, estimating, or measuring total daily energy needs, remember that the nutritional goal is appropriate total daily calories, neither underfeeding or overfeeding the patient. Whether the intake is spontaneous, supplemented, or completely controlled, physicians caring for the patient with respiratory disease should determine appropriate daily calories. Underfeeding the patient over a long period or during hypermetabolic states such as critical illness risks the adverse effects of malnutrition on thoracopulmonary function. Overfeeding the patient risks metabolic complications, especially nutritionally related hypercapnia.

Substrate Mix

Once total energy requirements are determined, the next question relates to the most appropriate substrate mix, that is, the percentage of total calories that are carbohydrate, fat, and protein. Protein (nitrogen) requirements in the patient with pulmonary disease are not significantly different from those in other patients. Optimal support would establish neutral or positive nitrogen balance depending on the need for repletion. Accomplish this in the critically ill patient with acute respiratory failure by giving 1 to 3 g of protein/kg/day.[37] Generally this amounts to approximately 20 percent of total calories being administered as protein. In patients with acute respiratory failure, higher levels of protein may increase the work of breathing and thus further fatigue the patient. Protein may need to be temporarily reduced. Protein has been shown to increase minute ventilation, oxygen consumption, and ventilatory response to hypoxia and hypercapnia.[27] Remember that prolonged lack of protein support contributes to nutritional deficiency.

The most appropriate carbohydrate-fat substrate mix for COPD patients is complicated and controversial. The precise substrate mix is largely an issue for respiratory disease patients in the intensive care unit (ICU), where nutritional support is totally controlled and adverse sequelae are theoretically more likely. Spontaneous oral intake is less problematic except when the intake is supplemented by prepared oral formulations.

Although the critically ill patient with respiratory failure does use lipid preferentially as a fuel source, glucose oxidation is not impaired, and lipid infusion probably does not change patterns of fuel oxidation.[43] Thus, there is no theoretical metabolic reason to choose one fuel over the other. There is also no benefit of glucose over lipids, and vice versa, in the sparing effect of proteins. Clear disadvantages of carbohydrate administration exist. Hyperglycemia, especially in diabetics or patients receiving corticosteroid therapy, can be exacerbated by high dextrose concentrations. Elevated blood glucose can negatively affect humoral immune function and potentiate the growth of *Candida albicans*.[44] The use of increased amounts of insulin can result in sodium and fluid retention, which may be especially undesirable in patients with cardiac or renal dysfunction. Excess glucose administration is not oxidized but stored as body fat. Clinically this can result in increased fatty deposition in the liver, as well as nutritionally associated hypercapnia.

Fat calories are required in nutritional support to provide essential fatty acids. Intravenous lipids, even during slow administration, may cause pulmonary hemodynamic changes in injured lungs.[45] The clinical significance of these changes may be small. Lipids, especially long-chain triglycerides, can impair reticuloendothelial clearance functions, even when hypertriglyceridemia is absent.[46] Hepatic steatosis is significantly influenced by the proportion of fat calories as well as glucose calories in excess of caloric needs.[47] Despite many disadvantages of intravenous lipids, fats in enteral feeding formulation are well tolerated with few adverse effects.

Although recommendations for an appropriate substrate mix of carbohydrates and fats vary, generally 60 to 70 percent carbohydrates are given with 20 to 30 percent fats (Table 28–4).

Complications

Multiple complications are associated with enteral nutrition and are of importance to the patient with respiratory disease (Table 28–5).

TABLE 28–4 Nutritional Recommendation for Patients with Respiration Disease

Determination of daily energy requirements (total calories)
Substrate mix
  Protein
    20% of total calories
    1–2 g/kg/day
  Carbohydrates
    60–70%
  Fats
    20–30%

TABLE 28–5 Complications of Enteral Nutritional Support

Mechanical
  Inadvertent tracheal intubation
  Clogging or obstruction of tube
  Aspiration of enteral feeding
Gastrointestinal
  Vomiting
  Abdominal distention
  Diarrhea
Metabolic
  Hyperglycemia
  Hypophosphatemia
  Hypercapnia

Complications can be generally classified into mechanical, infectious, GI, and metabolic types. Although of concern to all patients requiring enteral nutrition, patients with respiratory disease are particularly susceptible to adverse sequelae of pulmonary aspiration and the metabolic complication of nutritionally related hypercapnia.

Mechanical complications of enteral feeding relate to the size and position of the feeding tube and include inadvertent nasotracheal passage and clogging and obstruction of the tube.[48] Pleuropulmonary adverse sequelae that can potentially worsen respiratory disease include pneumothorax, pneumomediastinum, and subcutaneous emphysema; death may result. A common finding in these cases is the use of a wire stylet to assist passage of the flexible feeding tube. Neurologically impaired or pharmacologically sedated patients are at high risk. Radiographic confirmation of tube placement is essential.

Pulmonary aspiration of enteral feeding may have significant adverse sequelae in patients with respiratory disease. Large-volume aspiration of enteral feeding can precipitate or worsen respiratory failure; small-volume aspiration can cause nosocomial pneumonia with the potential for sepsis. The frequency of pulmonary aspiration is difficult to determine because the incidence of pulmonary aspiration reported with gastric intubation by feeding tubes varies widely, ranging from 0.8 to 77 percent.[49-51] In a review of 253 hospitalized patients treated with enteral nutritional support, only two patients (0.8 percent) were diagnosed as having aspiration pneumonia.[49] When aspiration was detected by glucose-positive endotracheal secretions, aspiration was diagnosed in 21 percent of mechanically ventilated patients.[50] Likewise, 77 percent of tracheally intubated patients were found to aspirate as determined by the presence of methylene blue in tracheal secretions.[51] It is difficult to draw general conclusions about the effect of feeding tubes from these studies because all differ in population studied, study design, method of diagnosing aspiration, and size of enteral feeding tube.

Multiple factors can affect the frequency and severity of aspiration. Clearly the presence of an endotracheal tube and the type of endotracheal tube influences the incidence of aspiration.[52] Other risk factors for aspiration include a reduced level of consciousness with consequential compromise in glottic closure, the presence of an artificial airway, and ileus or gastroparesis.[53]

Small-bore feeding tubes are generally recommended to decrease gastroesophageal reflux and ultimately pulmonary aspiration. Data supporting this recommendation are controversial. No aspiration of methylene blue–dyed tube feeding was found in 30 ventilated patients with small-bore (8 F) feeding tubes.[49] In contrast, bore size was not a significant variable in witnessed aspiration or aspiration pneumonia in hospitalized patients.[54] Recent data suggest that feeding tube size may not be an important variable in reflux. When reflux was assessed by gastroesophageal scintiscanning in healthy subjects, no difference was found in reflux between large-bore (14 F) and small-bore (8 F) nasogastric feeding tubes.[55] These data suggest additional factors may be more important in reflux. One of these clearly is patient's position. In early work, healthy volunteers with nasogastric tubes were studied in the supine, 10-, 30-, and 45-degree position as well as sitting upright. After a large volume of acid was instilled into the stomach, aspiration as detected by a fall in esophageal pH occurred only in the supine position.[56] More recent data confirm the importance of patient position with studies of pulmonary aspiration by scintiscanning tracheal secretions after isotopic labeling of enteral nutrition.[57] Radioactive count and therefore aspiration were four times higher in the supine position than in the semirecumbent position. Duration of supine position is also important. Aspiration increased 650 percent from 1 to 6 hours after placement in the supine position.[57]

These data confirm the presence of aspiration with enteral feeding. Documentation of aspiration is difficult. Recent data suggest that detection of aspiration by glucose determinations of tracheal secretions may be misleading.[58] Prevention of gastric content aspiration should be directed at minimizing the mechanical factors contributing to regurgitation such as patient elevation and improper tube placement. Gastric residuals should be checked frequently, especially in patients at risk for slowed gastric emptying.

GI complications of enteral feeding include vomiting, abdominal distention, and diarrhea. Alterations in GI motility occur primarily in the critically ill patient with acute respiratory failure.[59] Clinical manifestations of altered motility include ileus and diarrhea. Decreased bowel sounds and abdominal distention may occur in as many as 50 percent of ventilated patients.[59] Causes of ileus include electrolyte abnormalities such as hypokalemia and narcotic drugs such as morphine that reduce intestinal motility and enteral alimentation. Early aggressive correction of electrolyte abnormalities, reduction of narcotics, and suction from above and below will decrease the morbidity from progressive bowel dilation. Withholding enteral feeding in the presence of abdominal pain or distention or in the absence of bowel sounds is controversial. Jejunal tube feeding may result in less abdominal distention than feeding administered by the intragastric route.[60]

The incidence of diarrhea in acute respiratory failure patients may also approach 50 percent.[59] Causes can vary from infection, especially *Clostridium difficile,* to drugs such as antacids or cimetidine. Diarrhea is frequent in ventilated patients receiving enteral nutrition, although the precise cause is unknown. In addition to the known causes of diarrhea such as infection and antibiotics, severe diarrhea in enterally fed patients may also be a symptom of deranged metabolism; that is, luminal absorptive capacity may be affected by hypotension and reduced mesenteric circulation, toxemia, or the cellular derangement associated with multiple organ failure.[61] Hypoalbuminemia associated with volume expansion and severe catabolism has also been associated with diarrhea in critically ill patients.[62]

Multiple adverse effects ensue from diarrhea in patients with acute respiratory failure. Patient discomfort and embarrassment add to the distress of conscious patients.[63] Fecal incontinence in unconscious patients adds to the problems of skin care and allows bowel organisms to contaminate the skin and surrounding areas. The loss of nutrients, water, and electrolytes is obvious but difficult to measure. Cost is increased as nursing time. Treatment centers first around removal or treatment, whenever possible, of any known causes. Clostridial infection should always be ruled out. Although fiber in the enteral feeding may increase stool bulk and decrease diarrhea in nonseriously ill patients with respiratory disease, it does not appear to decrease diarrhea in critically ill patients.

Metabolic complications include electrolyte abnormalities. Hyperglycemia and hypophosphatemia are common.[64] Hypophosphatemia can worsen or precipitate acute respiratory failure.[22] Periodic evaluation of electrolyte levels should be undertaken in all patients fed enterally.

Nutritionally associated hypercapnia is an important metabolic complication of nutritional support in patients with respiratory disease. Nutritionally associated increases in carbon dioxide production can produce hypercapnia.[65] Clinical sequelae include worsening of dyspnea and exercise tolerance, precipitation of acute respiratory failure, and delayed weaning from mechanical ventilation.[66,67] Hypercapnia results from increase CO_2 production for two reasons. Glucose combustion causes more carbon dioxide production (VCO_2) than combustion of lipid in that an isocaloric substitution of all lipid for all glucose calories results in a 22 percent reduction in VCO_2.[65] More important, excess glucose calories result in lipogenesis and markedly increased respiratory quotient (RQ). The RQ of glucose is 1.0 and of fat is 0.7; however, the RQ of lipogenesis or fat production is approximately 8.0, reflecting the proportionally greater CO_2 production relative to oxygen consumption with lipogenesis. In healthy subjects, hypercapnia is avoided by increased ventilation. Patients with compromised ventilatory status such as COPD or those with fixed minute ventilation due to weak respiratory muscles may not be able to increase ventilation appropriately. Hypercapnia can result and precipitate respiratory distress, acute respiratory failure, and difficulty in weaning from mechanical ventilation.[66,67]

The cause of nutritionally related hypercapnia is generally thought to be excess carbohydrate (CHO) or glucose calories. Some confusion has existed, however, over whether those excess glucose calories relate to an excess proportion of CHO in a nutritional regimen or simple excess of total glucose calories. Prior data suggest that the cause of elevated VCO_2 and hypercapnia is simple excess total calories. A 62 percent increase in VCO_2 in surgical patients was found to precipitate respiratory distress.[68]

Total daily calories were 2.25 × REE. Acute respiratory failure was precipitated after the onset of total parenteral nutrition (TPN) in three elderly patients with COPD.[66] Total calories were greater than 2200/day in all. More recent data confirm increased VCO_2 production with stepwise increases in total calories.[69] CO_2 production increased in 10 mechanically ventilated patients receiving nutritional regimens at 1.0, 1.5, and 2.0 × REE with 60 percent CHO and 20 percent fat. The VCO_2 was significantly increased at 1.5 and 2.0 × REE compared with baseline. In contrast, when 10 additional patients were given isocaloric regimens that varied from 40 to 60 to 75 percent CHO, VCO_2 was not different.[69] These data suggest that total calories more clearly influence VCO_2 production than percentage of CHO calories when total calories are not excessive.

Quantitation of CO_2 production is accomplished by indirect calorimetry or by analyzing a timed collection of expired air. This problem can be avoided by identifying patients at risk, especially patients with respiratory disease, and by avoiding excessive total calories.

Enteral formulations with altered CHO:fat ratios have been developed and promoted especially for patients with COPD. These formulations commonly have lower CHO concentrations of calories with resultant higher fat concentrations. Data evaluating VCO_2 production from isocaloric administered nutritional regimens in COPD are limited. Eight postoperative patients received isocaloric nutritional regimens (1.5 × REE) of either 100 percent glucose or 50 percent glucose and 50 percent fat.[70] The VCO_2 increased in both nutritional regimens compared with basal values, although it was 11 percent higher with glucose alone compared with glucose and lipid. In a study of exercise gas exchange in healthy subjects, VCO_2 decreased from 290 ml/minute to 240 ml/minute with a low CHO (10 percent) concentration.[71] However, despite this decrease mean minute ventilation was not different during rest or exercise, suggesting that numerical decreases in VCO_2 from very low percentage CHO calories may not have a practical significance in decreasing minute ventilation. These data suggest that there is little value for special enteral formulations in COPD that decrease CHO calories when total calories are appropriate.

SUMMARY

The nutritional status of the patient with respiratory disease is an important consideration.

Adverse effects of malnutrition, especially those on respiratory muscle function, can impair respiratory function, increase symptoms, and worsen outcome. Physicians should evaluate nutritional status and intake in all patients with respiratory disease. When spontaneous oral intake is judged inadequate, consider supplementing oral intake with enteral nutritional formulations or, in cases of critical illness, providing complete nutritional support with enteral feeding. Total energy needs must be calculated or estimated to prevent underfeeding or overfeeding. Reducing carbohydrate calories, especially in supplemental nutritional formulations, appears to be of little value and not necessary when appropriate nutritional support is provided.

REFERENCES

1. Braun ST, Keim NL, Dixon RM et al: The prevalence and determinants of nutritional changes in chronic obstructive pulmonary disease. Chest 1984;86:558–563.
2. Hunter ABM, Carey MA, Larsh HW: The nutritional status of patients with chronic obstructive pulmonary disease. Am Rev Respir Dis 1981;124:376–381.
3. Driver AG, McAlevy MT, Smith JL: Nutritional assessment of patients with chronic obstructive pulmonary disease and respiratory failure. Chest 1982;82: 568–571.
4. Rochester DF, Esau SA: Malnutrition and the respiratory system. Chest 1984;85:411–415.
5. Braun NMT, Arora NS, Rochester DF: Respiratory muscle and pulmonary function in proximal myopathies. Thorax 1983;38:616–623.
6. Lands L, Desmond KJ, Demizio D et al: The effects of nutritional status and hyperinflation on respiratory muscle strength in children and young adults. Am Rev Respir Dis 1990;141:1506–1509.
7. Braun NMT, Arora NS, Rochester DF: Respiratory muscle and pulmonary function in proximal myopathies. Thorax 1983;38:616–623.
8. Rochester DF, Braun NMT: Determinant of maximal inspiratory pressure in chronic obstructive pulmonary disease. Am Rev Respir Dis 1985;132:42–47.
9. Cahill G: Starvation in man. N Engl J Med 1970;282: 668–675.
10. Long CL, Birkham RH, Geiger JW: Contribution of skeletal muscle protein in elevated rates of whole body protein catabolism in trauma patients. Am J Clin Nutr 1981;34:1087–1093.
11. Thurlbeck WM: Diaphragm and body weight in emphysema. Thorax 1978;33:483–487.
12. Arora NS, Rochester DF: Effect of body weight and muscularity on human diaphragm muscle mass, thickness and area. J Appl Physiol 1982;52:64–70.
13. Kelsen SG, Ference M, Kapoor S: Effects of prolonged undernutrition on structure and function of the diaphragm. J Appl Physiol 1985;58:1354–1359.
14. Lewis MI, Sieck GC, Fournier M et al: Effect of nutritional deprivation on diaphragm contractility and muscle fiber size. J Appl Physiol 1986;60:596–603.
15. Arora NS, Rochester DF: Respiratory muscle strength and maximal voluntary ventilation in undernourished patients. Am Rev Respir Dis 1982;126:5–8.
16. Kelly SM, Rosa A, Field S et al: Inspiratory muscle strength and body composition in patients receiving total parenteral nutrition therapy. Am Rev Respir Dis 1984;130:33–37.
17. Murciano D, Armengauk MH, Rigaud D et al: Diaphragmatic function in severely malnourished patients with anorexia nervosa. Am J Respir Crit Care Med 1994;150:1569–1574.
18. Gibson GJ, Pride NB, Newson DJ: Pulmonary mechanics in patients with respiratory muscle weakness. Am Rev Respir Dis 1978;118:373–376.
19. Weiner P, Suo J, Fernandez E, Cherniack RM: The effect of hyperinflation on respiratory muscle strength and efficiency in healthy subjects and patients with asthma. Am Rev Respir Dis 1990;141:1501–1505.
20. Wilson DO, Rogers RM, Sander MH et al: Nutritional intervention in malnourished patients with emphysema. Am Rev Respir Dis 1986;134:672–677.
21. Steinkamp G, von der Hardt H: Improvement of nutritional status and lung function after long-term nocturnal gastrostomy feeding in cystic fibrosis. J Pediatr 1994;124:244–249.
22. Aubier M, Murciano D, Lecoguic Y et al: Effect of hypophosphatemia on diaphragmatic contractility in patients with acute respiratory failure. N Engl J Med 1985;313:420–424.
23. Aubier M, Viires N, Piquet J et al: Effect of hypocalcemia on diaphragmatic strength generation. J Appl Physiol 1985;58:2053–2061.
24. Molloy DW, Dhingra S, Soven F et al: Hypomagnesia and respiratory muscle power. Am Rev Respir Dis 1984;129:497–498.
25. Doekel RC Jr, Zwillich CW, Scoggin CH: Clinical semistarvation: depression of hypoxic ventilatory response. N Engl J Med 1976;295:358–361.
26. Askanazi J, Rosenbaum SH, Hyman AI et al: Effects of parenteral nutrition on ventilatory drive. Anesthesiology 1980;53(suppl 1):185.
27. Askanazi J, Weissman C, La Sala PA et al: Effect of protein intake on ventilatory drive. Anesthesiology 1984; 60:106–110.
28. Chandra RK: Malnutrition. In Chandra RK (ed): Primary and Secondary Immunodeficiency Disorders. New York: Churchill Livingstone, 1983:187.
29. Shizgal HM: Nutrition and immune function. Surg Ann 1981;12:12–29.
30. Lewis MI, Belman MJ, Dorr-Uyemural L: Nutritional supplementation in ambulatory patients with COPD. Am Rev Respir Dis 1987;125:1062–1068.
31. Whittaker JS, Ryan CF, Buckley PA et al: The effects of refeeding on peripheral and respiratory muscle function in malnourished COPD patients. Am Rev Respir Dis 1990;142:283–288.
32. Layman DKM, Merdian-Bender M, Hegarty PVJ et al: Changes in aerobic and anaerobic metabolism in rat cardiac and skeletal muscles after total or partial dietary restrictions. J Nutr 1981;111:994–1000.
33. McRussel DR, Atwood HL, Whittaker JL et al: The effect of fasting and hypocaloric diets on the functional and metabolic characteristics of rat gastrocnemius muscles. Clin Sci 1984;82:895–991.
34. Pichard C, Vaughn C, Struk R et al: Effect of dietary manipulation (fasting, hypocaloric feeding and subsequent refeeding) on rat muscles energetics as assessed by nuclear magnetic resonance spectroscope. J Clin Invest 1988;82:895–901.
35. Sieck GC, Lewis ML, Banco CE: Effects of under-nutrition on diaphragm fiber size, SDH activity and fatigue resistance. J Appl Physiol 1989;66:2196–2205.

36. McRussel DR, Pendergast PJ, Daily PL et al: A comparison between muscle function and body composition in anorexia nervosa: the effect of refeeding. Am J Clin Nutr 1983;38:29–37.

37. DeBiasse MA, Wilmore DW: What is optimal nutritional support? New Horizons 1994;2:122–130.

38. Long CL, Schaffel N, Geiger JW et al: Metabolic response to injury and illness: estimates of energy and protein needs from indirect calorimetry and nitrogen balance. J Parenter Enter Nutr 1979;3:452–456.

39. Daly JM, Heymsfield SB, Head CA et al: Human energy requirements: overestimation by widely used prediction equations. Am J Clin Nutr 1985;42:1170–1174.

40. Liggett SB, St John RE, Lefrak SS: Determination of resting energy expenditure utilizing the thermodilution pulmonary artery catheter. Chest 1987;91:562–566.

41. Wilson DO, Rogers RM, Pennock B: Metabolic rate and weight loss in obstructive lung disease. J Parenter Enter Nutr 1990;14:7–11.

42. Donahoe M, Rogers RM, Wilson DO et al: Oxygen consumption of the respiratory muscles in normal and malnourished patients with chronic obstructive pulmonary disease. Am Rev Respir Dis 1989;149:385–391.

43. Cohen FJ: Glucose vs lipid calories. In Zaloga GP (ed): Nutrition in Critical Care. St. Louis: Mosby–Year Book, Inc, 1994:169–183.

44. Goldmann DA, Martin WT, Worthington JW: Growth of bacteria and fungi in total parenteral nutrition solutions. Am J Surg 1973;126:314–318.

45. Venus B, Smith RA, Patel C et al: Hemodynamic and gas exchange alterations during intralipid infusion in patients with adult respiratory distress syndrome. Chest 1989;95:1278–1281.

46. Seidner DL, Mascioli EA, Isfan NW et al: Effects of long-chain triglyceride emulsions in reticuloendothelial system function in humans. J Parenter Enter Nutr 1989;13:614–619.

47. Baker AL, Rosenberg IH: Hepatic complications of total parenteral nutrition. Am J Med 1987;82:489–497.

48. Bernard EA, Weser E: Complications and prevention. In Rombeau JL, Caldwell MD (eds): Enteral and Tube Feeding. Philadelphia: W.B. Saunders, 1984:542–570.

49. Cataldi-Betcher EL, Seltzer MH et al: Complications occurring during enteral nutrition support: a prospective study. J Parenter Enter Nutr 1983;7:546–552.

50. Kingston GW, Phang PT, Leathley MJ: Increased incidence of nosocomial pneumonia in mechanically ventilated patients with subclinical aspiration. Am J Surg 1991;161:589–592.

51. Elpern EH, Jacobs ER, Bone RC: Incidence of aspiration in tracheally intubated adults. Heart Lung 1987;16:527–531.

52. Andrews MJ, Pearson FG: Incidence and pathogenesis of tracheal injury following cuffed tube tracheostomy with assisted ventilation. Ann Surg 1971;173:249–263.

53. Mullan H, Robenoff RA, Robenoff R: Risk of pulmonary aspiration among patients receiving enteral nutrition support. J Parenter Enter Nutr 1992;16:160–164.

54. Metheny NA, Eisenberg P, Spies M: Aspiration pneumonia in patients fed through nasoenteral tubes. Heart Lung 1986;15:256–261.

55. Dotson R, Robinson R, Pingleton SK: The effect of nasogastric tube size on gastroesophageal reflux. Am J Respir Dis Crit Care Med 1994;149:1659–1662.

56. Nagler R, Spiro HM: Persistent gastroesophageal reflux induced during prolonged gastric intubation. N Engl J Med 1963;269:495–506.

57. Torres A, Serra-Batteles J, Rose E et al: Pulmonary aspiration of gastric contents in patients receiving mechanical ventilation: the effect of body position. Ann Intern Med 1992;116:540–543.

58. Kinsey GC, Murray MJ, Swensen SJ et al: Glucose content of tracheal aspirates: implications for the detection of tube feeding aspiration. Crit Care Med 1994;22:1524–1525.

59. Dark DS, Pingleton SK: Nonhemorrhagic gastrointestinal complications in acute respiratory failure. Crit Care Med 1989;17:755–758.

60. Montecalvo MA, Steger KA, Farber HW et al: Nutritional outcome and pneumonia in critical care patients randomized to gastric versus jejunal tube feeding. Crit Care Ed 1992;20:1377–1383.

61. Binder JH: Pathology of bile acid and fatty acid-induced diarrhea. In Field M, Fordtran JS, Schultz SC (eds): Secretory Diarrhea. Bethesda, MD: American Physiology Society, 1980.

62. Gottschlich MM, Warden GD, Micha M et al: Diarrhea in tube-fed burn patients: incidence, etiology, nutritional impact, and prevention. J Parenter Enter Nutr 1988;12:38–42.

63. Smith LE, Marien L, Brogdon C et al: Diarrhea associated with tube feeding in mechanically ventilated patients. Nurs Res 1990;39:148–152.

64. Heymsfield SB, Erbland M, Casper K et al: Enteral nutritional support: metabolic, cardiovascular, and pulmonary interrelations. Clin Chest Med 1986;7:41–69.

65. Silberman H, Silberman AW: Parenteral nutrition, biochemistry, and respiratory gas exchange. J Parenter Enter Nutr 1986;10:151–154.

66. Covelli HD, Black JW, Olsen MS et al: Respiratory failure precipitated by high carbohydrate loads. Ann Intern Med 1981;95:579–581.

67. Dark DS, Pingleton SK, Kerby GR: Hypercapnia during weaning: a complication of nutritional support. Chest 1985;88:141–143.

68. Askanazi J, Rosenbaum SH, Hyman AI et al: Respiratory changes induced by the large glucose loads of total parenteral nutrition. JAMA 1980;243:1444–1447.

69. Talpers SS, Romberger DJ, Bunce SB et al: Nutritionally associated increased carbon dioxide production. Excess total calories vs high proportion of carbohydrate calories. Chest 1992;102:551–555.

70. Delafosse B, Bouffard Y, Viale JP et al: Respiratory changes induced by parenteral nutrition in postoperative patients undergoing inspiratory pressure support ventilation. Anesthesiology 1987;66:393–396.

71. Sue DY, Chung MM, Gsosvenor M et al: Effect of altering the proportions of dietary fat and carbohydrate on exercise gas exchange in normal subjects. Am Rev Respir Dis 1989;139:1430–1434.

29

The Role of Enteral Nutrition in Organ and Cellular Transplantation

DOUGLAS G. FARMER
ROLANDO H. ROLANDELLI
ELISSA L. SMITH

The last two decades have witnessed the evolution of organ transplantation from a research endeavor to a successful therapeutic option for patients with organ failure. Today, commonly transplanted organs include the heart, lung, liver, kidney, pancreas, and small intestine, while common cellular transplants include pancreatic islets and bone marrow. In 1993, thousands of organ and cellular transplants were performed in the United States alone (Table 29–1).[1]

Nutrition, in general, is recognized as an important component of successful surgical outcome. There is a correlation between preoperative nutritional status and operative morbidity and mortality.[2,3] Preoperative nutritional support in the malnourished patient can reduce the morbidity and mortality associated with major surgical intervention.[4-6] However, total parenteral nutrition (TPN) has also been associated with septic complications.[6] Furthermore, early postoperative feeding with total enteral nutrition (TEN) has been shown to be safe and associated with fewer septic complications compared with TPN.[7,8]

The exact role of enteral nutrition (EN) in transplant recipients is still being defined. In this chapter, we will attempt to draw together data from both the surgical and transplant literature regarding nutritional status and outcome from surgical intervention. The impact of TEN on individual organ systems both in the normal and diseased states will be examined. Currently available work with specific organ and cellular transplants as it pertains to EN will be evaluated. From this review, we will draw rational conclusions for the role and use of EN in the organ and cellular transplant recipient.

SMALL INTESTINAL TRANSPLANTATION

Small intestinal transplantation (SIT) lags behind other major organ transplants in its clinical application. The first experimental SIT was performed by Alexis Carrel in 1901. However, long-term survival has only been achieved recently beginning in 1988 when a patient received a combined liver/small-bowel transplant in Ontario, Canada.[9] The main limitation in the clinical application of SIT is control of rejection. The small intestine is armed with a rich immune system to prevent microbes from passing from the lumen into the bloodstream. The combination of an unusually high load of immune cells within the parenchyma and the need for immunologic surveillance makes the

TABLE 29–1 Number of Transplants Performed in 1993

Organ	United States	Outside United States	Total
Small intestine	7	0	7
Liver	3062	2319	5381
Pancreas	118	22	140
Kidney-pancreas	538	163	701
Islet	6	7	13
Kidney	9851	10,308	20,159
Heart	1607	1490	3097
Lung	384	295	679
Heart-Lung	62	100	162
Bone Marrow	2326	2574	4900

Modified from Terasaki PI, Cecka JM (eds): Clinical Transplants 1993. Los Angeles: UCLA Tissue Typing Laboratory, 1993:601–731.

intestine a unique organ for transplantation. The dosing of immunosuppression is very difficult because of a very narrow margin between graft tolerance and barrier failure, which leads to bacterial translocation and sepsis. This section reviews the role of EN on the immune function of the intestine and on SIT.

Immune Function of the Intestine

The gut has evolved an elaborate system of immunity involving both specific and nonspecific barriers. Specific barriers include the gut-associated lymphoid tissue (GALT) and the secretion of immunoglobulin A (s-IgA). Nonspecific barriers include gastric acidity, duodenal alkalinization, digestive enzymes, motility, normal intestinal flora, and mucus production. Normally, the gut maintains a steady state between mucosal integrity, GALT, and enteric organisms.

An effective method to examine the role of enteral nutrients on gut barrier function uses a model of enterally deprived, parenterally fed (i.e., TPN) hosts. Alverdy and associates compared the rate of bacterial translocation to mesenteric lymph nodes in rats maintained on different feeding formulas.[10] Translocation rates were zero, 33, and 66 percent for animals fed standard chow orally, standard TPN solution by mouth, and standard TPN intravenously, respectively. Differences between intravenous and oral diets reached statistical significance, emphasizing that the presence of enteral nutrients diminishes translocation.

Interestingly, the presence of malnutrition alone is not sufficient to induce bacterial translocation. Deitch and coworkers demonstrated in mice that 72 hours of starvation or 21 days of protein depletion was not associated with spontaneous bacterial translocation.[11] However, the administration of intraperitoneal endotoxin induced higher translocation rates in protein-malnourished mice compared with their fed or starved counterparts. The results emphasized the importance of the host nutritional state during stress.

Enteral nutrients and the nutritional state of the host appear to affect GALT. Alverdy and coworkers examined the effects of enteral diets on s-IgA levels in bile.[12] No statistical difference was noted in the biliary s-IgA levels of rats fed either standard rat chow or TPN formula enterally. However, animals maintained on TPN had significantly lower s-IgA levels in the bile. Lichtman and associates examined antigen-stimulated mucosal s-IgA secretion in self-filling blind loops of intestine in undernourished rats.[13] Dietary restriction (50 percent caloric intake for 1 to 4 weeks) diminished total s-IgA production to half of normal but did not affect specific bacterial binding capacity of the s-IgA produced.

In a follow-up study, Alverdy and coworkers examined the effects of glutamine-supplemented TPN on gut immune cellularity as well as bile s-IgA and IgM production.[14] In the control group, rats were fed standard rat chow while the experimental group received glutamine-supplemented TPN. Again, TPN produced statistically significant decreases in biliary s-IgA as well as significant increases in biliary IgM production compared with controls. When lamina propria lymphocytes were examined, the experimental group manifested a statistically significant decrease in IgA-bearing plasma cells, T-helper cells, and T-suppressor cells while demonstrating a statistically significant increase in IgM-bearing lymphocytes compared with controls. These data further emphasize the impact of enteric nutrients on maintaining GALT.

It is not surprising that much attention has been directed toward enhancing gut function with intestinal fuels.

With regard to GALT, researchers in Chicago have examined the effect of TPN supplemented with 2 percent glutamine on translocation of bacteria, biliary s-IgA production, and immune cellularity in the lamina propria in rats.[14] Glutamine supplementation resulted in a statistically significant increase in bile s-IgA and IgM production and maintained the lamina propria IgA-bearing lymphocytes at control levels. Translocation rates were markedly reduced, and increased T-helper and suppressor cells were found in the lamina propria of animals who received glutamine. However, other authors have not been able to demonstrate an effect of glutamine on spontaneous translocation rates.

Rombeau and associates at the University of Pennsylvania have examined the effects of glutamine in a rat model of SIT.[15] Rats received orthotopic isograft SIT or sham operation with infusion of 2 percent glutamine intravenously or into the lumen of the small intestine for 14 days. Glucose absorption was measured by segmental perfusion of 14C-labeled glucose. The results were quite interesting insofar as both groups receiving glutamine had a similar degree of improvement in glucose absorption and cellularity, as measured by protein and DNA content and compared with the control groups.

Small Intestine Transplantation

Short-bowel syndrome (SBS) is the failure of the intestine to digest and absorb sufficient nutrients to maintain an adequate nutritional status.[16] The main clinical feature of SBS is malabsorptive diarrhea. SBS may be due to the lack of intestine resulting from congenital anomalies or surgical resection, or due to functional problems, such as chronic pseudo-obstruction. Patients with SBS quickly develop malnutrition unless they receive TPN. Resections of up to 50 percent of the small bowel are usually well tolerated. Resections of more than 80 percent of the small bowel are nearly always a cause of permanent SBS. In patients with resections between 50 percent and 80 percent, the remaining small bowel may adapt and compensate for the lack of absorptive surface.[17] Lifelong TPN can be fraught with devas-

tating complications such as liver failure and recurrent septicemia.[18] For this subset of patients, SIT offers an alternative option.

The surgical technique is quite straightforward, requiring arterial inflow from the abdominal aorta, venous outflow either into the portal vein or the inferior vena cava, and intestinal anastomoses proximally and distally (Fig. 29–1).[19] The terminal ileum of the transplanted intestine is vented out as an ileostomy to monitor rejection for the initial 6 months. The entire length of small bowel is transplanted from the ligament of Treitz to

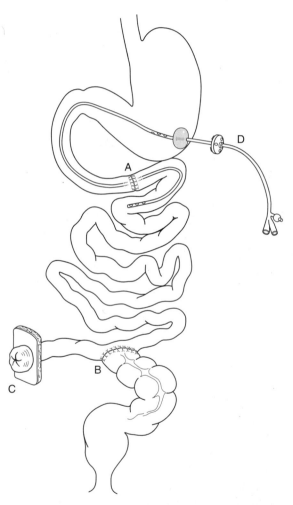

FIGURE 29–1   Small-bowel transplant. *A,* In isolated small-bowel transplants the jejunal end of the graft is anastomosed in an end-to-end fashion to the duodenum. *B,* Proximally to the end ileostomy the ileum is anastomosed in a side-to-end fashion to the colon. *C,* The ileal end of the graft is brought out as an end ileostomy. *D,* A transgastric jejunal tube is also placed to provide access to the small bowel while maintaining gastric decompression.

the ileocecal valve. The University of Pittsburgh experimented with adding large bowel as well. It was hoped that adding large bowel would reduce diarrhea, which it certainly does, but it also adds more immune tissue and bacteria, so rejection and infection are more likely.

All patients require a lengthy hospitalization. Most patients have one or more episodes of acute rejection that can be controlled by increasing the dose of immunosuppression. The greatest fear in SIT is chronic rejection, which develops in as many as 50 percent of recipients. Much controversy still exists concerning SIT, such as its indications and contraindications, the role of simultaneous liver transplantation, and the incidence of lymphoproliferative disorders. Until these controversies can be resolved, SIT will be considered an experimental procedure only used as a lifesaving measure in desperate situations.

Graft Function in SIT

The ultimate goal of SIT is to free the patient with SBS from TPN. This can only be done when the intestinal graft can absorb all the essential nutrients. A considerable amount of data exists regarding intestinal function and nutrition in various animal models of SIT.

Carbohydrate digestion and absorption was thoroughly investigated in a nonhuman primate model of SIT.[20] The absorption capacity for various forms of carbohydrates was studied in heterotopic allografts between 12 and 70 days after transplantation. These included monosaccharides such as sucrose and xylose, disaccharides such as sucrose and maltose, and polysaccharides such as the corn syrup and the tapioca starch in Progestemil. The absorption of all these carbohydrates was within normal levels in this animal model. The absorption of amino acids also seems to be well maintained after transplantation.[21]

During transplantation the lymphatic drainage of the small intestine is severed. This precludes administering long-chain triglycerides (LCTs). The lymphatic vessels of the transplanted intestine recanalize spontaneously into the recipient's lymphatic sumps. This process of lymphatic regeneration has been studied by several groups of investigators. On lymphangiography this process appears to take 3 to 4 weeks.[22]

Once lymphatic regeneration has occurred, fat absorption is also near normal. In canine orthotopic grafts treated with cyclosporin, the absorption of tritium-labeled oleic acid was comparable to autografts.[23] Cyclosporin is administered in a fatty vehicle (olive oil). Therefore, in subjects maintained on cyclosporin following SIT, immunosuppression depends on adequate fat absorption.

The absorption of nutrients across the transplanted intestine diminishes as the graft is rejected. This occurs uniformly for all nutrients. Therefore, it has been suggested to use absorption tests to monitor rejection. The test that has gained greatest acceptance is the D-xylose test.

One problem of SIT is the denervation of the intestine. Although denervation does not seem to interfere with absorption, it does affect the pattern of interdigestive myoelectrical complexes (IDMEC). The IDMEC is thought to be the "housekeeper" of the intestine, sweeping down to the colon any bacteria surviving in the small bowel. Autotransplantation disrupts the orderly migration of the IDMEC.[24] Similarly, in patients undergoing SIT at the University of Pittsburgh, the IDMEC were absent in three of nine patients and were either simultaneous, retrograde, or not propagated in the remaining six.[25]

Another problem associated with SIT is postoperative gastroparesis. In patients undergoing isolated SIT, delayed gastric emptying is seen in 20 percent of liquid studies and 25 percent of solid studies.[26] In patients receiving a combined liver/SIT, these abnormalities are present in 60 percent and 42 percent of patients, respectively. The exact cause of this complication is not known. Proposed mechanisms are a direct injury from dissection in the area of the vagi and the splachnic nerves or a cold injury from the graft's coming into the abdomen at very low temperatures.

Enteral Nutrition in SIT

Postoperative care after SIT is one of the most challenging endeavors in clinical practice. All these patients are expected to have major complications such as acute rejection, sepsis, and gastroparesis. The average hospital stay following SIT is 90 days. Experience in the nutritional management of these patients is still limited; however, some principles are already well-established.

The postoperative period after SIT can be divided into three phases: early, transitional, and late (Table 29–2). The early phase extends for 7 to 10 days. During this phase the intestinal graft recovers from ischemia, the anastomoses heal, and the native and grafted intestinal tract

TABLE 29–2   Phases Following Small Intestinal Transplantation

Early	Recovery from ischemia	Total parenteral nutrition
7–10 days	Anastomotic healing	Intestinal antisepsis
Transitional	Recovery gastric function	Jejunal feedings
4–6 weeks	Lymphatic regeneration	Low-TGC formula
Late	Normal absorption	Oral alimentation
> 6 weeks	Adequate barrier function	Low-sodium diet

recovers function. The mainstays of therapy are intravenous immunosuppression, intestinal antisepsis, and TPN.

The early postoperative period is associated with gastroparesis. Because access to the small bowel is crucial, we have found it useful to place a double-lumen transgastric jejunal tube.[27] This allows for gastric decompression until gastroparesis resolves and also allows for access to the small bowel for multiple purposes. These include diagnostic maneuvers, such as contrasted radiographs and permeability tests, and therapeutic measures, such as selective gut decontamination with antibiotics and EN.

The transitional phase begins when intestinal function has resumed, 7 to 10 days postoperatively, and lasts until gastric function is recovered, usually 4 to 6 weeks. During the intermediate phase EN is instituted and TPN is tapered. In the first month after SIT we use a diet free of LCTs and low in total fat, such as an elemental diet. Beyond the fourth week we introduce an oligomeric diet, based on short peptides and medium-chain triglycerides (MCTs), and later we introduce a polymeric diet.

The gastric port of the combined tube is maintained first on suction and then on gravity drainage. Once the output decreases, the tube is clamped and an oral diet is initiated. Because patients receiving immunosuppression tend to retain fluid, we prescribe a low-sodium diet. Adults may quickly regain their appetite so that EN can be discontinued. In children who are using the oral route for the first time in their lives, it may take several months before they can sustain their nutritional status by mouth.

Two reports from the University of Pittsburgh demonstrate the nutritional outcome of SIT patients.[28,29] In the first, 23 patients undergoing SIT were reviewed. Patients were maintained on TPN in the initial postoperative period followed by transition to EN. Absorption as measured by D-xylose testing and oral tacrolimus administration were normal in most recipients. Absorption of fat was, however, impaired in most patients but did improve over time. Serum total protein and albumin were maintained in a normal range in all but two patients. Normal growth was reported in all pediatric recipients, while eight of 11 adults gained weight after transplantation. Gut motility as measured by barium transit was normal in all but one patient. However, difficulties with EN were associated with graft rejection, systemic sepsis, and psychosocial factors.

In the second report, the nutritional management of 50 SIT recipients was reported with a mean follow-up time of 18.6 months. The mean time required to wean from TPN was 66.8 days in the pediatric recipients and 53.8 days in the adults. However, four pediatric and two adult patients still required TPN due to various complications. The pediatric recipients demonstrated a mean of 3.2 kg in weight gain; the adult recipients lost a mean of 2.4 kg. The authors noted that the majority of adults were overweight before transplantation.

Summary

Together, these studies have demonstrated SIT's potential to treat patients with SBS. TPN can generally be discontinued after SIT. Adequate perioperative nutritional intervention in patients undergoing SIT is crucial for success. In the early postoperative phase only TPN is used to allow the intestine to recover. EN is introduced in a second phase with very low fat content. The diet is changed from no fat to a diet based on MCT and finally on LCT. When gastroparesis subsides, the patient is allowed to eat. Children who acquired SBS at an early age have difficulty in developing an eating habit. The greatest limitation in the long-term success of SIT is chronic rejection, which occurs in as many as 50 percent of patients. Further work in the field is ongoing and holds promise for future advances.

LIVER TRANSPLANTATION

The development of liver transplantation is credited to Thomas Starzl, MD, who reported the first successful transplant in a human in 1963.[30] Refinements in techniques and postoperative management have allowed a gradual improvement in the survival rate, which presently averages 85 percent.[31] The main advances made in liver transplantation are the development of preservation solutions (University of Wisconsin), the discovery of new immunosuppressive agents, a better understanding of patient selection, and an expansion of the donor pool. The liver plays such a crucial role in nutrition and metabolism that malnutrition inexorably follows liver failure. In addition, liver failure can be due to nutritional interventions such as TPN (Table 29–3). In this section we review EN's effect on liver function and liver transplantation.

Enteral Nutrition and Liver Function

Luminal nutrients can influence the hepatic physiology directly by the presence of absorbed nutrients in the portal circulation and indirectly by releasing gastrointestinal (GI) hormones. Much of the evidence for EN's beneficial effect on hepatic function derives from studies in which enteral nutrients are absent, such as in starvation and during TPN.

In the starved state, the absence of enteral nutrients and enteral stimulation can profoundly affect hepatic structure and function. Several studies have reported histologic abnormalities associated with severe malnutrition in children. Most commonly, varying degrees of hepatic steatosis are seen pathologically. Other findings include cholestasis, nuclear enlargement, and mitochondrial swelling. These changes are reversible after nutritional repletion.

TABLE 29–3 Nutritional Disturbances Producing Liver Dysfunction

Prematurity
Low birth weight
Protein malnutrition
Starvation
Sepsis
Decreased portal inflow
Portal endotoxemia
Parenteral nutrition
   Excess calories
   Excess carbohydrates
   Amino acid deficiencies
   Contaminants
   High insulin:glucagon ratio
   Decreased cholecystokinin release

Hepatic dysfunction in the starved state is further demonstrated by studies on indocyanine green clearance.[32] Pigs were fasted to a weight loss of 20 percent below baseline and then were studied in both the fasted and refed states. Both the systemic and intrinsic clearances of indocyanine green were significantly reduced after fasting but returned to normal after refeeding. Because indocyanine green is exclusively excreted by the liver, the authors concluded that hepatic carrier–mediated transport is impaired in the fasting state and restored with enteral feeding. Whether this is secondary to malnutrition or to the absence of enteral stimulation remains to be answered.

TPN in the absence of enteral intake provides an ideal setting to investigate the effect of TPN on the liver in nutritionally balanced individuals. The detrimental effects of TPN on hepatic function have been established.[33] Serum levels of alanine aminotransferase (ALT), aspartate aminotransferase (AST), alkaline phosphatase (AP), and gamma-glutamyl transpeptidase (GGT) are the most sensitive indicators of TPN-induced hepatic dysfunction. Hyperbilirubinemia is less common, occurring in less than 46 percent of patients in most series.[34] Typically, elevations in liver function tests occur soon after TPN therapy is initiated and peak within four weeks. Elevations are usually transient and do not correlate with liver histology.

Histologically, several patterns are associated with TPN-induced liver dysfunction, with steatosis being the more common in adults.[35] A periportal distribution of fatty infiltration is seen initially, with more severe cases progressing to a centrilobular or panlobular distribution. Cholestasis is the predominant pattern among infants receiving TPN but can also be seen in adults. Typically, a centrilobular pattern of intracellular and canalicular cholestasis is seen.[36] Late histologic changes can include portal inflammation, bile duct proliferation, and portal fibrosis. Predisposing factors appear to be prematurity, low birth weight, sepsis, and lack of oral intake.

Chronic, irreversible liver disease is seen infrequently with long-term TPN. Periportal fibrosis, portal bridging, bile duct proliferation, and hepatic fibrosis are typical histologic changes associated with this state. The incidence of progression to irreversible liver failure is difficult to ascertain. Bowyer and coworkers[35] reported that 9 of 60 patients receiving TPN (average, 29 months) demonstrated persistent abnormalities in liver function tests. All had abnormal biopsies consisting of steatohepatitis

(8), centrilobular fibrosis (3), and cholestasis (3). Three patients eventually developed severe end-stage liver disease.

The etiology of TPN-induced liver failure remains speculative, with several theories offered. An excess in carbohydrate and lipid calories associated with TPN has been suggested.[38,39] Studies have implicated amino acid deficiencies, disturbances in the enterohepatic circulation, portal endotoxemia, and TPN contaminants.[17]

King and associates studied rats that were given identical TPN solutions (intravenous or intragastric) and were compared to chow-fed controls.[40] All animals achieved positive nitrogen balance and weight gain in a similar manner. Significantly, rats fed intravenous TPN demonstrated a 17 percent increase in liver weight and a 60 percent increase in hepatic lipid content compared with intragastric- or chow-fed animals. The results clearly demonstrated that the TPN solution, when administered intragastrically, failed to produce hepatic injury.

Whalen and colleagues addressed the possibilities that TPN itself may be hepatotoxic when administered intravenously, or, alternatively, a deficiency state created by the solution causes the hepatotoxic effect.[41] Using a rat model in which orally administered TPN solutions resulted in hepatic steatosis, the investigators fed rats for 10 days with oral TPN solution supplemented with either 0, 2, or 8 g of rat chow each day. Rats receiving at least 2 g of chow per day did not develop histologic evidence of hepatic steatosis.

Similarly, Waters and associates from the University of Tennessee investigated the effect of enteral nutrients in a indocyanine green clearance model similar to that discussed above.[42] Both nitrogen balance and indocyanine green clearance were significantly better in animals refed enterally compared with parenterally.

In addition to the direct effect of enteral nutrients on hepatic function, indirect hepatotrophic actions may play a role through GI hormones. Work by Starzl and associates on auxiliary liver transplantation demonstrated that atrophy rapidly ensued in livers subjected to total portal caval shunting or in grafts deriving portal flow from the systemic circulation.[43] Further work demonstrated that by diverting lobar portal inflow, differential atrophy and hypertrophy could be obtained in those hepatic lobes perfused with splanchnic blood.[44] In other experiments, Starzl was able to identify the proximal splanchnic circulation (i.e., that from the stomach, duodenum, and pancreas) as crucial to this hepatotrophic effect. Finally, using dogs subjected to total portocaval shunting followed by infusions of insulin, glucagon, or insulin plus glucagon, the group was able to identify insulin as the major hepatotrophic factor in the splanchnic circulation.

Work by Li and associates from the University of Cincinnati examined the effect of insulin and glucagon on hepatic morphology in TPN-fed rats.[45] Three experimental groups were fed increasing concentrations of glucose (15 percent, 20 percent, and 25 percent) by TPN and were compared with a group fed standard chow. At sacrifice, a strong correlation was found between increasing carbohydrate/dextrose intake and hepatic steatosis. More important, a significantly elevated portal insulin and insulin:glucagon ratio was noted in animals fed with higher glucose concentrations, leading the group to conclude that the insulin level in the portal circulation is directly affected by the concentration of dextrose in TPN and is directly related to the degree of hepatic steatosis.

Mok and Ming from Taiwan also examined GI hormones and TPN.[46] Rats were given nothing by mouth and sustained on standard TPN supplemented with glucagon, cholecystokinin, and secretin. Adding cholecystokinin had a beneficial effect on serum liver function tests, hepatic protein content, biliary content, and flow. The effects of secretin and glucagon were equivocal. The results suggested that cholecystokinin diminished TPN-induced hepatic impairment.

In summary, the impact of TEN on liver function is difficult to assess directly. Studies on states in which enteral nutrients are absent indicate that liver dysfunction is prevalent. Adding enteral nutrients can reverse and, in some cases, prevent this dysfunction. Whether the direct effect of enteric nutrients or the indirect effect through GI hormones is responsible is a matter of speculation. Until more data are available, we can conclude that the presence of enteral nutrients has a beneficial effect on hepatic function and the absence of enteral nutrients leaves the liver more susceptible to dysfunction.

Liver Transplantation

In liver transplantation the diseased liver is removed from the patient, and the donor liver is placed in the normal position (Fig. 29–2). This technique is named orthotopic liver trans-

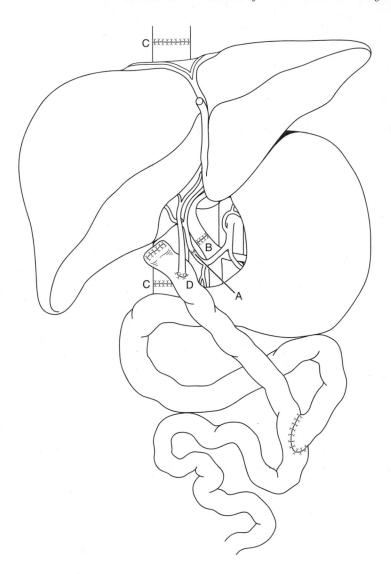

FIGURE 29–2   Liver transplant. *A,* The entire organ is placed in the orthotopic position. The arterial inflow is brought from the native hepatic artery. *B,* The portal vein is anastomosed in an end-to-end fashion recipient to donor. *C,* The venous outflow is directed through the recipient's inferior vena cava. *D,* The donor common bile duct can be connected to the recipient's distal common bile duct or to a Roux-Y limb of jejunum.

plantation (OLT). A recent refinement of the technique of liver transplantation is the use of reduced-size liver transplants for children. Instead of having a critically ill child wait in end-stage liver disease for a compatible donor, a segment of an adult liver is used. Because the liver has an enormous regeneration capacity, the long-term function of this liver is similar to a whole organ. This possibility has already reduced the mortality of pediatric patients awaiting liver transplants from 50 percent to 10 percent.[47] Success with using reduced-size liver transplants has led to another development— the use of living related donors.

The bile duct of the donor liver can be connected directly to the distal bile duct of the recipient (choledocholedocostomy or CDC) or into a Roux-Y limb of jejunum brought up to

the liver (choledocojejunostomy). Complications of these biliary anastomoses occur in as many as 29 percent of patients and have been termed the "Achilles' heel" of liver transplantation. Potential complications are bile leaks, biliary obstructions, and anastomotic leaks at the jejunojejunostomy performed to reconstruct the alimentary tract when a choledocojejunostomy is created. Other potential complications of liver transplantation are bleeding, vascular occlusions, wound complications, and bowel obstructions.

Enteral Nutrition and Liver Transplantation

Patients with liver failure represent a unique nutritional challenge. Malnutrition in one form or another is present in almost all patients with end-stage liver disease. This conclusion was borne out by Mendenhall and associates, who studied the nutritional state of 284 adults with alcohol-induced, chronic liver failure.[48] All patients demonstrated evidence of marasmus or kwashiorkor, and the severity of the malnutrition state correlated directly with the severity of the liver failure. Chin and associates examined the nutritional status of 27 children awaiting OLT.[49] Significant reductions in height, weight, head circumference, anthropometric measurements, and total body potassium level were noted. Both adults and children with liver failure are in a state of catabolism with increased protein breakdown, muscle wasting, and increased levels of insulin, glucagon, epinephrine, and cortisol.[50]

The nutritional assessment of these patients preoperatively is particularly difficult and has been reviewed extensively elsewhere.[51-53] Body weight analysis commonly leads to erroneous assessments due to frequent fluid accumulation. Serum proteins such as transferrin, albumin, and prealbumin are often abnormal in patients with liver failure, and it is difficult to determine the relative contribution of malnutrition to these abnormalities. Immunologic function tests are usually depressed in patients with chronic liver failure as well as those with malnutrition. However, despite these limitations, several groups have developed assessment methods and have demonstrated that preoperative malnutrition affects outcome after OLT.

The importance of preoperative nutritional assessment and supplementation before OLT is reinforced in a study by Shepherd and associates.[54] Thirty-two children accepted for liver transplantation underwent preoperative nutritional assessment based on weight and height. Data were expressed in terms of z score representing a ratio of the observed measurement compared with the mean of the standard obtained from growth charts. Despite receiving preoperative nutritional supplementation, undernourished children (z score < −1.0) demonstrated a significantly lower 1-year survival after OLT compared with their well-nourished counterparts (z score > −1.0) (33 percent vs 88 percent, P < 0.003). Furthermore, children who died after transplantation had significantly lower z scores for weight at evaluation compared with survivors (P < 0.02). The same group later corroborated these findings with a longer follow-up study.[49]

Moukarzel and colleagues used the z score for height as an indicator of the degree of mal-

nutrition to separate 102 pediatric OLT candidates into two groups.[53] Preoperative liver function indexes were not statistically different between the two groups. However, compared with the well-nourished group, the malnourished group (z score < −1.0 for height) demonstrated a statistically significant higher incidence of postoperative infections (61 percent vs 37 percent), surgical complications (46 percent vs 23 percent), retransplantation rate (15 percent vs 2 percent), and length of hospitalization and death rate (25 percent vs 9 percent).

Shaw and coworkers examined several preoperative variables in an attempt to develop a relative risk score for OLT candidates.[55] One of the six variables, malnutrition, was assessed preoperatively using a scoring system based on the clinical degree of muscle wasting and malnutrition. Patients with severe malnutrition and muscle wasting were assigned a score of 2, those with less severe malnutrition were assigned 1, and those with no evidence of malnutrition were assigned 0. Using two-way linear regression analysis, survival at six months was inversely correlated with degree of malnutrition (P = 0.025). Using multiple linear regression analysis, the combination of preoperative coma and malnutrition correlated with a lower 6-month survival. These findings led to renewed efforts to identify and maximize preoperative malnourished states.

Although relieving malnutrition before transplantation remains an important goal, delivering adequate nutrition represents a challenge in this group of patients. EN can be limited by malabsorption, impaired dietary intake, and poor patient compliance.[56] TPN can present problems with fluid and electrolyte balance as well as potentially worsen liver function. Standard amino acid mixtures can lead to a relative imbalance in the aromatic to branched chain amino acid (BCAA) ratio in the plasma. This imbalance has been implicated as a prime contributor to hepatic encephalopathy.

Successful nutritional supplementation in patients with chronic liver disease has been reported. Several studies have demonstrated improvement in nutritional parameters and short-term mortality from liver failure with enteral supplementation.[57-61] However, not all studies concur with these findings. These differences may be related to the variability of nutritional assessment parameters seen between different etiologies of liver failure. Potentially compounding the nutritional problem further are the tremendous metabolic demands of liver transplantation. Studies attempting to quantify these demands have been conflicting. Delafosse and colleagues demonstrated an increase in energy expenditure 50 percent to 75 percent above calculated levels, as well as increased nitrogen losses during the first two postoperative days after OLT.[62] Others have confirmed this increased resting energy expenditure (REE).[63]

In contrast, Plevak and associates evaluated 14 patients undergoing OLT.[64] No significant change in REE above preoperative levels was seen, but urinary nitrogen excretion was significantly increased and nitrogen balance was persistently negative, indicating continued protein catabolism. The number of patients was small, making definitive conclusions difficult.

Few studies exist evaluating the effect of postoperative nutritional supplementation after OLT. Reilly and associates administered TPN to patients with cirrhosis undergoing OLT and compared them with a similar group not receiving TPN after OLT.[65] Those receiving seven days of TPN achieved a better nitrogen balance, were weaned off the respirator sooner, and were transferred out of intensive care quicker than the controls. Implied in the results is a beneficial effect of posttransplant nutrition.

Wicks and associates compared the short-term outcome of ten patients given TPN and 14 patients given TEN after OLT.[66] No significant differences were noted between the two groups with regard to survival, ventilator dependence, length of hospital stay, infectious episodes, intestinal permeability or function, or anthropometric measurements.

More recently Hasse and coworkers at Baylor University conducted a study on early EN after liver transplantation.[67] Of 31 patients who completed the study, the 14 patients who received early EN had fewer infections than the 17 patients in the control group. Overall infections were 21.4 percent vs 47.1 percent, bacterial infections were 14.3 percent vs 29.4 percent, and viral infections were 0 percent vs 17.7 percent for the tube-fed and the control groups, respectively. Only the difference in viral infections was statistically significant.

Although it is becoming very clear that early EN is beneficial after liver transplantation, the main limiting factor is access to the GI tract for postoperative feeding. Although some support the use of jejunostomies in patients undergoing liver transplants,[68] most surgeons fear the risk of infection associated with tube enterostomies. Gastroparesis is also common, perhaps due to disturbance of the innervation of the stomach by surgical dissection. Therefore, the options are to place either two nasoenteric tubes or one dual-lumen nasoenteric tube for simultaneous gastric decompression and small-bowel feedings. Dual-lumen tubes commercially available are designed for placement under fluoroscopic or endoscopic guidance. Despite the exposure of the stomach, advancement of these tubes is difficult by manipulation over the serosa of the stomach and small bowel. In addition, it is difficult to ascertain where transition between the gastric portion and the enteric portion of the tube occurs by external palpation. There is a definite need for a tube that can be easily placed at surgery transnasally into the stomach and small bowel to allow simultaneous gastric decompression and small-bowel feedings.

Summary

TEN does directly affect hepatic function. Numerous studies have shown the effects on liver histology and function. The role of TEN in OLT is less well defined. Part of the problem lies in the ability to differentiate between clinical changes due to liver failure and those due to malnutrition. Currently, most efforts have been focused on identifying those transplant candidates who are malnourished and correcting that state. Significant impact on outcome has been demonstrated with this approach. More recently, the effect of postoperative nutritional supplementation has been investigated. Most results are still too preliminary for firm conclusions, but supplementation may be an effective therapy to improve outcome further after OLT.

ENTERAL NUTRITION AND RENAL TRANSPLANTATION

The kidney was the first solid organ transplanted successfully in humans. After a series of unsuccessful cadaveric and living donor transplants, the barrier of rejection was circumvented in 1955 by using identical twins as donors.[69] Since then renal transplantation has evolved to one of the most successful organ transplants. More than 20,000 kidney transplants were performed in 1993 alone, with projected overall 1- and 5-year graft survivals of 84 percent and 60 percent, respectively.[70] The primary indications for the procedure are end-stage renal disease secondary to diabetes mellitus and chronic glomerulonephritis.

Enteral Nutrition and Renal Function

The direct impact of enteral nutrients on renal function is difficult to ascertain. The effect of protein on renal function has drawn considerable attention and is worthy of mention. In animal models, the amount of protein in the diet affects renal mass and glomerular filtration rate (GFR). Using the rat model of chronic renal insufficiency, several studies have demonstrated reduced GFR and kidney size in animals maintained on low-protein diets.[71-73] Rabinowitz and associates[74] as well as other authors[75] have noted similar findings in sheep and dogs, respectively.

The data for humans are less straightforward. In healthy human volunteers, intravenous infusion of amino acids increases GFR.[76] Changes in dietary protein produced changes in GFR and effective renal plasma flow that were directly proportional to the amount of intake.[77-79] The situation becomes even more complex when the effect of protein loading is studied in those with abnormal kidney function. Bosch and associates studied the acute renal response to an oral protein load (70 to 80 g of protein/30 minutes) in patients with renal insufficiency.[80] A quantitatively but not qualitatively different response was noted compared with normal subjects. GFR and effective renal plasma flow increased significantly over baseline. Interestingly, those with renal insufficiency maintained on a low-protein diet before the testing had a higher renal reserve than those consuming a regular diet (19 ml/minute vs 5 ml/minute), but both groups demonstrated lower reserves than healthy subjects (29 ml/minute). Their data indicated that patients with renal insufficiency could respond to an oral protein load, although quantitatively less than healthy subjects. In addition, low-protein diets allowed maintenance of some renal reserve in abnormal kidneys.

In fact, low-protein diets are implicated in affecting the progression of renal failure. Acchiardo and associates studied the rate of deterioration of renal function as estimated by the reciprocal of serum creatinine in patients with renal insufficiency on a protein-restricted diet.[81] Significant changes in the progression of renal insufficiency were found with initiation of low-protein diets. These results have been confirmed by others.[76,82,83]

On the other hand, inadequate protein intake may adversely affect renal function. In studies of malnourished subjects, reduced GFR and renal plasma flow have been repeatedly demonstrated.[75,84] Both values returned to normal with protein repletion. Variability is probably related to the degree of renal insufficiency associated with malnutrition. Therefore, it is important to regulate protein intake based on the degree of renal insufficiency and renal reserve.

Renal Transplantation

Renal transplantation is usually performed in a heterotopic fashion with placement of the kidney in either iliac fossa. The inflow and outflow of blood is created through the iliac vessels, and the ureter is implanted into the bladder (Fig. 29–3). In cases of irreparable deformity of the bladder or neurogenic dysfunction, the ureter may be implanted into an ileal conduit created for this purpose.

In addition to the usual complications of any organ transplant, such as bleeding and vascular occlusions, complications of renal transplantation include ureteral leakage and obstruction and lymphoceles between the inferior pole of the kidney and the bladder. Those patients with an ileal conduit created for implantation of the ureter may develop anastomotic leakage and bowel obstruction.

Enteral Nutrition and Renal Transplantation

The nutritional cost of renal insufficiency and failure is high. Typically, renal patients are

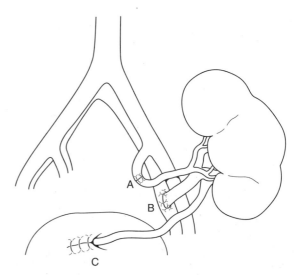

FIGURE 29–3 Renal transplantation. The entire donor kidney is placed in the iliac fossa. The inflow (*A*) and outflow (*B*) of blood is created through the iliac vessels. *C*, The ureter is implanted into the bladder.

malnourished. In one study of pediatric renal transplant recipients, 70 percent were below the third percentile for height and weight before transplantation.[85] In adults, Blumenkrantz and associates summarized their findings from the Veterans Administration Cooperative Dialysis Study of 79 uremic patients.[37] Compared with healthy controls, significantly lower values were noted in mean body weight, triceps skinfold thickness, percentage body fat, and midarm muscle circumference. Bansal and colleagues noted significant protein-calorie malnutrition in 19 percent of 52 uremic patients undergoing chronic maintenance hemodialysis.[86] Thurnberg and associates had similar findings in 72 percent of dialysis patients.[87] Similar nutritional problems are reported in children undergoing chronic peritoneal dialysis. Together, these studies indicate the nutritional problems encountered in this population.

The etiology of such malnourished states in this disease process are multifactorial (Table 29–4). Higher energy requirements have been advocated as one possible cause. Maintenance hemodialysis is associated with a high energy and protein cost due to losses in the dialysate as well as through blood loss.[88,89] Kluthe and associates quantified the amount of protein lost in maintenance hemodialysis and recommended protein supplementation based on these losses.[90] Salusky and associates felt that protein losses through the dialysate also contributed to malnourishment.[91]

However, Monteon and associates studied the energy expenditure by indirect calorimetry of healthy volunteers, patients with chronic renal failure, and those receiving hemodialysis.[92] No differences in energy expenditure were noted either at rest or with activity. Others concur with these findings.[93]

Insufficient caloric intake has been advocated by others as the etiology of malnourishment in patients with renal failure. Using dietary histories, Thurnberg and associates reported up to 50 percent of patients receiving maintenance hemodialysis consumed less than 15 percent of recommended caloric intake.[87] Grodstein and colleagues noted that seven of eight patients receiving chronic dialysis consumed adequate nitrogen intake.[94] Salusky and associates also reported significantly lower energy intake in children receiving peritoneal dialysis.[91]

The exact role of TEN in renal transplant recipients remains undefined. Little data exist on TEN and renal transplant recipients per se. However, the nutritional requirements of this

TABLE 29–4 Causes of Malnutrition in Patients with End-Stage Renal Disease

Increased energy expenditure (?)
Decrease energy intake
Increased protein losses:
    Losses in dialysate
    Blood losses
Gastrointestinal dysfunction
    Nausea, vomiting
    Diarrhea, malabsorption
Drug-nutrient interactions

group should not be ignored and should perhaps be examined from an adult/pediatric perspective.

In the pediatric population, growth and development are the standard yardstick of nutritional equilibrium. Most patients experience adequate oral intake after transplantation and require little supplementation. The exception is the younger child with end-stage renal disease undergoing renal transplantation. Jones and associates reported 79 renal transplant recipients less than 5 years old.[95] Forty-four percent required pretransplant enteral supplementation to sustain nutritional status, and 57 percent of those required further supplementation after transplantation. The standard deviation for height revealed growth retardation in all groups, with undialyzed patients having the most effect. Preoperative tube feeding appeared to improve catch-up growth after transplantation.

In adults, a report of nutritional status in long-term renal transplant survivors was published by Hiraga and associates.[96] Caloric intakes were unchanged over the 8-year study period. No mention of other nutritional parameters was made.

In general, patients do not have a problem with oral intake after renal transplantation. In those with postoperative complications imposed over preoperative malnutrition, nutritional support may be considered.

Summary

Direct effects of enteral nutrition on renal function are difficult to delineate. Attention has been focused on protein intake in relation to glomular filtration rate, effective renal blood flow, and renal reserve. This observation has been used to treat patients with progressive renal insufficiency more effectively to slow the deterioration of renal function.

Several points are important with regard to renal failure and insufficiency. First, renal insufficiency is present in malnourished individuals. Conversely, patients with renal insufficiency are typically malnourished. The etiology of this malnourishment is multifactorial but is related to diminished caloric intake, loss of proteins and amino acids through dialysis, and probable metabolic and hormonal derangements related to uremia.

Not withstanding, nutrition is an important factor in this patient population. Preoperative screening and nutrition support are probably needed to minimize transplant morbidity. However, scientific data are lacking to support such conclusions.

PANCREAS TRANSPLANTATION

The rationale for pancreatic transplantation is the replacement of the endocrine function in diabetic patients. The first pancreatic transplant was performed at the University of Minnesota in 1966.[97] In conjunction with kidney transplantation, pancreas transplantation is indicated most commonly for diabetic patients with renal failure.[98] The results have been excellent. Several studies report 1- and 3-year survival rates of approximately 90 percent and 80 percent, respectively.[99] In addition, serum glucose, insulin, glucagon, and hemoglobin A1c levels show prolonged improvement after successful engraftment.[98] Improvement in retinopathy, nephropathy, and neuropathy are less dramatic.

The outlook for islet cell transplantation remains guarded. There are few reports of successful islet allotransplant engraftment, and most of the success is short lived.[100,101] Autotransplantation of islets is a successful procedure achieving insulin independence and euglycemia consistently. The difference in allograft and autograft outcomes lies in both the rejection response and the islet-toxic effects of some immunosuppressant drugs.[98]

This section will review the role of TEN on pancreatic function. Up to this date no studies have been published addressing the role and effects of TEN on pancreatic or islet transplantation.

Enteral Nutrition and Pancreatic Function

The pancreatic gland produces two types of secretions: exocrine and endocrine. Exocrine secretions are digestive enzymes, such as amylase and lipase, and bicarbonate produced in the acini. Enzymes and bicarbonate are se-

creted into the duodenum in response to enteral nutrients. The effect of enteral nutrients on the exocrine function of the pancreas is mainly mediated by GI polypeptides such as cholecystokinin and secretin.[102]

Pancreatic transplants are placed in a heterotopic position (i.e., in the pelvis). The exocrine secretions are drained into the urinary bladder, through a short duodenal stump, while the arterial inflow and venous outflow are connected to the iliac vessels. Therefore, neither luminal nutrients nor the GI polypeptides produced in response to them can reach this auxiliary pancreas to stimulate acinar cells. However, the effect of nutrients on the endocrine function of the pancreas may be relevant to pancreatic transplantation.

McArdle and associates examined the pancreatic endocrine effects of enteral and parenteral delivery of identical nutritional formulas in humans.[103] Both groups had significant weight gain and positive nitrogen balance. Although serum glucagon levels remained normal in both groups, serum insulin levels were significantly elevated in the TPN group. This difference led to changes in body lipid metabolism and was probably mediated by altered hepatic glucose metabolism. Using a rat model, Track reported increases above basal levels for both insulin and glucagon during prolonged TPN administration.[104] The differences between the two studies probably represent species variation.

Similarly, Greenberg and associates studied the effect of TPN on GI hormonal secretion.[105] Nine patients with active inflammatory bowel disease were treated for a mean of 25 days with TPN and nil per os. Plasma levels of glucagon, insulin, and pancreatic polypeptide were assayed after the first meal taken by mouth as well as after a second test meal occurring a mean of 156 days after the first. Fasting and postprandial concentrations of both glucagon and pancreatic polypeptide were not significantly different between the first and second test meals. The same held true for fasting insulin levels. However, the peak postprandial serum insulin concentration was significantly lower after the first test meal compared with the second (88 ± 23 pM vs 187 ± 37 pM, $P < 0.001$). Serum glucose levels were maintained within a normal range after both meals. The results indicated a diminished overall response of insulin secretion after prolonged fast but one that appropriately maintained serum glucose.

From the data available on endocrine function there is no reason to favor one route of nutritional support over the other. However, as will be discussed, diabetic patients undergoing pancreatic transplantation are at high risk of developing infectious complications postoperatively. Therefore, it is preferable to eliminate any potential source of infection, such as intravenous lines, which would support EN in the few patients who require nutritional support after pancreatic transplantation.

Pancreatic Transplantation

The technique of whole-organ pancreas transplantation consists of isolating the pancreas in vascular pedicles and in conjunction with the duodenum from the donor, preparing the organ ex vivo in the "back table," and implanting it in the pelvis with inflow and outflow from the iliac vessels and drainage of the exocrine secretion into the bladder (Fig. 29–4). Most patients receive quadruple immunosuppression with cyclosporine, azathioprine, steroids, and OKT3 monoclonal antibody. Because in most cases the pancreas is transplanted in conjunction with one kidney, rejection is monitored by serum creatinine levels and renal biopsies. Pancreatic biopsies are rarely done. At least one episode of acute rejection occurs in approximately 80 percent of patients.[106]

Postoperative infections are very common after pancreatic transplantation, with rates as high as 80 percent. Some are related to the underlying diabetes and its complications, while others are technical in nature. Dehiscence of the duodenum with intraperitoneal leakage of pancreatic secretion and urine is the most feared complication.

After pancreatic transplantation carbohydrate metabolism immediately normalizes. Some of the systemic complications of diabetes, such as retinopathy and neuropathy, may improve. Pancreatic transplantation prevents the development of nephropathy in the transplanted kidney of diabetic patients.

Most patients have return of bowel activity in 2 to 3 days and resume oral diet. In some patients with diffuse neuropathy, postoperative gastroparesis and constipation may preclude resumption of oral alimentation. Any nutritional support is usually given as TPN. Occasionally, a patient with a complicated postoperative course may become a candidate for EN.

Summary

Enteral nutrients affect both exocrine and endocrine pancreatic function. Because of the heterotopic position of pancreatic transplants, en-

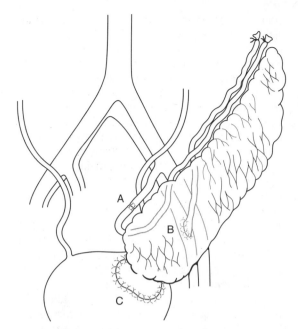

FIGURE 29–4 Pancreas transplantation. The donor pancreas with a stump of duodenum including the ampulla of Vater is placed in the iliac fossa. The arterial inflow (*A*) and venous outflow (*B*) are connected to the iliac vessels. *C*, The exocrine secretions are drained into the urinary bladder through the duodenal stump.

teral nutrients do not effect the exocrine function of the grafted pancreas. Circulating nutrients, supplied enterally or parenterally, will affect the endocrine function of the transplanted pancreas. Because of the underlying diabetes, and concomitant complications, patients undergoing pancreatic transplantation are at high risk of infection. Most patients do not need any form of nutritional support, but if nutritional support becomes necessary, EN is preferred because it avoids another potential source of infection.

CARDIAC TRANSPLANTATION

As with other organs, the success of cardiac transplantation is evident.[107] In 1993 there were 1607 heart transplants performed in the United States alone.[1] The results indicate the success of the procedure with 5-year survivals approaching 80 percent.[107] The most common indications continue to be cardiomyopathy and ischemic heart disease.

Enteral Nutrition and Cardiac Function

Adequate cardiac function is the basis for adequate function of all organs and systems.

On the other hand, patients with severe cardiac disease are frequently malnourished. This classic syndrome of "cardiac cachexia" was originally described by Pittman and Cohen and has been extensively reviewed elsewhere.[108,109]

This is particularly evident in infants and children with congenital heart defects who also manifest growth retardation.[110] The role of TEN in this setting was examined by Schwarz and associates.[111] Nineteen children were randomly assigned to receive continuous, partial, or no nasogastric nutritional supplementation and were followed an average of 5.25 months. All patients were malnourished at enrollment as manifested by reduced height/age and weight/height percentiles. Only those infants fed with continuous nasogastric nutrition achieved target caloric intake and demonstrated statistically significant improvements in both height and weight. Others have confirmed these findings in children[112] as well as in adults with congestive heart failure and cardiac cachexia.[113,114] Caution is warranted in these patients secondary to the phenomenon of refeeding edema related to the sudden increase in intravascular volume and metabolic demands, which outweigh cardiac compensatory mechanisms.[115]

The interrelationship between cardiac disease and malnutrition is magnified in the perioperative period. Several early studies delineated this relationship. Abel and associates first reported an increased mortality rate as well as complication rate in malnourished patients compared with well-nourished patients undergoing cardiac surgery.[116]

Gibbons and others were one of the first groups to demonstrate the efficacy of preoperative enteral supplementation in cardiac surgery patients.[117] Three patients with cardiac cachexia were evaluated preoperatively and found to be significantly malnourished based on standard anthropometric, visceral protein, and immunologic criteria. All received 3 weeks of preoperative and postoperative enteral nutritional supplementation followed by multivalve replacement. Surgery was tolerated well by the group with minimal morbidity. Likewise, Able and associates examined 44 malnourished patients before cardiac surgery and randomized them to receive or not receive five days of TPN. Little difference was noted between the groups, probably related to the short interval of supplementation. Although definitive studies documenting the efficacy of preoperative nutritional supplementation in patients with malnutrition are lacking, many authors currently recommend preoperative nutritional supplementation.

Cardiac Transplantation

Cardiac transplants are done in an orthotopic fashion after cardiectomy of the diseased heart. The atria of the donor heart are anastomosed to the recipient's atrial cuffs; then the pulmonary arteries and aorta are anastomosed in an end-to-end fashion (Fig. 29–5). Most patients regain a cardiac rhythm spontaneously; others may need cardioversion or pacing.[118]

Postoperative complications include donor heart failure and renal failure. The causes for heart failure are multiple, including depletion of energy stores in the donor heart, hyperacute rejection, and pulmonary hypertension. Occasionally, an external device for temporary mechanical circulatory support may be needed until the donor heart recovers. Renal failure can be due to hypoperfusion and nephrotoxicity of immunosuppression drugs.

Cardiac transplant recipients are also exposed to all the potential complications resulting from cardiopulmonary bypass, including central nervous system (CNS) dysfunction, ranging from disorientation and delirium to a

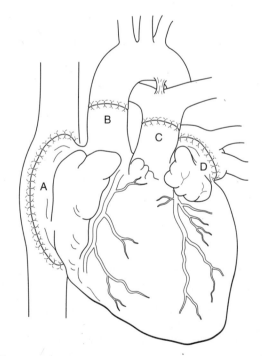

FIGURE 29–5 Cardiac transplantation. *A*, After cardiectomy the atria of the donor heart are anastomosed to the recipient's atrial cuffs. The aorta (*B*) and pulmonary artery (*C*) are anastomosed in an end-to-end fashion. *D*, The pulmonary veins are anastomosed to the left atrium.

full-blown stroke and pulmonary edema. More rarely, cardiac transplant recipients may also develop abdominal complications, usually resulting from low flow through the splachnic bed. These include mesenteric ischemia, pancreatitis, cholecystitis, and hepatic ischemia.

Enteral Nutrition and Cardiac Transplantation

As in nontransplant cardiac surgery, preoperative nutritional status may play a role in outcome after heart transplantation. The Texas Heart Institute reported the results of the first 52 patients undergoing transplantation.[119] Preoperatively, 10 were found to be severely malnourished and 13 marginally malnourished. Mortality correlated directly with preoperative nutritional state. Fifty percent of the malnourished patients died postoperatively compared with 23 percent of those with marginally compromised and 21 percent with adequate nutritional parameters.

However, controlled trials examining the role of preoperative nutritional status and supplementation in patients undergoing cardiac transplantation are lacking. A few studies have documented reversal of preoperative undernutrition based on improvements in anthropometric, somatic, and visceral protein measurements after transplantation.[120] Most studies continue to emphasize postoperative diet in relation to atherosclerosis. Definitive studies are needed to assess preoperative risk in association with nutritional status. Until that time, extrapolation from the non-transplant, cardiac surgical literature provides the only data.

Most patients undergoing cardiac transplantation will resume oral intake soon after surgery. Patients with CNS dysfunction may need nutritional support for as long as the CNS dysfunction lasts. To decide when to initiate tube feedings in these patients, monitor nasogastric tube output. When the output decreases to less than 200 ml/8 hours, or 600 ml/day, tube feedings can be initiated through the nasogastric tube with frequent monitoring of residuals.

Summary

Definitive changes in cardiac structure and function have been demonstrated in malnourished patients. Furthermore, congenital heart disease and chronic heart disease create a malnourished state that may render patients susceptible to increased morbidity and mortality. Preoperative maximization of nutritional status in undernourished cardiac patients is recommended until definitive studies documenting its efficacy are published.

LUNG TRANSPLANTATION

Successful lung transplantation was first reported in 1983 from the Toronto Lung Transplant Group.[121] Since that time, clinically successful lung transplantation has become increasingly more frequent. A decade later, the 1- and 3-year survival rates from the procedure are as high as 68 percent and 54 percent, respectively.[1] The most common indications for transplantation include chronic obstructive pulmonary disease (COPD), pulmonary fibrosis, and cystic fibrosis.[122] Additionally, the functional outcome from the procedure has been excellent.[123]

Enteral Nutrition and Pulmonary Function

An association between weight loss and COPD has long been noted.[124,125] Hunter and associates described nutritional depletion in hospitalized patients with COPD.[126] Fifty percent of patients had anthropometric measurements less than 60 percent of normal, while the majority of patients weighed less than their calculated ideal body weight. Openbrier and colleagues noted similar weight changes in COPD patients.[127]

In patients with COPD, malnourishment greatly affects pulmonary function. Wilson and associates used the data base from the National Institutes of Health Intermittent Positive-Pressure Breathing Trial to analyze pulmonary function in people with COPD and malnutrition;[128] 779 patients were classified according to the percent ideal body weight and pulmonary function. A significant direct correlation was found between percent ideal body weight and percent forced expiratory volume (FEV_1). In addition, survival was correlated with percent ideal body weight, with patients having body weight less than 90 percent of ideal manifesting poorer survival. This finding is similar to other reports in which mortality was higher and pulmonary function was lower in patients with COPD and weight loss compared with patients with COPD without weight loss.[129,130]

The etiology of weight loss in COPD is a matter of speculation and has been reviewed extensively elsewhere.[131,132] Some investigators feel it is related to increased REE. Wilson and Rogers showed that malnourished patients with COPD had a basal metabolic rate 1.38 to 1.79 times the basal energy expenditure as predicted by the Harris-Benedict equation.[133] Others have confirmed this finding.[134]

A higher work of breathing leading to an increased metabolic rate and energy expenditure has been postulated as the cause of weight loss in the COPD population. Donahoe and colleagues investigated this hypothesis by examining the oxygen consumption, oxygen cost of breathing, and pulmonary function in well-nourished and malnourished patients with COPD.[135] The mean resting oxygen consumption was higher in malnourished patients with COPD compared with well-nourished patients (4.20 ± 0.47 ml O_2/minute/kg vs 3.10 ± 0.53 ml O_2/minute/kg, $P < 0.001$), as was the oxygen cost. These data support the hypothesis that altered breathing mechanics in COPD produce increased energy needs that, if not met, lead to weight loss.

Alternatively, others feel the weight loss is related to decreased caloric intake. It is postulated that patients with COPD manifest a diminished appetite attributable to altered breathing patterns. In addition, semistarvation might in fact act as an adaptive mechanism by decreasing metabolic rate and oxygen demand. Most studies inventorying caloric intake in COPD patients fail to support this viewpoint, but the data collection is retrospective and susceptible to inaccuracies.[127,136]

In either case, the impact of EN on COPD patients is becoming obvious. Early encouraging results were reported from animal models[137] as well as the Minnesota experiment. Improvements in hypoxic drive was reported with refeeding.[138]

Wilson and associates subjected six patients with malnutrition (body weight < 90 percent ideal) and COPD to a 3-week, in-hospital regimen of controlled feeding to achieve caloric intake above that calculated for maintenance energy needs.[133] Significant improvements in body weight, triceps skinfold measurement, mid-arm muscle circumference, maximal inspiratory pressures, and maximal transdiaphragmatic pressures were observed. No differences in spirometry values or serum nutritional parameters were noted. Although not randomized or controlled, this study demonstrated the potential improvement in pulmonary function offered by correcting undernutrition.

In a similar study, Whittaker and associates randomly divided 10 patients with severe COPD and malnutrition in a group that re-ceived either 1000 kcal of Isocal (refed group) or 100 kcal of sham feedings (control group) above baseline intake.[139] All patients were treated in the hospital for a mean of 16 days followed by pulmonary function testing. The maximum static expiratory pressure and mean inspiratory mouth pressures were significantly improved in the refed group compared with the control group. No differences in pulmonary spirometry or maximum static inspiratory pressure were seen. These data supported the positive effect of refeeding on respiratory muscle function in patients with COPD and malnutrition. Other investigators have reported similar findings with respect to improvements in nutritional parameters and respiratory muscle strength using controlled dietary regimens.

The positive effects of nutrition have been seen in ventilatory-dependent patients. Bassili and Deitel retrospectively reviewed ventilator-dependent patients who received either isotonic intravenous support (control group) or supplemental nutrition support in the form of TPN or TEN (fed group).[140] Only 54.5 percent of patients in the control group were successfully weaned from the ventilator compared with 93 percent in the fed group ($P < 0.05$). This difference was even greater when only surgical patients were examined.

Exercise caution in refeeding pulmonary-compromised patients due to the reported negative effects of high-carbohydrate diets on CO_2 retention and weaning from mechanical ventilation.[141,142] Regardless, the positive effect of EN on pulmonary function is becoming obvious.

Lung Transplantation

Lung transplants can be performed unilaterally or bilaterally. Unilateral lung transplants are preferred in patients with emphysema, pulmonary fibrosis, and pulmonary hypertension. Bilateral lung transplants are preferred in patients with cystic fibrosis and bilateral bronchiectasis.[123] Unilateral lung transplants are performed through a posterolateral thoracotomy, while bilateral lung transplants are performed through a trans-sternal thoracotomy with a clamshell incision. The "Achilles heel" of lung transplantation is the bronchial anastomosis. Refinement in techniques has provided a safe method for performing this anastomosis by telescoping the donor bronchus into the recipient's bronchus. About one third of patients require cardiopulmonary bypass as part of the procedure.

Postoperatively these patients receive triple immunosuppression with cyclosporine, azathioprine, and corticosteroids, as well as antimicrobial prophylaxis (against bacteria, fungi, and viruses). The typical complications are rejection, infection, bleeding, and bronchial anastomotic problems.

Enteral Nutrition and Lung Transplantation

The nutritional aspects of lung transplantation, like those of many organs, are not well defined. Most patients with end-stage lung disease are malnourished, as highlighted above. However, controlled trials using preoperative and postoperative nutritional support are lacking.

The Toronto group has retrospectively reported on the nutritional status of a group of 35 patients who underwent lung transplantation.[143] Differences in the patient population were noted according to the etiology of lung disease. Using anthropometric data, the COPD and cystic fibrosis patients were considered malnourished preoperatively while the idiopathic pulmonary fibrosis, primary pulmonary hypertension, and bronchiectasis patients were considered adequately nourished. Improvement in nutritional status was seen in all malnourished patients by 6 months after transplantation without supplemental nutritional support.

The Loyola Lung Transplant Team mentions that it uses preoperative EN through a gastrostomy tube in malnourished patients undergoing lung transplantation.[123] The team also describes in the same paper a catastrophic complication due to intraperitoneal leakage from a percutaneous endoscopic gastrostomy and peritonitis, which resulted in one patient's death.

Clearly, more controlled trials are needed to elucidate the exact role of TEN in lung transplantation. The one study from Toronto demonstrates that some but not all patients with end-stage lung disease are malnourished preoperatively. Further investigation should be undertaken to determine if nutrition supplementation can affect outcome.

Summary

The association between nutritional states and lung function has long been recognized. Malnourished states are associated with not only changes in respiratory drive and pulmonary function but also morphologic changes in lung tissue and volumes. Furthermore, some patients with COPD are considered malnour-

ished and have been shown to have a worse prognosis. The etiology of this association between COPD and malnourishment is unclear.

Also unknown is the effect of preoperative nutritional support on patients with end-stage lung disease undergoing operative intervention and lung transplantation. It appears that those undergoing uncomplicated lung transplants regain a more normal nutritional status. Whether nutritional intervention can improve outcome after lung transplantation remains to be answered.

ENTERAL NUTRITION AND BONE MARROW TRANSPLANTATION

Bone marrow transplantation (BMT) is a commonly applied and successful procedure. Indications include both solid organ and hematologic malignancies, as well as abnormalities of white blood cell and red blood cell function. Outcomes are related to HLA typing and control of graft rejection, graft-versus-host disease, and infection. Survival is very much related to the underlying disease process. For patients with aplastic anemia undergoing HLA-identical marrow transplantation, 3-year survival rates are as high as 92 percent. The results for patients with hematologic malignancies are more variable, but disease-free survival rates of 30 to 60 percent have been reported. The results of unrelated, HLA-matched transplants are not as successful.[1]

Nutrition and Bone Marrow Transplant Recipients

On initial presentation, patients with hematologic malignancies who are candidates for BMT usually do not show signs of immunodeficiency or malnutrition. Patients with solid organ malignancies, or recurrences of hematologic malignancies, often present with malnutrition. In these patients, malnutrition may result in secondary immunodeficiency, which then compounds the effects of chemotherapy and radiation therapy.

Studies of cell-mediated immunity (CMI) reveal depressed responsiveness in malnourished patients.[144-147] Common indicators of CMI, like responses to tuberculin skin testing and reactions to 2,4-dinitrochlorobenzene, are frequently retarded or anergic in malnourished children. In vitro indicators such as response to phytohemagglutinin and concavalin A are depressed. Changes in the phenotype of circulating peripheral blood mononuclear cells have also been reported.[148-151]

Immunoglobulins are adversely effected by malnutrition. Although studies have demonstrated normal serum B-lymphocyte numbers as well as normal to elevated serum immunoglobulin levels in patients with protein-calorie malnutrition, depression in T-cell numbers and functions can lead to reductions in T-cell-derived help for B-cell proliferation.[146,152] Mucosal immunity is particularly impaired by reduced quantities of secretory IgA.[149] Levels of IgG may also be reduced. However, these data vary depending on the degree of malnutrition and type of antibody response elicited.[149,151]

Alteration in other immune functions, such as phagocytosis and complement, are frequently reported in patients with malnutrition. With phagocytic functions, variable results have been obtained but depression with prolonged malnutrition appears to be the trend.[151] Complement levels and function are also depressed in chronic malnourished states.[145,146,149,153]

Together, these alterations help explain the close association between malnutrition and infection. The exact mechanisms behind these observed alterations have not been fully elucidated. However, regardless of the organ transplanted, the relative immunosuppression created by the malnourished state can significantly affect outcome.

Bone Marrow Transplantation

Bone marrow transplantation is performed for bone marrow aplasia occurring spontaneously or in response to cytoxic chemotherapy as the treatment for malignancies. The methods of myeloablation are called "conditioning regimens" and include chemotherapy alone or chemoradiotherapy. The source of cells for BMT can be allogenic, related or unrelated donors, or autologous. Autologous BMT is really a reinfusion of previously aspirated cells rather than a transplant. The hematopoietic progenitor cells (stem cells) capable of repopulating the aplastic recipient marrow are recovered from the donor marrow. More recently stem cells have been harvested from peripheral blood by leukapheresis. Except in autologous and in syngeneic (identical twin donor) BMTs, all other BMTs (allogenic) require posttransplant immunosuppression.

Enteral Nutrition and Bone Marrow Transplantation

Nutrition is a critical aspect of successful BMT. Many candidates for the procedure are considered undernourished due to chronic illness, malignancy, or anorexia (Table 29–5). Pretransplantation regimens often include prolonged hospitalization and chemotherapy with its secondary GI side-effects, infection, and increased energy requirements. The degree of malnutrition in potential BMT candidates varies.

Energy requirements are significant after BMT. Szeluga and associates estimated the energy needs of 84 BMT recipients in the early postoperative period.[154] Predicted caloric requirements were highest in children (79 kcal/day) followed by adolescents (53 kcal/day) and adults (44 kcal/day). Actual energy intake in these groups of BMT recipients was 82 percent to 97 percent of the predicted needs, indicating the importance of nutritional monitoring and the substantial energy requirements after BMT.

Lenssen and associates[155] studied the long-term energy needs of 192 patients surviving more than 1 year after transplantation. Weight loss was the most commonly encountered nutritional-related problem, occurring in 28 percent of all patients and 33 percent of patients with extensive graft-versus-host disease. The number of patients with suboptimal anthropometric measurements (arm muscle area less than 25 percent and arm fat area greater than 75 percent) increased throughout the follow-up period. Dietary histories revealed that approximately one third of patients had nutritional intakes less than 85 percent of requirements. These data indicate that nutritional problems and needs are significant and long-term problems associated with BMT.

The efficacy of nutritional support as TPN is well documented. Multiple studies relate im-

TABLE 29–5 Mechanisms of Malnutrition in Bone Marrow Recipients

Hematologic malignancy
Cytoreductive therapy:
   Chemotherapy
   Radiation
   Immunotherapy
Graft-versus-host disease
   Acute (gastrointestinal tract, skin, liver)
   Chronic (gastrointestinal tract, skin, liver, lungs)
Graft-versus-host disease prophylaxis
Infection
   Bacterial
   Viral
   Fungal
Veno-occlusive disease of the liver

proved outcomes with administration of TPN during the acute transplantation period.[156-159]

However, administration of TEN has been limited. Most commonly, significant GI side-effects related to BMT exist. Stomatitis and esophagitis related to chemotherapy, immunosuppression, and neutropenia limit oral intake. Vomiting and anorexia occur often after administration of chemotherapeutic agents. Diarrhea related to infection, chemotherapeutic bowel toxicity, graft-versus-host disease, or enteral feeding itself can limit the role of TEN. Several studies have attempted to address the role of TEN in BMT.

Szeluga and associates prospectively compared a TPN regimen with an enteral feeding program in 65 patients undergoing BMT.[160] Preoperative nutrition status was good in most patients and comparable between groups. TPN was administered to supply 35 kcal/kg/day and was tapered according to the patients' simultaneous enteral intake. The EN program was tailored to achieve a similar caloric intake. Supplementation in the forms of oral protein-rich snacks and intravenous amino acids was used in those patients unable to achieve the goals. Seven of 30 enteral patients required crossover to the TPN group because of insufficient caloric intake. Four of 31 TPN patients required crossover to the EN group because of vascular access problems. Significant differences in body weight favoring the TPN group were noted by posttransplant day 28. TPN patients had significantly more hyperglycemia problems than their enteral counterparts, and the estimated cost of therapy was significantly higher in the TPN group. Time to hematologic recovery, length of hospitalization, and survival were not significantly different between groups. The authors concluded that TPN was not clearly superior to EN in BMT recipients.

A second study by Mulder and colleagues prospectively randomized 22 BMT recipients to receive either TPN alone or partial parenteral nutrition plus EN.[161] No significant differences in nutritional or clinical indexes were noted between the groups. Note that the weight/height index was significantly lower in the EN group before treatment was begun. The data indicated that EN support was a feasible way to administer calories in patients after BMT.

Summary

BMT is a clinically successful procedure associated with significant postoperative energy demands. At present, TPN is the standard method of nutrient administration used to achieve these demands. However, EN has been shown in several studies to be efficacious in certain patients. TEN offers several attractive advantages over TPN, such as eliminating central venous access, presence of nutrient in gut, and cost. Larger, prospective, randomized studies are required for definitive conclusions.

CONCLUSION

The clinical application of organ transplantation has exploded over the past decade. Many advances have been made in the techniques for harvesting, preserving, and implanting organs in recipient patients. The donor pool has expanded, although many patients in end-stage organ failure continue to die awaiting an organ. New drugs for immunosuppression have allowed the development of new transplants.

As the field of transplantation grows, more hospital beds are occupied with patients having complex problems resulting from transplantation. Modern techniques of nutritional assessment and support are now being applied for patients undergoing transplantation. Scientific data documenting the effectiveness of nutritional intervention in transplantation are still lacking.

Malnutrition is commonly associated with organ failure. The surgical procedures for organ transplantation are various orders of magnitude greater and more complex than traditional surgery. The addition of immunosuppression to these complex procedures raises the risk for life-threatening complications to the highest level. Any attempt should be made at reducing morbidity and mortality in these patients, even in the absence of conclusive data. Apply caution not to increase the risk of these delicate patients by adding invasive maneuvers to their care.

REFERENCES

1. Terasaki PI, Cecka JM (eds): Clinical Transplants 1993. Los Angeles: UCLA Tissue Typing Laboratory, 1993:601–731.
2. Mullen JL, Buzby GP, Matthews DC et al: Reduction in operative morbidity and mortality by combined preoperative and postoperative nutritional support. Ann Surg 1980;192:604–613.
3. Mullen JL, Buzby GP, Waldman MT et al: Prediction of operative morbidity and mortality by preoperative nutritional assessment. Surg Forum 1979;30:80–82.
4. Muller JM, Brenner U, Dienst C et al: Preoperative parenteral feeding in patients with gastrointestinal carcinoma. Lancet 1982;1:68–71.
5. Muller JM, Keller HW, Brenner U et al: Indications and effects of preoperative parenteral nutrition. World J Surg 1986;10:53–63.

6. The Veterans Affairs Total Parenteral Nutrition Cooperative Study Group: Perioperative total parenteral nutrition in surgical patients. N Engl J Med 1991;325: 525–532.

7. Moore FA, Moore EE, Jones TN et al: TEN versus TPN following major abdominal trauma—reduced septic morbidity. J Trauma 1989;29:916–922.

8. Moore FA, Feliciano DV, Andrassy RJ et al: Early enteral feeding, compared with parenteral, reduces postoperative septic complications. Ann Surg 1992; 216:172–183.

9. Grant D, Wall W, Mimeault R et al: Successful small-bowel/liver transplantation. Lancet 1990;335:181–184.

10. Alverdy JC, Aoys E, Moss GS: Total parenteral nutrition promotes bacterial translocation from the gut. Surgery 1988;104:185–190.

11. Deitch EA, Berg R, Specian R: Endotoxin promotes the translocation of bacteria from the gut. Arch Surg 1987;122:185–190.

12. Alverdy J, Sang H, Sheldon GF: The effect of parenteral nutrition on gastrointestinal immunity: the importance of enteral stimulation. Ann Surg 1985;202: 681–684.

13. Lichtman SN, Sherman PM, Forstner GG: Effect of dietary restriction on total and bacterium-specific mucosal secretory immunoglobulin A in bile-diverted intestinal self-filling blind loops. Infect Immun 1988; 56:395–399.

14. Alverdy JA, Aoys E, Weiss-Carrington P et al: The effect of glutamine-enriched TPN on gut immune cellularity. J Surg Res 1992;52:34–38.

15. Frankel W, Zhang W, Alfonso J et al: Glutamine enhances cellularity and function in transplanted small bowel. J Parenter Enter Nutr 1992;16(suppl 1):24S.

16. Rombeau JLR, Rolandelli RH: Enteral and parenteral nutrition in patients with enteric fistulas and short bowel syndrome. Surg Clin North Am 1987;67: 557–571.

17. Wilmore DW: Factors correlating with a successful outcome following extensive intestinal resection in newborn infants. J Pediatr 1972;80:88–95.

18. Sax HC, Bower RH: Hepatic complications of total parenteral nutrition. J Parenter Enter Nutr 1988;12: 615–618.

19. Tzakis AG, Todo S, Reyes J et al: Clinical intestinal transplantation: focus on complications. Transplant Proc 1992;24:1238–1240.

20. Hale DA, Waldorf KA, Kleinschmidt J et al: Small intestinal transplantation in nonhuman primates. J Pediatr Surg 1991;26:914–920.

21. Watson AJM, Lear PA, Montgomery A et al: Water, electrolyte, glucose and glycine absorption in rat small intestinal transplants. Gastroenterology 1988; 94:863–869.

22. Liu H, Teraoka S, Ota K et al: Successful lymphangiographic investigation of mesenteric lymphatic regeneration after orthotopic intestinal transplantation in the rat. Transplant Proc 1992;24:1113–1114.

23. Raju S, Didlake RH, Cayirli M et al: Experimental small bowel transplantation utilising Cyclosporin. Transplantation 1984;38:561–566.

24. Sarr MG, Kelly KA: Myoelectric activity of the autotransplanted canine jejuno-ileum. Gastroenterology 1981;81:303–310.

25. Hutson WR, Putnam PE, Todo S et al: The effects of small intestinal and multivisceral transplantation on gastric and small bowel motility in humans. Third International Symposium on Small Bowel Transplantation, Abstract O 70, 1993.

26. Furukawa H, Abu-Elmagd K, Hutson WR et al: Abnormal gastric emptying after intestinal transplantation. Third International Symposium on Small Bowel Transplantation, Abstract O 20, 1993.

27. Busuttil RW, Farmer DG, Shaked A et al: Successful combined liver and small intestine transplantation for short-gut syndrome and liver failure. West J Med 1993;158:184–188.

28. Reyes J, Tzakis AG, Todo S et al: Nutritional management of intestinal transplant recipients. Transplant Proc 1993;25:1200–1201.

29. Staschak-Chicko S, Altieri K, Funovits M et al: Eating difficulties in the pediatric small bowel recipient: the role of the nutritional management team. Transplant Proc 1994;26:1434–1435.

30. Starzl TE, Marchiaro TL, Von Kaulla K et al: Homotransplantation of the liver in humans. Surg Gynecol Obstet 1963;117:659–676.

31. Busuttil RW, Shaked A, Millis JM et al: One thousand liver transplants: lessons learned. Ann Surg 1994; 219:490–499.

32. Kudsk KA, Kisor DF, Waters B et al: Effect of nutritional status on organic anion clearance by the swine liver. Surgery 1992;111:188–194.

33. Quigley EMM, Marsh MN, Shaffer JL et al: Hepatobiliary complications of total parenteral nutrition. Gastroenterology 1983;104:288–301.

34. Moss RL, Das JB, Raffensperger JG: Total parenteral nutrition-associated cholestasis: clinical and histopathological correlation. J Pediatr Surg 1993;28: 1270–1275.

35. Bowyer BA, Fleming CR, Ludwig J et al: Does long-term home parenteral nutrition in adult patients cause chronic liver disease? J Parenter Enter Nutr 1985;9:11–17.

36. Hughs CA, Talbot IC, Ducker DA et al: Total parenteral nutrition in infancy: effect on the liver and suggested pathogenesis. Gut 1983;24:241–248.

37. Blumenkrantz MJ, Kopple JD, Gutman RA et al: Methods for assessing nutritional status of patients with renal failure. Am J Clin Nutr 1980;33:1567–1585.

38. Hall RI, Grant JP, Ross LH et al: Pathogenesis of hepatic steatosis in the parenterally fed rat. J Clin Invest 1984;74:1658–1668.

39. Kaminski DL, Adams A, Jellinek M: The effect of hyperalimentation on hepatic lipid content and lipogenic enzyme activity in rats and man. Surgery 1980;88:93–100.

40. King WWK, Boelhouwer RU, Kingsnorth AN et al: Nutritional efficacy and hepatic changes during intragastric, intravenous, and prehepatic feeding in rats. J Parenter Enter Nutr 1983;7:443–446.

41. Whalen GF, Shamberger RC, Perez-Atayde A et al: A proposed cause for the hepatic dysfunction associated with parenteral nutrition. J Pediatr Surg 1990; 25:622–626.

42. Waters B, Kudsk KA, Jarvi EJ et al: Effect of route of nutrition on recovery of hepatic organic anion clearance after fasting. Surgery 1994;115:370–374.

43. Marchioro TL, Porter KA, Dickinson TC et al: Physiologic requirements for auxiliary liver homotransplantation. Surg Gynecol Obstet 1965;121:17–31.

44. Starzl TE, Watanabe K, Porter KA et al: Effects of insulin, glucagon, and insulin/glucagon infusions on liver morphology and cell division after complete portacaval shunt in dogs. Lancet 1976;1:821–825.

45. Li S, Nussbaum MS, Teague D et al: Increasing dextrose concentrations in total parenteral nutrition (TPN) causes alterations in hepatic morphology and

plasma levels of insulin and glucagon in rats. J Surg Res 1988;44:639–648.

46. Mok K-T, Meng HC: Intestinal, pancreatic, and hepatic effects of gastrointestinal hormones in a total parenteral nutrition rat model. J Parenter Enter Nutr 1993;17:364–369.

47. Wood RP, Ozaki CF, Katz SM et al: Liver transplantation: the last ten years. Surg Clin North Am 1994; 74(5):1133–1154.

48. Mendenhall CL, Anderson S, Weesner RE et al: Protein-calorie malnutrition associated with alcoholic hepatitis: Veterans Administration Cooperative Study Group on Alcoholic Hepatitis. Am J Med 1984;76: 211–222.

49. Chin SE, Shepherd RW, Cleghorn GJ et al: Survival, growth and quality of life in children after orthotopic liver transplantation: a 5 year experience. J Pediatr Child Health 1991;27:380–385.

50. Latifi R, Killam RW, Dudrick SJ: Nutritional support in liver failure. Surg Clin North Am 1991;71:567–578.

51. Goulet OJ, de Ville de Goyet J, Otte JB et al: Preoperative nutritional evaluation and support for liver transplantation in children. Transplant Proc 1987;19: 3249–3255.

52. Hehir DJ, Jenkins RL, Bistrian B et al: Nutrition in patients undergoing orthotopic liver transplant. J Parenter Enter Nutr 1985;9:695–700.

53. Moukarzel AA, Najm I, Vargas J et al: Effect of nutritional status on outcome of orthotopic liver transplantation in pediatric patients. Transplant Proc 1990;22:1560–1563.

54. Shepherd RW, Chin SE, Cleghorn GJ et al: Malnutrition in children with chronic liver disease accepted for liver transplantation: clinical profile and effect on outcome. J Pediatr Child Health 1991;27:295–299.

55. Shaw BW Jr, Wood RP, Gordon RD et al: Influence of selected patient variables and operative blood loss on six-month survival following liver transplantation. Semin Liver Dis 1985;5:385–393.

56. Silk DBA, O'Keefe SJD, Wicks C: Nutritional support in liver disease. Gut Supplement 1991: S29–S33.

57. Cabre E, Gonzalez-Huix F, Abad-Lacruz A et al: Effect of total enteral nutrition on the short-term outcome of severely malnourished cirrhotics: a randomized controlled trial. Gastroenterology 1990;98:715–720.

58. Charlton CPJ, Buchanan E, Holden CE et al: Intensive enteral feeding in advanced cirrhosis: reversal of malnutrition without precipitation of hepatic encephalopathy. Arch Dis Child 1992;67:603–607.

59. DiCecco SR, Wieners EJ, Wiesner RH et al: Assessment of nutritional status of patients with end-stage liver disease undergoing liver transplantation. Mayo Clin Proc 1989;64:95–102.

60. Nasrallah SM, Galambos JT: Amino acid therapy of alcoholic hepatitis. Lancet 1980;ii:1276–1277.

61. Naveau S, Pelletier G, Poynard T et al: A randomized clinical trial of supplementary parenteral nutrition in jaundiced alcoholic cirrhotic patients. Hepatology 1986;6:270–274.

62. Delafosse B, Faure JL, Bouffard Y et al: Liver transplantation—energy expenditure, nitrogen loss, and substrate oxidation rate in the first two postoperative days. Transplant Proc 1989;21:2453–2454.

63. Hasse JM: Nutritional implications of liver transplantation. Henry Ford Hosp Med J 1990;38:325–340.

64. Plevak DJ, DiCecco SR, Wiesner RH et al: Nutritional support for liver transplantation: identifying caloric and protein requirements. Mayo Clin Proc 1994;69: 225–230.

65. Reilly J, Mehta R, Teperman L et al: Nutritional support after liver transplantation: a randomized prospective study. J Parenter Enter Nutr 1990;14:386–391.

66. Wicks C, Somasundaram S, Bjarnason I et al: Comparison of enteral feeding and total parenteral nutrition after liver transplantation. Lancet 1994;344: 837–840.

67. Hasse JM, Blue LS, Liepa GU et al: Early enteral nutrition support in patients undergoing liver transplantation. J Parenter Enter Nutr 1995;19:437–443.

68. Pescovitz MD, Mehta PL, Leapman SB et al: Tube jejunostomy in liver transplant recipients. Surgery 1995;117(6):642–647.

69. Merrill JP, Murray JE, Harrison JH et al: Successful homotransplantation of the human kidney between identical twins. JAMA 1956;160:277.

70. Suthanthiran M, Strom TB: Renal transplantation. N Engl J Med 1994;331:365–376.

71. Ichikawa I, Purkerson ML, Klahr S et al: Mechanism of reduced glomerular filtration rate in chronic malnutrition. J Clin Invest 1980;65:982–988.

72. Pennell JP, Sanjana V, Frey NR et al: The effect of urea infusion on the urinary concentrating mechanism in protein-depleted rats. J Clin Invest 1975;55:399–409.

73. Schoolwerth AC, Sandler RS, Hoffman PM et al: Effects of nephron reduction and dietary protein content on renal ammoniagenesis in the rat. Kidney Int 1975;7:397–404.

74. Rabinowitz L, Gunther RA, Shoji ES et al: Effects of high and low protein diets on sheep renal function and metabolism. Kidney Int 1973;4:188–207.

75. Klahr S, Tripathy K: Evaluation of renal function in malnutrition. Arch Intern Med 1966;118:322–325.

76. Brenner BM, Meyer TW, Hostetter TH: Dietary protein intake and the progressive nature of kidney disease: the role of hemodynamically mediated glomerular injury in the pathogenesis of progressive glomerular sclerosis in aging, renal ablation, and intrinsic renal disease. N Engl J Med 1982;307:652–659.

77. Bosch JP, Saccaggi A, Lauer A et al: Renal functional reserve in humans: effect of protein intake on glomerular filtration rate. Am J Med 1983;75:943–950.

78. Bosch JP, Lauer A, Glabman S: Short-term protein loading in assessment of patients with renal disease. Am J Surg 1984;77:873–879.

79. Pullman TN, Alving AS, Dern RJ et al: The influence of dietary protein intake on specific renal functions in normal man. J Lab Clin Med 1954;44:320–332.

80. Bosch JP, Lew S, Glabman S et al: Renal hemodynamic changes in humans: response to protein loading in normal and diseased kidneys. Am J Med 1986;81:809–815.

81. Acchiardo SR, Moore LW, Cockrell S: Does low protein diet halt the progression of renal insufficiency? Clinical Nephrol 1986;25:289–294.

82. Rosman JB, Ter Wee PM, Meijer S et al: Prospective randomized trial of early dietary protein restriction in chronic renal failure. Lancet 1984;2:1291–1295.

83. Oldrizzi L, Rugiu C, Valvo E et al: Progression of renal failure in patients with renal disease of diverse etiology on protein-restricted diet. Kidney Int 1985;27: 553–557.

84. Gordillo G, Soto RA, Metcoff J et al: Intracellular composition and hemostatic mechanisms in severe chronic infantile malnutrition, III. Renal adjustments. Pediatrics 1957;20:303–316.

85. Valdes R, Munoz R, Bracho E et al: Surgical complications of renal transplantation in malnourished children. Transplant Proc 1994;26:50–51.

86. Bansal VK, Popli S, Pickering J et al: Protein-calorie malnutrition and cutaneous anergy in hemodialysis maintained patients. Am J Clin Nutr 1980;33: 1608–1611.

87. Thurnberg B, Swamy AP, Cestero RVM: Cross-sectional and longitudinal nutritional measurements in maintenance hemodialysis patients. Am J Clin Nutr 1981;34:2005–2012.

88. Kopple JD: Abnormal amino acid and protein metabolism in uremia. Kidney Int 1978;14:340–348.

89. Varella L: Nutritional support for the patient with renal failure. Crit Care Nurs Clin North Am 1993;5: 79–96.

90. Kluthe R, Luttgen FM, Capetianu T et al: Protein requirements in maintenance hemodialysis. Am J Clin Nutr 1978;31:1812–1820.

91. Salusky IB, Fine RN, Nelson P et al: Nutritional status of children undergoing continuous ambulatory peritoneal dialysis. Am J Clin Nutr 1983;38:599–611.

92. Monteon FJ, Laidlaw SA, Shaib JK et al: Energy expenditure in patients with chronic renal failure. Kidney Int 1986;30:741–747.

93. Compher C, Mullen JL, Barker CF: Nutritional support in renal failure. Surg Clin North Am 1991;71: 597–608.

94. Grodstein GP, Blumenkrantz MJ, Kopple JD: Nutritional and metabolic response to catabolic stress in uremia. Am J Clin Nutr 1980;33:1411–1416.

95. Jones JW, Nevins T, McHugh L et al: Nutrition and growth in pediatric renal transplant recipients. Transplant Proc 1994;26(1):62–63.

96. Hiraga S, Kitamura M, Kobayashi D et al: Long-term follow-up study of renal transplant recipients. Transplant Proc 1994;26:2090–2093.

97. Kelly WD, Lillehei RC, Merkel FK et al: Allotransplantation of the pancreas and duodenum along with the kidney in diabetic nephropathy. Surgery 1967;61: 827–837.

98. Robertson RP: Pancreatic and islet transplantation for diabetes cures or curiosities? N Engl J Med 1992;327: 1861–1868.

99. Sollinger HW, Ploeg RJ, Eckhoff DE et al: Two hundred consecutive simultaneous pancreas-kidney transplants with bladder drainage. Surgery 1993;114: 736–744.

100. Ricordi C, Tzakis A, Carroll P et al: Human islet allotransplantation in 18 diabetic patients. Transplant Proc 1992;24:961.

101. Scharp DW, Lacy PE, Santiago JV et al: Results of our first nine intraportal islet allografts in type 1, insulin-dependent diabetic patients. Transplantation 1991; 51:76–85.

102. Fine H, Levine GM, Shiau Y-F: Effects of cholecystokinin and secretin on intestinal structure and function. Am J Physiol 1983;245:G358–G363.

103. McArdle AH, Palmason C, Morency I et al: A rationale for enteral feeding as the preferable route for hyperalimentation. Surgery 1981;90:616–621.

104. Track NS: Mechanisms of release of gastro-enteropancreatic endocrine cells. World J Surg 1979;3: 457–461.

105. Greenberg GR, Wolman SL, Christofides ND et al: Effect of total parenteral nutrition on gut hormone release in humans. Gastroenterology 1981;80:988–993.

106. Sollinger HW, Geffner SR: Pancreas transplantation. Surg Clin North Am 1994;74(5):1183–1195.

107. Kaye MP: The registry of the International Society for Heart Transplantation: fourth official report—1987. J Heart Transplant 1987;6:63–67.

108. Webb JG, Kiess MC, Chan-Yan CC: Malnutrition and the heart. CMAJ 1986;135:753–758.

109. Heymsfield SB, Smith J, Redd S et al: Nutritional support in cardiac failure. Surg Clin North Am 1981;61: 635–652.

110. Mehrizi A, Drash A: Growth disturbance in congenital heart disease. J Pediatr 1962;61:418–429.

111. Schwarz SM, Gewitz MH, See CC et al: Enteral nutrition in infants with congestive heart disease and growth failure. Pediatrics 1990;86:368–373.

112. Vanderhoof JA, Hofschire PJ, Baluff MA et al: Continuous enteral feedings: an important adjunct to the management of complex congenital heart disease. Am J Dis Child 1982;136:825–827.

113. Heymsfield SB, Casper K: Congestive heart failure: clinical management by use of continuous nasoenteric feeding. Am J Clin Nutr 1989;50:539–544.

114. Poindexter SM, Dear WE, Dudrick SJ: Nutrition in congestive heart failure. Nutr Clin Pract 1986;1: 83–88.

115. Quinn T, Askanazi J: Nutrition and cardiac disease. Crit Care Clin 1987;3:167–185.

116. Abel RM, Fischer JE, Buckley MJ et al: Malnutrition in cardiac surgical patients: results of a prospective, randomized evaluation of early postoperative parenteral nutrition. Arch Surg 1976;111:45–50.

117. Gibbons GW, Blackburn GL, Harken DE et al: Pre- and postoperative hyperalimentation in the treatment of cardiac cachexia. J Surg Res 1976;20:439–444.

118. Frazier OH, Macris MP: Progress in cardiac transplantation. Surg Clin North Am 1994;74(5): 1169–1182.

119. Frazier OH, Van Buren CT, Poindexter SM et al: Nutritional management of the heart transplant recipient. J Heart Transplant 1985;4:450–452.

120. Grady KL, Herold LS: Comparison of nutritional status in patients before and after heart transplantation. J Heart Transplant 1988;7:123–127.

121. Toronto Lung Transplant Group: Unilateral lung transplantation for pulmonary fibrosis. N Engl J Med 1986;314:1140–1145.

122. Low DE, Trulock EP, Kaiser LR et al: Morbidity, mortality, and early results of single versus bilateral lung transplantation for emphysema. J Thorac Cardiovasc Surg 1992;103:1119–1126.

123. Montoya A, Mawulawde K, Houck J et al: Survival and functional outcome after single and bilateral lung transplantation. Surgery 1994;116:712–718.

124. Dornhorst AC: Respiratory insufficiency. Lancet 1955;268:1185–1187.

125. Filley GF, Beckwitt HJ, Reeves JT et al: Chronic obstructive bronchopulmonary disease, II. Oxygen transport in two clinical types. Am J Med 1968;44: 26–38.

126. Hunter AMB, Carey MA, Larsh HW: The nutritional status of patients with chronic obstructive pulmonary disease. Am Rev Respir Dis 1981;124:376–381.

127. Openbrier DR, Irwin MM, Cauber JH et al: Factors affecting nutritional status and the impact of nutritional support in patients with emphysema. Chest 1984;85 (suppl):67S–69S.

128. Wilson DO, Rogers RM, Wright EC et al: Body weight in chronic obstructive pulmonary disease: the National Institutes of Health Intermittant Positive-Pressure Breathing Trial. Am Rev Respir Dis 1989;139: 1435–1438.

129. Renzeti AD Jr, McClement JH, Litt BD: The Veterans Administration Cooperative Study of Pulmonary Function, III. Mortality in relation to respiratory func-

tion in chronic obstructive pulmonary disease. Am J Med 1966;41:115–129.

130. Grant JP: Nutrition care of patients with acute and chronic respiratory failure. Nutr Clin Pract 1994;9: 11–17.

131. Wilson DO, Rogers RM, Hoffman RM: Nutrition and chronic lung disease. Am Rev Respir Dis 1985;132: 1347–1365.

132. Mowatt-Larssen C, Brown RO: Specialized nutritional support in respiratory disease. Clin Pharm 1993;12: 276–292.

133. Wilson DO, Rogers RM: Basal O_2 consumption and metabolic rate is elevated in severe COPD. Chest 1986;89(suppl):517S.

134. Goldstein S, Askanazi J, Weissman C et al: Energy expenditure in patients with chronic obstructive pulmonary disease. Chest 1987;91:222–224.

135. Donahoe M, Rogers RM, Wilson DO et al: Oxygen consumption of the respiratory muscles in normal and malnourished patients with chronic obstructive pulmonary disease. Am Rev Respir Dis 1989;140: 385–391.

136. Braun SR, Keim NL, Dixon RM et al: The prevalence and determinants of nutritional changes in chronic obstructive pulmonary disease. Chest 1984;86: 558–563.

137. Sahebjami H, Vassallo CL: Effects of starvation and refeeding on lung mechanics and morphometry. Am Rev Respir Dis 1979;119:443–451.

138. Doekel RC Jr, Zwillich CW, Scoggins CH et al: Clinical semi-starvation: depression of hypoxic ventilatory response. N Engl J Med 1976;295:358–361.

139. Whittaker JS, Ryan CF, Buckley PA et al: The effects of refeeding on peripheral and respiratory muscle function in malnourished chronic obstructive pulmonary disease patients. Am Rev Respir Dis 1990;142: 283–288.

140. Bassili HR, Deitel M: Effect of nutritional support on weaning patients off mechanical ventilators. J Parenter Enter Nutr 1981;5:161–163.

141. Van den Berg B, Stam H: Metabolic and respiratory effects of enteral nutrition in patients during mechanical ventilation. Intensive Care Med 1988;14:206–211.

142. DeMeo MT, Van De Graaff W: The hazards of hypercaloric nutritional support in respiratory disease. Nutr Rev 1991;49:112–114.

143. Madill J, Maurer JR, De Hoyos A: A comparison of preoperative and postoperative nutritional states of lung transplant recipients. Transplantation 1993;56: 347–350.

144. Dowd PS, Heatley RV: The influence of undernutrition on immunity. Clin Sci 1984;66:241–248.

145. Smythe PM, Schonland M, Brereton-Stiles GG et al: Thymolymphatic deficiency and depression of cell-mediated immunity in protein-calorie malnutrition. Lancet 1971;2:939–943.

146. Chandra RK: Immunocompetence in undernutrition. J Pediatr 1972;81:1194–1200.

147. McMurray DN, Loomis SA, Casazza L et al: Development of impaired cell-mediated immunity in mild and moderate malnutrition. Am J Clin Nutr 1981;34: 68–77.

148. Chandra RK, Gupta S, Singh H: Inducer and suppressor T cell subsets in protein-energy malnutrition: analysis by monoclonal antibodies. Nutr Res 1982; 2:21–26.

149. Chandra RK: Nutrition, immunity, and infection: present knowledge and future directions. Lancet 1983; 1:688–691.

150. Chandra RK: Numerical and functional deficiency in T helper cells in protein energy malnutrition. Clin Exp Immunol 1983;51:126–132.

151. Garre MA, Boles JM, Youinou PY: Current concepts in immune derangement due to undernutrition. J Parenter Enter Nutr 1987;11:309–313.

152. Steihm ER: Humoral immunity in malnutrition. Federation Proc 1980;39:3093–3097.

153. Haller L, Zubler RH, Lambert PH: Plasma levels of complement components and complement haemolytic activity in protein-energy malnutrition. Clin Exp Immunol 1978;34:248–252.

154. Szeluga DJ, Stuart RK, Brookmeyer R et al: Energy requirements of parenterally fed bone marrow transplant recipients. J Parenter Enter Nutr 1985;9: 139–143.

155. Lensson P, Sherry ME, Cheney CL et al: Prevalence of nutrition-related problems among long-term survivors of allogeneic marrow transplantation J Am Diet Assoc 1990;90:835–842.

156. Herrmann VM: Nutrition support in bone marrow transplant recipients. Nutr Clin Pract 1993;8: 19–27.

157. Weisdorf SA, Lysne J, Wind D et al: Positive effect of prophylactic total parenteral nutrition on long-term outcome of bone marrow transplantation. Transplantation 1987;43:833–838.

158. Uderzo C, Rovelli A, Bonomi M et al: Total parenteral nutrition and nutritional assessment in leukaemic children undergoing bone marrow transplantation. Eur J Cancer 1991;27:758–762.

159. Geibeg CB, Owens JP, Mirtallo JM et al: Parenteral nutrition for marrow transplant recipients: evaluation of an increased nitrogen dose. J Parenter Enter Nutr 1991;15:184–188.

160. Szeluga DJ, Stuart RK, Brookmeyer R et al: Nutritional support of bone marrow transplant recipients: a prospective, randomized clinical trial comparing total parenteral nutrition to an enteral feeding program. Cancer Res 1987;47:3309–3316.

161. Mulder POM, Bouman JG, Gieterna JA: Hyperalimentation in autologous bone marrow transplantation for solid tumors: comparison of total parenteral versus partial parenteral plus enteral nutrition. Cancer 1989; 64:2045–2052.

BIBLIOGRAPHY

Chin SE, Shepard RW, Thomas BJ et al: The nature of malnutrition in children with end-stage liver disease awaiting orthotopic liver transplantation. Am J Clin Nutr 1992;56:164–168.

Deeg HJ, Kingemann HG, Philips GL: Bone marrow transplantation, 2nd. edition. Berlin-Heidelberg: Springer-Verlag, 1992.

Iwatsuki S, Starzl TE, Todo S et al: Experience in 1,000 liver transplants under cyclosporine-steroid therapy: a survival report. Transplant Proc 1988;20:498–504.

Klahr S, Purkerson ML: Effects of dietary protein on renal function and on the progression of renal disease. Am J Clin Nutr 1988;47:146–152.

Sutherland DER, Dunn DL, Goetz FC et al: A 10-year experience with 290 pancreas transplants at a single institution. Ann Surg 1989;210:274–288.

Wilson DO, Rogers RM, Sanders MH et al: Nutritional intervention in malnourished patients with emphysema. Am Rev Respir Dis 1986;134:672–677.

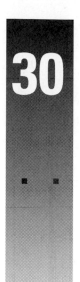

30

Home Enteral Nutrition in Adults

LYN HOWARD
MARGARET MALONE
BRUCE M. WOLF

Although enteral tube feeding has been available for decades, recent advances in infusion equipment and formulas have greatly expanded the potential use of this form of artificial nutrition support, particularly in nonhospital settings.

This chapter reviews the factors to take into account in initiating home enteral nutrition (HEN), the prevalence and growth of HEN, and the clinical outcome of patients receiving HEN for different primary diagnoses.

INITIATING HOME ENTERAL NUTRITION

Considerations

Tube feeding at home is appropriate if the patient and family accept it and meet the following criteria:

1. The patient cannot be nutritionally sustained through dietary adjustment or oral supplementation alone.
2. The patient has severe dysphagia due to an anatomic and functional impairment or impaired small bowel absorption that can be overcome by tube feeding delivered slowly and over a prolonged time.
3. The patient can experience sufficient nutritional benefit and rehabilitation to

justify the potential discomfort and hazards of the treatment.
4. The patient has sufficient home support and is medically stable enough to be managed effectively and safely at home.

It is controversial whether patients with moderate (15 to 25 percent weight loss) or severe (>25 percent weight loss) malnutrition, secondary to an inadequate oral intake but without primary dysphagia or a major absorption problem, should also qualify for tube enteral nutrition. This category includes patients with dementia or metabolic disorders leading to profound anorexia. Probably the issue is best resolved by studies that determine if the tube enteral support in such clinical situations enhances quality of life and reduces nutrition-related complications and hence medical cost.

Technical Aspects

The home enteral patient frequently receives treatment for months or years and may plan to return to the work force while receiving tube feedings on a full- or part-time basis. In such circumstances the technical aspects of the treatment must be cosmetically acceptable, comfortable, and compatible with normal activity.

HEN patients who are sustained by overnight intragastric feeding may elect to intubate themselves each evening with a nasogastric tube.[1-4] Such an approach requires a simple, small-bore tube that can easily be slipped in and out, washed, and reused. For this purpose an 8-F polyvinyl chloride tube that stiffens modestly with ice water is usually superior to a weighted Silastic tube that depends on a wire introducer. Learning the self-intubation technique requires the support of an experienced professional. Most patients feel competent after inserting their tube successfully three or four times.

The majority of long-term HEN patients prefer permanent access through a tube placed percutaneously intragastrically, through the stomach into the jejunum or directly into the jejunum. Such tubes may be inserted surgically, endoscopically, or radiologically, and once the enterocutaneous tract is well established, the enteral access tube can frequently be replaced by a "button," a device that lies flush with the abdominal wall (Fig. 30–1) and is more comfortable and cosmetically acceptable to the long-term patient.[5,6] The gastric button has been widely used, but accessing the jejunum through a "button" is relatively new. Gorman and colleagues[7] recently reported a randomized study comparing 21 patients fed through a jejunostomy button with 21 patients fed through a traditional red rubber jejunostomy catheter. The mean follow-up time was 39 ± 7 days for the button group and 43 ± 13 days for the standard jejunostomy group. There were significantly fewer problems in the button group (n = 1) compared with the tube group (n = 8). The problems related chiefly to tube dislodgment or occlusion; one patient in each group had a peritubular leak.

For home use, compact portable home pumps allow the greatest mobility. Some examples are listed in Table 30–1, however, this is an evolving technology, and simpler models with lighter rechargeable batteries can be expected. The nutrient formulas and infusion pump can be carried in a small back or waist pack, allowing the patient unfettered mobility. With such equipment, tube enteral feeding can be delivered around the clock and at the work site if necessary.

With increasing pressures for rapid, early hospital discharge, patients are often sent home for tube feeding with inadequate instruction, which can lead to costly readmissions. Many hospitals are developing a patient learning service[8,9] where the patient and family receive instruction in a range of complex technologies now delivered at home. Many such services have developed an array of good teaching materials that they are willing to share with other professionals. A list of materials collated by Evans and coworkers,[10] which are pertinent to patients and families learning about HEN, are listed in Table 30–2.

PSYCHOSOCIAL SUPPORT FOR HEN PATIENTS

Despite many user-friendly improvements in the equipment and technology for delivering effective HEN, it is still psychologically and physically a very stressful undertaking for patients and their families. There is often the social loss of normal eating, discomfort from the tube, and gastrointestinal (GI) symptoms of nausea, bloating, and cramping, which may lead to vomiting and diarrhea. Using a disturbed gut is in many ways more of a challenge than parenteral feeding, albeit safer and much less expensive. In addition, for young patients there is a disruption of body image, since feeding tubes are seen in many respects as akin to an ostomy.

Patient-to-patient support, first receiving it and then giving it, can make a substantial difference. This grass-roots support may be available in large nutrition support programs and is available nationally through the Oley Founda-

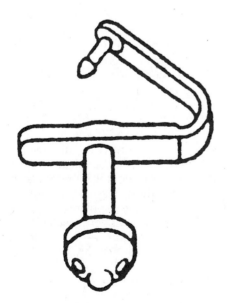

FIGURE 30–1 Example of an enteral feeding tube button, which can be used for both gastrostomy and jejunostomy access.

TABLE 30–1   Examples of Enteral Feeding Pumps

Name	Flow Rate (ml/hour)	Manufacturer	Comments
Clintec 2200 volume	1–295	Clintec Nutrition	Memory for flow rate, dose, delivered, alarm for low battery, battery on, dose complete, occlusion/empty
Corflo 300	1–300	Corpak Inc	Tracks volume infused on each shift, rates and amounts stored in memory for 24 hours, alarms for free flow, dose limit, low battery, occlusion/empty
EP85	1–295	Elan Pharma	Records and displays accumulated amount of formula delivered over several feedings, alarms for free flow, occlusion/empty, dose complete, low battery
Rate Saver Plus	0–300	EntraCare Corp	Has set detection and set security features, alarms for no flow, set out, dose complete, system error, low battery
Flexiflo 111	1–300	Ross Products Division, Abbott	Easy to use touch controls. Flexiflo Companion available for portable use. Flexiflo Quantum has automatic flushing feature
Compat	1–295	Sandoz Nutrition	Model #199235: memory for infusion rate, dose limit, volume delivered and accumulated, alarms for low battery, occlusion/empty, dose complete, free flow, rate change Model #199225: infusion rate and volume constantly displayed. Alarm features as above

tion, which supports patients receiving home parenteral and enteral nutrition[11] through the *Lifeline Letter,* a regional coordinator network and annual consumer conference.

PREVALENCE AND GROWTH OF HEN IN THE UNITED STATES

This information is not accurately known for the general population, since there are no national requirements to report to some central source all patients initiated on HEN.

Nonetheless prevalence and growth can be estimated from two large data bases, the Medicare common working file and the North American Home Parenteral and Enteral Nutrition Patient Registry.[12] In 1989 there were 34,000 Medicare HEN patients, and this number increased 25 percent per year so that by 1992 there were 73,000 Medicare HEN patients. In 1992 Medicare was the primary payor for 48 percent of the HEN patients reported to the Registry; therefore the total HEN population that year was about 152,000 patients.

Between 1989 and 1992 the yearly Medicare HEN prevalence averaged 1660 per million

Medicare population.[13] However, Medicare prevalence exaggerates the prevalence in the general population, for although about half of all HEN patients have Medicare as their primary payor, Medicare beneficiaries represent only 13 percent of the population.[14] In other words, Medicare prevalence overestimates HEN prevalence in the general population by a factor of four. This means that between 1989 and 1992 HEN prevalence in the general population was about 415 per million.[13]

A rather similar usage frequency was found in a farming community in Minnesota.[15] In Olmsted County all endoscopically and surgically placed enteral feeding tubes must be reported. In 1988 there were 550 enterostomy procedures per million population.

HEN prevalence has been reported by only one other western country—Great Britain. The British Association for Parenteral and Enteral Nutrition estimates an HEN prevalence of 50 to 60 per 1 million population in 1992, and this use appears to be growing about 20 percent per year.[16] The much higher U.S. prevalence may reflect in part a methodologic difference. In the United States the Medicare data mea-

TABLE 30–2   HEN Patient Education Materials

Name of Publication	Source	Comment
ALS: Maintaining Nutrition	MD Anderson ALS Center, Houston, TX	Audience: general $6/copy
Care of the Pediatric Nasogastric Tube	Cooper Hospital/University Medical Center, Camden, NJ	Audience: pediatric $5/copy
Caring for your Child with a Gastrostomy	University of Wisconsin Hospital & Clinics, Madison	Audience: pediatric $5/copy
Giving Tube Feeds at Home	Nebraska Methodist Hospital,	Audience: general $10/copy
Home Enteral Nutrition Training Manual	Virginia Mason Medical Center, Seattle, WA	Audience: RD, Adult HEN $25/copy
Home Tube Feeding Guide	Food & Nutriton Dept, University of Washington Medical Center, Seattle	Audience: general $3.50/copy
Home Tube Feeding in Five Steps	Nutrition Support Services, LDS Hospital, Salt Lake City	Audience: adult $75/kit
Home Tube Feeding Manual	Cooper Hospital/University Medical Center, Camden, NJ	Audience: general $5/copy
Home Tube Feeding Patient Information	Foothills Hospital, Calgary, Alberta, Canada	Audience: general $15/copy
Home Tube Feedings	Emory University Hospital, Altanta, GA	$12.50/copy
Kangaroo Home Tube Feedings: Practical Tips and Techniques	Sherwood Medical Company, St Louis, MO	Complimentary
Mastering the Technique of Tube Feeding at Home	Ross Laboratories, Columbus OH	Call for information, 800-227-5767
Nasogastric Feeding	UC Davis Medical Center, Sacramento, CA	$2/copy
Nasogastric Intubation	Bristol Myers Company, Mead Johnson Nutritionals, Evansville, IN	Complimentary
Patient Care Manual	Wilson Cook Medical Co, Winston-Salem, NC	Call for information, 800-245-4717
Trouble Shooting Guide	Sandoz Nutrition, East Hanover, NJ	Call for information, 800-321-3559. Video also available
Tube Feeding at Home	Bristol Myers Company, Mead Johnson Nutritonals, Evansville, IN	Complimentary
Tube Feeding Instructions for Home	Cleveland Clinic Foundation, Cleveland, OH	Audience: general $9.75/copy
Tube Feeding Your Child at Home	Ross Laboratories, Columbus, OH	Call for information, 800-227-5767
What is Enteral Nutrition	ASPEN	Audience: general $35/100 members, $45/100 non members
Your Guide to Home Tube Feeding	Clintec Nutrition Company, Deerfield, IL	Audience: general Complimentary

Adapted from Evans MA, Czopek S: Home nutrition support materials. Nutr Clin Pract 1995;10:37–39. With permission.

sured "period" prevalence, or the number of HEN patients per year. The British study measured "point" prevalence, or the number of HEN patients during a specific month. Since data show that the average Medicare patient stays on HEN only 70 days, "point" prevalence would be four or five times lower than "period" prevalence. This adjustment would bring the British use much closer to the U.S. use.

COST OF HEN THERAPY

Although HEN costs approximately one tenth of home parenteral nutrition (HPN),[13] until the late 1980s HEN was often inadequately reimbursed while HPN was generously reimbursed. The reason for this discrepancy may have been that classic tube feeding, done for many decades with a large-bore rubber catheter using boluses of home-blended tube feed, was relatively inexpensive, and the cost of more modern equipment, commercial nutrient solutions, and portable infusion pumps may have been deemed unnecessarily expensive and elaborate by the payors. However, once it became clear that this improved technology was associated with more substantial rehabilitation and could sometimes substitute for more costly HPN, HEN reimbursement significantly improved.

Between 1989 and 1992 the number of Medicare HEN beneficiaries doubled (34,000 to 73,000) but the dollars paid for HEN by Medicare almost tripled, increasing from $47 million to $137 million. These dollars paid were 80 percent of the allowable charge. As shown in Table 30–3, in 1992 the Medicare allowable charge for HEN ranged from $25 to $50 a day, depending on the formula prescribed. The average allowable charge was $33 a day, which included the nutrient formula, dressing kit, administration set, and pump loan. A HEN therapy cost of $33 a day translates into a yearly cost of $12,000/patient/year.

Although parenteral nutrition delivered at home saves 50 to 75 percent of the cost of providing parenteral nutrition in hospital, enteral nutrition at home saves 90 to 95 percent of the in-hospital cost. Because these major savings are reaped by shifting care and support from the expensive hospital setting to the patient's home and family, some nursing support in the home and respite care in long-term situations are probably cost-effective considerations.

TABLE 30–3 Medicare Allowable Charges (Dollars per Day) for HEN Therapy in 1992*

Tube-feeding formula	10–35
Dressing kit	0.5–2.0
Administration set	11
Pump loan	3.6
Mean[†] (Range)	33 (25–50)

*Medicare paid 80% of these allowable charges.
[†]The mean daily Medicare allowable charge was calculated from actual Medicare reimbursement of 1000 Medicare HEN patient days to five large nutrition support programs. This mean daily reimbursement was increased from 80 to 100% to derive the mean daily Medicare allowable charge.

If one assumes that the Medicare allowable charge was an average reimbursement from all primary insurance payors in the United States, then the national cost of all HEN in 1992 was about one third of $1 billion. These dollars only covered direct therapy costs and did not cover costs related to home nursing, physician supervision, laboratory monitoring, or the cost of treatment related to therapy complications. Nor did they include tube enteral feeding costs in nursing homes, where there were approximately an equal number of tube-fed patients.

DISEASE SPECTRUM OF PATIENTS USING HEN

Although involvement in the national Registry is voluntary and hence the reported clinical experience is not drawn from a randomized sample of patients, the experience described comes from a large and widely dispersed geographic sample.[12] Over 8 years (1985 to 1992) 217 nutrition support programs across the United States have described the longitudinal outcome of more than 12,000 patients receiving home nutrition support. Only patients entered in the Registry at the beginning of their therapy were used for outcome analysis, since with these patients their entire clinical course was known, through to their last follow-up report. The Registry has 9565 such patients, 4084 receiving HEN and 5481 receiving HPN. The higher fraction of HPN patients in the Registry sample is contrary to estimates of national HEN/HPN prevalence in which HEN patients are three to four times more common.[13] This discrepancy may reflect the fact that HEN therapy is prescribed and supervised by many physician specialists, while HPN therapy is more commonly under the jurisdiction of medical nutrition specialists, who have been the chief source of Registry information.

As shown in Figure 30–2, the two largest disease categories in which HPEN was used were neoplasm (43 percent) and neuromuscular swallowing disorders (29 percent). The different diagnoses resulting in small bowel disease and malabsorption collectively accounted for 12 percent, while all other diseases accounted for 16 percent. This latter category included many patients whose nutritional depletion was secondary to an inadequate oral intake rather than primary dysphagia or a major absorption problem. Examples were patients with a psychological or cognitive disorder such as anorexia nervosa or dementia, patients with a severe metabolic disturbance leading to anorexia such as

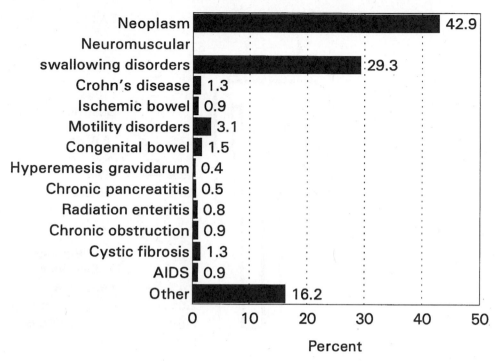

FIGURE 30–2 The distribution of diagnoses in new patients on HEN reported to the North American HPEN Registry from 1985 to 1992. The values shown were percentages of the total for each category (N = 4084).

renal or liver failure, and patients whose food intake was inadequate due to extreme dyspnea as in chronic obstructive pulmonary disease.

CLINICAL OUTCOME WITH HEN THERAPY

The single most important factor influencing the clinical outcome for any patient receiving HEN is the primary underlying disease, because fewer than 5 percent of deaths of patients receiving HEN are attributed to a complication of the nutrition therapy.[17]

The following sections focus on disease-specific outcome studies from both the Registry and other sources. In the Registry, clinical outcome was assessed by four parameters: (1) survival during therapy, (2) status 1 year after starting HEN, (3) rehabilitation status as judged by the supervising professional, and (4) complication rates per patient year that resulted in rehospitalization.

HEN in Cancer Patients

The Registry has outcome information on 1644 HEN patients with a neoplasm (Table 30–4). As shown in Figure 30–3, most neo-

TABLE 30–4 HEN Clinical Outcome in Patients of All Ages with Cancer

Number of patients	1644
Average (SD) age in years	61 (17)
Survival on HEN*	
Percentage at 12 months ± SEM	25 ± 2
Expected survival	
Percentage at 12 months	97
Rehabilitation status	
Percentage at 12 months ± SEM	
Complete	21 ± 3
Partial	59 ± 3
Minimal	21 ± 3
HEN therapy status	
Percentage at 12 months ± SEM	
Resume oral intake	30 ± 2
Continue HEN	6 ± 1
Died	59 ± 2
Complication rates	
Rehospitalizations/patient year	
HEN related	0.4
Non-HEN related	2.7

SD = standard deviation; SEM = standard error of the mean.
*Survival rates on therapy are values at 1 year, calculated by the life-table method.
Data from Oley Foundation, Albany, NY.

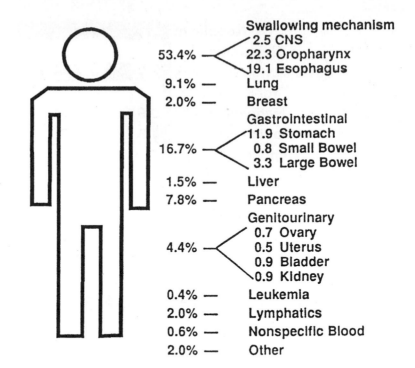

FIGURE 30–3 The primary tumor sites of active cancer patients receiving HEN. The frequency of tumor site is reported as a percent.

Swallowing mechanism
53.4% — 2.5 CNS / 22.3 Oropharynx / 19.1 Esophagus
9.1% — Lung
2.0% — Breast
Gastrointestinal
16.7% — 11.9 Stomach / 0.8 Small Bowel / 3.3 Large Bowel
1.5% — Liver
7.8% — Pancreas
Genitourinary
4.4% — 0.7 Ovary / 0.5 Uterus / 0.9 Bladder / 0.9 Kidney
0.4% — Leukemia
2.0% — Lymphatics
0.6% — Nonspecific Blood
2.0% — Other

plasms interfered with chewing, swallowing, or gastric outflow. For those who stayed on therapy, half were dead at 4 months but 25 percent lived beyond 1 year (Fig. 30–4). After 1 year, 30 percent of those who started treatment had resumed full oral nutrition. The majority of surviving patients experienced partial rehabilitation, which implied some limitation of age-appropriate activities.

Rehospitalization was common but principally for non-HEN related complications. Information provided to the Registry about tumor type and specifics of the oncologic therapy received by these patients was limited. However, Figure 30–5 compares the therapy status for different tumor sites at 1 year and shows that patients with leukemias and lymphomas had the best survival.[17] In fact, many patients probably had treatable disease and HEN was required only through a period of aggressive oncologic treatment. Szeluga and associates showed that enteral nutrition in hospitalized bone marrow transplant patients can be as effective as total parenteral nutrition (TPN).[18] Some bone marrow transplant patients must continue enteral tube feeding at home while their bowel slowly recovers.

Most cancer patients with upper GI obstruction can be fed by a gastrostomy, but others have gastric outlet obstruction and require a jejunostomy. In experienced centers percutaneous endoscopic gastrostomies (PEGs) and jejunostomies (PEJs) can be performed under local anesthetic in an endoscopy suite, avoiding hospitalization, abdominal surgery, or the discomfort of a nasogastric tube.[19-21] In 42 patients with head and neck cancers and severe dysphagia, Shike and colleagues[20] were successful in placing a feeding PEG or PEJ in 39 patients. In three patients the procedure was technically impossible. The only complications were local skin site infections, all of which responded to antibiotics. None of the patients developed peritonitis, and just one patient experienced aspiration pneumonia. Shike's group also described bypassing obstructive esophageal or gastric outlet tumors with an external shunt.[22] Such patients may tolerate an oral liquid diet, making home management relatively simple.

Gibson and Wenig[19] described the benefit of routine preoperative placement of a PEG in 89 patients with advanced (stage III and IV) head and neck cancer who were undergoing primary resection. The complication rate associated with the PEG was 5 percent. The hospital stay of the PEG patients was reduced by 61 percent compared with control patients receiving standard nasogastric feedings. This difference reached statistical significance for tumors involving the larynx and pharynx.

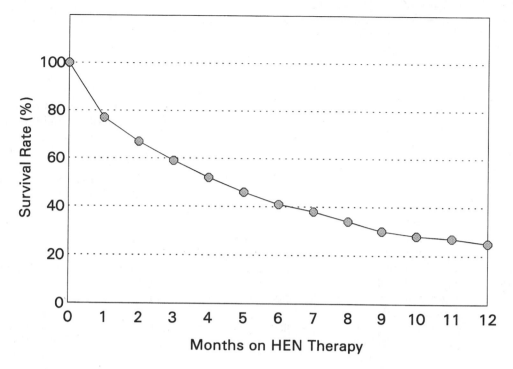

FIGURE 30–4 Survival rates on HEN for patients with active cancer. The expected survival rate at 12 months for age- and sex-matched individuals in the general U. S. population is 97 percent.

Tumor type

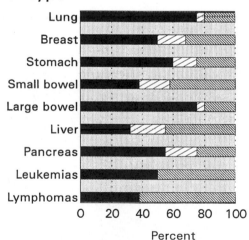

FIGURE 30–5 Therapy status of HEN patients with active cancer of different primary sites 12 months after starting HEN. Each horizontal bar shows the percent of patients who resumed oral intake (▨), remained on HEN (▨), or died (■).

Campos and colleagues[23] described the EN outcome in 39 patients with advanced upper GI head and neck cancer. Ten patients (25 percent) died of their disease before they could be discharged. Median survival was 5.5 months, and median HEN support was for 3 months. Four patients (10 percent) resumed full oral nutrition, and their gastrostomies were removed. A quarter of the patients were never readmitted, a quarter were readmitted once, and half were readmitted twice or more.

Sami and colleagues described HEN in 12 patients, 10 with head and neck cancer and 2 with traumatic esophageal perforation who were followed for 30 to 435 days.[24] During this period most patients felt they had an improved quality of life related to their nutrition support, and there were no therapy-related readmissions.

The decision whether to offer some form of nutrition to patients whose swallowing or bowel function is compromised by an untreatable, rapidly progressive tumor is difficult.[25] A recent report evaluated the role of nutrition and hydration in 32 patients with a life expectancy of 3 months or less and found that they rarely experienced hunger and thirst. There was no evidence that food and fluid, beyond that requested by the patient, contributed to the patient's comfort.[26]

To most physicians, nutrition support in untreatable cancer is appropriate if the patient wants such treatment and it seems likely that the patient will survive beyond 3 months and experience a reasonable quality of life. Since HEN is safer than HPN, such an approach is easier to justify.

HEN in Patients with a Neuromuscular Disorder of Swallowing

The Registry has outcome information on 1134 patients with dysphagia due to neuromuscular disorders unrelated to cancer. For most of these patients the dysphagia was secondary to a cerebrovascular accident or stroke. However a few adult patients had other diseases such as muscular dystrophy, motor neuron disease, and sclerodema, whereas young adults and children had developmental disabilities such as pharyngeal dysfunction associated with cerebral palsy or a syndrome of cricopharyngeal incoordination or micrognathia.

Because dysphagia due to a neuromuscular disorder is a classic indication for tube enteral nutrition, the quality of the clinical outcome in this setting has important implications. In this respect the overall measures of HEN outcome documented by the Registry were disappointing; the median survival was

18 months, with only 19 percent of patients resuming full oral nutrition and 75 percent experiencing minimal rehabilitation.[12] Since two thirds of these patients were 65 years or older, a group in whom the stroke diagnosis predominated, it seemed probable that extensive neurologic damage accompanied the dysphagia, limiting overall rehabilitation.

To evaluate the outcome for younger patients with perhaps a greater rehabilitation potential, a separate analysis was undertaken of patients under 25 years. This cohort was compared with patients 65 years and over (Figure 30–6, Table 30–5). As this breakdown shows, younger patients have a more encouraging prognosis, with 89 percent surviving beyond 1 year on therapy and 54 percent experiencing complete or partial rehabilitation. This better outcome occurred despite the fact that these younger individuals also had a continuing need for HEN. The HEN therapy complications resulting in rehospitalization were infrequent and similar in both young and old patients, reemphasizing the relative safety of this therapy. For patients 65 years and older the clinical outcome was sufficiently dismal that more in-depth quality of life studies are needed to determine when HEN is really a

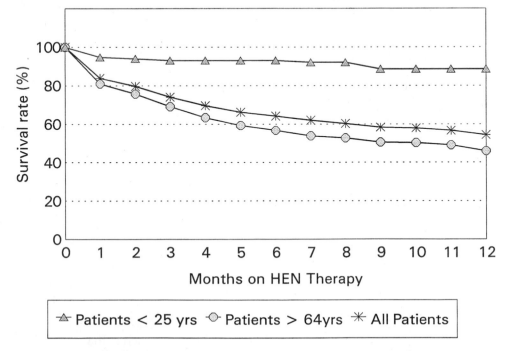

FIGURE 30–6 Survival rates on HEN for patients with neuromuscular disorders of swallowing. The three survival curves represent all age groups (*), patients less than 25 years old (△), and patients greater than 64 years old (○). The expected survival rate at 12 monhts for age- and sex-matched individuals in the general U.S. population for these three groups is 95 percent, 99.6 percent, and 93 percent, respectively.

TABLE 30–5 Neuromuscular Disorders of Swallowing: HEN Clinical Outcome Measures by Age Group

	All Ages	Under 25	65 and Over
Number of patients	1134	146	787
Female:Male	587:547	60:86	436:351
Average (SD) age in years	65 (26)	6 (6)	79 (8)
Survival on HEN*			
Percentage at 12 months ± SEM	54 ± 2	89 ± 4	46 ± 3
Expected survival (%)	95	99	93
Rehabilitation status			
Percentage at 12 months ± SEM			
Complete	4 ± 1	15 ± 1	2[†]
Partial	20 ± 3	39 ± 1	12 ± 3
Minimal	76 ± 3	46 ± 1	86 ± 3
HEN therapy status			
Percentage at 12 months ± SEM			
Resume oral intake	19 ± 1	23 ± 5	17 ± 2
Continue HEN	27 ± 2	59 ± 5	21 ± 2
Died	46 ± 2	14 ± 4	53 ± 2
Complication rates			
Rehospitalizations/patient year			
HEN related	0.29	0.27	0.34
Non-HEN related	0.91	0.95	0.94

SD = standard deviation; SEM = standard error of the mean.
*Survival rates on therapy are values at 1 year, calculated by the life-table method.
[†]Numbers too small to calculate SEM.
Data from Oley Foundation, Albany, NY.

sound recommendation to these patients and their families.

Other investigators have arrived at similar conclusions. Wolfsen and colleagues[27] described the outcome and long-term survival of 191 patients undergoing PEG or PEJ using a retrospective chart review. The majority of the patients (64 percent) had neuromuscular disorders of swallowing, usually due to a stroke, and the rest had cancer. One third of the patients were dead within 60 days, and 50 percent were dead after 6 months. None of the mortality was related to the tube feeding. These authors question the appropriateness of initiating tube feeding in these patients given their limited survival.

The follow-up study of Olmsted County, MN, residents with PEGs and PEJs[15,28] also found that 50 percent of patients with dysphagia and stroke were dead in 4 months. Again, most deaths were due to the underlying disease, not to a complication of HEN.

In contrast, Moran and Frost[29] described the outcome in 41 patients referred for a PEG; 75 percent of these patients had a neuromuscular disorder of swallowing. There were two therapy-related complications, one failed insertion and one peritubular infection. A third of the patients died at a mean of 3 months, but a third resumed oral nutrition, allowing tube removal. These authors felt the gastrostomy feedings may have speeded the recovery of speech and swallowing in those patients who recovered from their stroke.

HEN in Patients with Impaired Small Bowel Absorption

One in eight of the HEN patients reported to the Registry had small-bowel disease and severe malabsorption rather than a swallowing disorder. This is clearly a somewhat different challenge and it therefore seemed important to examine the clinical outcome for this group of patients. Because the number of patients in a particular diagnostic group was relatively small, HEN patients with Crohn's disease (52), ischemic bowel disease (37), motility disorders (120), congenital bowel defects (61), radiation enteritis (30), and other nonmalignant causes of short-bowel syndrome (29) were combined for this analysis. The total number was 329 patients, with an average age of 36 years. For those who stayed on therapy, over 80 percent survived 1 year (Fig. 30–7). At 1 year 45 percent of those who started treatment had resumed full oral nutrition and 85 percent had experienced complete or partial rehabilita-

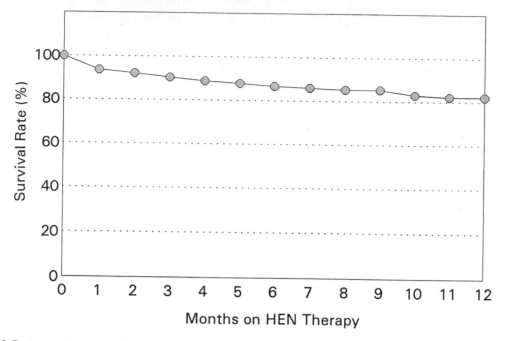

FIGURE 30–7   Survival rates on HEN for patients with impaired small-bowel absorption. The expected survival rate at 12 months for age- and sex-matched individuals in the general U.S. population is 99 percent.

tion. A HEN-related complication resulted in re-hospitalization once every 2 years on average. Rehospitalization for a disease-related complication was two to three times a year (Table 30–6).

In summary, patients with malabsorption requiring HEN had a good prognosis. Patients in these same disease categories also have good survival when they require HPN.[13] However, HPN was associated with double the frequency of nutrition support complications and was ten times more expensive. For these reasons enteral therapy appears superior to parenteral therapy when medically feasible.

For the patient with short-bowel syndrome who is receiving long-term HEN, concerns exist not only about absorption of fluids and major substrates (calories and protein) but also about divalent cations (calcium, magnesium, copper, zinc), fat-soluble vitamins (vitamins A, D, E, and K) and vitamin B_{12}. The patient's mineral and vitamin status must be monitored once or twice a year.

Tamura et al[30] described a case report of a patient who, after receiving a defined formula diet for 19 months, developed normocytic anemia and neutropenia due to copper deficiency. The tube feeding provided 2.6 to 5.1 µmol copper/day. When the patient's copper intake was increased to 34 µmol/day his hematological abnormalities resolved.

Normal vitamin levels were reported from 8 patients receiving long-term enteral feeding

TABLE 30–6   HEN Clinical Outcome for Patients of All Ages with Impaired Small Bowel Absorption

Number of patients	329
Average (SD) age in years	36 (17)
Survival on HEN*	
Percentage at 12 months ± SEM	82 ± 4
Expected survival	
Percentage at 12 months	99
Rehabilitation status	
Percentage at 12 months ± SEM	
Complete	43 ± 6
Partial	42 ± 6
Minimal	15 ± 4
HEN therapy status	
Percentage at 12 months ± SEM	
Resume oral intake	45 ± 3
Continue HEN	28 ± 3
Died	17 ± 3
Complication rates	
Rehospitalizations/patient year	
HEN related	0.4
Non-HEN related	2.7

SD = standard deviation; SEM = standard error of the mean.
*Survival rates on therapy are values at 1 year, calculated by the life-table method.
Data from Oley Foundation, Albany, NY.

when the level of vitamin supplementation provided by the enteral formula was modestly in excess of the recommended daily intake.[31]

HEN Therapy for Other Disorders

Cystic Fibrosis

Cystic fibrosis is commonly associated with undernutrition and failure to thrive. The malnutrition has multiple causes, but primarily relates to an inadequate nutrient intake in relation to the increased metabolic requirements associated with the disease. Chronic undernutrition leading to loss of muscle mass and impaired immunocompetence may contribute to worsening of pulmonary function.[32] A number of reports describe a positive outcome associated with supplemental HEN feeding in this patient population.[32-38]

Acquired Immunodeficiency Syndrome

Weight loss is a common presenting complaint in individuals infected with the human immunodeficiency virus (HIV). Because disease involvement of the GI tract either with the virus itself or with opportunistic organisms is frequent, enteral nutrition support, although safer than parenteral feeding, presents a major technical challenge. Kotler and colleagues[39] described the outcome of a prospective study in 8 acquired immunodeficiency syndrome (AIDS) patients designed to assess the feasibility, tolerance, and efficacy of enteral feeding. These patients received a defined formula diet (Reabilan, O'Brien Pharmaceuticals Inc.) through an endoscopically placed gastrostomy tube. During the first month of therapy they received 500 kcal/day above their predicted basal energy expenditure, adjusted for a 20 percent stress factor. Subsequently the feeding was increased by 150 kcal every other day to the limit of their tolerance for a 1-month period. Five patients continued enteral feeding for 4 to 32 weeks. In the first month three stopped feeding and returned to oral intake. The survival probability at 6 months was 50 percent, and three patients were alive at 14 months. Enteral feeding was well tolerated and was associated with a 14 percent increase in total body potassium. Serum albumin, transferrin, and body fat also increased. Patients noted an overall improvement in their health status, particularly their mental function, which they attributed to tube feeding.

AIDS is a very costly disease, and thus a randomized study of enteral support early in the weight-loss phase seems justified to address more clearly issues of HEN feasibility and effectiveness.

Chronic Renal Failure

Severe malnutrition occurs in at least 15 percent of patient receiving chronic dialysis. This is a multifactorial problem, but principal issues are impaired intake and increased losses into the dialysate. Poor intake is chiefly due to a profound anorexia caused by the metabolic derangements of renal failure. A few patients have a motility disturbance, leading to bacterial overgrowth and malabsorption that may respond to cyclic antibiotics. The motility disturbance may be due to uremia and underdialysis or to a visceral neuropathy or ischemia related to underlying diabetes or some other primary disease.

HEN is one of many strategies used to improve nutritional depletion in these patients. The reports of successful HEN are chiefly in children, in whom chronic malnutrition also leads to distressing growth failure.[40-43] A gastrostomy tube has been used in children receiving both hemodialysis and continuous cycling peritoneal dialysis. In these children HEN not only restored growth,[41] it also reduced the frequency of peritonitis[42] and improved the outcome for renal transplantation.[43,44] Reports have examined the special hazards of HEN in this population.[45,46]

ETHICAL ISSUES

Ethical issues regarding the provision or withdrawal of enteral nutrition support are often difficult. It has been legally determined that tube enteral nutrition is active treatment and not just supportive care. Because tube enteral nutrition is active medical treatment, it can be withheld if providing such treatment is deemed inappropriate[47] and not beneficial to the patient. Some of these difficult decisions can be made easier for the patient, family, and health care provider if the patient has an advance medical directive or living will.

REFERENCES

1. Fitzpatrick WW Sr: Profile: William W. Fitzpatrick, Jr. Part I Lifeline Letter XV:(1):3. Part 2 Lifeline PS 3:(1): 2–3. Albany, NY: Oley Foundation, 1994.
2. Fitzpatrick WW Jr: The pros and cons of tube feeding. Lifeline Letter. Albany, NY: Oley Foundation, 1994;XV: 5–4.
3. Howard L, Bigaouette J, Goodman AD et al: Enhanced calcium requirements in a child with type I glycogen storage disease on frequent enteral feeding therapy. The Proceedings of the International Society of Parenteral Nutrition, Acta Chir Scand, 1979;494(suppl):88–91.
4. Aiges H, Markewitz J, Rosa J et al: Home nocturnal supplemental nasogastric feedings in growth retarded adolescents with Crohn's disease. Gastroenterology 1989;97:905–910.
5. Baskin WN: Advances in enteral nutrition techniques. Am J Gastroenterol 1992;87(11):1547–1553.
6. Payne J: Enteral nutrition: accessing patients. Nutrition 1992;8:223–231.
7. Gorman RC, Morris JB, Metz CA et al: The button jejunostomy for long term jejunal feeding: results of a prospective randomized trial. J Parenter Enteral Nutr 1993;17:428–431.

8. Sumpmann M: An education center for patient's high-tech learning needs. Patient Ed Counsel 1989;13:309–323.

9. Goldstein N: Patient learning center reduces patient readmissions. Patient Ed Counsel 1991;17:177–190.

10. Evans MA, Czopek S: Home nutrition support materials. Nutr Clin Pract 1995;10:37–39.

11. Oley Foundation for Home Parenteral and Enteral Nutrition: 214 Hun Memorial, A-23, Albany Medical Center, Albany, NY 12208. (518)262-5079,(800)776-OLEY.

12. North American Home Parenteral and Enteral Nutrition Patient Registry Annual Reports 1985–1992, published 1988 to 1994. Albany, NY: Oley Foundation.

13. Howard L, Ament M, Fleming CR et al: Current use and clinical outcome of home parenteral and enteral nutrition therapies in the United States. Gastroenterology 1995;109:355–365.

14. US Bureau of the Census Statistical Abstract of the United States 1994, 114th edition. Washington, DC: US Government Printing Office, 1994.

15. Bergstrom L, Larson D, Zinsmeister A et al: Utilization and outcomes of surgical gastrostomies and jejunostomies in an era of percutaneous endoscopic gastrostomy: a population-based study of outcome. 19th Clinical ASPEN Congress. 1995;19(1, suppl):52.

16. Elia M (chairman and editor): Enteral and Parenteral Nutrition in the Community. A Report by a Working Party of the British Association for Parenteral and Enteral Nutrition (BAPEN). BAPEN POB 922 Maidenhead Berks SL6 4 SH, 1994.

17. Howard L: Home parenteral and enteral nutrition in cancer patients. Cancer 1993;72(11, suppl):3531–3541.

18. Szeluga DJ, Stuart RK, Brook Meyer R et al: Nutritional support of bone marrow transplant recipients. A prospective randomized clinical trial comparing total parenteral nutrition to an enteral nutrition program. Cancer Res 1987;47:3309–3316.

19. Gisbon S, Wenig BL: Percutaneous endoscopic gastrostomy in the management of head and neck carcinoma. Laryngoscope 1992;103(9):977–980.

20. Shike M, Berner YN, Gerdes H et al: Percutaneous endoscopic gastrostomy and jejunostomy in patients with cancer of the head and neck. Otolaryngol Head Neck Surg 1989;101(5):549–554.

21. Shike M, Schroy P, Morse R et al: Percutaneous endoscopic jejunostomy in cancer patients with previous gastric resection. Gastrointest Endosc 1987;33:373–374.

22. Shike M, Wallach C, Bloch A: Combined gastric drainage-jejunal feeding through a percutaneous endoscopic stoma. Gastrointest Endosc 1990;36:290–299.

23. Campos AC, Butters M, Meguid MM: Home enteral nutrition via gastrostomy in advanced head and neck cancer patients. Head Neck 1990;12(2):137–142.

24. Sami H, Saint-Aubert B, Szawlowski AW et al: Home enteral nutrition system: one patient, one daily ration of an "all in one" sterile and modular formula in a single container. J Parenter Enteral Nutr 1990;14:173–176.

25. Howard L, Malone M: What factors determine the appropriateness of home parenteral and enteral nutrition in the cancer patient? Home Care Consult 1994;1:18–27.

26. McCann RM, Hall WJ, Groth-Juncker A: Comfort care for terminally ill patients. The appropriate use of nutrition and hydration. JAMA 1994;272:1263–1266.

27. Wolfsen HC, Kozarek RA, Ball TJ et al: Long term survival in patients undergoing percutaneous endoscopic gastrostomy and jejunostomy. Am J Gastroenterol 1990;85(9):1120–1122.

28. Taylor CA, Larson DE, Ballard DJ et al: Predictors of outcome after percutaneous endoscopic gastrostomy: a community-based study. Mayo Clin Proc 1992;67:1042–1049.

29. Moran BJ, Frost RA: Percutaneous endoscopic gastrostomy in 41 patients: indications and clinical outcome. J R Soc Med 1992;85(6):320–321.

30. Tamura H, Hirose S, Watanabe O et al: Anemia and neutropenia due to copper deficiency in enteral nutrition. J Parenteral Enteral Nutr 1994;18:185–189.

31. Berner Y, Morse R, Frank O et al: Vitamin plasma levels in long term enteral feeding patients. J Parenter Enteral Nutr 1989;13(5):525–528.

32. Durie PR, Pencharz PB: Cystic fibrosis: nutrition. Br Med Bull 1992;48:823–846.

33. Park RH, Galloway A, Russell RI et al: Home Sweet HEN—a guide to home enteral nutrition. Br J Clin Pract 1992;46(2):105–110.

34. Dalzell AM, Shepherd RW, Dean B et al: Nutritional rehabilitation in cystic fibrosis: a 5 year follow-up study. J Pediatr Gastroenterol Nutr 1992;15(2):141–145.

35. Booth IW: The nutritional consequences of gastrointestinal disease in adolescence. Acta Pediatr Scand Suppl 1991;373:91–102.

36. MacDonald A, Holden C, Harris G: Nutritional strategies in cystic fibrosis: current issues. J Royal Soc Med 1991;84(suppl 18):28–35.

37. Steinkamp G, Rodeck B, Seidenberg J et al: Stabilization of lung function in cystic fibrosis during long term feeding via a percutaneous endoscopic gastrostomy. Pneumologie 1990;44(10):1151–1153.

38. Gaskin KJ, Waters DL, Baur LA et al: Nutritional status, growth and development in children undergoing intensive treatment for cystic fibrosis. Acta Pediatr Scand Suppl 1990;366:106–110.

39. Kotler DP, Tierney AR, Ferraro R et al: Enteral alimentation and repletion of body cell mass in malnourished patients with acquired immunodeficiency syndrome. Am J Clin Nutr 1991;53(1):149–154.

40. Enia G, Sicuso C, Alati G et al: Subjective global assessment of nutrition in dialysis patients. Nephrol Dial Transplant 1993;8(10):1094–1098.

41. Watson AR, Coleman JE, Taylor EA: Gastrostomy buttons for feeding children on continuous cycling peritoneal dialysis. Adv Periton Dial 1992;8:391–395.

42. Dabbagh S, Fassinger N, Clement K et al: The effect of aggressive nutrition on infection rates in patients maintained on peritoneal dialysis. Adv Periton Dial 1991;7:161–164.

43. Brewer ED: Growth of small children managed with chronic peritoneal dialysis and nasogastric tube feedings: 203 month experience in 14 patients. Adv Periton Dial 1990;6:269–272.

44. Jones JW, Nevins T, McHugh L et al: Nutrition and growth in pediatric renal transplant recipients. Transplant Proc 1994;26(1):62–63.

45. Murugasu B, Conley SB, Lemire JM et al: Fungal peritonitis in children treated with peritoneal dialysis and gastrostomy feeding. Pediatr Nephrol 1991;5(5):620–621.

46. Wood EG, Bunchman TE, Khurana R et al: Complications of nasogastric and gastrostomy tube feedings in children with end stage renal disease. Adv Periton Dial 1990;6.

47. ASPEN Board of Directors: Section IX: Ethical and legal issues in specialized nutritional support. J Parenter Enteral Nutr 1993;17:50SA–52SA.

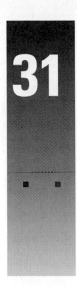

31

Nutrient-Drug Interactions

CYNTHIA A. THOMSON
CAROL J. ROLLINS

As the role of enteral feeding in the care of patients evolves, it has become evident that nutrient-medication interactions can affect the quality and the cost effectiveness of health care. A recent case report cited a patient who required 36 days of additional hospitalization for uncontrollable diarrhea that, after a $4250 medical evaluation, was found to be due to a high-sorbitol liquid medication.[1] Clearly, nutrient-drug interactions can result in a variety of clinically significant problems including inadequate nutrient or drug absorption, altered tolerance to enteral feeding, altered metabolism, physical incompatibilities resulting in clogged feeding tubes, drug antagonistic activity, and altered drug elimination.[2,3]

TYPES OF NUTRIENT-DRUG INCOMPATIBILITIES

To classify the nutrient-drug interactions, specific incompatibilities have been described in the literature[4] and consist of physical, pharmaceutical, pharmacologic, physiologic, and pharmacokinetic incompatibilities. Most drugs appear to be compatible with enteral feeding solutions and administration protocols; however, when present, incompatibilities can result in notable problems. Keep in mind that most nutrient-drug interactions involve a single incompatibility that can be effectively resolved; only rarely are the interactions complex enough to consist of two or more incompatibilities.

Physical Incompatibilities

Physical incompatibilities occur when mixing of a medication and enteral formula results in a change in formula texture (granulation or gel formation), flow rate, viscosity, separation, precipitation, or breaking of an emulsion. Table 31–1 provides examples of the types of physical incompatibilities that occur when selected medications are administered with enteral

TABLE 31–1 Physical Incompatibilities Between Medications and Enteral Formulas

Type	Medication(s)
Granulation	Cibalith-S syrup, Mellaril oral solution, Thorazine concentrate, Organidin elixir
Gel formation	Feosol elixir, Neo-calglucon syrup, Dimetane elixir, Sudafed syrup, Klorvess syrup
Separation	Kaopectate
Precipitation	Robitussin expectorant

Adapted with permission from Cutie AJ, Altman E, Lenkel L: Compatibility of enteral products with commonly employed drug additives. J Parenter Enter Nutr 1983;7(2): 186–191.

feeding products.[5] Limited data are currently available on the physical compatibility of medications with enteral formulas, particularly with newer enteral products and medications developed within the past decade. In general, formulas with intact protein are more prone to break the emulsion than are peptide or free amino acid–based enteral products.[6] Avoiding acidic pharmaceutical syrups will reduce the risk for physical incompatibilities.

A major complication of physical incompatibility is the clogging of enteral feeding tubes. In a recent study by Davidson and colleagues,[7] 33 percent of patients receiving psyllium hydrophilic mucilloid treatment to prevent diarrhea demonstrated clogged feeding tubes, requiring tube replacement. Infusion rate or interruptions in feeding schedules did not seem to alter this result; however, formula temperature can affect tube patency. Administering refrigeration-temperature formula with psyllium increases the likelihood of feeding tube blockage. Mixing psyllium with room-temperature formula to prevent feeding tube obstruction is recommended.

Pharmaceutical Incompatibility

Pharmaceutical incompatibility is a change in medication dosage form that results in altered enteral formula or drug potency, efficacy, or tolerance. The classic example of pharmaceutical incompatibility is the crushing of enteric-coated tablets or the opening of slow-release capsules in an effort to reduce the risk of clogging the enteral feeding tube. A list of oral medication dosage forms that should not be crushed is published periodically in *Hospital Pharmacy*.[8] Information from the 1994 listing is provided in Table 31–2. To avoid pharmaceutical incompatibilities, use an interdisciplinary approach that includes consultation by dietitians, nursing staff, and pharmacists working together to determine the most effective route for mediation administration (i.e., liquid vs tablet, need to administer with food to reduce gastrointestinal [GI] distress). Occasionally, crushing or opening a medication is not advised because of the unacceptable taste. In this case, opening or crushing the medication for administration through an enteral feeding tube is permissible.

Pharmacologic Incompatibility

Pharmacologic incompatibility is the most frequently encountered drug-nutrient interaction in clinical practice.[9] This incompatibility centers around a medication's mechanism of action leading to enteral feeding intolerance, as manifested by diarrhea, GI distention, nausea, emesis, altered taste perceptions, altered biochemical levels, or antagonistic activity. Examples of pharmacologic incompatibilities are included in Table 31–3.

One of the more common pharmacologic incompatibilities is related to vitamin K and warfarin.[10,11,12] To avoid problems with warfarin activity and vitamin K, the clinician must review the vitamin K content of the enteral products on formulary. Table 31–4 provides a list of enteral formulas and the vitamin K content/1000 kcal of formula. Oral anticoagulant therapy can be stabilized for a given level of vitamin K intake (within reason), but significant changes in vitamin K intake, as can occur when an enteral formula is being progressed toward goal rate, can have a significant effect on anticoagulation. Therefore, it is best to avoid formulas containing greater than 75 to 80 mg of vitamin K/1000 kcal when a patient is receiving oral anticoagulation therapy.

Biochemical alterations associated with medication use are another common clinical problem. Table 31–5 lists some of the more frequently diagnosed biochemical alterations and the medication(s) associated with each alteration in biochemical values. Those alterations classified as pharmacologic incompatibility are also indicated in Table 31–5.

Physiologic Incompatibility

Physiologic incompatibility involves the nonpharmacologic actions of a medication that result in altered tolerance to nutrition support. Diarrhea related to increased osmolality is the most common physiologic incompatibility.[13,14] Generally, physiologic incompatibilities can be avoided by changing the administration route (i.e., changing oral medications to an intravenous or intramuscular route) or, in the case of osmolality, by reducing the osmolality by diluting the medication with water before administration through the feeding tube. Lowering the dosage level or changing to an alternative medication, if medically feasible, can also reduce symptoms. Finally, symptoms such as diarrhea can be treated or prevented with other medications. Table 31–6 provides a list of hypertonic medications frequently prescribed to enterally fed patients.

Another common cause of diarrhea in enterally fed patients is related to the excipients

Text continued on page 531.

TABLE 31–2 Oral Dosage Forms Not for Crushing

Drug Product	Distributor/Marketing Company	Dosage Forms	Reasons/Comments
Acutane	Roche	Capsule	Mucous membrane irritant
Actifed 12 Hour	Burroughs Wellcome	Capsule	Slow release[†]
Acutrim	Ciba Consumer	Tablet	Slow release
Aerolate SR, JR, III	Fleming & Co.	Capsule	Slow release[*†]
Afrinol Repetabs	Schering	Tablet	Slow release
Allerest 12 Hour	Fisons	Caplet	Slow release
Artane Sequels	Lederle	Capsule	Slow release[*†]
Arthritis Bayer Time Release	Glenbrook	Capsule	Slow release
ASA Enseals	Lilly	Tablet	Enteric-coated
Asbron G Inlay	Sandoz	Tablet	Multiple compressed tablet[†]
Atrohist Plus	Adams	Tablet	Slow release
Atrohist Sprinkle	Adams	Capsule	Slow release[*]
Azulfidine Entabs	Pharmacia Labs	Tablet	Enteric-coated
Baros	Lafayette	Tablet	Effervescent tablet[¶]
Bayer Extra Strength Enteric 500	Sterling Health	Tablet	Slow release
Bayer Low Adult 81 mg Strength	Sterling Health	Tablet	Enteric-coated
Bayer Regular Strength 325 mg Caplet	Sterling Health	Tablet	Enteric-coated
Betachron E-R	Inwood	Capsule	Slow release
Betapen-VK	Apothecon	Tablet	Taste[‖]
Biohist-LA	Wakefield	Tablet	Slow release[††]
Biphetamine	Fisons	Capsule	Slow release
Bisacodyl	(various)	Tablet	Enteric-coated[†]
BiscoLax	Raway	Tablet	Enteric-coated[†]
Bontril SR	Carnrick	Capsule	Slow release
Breonesin	Sanofi Winthrop	Capsule	Liquid filled[§]
Brexin LA	Savage	Capsule	Slow release
Bromfed	Muro	Capsule	Slow release[†]
Bromfed PD	Muro	Capsule	Slow release[†]
Calan SR	Searle	Tablet	Slow release[††]
Cama Arthritis Pain Reliever	Sandoz Consumer	Tablet	Multiple compressed tablet
Carbiset-TR	Nutripharm	Tablet	Slow release
Cardizem	Marion-Merrell Dow	Tablet	Slow release
Cardizem CD	Marion-Merrell Dow	Capsule	Slow release[*]
Cardizem SR	Marion-Merrell Dow	Capsule	Slow release[*]
Carter's Little Pills	Carter-Wallace	Tablet	Enteric-coated
Cefal Filmtab	Abbott	Tablet	Enteric-coated
Charcoal Plus	Kramer Laboratories	Tablet	Enteric-coated
Chloral Hydrate	(various)	Capsule	**Note:** product is in liquid form within a special capsule[†]
Chlorpheniramine Maleate Time Release	(various)	Capsule	Slow release
Chlor-Trimeton Repetab	Schering	Tablet	Slow release[†]
Choledyl SA	Parke-Davis	Tablet	Slow release[†]
Cipro	Miles	Tablet	Taste[‖]
Codimal LA	Central	Capsule	Slow release
Colace	Mead Johnson	Capsule	Taste[‖]
Comhist LA	Norwich Eaton	Capsule	Slow release[*]
Compazine Spansule	SmithKline Beecham	Capsule	Slow release[†]
Congress SR, JR	Fleming & Co.	Capsule	Slow release
Constant T	Geigy	Tablet	Slow release[*]
Contac	SmithKline Beecham	Capsule	Slow release[*]
Cotazym S	Organon	Capsule	Enteric-coated[*]

Table continued on following page.

TABLE 31–2   Oral Dosage Forms Not for Crushing   *Continued*

Drug Product	Distributor/Marketing Company	Dosage Forms	Reasons/Comments
Creon 10, 20	Solvay	Capsule	Enteric-coated*
Cystospaz-M	Schwartz Pharma	Capsule	Slow release
Cytoxan	Bristol-Myers	Tablet	**Note:** drug may be crushed but maker recommends using inj.
Dallergy	Laser	Capsule	Slow release
Dallergy-D	Laser	Capsule	Slow release
Dallergy-JR	Laser	Capsule	Slow release
Deconamine SR	Berlex	Capsule	Slow release†
Deconsal II	Adams	Tablet	Slow release
Deconsal Sprinkle	Adams	Capsule	Slow release*
Defen-LA	Horizon	Tablet	Slow release††
Demazine Repetabs	Schering	Tablet	Slow release†
Depakene	Abbott	Capsule	Slow-release-mucous membrane irritant†
Depakote	Abbott	Capsule	Enteric-coated
Desoxyn Graduments	Abbott	Tablet	Slow release
Desyrel	Mead Johnson	Tablet	Taste‖
Dexatrim, Max. Strength	Thompson Medical	Tablet	Slow release
Dexedrine Spansule	SmithKline Beecham	Capsule	Slow release
Diamox Sequels	Lederle	Capsule	Slow release
Dilatrate SR	Reed & Carnrick	Capsule	Slow release
Dimetane Extentab	A.H. Robins	Tablet	Slow release†
Disobrom	Geneva	Tablet	Slow release
Disophrol Chronotab	Schering	Tablet	Slow release
Dital	UAD	Capsule	Slow release
Donnatal Extentab	A.H. Robins	Tablet	Slow release†
Donnazyme	A.H. Robins	Tablet	Enteric-coated
Drisdol	Sanofi Winthrop	Capsule	Liquid filled§
Drixoral	Schering	Tablet	Slow release†
Drixoral Sinus	Schering	Tablet	Slow release
Dulcolax	Boehringer Ingelheim	Tablet	Enteric-coated‡
Dynabac	Bock Pharmacal	Tablet	Enteric-coated
Easprin	Parke-Davis	Tablet	Enteric-coated
Ecotrin	SmithKline Beecham	Tablet	Enteric-coated
E.E.S. 400	(various)	Tablet	Enteric-coated†
Elixophyllin SR	Forest	Capsule	Slow release*†
E-Mycin	Boots	Tablet	Enteric-coated
Endafed	UAD	Capsule	Slow release
Entex LA	Norwich Eaton	Tablet	Slow release†
Entozyme	A.H. Robins	Tablet	Enteric-coated
Equanil	Wyeth-Ayerst	Tablet	Taste‖
Ergostat	Parke-Davis	Tablet	Sublingual form**
Eryc	Parke-Davis	Capsule	Enteric-coated*
Ery-tab	Abbott	Tablet	Enteric-coated
Erythrocin Stearate	(various)	Tablet	Enteric-coated
Erythromycin Base	(various)	Tablet	Enteric-coated
Eskalith CR	SmithKline Beecham	Tablet	Slow release
Fedahist Timecaps	Schwarz Pharma	Capsule	Slow release†
Feldene	Pfizer	Capsule	Mucous membrane irritant
Feocyte	Dunhall	Tablet	Slow release
Feosol	SmithKline Beecham	Tablet	Enteric-coated†
Feosol Spansule	SmithKline Beecham	Capsule	Slow release*†
Feratab	Upsher-Smith	Tablet	Enteric-coated†
Fergon	Sanofi Winthrop	Tablet	Slow release*
Fero-Grad 500 mg	Abbott	Tablet	Slow release

TABLE 31–2 Oral Dosage Forms Not for Crushing *Continued*

Drug Product	Distributor/Marketing Company	Dosage Forms	Reasons/Comments
Fero-Gradumet	Abbott	Tablet	Slow release
Ferralet SR	Mission	Tablet	Slow release
Festal II	Hoechst-Roussel	Tablet	Enteric-coated
Feverall Sprinkle Caps	Upsher-Smith	Capsule	Taste* **Note:** capsule contents intended to be placed in a teaspoonful of water or soft food.
Fumatinic	Laser	Capsule	Slow release
Gastrocrom	Fisons	Capsule	**Note:** contents may be dissolved in water for administration.
Geocillin	Roerig	Tablet	Taste
Glucotrol XL	Pratt	Tablet	Slow release
Gris-Peg	Herbert Laboratories	Tablet	**Note:** crushing may result in precipitation as larger particles.
Guaifed	Muro	Capsule	Slow release
Guaifed-PD	Muro	Capsule	Slow release
Guaifenex LA	Ethex	Tablet	Slow release††
Guaifenex PSE 120	Ethex	Tablet	Slow release††
Humabid DM	Adams	Tablet	Slow release
Humabid DM Sprinkle	Adams	Capsule	Slow release*
Humabid LA	Adams	Tablet	Slow release
Humabid Sprinkle	Adams	Capsule	Slow release*
Hydergine L-C	Sandoz	Capsule	**Note:** product is in liquid form within a special capsule†
Hydergine Sublingual	Sandoz	Tablet	Sublingual route†
Hytakerol	Sanofi Winthrop	Capsule	Liquid filled§†
Iberet	Abbott	Tablet	Slow release†
Iberet 500	Abbott	Tablet	Slow release†
ICaps Time Release	LaHaye Labs	Tablet	Slow release
ICaps Plus	LaHaye Labs	Tablet	Slow release
Ilotycin	Dista	Tablet	Enteric-coated
Imdur	Key	Tablet	Slow release††
Inderal LA	Wyeth-Ayerst	Capsule	Slow release
Inderide LA	Wyeth-Ayerst	Capsule	Slow release
Indocin SR	MSD	Capsule	Slow release*†
Ionamin	Fisons	Capsule	Slow release
Isoclor Timesule	Fisons	Capsule	Slow release†
Isoptin SR	Knoll	Tablet	Slow release
Isordil Sublingual	Wyeth-Ayerst	Tablet	Sublingual form**
Isordil Tembid	Wyeth-Ayerst	Tablet	Slow release
Isosorbide Dinitrate Sublingual	(various)	Tablet	Sublingual form**
Isosorbide Dinitrate SR	(various)	Tablet	Slow release
Isuprel Glossets	Sanofi Winthrop	Tablet	Sublingual form**
K + 8	Alra	Tablet	Slow release†
K + 10	Alra	Tablet	Slow release†
Kaon-CL 6.7 mEq	Adria	Tablet	Slow release†
Kaon CL 10	Adria	Tablet	Slow release†
K + Care	Alra	Tablet	Effervescent tablet¶†
K-Lease	Adria	Capsule	Slow release*†
Klor-Con	Upsher-Smith	Tablet	Slow release†
Klor-Con/EF	Upsher-Smith	Tablet	Effervescent tablet¶†

Table continued on following page.

TABLE 31–2   Oral Dosage Forms Not for Crushing   *Continued*

Drug Product	Distributor/Marketing Company	Dosage Forms	Reasons/Comments
Klorvess	Sandoz	Tablet	Effervescent tablet¶†
Klotrix	Mead Johnson	Tablet	Slow release†
K-Lyte	Mead Johnson	Tablet	Effervescent tablet¶
K-Lyte CL	Mead Johnson	Tablet	Effervescent tablet¶
K-Tab	Abbott	Tablet	Slow release†
Levsinex Timecaps	Schwarz Pharma	Capsule	Slow release
Lithobid	Ciba	Tablet	Slow release†
Lodrane LD	ECR Pharmaceutical	Capsule	Slow release*
Mag-Tab	Niche	Tablet	Slow release
Meprospan	Wallace	Capsule	Slow release*
Mestinon Timespan	ICN Pharmaceutical	Tablet	Slow release†
MI-Cebrin	Dista	Tablet	Enteric-coated
MI-Cebrin T	Dista	Tablet	Enteric-coated
Micro K	A.H. Robins	Capsule	Slow release*†
Motrin	Upjohn	Tablet	Taste‖
MS Contin	Purdue Frederick	Tablet	Slow release†
MSC Triaminic	Sandoz	Tablet	Enteric-coated
Muco-Fen-LA	Wakefield	Tablet	Slow release††
Naldecon	Bristol Labs	Tablet	Slow release†
Nasatab LA	ECR Pharmaceutical	Tablet	Slow release††
Nico 400	Jones Medical	Capsule	Slow release
Nicobid	Rhone-Poulenc Rorer	Capsule	Slow release
Nitro Bid	Marion-Merrell Dow	Capsule	Slow release*
Nitrocine Timecaps	Schwarz Pharma	Capsule	Slow release
Nitroglyn	Kenwood	Capsule	Slow release*
Nitrostat	Parke-Davis	Tablet	Sublingual route**
Nitro-Time	Time-Cap Labs	Capsule	Slow release
Nitrong	Rhone-Poulenc Rorer	Tablet	Slow release**
Noctec	Apothecon	Capsule	**Note:** product is in liquid form within a special capsule†
Nolamine	Carnrick	Tablet	Slow release
Nolex LA	Carnrick	Tablet	Slow release
Norflex	3M Pharmaceuticals	Tablet	Slow release
Norpace CR	Searle	Capsule	Slow release form within a special capsule
Novafed	Marion-Merrell Dow	Capsule	Slow release
Novafed A	Marion-Merrell Dow	Capsule	Slow release
Ondrox	Unimed	Tablet	Slow release
Optilets 500 filmtab	Abbott	Tablet	Enteric-coated
Optilets M 500 filmtab	Abbott	Tablet	Enteric-coated
Oragrafin	Squibb Diagnostics	Capsule	**Note:** product is in liquid form within a special capsule
Oramorph SR	Roxane	Tablet	Slow release†
Ornade Spansule	SmithKline Beecham	Capsule	Slow release
Pabalate	A.H. Robins	Tablet	Enteric-coated
Pabalate SF	A.H. Robins	Tablet	Enteric-coated
Pancrease	Ortho McNeil	Capsule	Enteric-coated*
Pancrease MT	Ortho McNeil	Capsule	Enteric-coated*
Panmycin	Upjohn	Capsule	Taste
Papaverine Sustained Action	(various)	Capsule	Slow release
Pathilon Sequels	Lederle	Capsule	Slow release*
Pavabid Plateau	Marion-Merrell Dow	Capsule	Slow release*
PBZ-SR	Geigy	Tablet	Slow release†
Perdiem	Rhone-Poulenc Rorer	Granules	Wax coated

TABLE 31–2   Oral Dosage Forms Not for Crushing   *Continued*

Drug Product	Distributor/Marketing Company	Dosage Forms	Reasons/Comments
Peritrate SA	Parke-Davis	Tablet	Slow release[††]
Permitil Chronotab	Schering	Tablet	Slow release[†]
Phazyme	Reed & Carnrick	Tablet	Slow release
Phazyme 95	Reed & Carnrick	Tablet	Slow release
Phenergan	Wyeth-Ayerst	Tablet	Taste[‖†]
Phyllocontin	Purdue Frederick	Tablet	Slow release
Plendil	Astra Merck	Tablet	Slow release
Polaramine Repetabs	Schering	Tablet	Slow release[†]
Pneumonist	ECR Pharmaceutical	Tablet	Slow release[††]
Prelu-2	Boehringer Ingelheim	Capsule	Slow release
Prevacid	TAP Pharmaceutical	Capsule	Slow release
Prilosec	Astra Merck	Capsule	Slow release
Pro-Banthine	Schiapparelli Searle	Tablet	Taste
Procainamide HCL SR	(various)	Tablet	Slow release
Procan SR	Parke-Davis	Tablet	Slow release
Procardia	Pfizer	Capsule	Delays absorption[#§]
Procardia XL	Pfizer	Tablet	Slow release
			Note: AUC is unaffected.
Profen II	Wakefield	Tablet	Slow release[††]
Profen-LA	Wakefield	Tablet	Slow release[††]
Pronestyl SR	Bristol-Myers Squibb	Tablet	Slow release
Proventil Repetabs	Schering	Tablet	Slow release[†]
Prozac	Dista	Capsule	Slow release[*]
Quadra Hist	Schein	Tablet	Slow release
Quibron-T SR	Bristol-Myers Squibb	Tablet	Slow release[†]
Quinaglute Dura Tabs	Berlex	Tablet	Slow release
Quinalan Lanatabs	Lannett	Tablet	Slow release
Quinalan SR	Lannett	Tablet	Slow release
Quinidex Extentabs	A.H. Robins	Tablet	Slow release
Respa-1st	Respa	Tablet	Slow release[††]
Respa-DM	Respa	Tablet	Slow release[††]
Respa-GF	Respa	Tablet	Slow release[††]
Respahist	Respa	Capsule	Slow release[*]
Respaire SR	Laser	Capsule	Slow release
Respid	Boehringer Ingelheim	Tablet	Slow release
Ritalin SR	Ciba	Tablet	Slow release
Robimycin Robitab	A.H. Robins	Tablet	Enteric-coated
Rondec TR	Dura	Tablet	Slow release[†]
Roxanol SR	Roxane	Tablet	Slow release[†]
Ru-Tuss	Boots	Tablet	Slow release
Ru-Tuss DE	Boots	Tablet	Slow release
Sinemet CR	DuPont Pharm	Tablet	Slow release[††]
Singlet	Marion-Merrell Dow	Tablet	Slow release
Slo-Bid Gyrocaps	Rhone-Poulenc Rorer	Capsule	Slow release[*]
Slo-Niacin	Upsher Smith	Tablet	Slow release
Slo-Phyllin GG	Rhone-Poulenc Rorer	Capsule	Slow release[†]
Slo-Phyllin Gyrocaps	Rhone-Poulenc Rorer	Capsule	Slow release[*†]
Slow-FE	Ciba Consumer	Tablet	Slow release[†]
Slow-FE with Folic Acid	Ciba Consumer	Tablet	Slow release
Slow-K	Summit	Tablet	Slow release[†]
Slow-Mag	Searle	Tablet	Slow release
Sorbitrate SA	ICI Pharma	Tablet	Slow release
Sorbitrate Sublingual	ICI Pharma	Tablet	Sublingual route
Sparine	Wyeth-Ayerst	Tablet	Taste[‖]
S-P-T	Fleming	Capsule	**Note:** Liquid gelatin thyroid suspension.

Table continued on following page.

TABLE 31–2 Oral Dosage Forms Not for Crushing *Continued*

Drug Product	Distributor/Marketing Company	Dosage Forms	Reasons/Comments
Sudafed 12 hour	Burroughs Wellcome	Capsule	Slow release[†]
Sudex	Atley	Tablet	Slow release[††]
Sustaire	Pfizer	Tablet	Slow release[†]
Syn-RX	Adams Lab	Tablet	Slow release
Tavist-D	Sandoz	Tablet	Multiple compressed tablet
Tedral SA	Parke-Davis	Tablet	Slow release
Teldrin	SmithKline Beecham	Capsule	Slow release[*]
Temaril Spansules	Allergan Herbert	Capsule	Slow release[†]
Tepanil Ten-Tab	3M Pharmaceuticals	Tablet	Slow release
Tessalon Perles	Forest	Capsule	Slow release
Theo-24	Searle	Tablet	Slow release[†]
Theobid	Russ	Capsule	Slow release[*†]
Theobid Jr.	Russ	Capsule	Slow release[*†]
Theochron	(various)	Tablet	Slow release
Theoclear LA	Central	Capsule	Slow release[†]
Theo-Dur	Key	Tablet	Slow release[†]
Theo-Dur Sprinkle	Key	Capsule	Slow release[*†]
Theo-Sav	Savage	Tablet	Slow release[††]
Theolair SR	3M Pharmaceuticals	Tablet	Slow release[†]
Theovent	Schering	Capsule	Slow release[†]
Theox	Carnrick	Tablet	Slow release
Therapy Bayer	Glenbrook	Caplet	Enteric-coated
Thorazine Spansule	SmithKline Beecham	Capsule	Slow release
T-Phyl	Purdue Frederick	Tablet	Slow release
Trental	Hoechst-Roussel	Tablet	Slow release
Triaminic	Sandoz	Tablet	Enteric-coated[†]
Triaminic 12	Sandoz	Tablet	Slow release[†]
Triaminic TR	Sandoz	Tablet	Multiple compressed tablet[†]
Trilafon Repetabs	Schering	Tablet	Slow release[†]
Triptone Caplets	Commerce	Tablet	Slow release
Toprol XL	Astra	Tablet	Slow release[††]
Tuss LA	Hyrex	Tablet	Slow release
Tuss Ornade Spansule	SmithKline Beecham	Capsule	Slow release
Tylenol Extended Relief	McNeil	Capsule	Slow release
Uniphyl	Purdue Frederick	Tablet	Slow release
ULR-LA	Geneva	Tablet	Slow release
Valrelease	Roche	Capsule	Slow release
Verelan	Lederle	Capsule	Slow release[*]
Volmax	Muro	Tablet	Slow release[†]
Wellbutrin	Burroughs Wellcome	Tablet	Anesthetizes mucous membrane
Wyamycin S	Wyeth-Ayerst	Tablet	Slow release
Wygesic	Wyeth-Ayerst	Tablet	Taste
Zorprin	Boots	Tablet	Slow release
Zymase	Organon	Capsule	Enteric-coated

[*]Capsule may be opened and the contents taken without crushing or chewing; soft food such as applesauce or pudding may facilitate administration; contents may generally be administered via nasogastric tube using an appropriate fluid provided entire contents are washed down the tube.
[†]Liquid dosage forms of the product are availabe; however, dose, frequency of administration, and manufacturers may differ from that of the solid dosage form.
[‡]Antacids and/or milk may prematurely dissolve the coating of the tablet.
[§]Capsule may be opened and the liquid contents removed for administration.
[∥]The taste of this product in a liquid form would likely be unacceptable to the patient; administration via nasogastric tube should be acceptable.
[¶]Effervescent tablets must be dissolved in the amount of diluent recommended by the manufacturer.
[#]If the liquid capsule is crushed or the contents expressed, the active ingredient will be, in part, absorbed sublingually.
[**]Tablets are made to disintegrate under the tongue.
[††]Table is scored and may be broken in half without affecting release characteristics.
Reprinted with permission from Mitchell JF: Oral dosage forms that should not be crushed. Hosp Pharm 1996;31:27–37.

TABLE 31–3 Pharmacologic Incompatibilities Between Medications and Enteral Formulas

Nausea or Emesis	Antibiotics—erythromycin Antiparkinson's agents Anti-inflammatory agents Chemotherapeutic agents Opiates
Diarrhea	Antibiotics Laxatives Cathartics Metoclopramide Doxorubicin Etoposide Cholinergics Chemotherapeutic agents
Antagonistic activity	Warfarin—vitamin K antagonist Methotrexate, trimethoprim, pyrimethamine—folate antagonists

TABLE 31–4 Vitamin K Content of Selected Enteral Formulas

Formula	Vitamin K Content/1000 kcal (µg)
Vivonex TEN	22
Ensure Plus	39
Ensure	39
Osmolite	39
Isosource HN	40
Two Cal HN	42
Vivonex Plus	44
Isotein HN	48
Vital HN	54
Glucerna	57
Pulmocare	57
Jevity	59
Ultracal	59
Liposorb	60
Compleat Modified	63
Impact	67
Isosource VHN	80
Nutren 1.0	80
Peptamen	80
Promote with fiber	80
Replete	80
Criticare HN	117
Isocal HCN	118
Isocal	123
Sustacal HC	138
Magnacal	150

Revised (1995) from Thomson CA, Rollins CJ: Enteral feeding and medication incompatibilities. Support Line 1991; 8(3):9–11.

(additives) used in medication manufacturing. Sorbitol is the most common diarrhea-inducing excipient, yet its presence is seldom included on the label or in the product information.[15,16] Table 31–7 provides data on some medications that contain sorbitol. Some sweeteners such as mannitol, lactose, saccharin, and sucrose also contribute to diarrhea. If patients have diarrhea of unknown etiology, excipients in medications may be the cause. Clinicians should contact manufacturers for specific information. Patients with food allergies such as gluten sensitivity or lactose intolerance will need close monitoring for this problematic situation.

Other adverse reactions such as urticaria, asthma, belching, nausea, or even anaphylactic shock can also occur in patients sensitive to sweeteners, flavorings, or dyes that may be added to medications in the manufacturing process. Table 31–8 outlines the currently published data regarding sweetener content of commonly prescribed antimicrobial medications.[17]

Pharmacokinetic Incompatibility

The final type of incompatibility between medications and nutrients occurs when the enteral feeding alters the bioavailability, distribution, metabolism, or elimination of the medications, or the reverse, when the medication alters nutrient function. The most thoroughly studied of the pharmacokinetic incompatibilities associated with enteral feeding is phenytoin. Several studies have indicated that administration of phenytoin concurrent with enteral feeding will result in reduced bioavailability of phenytoin.[18,19] This observation has led to the recommendation that patients receiving enteral feeding and oral phenytoin should have the feeding held for 1 to 2 hours before and after the phenytoin dose.[20] However, this approach has not always been shown to be effective;[21] therefore, other investigators have recommended increases in phenytoin dose until therapeutic drug levels are achieved and maintained. Another option is to provide the phenytoin intravenously[22] or in capsule form[23] to enhance absorption.

Other medications, such as ciprofloxacin, have shown improved absorption when administered nasoduodenally rather than nasogastrically.[24] Still other medications, such as hydralazine, may be more efficiently absorbed using continuous enteral feeding rather than intermittent, bolus feedings.[25] Finally, the nutrient composition of the enteral formula selected can also significantly affect intestinal drug metabolism, particularly if the formula is low in lipid content and the drug is metabolized hepatically.[26] To date, the available clinical data regarding the impact of enteral formulas on drug bioavailability remain limited; how-

TABLE 31–5 Common Biochemical Abnormalities Associated with Medications Prescribed for Enterally Fed Patients

Serum glucose	
Hyperglycemia	Morphine, phenytoin, thiazides,* corticosteroids,* estrogen,* phenothiazine,* probenecid,* clonidine,* chemotherapeutic agents
Hypoglycemia	Acetaminophen,* monoamine oxidase inhibitors,* sulfamides,* phenylbutazone,* propranolol,* barbiturates*
Serum potassium	
Hyperkalemia	Spironolactone,* penicillin G potassium
Hypokalemia	Ampicillin, carbenicillin, piperacillin, ticarcillin, amphotericin,* thiazides,* furosemide,* diuretics,* laxatives*
Serum sodium	
Hypernatremia	Penicillin G sodium, mediations with large volume normal saline
Hyponatremia	Laxatives,* diuretics,* probenecid,* amphotericin, potassium-sparing diuretics,* thiazides,* furosemide*
Serum magnesium	
Hypermagnesemia	Magnesium-containing antacids in patients with renal dysfunction
Hypomagnesemia	Amphotericin, cyclosporin, thiazides,* furosemide,* cisplatin, ciprofloxacin, probenecid, carbenicillin, pentamidine
Serum phosphorus	
Hyperphosphatemia	Chemotherapeutic agent–induced cell lysis,* excess glucose administration with medications
Hypophosphatemia	Sucralfate, corticosteroids, furosemide,* thiazides*
Calcium losses	Furosemide,* triamterene,* probenecid, corticosteroids, indomethacin
Serum lipids	
Hypertriglyceridemia	Cyclosporin,* corticosteroids, thiouracil, chlorpromazine

*Classified as pharmacologic incompatibility.

ever, if drug efficacy appears to be reduced during enteral feeding, the clinician should consider altering the formula, feeding route, or feeding regimen to resolve the problem.

The intestinal absorption of nutrients can be altered by administering specific medications as well. Table 31–9 lists some of the common drug-induced nutrient absorption defects.[27]

CORRECTING VITAMIN, MINERAL, AND ELECTROLYTE DEFICIENCIES

When deficiencies in vitamins, minerals, or electrolytes are diagnosed, replacement therapy should be initiated. Replacement therapies available that are known to be compatible with enteral feeding include liquid multivitamin preparations, potassium acetate, chloride or phosphorus injections, potassium phosphate preparations (e.g., Neutra-Phos and Phospho-soda), magnesium oxide, sodium chloride, acetate or phosphate injection, and water-based fat-soluble vitamins.[28]

AVOIDING MEDICATION AND ENTERAL FEEDING INCOMPATIBILITIES

Table 31–10 illustrates possible solutions to the common enteral feeding–medication in-

compatibilities outlined in this chapter.[29] Keep in mind that preventing these incompatibilities results in the most cost-effective care. Review medications before initiating enteral feedings and reevaluate the patient's medications on a regular basis to avoid incompatibilities whenever possible.

MEDICATION ADMINISTRATION THROUGH ENTERAL FEEDING TUBES

Avoid administering medications through enteral feeding tubes if possible. In many instances an alternative medication route, such as oral, intravenous, or even intramuscular, is available. Reducing the frequency and duration of enteral feeding tube use to provide medications to the patient results in reduced risk for tube occlusion. When medications must be administered through the enteral feeding tube, the following guidelines should serve to reduce the incidence of clogged feeding tubes.[30,31]

1. Flush the feeding tube with 15 to 30 ml of warm tap water before and after administering any single medication.
2. If a medication is to be given on an empty stomach, check gastric residuals

TABLE 31–6 Frequently Prescribed Hypertonic Medications

Product	Manufacturer	Average Osmolality (mOsm/kg)
Acetaminophen elixir, 65 mg/ml	Roxane	5400
Acetaminophen with codeine elixir	Wyeth	4700
Aminophylline liquid, 21 mg/ml	Fisons	450
Amoxacillin suspension, 50 mg/ml	Squibb	2250
Ampicillin suspension, 50 mg/ml	Squibb	2250
Ampicillin suspension, 100 mg/ml	Bristol	1850
Calcium glubionate syrup, 0.36 g/ml	Sandoz	2550
Cephalexin suspension, 50 mg/ml	Dista	1950
Cimetidine solution, 60 mg/ml	Smith Kline & French	5550
Cotrimoxazole suspension	Burroughs	2200
Dexamethasone elixir, 0.1 mg/ml	Organon	3350
Dexamethasone solution, 1 mg/ml	Roxane	3100
Dextromethorphan hydrobromide syrup, 2 mg/ml	Parke-Davis	5950
Digoxin elixir, 50 µg/ml	Burroughs	1350
Diphenydramine hydrochloride elixir, 2.5 mg/ml	Roxane	850
Diphenoxylate hydrochloride-atropine sulfate	Roxane	8800
Docusate sodium syrup, 3.3 mg/ml	Roxane	3900
Erythromycin ethylsuccinate suspension, 40 mg/ml	Abbott	1750
Ferrous sulfate liquid, 60 mg/ml	Roxane	4700
Fluphenazine hydrochloride elixir, 0.5 mg/ml	Squibb	1750
Furosemide solution, 10 mg/ml	Hoechst-Roussel	2050
Kaolin-pectin suspension	Roxane	900
Haloperidol concentrate, 2 mg/ml	McNeil	500
Hydroxyline hydrochloride syrup, 2 mg/ml	Roerig	4450
Lactulose syrup, 0.67 mg/ml	Roerig	3600
Lithium citrate syrup, 1.6 mEq/ml	Roxane	6850
Methyldopa suspension, 50 mg/ml	Merck, Sharp & Dohme	2050
Metoclopramide hydrochloride syrup, 1 mg/ml	Robins	8350
Multivitamin liquid	Upjohn	5700
Nystatin suspension, 100,000 units/ml	Squibb	3300
Paregoric tincture	Roxane	1350
Phenytoin sodium suspension, 6 mg/ml	Parke-Davis	2000
Phenytoin sodium suspension, 25 mg/ml	Parke-Davis	1500
Potassium chloride liquid, 10%	Adria	3000
Potassium chloride liquid, 10%	Roxane	3300
Potassium iodide saturated solution, 1 g/ml	Upsher Smith	10,950
Prochlorperazine syrup, 1 mg/ml	Smith Kline & French	3250
Promethazine hydrochloride syrup, 1.25 mg/ml	Wyeth	3500
Sodium citrate liquid	Willen	2050
Sodium phosphate liquid, 0.5 g/ml	Fleet	7250
Theophylline solution, 5.33 mg/ml	Berlex	800
Thiabendazole suspension, 100 mg/ml	Merck, Sharp & Dohme	2150
Thioridazine suspension, 20 mg/ml	Sandoz	2050
Trace element injection	Lyphomed	500

Adapted from Dickerson RN, Melnick G. Osmolality of oral drug solutions and suspensions. Am J Hosp Pharm 1988;45:832–834. Copyright 1988, American Society of Hospital Pharmacists, Inc. Reprinted with permission. (R9634) ASHP assumes no responsibility for the accuracy of the translation.

before medication administration of all gastric feedings.

3. Use only water to flush feeding tubes, because other liquids (e.g., cranberry juice, colas) will not only significantly increase osmolality but may also result in tube occlusion.

4. When ordering medications for enteral feeding tube administration, provide this information to the dispensing pharmacist so that the most appropriate solution or suspension can be used.

5. Administer medications as liquid, crushed tablets, or opened capsules di-

Text continued on page 538.

TABLE 31–7   Sorbitol Content of Selected Oral Medications

Active Ingredients or Brand Name	Manufacturer	Sorbitol Content per Common Dosage (g/dose)*
Acetaminophen USP	Roxane Laboratories, Inc.	5.47 g/500 mg
Acetaminophen, Codeine	Carnrick Laboratories, Inc.	0.62 g/10 ml
Acyclovir	Burroughs Wellcome Co.	†
Aluminum hydroxide gel	Roxane Laboratories, Inc.	0.53 g/5 ml
Amantadine	Du Pont Pharmaceuticals	6.4 g/100 mg
Aminocaproic acid	Lederle Laboratories	5.2 g/5 g
Aminophylline	Roxane Laboratories, Inc.	1.3 g/200 mg
Atropine sulfate, Phenobarbital	(Poythress Laboratories)	2.5 g/5 ml
Betamethasone	Schering Laboratories	1 g/0.6 mg
Dimetane DX	Wyeth-Ayerst Laboratories	1.75 g/5 ml
Carbamazepine	Geigy Pharmaceuticals	1.7 g/200 mg
Calcium carbonate	Roxane Laboratories, Inc.	1.4 g/500 mg
Chloral hydrate USP	Roxane Laboratories, Inc.	1.4 g/500 mg
Chlorpromazine	Roxane Laboratories, Inc.	0.04 g/100 mg
Chlorprothixene	Roche Laboratories	0.72 g/50 mg
Cimetidine	SmithKline Beecham	2.52 g/300 mg
Colistin sulfate	Parke-Davis	0.25 g/350 mg
Codeine phosphate	Roxane Laboratories, Inc.	1.4 g/15 mg
Dexamethasone	Organon Inc.	3.86 g/0.75 mg
	Roxane Laboratories, Inc.	1.84 g/0.75 mg
Dexchlorpheniramine	Schering Laboratories	1 g/2 mg
Dextromethorphan, Guaifenesin	(Bristol Laboratories)	1.4 g/5 mg
Diazepam	Roxane Laboratories, Inc.	1.05 g/5 mg
Digoxin USP	Roxane Laboratories, Inc.	1.05 g/0.25 mg
Diphenoxylate, Atropine	Roxane Laboratories, Inc.	1.82 g/4 ml
Doxepin	Warner Chilcott Laboratories	1.93 g/75 mg
Doxycycline	Pfizer Laboratories	7 g/100 mg
Dyphylline, Guaifenesin	Savage Laboratories	0.9 g/15 ml
Furosemide	Hoeschst-Roussel Pharmaceuticals, Inc.	1.4 g/40 mg
	Pharmaceuticals Basics, Inc.	†
	Roxane Laboratories, Inc.	0.49 g/40 mg
Guaifenesin	(Bristol Laboratories)	1.4 g/5 ml
	Scot-Tussin Pharmacal Co.	1.44 g/5 ml
	Roxane Laboratories, Inc.	0.53 g/5 ml
Guaifenesin, Codeine	Wyeth-Ayerst Laboratories	1.75 g/5 ml
Hydroxyzine	Pfizer Laboratories	5.8 g/5 ml
Hydromorphone	Knoll Pharmaceuticals	2.6 g/4 mg
Indomethacin	Merck Sharp & Dohme	1.75 g/25 mg
Iodinated glycerol, Dextromethorphan	Everett Laboratories, Inc.	1.93 g/5 ml
Iodinated glycerol, Codeine	Wallace Laboratories	1 g/5 ml
Vitafol (liquid vitamin preparation)	Everett Laboratories	13.88 g/15 ml
Vitalize-SF (liquid vitamin preparation)	Scot-Tussin Pharmacal Co.	5.4 g/15 ml
Lithium	Ciba Pharmaceutical Company	3.86 g/300 mg
Magaldrate	Roxane Laboratories, Inc.	0.88 g/5 ml
Magnesia, Alumina USP	Roxane Laboratories, Inc.	3.15 g/30 ml
Meperidine	Roxane Laboratories, Inc.	1.4 g/50 mg
Metaproterenol	Boehringer Ingelheim	1.08 g/10 mg
	Roxane Laboratories, Inc.	1.4 g/10 mg
	Pharmaceuticals Basics, Inc.	†
Methadone	Roxane Laboratories, Inc.	0.7 g/10 mg
Methionine	Forest Pharmaceuticals, Inc.	2.33 g/500 mg
Metoclopramide	Wyeth-Ayerst Laboratories	3.5 g/10 mg
	Biocraft Laboratories, Inc.	4.2 g/10 mg
	Warner Chilcott Laboratories	4.2 g/10 mg
	Roxane Laboratories, Inc.	2.8 g/10 mg
	Pharmaceuticals Basics, Inc.	

TABLE 31–7   Sorbitol Content of Selected Oral Medications   *Continued*

Active Ingredients or Brand Name	Manufacturer	Sorbitol Content per Common Dosage (g/dose)*
Milk of Magnesia	Roxane Laboratories, Inc.	6.09 g/30 ml
Milk of Magnesia, Cascara	Roxane Laboratories, Inc.	0.53 g/5 ml
Minocycline	Lederle Laboratories	1.03 g/100 mg
Molindone	Du Pont Pharmaceuticals	0.65 g/50 mg
Morphine	Roxane Laboratories, Inc.	0.42 g/10 mg
	Roxane Laboratories, Inc.	0.53 g/20 mg
Nalidixic acid	Winthrop Pharmaceuticals	7 g/500 mg
Naproxen	Syntex Laboratories, Inc.	0.9 g/250 mg
Nitrofurantoin	Proctor & Gamble Pharm.	†
	(Norwich Eaton Pharmaceuticals)	‡
Nortriptyline	Eli Lilly and Company	8 g/25 mg
Oxtriphylline	Parke-Davis	2.9 g/300 mg
Oxybutynin	Marion Merrell Dow, Inc.	1.3 g/5 mg
Oxycodone	Roxane Laboratories, Inc.	0.7 g/5 mg
Perphenazine	Schering Laboratories	0.5 g/4 mg
Pseudoephedrine,	(Reid-Rowell)	1.88 g/5 ml
Chlorpheniramine	Scot-Tussin Pharmacal Co.	1.75 g/5 ml
Scot-Tussin Sugar-Free Original	Scot-Tussin Pharmacal Co.	1.22 g/5 ml
Tussirex Sugar-Free	Scot-Tussin Pharmacal Co.	1.13 g/5 ml
Promethazine VC w/Codeine	Warner Chilcott Laboratories	0.003 g/5 ml
P-V Tussin	(Reid-Rowell)	1.67 g/5 ml
Tuss-Ornade	SmithKline Beecham	2.61 g/5 ml
Triaminic Expectorant w/Codeine	Sandoz Pharmaceuticals	§
Naldecon DX Adult	(Bristol Laboratories)	1.4 g/5 ml
Naldecon DX Pediatric	(Bristol Laboratories)	0.16 g/1 ml
Naldecon EX Children's	(Bristol Laboratories)	2.8 g/5 ml
Naldecon EX Pediatric	(Bristol Laboratories)	0.16 g/1 ml
Naldecon Pediatric Drops	Bristol Laboratories	0.11 g/1 ml
Naldecon Pediatric Syrup	Bristol Laboratories	2.73 g/5 ml
Naldecon Syrup	Bristol Laboratories	2.73 g/5 ml
Ru-Tuss with Hydrocodone	Boots Pharmaceuticals, Inc.	0.97 g/30 ml
Triaminic Expectorant DH	Sandoz Pharmaceuticals, Corp.	§
Potassium gluconate, Potassium chloride liquid	Fisons Corp.	8.1 g/15 ml
Potassium gluconate, Potassium chloride powder	Fisons Corp.	0.6 g/20 mEq
Potassium chloride	Fleming and Company	0.45 g/10 mEq
Prednisolone	Fisons, Corp.	0.36 g/5 mg
Prednisone	Muro Pharmaceutical, Inc.	≈2 g/5 mg
Propranolol	Roxane Laboratories, Inc.	3.15 g/20 mg
		3.15 g/40 mg
Rondec syrup	Ross Laboratories	2.9 g/5 ml
Rondec-DM	Ross Laboratories	2.9 g/5 ml
Novahistine DH	Marion Merrell Dow	0.94 g/5 ml
Tussar-SF	Rorer Pharmaceuticals	4.3 g/5 ml
Novahistine Expectorant	Marion Merrell Dow, Inc.	1.02 g/5 ml
Nucofed	Roberts Pharmaceutical Corp.	1.4 g/5 ml
Robitussin DAC	Wyeth-Ayerst Laboratories	1.75 g/5 ml
Saliva substitute	Roxane Laboratories, Inc.	0.03 g/1 ml
Sodium polystyrene, Sulfonate	Roxane Laboratories, Inc.	14.7 g/15 g
		49 g/50 g
Sulfamethoxazole	Roche Laboratories	0.72 g/500 mg
Theophylline		
Theostat 80	Laser, Inc.	3.4 g/300 mg
Slo-Phyllin80	Rorer Pharmaceuticals	22.6 g/300 mg
Accurbron	Marion Merrell Dow	6.75 g/300 mg
	Roxane Laboratories, Inc.	25.6 g/300 mg

Table continued on following page.

TABLE 31–7   Sorbitol Content of Selected Oral Medications   *Continued*

Active Ingredients or Brand Name	Manufacturer	Sorbitol Content per Common Dosage (g/dose)*
Theolair	3M Pharmaceuticals	22.67 g/300 mg
Aerolate	Fleming and Company	9.12 g/30 ml
Theophylline, Guaifenesin		
Quibron	Bristol Laboratories	1.05 g/30 ml
Slo-Phyllin GG	Rorer Pharmaceuticals	3.7 g/30 ml
Synophylate GG	Central Pharmaceuticals, Inc.	5.76 g/30 ml
Theophylline, Guaifenesin		
Asbron-G	Sandoz Pharmaceuticals, Corp.	§
Elixophyllin-GG	Forest Pharmaceuticals, Inc.	14.45 g/45 ml
Thiabendazole	Merck, Sharp & Dohme	1.4 g/500 ml
Trihexyphenidyl	Lederle Laboratories	4.15 g/2 mg
Trimethoprim, Sulfamethoxazole		
Bactrim	Roche Laboratories	1.4 g/20 ml
Septra Grape Suspension	Burroughs Wellcome Co.	†
Septra Suspension	Burroughs Wellcome Co.	†
	Biocraft Laboratories	2 g/20 ml
	Lederle Laboratories	2 g/20 ml
Thioridazine	Sandoz Pharmaceuticals	§
	Warner Chilcott Laboratories	0.13 g/30 mg
		0.13 g/100 mg
	Roxane Laboratories, Inc.	0.21 g/30 mg
		0.14 g/100 mg
Thiothixene	Roerig Div., Pfizer, Inc.	0.6 g/5 mg
	(Lemmon Company)	0.5 g/5 mg

*Multiple ingredient doses listed in ml volume.
†Manufacturer refused to provide requested information.
‡Contains sorbitol; manufacturer requested information remain confidential.
§Contains sorbitol; manufacturer did not supply information before manuscript submission.
Manufacturer's in parentheses produced product indicated at time of survey but are no longer the manufacturer of record.
References: *American Drug Index,* 1990; *Drug Facts and Comparisons* 1993; *Physicians' Desk Reference,* 1993.
Reprinted by permission of the publisher from Johnston KR, Govel LA, Andritz MH: Gastrointestinal effects of sorbitol as an additive in liquid medications. Am J Med 1994;97:185–191. Copyright 1994 by Excerpta Medica Inc.

TABLE 31–8   Sweetner Content of Selected Antimicrobials

Sweetner	Antimicrobials							
	Amox	Amp	Pen	Ceph	Eryth	Sulf	Other	Total
	(11)	(10)	(12)	(19)	(18)	(10)	(11)	
Mannitol	5	1	0	0	1	0	0	7
Lactose	0	0	0	1	2	1	3	7
Saccharin	5	4	11	0	1	4	5	30
Sorbitol	0	0	0	0	1	3	3	7
Sucrose	8	9	12	18	14	7	6	74
Unspecified	0	0	0	0	3	1	0	4

Amox = amoxicillin; Amp = ampicillin; Pen = penicillin; Ceph = cephalosporins; Eryth = erythromycin; Sulf = sulfonamides. Number of preparations for which data were collected are listed in parentheses.
Reproduced by permission from Kumar A, Weatherly MR, Beaman DC: Sweeteners, flavorings, and dyes in antibiotic preparations. Pediatrics 1991;87:352–360. Copyright 1991.

TABLE 31–9   Nutrient Absorption Defects Induced By Medications

Drug	Nutrients Lost	Mechanism	Notes on Nutritional Care
Antacids (containing magnesium)	Riboflavin	Increases pH	Monitor serum riboflavin
Anticonvulsant (Phenytoin, primidone, phenobarbital)	Folate, vitamin B_{12}, Ca	Accelerates vitamin D metabolism in liver; mechanism in folate absorption unclear	Monitor nutrient levels; supplement as necessary
Antihypertensive (Methyldopa)	Folate, vitamin B_{12}, Fe	Autoimmune	
Anti-infectives			
Neomycin, cycloserine, erythromycin, kanamycin	Nitrogen, fat, Ca, Na, K, Mg, Fe, vitamins A, B_{12}, folate	Structural defect; bile acid sequestration	Monitor nutrient levels; supplement as necessary
Sulfasalazine	Folate	Mucosal block	Monitor for anemia (uncommon)
Tetracyclines		Forms chelates with di- and trivalent cations (effect on Fe absorption not clinically significant)	Take medication 1 hour a.c. or 2 hours p.c.
Anti-inflammatory (gout) (Colchicine)	Fat, carotene, Na, K, vitamin B_{12}	Mitotic arrest; structural defect; enzyme damage	Monitor vitamins A and B_{12} and electrolyte status; supplement as necessary
Antineoplastic (methotrexate)	Folate, vitamin B_{12}, Ca	Mucosal damage	Monitor folate and B_{12} status
Antitubercular (para-aminosalicylic acid)	Fat, Ca, Mg, Fe, folate, vitamin B_{12}	Mucosal block in B_{12} uptake; can cause megaloblastic anemia; mechanism in fat absorption unclear	Monitor nutrient levels; supplement as necessary
Contraceptive (Estrogen containing)	Vitamin C		
Glucocorticoid (Dexamethaxone)	Folate		Megaloblastic anemia
Hypocholesterolemic Cholestyramine	Fat, fat-soluble vitamins, carotene, vitamin B_{12}, Fe	Binding of bile acids, salts and nutrients	Monitor B_{12}, A and Fe sttus; supplement as necessary
Clofibrate	Vitamins A, D, E, B_{12}	Unknown action on liver	Monitor nutrients; supplement as necessary
Colestipol	Fat, fat-soluble vitamins	Binds and promotes excretion of bile acids	Monitor nutrient levels
Laxatives			
Castor oil	Ca, K		Ca and K supplements
Milk of magnesia	Ca, K		Ca and K supplements
Mineral oil	Carotene, vitamins A, D, K	Physical barrier; nutrients dissolve in oil and are lost	Avoid use near mealtimes
Phenolphthalein	Vitamins D, Ca	Intestinal "hurry," K depletion; structural changes	Monitor serum K and Ca; supplement K and Ca
Potassium repletion (KCl)	Vitamin B_{12}	Change in ileal pH to inhibit B_{12} absorption	Monitor B_{12} status
Sedative (Glutethimide)	Ca		Acute folacin deficiency

Compiled from Roe, DA, *Drug-Induced Nutritional Deficiencies.* Westport, Conn.: AVI, 1976; Utah Dietetic Association, *Handbook of Clinical Dietetics,* 1977; Bernard, MA, Jacobs, DO, Rombeau JL, *Nutritional and Metabolic Support of Hospitalized Patients.* Philadelphia: W B Saunders, 1986; Holtzapple PG, Schwartz SE, Drug-induced maldigestion and malabsorption. In Roe DA, Campbell TC eds, *Drugs and Nutrients. The Interactive Effects.* New York: Dekker, 1984; Grant A, *Nutritional Assessment Guidelines,* 2nd ed. Seattle: Anna Grant, 1979; and Moore AO, Powers DE, *Food-Medication Interactions,* 3rd ed. Tempe, Ariz: Food-Medication Interactions, 1981.
From Zeman FJ: Drugs and nutritional care. In Clinical Nutrition and Dietetics, 2nd edition. © 1991. Reprinted by permission of Prentice-Hall, Inc., Upper Saddle River, NJ.

TABLE 31–10 Clinical Alternatives to Avoid Enteral Nutrition-Medication Incompatibilities

Action	Type of Incompatibility				
	Physical	Pharmaceutical	Pharmacologic	Physiologic	Pharmacokinetic
Do not mix medication with enteral formula	✗				✗
Try another enteral formula	✗			✗	✗
Use alternate dosage form	✗	✗		✗	✗
Use alternate route for administration	✗	✗		✗	✗
Use a therapeutic equivalent	✗	✗	✗	✗	✗
Check dosing for appropriateness	✗		✗	✗	✗
Use adjunct medication to treat adverse effect			✗	✗	
Dilute medication				✗	

Reprinted with permisstion from Thomson CA, Rollins CJ: Enteral feeding and medication incompatibilities. Support Line 1991;13(3):12–14.

luted in 10 to 15 ml of room temperature tap water. Be aware which medications should not be crushed or opened.

6. Administer each medication separately.
7. Dilute hypertonic medications with water.
8. Administer medications known to cause GI irritation when formula remains in the GI tract.
9. Avoid potential food-drug interactions by using alternate administration routes, alternate formulas or medications, altered feeding or medication schedule as indicated, and multidisciplinary team input.
10. Ongoing monitoring and documentation is essential for diagnosis and effective treatment of potential medication-enteral feeding interactions.

CONCLUSIONS

Several different types of medication-enteral feeding interactions or incompatibilities can affect the quality of care provided to enterally fed patients—physical, pharmaceutical, pharmacologic, physiologic, and pharmacokinetic incompatibilities. Clinicians should be aware of the potential for these interactions as well as the appropriate methods to prevent or avoid them. A cooperative, team approach involving the expertise of the physician, pharmacist, clinical dietician, and nurse is essential to providing optimal care.

REFERENCES

1. Hill DB, Henderson LM, McClain MD: Osmotic diarrhea induced by sugar-free theophylline solution in critically ill patients. J Parenter Enter Nutr 1991;15: 332–336.
2. Fagerman KE, Ballou AE: Drug compatibilities with enteral feeding solutions co-administered by tube. Nutr Supp Serv 1988;8:31–32.
3. Wright B, Robinson L: Enteral feeding tubes as drug delivery systems. Nutr Supp Serv 1986;6:33–48.
4. Thomson CA, Rollins CR: Enteral feeding and medication incompatibilities. Support Line 1991;8(3):9–11.
5. Cutie AJ, Altman E, Lenkel L: Compatibility of enteral products with commonly employed drug additives. J Parenter Enter Nutr 1983;7(2):186–191.
6. Burns PE, McCall L, Wirsching R: Physical compatibility of enteral formulas with various common medications. J Am Diet Assoc 1988;88(9):1094–1096.
7. Davidson LJ, Belknap DC, Flournoy DJ: Flow characteristics of enteral feeding with psyllium hydrophilic mucilloid added. Heart Lung 1991;20(4):405–408.
8. Mitchell JF, Pawlicki KS: Oral dosage forms that should not be crushed. Hosp Pharm 1994;29:666–668, 670–675.
9. Roe DA: Handbook on Drug and Nutrient Interactions, 5th edition. Chicago: The American Dietetic Association, 1994.
10. Lee M, Schwartz RN, Sharifi R: Warfarin resistance and vitamin K. Ann Intern Med 1981;94:140–141.
11. Parr MD, Record KE, Griffith GL et al: Effect of enteral nutrition on warfarin therapy. Clin Pharmacol 1982;1:274–276.

12. Howard PA, Hannaman KN: Warfarin resistance linked to enteral nutrition products. J Am Diet Assoc 1985;85:713–714.

13. Dickerson RN, Melnik G: Osmolality of oral drug solutions and suspensions. Am J Hosp Pharm 1988;45:832–834.

14. Niemiec PW, Vanderveen TW, Morrison JL: Gastrointestinal disorders caused by medication and electrolyte solution osmolality during enteral nutrition. J Parenter Enter Nutr 1983;7:387–389.

15. Lutomski DM, Gora ML, Wright SM et al: Sorbitol content of selected oral liquids. Ann Pharmacother 1993;27:269–273.

16. Edes TE, Walk, BE, Austin JL: Diarrhea in tube-fed patients: feeding formula not necessarily the cause. Am J Med 1990;88:91–93.

17. Kumar A, Weatherly MR, Beaman DC: Sweeteners, flavorings and dyes in antibiotic preparations. Pediatrics 1991;87:352–360.

18. Saklad JJ, Graves RH, Sharp WP: Interaction of oral phenytoin absorption from tube feedings. J Parenter Enter Nutr 1986;10:322–323.

19. Maynard GA, Jones KM, Guidry JR: Phenytoin absorption from tube feedings. Arch Intern Med 1987;147:1821–1823.

20. Bauer LA: Interference of oral phenytoin absorption by continuous infusion nasogastric feedings. Neurology 1982;32:570–572.

21. Ozuna J, Friel P: Effect of enteral tube feeding on serum phenytoin levels. J Neurosurg Nurs 1984;16(6):289–291.

22. Holtz L, Milton J, Sturek JK: Compatibility of medications with enteral feedings. J Parenter Enter Nutr 1987;11(2):183–186.

23. Nishimura LY, Armstrong EP, Plezia PM et al: Influence of enteral feedings on phenytoin sodium absorption from capsules. Drug Intell Clin Pharm 1988;22:130–133.

24. Yuk JH, Nightingale CH, Quintiliani R et al: Absorption of ciprofloxacin administered through a nasogastric or nasoduodenal tube in volunteers and patients receiving enteral nutrition. Diagn Microbiol Infect Dis 1990;13:99–102.

25. Semple HA, Koo W, Tam YK et al: Interactions between hydrazaline and oral nutrients in humans. Ther Drug Monit 1991;13:304–308.

26. Knodell RG: Effects of formula composition on hepatic and intestinal drug metabolism during enteral nutrition. J Parenter Enter Nutr 1990;14:34–38.

27. Zeman FJ: Drugs and nutritional care. In Clinical Nutrition and Dietetics, 2nd. edition. New York: Macmillan Publishing Company, 1993;97–108.

28. Page CP, Hardin TC: Nutritional Assessment and Support: A Primer. Baltimore: Williams & Wilkens, 1993.

29. Thomson CA, LaFrance RJ: Pharmacotherapeutics. In Gottschlich MM, Matarese LE, Shronts EP (eds): Nutrition Support Dietetics Core Curriculum, 2nd. edition. Rockville, MD: Aspen, 1993;452–453.

30. Barber JR: Inquire here: drug-nutrient interactions and enteral feeding. Support Line 1990;12:12–14.

31. Speerhas RA: Administering medications with enteral feedings. Support Line 1994;16(5):1–9.

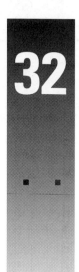

32

Diarrhea and Enteral Nutrition

TIMOTHY E. BOWLING
DAVID B. A. SILK

Enteral feeding has become an invaluable therapeutic tool in both the hospital and home setting. However, it is not without its complications, the most common of which is diarrhea. This occurs in up to 25 percent of patients in general hospital units[1-3] and 63 percent of patients in intensive care units (ICUs).[4,5]

According to basic physiologic principles, which take into account the capacity of the normal small and large intestine to assimilate fluid and electrolytes, diarrhea can be defined as the passage of more than 200 g of stool/24-hour period.[6] It follows that this definition of diarrhea depends on accurate measurement of stool output. Unfortunately, this is often not a feasible option in patients who may be bed bound, fecally incontinent, or uncooperative. There has thus been little agreement on the definition of enteral feeding–related diarrhea, with as many as 14 different definitions having been used; some studies do not specify a definition at all.[7] This lack of agreement accounts for the large variation of reported incidences of enteral feeding–related diarrhea, ranging from 2.3 percent[3] to 63 percent.[8] However, despite this, there is no disagreement among these studies that diarrhea is the most common complication of enteral feeding.

The clinical implications of enteral feeding–related diarrhea are significant. It undoubtedly limits the efficacy of the feeding process; it adds to potential complications, such as in-fected sacral pressure sores and altered fluid and electrolyte balance[5]; it causes considerable distress to both patients and nursing staff; and it increases the cost of patient care.[9] Occasionally it is so severe that enteral feeding must be stopped and parenteral feeding started, with all its potential complications.[1-3,5,10]

ETIOLOGY

Many causes have been reported (Table 32–1), but as yet no definitive answer exists.

Antibiotics

There is a recognized association between enteral feeding–related diarrhea and concomitant antibiotic therapy.[4,11-15] However, the incidence of diarrhea in enterally fed patients taking antibiotics far exceeds the incidence in normally fed patients taking the same antibiotics.[4]

TABLE 32–1 Proposed Causes of Enteral Feeding–Related Diarrhea

Concomitant antibiotic therapy
Infected diets
Diet osmolality
Lactose intolerance
Hypoalbuminemia
Osmotically active medications

Thus there appears to be a synergistic relationship between enteral feeding and antibiotic treatment that accounts for the high incidence of diarrhea.[16]

The diarrheagenic nature of antibiotics has been recognized for decades.[4,13,17-20] Many believe that it arises from toxic actions of the antibiotics on the normal intestinal flora with bacterial overgrowth of certain undesirable strains, such as enterobacteria (*Klebsiella, Proteus, Pseudomonas*) or virulent strains of *Staphylococcus* not affected by the antibiotic in use.[21] Other evidence implicates *Clostridium difficile* proliferation as a significant mediator of antibiotic-related diarrhea.[22-25]

C. difficile is isolated in 20 to 30 percent of patients with antibiotic-associated diarrhea and about 95 percent of cases of pseudomembranous colitis.[26,27] However, it is also found in about 4 percent of healthy adults.[26,28] *C. difficile* produces at least three toxins that may cause diarrhea. Toxin A is an enterotoxin that damages the villous tips and brush border membrane, leading to mucosal erosion and exudation and secretion of fluid into the gut lumen.[29] There is no available toxin assay. Toxin B is a potent cytotoxin for which there is an assay; it decreases protein synthesis[30] and disrupts cellular actin fibers.[31] There is also evidence of a motility factor, which alters intestinal motor activity, but its role remains unknown.[32]

Although its role in pseudomembranous colitis has been clearly established, the role of *C. difficile* in less severe antibiotic-related gastrointestinal (GI) illness is unclear. Even when the toxins are present they may not cause the symptoms, although at present patients with antibiotic-associated diarrhea and a positive toxin assay are considered to have *C. difficile* disease.

Studies have demonstrated positive cytotoxin in about 20 percent of patients with antibiotic-associated diarrhea and in 7 to 25 percent of patients who are receiving antibiotics but who do not have diarrhea.[15,27,33] These figures imply that additional mechanisms are involved in antibiotic-associated diarrhea. Several studies have identified an association between antibiotic-associated diarrhea and decreased concentrations of fecal short-chain fatty acids (SCFAs), occurring as a result of diminished colonic carbohydrate fermentation.[15,34,35] This is an important observation and likely to be a vital link between antibiotic-associated diarrhea and enteral feeding. This topic is discussed in more detail later in this chapter.

Infected Diets

A number of investigators have documented that bacterial colonization and infectious complications develop due to contamination of the enteral diet.[36-39] Enteral diets are often ideal culture media, with rapid bacterial proliferation taking place once contamination has occurred.[40,41] Various studies have demonstrated gross contamination of both commercial and hospital-prepared feeds, with microbial numbers ranging up to 10^9 organisms/ml.[36,37,42-47] The micro-organisms that have been isolated from these enteral feeds have included *Klebsiella* spp, *Escherichia coli, Enterobacter* spp, *Salmonella enteritidis, Pseudomonas aeruginosa, Staphylococcus aureus, Staphylococcus epidermidis, Bacillus* spp, *Proteus* spp, β-hemolytic streptococcus, and yeasts.

Several studies have looked at the rate of bacterial growth once contamination has occurred. In a preliminary study, White and colleagues inoculated a commercial feed with one *S. aureus* organism per milliliter and obtained, after 24 hours at 37°C, a viable count of 8.2×10^5 organisms/ml.[48] Simmons inoculated 20-ml portions of a hospital-prepared feed with 1×10^3 *S. aureus* or *E. coli*/ml and reported that the counts exceeded 1×10^5/ml after only 8 hours at 23°C.[49] Anderton looked at the rate of *E. coli* multiplication in an in vitro study designed to simulate hospital conditions.[41] They found that in a commercially prepared diet inoculated with 10^2 colony-forming units (CFUs)/ml of *E. coli* that this colonization figure had doubled within 8 hours. In the recipient flask (patient's stomach) there were 10^8 CFU/ml in the same period. Even contamination with 10^{-1} CFU/ml produced a growth of 10^3 CFU/ml within 3 hours. It appears that the level of initial contamination greatly influences the final bacterial load.

Contaminated diets entering the patient containing as little as 10^3 CFU/ml can cause not only diarrhea but also sepsis, pneumonia, and urinary tract infections.[37-39,50] But where do these organisms originate? In the days when enteral diets were made up in the hospital kitchens, problems of contamination were much more commonplace,[36,41,44,51] and there is no doubt that the use of commercially prepared diets has been a major factor in reducing the incidence of diet contamination. But there has been considerable variation in the literature in the incidences of contamination of commercially prepared diets. Curtis and colleagues found a 15 percent incidence,[52] Thurn and associates a 21 percent incidence,[50] and

Fernandez-Crehuet Navajas a 25 percent incidence,[53] but Bastow[44] and Keighley[46] found these diets to be entirely sterile. However, where the diets are sterile at the commencement of feeding, they are usually contaminated by the end of the administration.[54]

Payne-James performed a prospective clinical study examining whether organisms can ascend retrogradely from the enteral tube through the giving set.[55] The study was carried out on patients being enterally fed over a 48-hour period. There were three designs of giving set: one with no drip chamber (group I; n = 18), one with a drip chamber (group II; n = 17), and one with a drip chamber and an antireflux ball valve (group III; n = 18). Samples of diet were taken before the study and at 12 hourly intervals both from the giving sets and from the diet containers. Colonization occurred in the giving sets by 24 hours in groups I and III but in the diet container only in group I. The conclusions drawn were that retrograde spread of organisms from the patient to the diet container did occur, but the insertion of a drip chamber (but not an antireflux valve) prevented this problem, presumably by interrupting continuity of flow and by acting as a physical barrier to the proximal progression of the organisms.

In addition to organisms ascending into the diet container, scanning electron microscopy of the internal walls of feeding tubes has shown that these also can become colonized.[56] In a recent study of 48 cancer patients the feeding tubes were meticulously cultured before and after 1 day of feeding. The investigators found 16 of the 48 tubes contaminated with a median concentration of 10^6 CFU/ml of 102 different strains. There was no difference whether the diet was reconstituted in the hospital or commercially prepared.[57]

These colonizing organisms mainly come from the patient, but some originate from staff setting up the feed, as evidenced by large numbers of contaminating *Klebsiella* and *Enterobacter* spp.[57] This problem of infection from staff handling is, as already mentioned, no longer as common now that most diets are commercially prepared. However, as a result of these various studies, we recommend avoiding "hanging time" of enteral feeding resevoirs of longer than 24 hours.[55,58]

Once the diet is contaminated, bacteria multiply to potentially pathogenic levels and are then placed directly into the GI tract. In the healthy adult, stomach pH and enzyme activity may reduce bacterial multiplication, but many patients, especially those in ICUs, are receiving antacids or H_2 blockers, which raise the pH and therefore negate this physiologic effect.[59] Alternatively the patients may be receiving antibiotics, which may predispose to infection by gram-negative bacilli.[60] Patients already at risk of infection, such as those immunocompromised for whatever reason, are particularly prone to the adverse effects of gut colonization. A number of investigators have shown that such episodes can be causally related to the administration of contaminated enteral diet.[36,37,39,61]

This influx of large quantities of bacteria into the GI tract, even if they did originate from the patient, albeit at much smaller concentrations, will inevitably alter the intestinal flora. Fernandez-Crehuet Navajas found that 36 percent of 117 patients receiving an enteral diet developed GI symptoms (fever, vomiting, abdominal pain, or diarrhea) in the first 24 hours of feeding.[53] Sixty-seven percent of these patients had received a contaminated diet; 32 percent, a sterile one. The diarrhea could occur either as a straightforward gastroenteritic illness or by altering the metabolism of carbohydrates to SCFAs further down the GI tract (see below).

Diet Osmolality

Up until 1984 it was believed that undiluted hypertonic diets were a major factor in the pathogenesis of enteral side-effects, such as diarrhea.[62,63] For this reason "starter" regimens were used for the first few days of enteral feeding, where the diet was diluted and the tonicity subsequently increased over 3 to 5 days to full strength.[62-64] The hypothesis underlying this assumption was that introducing a high osmolar load into the duodenum would cause such a large movement of water into the lumen to achieve isotonicity that the normal absorptive capacity of the small and large intestine would be overwhelmed.[62,65] However, the rate of gastric emptying during the intragastric infusion of diet, as opposed to bolus feeding, is controlled and regulated by the energy content and not the osmolality of gastric contents.[66,67] Keohane and associates performed a study randomizing patients to receive, by 24-hour nasogastric infusion, either a hypertonic diet (430 mOsm/kg), the same diet with a starter regimen (osmolality increasing from 145 to 430 mOsm/kg over 4 days) or an isotonic diet (300 mOsm/kg).[14] No differences in side-effects were noted between any of the groups, and the main advantage of the hypertonic group was that 60 percent more nutrients could be administered in the first 3 days. As a result of this study the use of hypertonic diets has not been discontinued, and starter regimens in intragastrically fed patients are no longer felt to be necessary.

There are no similar controlled data, however, on patients fed postpylorically, and some investigators still advocate the use of starter regimens in these patients.[68] Although the volume of fluid entering the colon (colonic inflow) has been shown to be increased during intraduodenal infusion, the amounts are well within the absorptive capacity of the colon,[69] and therefore there is probably no need for starter regimens in these patients either.

Lactose Intolerance

Walike and Walike were the first to suggest that the lactose content was the cause of enteral feeding related diarrhea,[70] and it has been demonstrated that diarrhea occurs when patients with biochemically proved lactose malabsorption are bolus fed lactose-containing enteral diets.[71] However, in another study, enterally fed patients with biochemically proved lactose malabsorption did not have a higher incidence of GI side-effects when fed a lactose-containing enteral diet compared with a lactose-free formulation.[12] The explanation for this apparent discrepancy lies in the load (concentration × rate) of lactose administered to "lactose-intolerant" patients. Lactase, or β-galactosidase, is a brush border hydrolase, the specific activity of which is reduced (but not absent) in patients and subjects with lactose malabsorption. If 2 to 3 L of a lactose-containing diet is infused constantly over 24 hours, the load of lactose administered per unit of time is low and usually within the capacity of the brush border hydrolases, and hence symptoms will not occur.[14] However, if high loads of lactose are administered by bolus feeding, the lactose load will overwhelm the hydrolases and symptoms will consequently develop.[71] There is therefore, on the basis of the current literature, no evidence that lactose malabsorption is a cause of enteral feeding–related diarrhea.

Hypoalbuminemia

Several clinical studies have suggested a relationship between hypoalbuminemia and enteral feeding–related diarrhea.[72-75] Some animal data suggest that hypoalbuminemia is associated with impaired intestinal fluid absorption.[76] Brinson and coworkers found

that inducing hypoproteinemia in rats by volume expansion caused a fourfold to fivefold increase in lymph flow, a fall in capillary albumin clearance, and an increase in mucosal albumin clearance.[77] These findings agreed with other experiments, where volume expansion resulted in elevated intestinal interstitial hydrostatic pressure and exudation of protein into the intestinal lumen.[78,79] In addition to protein exudation, net transmucosal water movement converted from a net absorptive state to a net secretory state as plasma protein levels fell below 40 g/L—equivalent to an albumin of about 26 g/L.[77] In earlier work the same investigators had noted a correlation between intolerance of standard enteral diets and diarrhea with serum albumin levels of less than 25 g/L.[74]

Contrary to the intolerance of hypoproteinemic patients to standard enteral diets, it has been noted that dipeptide and tripeptide diets are well tolerated in patients with kwashiorkor-like hypoalbuminemia.[80] Animal studies have also confirmed that a peptide enteral formula results in enhanced intestinal absorption and reduced intestinal albumin clearance in rats subjected to acute hypoproteinemia.[77,81] These observations have been attributed to the efficient peptide transport mechanisms, specific to dipeptides and tripeptides, present in the intestinal mucosa.[82-84] It has subsequently been hypothesized that when the intestinal absorptive capacity is compromised by intestinal mucosal edema associated with acute hypoalbuminemia, enteral alimentation enriched with small-molecular-weight peptides may "protect" the intestinal mucosa by promoting intestinal absorption.[85]

In the human clinical studies that have indicated a positive association between enteral feeding–related diarrhea and hypoalbuminemia, it was not clearly stated whether these patients had other "risk factors" for enteral feeding–related diarrhea, namely, concomitant antibiotic therapy.[72,74,75] Other studies, however, have found no association[86,87] between these two factors. Despite experimental and animal evidence confirming better absorption of peptide diets in hypoproteinemic patients, no controlled clinical trial in humans has been performed. Hypoalbuminemia may contribute to enteral feeding related–diarrhea, but further in vivo studies are needed.

Osmotically Active Medication

Sorbitol is commonly added to medicinal elixirs to improve palatability and is contained in a wide variety of solutions including theo-phylline, paracentomol, cough preparations, cimetidine, isoniazid, lithium, and vitamins. It Is, however, an osmotically active substance, and several investigators have identified sor-bitol-containing elixirs as a cause of enteral feeding–related diarrhea.[88-90]

Additional Factors

Of the various proposed mechanisms for en-teral feeding related–diarrhea discussed above, only antibiotic therapy, infected diets, osmoti-cally active elixir medications, and possibly hy-poalbuminemia stand up to critical analysis. However, despite careful attention to these fac-tors, enteral feeding–related diarrhea still oc-curs in approximately 15 percent of patients (Silk DBA, personal communication). Some other factor(s) must therefore contribute to the pathogenesis of enteral feeding–related diar-rhea.

Small Intestinal Responses to Enteral Feeding

In 1978, Wright and colleagues perfused the human duodenum in vivo with a nutrient mix-ture and found a secretion of water and elec-trolytes in the jejunum, which was separated from the duodenum by an occluding balloon.[91] These results implied that a mediator or medi-ators were responsible for the distal secretory effect, and the most likely candidate was a hor-monal mechanism. Further support of hor-monal involvement was provided by the demonstration of a jejunal secretion of water and electrolytes in response to the intravenous infusion of a physiologic mixture of gastrin, se-cretin, cholecystokinin, glucagon, and gastroin-testinal polypeptide (GIP) similar to that found in the normal postprandial state.[92] However, re-cently several studies have demonstrated a proabsorptive response in the jejunum to a meal stimulus that appears to be induced by nutrient osmolality.[93-99] These studies therefore appear to contradict Wright's results. However, the latter study had methodologic problems: first, the measurement of jejunal water and ion transport was performed at a level of only 55 percent recovery of ^{14}C PEG, a level not at a steady state. Second, ionic transport was mea-sured by a luminal perfusate solution lacking glucose and amino acids, thereby eliminating the possibility of sodium absorption coupled to one of these organic solutes. Third, a balloon was inflated intraluminally to partition the duo-denum from the jejunum during the nutrient infusions. Such balloon distention can serve as

an intraluminal tactile stimulus, which as been shown to initiate a secretory response in more distal bowel.[100]

Because of the resulting uncertainty over the small intestinal responses to enteral feeding, Raimundo and colleagues carried out a series of in vivo perfusion studies in healthy volunteers to investigate the small intestinal response to both intragastric and intraduodenal enteral feeding.[69,101] Two parameters were looked at: the motor activity of the small intestine, and the volume of fluid entering the cecum (colonic in-flow). During postpyloric feeding the small in-testinal motility appropriately converted to the normal postprandial pattern and the colonic in-flow volumes were increased from fasting lev-els.[69] During intragastric feeding both motility and inflow volumes remained similar to that ob-served during the fasting state.[101] The diet infu-sion rate during these studies was the same as that used to provide 2000 kcal or 2 L/24 hours, which is what most patients will receive in the hospital, and only provides 60 kcal/hour. As the receptors controlling the small intestinal re-sponses to diet appear to be located in the prox-imal small intestine,[93-99] this may explain why diet infused directly into the duodenum is able to initiate the fed response, whereas the same rate of infusion into the stomach, which will gradually release its contents through the py-lorus, is insufficient to initiate the normal post-prandial responses.

Taking these studies together, it appears that the small intestine responds predictably to en-teral feeding, both in terms of motility and fluid movement, irrespective of the site of diet infu-sion. However, during Raimundo's studies those subjects fed intragastrically invariably de-veloped diarrhea,[101] despite the lack of any nor-mal postprandial response, whereas those fed intraduodenally did not develop diarrhea. This led to the hypothesis that enteral feeding–re-lated diarrhea may occur due to a colonic func-tion disorder.

Colonic Responses to Enteral Feeding

To examine the colonic response to enteral feeding, two sets of experiments were carried out—one to look at colonic water and elec-trolyte transport and the second to look at motility responses. A new technique of in vivo colonic perfusion was designed to en-able assessment of water and electrolyte movement simultaneously in the ascending and distal colon in response to the intragas-tric and intraduodenal infusion of a standard polymeric enteral diet.[102] The distal colonic motor activity was measured with an established technique: using four water-perfused catheters inserted in the descending, proximal, and distal sigmoid and in the rectum and monitoring activity before and during enteral feeding.[103,104] In all these studies two different strengths of a polymeric diet were infused either intragastrically or intraduodenally: a low-load diet infused at 1.4 ml/minute (1.4 kcal/min; 8.75 mg of N/minute) and a high-load diet infused at 2.8 ml/minute (4.2 kcal/minute; 26.1 mg of N/minute). The low-load diet corresponded clinically to the administration of 2 L (2000 kcal)/24 hours (equivalent to 2 L/day)—the same used in Raimundo's studies.[101] Catabolic patients or those being fed cyclically over 12 to 14 hours/day, a common situation especially in the home setting, require higher dietary loads—the high-load diet in our studies corresponded to this type of feeding.

A marked secretion of water, sodium, and chloride was demonstrated in the ascending colon during the intragastric infusion of the low- and high-load diets and during the intraduodenal infusion of the high-load diet[105] (Fig. 32–1). This secretion amounted to approximately 120 ml/hour or, if equated over 24 hours, almost 3 L/day. The distal colon showed absorption during fasting and feeding in all the groups (Fig. 32–2).

The distal colonic segmental motor activity was unchanged from fasting during the low-load diet infusions,[106] but during the high-load infusions activity was suppressed significantly immediately after intragastric infusion began

LOW LOAD DIET

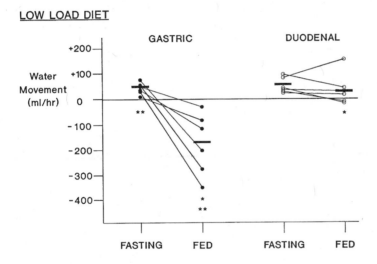

HIGH LOAD DIET

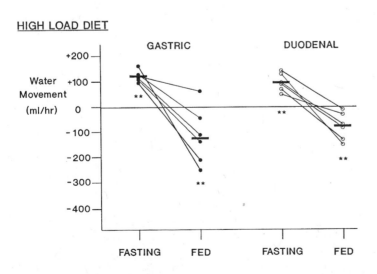

FIGURE 32–1 Water movement in the ascending colon. Each point represents a subject; the thick lines are the medians. ● = gastric feeding; ○ = duodenal feeding; + = net absorption; – = net secretion; * = gastric vs duodenal; $P = <0.05$; ** = fasting vs fed, $P < 0.05$. (From Bowling TE, Raimundo AM, Grimble GK, Silk DBA: Colonic secretory effect in response to enteral feeding in man. Gut 1994;35:1734–1741. Published by BMJ Publishing Group.)

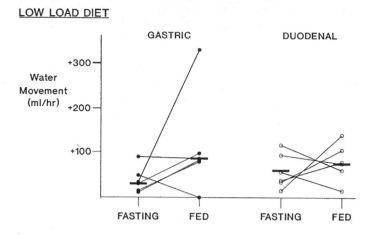

LOW LOAD DIET

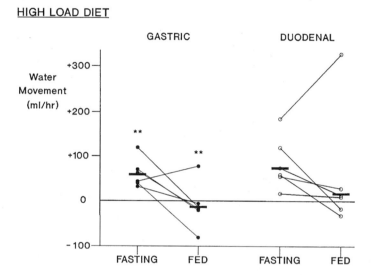

HIGH LOAD DIET

FIGURE 32-2 Water movement in the distal colon. Each point represents a subject; the thick lines are the medians. ● = gastric feeding; ○ = duodenal feeding; + = net absorption; − = net secretion; ** = fasting vs fed, *P* < 0.05. (From Bowling TE, Raimundo AM, Grimble GK, Silk DBA: Colonic secretory effect in response to enteral feeding in man. Gut 1994;35: 1734–1741. Published by BMJ Publishing Group.)

and within 3 hours after intraduodenal infusion began (Fig. 32–3).[107]

Possible Mechanisms of Abnormal Colonic Response to Enteral Feeding

These studies are the first to examine the in vivo human colonic response to enteral feeding and have demonstrated a colonic secretion of water and electrolytes, predominantly in the ascending colon, during both intragastric and intraduodenal feeding, and a suppression of distal colonic segmental motor activity during both the high-load diet infusions. The secretion amounted to an overall colonic load of up to 2.24 ml/minute (in the high-load intragastric group) during a perfusion period of 6 hours. If it is possible to extrapolate this over a 24-hour period, the additional colonic volume would amount to 3.2 L/day. This secretion, we feel, is

likely to be important in the pathogenesis of enteral feeding–related diarrhea.

The human colon's normal absorptive capacity is 5700 ml/day,[108] and it may therefore be supposed that the colon should be able to absorb this extra fluid. In the above study the cecum of volunteers was intubated and fluid infused at rates sufficient to cause an increase in stool frequency and volume.[108] The figure of 5700 ml/day was derived from the volume of fluid required to cause diarrhea (stool weight > 200 g/day) plus the assumed cecal inflow volumes and therefore reflected the entire colon's absorptive capacity. In our studies the ascending colon, which in normal circumstances is the site of maximal fluid absorption, secreted water and electrolytes, and therefore the colon's absorptive capacity would have been seriously impaired, such

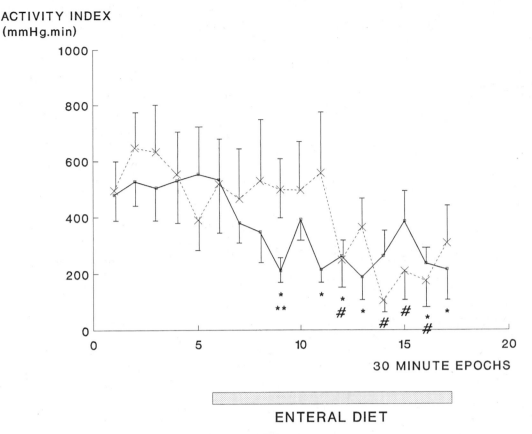

FIGURE 32–3 Distal colonic segmental motor activity during high load enteral feeding: Mean activity index + / – standard error of the mean. ——□——gastric feeding; ----✗---- duodenal feeding; * = fasting vs fed (gastric group), $P < 0.05$; # = fasting vs fed (duodenal group), $P < .05$; ** = gastric vs duodenal, $P < 0.05$. (From Bowling TE, Raimundo AM, Jameson JS, Rogers J, Silk DBA: The effect of enteral feeding on colonic motility in man. Gut [in press].)

that an increased colonic load of 2.24 ml/minute could cause diarrhea. To compound matters, the suppression of segmental colonic motor activity, which results in accelerated transit of colonic contents,[109] is likely to diminish further the colon's absorptive capacity.

In our studies diarrhea occurred more commonly when subjects were fed intragastrically with a high-load enteral diet. This group has the greatest secretion and most profound suppression of motility. In the low-load groups, where motility remained unchanged from the fasting state and secretion only occurred in those fed intragastrically, diarrhea was not observed; in the high-load duodenal group, where there was an overall secretion of 1 ml/minute, predominantly in the ascending colon, and a delayed suppression of colonic motor activity, diarrhea occurred in only one subject. Therefore, the clinical observations (i.e., the incidence of diar-

rhea) are supported by the experimental results.

In these colonic studies, abnormal colonic responses are observed with lower loads of intragastric diet than with intraduodenal diet. The resulting secretion cannot be locally mediated in the colon because of the differences in fluid transport between the intragastric and intraduodenal groups. The changes in segmental colonic motor activity may be associated with the alterations in fluid transport. However, the relationship between these two is not clear-cut. In the low-load groups no changes in motor activity are observed, whereas in the high-load groups there is significant suppression of activity. This suppression is unlikely to occur only as a direct result of the colonic fluid secretion, because the overall secretion in the low-load intragastric group (1.4 ml/minute) exceeds that in the high-load intraduodenal group (1 ml/minute) and because the suppression of motor activity in the high-load intragastric group starts immediately after feeding, that is, before there is any volume effect from the secretion.

The most likely explanation for these colonic responses is some kind of neurohumoral response initiated from the proximal GI tract during feeding. During all our studies, serum was stored to estimate a variety of GI polypeptide hormones. One such hormone appears to be involved: peptide YY. In humans this hormone is found predominantly in the colon and terminal ileum[110] and has been demonstrated to inhibit intestinal secretion in animals in vitro and in vivo models.[111,112] In our studies circulating peptide YY levels were significantly raised during intraduodenal feeding but remained unchanged from fasting during intragastric feeding (Fig. 32–4).[113] What can be hypothesized is that during intraduodenal feeding the increase in peptide YY levels inhibits colonic secretion but during intragastric feeding there is the loss of this negative feedback loop and hence the secretion is not inhibited. This clearly is not the whole story. To prevent the secretion the peptide YY must be inhibiting

another secretory agent—presumably another hormone. We have also assayed vasoactive intestinal polypeptide (VIP), pancreatic glucagon, and neurotensin, but none of these alter during enteral feeding.

Fiber and Diarrhea

Nonstarch polysaccharide, or fiber, passes through the small intestine and enters the colon where it is metabolized anerobically by endogenous bacteria.[114] One of the major breakdown products of this process is SCFAs—acetate, propionate, and butyrate. SCFAs have several biologic functions. They play an important role in maintaining colonic epithelial integrity[115] and in stimulating mucosal proliferation.[116] They are also avidly absorbed in the colon[117] and therefore enhance water and electrolyte absorption.[115,118-120] It is through this effect that they are likely to be important in the pathogenesis of diarrhea.

Ruppin and colleagues performed some in vivo human colonic perfusion studies to examine water and electrolyte movement in response to SCFAs in detail.[118] They perfused the

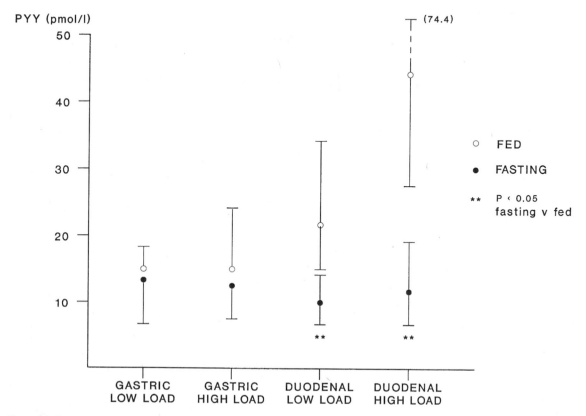

FIGURE 32–4 Peptide YY levels during perfusion studies (median + range). ● = fasting; o = fed; ** = fasting vs fed, *P* < 0.05.

entire colon with an isotonic solution containing 0, 30, 60, or 90 mM of one SCFA (but no solutions containing all three) directly into the cecum. They found that all three SCFAs enhanced water, sodium, and potassium absorption and bicarbonate secretion, mainly in a dose-dependent fashion.

Recently antibiotics have been shown to alter colonic flora and inhibit the bacterial fermentation of fiber and hence the production of SCFAs.[121,122] With a smaller colonic concentration of SCFAs there will be a diminished stimulus to salt and water absorption. It is through this mechanism that antibiotics could mediate diarrhea. It is also the theoretical reason why supplementing an enteral diet with fiber may be of benefit in patients with enteral feeding–related diarrhea.[123] Most commercially available polymeric enteral diets do not contain a fiber source, and hence there will be little colonic SCFA production. In patients receiving both enteral feeding and antibiotics two possible mechanisms may account for the apparent synergistic effect between enteral feeding and antibiotics in producing a higher than expected incidence of diarrhea:[19] first, the diets are producing relatively smaller amounts of SCFAs; second, the antibiotics will influence the metabolism of any potential source of SCFA.

A number of clinical studies have investigated whether fiber supplementation of enteral diets results in a decreased incidence of enteral feeding–related diarrhea.[12,124-126] All were carried out in ICUs, and none showed any benefit. We believe the reason for this is twofold. First, the amount of fermentable soluble fiber in soy polysaccharide, the most common fiber source used in enteral diets, ranges from 5 to 27 percent (depending on the analytical method used),[127,128] and therefore the amount of SCFAs produced is limited.[129] Second, the patients studied were in the ICU; confounding factors in both the control and study groups, such as concomitant antibiotics or hypoalbuminemia, were not taken into account and would affect the outcome. Indeed, in two of the studies there was a correlation between diarrhea and the administration of antibiotics.[12,123] These studies therefore do not accurately reflect the possible beneficial effects of fiber or its metabolic products (i.e., SCFAs) on the incidence of enteral feeding–related diarrhea.

We have demonstrated a secretion of water and electrolytes in the ascending colon during enteral feeding. Because the ascending colon is the primary site of action of SCFAs, it was an obvious extension to our studies to examine the effects of SCFAs on this secretory effect. This was done using an identical in vivo human colonic perfusion technique as used in our earlier studies[102] except that a physiologic solution of SCFAs was infused directly into the cecum during the intragastric administration of a low-load polymeric enteral diet (1 kcal/minute). During a control period of feeding there was an ascending colonic secretion, which was reversed to a net absorption during the cecal infusion of the SCFA solution (Fig. 32–5).[129] SCFAs' ability to reverse the colonic secretion may well have implications in the management of enteral feeding–related diarrhea.

MANAGING ENTERAL FEEDING–RELATED DIARRHEA

Having discussed at length the various possible mechanisms underlying the pathogenesis of enteral feeding–related diarrhea, how should this common problem be managed in a clinical setting?

It is reasonable to conclude from the various studies discussed above that the secretion of water and electrolytes in the ascending colon is a genuine response to enteral feeding and that this is likely to be of primary importance in the pathogenesis of enteral feeding–related diarrhea. The consistent finding that intragastric feeding leads to more profound changes in both water and electrolyte secretion and in the suppression of colonic motor activity and, more important, to an increased incidence of diarrhea suggests that perhaps patients should preferentially be fed postpylorically. It could also be argued that the continuous intragastric infusion of an enteral diet is not a physiologic way of feeding in that it does not resemble normal eating. Intraduodenal diet infusion, on the other hand, is more physiologic because it is not dissimilar to the gradual release of gastric contents through the pylorus. It would, however, not be right to advocate the routine use of postpyloric feeding in the absence of controlled clinical trials comparing the effects of prepyloric and postpyloric feeding.

We recommend the following for a patient with troublesome diarrhea:

1. Review antibiotic therapy and stop if possible.
2. Review H_2 antagonist therapy and stop if possible.
3. Stop laxatives or osmotically active elixir medications.
4. Try loperamide or codeine phosphate.

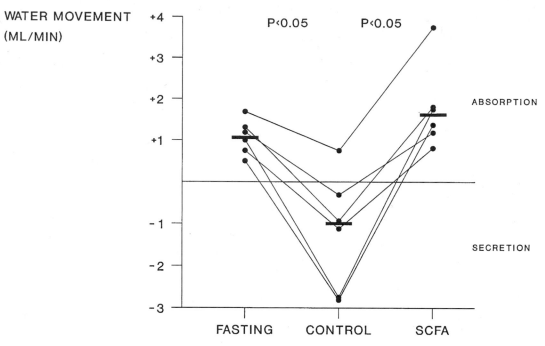

FIGURE 32–5   Water movement in the ascending colon during intragastric feeding before and during the intra-caecal infusion of short-chain fatty acids (SCFAs). (From Bowling TE, Raimundo AM, Grimble GK, Silk DBA: Reversal by short-chain fatty acids of colonic fluid secretion induced by enteral feeding. Lancet 1993;342:1266–1268. © by The Lancet Ltd., 1993.)

5. Consider a fiber-containing diet.
6. Consider postpyloric feeding.

Most patients should improve sufficiently on steps 1 to 4; 5 and 6, as discussed, are based on theoretical and anecdotal evidence, and clinical trial data are awaited. If despite these steps the diarrhea is still difficult to manage, enteral feeding should be stopped and total parenteral feeding instituted.

THE FUTURE

There is considerable scope for further investigation. Clearly the experimental findings in healthy volunteers described in this chapter must be evaluated in patients. Prospective randomized controlled clinical trials comparing prepyloric and postpyloric feeding; fiber- and nonfiber-containing diets, stratified for confounding factors such as antibiotics and hypoalbuminemia; and bolus vs continuous feeding on the incidence of diarrhea and other complications are all needed. As discussed earlier, fiber-containing diets may not be the optimal way to achieve increased concentrations of SCFAs in the colon, and therefore ways of incorporating SCFAs into enteral diets, such as microencapsulation, must be found so that

they arrive in the cecum unaffected by their passage through the small intestine. Also, further studies examining the hormonal responses to enteral feeding are needed to elucidate the pathways that lead to the abnormal colonic responses.

The solution to enteral feeding–related diarrhea is nearer now that we have begun to find vital clues to the underlying mechanisms. One hopes that before long clinicians will have learned enough about this common problem to combat it successfully in the majority of patients.

REFERENCES

1. Heymsfield SB, Bethel RA, Ansley JD et al: Enteral hyperalimentation: an alternative to central venous hyperalimentation. Ann Intern Med 1979;90:63–71.
2. Heibert JM, Brown A, Anderson RG et al: Comparison of continuous vs intermittent tube feedings in adult burn patients. J Parenter Enter Nutr 1981;5:73–75.
3. Cataldi-Betcher EL, Seltzer MH, Slocum BA et al: Complications occurring during enteral nutrition support: a prospective study. J Parenter Enter Nutr 1983;7:546–552.
4. Keohane PP, Attrill H, Love M et al: Relation between osmolality and gastrointestinal side effects in enteral nutrition. Br Med J 1984;288:678.
5. Kelly TW, Patrick MR, Hillman KM: Study of diarrhoea in critically ill patients. Crit Care Med 1983;11:7–9.

6. Turnberg LA: Mechanisms of diarrhoea. Curr Conc Gastroenterol 1986 (Spring):3–9.

7. Zimmaro Bliss D, Guenter PA, Settle RG: Defining and reporting diarrhoea in tube-fed patients—what a mess! Am J Clin Nutr 1992;55:753–759.

8. Smith CE, Marien L, Brogdon C et al: Diarrhoea associated with tube feeding in mechanically ventilated critically ill patients. Nurs Res 1990;39:148–152.

9. Dobb GJ: Diarrhoea in the critically ill. Intensive Care Med 1986;12:113–115.

10. Larkin JM, Moylan JA: Complete enteral support to the thermally impaired patient. Am J Surg 1976;131:722–724.

11. Bastow MD: Complications of enteral feeding. Gut 1986;27(suppl 1):51–55.

12. Guenter PA, Settle RG, Perlmutter S et al: Tube feeding related diarrhoea in acutely ill patients. J Parenter Enter Nutr 1990;14:277–280.

13. Jones BJM, Lees R, Andrews J et al: Comparison of an elemental and polymeric enteral diet in patients with normal gastrointestinal function. Gut 1983;24:78–84.

14. Keohane PP, Attrill H, Jones BJM et al: The roles of lactose and *Clostridium difficile* in the pathogenesis of enteral feeding associated diarrhoea. Clin Nutr 1983;1:259–264.

15. Surawicz CM, Elmer GW, Speelman P et al: Prevention of antibiotic associated diarrhoea by *Saccharomyces boulardii:* a prospective study. Gastroenterology 1989;96L:981–988.

16. Silk DBA: Towards the optimization of enteral nutrition. Clin Nutr 1987;6:61.

17. Woolfson AMJ, Ricketts CR, Hardy SM et al: Prolonged nasogastric tube feeding in critically ill and surgical patients. Postgrad Med J 1976;52:678–682.

18. Levine HG, Lamont JT: Diarrhoea we can treat: antibiotic-associated colitis. Compr Ther 1982;8:36–43.

19. Jacobson ED, Falçon WW: Malabsorptive effects of neomycin in commonly used doses. JAMA 1961;175:187–190.

20. Broom J, Jones K: Causes and prevention of diarrhoea in patients receiving enteral nutritional support. J Human Nutr 1981;35:123–127.

21. Editorial: Tetracycline diarrhoea. Br Med J 1968;402.

22. Bartlett JG, Chang TU, Gurwith M et al: Antibiotic associated psudomembranous colitis due to toxin-producing clostridia. N Engl J Med 1978;298:531–534.

23. Burdon DW, Thompson H, Candy DCA et al: Enterotoxins of *Clostridium difficile.* Lancet 1981;2:258–259.

24. George WL, Sutter VL, Finegold SM: Toxicity and antimicrobial susceptibility of *Clostridium difficile,* a cause of antimicrobial agent-associated colitis. Curr Microbiol 1978;1:55–58.

25. Grube BJ, Heimbach DM, Marvin JA: *Clostridium difficile* diarrhoea in critically ill burned patients. Arch Surg 1987;122:655–661.

26. Bartlett JG: Antibiotic-associated pseudomembranous colitis. Rev Infect Dis 1979;1:530–539.

27. George WL, Rolfe RD, Finegold SM: *Clostridium difficile* and its cytotoxin in faeces of patients with antimicrobial agent associated diarrhoea and miscellaneous conditions. J Clin Microbiol 1982;15:1049–1053.

28. George WL, Rolfe RD, Sutter VL et al: Diarrhoea and colitis associated with antimicrobial therapy in man and animals. Am J Clin Nutr 1979;32:251–257.

29. Lyerly DM, Krivan HC, Wilkins TD. *Clotridium dificile:* its disease and toxins. Clin Microbiol Rev 1988;1:1–18.

30. Pothoulakis C, Triadafilopoulos G, Clark M et al: *Clostridium difficile* cytotoxin inhibits protein synthesis in fibroblasts and intestinal mucosa. Gastroenterology 1986;91:1147–1153.

31. Thelestam M, Bronnegard M: Interaction of cytopathogenic toxin from *Clostridium difficile* with cells in tissue culture. Scand J Infect Dis 1980;22(suppl):16–29.

32. Justus PG, Martin JL, Goldberg DA et al: Myoelectric effects of *Clostridium difficile:* motility altering factors distinct from its cytotoxin and enterotoxin in rabbits. Gastroenterology 1982;83:836–843.

33. Viscidi R, Willey S, Bartlett JG: Isolation rates and toxigenic potential of *Clostridium difficile* isolates from various patient populations. Gastroenterology 1981;81:5–9.

34. Raimundo AH, Wilden S, Rogers J et al: Influence of metronidazole on volatile fatty acid (VFA) production from soy polysaccharide—relevence to enteral feeding related diarrhoea. Gastroenterology 1990;99:A197.

35. Clausen MR, Bonnen H, Tvede M et al: Colonic fermentation to short chain fatty acids is decreased in antibiotic-associated diarrhea. Gastroenterology 1991;101:1497–1504.

36. Casewell MW, Cooper JE, Webster M: Enteral feeds contaminated with *Enterobacter cloacae* as a cause of septicaemia. Br Med J 1981;282:973.

37. Pottecher B, Goetc ML, Jacquemaire MA et al: Enterocolites infectieuses chez des malades de reanimation alimentes par sonde nasogastrique. Ann Anesth Franc 1979;20:595.

38. Casewell MW, Phillips I: Food as a source of *Klebsiella* species for colonisation and infection of intensive care patients. J Clin Path 1978;31:845–849.

39. Levy J, van Laethem Y, Verhaegen G: Contaminated enteral nutrition solutions as a cause of nosocomial bloodstream infection: a study using plasmid fingerprinting. J Parenter Enter Nutr 1989;13:228–234.

40. Anderton A: Microbiological aspects of the preparation and administration of nasogastric and nasoenteric tube feeds in hospital—a review. Hum Nutr Appl Nutr 1983;37A:426–440.

41. Anderton A: The potential of *Escherichia coli* in enteral feeds to cause food poisoning: a study under simulated ward conditions. J Hosp Infect 1984;5:155–163.

42. Fason MF: Controlling bacterial growth in tube feeding. Am J Nurs 1967;67:1246–1247.

43. Schreiner RL, Eitzen H, Gfell MA et al: Environmental contamination of continuous drip feedings. Pediatrics 1979;63:232–237.

44. Bastow MD, Greaves P, Allison SP: Microbial contamination of enteral feeds. Hum Nutr Appl Nutr 1982;36A:213–217.

45. Gill KJ, Gill P: Contaminated enteral feeds. Br Med J 1982;282:1971.

46. Keighley MRB, Mogg B, Bentley S et al: "Home-brew" compared with commercial preparations for enteral feeding. Br Med J 1982;284:163–165.

47. Gibbs J: Bacterial contamination of nasogastric feeds. Nurs Times 1982;79:41–47.

48. White WT, Acuff TE, Sikes TR et al: Bacterial contamination of enteral nutrient solution: a preliminary report. J Parenter Enter Nutr 1979;3:459–461.

49. Simmons NA: Hazards of naso-enteric feeds. J Hosp Infect 1981;2:276–278.

50. Thurn J, Crossley K, Gerdts A et al: Enteral hyperalimentation as a source of nosocomial infection. J Hosp Infect 1990;15:203–217.

51. Fagerman KE, Paauw JD, McCamish MA et al: Effects of time, temperature, and preservative on bacterial growth in enteral nutrient solutions. Am J Hosp Pharm 1984;41:1122–1126.

52. Curtis P, Freedland DO, Robert D et al: Microbial contamination of continuous drip feedings. J Parenter Enter Nutr 1989;12:18–22.

53. Fernandex-Crehuet Navajas M, Chacon DJ, Solvas JF et al: Bacterial contamination of enteral feeds as a possible risk of nosocomial infection. J Hosp Infect 1992;21:111–120.

54. Anderson KR, Norris DJ, Godfrey LB et al: Bacterial contamination of tube-feeding formulas. J Parenter Enter Nutr 1984;8:673–678.

55. Payne-James JJ, Rana SK, Bray MJ et al: Retrograde (ascending) bacterial contamination of enteral diet administration systems. J Parenter Enter Nutr 1992; 16:369–373.

56. Anderton A: Scanning electron microscopy of the internal wall topography of enteral feeding tubes. Clin Nutr 1984;3:171–176.

57. Bussy V, Marechal F, Nasca S: Microbial contamination of enteral feeding tubes occurring during nutritional treatment. J Parenter Enter Nutr 1992;16: 552–557.

58. Anderton A: Microbiological quality of products used in enteral feeds. J Hosp Infect 1986;7:68–73.

59. du Moulin GC, Paterson DG, Hedley-White J et al: Aspiration of gastric bacteria in antacid-treated patients: a frequent cause of post-operative colonisation of the airway. Lancet 1982;i:570–578.

60. Pollack M, Charrache P, Nieman RE et al: Factors affecting colonisation and antibiotic resistance patterns of Gram negative bacteria in hospital patients. Lancet 1972;2:668–670.

61. Pingleton SK: Enteral nutrition as a risk factor for nosocomial pneumonia. Eur J Clin Microbiol Infect Dis 1989;8:51–55.

62. Masterson JP, Dudley H, Macrae S: Design of tube feeds for surgical patients. Br Med J 1963;ii;909–913.

63. Lee HA: Why enteral nutrition? Res Clin Forums 1979;1:16–24.

64. Silk DBA: Enteral nutrition. Med Int UK 1982;15: 668–673.

65. Abbott WE, Krieger H, Levey S: Nutrition for the non-ingesting patient. NY State J Med 1959;15: 2911–2922.

66. Meeroff J, Vayliang W, Go M et al: Control of gastric emptying by osmolality of duodenal contents in man. Gastroenterology 1975;68:1144–1151.

67. McHugh P, Moran T: Calories and gastric emptying: a regulatory capacity with implications for feeding. Am J Physiol 1979;236:254–260.

68. Sagar S, Harland P, Shields R: Early post-operative feeding with elemental diet. Br Med J 1979;i: 293–295.

69. Raimundo AH, Rogers J, Spiller RC et al: Colonic inflow and small bowel motility during intraduodenal enteral nutrition. Gut 1988;29:A1469–A1470.

70. Walike BC, Walike JW: Relative lactose intolerance: a clinical survey of tube-fed patients. JAMA 1977;238: 948–955.

71. O'Keefe SJD, Adam JK, Cakata E et al: Nutritional support of malnourished lactose intolerance in African patients. Gut 1984;25:942–947.

72. Ford EG, Jennings M, Andrassy RJ: Serum albumin (oncotic pressure) correlates with enteral feeding tolerance in the pediatric surgical patient. J Pediatr Surg 1987;22:597.

73. Waitzberg D, Teixera de Silva ML, Borges VC et al: Factors associated with diarrhoea in tube fed patients. Role of serum albumin concentration. Clin Nutr 1988;7(suppl 1):58.

74. Brinson RR, Kolts BE: Hypoalbuminaemia as an indicator of diarrhoeal incidence in critically ill patients. Crit Care Med 1987;15:506–509.

75. Brown RO, Powers DA, Luther RW: Serum albumen concentration as a predictor of adult patients who develop diarrhoea associated with enteral feeding. J Parenter Enter Nutr 1988;12:20S.

76. Moss G: Post-operative metabolism: the role of plasma albumen in the enteral absorption of water and electrolytes. Pac Med Surg 1967;75:355–359.

77. Brinson RR, Pitts VL, Taylor SA: Intestinal absorption of peptide enteral formulas in hypoproteinaemic (volume expanded) rats: a paired analysis. Crit Care Med 1989;17:657–660.

78. Paving HH, Rossing N, Nielsen SL et al: Increased transcapillary escape rate of albumin, Ig G, and Ig M after plasma volume expansion. Am J Physiol 1974; 227:245–250.

79. Duffy PA, Granger DN, Taylor AE: Intestinal secretion induced by volume expansion in the dog. Gastroenterology 1978;75:413–418.

80. Brinson RR, Kolts BE: Diarrhoea associated with severe hypoalbuminaemia: a comparison of a peptide-based chemically defined diet and standard enteral alimentation. Crit Care Med 1988;16:130–137.

81. Granger DN, Brinson RR: Intestinal absorption of elemental and standard enteral formulas in hypoproteinaemic (volume expanded) rats. J Parenter Enter Nutr 1988;12:278–281.

82. Fairclough PD, Silk DBA, Clark ML et al: New evidence for intact di- and tri-peptide absorption. Gut 1975;16:843A.

83. Silk DBA, Fairclough PD, Clark ML et al: Uses of a peptide rather than free amino acid nitrogen source in chemically defined elemental diets. J Parenter Enter Nutr 1980;4:548–551.

84. Hegarty JE, Fairclough PD, Moriarty KJ et al: Effects of concentration on in vivo absorption of a peptide containing protein hydrolysate. Gut 1982;23: 304–309.

85. Fairclough PD, Hegarty JE, Silk DBA et al: A comparison of the absorption of the absorption of two protein hydrolysates and their effects on water and electrolyte movements in the human jejunum. Gut 1980;21:829–834.

86. Patterson ML, Dominguez JM, Lyman B et al: Enteral feeding in the hypoalbuminaemic patient. J Parenter Enter Nutr 1990;14:362–365.

87. Jorgensen L, Trautner F, Engquist A: Microbial contamination of tube feeding solutions. Ugeskr Laeger 1990;152:1824–1827.

88. Hyams JS: Sorbitol intolerance: an underappreciated cause of functional gastrointestinal complaints. Gastroenterology 1983;84:30–33.

89. Edes TE, Walk BE, Austin JL: Diarrhea in tube-fed patients: feeding formula not necessarily the cause. Am J Med 1990;88:91–93.

90. Heimburger DC, Sockwell DG, Geels WJ: Diarrhea with enteral feeding; prospective reappraisal of putative causes. Nutrition 1994;10:392–396.

91. Wright JP, Barbezat GO, Clain JE: Jejunal secretion in response to a duodenal mixed nutrient perfusion. Gastroenterology 1978;76:94–98.

92. Poitras P, Modigliani R, Bernier JJ: Effects of gastrin, secretin, cholecystokinin, glucagon and gastric inhib-

itory polypeptide on jejunal absorption in man. Gut 1980;21:299–304.

93. Sarr MG, Kelly KA, Phillips SF: Canine jejunal absorption and transit during interdigestive and digestive motor states. Am J Physiol 1980;239:G167–172.

94. Sarr MG, Kelly KA, Phillips SF: Feeding augments canine jejunal absorption via a hormonal mechanism. Dig Dis Sci 1981;26:961–965.

95. McFadden DW, Jaffe BM, Ferrara BA et al: Jejunal absorptive response to a test meal and its modification by cholinergic and calcium channel blockade in the awake dog. Surg Forum 1984;35:174–176.

96. Bastidas JA, Yeo CJ, Schmieg RE et al: Endogenous opiates in the mediation of early meal-induced jejunal absorption of water and electrolytes. Am J Surg 1989;157:27–32.

97. Bastidas JA, Orandle MS, Zinner MJ et al: Small bowel origin of the signal for meal-induced jejunal absorption. Surgery 1990;108:376–383.

98. Yeo CJ, Bastidas JA, Schmieg RE et al: Meal-stimulated absorption of water and electrolytes in canine jejunum. Am J Physiol 1990;259:G402–G409.

99. Anthone GJ, Mavrophilipos ZV, Zinner MJ et al: Meal-stimulated canine jejunal ionic absorption: effect of direct jejunal meal delivery and premeal intravenous hydration. Dig Dis Sci 1992;37:842–848.

100. Caren JF, Meyer JH, Grossman MI: Canine intestinal secretion during and after rapid distension of the small bowel. Am J Physiol 1974;227:183–188.

101. Raimundo AH, Rogers J, Silk DBA: Is enteral feeding related diarrhoea initiated by an abnormal colonic response to intragastric diet infusion? Gut 1990;31:A1195.

102. Bowling TE, Raimundo AH, Silk DBA: In vivo segmental colonic perfusion in man: a new technique. Eur J Gastroenterol Hepatol 1993;5:809–815.

103. Rogers J, Henry MM, Misiewicz JJ: Increased segmental activity and intraluminal pressures in the sigmoid colon of patients with the irritable bowel syndrome. Gut 1989;30:634–641.

104. Rogers J, Misiewicz JJ: Fully automated computer analysis of intracolonic pressures. Gut 1989;30:642–649.

105. Bowling TE, Raimundo AH, Silk DBA: Colonic secretory effect in response to enteral feeding in man. Gut 1995;35:1734–1741.

106. Raimundo AH, Jameson JS, Rogers J et al: The effect of enteral nutrition on distal colonic motility. Gastroenterology 1992;102:A573.

107. Bowling TE, Raimundo AH, Jameson JS et al: Suppression of colonic motility in response to enteral feeding in man. Gastroenterology 1993;104:A610.

108. Debongnie JC, Phillips SF: Capacity of the human colon to absorb fluid. Gastroenterology 1978;74:698–703.

109. Williams NS, Meyer JH, Jehn D et al: Canine intestinal transit and digestion of radiolabelled liver particles. Gastroenterology 1984;86:1451–1459.

110. Tatemoto K, Nakano G, Makk P et al: Isolation and primary structure of human peptide YY. Biochem Biophys Res Commun 1988;157:713–717.

111. Bilchik AJ, Hines OJ, Adrian TE et al: Peptide YY is a physiological regulator of water and electrolyte absorption in the canine small bowel in vivo. Gastroenterology 1993;105:1441–1448.

112. Okuno M, Nakanishi Y, Shinomura Y et al: Peptide YY enhances NaCl and water absorption in the rat colon in vivo. Experientia 1992;48:47–50.

113. Bowling TE, Bloom SR, Silk DBA: Is an abnormal Peptide YY response the cause of enteral feeding related diarrhea? Gastroenterology 1995;108:A718.

114. Cummings JH, Branch WJ: Fermentation and production of short chain fatty acids in the human large intestine. In Vahouny GB, Kritchevsky D (eds): Dietary Fibre: Basic and Clinical Aspects, New York: Plenum Press, 1986;131–152.

115. Roediger WEW: Role of anaerobic bacteria in the metabolic welfare of the colonic mucosa in man. Gut 1980;21:793–798.

116. Jacobs LR: Effects of dietary fiber on mucosal growth and cell proliferation in the small intestine of the rat: a comparison of oat bran, pectin and guar with total fiber deprivation. Am J Clin Nutr 1983;37:954–960.

117. Cummings JH: Short chain fatty acids in the human colon. Gut 1981;22:763–779.

118. Ruppin H, Bar-Meir S, Soergel KH et al: Absorption of short chain fatty acids by the colon. Gastroenterology 1980;78:1500–1507.

119. Binder HJ, Mehta P: Short chain fatty acids stimulate active sodium and chloride absorption in vitro in the rat distal colon. Gastroenterology 1989;96:989–996.

120. Holtug K, Clausen MR, Hove H et al: The colon in carbohydrate malabsorption: Short chain fatty acids, pH, and osmotic diarrhoea. Scand J Gastroenterol 1992;27:545–552.

121. Raimundo AH, Kapadia S, Terry DL et al: The effect of fibre-free enteral diets and the addition of soy polysaccharide on human bowel function and short chain fatty acid (SCFA) production. J Parenter Enter Nutr 1992;16:29S, 69.

122. Clausen MR, Bonnen H, Tvede M et al: Colonic fermentation to short chain fatty acids is decreased in antibiotic-associated diarrhea. Gastroenterology 1991;101:1497–1504.

123. Roediger WEW, Moore A: Effect of short chain fatty acids on sodium absorption in isolated human colon perfused through the vascular bed. Dig Dis Sci 1981;26:100–106.

124. Hart G, Dobb GJ: Effect of a fecal bulking agent on diarrhoea during enteral feeding in the critically ill. J Parenter Enter Nutr 1988;12:465–168.

125. Frankenfield DC, Beyer PL: Soy-polysaccharide fiber: effect on diarrhoea in tube-fed, head-injured patients. Am J Clin Nutr 1989;50:533–538.

126. Dobb GJ, Towler SC: Diarrhoea during enteral feeding in the critically ill: a comparison of feeds with and without fibre. Intensive Care Med 1990;16:252–255.

127. Englyst HN, Hudson GJ: Colorimetric method for routine measurement of dietary fibre as nonstarch polysaccharides: a comparison with gas-liquid chromatography. Food Chem 1987;24:63–76.

128. Spiller GA, Chernoff MC, Hill RA et al: Effect of purified cellulose, pectin and a low-residue diet on fecal volatile fatty acids, transit time and fecal weight in humans. Am J Clin Nutr 1980;33:754–759.

129. Bowling TE, Raimundo AH, Grimble GK et al: Colonic fluid secretion induced by enteral feeding in man is reversed by short chain fatty acids. Lancet 1993;342:1266–1268.

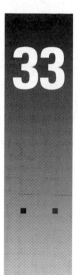

33

Complications of Enteral Feeding and Their Prevention

ELIE HAMAOUI
ROBERT KODSI

The aim of tube feeding is generally to compensate for or bypass some dysfunction of the alimentary canal. The complications of such nutritional support generally result from inadequate compensation for the deficit or from the invasiveness of a technique that often violates physiologic defense mechanisms. Not infrequently, however, a perceived complication of tube feeding is in fact caused not by the nutritional support but by the underlying disease or by its therapy. In such a situation, addressing the wrong etiology can only compound the problem.

Accordingly, this chapter addresses the pathogenesis of the various reported complications of tube feeding to define a rational approach to prevention and treatment. To facilitate the discussion, a brief overview of gastrointestinal (GI) physiology, particularly as related to tube feeding, is in order. (See Chapters 2 and 22 for a fuller discussion.)

In the normal state of affairs, the body's nutrient needs, as translated by hunger and satiety, result in feeding behavior, which is remarkably safe and effective and exquisitely well coordinated. Every swallow demands airway protection. Gastric filling signals the end of a meal, regardless of how many previous meals the individual may have missed; so does intestinal distention (of any cause, including that

due to a fecal impaction). Food, passing along the alimentary canal, stimulates mucosal growth and function, which are integral for the defense of the internal milieu against noxious factors that may accompany eaten foods. The secretory products of one segment of the gut often function not only in digestion and absorption but also as stimulants and trophic factors for the next segment of gut.

The placement of a nasogastric feeding tube in a patient with neurogenic dysphagia does indeed protect the airway from (liquid) food in transit to the stomach. However, by bypassing the oropharynx, one also forgoes the benefits of food-stimulated salivary and oropharyngeal secretions, which not only begin the digestive and antimicrobial processing of foods—through the action of salivary amylase, secretory immunoglobulins, mucus, etc.—but also help maintain the oropharyngeal mucosa's integrity and function. A dry oropharyngeal mucosa is more susceptible to ulceration and infection and, by being less sensitive to touch, may further depress the gag reflex and thus predispose to aspiration.

Similarly, feeding into the jejunum reduces the risk of regurgitation and aspiration of feed, but it also bypasses even more of the beneficial interactions between food and the upper GI tract. Additional complications may therefore include increased risk of stress gastritis,[1] bacterial overgrowth,[1] and impaired nutrient absorption.[2]

Another potential source of problems in tube feeding is that the content and timing of feeding are not under the control of physiologic needs and tolerances. Thus, whereas a healthy subject can stop eating when he or she feels full and can respond to osmoreceptors and drink an extra glass of water to quench perceived thirst, the tube-fed patient, particularly one who cannot communicate needs or discomfort, is at the mercy of whatever deficits or excesses might come down the tube.

Successful tube feeding requires the clinician to do the following:

1. Establish and maintain safe access to the GI tract for nutrient delivery.
2. Deliver nutrients in a form and regimen appropriate to the level of available GI function and in quantities consistent with metabolic requirements and limitations.
3. Compensate for violated or bypassed physiologic safeguards.

At any of these steps, a variety of complications can frustrate the nutrition effort. Although these complications can be categorized as primarily mechanical, septic, or metabolic, when they occur they do not announce their etiology, and some diagnostic work-up is usually required. As a practical approach, we shall consider them in the order in which they may occur.

ACCESS PROBLEMS

Feeding tubes can be placed transnasally, transorally, or percutaneously into the esophagus, the stomach, or small bowel by various operative and nonoperative techniques. The insertion techniques and their immediate complications are described in Chapters 11, 12, and 14. The problems discussed here are those encountered during the chronic maintenance of such access.

Pressure Necrosis and Its Complications

The presence of a tube or any foreign body pressing against a mucosal surface can cause necrosis, ulceration, abscess formation, and even perforation of that viscus. This can affect nasopharyngeal, esophageal, gastric, and duodenal points of contact with a feeding tube. In patients with both esophageal and endotracheal tubes, pressure necrosis can lead to fistula formation between the esophagus and the trachea. The extent of necrosis is proportional to the amount of tissue exposed, the duration of the exposure, and the amount of pressure to which the tissue is exposed. To reduce this risk, small-bore soft feeding tubes are used. When long-term feeding is anticipated a nasoenteral tube is replaced by a gastrostomy tube. In treating the complications of pressure necrosis, one must remove the cause of the pressure and protect the injured area until it can heal.

Nasal Pressure Necrosis

When the nasogastric tube is taped under pressure to the naris, deforming ulceration of the nose can develop. Use of a soft, small-bore feeding tube can reduce this complication. Correct taping of the tube to the nose (Fig. 33–1*A*) and avoiding extreme angulation of the tube as it exits the nose (Fig 33–1*B*) will help prevent pressure necrosis. If the nasogastric tube becomes displaced, reinsertion in the contralateral naris will reduce the amount of exposure time for each side. Patients with facial fractures, especially mechanically ventilated patients, are also at high risk for other, less common complications of pressure necrosis, including sinusitis, abscess formation, and cartilage damage.[3] If these complications occur, remove the feeding tube and use another feeding route.

Esophageal Pressure Necrosis

The majority of mucosal surface exposed to nasoenteral feeding tubes is esophageal. Although esophageal ulceration is a common complication of large-bore nasogastric tubes, the incidence of ulceration is believed to be reduced with flexible small-bore tubes. Patients with underlying esophageal disorders are at especially increased risk for pressure necrosis.[4] This may be due to lack of normal esophageal motility and consequent immobility of the nasogastric tube. As noted above, the dreaded and thankfully uncommon tracheoesophageal fistula occurs when contiguous tracheal and esophageal walls are compressed between an endotracheal balloon on one side and a rigid nasogastric tube on the other. Symptoms of this type of fistula include recurrent aspiration and leakage of air into the GI tract of patients on positive pressure ventilators. Radiologic studies with barium and endoscopic or bronchoscopic visualization are the primary methods of diagnosis. In patients on positive pressure ventilators, the analysis of

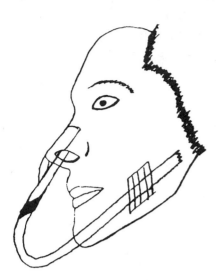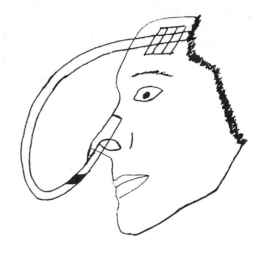

FIGURE 33–1   *A,* Correct taping of the nasogastric tube to avoid pressure necrosis on the anterior nairs. *B,* Incorrect taping of the nasogastric tube.

gastric gas for oxygen content may help in the diagnosis.[5]

The goal of medical therapy is to allow the fistulous tract to close by removing the foreign body that causes the pressure. The fistulous tract must then be protected to facilitate healing. This can be accomplished by removal of the nasogastric tube and placement of a percutaneous endoscopic gastrostomy (PEG) tube for drainage and of a separate gastrojejunostomy tube for feeding. In addition, the endotracheal balloon should be repositioned below the fistula to relieve pressure and protect against aspiration. Other therapies including stent placement and fibrin glue have been employed with varying results.[6,7] Unfortunately, many patients ultimately require surgical repair for this relatively rare complication.

Gastric Pressure Necrosis

When a PEG tube is placed under tension, pressure by the PEG bumper can cause mucosal ulcer formation and bumper erosion into the mucosal layer of the stomach.[8-11] In severe cases, bleeding[8] and further erosion into the muscular layer and abdominal wall can occur. This complication has been called the "buried bumper syndrome." Suspect a buried bumper with blockage of feeding or inability to rotate or freely move a PEG tube. Perform endoscopy if a tube becomes fixed or immobile. If a buried bumper is discovered, remove it, even if it is functional and asymptomatic. If it is left in place, further migration, obstruction, and perforation may occur.[9-11]

Methods for removing a buried bumper include surgical exploration, blunt external instrument dissection under local anesthesia, and endoscopic removal with adjuvant Savory dilator.[12] Degree of impaction, underlying medical condition, and physician familiarity with removal procedures determine the method chosen to extract the bumper. To avoid the buried bumper syndrome, ensure that the PEG tube is not placed under excessive tension. Foutch and colleagues have suggested rotation and 5-mm advancement of the PEG tube after fistula tract formation to help prevent this complication.[11]

Feeding Tube Displacement and Migration

When a tube is displaced, feeding may be delivered to a location other than the one intended. This can lead to aspiration, diarrhea, or, in the case of gastrostomy or jejunostomy tubes, peritonitis. After initial tube placement is confirmed, marking the tube at skin level, although subject to error, helps verify that the tube remains in place. Verify tube placement before the daily routine of feeding. In addition, insufflation of air while the clinician ausculates the abdomen, although also subject to misinterpretation, can be useful if done routinely. If the tube's position is unclear, x-ray examination or fluoroscopy can be used but are impractical on a daily basis.

Small-bore soft nasogastric tubes are the most commonly displaced, with 40 to 68 percent of patients experiencing displacement during nasoenteral feeding.[13-18] Most occur when patients pull their tubes out. Associated risk factors include patient agitation,[14-16] frequent coughing,[15,16] endotracheal intubation,[16] and nasotracheal suctioning.[16] A few studies suggest that weighted tubes stayed in place better,[16] but most studies find that weighted tubes, including those placed into the duodenum, are not less prone to displacement.[19] Because nasoenteral tubes are the most frequently displaced, when long-term nasoenteral feeding is needed, nasal bridals have proved effective. Experience at our institution (Weiss A, personal communication) with over 1000 bridals inserted during the last 12 years shows that although the incidence of occlusion is unchanged, there were only two or three cases of significant nasal trauma or sinusitis.

PEG tube displacement is a less common occurrence than nasoenteral tube displacement. Forward migration of the PEG tube can lead to bowel obstruction,[20] ulceration, or pancreatitis secondary to blockage of the papilla of Vater.[21] Fortunately these complications are rare. More commonly PEG tubes are inadvertently removed by an agitated patient. This is most dangerous when the tube is pulled out before a mature fistula tract has formed (<2 weeks), because of the risk of leakage into the peritoneal cavity. In a study by Galat, 2 percent of the tubes were pulled out within the first week.[22] When the tube is removed during the first 2 weeks, replacement must be performed under endoscopic guidance after the old tract has closed. If a replacement tube is placed by pushing it through an immature fistula tract, the stomach can become detached from the abdominal wall, and intraperitoneal leakage or misplacement of the tube in the abdominal cavity can occur. To reduce the incidence of PEG tube displacement in agitated patients, use a shortened extra-abdominal tube length coupled with patient restraints and mittens. When the fistula tract matures, the PEG tube can be changed to a button, which the patient is less likely to dislodge. Initial placement of the PEG button has had too high a complication rate to be recommended, but improving techniques may lead to a PEG button that can be placed initially.

Tube Obstruction

Obstruction of the feeding tube is one of the most common complications of enteral feeding.[23,24] Most obstructions are secondary to coagulation of formula;[25] other causes include obstruction by pill fragments, tube kinking, and precipitation of incompatible medications. The rate of tube obstruction varies with tube diameter, quality of nursing care, the type of tube (jejunostomy vs gastrostomy), and the duration of tube placement. Tube obstruction also depends on whether gastric residuals are checked through the feeding tube. Up to 80 percent of all obstructions are caused by coagulation of formula, with the incidence of obstruction up to 10 times greater for patients whose residuals are checked through the feeding tube.[26] Obstruction also occurs up to three times more frequently in patients fed by continuous vs bolus feeding,[27] but this benefit must be weighed against the risks of bolus feeding (see below). Sucralfate and antacids have also been reported to cause tube obstruction by precipitating with enteral formulas.[27-31] This interaction is generally reported in patients with underlying neurologic disorders affecting esophageal and gastric motility[29,30] but has also been reported in patients with no underlying motility disorder.

When a tube becomes obstructed during enteral feeding, it is usually preferable to dislodge the obstruction rather than replace the tube. The use of warm water alternating with gentle pressure and suction will relieve most obstructions. If this fails, we instill carbonated water, let it sit for 1 hour, and then try pressure and suction again. Some[24] have recommended infusing pancreatic enzyme to dissolve the obstruction; however, we have rarely found this necessary except in needle catheter jejunostomy tubes, because of their small diameter and the difficulty in replacing them.

When a PEG tube becomes blocked, check for the ability to rotate the tube freely. If the tube is fixed and immobile, suspect a buried bumper and perform endoscopy. If the PEG tube freely rotates and the above measures fail to dislodge the obstruction, carefully passing a closed endoscopic biopsy forceps, which is designed to coil before penetrating the gastric wall, through the PEG tube usually provides adequate force to dislodge the obstruction.

The following strategies may help prevent tube obstruction in patients who are fed enterally:

1. Use elixir forms of medications rather than crushed pill forms. If the elixir is not available, crush and dissolve the pills before administration.
2. Flush the feeding tube with water before and after administering medica-

tions or enteral feedings. Take special care with sucralfate and antacids.

3. Flush the feeding tube with water after each check of gastric residuals, since acid pH will cause the formula to coagulate, thus obstructing the tube.

Leakage Through Ostomy Sites

Leakage at a stoma site may indicate tube dysfunction, infection of the stoma site, or a stoma diameter greater than necessary for the tube. If tube dysfunction is the cause, replacement is usually necessary. If infection is the cause, antibiotics, debridement, and tube removal are sometimes necessary. If the stoma has enlarged, as in the case of PEG tube leakage, then the diameter must be reduced. As with all fistula tracts, removal of the foreign body, and measures to decrease fistula output are the best initial steps to lead to closure. This is accomplished by removing the PEG tube and close observation every few hours, until the stoma has contracted to the point where a replacement tube will fit with no leak. During this time no feeding is given into the stomach, and prokinetic agents coupled with H_2 blockers are given to reduce stoma output.[32] To manage more persistent leaks, which may need days to heal, a sump tube, attached to low suction, is placed either nasogastrically or through the stoma as described by Mushin.[33] The patient can be fed through a small-bore feeding tube passed through the nose or stoma and into the jejunum by fluoroscopy or endoscopy.

Complications Unique to Needle Catheter Jejunostomies

Needle catheter jejunostomy (NCJ) feedings bypass more of the protective physiologic barriers than any other type of enteral feeding. Despite this, in select groups of patients, NCJ has well-accepted advantages. NCJ is placed incidentally to a major abdominal operation to allow earlier postoperative feeding while minimizing the risks of aspiration. Three complications are unique to NCJ: small bowel ischemia, pneumatosis intestinalis, and small bowel obstruction. Other complications such as catheter dislodgment, leakage, tube obstruction, and diarrhea are covered elsewhere.

Small Bowel Ischemia

The jejunum is not designed as a reservoir and responds poorly to distention. If the feeding rate through the jejunostomy exceeds the ability of the local jejunal segment to process it, distention can occur with pathologic results. Jejunal infarction of the gut wall has been reported in a series of patients with needle catheter jejunostomies.[34-37] In separate papers covering different time periods in the same institution, Choban and Gaddy reported that 10 of 203 (5 percent) patients developed ischemic small bowel with needle catheter jejunostomies feedings. The actual incidence is probably much lower.[37-40] In all patients there were risk factors for hypoperfusion of the gut. However, there are case reports of intestinal ischemia despite lack of risk factors for hypoperfusion.[36] Ratliff and colleagues in 1987 described a case where distention of the jejunum by feedings caused ischemia to the proximal jejunum.[35] After surgical decompression of the jejunum, viability was restored immediately. This suggests that some of the ischemic complications noted with jejunostomy feedings are secondary to overdistention of the jejunal segment from feedings. Other contributing factors may be increased metabolic rate from actively fed gut[34,37] or high osmolality of the enteral feeding.

Patients with jejunostomies should have routine examinations for abdominal distention. Enteral feedings should be held in patients at acute risk for bowel ischemia. These include hypotensive patients and patients receiving vasopressors.[36,41] Early recognition may prevent a potentially fatal outcome.

Pneumatosis Intestinalis

Pneumatosis intestinalis, found in a wide spectrum of clinical conditions,[42,43] is a relatively rare complication of needle catheter jejunostomy, with an incidence of less than 1 percent. The underlying etiology in NCJ patients has not been fully elucidated but is probably multifactorial, including gut hypoxia, mucosal compromise by pathogenic organisms, lymphatic obstruction, and dissection of intraluminal air through the catheter defect in the mucosa. If this relatively rare complication does occur and the patient is hemodynamically stable, conservative management with close observation appears prudent. However, if the patient develops metabolic acidosis, peritoneal signs, or other clinical deterioration, early surgical intervention is usually warranted. Most reported cases of pneumatosis intestinalis secondary to NCJ have been successfully managed with conservation methods using parenteral nutrition, broad-spectrum antibiotics, high-flow oxygen and ensuring adequate hemoglobin concentration. Catheter removal was not necessary in these patients. No specific recommendations have been proposed to prevent this complication, so a high index of suspicion is necessary for early diagnosis and treatment.

Bowel Obstruction

Bowel obstruction can occur when the jejunum rotates around the loop of jejunum fixed to the abdominal wall. This can eventually form an obstruction with similar pathology to a sigmoid volvulus. Fortunately, the incidence of this complication is less than 1 percent.

PROBLEMS ENCOUNTERED DURING ADMINISTRATION OF FEEDING

In the healthy individual, oral intake that is not tolerated by the gut usually causes GI symptoms such as abdominal discomfort and nausea and is often returned promptly as vomitus or rapidly expelled as diarrhea. Pavlovian associations help one avoid too many "rechallenges" with the noxious food, and the problem mercifully resolves. Similar intolerance symptoms often occur in the tube-fed patient, but here the associations are more difficult to tease out because of the confounding presence of diseases and therapies, not just the feeding formula and its possible contaminants.

Regurgitation

Feeding that cannot be absorbed or moved downstream and instead accumulates within the gut lumen will eventually back up and be regurgitated, actively or passively, and may lead to aspiration pneumonia as its most dreaded complication. Warning signs in the conscious patient include abdominal discomfort or a sense of bloating and nausea. In the noncommunicative patient, frank abdominal distention or a high gastric residual may be the first sign of trouble. These signs and symptoms, singly or in combination, occur in 10 to 20 percent of tube-fed patients.[44-46]

When any of the above warning signs occur, stop or at least slow tube feeding while investigating the cause. Look for some form of obstruction, either anatomic or functional. Common anatomic obstructions in such patients include gastric outlet obstruction due to peptic ulcer disease or due to displacement of a PEG tube and bumper into the pyloric channel;[47] small bowel obstruction due to adhesions or internal hernias; and large bowel obstruction, often by a fecal impaction. Functional obstruc-

tions are caused by gut dysmotility. These may be localized to one part of the gut, such as diabetic gastroparesis, or involve most or all of the gut, as in severe sepsis or electrolyte imbalance. As elsewhere in medicine, a rational approach to the problem requires a proper assessment—through history, physical examination, and appropriate laboratory tests—before deciding on therapy.

Regardless of the type of obstruction, continuing the feeding will inevitably lead to excessive accumulation and eventual regurgitation, even if the feeding is administered distal to the stomach. (If there is any doubt on this point, consider the fact that the presentation of patients with small bowel obstruction or even large bowel obstruction almost always includes vomiting.[48]) Thus switching from gastric to jejunal feeding, a commonly recommended remedy for patients with recurrent aspiration, will not stop the regurgitation if the problem is a fecal impaction. In fact, in such a patient the mistake would be to start the feeding before clearing the obstruction.

How does one detect an obstruction that develops after tube feeding has been started and initially well tolerated? By looking for the above warning signs of excessive accumulation within the GI tract. In the conscious and communicative patient, take advantage of the patient's physiologic indicators and pay attention to complaints of bloating, abdominal discomfort, or constipation even if gastric residuals are not yet excessively high. In the noncommunicative patient, monitoring the bowel record and careful periodic exams must replace the muted physiologic signs. At a minimum, check the abdomen daily for distention and measure gastric residuals whenever feeding is added to the bag.

Aspiration

Pulmonary aspiration is a common complication of enteral feeding,[49,50,51] with a reported incidence ranging from <5 to 95 percent.[49-57] This wide range is due to lack of consistency in how aspiration is defined and underlines the need to standardize the definition. The incidence of clinically significant pneumonia from these events is just as varied. One large trial conducted in patients with PEGs cites the incidence of pneumonia in these patients as 23 percent over 1 year.[58] Other studies, using varied patient populations, have an incidence of pneumonia ranging from <1 to 50 percent.[18,50-57,59-61] Identifiable patient risk factors for aspiration include previous aspiration pneumonia,[8,58,59,61,62] impaired mental status,[56] neurologic injury,[63,64] absence of a cough or gag reflex, mechanical ventilation,[50,60,65] and age.[49,52,60]

In devising strategies to prevent aspiration pneumonia, first determine the source of the aspirated material. If a patient aspirates oropharyngeal secretions, withholding gastrostomy feedings will do nothing except lead to malnutrition, and placement of a feeding jejunostomy may only add the complications of a jejunostomy tube. Methods of distinguishing aspirated gastric feedings from oropharyngeal secretions include adding colored dye to the feedings[51,52,55,57] or oropharynx[66] and performing glucose oxidase strip testing of tracheal aspirate.[49-51] The latter is felt to be more sensitive[51-55] but is probably less specific. Feedings and oral secretions[67] have been radiolabeled in the research setting, but this is of limited practical use due to cost and procedural complexity. If tube feeding is being aspirated into the lungs, take steps to prevent aspiration.

Strategies to reduce the risk of aspiration include elevating the head of the bed, checking gastric residuals, using small-bore feeding tubes, continuous feedings, direct gastric feeding (PEG), postpyloric feeding, and surgical procedures. Although a consensus is lacking about how effective the above strategies are in reducing the risk of aspiration pneumonia, there is agreement that elevating the head of the bed at 30 to 45 degrees,[51,68,69] closely monitoring gastric residuals every 4 to 6 hours, and holding the feeding if the residuals are "excessive" may be helpful. The definition of "excessive" gastric residuals is a subject of debate. In our experience, patients who are fed by continuous drip into the stomach and tolerate the feeding rarely have gastric residuals over 10 to 30 ml. Most authors recommend holding the feeding whenever the residual exceeds 100 ml[53,63,70-73] or 150 ml.[74-76]

McClave et al[77] studied nasogastrically fed healthy volunteers, critically ill patients, and stable gastrostomy tube-fed patients, in all of whom gastric residuals were measured every 2 hours during an 8-hour continuous intragastric infusion of a semielemental formula given at a rate to provide 25 kcal/kg/day. They found that although no subject was "clearly intolerant (i.e., vomiting, aspiration)," residuals up to 165 ml were measured in the healthy volunteers, up to 375 ml in the critically ill, and up to 104 ml in the stable gastrostomy patients. (The lower residual in the gastrostomy patients was attributed to the fact that the position of the gastrostomy tube in the anterior stomach wall does not permit as complete an aspiration of gastric content as does a nasogastric tube.) Based on their findings, these authors recommend accepting gastric residuals up to 200 ml in nasogastrically fed patients (100 ml in patients fed through a gastrostomy tube) before even considering holding the feeding.

However, if one's concern is to minimize the risk of regurgitation and aspiration, it seems prudent to avoid even a "tolerable" level of gastric filling. We hold the feeding (and reexamine the patient) when the residual is 100 ml or greater. This cut off has not limited our capacity to provide adequate feeding to our patients. Instead, it often guides us to otherwise unsuspected electrolyte abnormalities, constipation, or early sepsis.

Unfortunately, compliance with checking gastric residuals is poor. In a study by Breach in 1988, only 55 to 60 percent of the time were gastric residuals noted as recommended by protocol,[75] and others have confirmed irregular compliance with checking residuals and bed elevation.[78] It is important to distinguish complications that result from poor compliance from those that occur due to ineffective preventive methods. The first type is addressed by more focused education; the other demands creation of a new methodology.

It is common practice to reinject nonexcessive gastric residuals to prevent electrolyte abnormalities and loss of nutrients.[53]

Continuous vs Bolus Feedings

The use of continuous vs bolus feedings is a double-edged sword in protecting against aspiration. Continuous feeding has been shown to induce less gastroesophageal reflux than bolus feedings,[79] but it may increase the incidence of gastric colonization and subsequent pneumonia in patients not receiving acid-neutralizing medication (see below). Coben demonstrated decreased lower esophageal sphincter (LES) pressures and increased gastroesophageal reflux in bolus feeding compared with continuous feeding.[79] In a prospective randomized study of 60 patients, Ciocon[25] found a 33 percent rate of pneumonia in the bolus-fed group compared with 17 percent in the continuously fed group. Although the difference was not statistically significant, this author as well as others recommended nonbolus feeding to reduce the incidence of aspiration pneumonia.

Size of Feeding Tube

Smaller-bore feeding tubes were thought to induce less LES relaxation and hence less risk of regurgitation and aspiration. However, controlled studies have failed to demonstrate a consistent advantage. In a recent study, small-bore feeding tubes had an equal incidence of reflux as detected by radiolabeling of gastric contents in healthy subjects.[19] This, however, may not be applicable to enterally fed patients who have underlying medical or neurologic disorders. In a limited study of 25 patients, Sands failed to demonstrate a reduced incidence of pneumonia in patients with small-bore feeding tubes.[54] Other studies, not specifically designed to compare aspiration risks with different-sized feeding tubes, did not show a protective effect on patients who were fed with small-bore tubes.[52,56] In conclusion, it has not yet been convincingly demonstrated that the use of small-bore feeding tubes reduces the risk of aspiration, although for other reasons, including patient comfort and reduced nasopharyngeal and esophageal injury, their use is justifiably recommended.

Direct Gastric Feeding (PEG)

Removing the nasogastric feeding tube, thereby reducing reflux through the LES, may reduce the incidence of aspiration pneumonia. Although some studies have demonstrated a small short-term decrease in the rate of aspiration in patients with PEG tubes,[80] prospective randomized trials have failed to show any significant difference in the rate of aspiration with PEG tubes vs nasogastric tubes.[81] In contrast, postpyloric feeding has had greater success in reducing the rate of aspiration pneumonia in enterally fed patients.

Post-Pyloric Feeding

Although no method of feeding has eliminated the risk of aspiration pneumonia, the concept that feeding a patient beyond the pylorus will reduce this risk is a logical one. Feedings would have to traverse both the pyloric sphincter and LES to reach the lung. In addition, gastric distention and its effect on LES pressure would be reduced. Three methods of postpyloric feeding that have been studied are nasoenteral, transgastric, and direct jejunal feedings through jejunostomy.

Nasoenteral Feeding. Although nasoenteral feeding has been shown in most studies to reduce the incidence of aspiration pneumonia,[56,82] agreement has not been universal.[83] Difficulties associated with initial tube insertion[84] and maintenance of placement[82] makes this route impractical for most patients. Conservative methods, prokinetic agents, and patient positioning on the right side have failed to consistently produce nasoduodenal placement in most patients.[84] Fluoroscopic or endoscopic guidance has had greater success but at a substantially increased cost. In addition, when postpyloric placement is achieved, the tube may fall back into the stomach and require repositioning.

Transgastric Feedings. As with all studies with postpyloric feeding, some find a reduced incidence of aspiration with transgastric (percutaneous endoscopic jejunostomy [PEJ]) feedings,[85,86] while others have found no protection in feeding patients by this route.[8,87-89] The high mechanical failure rate of these tubes coupled with the lack of consistent protection from aspiration prevents PEJ tubes from being useful in preventing aspiration pneumonia. By contrast, direct jejunal feedings though jejunostomy have had a more consistent effect in protecting patients against aspiration pneumonia.[90]

Direct Jejunal Feedings. By infusing feedings distal to the ligament of Treitz, direct jejunal feedings provide the most protection against aspiration. It is, however, the most technically difficult to establish and bypasses more protective barriers than any other type of feeding. The jejunostomy is usually created as an adjunctive procedure to another abdominal surgery and allows early postoperative feeding. The protection against postoperative aspiration is well documented.[90] The placement of a jejunostomy as an independent procedure to protect against aspiration has also been successful but is associated with the highest incidence of morbidity and mortality of any feeding device placement. The 30-day postoperative mortality is 20 percent, usually secondary to the patient's underlying medical condition. As mentioned above, jejunostomy feeding will do nothing to prevent aspiration of oropharyngeal content, and this source of aspiration should be considered before the decision to place a jejunostomy tube. If, however, gastric feedings are being aspirated, then placement of a jejunostomy may help. When a jejunostomy fails to prevent recurrent severe aspiration of enteral feedings, surgical therapy may be indicated.

Surgical Procedures

In carefully selected patients, surgical procedures may prevent recurrent aspiration. Surgical techniques attempt to prevent both reflux and aspiration of refluxed material. To prevent reflux, fundoplication is the procedure of choice but has limited success.[91] Modified epiglottoplasty,[92] closure of the larynx at the level of the false cords,[93] total laryngectomy, and other surgical therapies have been successful in preventing recurrent aspiration. In some cases, the alert but dysphagic patient may be able to return to an oral diet.[94] Candidate patients require evaluation by both the surgeon and the speech pathologist.

In short, although there is no unanimous agreement on the most efficacious regimen for preventing aspiration pneumonia, we consider the following to help reduce risk:

1. Monitor the patient daily for GI symptoms (nausea, abdominal discomfort, bloating, obstipation).
2. Check gastric residuals every 4 to 6 hours. Hold feeding for 2 hours if the residual is greater than 100 ml, then recheck. If high residuals persist, perform a GI work-up. Prokinetic agents such as cisapride may play a role in reducing gastric residuals, especially in patients with autonomic dysfunction such as diabetic gastroparesis.
3. Elevate the head of the bed 30 to 45 degrees throughout the feeding period. Before placing the patient in the recumbent position, stop the feeding and aspirate the gastric residual into a syringe.
4. Use continuous rather than bolus feeding to minimize gastric distention.
5. Verify tube placement, initially by x-ray study and daily by checking position marker and auscultation. (The latter methods are not completely reliable but provide some degree of protection.)
6. Avoid administering drugs that might decrease LES tone.
7. Avoid paralytic and sedative drugs or use sparingly.
8. Use jejunostomy feeding in patients with recurrent aspiration of gastric feedings despite above measures.
9. Consider surgical therapy in carefully selected patients, particularly those who might be able to return to an oral diet.

Diarrhea

At least 14 different definitions of diarrhea can be found in the literature of enteral feeding.[95] These range from 1 liquid stool/day[96] to more than 500 ml of soft or liquid stools/day for 2 days.[97] Depending on how diarrhea is de-

fined and quantitated, its reported incidence in tube-fed patients ranges from 2.3 to 68 percent of patients.[53,78,95,97-104] Given the wide range of what is considered normal bowel frequency—three times a week to three times a day.[105]—the suggestion that only a significant worsening of previous bowel habits be considered diarrhea[106] seems reasonable as a working definition. (Chapter 32 also discusses diarrhea and enteral nutrition.)

However, regardless of what definition one adopts, the basic approach to this problem should not change. In essence, what is needed is the same type of diagnostic thinking that physicians must bring to any ailment and is no different from the approach to diarrhea[105] in a patient fed by mouth. It is a mistake to assume that diarrhea "normally" accompanies tube feeding or to think that it can be prevented by use of continuous drip (rather than bolus) feeding or by the prophylactic addition of anticholinergic medication to the formula. To be sure, tube feeding can cause diarrhea, especially when inappropriately chosen or administered, but do not automatically assume it is the culprit. In fact, in most situations, tube feeding does not cause the diarrhea.[97,107,108]

In dealing with a complaint of diarrhea, first ascertain that diarrhea is indeed the problem. It is not uncommon, especially in bed-bound or elderly patients, for constipation to be mistaken for diarrhea, because of the frequent oozing around a fecal impaction.[105] The tip off is an incongruously distended abdomen—in a patient who should have been "emptied" by the alleged diarrhea—and the normal or hyperactive sounds of a bowel working against an obstruction. Rectal examination often confirms the diagnosis and may indicate the need for digital disimpaction if the stools are hard. Occasionally, an abdominal x-ray film is required to diagnose a fecal impaction in the sigmoid or above. Needless to say, antidiarrheal agents are the wrong therapy in this situation. Rather, after treating the acute constipation, resume the feeding using a formula that contains more fiber and water to soften to stools and facilitate evacuation. For those patients who then develop "soft stool" impactions, which are not uncommon in patients with multiple sclerosis, Parkinsonism, cerebrovascular accidents, or lumbosacral spine or sacral nerve disease, periodic tap water enemas or a stimulant cathartic such as bisacodyl may be necessary.

True diarrhea should also be distinguished from fecal incontinence, which is the involuntary release of rectal content.[105] Here, because the incontinence is worse when the stools are liquid,[105] adding fiber (the nonsoluble, bulk-forming type) to produce less liquid stools may be helpful.

Pathophysiologically, diarrhea can be of two basic types, osmotic or secretory.[105] An osmotic diarrhea ceases when that which cannot be absorbed by the gut is discontinued. In contrast, a secretory diarrhea continues even after all intake has been stopped. When tube feeding per se causes diarrhea in a given patient, it does so by an osmotic mechanism, either because it contains one or more components that cannot be absorbed by the patient's gut or because the feeding is hypertonic and is being infused too rapidly into the intestine, causing dumping syndrome. Stopping such feeding cures the diarrhea, usually within 24 hours. If the diarrhea continues unabated, it is unrelated to the feeding and will not respond to diluting or changing the feeding. Seek and address other causes of diarrhea, especially drugs[97,104,105,107-109] (see Table 33–1). Frequent offenders include magnesium-containing antacids, sorbitol-dissolved drugs, cathartics (e.g., for hepatic encephalopathy, hyperkalemia, or previous constipation), and antibiotics. The latter suppress normal gut flora and may thus lead to the overgrowth of enteropathogenic organisms (especially *Clostridium difficile*), causing colitis and diarrhea.[110] In addition, as discussed below, antibiotics may cause loose stools by suppressing the bacterial fermentation of dietary fiber into short-chain fatty acids (SCFAs), which fuel sodium and water absorption by colonocytes.

Even when the tube feeding itself appears to be the cause of the diarrhea, such as when stopping the feeding stops the diarrhea, it is important to understand the mechanism. If a hypertonic formula was being used for bolus feeding through a jejunostomy, suspect dumping syndrome. In such a case, diluting the feeding to isotonicity and giving it by slow drip (i.e., performing those functions that the stomach normally carries out when it receives a meal) would quickly solve the problem. However, if the patient is already receiving isotonic drip feeding, then diluting the feeding—a commonly recommended remedy for "tube-feeding diarrhea"—would accomplish little more than give the patient extra water and less feeding, which is often the opposite of what is needed.

In such a situation, the problem is likely to be some form of maldigestion or malabsorption. For example, in a lactase-deficient individual, a lactose-containing formula can cause diarrhea; switching to a lactose-free formula will cure the diarrhea. A patient with a history

TABLE 33–1 Common Drug-Induced Diarrheas in Tube-Fed Patients

Osmotic
Magnesium-containing antacids
Sorbitol-containing medications (e.g., certain elixirs of theophylline, acetaminophen, vitamins)
Potassium supplements
Phosphorus supplements
Magnesium supplements
Osmotic laxatives (e.g., lactulose, milk of magnesia)

Nonosmotic
Quinidine
Stimulant laxatives (e.g., bisacodyl, castor oil)
Antibiotics
Prokinetic drugs (e.g., metoclopramide, cisapride, erythromycin)

of exocrine pancreatic insufficiency will maldigest and hence malabsorb a polymeric formula; here, an elemental formula would be a more rational choice. Similarly, in patients with extensive mucosal atrophy or damage (such as in kwashiorkor malnutrition,[111] folate deficiency,[112] acquired immunodeficiency syndrome [AIDS] enteropathy,[113] or radiation enteritis[105]) an elemental formula may be better tolerated than a polymeric one, at least until mucosal recovery has occurred.

Hypoalbuminemia has been associated with a high incidence of diarrhea in tube-fed patients.[100,104,114-117] The approach to this diarrhea is a matter of intense debate. First, a number of studies have failed to confirm that such a relationship exists.[99,118-120] Second, even where there appears to be a relationship, some argue that the correlation is not with the hypoalbuminemia but rather with what the lower albumin reflects, namely, more severe disease that is likely to require more antibiotics or other diarrhea-producing drugs.[121,122]

Nevertheless, note that in those studies that did demonstrate a correlation of diarrhea with hypoalbuminemia and not with other known factors, two different approaches appeared effective. The first postulates that the reduced serum albumin level leads to diarrhea because the resulting low oncotic pressure in intestinal capillaries fails to draw fluid (and nutrients) from the mucosal interstitium and ultimately from the intestinal lumen. Acute plasma dilution in the dog does indeed change intestinal function from net absorption to net secretion.[123] Ford and coworkers[116] showed in pediatric surgical patients that correcting hypoalbuminemia with albumin infusions (raising serum albumin from 23.1 g/L to 34.1 g/L) improved their tolerance of enteral feeding from 51 to 87 percent of their nutritional requirement.

The other approach rests on the premise that the hypoalbuminemia reflects protein-calorie malnutrition, which causes a maldigestive-malabsorptive diarrhea because of the associated loss of brush border enzymes and intestinal villus atrophy.[100] Given this digestive and absorptive deficit, an elemental formula would appear to be a logical choice. However, in one study[124] such a formula was poorly tolerated due to its high osmolality. Brinson and colleagues,[125] therefore, tested a semielemental, peptide-based formula. They found that the diarrhea (> 300 ml stools/day) improved when the hypoalbuminemic patients (serum albumin < 2.6 g/L) were switched from an isotonic polymeric formula to the peptide-based formula. Meredith and colleagues[126] also observed less diarrhea in trauma patients given a peptide formula than in those receiving an intact protein formula.

Other investigators, however, failed to confirm the benefit of either albumin infusions[127] or use of a peptide-based formula[119,128] in reducing the incidence of diarrhea, although the confounding presence of antibiotics was acknowledged in at least one study.[127]

Although the above data on hypoalbuminemia and diarrhea appear confusing and conflicting, perhaps they are not unexplainable. Hypoalbuminemia can result from decreased synthesis, increased losses or catabolism, dilution, or redistribution (from intravascular to extravascular space). To the extent that, in a given patient, hypoalbuminemia is the result of an inadequate nutrient intake to support protein synthesis in the liver, one would expect the gut mucosa to be similarly hampered in its protein synthesis (including brush border enzymes) and cell multiplication. This would result in an atrophic gut mucosa with impaired digestive and absorptive capabilities. In this type of hypoalbuminemic patient (i.e., where the hypoalbuminemia was caused by malnutrition), and provided other causes of diarrhea have been ruled out, there is a scientific basis to expect that switching to a predigested formula will alleviate the diarrhea. Our experience with this type of patient agrees with that of Brinson and colleagues.[125] By contrast, albumin infusions in this situation, even with full correction of the oncotic pressure, would not be expected to help, since digestion and absorption would remain impaired.

On the other hand, where the hypoalbuminemia is the result of albumin losses (e.g., through hemorrhage, nephrotic syndrome) or due to hepatocellular dysfunction, and where there is no gut mucosal dysfunction, diarrhea may indeed be related to a reduced oncotic pressure favoring extravasation of fluid and solute from capillary to interstitium and perhaps to gut lumen and thus interfering with the uptake of otherwise absorbable nutrients. For such a patient (and assuming that other causes of diarrhea have been ruled out), albumin infusions to correct the oncotic pressure and turn the tide would seem to make the most sense. By contrast, monomeric formulas would not be expected to reverse the pathophysiologic process here and they might make it worse if they are hypertonic.

Based on the above analysis, one would predict that if elemental or semielemental formulas are of value in stopping diarrhea in hypoalbuminemic patients, it would be in those whose low albumin level reflects chronic protein malnutrition, whereas albumin infusions would be most effective where the hypoalbuminemia is solely the result of plasma protein losses. Also, it should be evident that unless other causes of diarrhea are ruled out, no treatment is likely to be predictably effective.

It is therefore of note that the Brinson study[125] supporting the use of peptide formulations was obtained in medical ICU patients whose hypoalbuminemia is more often a sign of true kwashiorkor than a result of acute losses of plasma protein. In contrast, the Ford study[116] showing the benefit of albumin infusions was done in surgical patients, whose low albumin level is most often the result of acute perioperative net plasma losses than a sign of true malnutrition. Furthermore, in both these studies drugs and other causes of diarrhea were excluded. In contrast, among the studies that reported no benefit of these treatment modalities, none focused (by plan or by chance) on any subgroup of hypoalbuminemics, and few could effectively rule out other contributing factors in the diarrhea.

The role of fiber in preventing diarrhea in the tube-fed patient appears to be as a precursor for SCFA production by the colonic bacteria.[129] SCFAs are the preferred fuel of colonocytes[130] and appear to potentiate sodium and water absorption in the colon.[131-134] In the absence of such fiber, healthy subjects given standard isotonic tube feeding tend to have liquid (though not more frequent) stools.[135] Adding fiber (pectin) corrects the problem.[135] However, in studies of acutely ill tube-fed patients, including fiber in the tube feeding produced conflicting results. Some found it of little[104] or no[136,137] use in preventing diarrhea; others[138,139] reported significant improvement.

This discrepancy may be related in part to the type of fiber used (i.e., soluble fiber such as pectin[135] and partially hydrolyzed guar gum[139] may be more completely fermented to SCFA than insoluble fiber such as soy polysaccharides).[136] However, a more important difference pertains to the concomitant use of antibiotics, since these can reduce gut flora and may thus markedly impair bacterial production of SCFAs from whatever fiber is added to the formula. Thus in the Homann study,[139] where patients receiving antibiotics were excluded, adding fiber reduced the incidence of diarrhea. By contrast, in the Dobb study,[136] where patients were concomitantly receiving two antibiotics on average, adding fiber offered no advantage. Thus even without favoring the overgrowth of *C. difficile* or other pathogen causing colitis, antibiotics can cause loose stools by interfering with SCFA production and thereby with water extraction by coloncytes. Whether reinoculation of the gut with beneficial bacteria can overcome the effect of antibiotics and restore the benefits of fiber remains to be tested.

Our recommended approach to diarrhea in the tube-fed patient consists of the following steps:

1. Examine the patient to rule out the possibility that constipation or stool incontinence is masquerading as "diarrhea."
2. Review the patient's medication regimen for diarrhea-producing drugs (especially hypertonic medications and antibiotics). Discontinue any unnecessary medication; substitute with non-diarrhea-producing alternates wherever feasible.
3. If the patient is taking or recently took antibiotics, send stools for *C. difficile* toxin and for culture.
4. If pseudomembranous colitis is suspected, give the patient enteral metronidazole or vancomycin and use Kaopectate rather than an antiperistaltic agent for diarrhea control, so as not to predispose to toxic megacolon.
5. If diarrhea persists, measure stool electrolytes and osmolality if available, to determine osmotic gap, or hold the feeding for 24 hours and monitor the effect on stool output. The diarrhea is considered osmotic if the osmotic gap ([stool osmolality]—2 × [the sum of concentrations of stool sodium + stool potassium]) is greater than 140 mmol/L,[97] or if the diarrhea improves when intake is discontinued.
6. If a digestive/absorptive impairment exists or is suspected (e.g., due to mucosal atrophy or enteritis), be sure the patient is receiving an elemental or semielemental formula. If no such intrinsic impairment is present but the patient is hypoalbuminemic, and assuming drug-induced diarrhea has been ruled out, then infuse albumin to raise the serum albumin level to 30 g/L, while continuing a polymeric fiber–containing formula.
7. If despite the above measures an osmotic diarrhea persists, or if a secretory diarrhea is diagnosed, begin parenteral nutrition at this point (or sooner if the patient was already malnourished), being sure to compensate for the diarrheal losses of fluid, electrolytes, and zinc.

MICROBIAL CONTAMINATION OF TUBE-FEEDING FORMULAS

For a healthy individual, ingestion of nonsterile foods is generally of little concern. In the tube-fed patient, however, the administration of contaminated formula may have serious consequences, including diarrhea, pneumonia, and septicemia.[140-148] The difference is related both to a high bacterial load that may develop during the administration of the tube-feeding formula (greater bacterial proliferation with increasing "hang time")[142,145,146,149-153] and to the fact that the patient's defense system may be weakened by such factors as severe illness, stress, tracheal intubation, antacids, antibiotic treatment,[154-159] or even by the mere fact of bypassing part of the gut and its defenses (as described above.)

Of the various types of pneumonias that may develop in tube-fed patients, two types should be distinguished from each other. The first is referred to above as "aspiration pneumonia." It can result from the regurgitation and aspiration of gastric content or from the inadvertant administration of tube feeding directly into the tracheobronchial tree. The other type of pneumonia is related not to aspiration of feeding but to a gastropulmonary route of bacterial colonization. To prevent this type of pneumonia, it is necessary to avoid bacterial contamination of enteral feeding and especially to prevent bacterial proliferation in the stomach. Because gastric acid exerts a physiologic check on bacterial survival in the upper GI tract, antacids and inhibitors of acid production, which are commonly used for stress ulcer prophylaxis, increase the risk of pneumonia.[156,160,161] To the extent that feeding can neutralize gastric acid and prevent gastric pH from falling, it can likewise favor unchecked microbial growth, leading to significant gastropulmonary colonization and eventually pneumonia.[59] For this reason intermittent feeding may be more advantageous than round-the-clock tube feeding,[162] although of course not if antacid therapy is used to keep gastric pH alkaline when the feeding is not being adminstered.[163]

Contaminating organisms have included *Klebsiella, Enterobacter cloacae, Escherichia coli, Pseudomonas aeruginosa, Acinetobacter baumannii, Serratia marcescens, Salmonella enteritidis, Moraxella* spp, *Bacillus cereus, Staphylococcus aureus, Staphylococcus epidermidis,* β-hemolytic streptococci, *Enterococcus faecalis,* and yeasts.[140,141,144,145,164-174] Contamination may originate from nonsterile ingredients, additives, dilutants, mixing utensils, reservoir bags, and nonaseptic manipulation of the feeding by the patient or caretaker.[141,143,144,147,166,172,175-181] Prolonged hang time at room temperature allows even minimal bacterial contamination to proliferate into a heavy bacterial load,[149,153,182] particularly since most formulas are an excellent culture medium.[141,150,159,183]

To reduce the risk of microbial contamination and its adverse effects, many recommend the following:

1. Use commercially prepared sterile formulas rather than those prepared at home or in the hospital kitchen.[106,142,147,184,185]
2. Any mixing or other formula preparation should be done under aseptic conditions in the dietary department.[144,147,185] Blenders and other kitchen utensils used for this purpose should be meticulously cleaned[147] and soaked in bactericidal cleansing solution.[184] Whether tap water[186] or only sterile water[187] should be used for reconstitution of powdered formulas is controversial. The extra care may be indicated in feeding the immunocompromised patient.[185,188,189]
3. To avoid contaminating formula during the transfer from can or bottle to the administration bag, use prefilled, ready-to-use containers of formula.[147,184,190] These 1-L bags require only that the delivery set be inserted through a sterile entry site on the bag, thus allowing direct infusion from the manufacturer's container. If the prefilled, ready-to-use system is not available, transfer formula to the feeding bag by a "no touch" technique. This avoids formula's being poured over the contaminated surface of can, bottle, or carton, or the opening of such containers with contaminated openers.[166,184,188]
4. Once it is set up, treat the enteral diet delivery system as a "closed system" to avoid introducing contaminants, whether airborne or with additives.[183,184,189]
5. Commercially prepared sterile formulas, administered from prefilled, ready-to-use containers, can be left hanging at room temperature and used for at least 24 hours.[147,171,184,190,191] Do not leave nonsterile formulas for more than 8 to 12 hours.[184,185,189,190,192]
6. Do not use the delivery set for longer than 24 hours.[106,181,184] Change or at least rinse the reservoir between additions of formula.[190,192]
7. Vigorous hand washing, preferably with a bacteriostatic soap, should precede any handling of the formula (during preparation or administration) or of the feeding system.[144,190,192]
8. Intermittent feeding is preferable to continuous, round-the-clock feeding, so as to allow gastric pH to fall periodically, thus maintaining relative sterility in the upper gut.[193] Where pharmacologic stress ulcer prophylaxis is necessary, sucralfate may be preferable to antacids or H_2 receptor blockers, since sucralfate allows a lower gastric pH.[194] The patient should be monitored by hypophosphatemia, however, since sucralfate binds phosphate.

NUTRITIONAL-METABOLIC COMPLICATIONS

Refeeding Syndrome

The refeeding syndrome is not unique to the enteral route of nutritional support. It can also occur during oral and parenteral alimentation and results from excessively rapid repletion or from failure to anticipate and meet specific nutrient requirements of the reexpanding body cell mass. Potential complications include generalized muscle weakness, tetany, myocardial dysfunction, arrhythmias, seizures, excessive sodium and water retention, hemolytic anemia, phagocyte dysfunction, and death from cardiac or respiratory failure. Although various aspects of this syndrome have been described by several authors during the past 50 years,[195-205] the most complete review of this topic is probably the one published in 1990 by Solomon and Kirby[206] (although some have found it too inclusive[207]).

To avoid the complications of the refeeding syndrome, one must understand its pathogenesis. This requires understanding the body's adaptations to a state of famine.[111] In addition to a slower metabolic rate, these include a reduction in the functional reserve of most if not all organ systems. Thus significant reductions occur in cardiac output, hemoglobin level (and hence in oxygen-carrying capacity), renal concentration capacity, and so on. These reductions per se are not severe enough to cause failure of any organ system during the state of starvation. However, during recovery from starvation, excessively rapid refeeding can overwhelm the patient's limited functional reserves and thus cause death from congestive failure.

Another potential cause of fluid overload, edema, and congestive failure during refeeding pertains to the reintroduction of carbohydrate intake and metabolism. For one thing, carbohydrate intake stimulates the release of insulin, one of whose actions is to reduce salt and water excretion.[206] If carbohydrates are reintroduced too suddenly, the resulting fluid retention may overwhelm the patient's limited cardiac reserve and thus cause heart failure. Second, the return of carbohydrate metabolism may unmask a latent deficiency of thiamine, leading to "high output" failure or "wet beriberi" (and Wernicke's encephalopathy).[206,208]

Perhaps the most important pathogenic aspect of the refeeding syndrome relates to electrolyte shifts from the extracellular to the intracellular compartment. The reexpansion of body cell mass requires not just "protein and energy" but all the components of intracellular space.[209] Of particular clinical concern are the predominant intracellular ions, potassium, magnesium, and phosphate. During the catabolism of starvation, as body cell mass shrinks, these ions (together with up to 300 ml of intracellular fluid/day)[210] pass into the extracellular space. They are then excreted through the kidneys as they reach the renal threshold for excretion. Not surprisingly, therefore, the serum level of these ions remains deceptively normal or even high despite the worsening depletion.

During refeeding, these ions (whatever has not been excreted) are avidly reabsorbed by the reexpanding intracellular compartment, and their serum levels can fall dangerously low within days, unless closely monitored and supplemented.[206] In our experience, such supplementation may be necessary even in a patient with severe renal insufficiency and generally correlates with the severity of the cachexia and with the rapidity of protein-calorie repletion. Thus the initially "normal" laboratory values must not lull one into a false sense of security, and close monitoring and careful anticipant therapy remain indispensable to avoid disaster.

Another cause of electrolyte shifts is the resumption of exogenous carbohydrate metabolism. This affects primarily potassium and phosphate, which are driven intracellularly together with glucose,[206] causing hypokalemia and hypophosphatemia. Treatment of the uncontrolled diabetic with insulin also allows resumption of glucose use and leads to identical electrolyte shifts.[211] It follows that in refeeding a cachectic diabetic patient requiring insulin one must be doubly careful.

An important point to keep in mind during the management of electrolyte abnormalities during refeeding pertains to two secondary effects of hypomagnesemia.[212] First, hypomagnesemia causes an inappropriately high urinary excretion of potassium, thus exacerbating the hypokalemia and preventing its correction by even large doses of potassium supplements. This occurs because the sodium-potassium pump adenosine triphosphatase (ATPase), which is required for tubular reabsorption of potassium, is magnesium dependent.[212]

The second effect of hypomagnesemia is hypocalcemia,[212] which also remains resistant to supplementation until magnesium is repleted. Here the problem is that in the presence of magnesium depletion, parathyroid hormone (PTH) fails to elicit calcium efflux from bone.[212] Furthermore, although increasing amounts of PTH are initially secreted by the parathyroid gland in response to the falling calcium level, the continued decrease in magnesium level eventually inhibits PTH secretion. Thus a patient who is hypocalcemic because of magnesium depletion may have a high, normal, or low PTH level, and attention to this aspect of the refeeding syndrome can avoid the expense of an unnecessary endocrine work-up.

Recommendations for avoiding refeeding syndrome complications include the following:

1. Anticipate the problem whenever a "patient at risk" (one who has lost weight and is expected to regain it) is being fed.[206]
2. Initial nutritional goals should not exceed 20 to 30 kcal/kg/day[213] or about 1000 kcal/day,[206,213] and 1.0 to 1.2 g of protein/kg/day.[213] These can be increased to stress requirements of 25 to 35 kcal/kg/day and 1.5 g protein/kg/day over 1 to 2 weeks, as tolerated.[213]
3. Even if the initial serum levels of potassium, magnesium, and phosphate are normal or high, monitor them closely, especially during the first week,[206] and supplement them as needed. We recommend aiming for a serum level in the middle to upper range of normal.
4. Provide supplemental vitamins, especially thiamine.[213]
5. Monitor even young patients (and certainly elderly ones) for signs of fluid overload and congestive failure,[202,203] since digoxin and diuretics may be required.[214]

Drug-Feeding Interactions

The requirement that all medications be administered through the feeding tube demands that alternatives be found for sustained-release medicines and for medicines that are specially coated to withstand stomach acid. The function, bioavailability, pharmacokinetics, and toxicity of many medications can be altered dramatically by pulverizing or dissolving them. Assuming the physical properties of the medication allow passage through a tube, physiochemical interactions with the tube and with other substances within the tube must be considered. For example, phenytoin and warfarin absorption can be reduced when administered with enteral feedings. The exact mechanism of this interaction has not been identified. In the case of phenytoin, changes in bioavailability may be related to adsorption of the drug along the wall of the feeding tube,[215] although this is probably of less clinical significance than is the binding of the drug to other medications or to components of the feeding formula.[216-220]

Administration through jejunostomy may decrease bioavailability due to lack of time for dissolution and absorption. Warfarin interaction may be related to vitamin K content of the feeding formula.[221,222] However, resistance has been noted even with enteral formulas containing low levels of vitamin K.[223,224] Lipid content of the feedings may also influence the activity of the hepatic P-450 enzymes and consequently the pharmacokinetics and bioavailability of medications metabolized this way.[225]

It is therefore important to monitor closely drug levels when starting, stopping, or switching enteral formulas or routes. Because generic drugs may vary in drug base and consequently in drug interaction with feeding, erratic drug levels may require a switch to brand name medications.

To reduce adverse drug-feeding interactions in the tube-fed patient, the following guidelines may be helpful:

1. Do not crush "sustained-release" or enterically coated medications. Use alternative preparations.
2. Administer each drug in a separate syringe to avoid drug-drug interactions.
3. Flush the feeding tube with water before and after administering each drug to prevent binding of drug to the tube, to other drugs, or to the feeding formula.
4. Use brand name drugs when drug level is crucial to therapy.
5. Be consistent with drug administration. Administer each drug at the same time of day and either with or without feedings.
6. Monitor drug levels when changing enteral feeding formulas or regimens. Be especially careful with warfarin and phenytoin levels.
7. Do not give phenytoin with feeding. We hold the feeding for at least 30 minutes before and after each dose. The same approach may prove helpful for other drugs when levels appear erratic or persistently low.

REFERENCES

1. Rolandelli RH, De Paula JA, Guenter P et al: Critical illness and sepsis. In Rombeau JL, Caldwell MD (eds): Clinical Nutrition: Enteral and Tube Feeding. 2nd edition, Philadelphia: WB Saunders Co., 1990.
2. Curet-Scot M, Shermeta DW: A comparison of intragastric and intrajejunal feedings in neonatal piglets. J Pediatr Surg 1986;21:552–555.
3. Caplan ES, Hoyt NJ: Nosocomial sinusitis. JAMA 1982;249:639–645.
4. Bell MD, Tate LG, Hensley GT: Esophageal-atrial fistula resulting in systemic "meat and vegetable" emboli. Am J Forensic Med Pathol 1992;13(2):137–141.
5. Kovitz KL, Siebens A, Brower RG: Diagnosis of tracheoesophageal fistula by analysis of gastric air. Chest 1993;104(2):641–642.
6. Nelson DB, Silvis SE, Ansel HJ: Management of tracheoesophageal fistula with a silicone covered self

expanding metal stent. Gastrointest Endosc 1994; 40(4):497–499.

7. Bouchi J: Closure of a tracheoesophageal fistula by bronchoscopic application of tissue glue. Chest 1993;103(3):980.

8. DiSario JA, Foutch PG, Sanowski RA: Poor results with percutaneous endoscopic jejunostomy. Gastrointest Endosc 1990;36(3):257–260.

9. Shallman RW, Norfleet RG, Hardach JM: Percutaneous endoscopic gastrostomy feeding tube migration and impaction in the abdominal wall. Gastrointest Endosc 1988;34:367.

10 Gluck M, Levant JA, Drennan F et al: Retraction of Sacks-Vine gastrostomy tubes into the gastrointestinal wall: report of seven cases. Gastrointest Endosc 1988;34:215.

11. Foutch PG, Woods CA, Sawyer RL et al: Push and pull techniques for placement of percutaneous endoscopic gastrostomy tubes: a comparison of methods. Gastrointest Endosc 1988;34:176 (abstract).

12. Klein S, Heare BR, Soloway RD: The "Buried Bumper Syndrome": a complication of percutaneous endoscopic gastrostomy. Am J Gastroenterol 85(4): 448–451.

13. Jeffers SL, Door LA, Meguid MM: Mechanical complications of enteral nutrition: prospective study of 109 consecutive patients (abstract). Clin Res 1984;32:233A.

14. Meer JA: Inadvertent dislodgement of nasoenteral feeding tubes: incidence and prevention. J Parenter Enter Nutr 1987;11(2):187–189.

15. Gutierrez LD, Balfe DM: Fluoroscopically guided nasoenteral feeding tube placement: results of a 1-year study. Radiology 1991;178:759–762.

16. Metheny NA, Spies M, Eisenberg P: Frequency of nasoenteral tube displacement and associated risk factors. Res Nurs Health 1986;9:241–247.

17. Crocker K, Krey S, Steffee W: Performance evaluation of a new nasogastric feeding tube. J Parenter Enter Nutr 1981;1:80–82.

18. Ciocon JO, Silverstone FA, Graver LM et al: Tube feeding in elderly patients. Indications, benefits, and complications. Arch Intern Med 1990;148(2):523–528.

19. Keohane PP, Attrill H, Silk DB: Clinical effectiveness of weighted and unweighted nasogastric feeding tubes in enteral nutrition: a controlled clinical trial. J Clin Nutr Gastroenterol 1986;1:189.

20. Wolf EL, Frager D, Beneventano TC: Radiologic demonstration of important gastrostomy tube complications. Gastrointest Radiol 1986;11:20–26.

21. Barthel JS, Mangum D: Recurrent acute pancreatitis in pancreas divisum secondary to minor papilla obstruction from a gastrostomy feeding tube. Gastrointest Endosc 37(6):638–640.

22. Galat SA, Gerig KD, Porter JA et al: Management of premature removal of the percutaneous gastrostomy. Am Surg 1990;56(11):733–736.

23. Lipman TO: The fate of enteral feeding tubes. Nutr Supp Serv1983;3:71.

24. Marcuard SP, Stegall KS: Unclogging feeding tubes with pancreatic enzyme. J Parenter Enter Nutr 1990; 14:198–200.

25. Ciocon JO, Ciocon DJ, Tiessen C et al: Continuous compared with intermittent tube feeding in the elderly. J Parenter Enter Nutr 1992;16(6):525–532.

26. Powell KS, Marcuard SP, Farrior ES et al: Aspirating gastric residuals causes occlusion of small bore feeding tubes. J Parenter Enter Nutr 1993;17(3):243–246.

27. Carrougher JG, Barrilleaux CN: Esophageal bezoars: the sucralith. Crit Care Med 1991;19(6):837–839.

28. Rowbottom SJ, Wilson J, Grant IS: Total oesophageal obstruction in association with combined enteral feed and sucralfate therapy. Anaesth Int Care 1993; 21(3):372–374.

29. Anderson W, Weatherstone G, Veal C et al: Esophageal medication bezoar in a patient receiving enteral feedings and sucralfate. Am J Gastroenterol 1989; 84(2):205–206.

30. Algozzine GH, Hill G, Scoggins WG et al: Sucralfate bezoar. N Engl J Med 1983;309:1387.

31. Valli C, Schulthess HK, Asper R: Interaction of nutrients with antacids: a complication during enteral feeding. Lancet 1986;1:747–748.

32. Sriram K, Hammond J: Leakage of feedings and gastric contents through ostomy sites. J Parenter Enter Nutr 1986:437.

33. Mushin U, Kite CJ: Gastrostomy tube leakage: a new way of successful conservative management. J Parenter Enter Nutr 1985;9(5):630–631.

34. Gaddy MC, Max MH, Schwab C et al: Small bowel ischemia: a consequence of feeding jejunostomy? South Med J 1986;79(2):180–182.

35. Ratliff JL, Keisler DS: Jejunal distention with elemental feedings following duodenal injury. J Trauma 1987;27(12):1370–1371.

36. Odom JW, Pastena JA, Ritota P et al: Enteral nutrition supplied by jejunostomy can result in jejunal infarction. NYS J Med 1992;92(1):25.

37. Choban PS, Max MH: Feeding jejunostomy: a small bowel stress? Am J Surg 1988;155:112–117.

38. Jones TN, Moore FA, Moore EE et al: Gastrointestinal symptoms attributed to jejunostomy feeding after major abdominal trauma-A critical analysis. Crit Care Med 1989;17(11):1146–1150.

39. Smith DC, Sarr MG: Clinically significant pneumatosis intestinalis with postoperative enteral feedings by needle catheter jejunostomy: an unusual complication. J Parenter Enter Nutr 1991;15(3):328–331.

40. Page CP, Carlton PK, Andrassy RJ et al: Safe, cost effective postoperative nutrition. Defined formula diet via needle catheter jejunostomy. Am J Surg 1979;138:939–945.

41. Kudsk KA, Minard G: Enteral nutrition. In Zaloga GP (ed): Nutrition in Critical Care. St Louis: Mosby, 1994.

42. Dickey K, Fenwick J, Sussman B et al: Pneumatosis intestinalis in patients with Crohn's disease. Dig Dis Sci 1992;37(6):813–817.

43. Balthazar EJ, Stern J: Necrotizing Candida enterocolitis in AIDS: CT features. J Comput Assist Tomogr 1994;18(2):298–300.

44. Heymsfield SB, Bethel RA, Ansley JD et al: Enteral hyperalimentation: an alternative to central venous hyperalimentation. Ann Intern Med 1979;90:63–71.

45. Keohane PP, Attrill H, Love M et al: Relation between osmolality of diet and gastrointestinal side effects in enteral nutrition. Br Med J 1984;288:678–681.

46. Jones BJM, Lees R, Andrews J et al: Comparison of an elemental and a polymeric enteral diet in patients with normal gastrointestinal function. Gut 1983;24: 78–84.

47. Shellito PC, Malt RA: Tube gastrostomy: technique and complications. Ann Surg 1985;201:180–185.

48. Silen W: Acute intestinal obstruction. In Isselbacher KJ, Braunwald E, Wilson JD et al (eds): Harrison's Principles of Internal Medicine, 13th edition. New York: McGraw-Hill, 1994.

49. Winterbauer RH, Durning RB, Barron E et al: Aspirated nasogastric feeding solution detected by glucose strips. Ann Intern Med 1986;95(1):67–68.

50. Kingston GW, Phang PT, Leathley MJ: Increased incidence of nosocomial pneumonia in mechanically ventilated patients with subclinical aspiration. Am J Surg 1991;161:589–592.

51. Potts RG, Zaroukian MH, Guerrero PA et al: Comparison of blue dye visualization and glucose oxidase test strip methods for detecting pulmonary aspiration of enteral feedings in intubated adults. Chest 1993; 103(1):117–121.

52. Mullan H, Roubenoff RA, Roubenoff R: Risk of pulmonary aspiration among patients receiving enteral nutritional support. J Parenter Enter Nutr 1992;16(2): 160–164.

53. Cataldi-Becher EL, Seltzer MH, Slocum BA et al: Complications occurring during enteral nutrition support: a prospective study. J Parenter Enter Nutr 1983;7: 546–552.

54. Sands JA: Incidence of pulmonary aspiration in intubated patients receiving enteral nutrition through wide and narrow bore nasogastric tubes. Heart Lung 1991;20:75–80.

55. Liu DW, McIntyre RW, Watters JM: Pulmonary aspiration in critically ill patients receiving enteral feeding. Clin Invest Med 1989;12:R105.

56. Metheny N, Eisenberg P, Spies M: Aspiration pneumonia in patients fed through nasoenteral tubes. Heart Lung 1986;15(3):256–261.

57. Medley F, Stechmiller J, Field A: Complications of enteral nutrition in hospitalized patients with artificial airways. Clin Nurs Res 1993;2(2):212–223.

58. Cogen R, Weinryb J: Aspiration pneumonia in nursing home patients fed via gastrostomy tubes. Am J Gastroenterol 1989;84(12):1509–1512.

59. Jacobs S, Chang RWS, Lee B et al: Continuous enteral feeding: a major cause of pneumonia among ventilated intensive care unit patients. J Parenter Enter Nutr 1990;14:353–356.

60. Elpern EH, Scott MG, Petro L et al: Pulmonary aspiration in mechanically ventilated patients with tracheostomies. Chest 1994;105(2):563–566.

61. Cogen R, Weinryb J, Pomerantz C et al: Complications of jejunostomy tube feeding in nursing facility patients. Am J Gastroenterol 1991;86(11):1610–1613.

62. Torres A, Aznar R, Gatell JM et al: Incidence, risk, and prognosis factors of nosocomial pneumonia in mechanically ventilated patients. Am Rev Resp Dis 1990;142(3):523–528.

63. Norton J, Ott L, McClain C et al: Intolerance to enteral feeding in the brain injured patient. J Neurosurg 1988;68:62–66.

64. Kidd D, Lawson J, Nesbitt R et al: Aspiration in acute stroke: a clinical study with videofluoroscopy. Q J Med 1993;86(12):825–829.

65. Atherton ST, White DJ: Stomach as a source of bacteria colonizing respiratory tract during artificial ventilation. Lancet 1978;1978(2):968–969.

66. Spray SB, Zuidema GD, Cameron JL: Incidence of aspiration with endotracheal tubes. Am J Surg 1976; 131:701–703.

67. Silver KH, Van Nostrand D: Scintigraphic detection of salivary aspiration: description of a new diagnostic technique and case reports. Dysphagia 1992;7(1):45–49.

68. Anderson B: A theoretical protocol for nutritional maintenance of head-injured patients. J Neurosurg Nurs 1984;16:50.

69. Torres A, Serra-Batlles J, Ros E et al: Pulmonary aspiration of gastric contents in patients receiving mechanical ventilation: the effect of body position. Ann Intern Med 1992;116(7):540–543.

70. Newmark SR, Koelzer C, McCown MH: Current concepts in nutrition: enteral tube feeding. J Okla State Med Assoc 1987;80:163–165.

71. Heitkemper MM, Williams S: Prevent problems caused by enteral feeding. J Gerontol Nurs 1985; 11:25–30.

72. Metheny NM: Twenty ways to prevent tube-feeding complications. Nursing 1985;15:47–50.

73. Payne-James J, Silk D: Enteral nutrition: background, indications, and management. Baillieres Clin Gastroenterol 1988;2:815–847.

74. Rombeau JL, Barot LR: Enteral nutritional therapy. Surg Clin N Am 1981;61:605–620.

75. Breach CL, Saldanha LG: Tube feedings: a survey of compliance to procedures and complications. Nutr Clin Pract 1988;3:230–234.

76. Irwin MM: Enteral and parenteral nutrition support. Semin Oncol Nurs 1986;2:44–54.

77. McClave SA, Snider HL, Lowen CC et al: Use of residual volume as a marker for enteral feeding intolerance: prospective blinded comparison with physical examination and radiographic findings. J Parenter Enter Nutr 1992;16:99–105.

78. Flynn KT, Norton CC, Fisher RL: Enteral tube feeding: indications, practices, and outcomes. Image: J Nurs Scholarship 1987;19:16–19.

79. Coben RM, Weintraub A, DiMarino AJ et al: Gastroesophogeal reflux during gastrostomy feedings. Gastroenterology 1994;106:13–18.

80. Fay DE, Poplausky M, Gruber M et al: Long term feeding: a retrospective comparison of delivery via percutaneous endoscopic gstrostomy and nasoenteric tubes. Am J Gastroenterol 1991;86(11):1604–1609.

81. Baeten C, Hoefnagles J: Feeding via nasogastric tube or percutaneous endoscopic gastrostomy. A comparison. Scan J Gastroenterol 1992;194 (suppl):95–98.

82. Montecalvo MA, Steger KA, Farber HW et al: Nutritional outcome and pneumonia in critical care patients randomized to gastric versus jejunal feedings. Crit Care Med 1992;20(10):1377–1387.

83. Strong R, Condon S, Solinger M et al: Equal aspiration rates from post pylorus and intragastric placed small bore nasoenteric feeding tubes: a randomized prospective study. J Parenter Enter Nutr 1992;16: 59–63.

84. Marian M, Rappaport W, Cunningham D et al: The failure of conventional methods to promote spontaneous transpyloric feeding tube passage and the safety of intragastric feeding in the critically ill patient. Surg Gynecol Obstet 1993;176:475–479.

85. Kaplan DS, Murthy UK, Linscheer WG: Percutaneous endoscopic jejunostomy: long term follow-up of 23 patients. Gastrointest Endosc 1989;35(5): 403–406.

86. Henderson JM, Strodel WE, Gilinsky NH et al: Limitations of percutaneous jejunostomy. J Parenter Enter Nutr 1993;17(6):546–550.

87. Lazarus B, Murphy J, Culpepper L et al: Aspiration associated with long term gastric versus jejunal feedings: a critical analysis of the literature. Arch Phys Med Rehabil 1990;71:46–52.

88. Kadakia SC, Sullivan HO, Starns E et al: Percutaneous endoscopic gastrostomy or jejunostomy and the incidence of aspiration in 79 patients. Am J Surg 1992; 164:114–118.

89. Wolfson HC, Kozarek RA, Ball TJ et al: Tube dysfunction following percutaneous endoscopic gastrostomy and jejunostomy. Gastrointest Endosc 1990;36: 261–263.

90. Weltz CR, Morris JB, Mullen JL: Surgical jejunostomy in aspiration risk patients. Ann Surg 1992;215(2): 140–145.

91. Bui HD, Dang CV, Chaney RH et al: Does gastrostomy and fundoplication prevent aspiration pneumonia in mentally retarded patients? Am J Ment Retard 1989; 94(1):16–19.

92. Meiteles LZ, Kraus W, Shemen L: Modified epiglottoplasty for the prevention of aspiration. Laryngoscope 1993;103(12):1395–1398.

93. Kitahara S, Ikeda M, Ohmae Y et al: Laryngeal closure at the level of the false cord for the treatment of aspiration. J Laryngol Otol 1993;107(9):826–828.

94. Mendelsohn M: A guided aproach to surgery for aspiration: two case reports. J Laryngol Otol 1993;107(2): 121–126.

95. Zimmaro Bliss D, Guenter PA, Settle RG: Defining and reporting diarrhea in tube fed patients—what a mess! Am J Clin Nutr 1992;55:753–759.

96. Schwartz DB, Darrow AK: Hypoalbuminemia-induced diarrhea in the enterally alimented patient. Nutr Clin Pract 1988;3:235–237.

97. Edes TE, Walk BE, Austin JL: Diarrhea in tube-fed patients: feeding formula not necessarily the cause. Am J Med 1990;88:91–93.

98. Kelly TWJ, Patrick MR, Hillman KM: Study of diarrhea in critically-ill patients. Crit Care Med 1983;11: 7–9.

99. Pesola GR, Hogg JE, Yonnios T et al: Isotonic nasogastric tube feedings: do they cause diarrhea? Crit Care Med 1989;17:1151–1155.

100. Dark DS, Pingleton SK: Nonhemorrhagic gastrointestinal complications in acute respiratory failure. Crit Care Med 1989;17:755–758.

101. Woolfson AMJ, Ricketts CR, Saour JN et al: Prolonged nasogastric tube feeding in critically ill and surgical patients. Postgrad Med J 1976;52:678–682.

102. Smith CE, Marien L, Brogdon C et al: Diarrhea associated with tube feeding in mechanically ventilated critically ill patients. Nurs Res 1990;39:148–152.

103. Benya R, Layden TJ, Mobarhan S: Diarrhea associated with tube feeding: the importance of using objective criteria. J Clin Gastroenterol 1991;13:167–172.

104. Guenter PA, Settle RG, Perlmutter S et al: Tube-feeding related diarrhea in acutely ill patients. J Parenter Enter Nutr 1991;15:277–280.

105. Friedman LS, Isselbacher KJ: Diarrhea and constipation. In Isselbacher KJ, Braunwald E, Wilson JD et al (eds): Harrison's Principles of Internal Medicine, 13th edition. New York: McGraw-Hill, 1994.

106. Cabre E, Gassull MA: Complications of enteral feeding. Nutrition 1993;9:1–9.

107. Heimburger DC: Diarrhea with enteral feeding: will the real cause please stand up? Am J Med 1990; 88:89–90.

108. Heimburger DC, Sockwell DG, Geels WJ: Does tube feeding cause diarrhea? Am J Clin Nutr 1991;53:19.

109. Hamaoui E, Krasnopolsky-Levine E, Lefkowitz R: Nutritional support in AIDS patient (Case report). Nutr Clin Pract 1990;5:63–67.

110. Kasper DL, Zaleznik DF: Gas gangrene and other clostridial infections. In Isselbacher KJ, Braunwald E, Wilson JD et al (eds): Harrison's Principles of Internal Medicine, 13th edition. New York: McGraw-Hill, 1994.

111. Torun B, Chew F: Protein-energy malnutrition. In Shills ME, Olson JA, Shike M (eds): Modern Nutrition in Health and Disease. Philadelphia: Lea & Febiger, 1994.

112. Herbert V, Das KC: Folic acid and B$_{12}$. In Shills ME, Olson JA, Shike M (eds): Modern Nutrition in Health and Disease. Philadelphia: Lea & Febiger, 1994.

113. Fauci AS, Lane HC: Human immunodeficiency virus (HIV) disease: AIDS and related disorders. In Isselbacher KJ, Braunwald E, Wilson JD et al (eds): Harrison's Principles of Internal Medicine, 13th edition. New York: McGraw-Hill, 1994.

114. Brinson RR, Kolts BE: Hypoalbuminemia as an indicator of diarrheal incidence in critically ill patients. Crit Care Med 1987;15:506–509.

115. Moss G: Malabsorption associated with exteme malnutrition: importance of replacing plasma albumin. J Am Coll Nutr 1982;1:89–92.

116. Ford EG, Jennings LM, Andrassy RJ: Serum albumin (oncotic pressure) correlates with enteral feeding tolerance in the pediatric surgical patient. J Pediatr Surg 1987;22:597–599.

117. Waitzberg D, Teixera de Silva ML, Borges VC et al: Factus associated diarrhoea in tube fed patients. Role of serum albumin concentration. Clin Nutr 1988; 7(suppl):58.

118. Gottschlich MM, Warden GD, Michel MA et al: Diarrhea in tube-fed burn patients: incidence, etiology, nutritional impact, and prevention. J Parenter Enter Nutr 1988;12:338–345.

119. Mowatt-Larssen CA, Brown RO, Wojtysiak SL et al: Comparison of tolerance and nutritional outcome between a peptide and a standard enteral formula in critically ill, hypoalbuminemic patients. J Parenter Enter Nutr 1992;16:20–24.

120. Patterson ML, Dominguez JM, Lyman B et al: Enteral feeding in the hypoalbuminemic patient. J Parenter Enter Nutr 1990;14:362–365.

121. Hensrud D, Heimburger DC: Tube feeding-related diarrhea. J Parenter Enter Nutr 1992;16:192–193.

122. Chantker S, Parrish C, Morse JH: Hypoalbuminemia may not be the cause of diarrhea in tube-fed patients admitted to the University of Virginia Health Sciences Center. Abstract #124, ASPEN 19th Clinical Congress program. Miami: 1995:591.

123. Duffy PA, Granger DN, Taylor AE: Intestinal secretion induced by volume expansion in the dog. Gastroenterology 1978;75:413–418.

124. Cobb LM, Cartmill AM, Gilsdorf RB: Early postoperative nutritional support using the serosal tunnel jejunostomy. J Parenter Enter Nutr 1981;5: 397–401.

125. Brinson RR, Kolts BE: Diarrhea associated with severe hypoalbuminemia: a comparison of a peptidebased chemically defined diet and standard enteral alimentation. Crit Care Med 1988;16:130–136.

126. Meredith JW, Ditesheim JA, Zaloga GP: Visceral protein levels in trauma patients are greater with peptide diet than with intact protein diet. J Trauma 1990;30: 825–829.

127. Foley EF, Borlase BC, Dzik WH et al: Albumin supplementation in the critically ill. Arch Surg 1990;125: 739–742.

128. Viall C, Porcelli D, Teran JC et al: A double-blind clinical trial comparing the gastrointestinal side effects of two enteral feeding formulas. J Parenter Enter Nutr 1990;14:265–269.

129. Rombeau JL, Kripke SA: Metabolic and intestinal effects of short chain fatty acids. J Parenter Enter Nutr 1990;14(suppl):181S–185S.

130. Roediger WE: Role of anaerobic bacteria in the metabolic welfare of the colonic mucosa in man. Gut 1980;21:793–798.

131. Roediger WE, Moore A: Effect of short-chain fatty acids on sodium absorption in isolated human colon perfused through the vascular bed. Dig Dis Sci 1981;26:100–106.

132. Ruppin H, Bar-Meir S, Soergel KH et al: Absorption of short chain fatty acids by the colon. Gastroenterology 1980;78:1500–1507.

133. Binder HJ, Mehta P: Short chain fatty acids stimulate active sodium and chloride absorption *in vitro* in the rat distal colon. Gastroenterology 1989;96:989–996.

134. Bowling TE, Raimundo AH, Grimble GK et al: Reversal by short-chain fatty acids of colonic fluid secretion induced by enteral feeding. Lancet 1993;342:1266–1268.

135. Zimmaro DM, Rolandelli RH, Koruda MJ et al: Isotonic tube feeding formula induces liquid stool in normal subjects: reversal by pectin. J Parenter Enter Nutr 1989;13:117–123.

136. Dobb GJ, Towler SC: Diarrhoea during enteral feeding in the critically ill: a comparison of feeds with and without fibre. Intensive Care Med 1990;16:252–255.

137. Hart GK, Dobb GJ: The effect of a fecal bulking agent on diarrhea during enteral feeding in the critically ill. J Parenter Enter Nutr 1988;12:465–468.

138. Heather DJ, Howell L, Montana M et al: Effect of a bulk-forming cathartic on diarrhea in tube-fed patients. Heart Lung 1991;20:409–413.

139. Homann HH, Kemen M, Fuessenich C et al: Reduction in diarrhea incidence by soluble fiber in patients receiving total or supplemental enteral nutrition. J Parenter Enter Nutr 1994;18:486–490.

140. Casewell MW, Cooper JE, Webster M: Enteral feeds contaminated with Enterobacter cloacae as a cause of septicaemia. Br Med J 1981;282:973.

141. De Vries EGE, Mulder NH, Houven B et al: Enteral nutrition by nasogastric tube in adult patients treated with intensive chemotherapy for acute leukemia. Am J Clin Nutr 1983;35:1490–1496.

142. Keighley MRB, Mogg B, Bentley S et al: "Home brew" compared with commercial preparation for enteral feeding. Br Med J 1982;284:163.

143. Anderson KR, Norris DJ, Godfrey LB et al: Bacterial contamination of tube-feeding formulas. J Parenter Enter Nutr 1984;8:673–678.

144. Thurn J, Crossley K, Gerdts A et al: Enteral hyperalimentation as a source of nosocomial infection. J Hosp Infect 1990;15:203–217.

145. Levy Y, Caethem JV, Verhaegan G et al: Contaminated enteral nutrition solutions as a cause of nosocomial bloodstream infection: a study using plasmid fingerprinting. J Parenter Enter Nutr 1989;13:228–234.

146. Fernandez-Crehuet Navajaz M, Jurado Chacon D, Guillan Sohas JF et al: Bacterial contamination of enteral feeds as a possible risk of nosocomial infections. J Hosp Infect 1992;21:111–120.

147. Belknap Mickschl D, Davidson LT, Flournoy DJ et al: Contamination of enteral feedings and diarrhea in patients in intensive care units. Heart Lung 1990;19:362–370.

148. Baldwin BA, Zagoren AJ, Rose N: Bacterial contamination of continuous infused enteral alimentation with needle catheter jejunostomy. J Parenter Enter Nutr 1983;8:30–33.

149. Hartemann P, Blech MF, Paqun JL et al: Etude de differents fateurs de contamination et de la proliferation bacterienne ds aliments sondes, de la preparation a l'administration au malade. Techniques Hospitalieres 1984;464:45–50.

150. Simmons NA: Hazards of naso-enteric feeds. J Hosp Infect 1981;2:276–278.

151. Schroeder P, Fisher D, Voltz M et al: Microbial contamination of enteral feeding solutions in a community hospital. J Parenter Enter Nutr 1983;7:364–368.

152. Bengoa JM, Hyde AL, Ducel G et al: Surete bacteriologique de la nutrition enteral a debit continue. Scheiz Med Wschr 1985;115:903–906.

153. Fagerman KE, Paauw JD, McCamaish MA et al: Effects of time, temperature, and preservative on bacterial growth in enteral nutrition solutions. Am J Hosp Pharm 1984;41:1122–1126.

154. Van der Waaij D, Berghuis JM, Lekkekerk JEC: Colonization resistance of the digestive tract to mice during systemic antibiotic treatment. J Hyg (Camb) 1972;70:605–610.

155. Driks MR, Craven DE, Celli BR et al: Nosocomial pneumonia in intubated patients given sucralfate vs antacids or histamine type 2 blockers: the role of gastric colonization. N Engl J Med 1987;317:1376–1382.

156. Du Moulin GC, Paterson DG, Hedley-White J et al: Aspiration of gastric bacteria in antacid-treated patients: a frequent cause of postoperative colonization of the airway. Lancet 1982;1:242–245.

157. Pingleton S, Hinthorn DR, Lin C: Enteral nutrition in patients receiving mechanical ventilation. Multiple sources of tracheal colonization include the stomach. Am J Med 1986;80:827–832.

158. Tryba M: The risk of acute stress bleeding and nosocomial pneumonia in ventilated ICU-patients: sucralfate vs antacids. Am J Med 1987;83:117–124.

159. Pottecher B, Goete ML, Jaquemaire MA et al: Enterocolites chez des malades alimentes par sonde nasogastrique. Ann d'Anesth Franc 1979;20:595.

160. Tryba M: The gastropulmonary route of infection—fact or fiction? Am J Med 1991;91:135S–146S.

161. Apte NM, Karnad DR, Medhekar TP et al: Gastric colonization and pneumonia in intubated critically ill patients receiving stress ulcer prophylaxis: a randomized, controlled trial. Crit Care Med 1992;20:590–593.

162. Lee B, Chang RWS, Jacobs S: Intermittent nasogstric feeding: a simple and effective method to reduce pneumonia among ventilated ICU patients. Clin Int Care 1990;1:100–102.

163. Tryba M: Pneumonia and continuous enteral feeding [letter]. J Parenter Enter Nutr 1991;15:582.

164. De-Leauw IH, Vanderwoude MF: Bacterial contamination of enteral diets. Gut 1986;27(suppl 1):56–57.

165. Gill K, Gill P: Contaminated enteral feeds. Br Med J 1971, 1981;282.

166. Bastow D, Greaves P, Allison SP: Microbial contamination of enteral feeds. Hum Nutr Appl Nutr 1982;36A:213–217.

167. Anderton A: Microbiological quality of products used in enteral feeds. J Hosp Infect 1986;7(suppl A):68–73.

168. White WT, Acuff TE, Sykes TR et al: Bacterial contamination of enteral nutrient solution: a preliminary report. J Parenter Enter Nutr 1979;3:459–461.

169. Casewell MW: Bacteriological hazards of contaminated enteral feeds. J Hosp Infect 1982;3:329–331.

170. Allwood MC: Microbial contamination of parenteral and enteral nutriton. Acta Chir Scand 1981;507:383–387.

171. Schreiner RL, Eitzen N, Gfele MA et al: Environmental contamination of continuous drip feeding. Pediatrics 1979;63:232–237.

172. Casewell M, Phillips I: Food as a source of Klebsiella species for colonization and infection of intensive care patients. J Clin Path 1978;31:845–849.

173. Beyer PL, Parrish-Zepeda A, Furtado D: A prospective survey of contamination of enteral feeding solutions

in the clinical setting. In Proceedings of the Ross Laboratories Workshop on Contamination of Enteral Feeding Products During Clinical Usage. Columbus, OH: Ross Laboratories, 1983:27–32.

174. Gutman LT, Idriss ZH, Gehlbach S et al: Neonatal staphylococcal enterocolitis: association with indwelling feeding catheters and S. aureus colonization. J Pediatr 1976;88:836–869.

175. Anderton A: Microbiological aspects of the preparation and administration of nasogastric and nasoenteric feeds in hospitals. Hum Nutr Appl Nutr 1983; 37A:426–440.

176. Casewell MW, Phillips I: Hands as a route of transmission for Klebsiella species. Br Med J 1977;2:1315.

177. Freedland CP, Roller RD, Wolfe BM et al: Microbiological contamination of continuous drip feedings. J Parenter Enter Nutr 1989;13:18–22.

178. Keohane PP, Attrill H, Love M et al: Controlled trial of aseptic enteral diet preparation—significant effect on bacterial contamination and nitrogen balance. Clin Nutr 1990;2:362–370.

179. Muytjens HL, Roelofs-Willhelms H, Jaspar GH: Quality of powdered substitutes for breast milk with regards to members of the family enterobacteriacae. J Clin Micro 1988;26:743–746.

180. Simmons BP, Gelfand MS, Haas M et al: Enterobacter sakazakii: infections in neonates associated with intrinsic contamination of a powdered infant formula. Infect Control Hosp Epidermiol 1989;10:398–401.

181. Kohn CL: The relationship between enteral formula contamination and length of enteral delivery set usage. J Parenter Enter Nutr 1987;6:21–24.

182. Fagerman KE, Paauw JA, Dean RE: Bacterial contamination of enteral solutions. J Parenter Enter Nutr 1985;9:378.

183. Iannini PB, Mumford F, Buckalew F: Microbial contamination of enteral liquid nutritional systems. In Proceedings of the Ross Laboratories Workshop on Contamination of Enteral Feeding Products During Clinical Usage. Columbus, OH: Ross Laboratories, 1983: 11–15.

184. Silk DBA, Payne-James JJ: Complications of enteral nutrition. In Rombeau JL, Caldwell MD (eds): Enteral and Tube Feeding, 2nd edition. Philadelphia: WB Saunders, 1990.

185. Lenssen P, Cheney C: Enteral feeding of the immunocompromised patient. In Rombeau JL, Caldwell MD (eds): Enteral and Tube Feeding, 2nd. edition. Philadelphia: WB Saunders, 1990;361–385.

186. Nugent M, Hansell DT, Gray GR: Bacterial contamination of reconstituted and commercially prepared enteral feeds. Clin Nutr 1987;6:232–235.

187. Hoestetler C, Lipman TO, Gerachty M et al: Bacterial safety of reconstituted continuous drip tube feeding. J Parenter Enter Nutr 1982;6:232–235.

188. Workshop Summary: In Report of the Ross Workshop on Contamination of Enteral Feeding Products During Clinical Usage. Columbus, Ohio: Ross Laboratories, 1983:38–39.

189. Moe G: Enteral feeding and infection in the immunocompromised patient. Nutr Clin Pract 1991;6:55–64.

190. Eisenberg PG: Causes of diarrhea in tube-fed patients: a comprehensive approach to diagnosis and management. Nutr Clin Pract 1993;8:119–123.

191. Crocker KS, Krey SH, Markovic M et al: Microbial growth in clinically used enteral delivery systems. Am J Infect Control 1986;14:250–256.

192. Guidelines for preventing contamination of enteral feedings. In Report of the Ross Workshop on Contamination of Enteral Feeding Products During Clinical Usage. Columbus, Ohio: Ross Laboratories, 1983; 40–41.

193. Lee B, Chang RWS, Jacob S: Intermittent nasogastric feeding: a simple and effective method to reduce pneumonia among ventillated ICU patients. Clin Int Care 1990;1:100–102.

194. Prod'hom G, Leuenberger P, Koerfer J et al: Nosocomial pneumonia in mechanically ventilated patients receiving antacid, ranitidine, or sucralfate as prophylaxis for stress ulcer. A controlled trial. Ann Intern Med 1994;120:653–662.

195. Keys A, Henschel A, Tayor HL: The size and function of the human heart at rest in semi-starvation and in subsequent rehabilitation. Am J Physiol 1947;150: 153–169.

196. Brozek J, Chapman CB, Keys A: Drastic food restriction: effect on cardiovascular dynamics in normotensive and hypertensive conditions. JAMA 1948;137: 1569–1574.

197. Burger GCE, Drummond JC, Sandstead HR: Malnutrition and Starvation in Western Netherlands, September 1944–July 1945. Parts 1 and 2. The Hague: General State Printing Office, 1948.

198. Schnitker MA, Mattman PE, Bliss TL: A clinical study of malnutrition in Japanese prisoners of war. Ann Intern Med 1951;35:69–96.

199. Katz AL, Hollingsworth DR, Epstein FH: Influence of carbohydrate and protein on sodium excretion during fasting and refeeding. J Lab Clin Med 1968; 172:93–104.

200. Silvis SE, Paragas PD Jr: Parasthesias, weakness, seizures, and hypophosphatemia in patients receiving hyperalimentation. Gastroenterology 1972;62: 513–520.

201. Craddock PR, Yawata Y, Van Santen L et al: Acquired phagocyte dysfunction: a complication of the hypophosphatemia of parenteral hyperalimentation. N Engl J Med 1974';290:1403–1407.

202. Patrick J: Death during recovery from severe malnutrition and its possible relationship to sodium pump activities in the leukocyte. Br Med J 1977;1: 1051–1054.

203. Heymsfield SB, Bethel RA, Ansley JD et al: Cardiac abnormalities in cachectic patients before and during nutritional repletion. Am Heart J 1978;95:584–594.

204. Weinsier RL, Krundieck CL: Death resulting from overzealous total parenteral nutrition: the refeeding syndrome revisited. Am J Clin Nutr 1981;34: 393–399.

205. Mattioli S, Miglioli M, Montagna P et al: Wernicke's encephalopathy during total parenteral nutrition: observation in one case. J Parenter Enter Nutr 1988;12: 626–627.

206. Solomon SM, Kirby DF: The refeeding syndrome: A review. J Parenter Enter Nutr 1990;14:90–97.

207. Faintuch J: The refeeding syndrome: a review [letter; comment]. J Parenter Enter Nutr 1990;14:667–668.

208. Tanphaichitr V: Thiamin. In Shils ME, Olson JA, Shike M (eds): Modern Nutrition in Health and Disease. Philadelphia: Lea & Febiger, 1994.

209. Rudman D, Millikan WJ, Richardson TJ et al: Elemental balances during intravenous hyperalimentation of underweight adult subjects. J Clin Invest 1975; 55:94–104.

210. Grant JP: Handbook of Total Parenteral Nutrition, 2nd edition. Philadelphia: WB Saunders Co., 1992;179.

211. Matz R: Parallels between treated uncontrolled diabetes and the refeeding syndrome with emphasis on fluid and electrolyte abnormalities. Diabetes Care 1994;17:1209–1213.

212. Shils ME: Magnesium. In Shils ME, Olson JA, Shike M (eds): Modern Nutrition in Health and Disease. Philadelphia: Lea & Febiger, 1994.

213. Bowling TE, Silk DBA: Refeeding remembered. Nutrition 1995;11:32–34.

214. Schlictig R, Ayres SM: The refeeding syndrome. In Nutritional Support of the Critically Ill. Chicago: Year Book Medical Publishers, 1988:181.

215. Fleisher D, Sheth N, Kou JH: Phenytoin interaction with enteral feedings administered through nasogastric tubes. J Parenter Enter Nutr 1990;14(5):613–616.

216. Bauer LA: Interference of oral phenytoin absorption by continuous nasogastric feedings. Neurology 1982;32:570–572.

217. Maynard GA, Jones KM, Guidry JR: Phenytoin adsorption from tube feedings. Arch Intern Med 1987;147:1821.

218. Hooks MA, Longe RL, Taylor AT et al: Recovery of phenytoin from an enteral formula. Am J Hosp Pharm 1986;43:685–688.

219. Longe R, Smith O: Phenytoin interaction with an oral feeding results in loss of seizure control. J Am Geriatr Soc 1988;36:542–544.

220. Olson KM, Hiller CH, Ackerman BH et al: Effect of enteral feedings on oral phenytoin absorption. Nutr Clin Pract 1989;4:176–178.

221. O'Reilly RA, Rytand DA: Resistance to warfarin due to unrecognized vitamin K supplementation. N Engl J Med 1980;303:160–161.

222. Zallman JA, Lee DP, Jeffrey PL: Liquid nutrition as a cause of warfarin resistance. Am J Hosp Pharm 38:1174–1181.

223. Martin JE, Lutomski MS: Warfarin resistance and enteral feedings. J Parenter Enter Nutr 1989;13(2):206–208.

224. Parr MD, Record KE, Griffith GL et al: Effects of enteral nutrition on warfarin therapy. Clin Pharm 1982;l:274–276.

225. Knodell RG: Effects of formula composition on hepatic and intestinal drug metabolism during enteral nutriton. J Parenter Enter Nutr 1990;14(1):34–38.

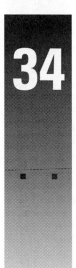

34

Short-Bowel Syndrome

MARY F. CHAN
SAMUEL KLEIN

Short-bowel syndrome refers to the nutritional and metabolic consequences of extensive small intestinal resection. Patients who have had massive intestinal resection present the most challenging nutritional management problems for the clinician. Fortunately, this syndrome occurs infrequently. However, the principles used in managing patients with short-bowel syndrome are applicable to other patients with severe malabsorption.

ETIOLOGY

The major causes of massive small-bowel resection differ in adults and children. In adults extensive resection is most often performed for vascular insults to the small bowel.[1,2] Risk factors for vascular compromise include old age, long-standing congestive heart failure, atherosclerosis, valvular heart disease, chronic diuretic use, hypercoagulable states, and oral contraceptive use. Less common causes of short-bowel syndrome in the adult include regional enteritis, abdominal trauma, primary or metastatic carcinoma, and radiation enteropathy. The majority of underlying conditions associated with short-bowel syndrome in children have their origin in intrauterine life. Antenatal vascular accidents resulting in intestinal atresia are a common cause of this syndrome. Necrotizing enterocolitis and midgut segmental volvulus secondary to malrotation are frequent postnatal causes. Trauma, mesenteric vascular

embolism or thrombosis secondary to hypercoagulable states or cardiac valvular lesions, and Hirshsprung's disease are less common.[3-5]

ADAPTATION

Massive intestinal resection causes morphologic and functional adaptive changes in the residual small bowel. The intestine dilates, and hyperplasia occurs in both the villi and crypts.[6-8] The net result of these changes is that absorption per unit length of intestine increases even though the absorptive capacity of the individual enterocyte does not change. Adaptation can continue for years. Therefore, absorption improves with time, and some patients may be successfully weaned off total parenteral nutrition (TPN) 4 or 5 years after resection.

Stimulation of small-bowel adaptation may involve one or more of the following mechanisms: (1) exposure to luminal nutrients, (2) stimulation by endogenous gastrointestinal (GI) secretions, (3) trophic effects of gut hormones, such as epidermal growth factor or gastrin, (4) stimulation by polyamines, (5) neural factors, and (6) changes in blood flow to the residual bowel.[6,7,9-14] The presence of luminal nutrients, particularly fat, is probably the most important factor and has a profound effect on enterocyte growth, villus morphology, mucosal enzyme activity, and segmental absorptive function.[13] Maintaining normal intestinal structure and function depends on regular food intake, and the absence of ingested nutrients causes intestinal atrophy and loss of brush border enzymes.[6,15,16] Recent data raise the possibility that providing trophic factors, such as growth hormone, glutamine, and fiber, can increase intestinal mass and enhance absorption.[17]

CLINICAL CONSIDERATIONS

The normal GI tract has considerable absorptive capacity. Usually, more than 8 L of fluid enters the upper small intestine daily from the diet and from salivary gland, stomach, biliary tree, pancreas, and intestinal secretions. Most of this fluid is absorbed in the small bowel by solvent drag, and 1 to 1.5 L enter the colon. Sodium ions are actively absorbed in the jejunum, whereas other electrolytes are absorbed passively down a concentration gradient. Most ingested macronutrients are absorbed within the first third of the small intestine.[18]

The terminal ileum has several specialized functions. It contains specific receptors for vitamin B_{12} and bile salt absorption. The presence of lipid or protein in the terminal ileum enhances upper intestinal nutrient absorption by slowing gastric emptying and jejunal transit, the so-called ileal brake.[19] The terminal ileum and "ileocecal valve" also prevent bacterial overgrowth by limiting the reflux of colonic bacteria into the small bowel.

The colon can enhance small-bowel absorption by normalizing early gastric emptying of liquids after massive small intestinal resection.[20] The colon can also compensate for small-bowel malabsorption. Although the colon normally absorbs approximately 1 L of effluent emptied from the small intestine each day, it can absorb up to 5 L/day.[21] In addition, the colon can salvage approximately 500 kcal of unabsorbed carbohydrates by bacterial fermentation of carbohydrate to short-chain fatty acids (SCFAs).[22-25] SCFAs serve as both a systemic and colonocyte fuel and enhance colonic water and electrolyte absorption.[26]

Initial Clinical Assessment

A careful medical history and review of the medical records, operative reports, and radiologic studies are needed to evaluate the extent and site of resection and to determine the presence of diseases that affect nutrient absorption. The amount of small bowel remaining and the site of intestinal resection help determine the patient's absorptive capacity. However, the variability in absorptive function makes it difficult to predict accurately the clinical prognosis in each patient.

In general jejunal resection is better tolerated than ileal resection because the ileum undergoes intense mucosal hyperplasia and can assume most of the jejunum's absorptive functions. In contrast, the jejunum cannot assume the specialized functions of the ileum, such as bile salt and vitamin B_{12} absorption.[11,27,28] Patients who have had jejunal resections alone can usually maintain normal nutritional status with a regular diet. Resection of up to 50 percent of small intestine causes little nutrient malabsorption when at least 150 cm of terminal ileum and the colon are left intact.

Limited (less than 50 cm) ileal resection is usually well tolerated. However, removal of 50 to 100 cm of terminal ileum can significantly impair vitamin B_{12} and bile salt absorption. In patients who have most of the colon intact, bile salt–induced diarrhea ("cholerheic" diarrhea) might occur because of the increased delivery of unabsorbed bile acids to the colon. Bile salts inhibit colonic water and electrolyte absorption and stimulate colonic motility.[29] More extensive ileal resection (more than 100 cm) often causes fat malabsorption and steatorrhea. In this situation, the rate of bile salt loss exceeds the liver's capacity for synthesis, resulting in bile salt depletion and insufficient intraluminal bile salts for micelle formation. Furthermore, the loss of the "ileal brake" can also impair absorption because of the faster transit time.

When more than 75 percent of the small intestine is resected, serious malabsorption occurs. Jejunal length is an important determinant of sodium and water absorption; usually patients with less than 100 cm of small bowel have negative balances while those with more than 100 cm can achieve positive balances.[30] Patients who have a jejunostomy with less than 100 cm of jejunum have large stomal outputs, absorb less than 35 percent of their energy intake, and require intravenous fluid and electrolyte supplementation.[30,31] Patients who have a jejunostomy and less than 60 cm of intestine often require permanent TPN. The presence of a functioning colon becomes a critical factor in patients with very short lengths of remaining small intestine. Patients who have 30 to 60 cm of jejunum and an intact colon may need regularly scheduled infusions of fluid and electrolytes but often can be managed without long-term TPN. However, when jejunal length is less than 30 cm, colonic fluid and electrolyte absorption is usually not able to compensate

TABLE 34–1 Electrolyte Concentrations in Gastrointestinal Fluids

	Na (mEq/L)	K (mEq/L)	Cl (mEq/L)	HCO₃ (mEq/L)
Stomach	65	10	100	—
Bile	150	4	100	35
Pancreas	150	7	80	75
Duodenum	90	15	90	15
Mid-small bowel	140	6	100	20
Terminal ileum	140	8	60	70
Rectum	40	90	15	30

Adapted from Klein S: Nutritional assessment and nutrient requirements in hospitalized patients. In Sachar DB, Waye JD, Lewis BS (eds): Gastroenterology for the House Officer. Baltimore: Williams & Wilkins, 1989.

adequately for the severe impairment in small intestinal function, and chronic TPN is necessary.

An assessment of fluid losses through diarrhea, ostomy output, and fistula volume should be made to help determine fluid requirements. Knowledge of fluid losses is also useful in calculating intestinal mineral losses by multiplying volume loss by the measured or estimated electrolyte concentrations in intestinal fluid (Table 34–1). The physician must also be aware of potential drug-nutrient interactions that would increase nutritional requirements by decreasing nutrient absorption or increasing nutrient excretion. In patients who do not respond to treatment as predicted, dynamic studies of intestinal fat and nitrogen absorption and evaluation of ostomy, fecal, or fistula mineral and fluid losses may help in adjusting the treatment program.

Is Medical Intervention Necessary?

The urgency for medical intervention is determined by the severity of hemodynamic and nutritional abnormalities. Therefore, it is important to perform a careful history and physical examination to evaluate for symptoms and signs of dehydration and specific nutrient deficiencies (Tables 34–2 and 34–3). A dietary history or food record is useful in determining nutrient requirements in nutritionally stable patients and in identifying dietary inadequacies in those with nutrient deficiencies. Laboratory tests are used to screen for complications of specific nutrient deficiencies with special attention to anemia, coagulopathy, electrolyte abnormalities, and osteoporosis or osteomalacia. Screening laboratory studies should include blood tests to determine hemoglobin concentration and red blood cell (RBC) indexes, white blood cell (WBC) count, prothrombin time, and serum levels of urea nitrogen, creati-

nine, albumin, calcium, phosphorus, sodium, potassium, bicarbonate, and magnesium. A 24-hour urine collection to determine calcium and oxalate excretion should be performed in patients at high risk for bone disease or hyperoxaluria. More extensive blood studies and bone mineral densitometry may be necessary in many patients after the initial evaluation has been completed. Table 34–4 lists the laboratory tests available to determine potential vitamin and mineral deficiencies.

MANAGEMENT STRATEGIES

The clinical course of a patient with massive bowel resection passes through several phases.[12,32,33] In the immediate postoperative period there can be considerable fluid and electrolyte losses. The GI tract cannot be used, so fluids, electrolytes, and nutrients must be delivered parenterally. In the next phase oral intake is initiated and gradually advanced. This period may last from a few months to years until maximal adaptation has been achieved and

TABLE 34–2 Symptoms and Signs of Dehydration

Symptoms
Thirst
Dry mouth
Decreased urination
Nausea and vomiting
Mental confusion
Weakness

Signs
Systolic hypotension or tachycardia with postural changes
Decreased skin turgor
Sunken eyes
Mucosal xerosis
Swollen tongue

TABLE 34–3   Selected Symptoms and Signs of Nutritional Deficiencies

	Symptoms or Signs	Possible Nutrient Deficiency
General	Weakness, weight loss, muscle wasting	Protein, calorie
Skin	Pallor	Folate, iron, vitamin B_{12}
	Follicular hyperkeratosis	Vitamin A, vitamin C
	Perifollicular petechiae	Vitamin C
	Dermatitis	Protein, calorie, niacin, riboflavin, zinc, vitamin A, essential fatty acids
	Bruising, purpura	Vitamin C, vitamin K
Hair	Easily plucked, alopecia	Protein, zinc, biotin
	Corkscrew hairs, coiled hair	Vitamin C, vitamin A
Eyes	Night blindness, keratomalacia, photophobia	Vitamin A
	Conjunctival inflammation	Vitamin A, riboflavin
Mouth	Glossitis	Riboflavin, niacin, folate, vitamin B_{12}, protein
	Bleeding or receding gums, mouth ulcers	Vitamin A, vitamin C, vitamin K, folate
	Decreased taste	Zinc, vitamin A
	Burning or sore mouth/tongue	Vitamin B_{12}, vitamin C, niacin, folate, iron
	Angular stomatitis or cheilosis	Riboflavin, niacin, pyridoxin, iron
Neurologic	Tetany	Calcium, magnesium
	Paresthesias	Thiamine, pyridoxine
	Loss of reflexes, wrist drop, foot drop, loss of vibratory and position sense	Vitamin B_{12}, vitamin E
	Dementia, disorientation	Niacin, vitamin B_{12}
	Ophthalmoplegia	Vitamin E, thiamine
	Depression	Biotin, folate, vitamin B_{12}

long-term therapeutic options are better defined.

The long-term goals of therapy are to control diarrhea; maintain fluid, electrolyte, and nutritional homeostasis; treat and prevent medical complications; and maximize quality of life. The therapeutic approach depends on (1) GI tract function, (2) the presence of macronutrient, micronutrient, electrolyte, and fluid deficits, (3) identification of risk factors for future medical complications, (4) the presence of coexisting diseases that affect the ability to provide nutritional therapy, and (5) an evaluation of factors affecting the patient's activities of daily living and quality of life. Initial therapy often requires subsequent modification because of individual variability in absorptive function, continued intestinal adaptation, and the development of new medical complications or disease progression. Close clinical monitoring is critical so that adjustments in medical and nutritional therapy can be made as necessary.

Control of Diarrhea

Diarrhea is often caused by a combination of factors, including decreased absorption of in-testinal secretions, rapid intestinal transit, and consumption of unabsorbed foods and additives. Therefore, therapy for diarrhea involves limiting endogenous secretions, slowing motility, and improving solute absorption.

Gastric secretion and transient gastric hypersecretion may contribute to diarrhea. Decreasing gastric secretions with an H_2-receptor antagonist or with a proton pump inhibitor may be beneficial in a subgroup of patients, especially in the early postoperative period.[34-38] The presence of acidic jejunostomy or ileostomy effluent is a clear indication for acid-reduction therapy.[39] Large doses, twice the usual amount used for ulcer healing, may be required for adequate control in certain patients.

Opiates are the most effective means for slowing intestinal motility and act by delaying gastric emptying, decreasing peristalsis of the small and large intestine, and increasing anal sphincter tone. Try loperamide (Imodium) first because it is metabolized on first pass by the liver and does not easily cross the blood-brain barrier, thereby limiting its side-effects and potential for drug dependence. If loperamide is not effective, other opiates, such as codeine or

TABLE 34–4 Laboratory Tests for Detection of Selected Vitamin and Mineral Deficiencies

Vitamin	Test	Reference Range*		Comment
		Marginal	Deficient Units	
Folate	Folic acid (serum)	2–5.9	< 2 (ng/ml)	Reflects body stores and recent intake
	Folic acid (RBC)	150–300	< 150 (ng/ml)	Reflects body stores
B_{12}	Cobalamin (serum)	180–350[†]	< 180 (pg/ml)	Reflects body stores
B_{12} or folate	Homocysteine (serum)	—	> 20 (μmol/L)	Tests functional block in enzyme activity
B_{12}	Methylmalonic acid (serum)	> 390–500	> 500 (mmol/L)	Tests functional block in enzyme activity
A	Retinol (serum)	35–70	< 35 (μg/dl)	Reflects recent intake and body stores
D	25-hydroxy vitamin D (serum)	10–20	< 8–10 (ng/ml)	Reflects body stores
E	Tocopherol (serum)	120–150	< 120 (μg/dl)	Reflects body stores
	Tocopherol/total lipid (serum)	0.6–1.0	< 0.6 (ratio mg/g)	Ratio is preferred
K	Prothrombin time	—	> 2 sec over control	Not specific for vitamin K
	Vitamin K_1 (serum)	0.1–0.3	< 0.1 (nmol/L)	Reflects body stores
Calcium	24-hour urinary calcium	—	< 2 mg/kg/24 hours	Reflects recent intake
	Bone densitometry	—	> 2 SD below the mean	Reflects bone calcium content, not osteoid matrix
Magnesium	Magnesium (serum)	—	—	May not represent body stores
Zinc	Zinc (serum)	—	—	May not represent body stores

SD = standard deviation.
*Values may vary in different laboratories.
[†]Neuropathy may be seen with serum levels of cobalamin less than 350 pg/ml.

deodorized tincture of opium (10 to 25 drops/6 hours), can be added to the regimen. Alternatively, adding an anticholinergic agent to an opiate may be beneficial. Diphenoxylate with atropine (Lomotil) is one option, but it is expensive and inconvenient if large doses are needed. We have found that capsules containing 25-mg powdered opium and 15-mg powdered belladonna are less expensive and more potent than Lomotil. However, these capsules are not commercially available and require a willing pharmacist to make them.

Therapy with the somatostatin analog, octreotide acetate (Sandostatin), has been shown to decrease ostomy or stool volume (by 500 to 4000 g/day), decrease sodium and chloride loss, and prolong small-bowel transit in patients with short-bowel syndrome.[40-42] Drawbacks of this therapy include the drug's cost, the need for subcutaneous injections, and its side-effects. Octreotide can decrease appetite, impair fat absorption,[43] increase the risk of gallstones,[44] decrease the use of amino acids for splanchnic protein synthesis,[45] and inhibit intestinal adaptation.[46] Nevertheless, in patients who have persistent large-volume intestinal output despite standard antidiarrheal therapy, a trial of 100 μg injected subcutaneously three times a day with meals may be useful.

Foods and medications that cause diarrhea should be avoided. Traditionally, it has been recommended to decrease or eliminate lactose-containing foods because of the reduction in intestinal lactase in patients who have had intestinal resection. However, recent data have shown that patients with jejunostomies and between 15 cm and 150 cm of jejunum can tolerate 20-g lactose loads as milk or yogurt.[47] Although lactose was better absorbed from yogurt than from milk, there was no difference in clinical symptoms. Foods that have laxative effects, such as caffeine-containing drinks and dietetic products containing osmotically active sweeteners (sorbitol, xylitol, and mannitol), should be avoided. Medications that contain magnesium or sorbitol can also contribute to diarrhea.[48] Table 34–5 provides a list of commonly prescribed medications that can cause osmotic diarrhea.

Enteral Feeding

Patients who require parenteral nutrition in the immediate postoperative period can be weaned as enteral or oral feedings are advanced. The ability to use the enteral route to provide all nutrient requirements is determined by intestinal absorptive function and the presence of adverse symptoms caused by feeding. Patients with nausea, vomiting, abdominal pain, or severe diarrhea may be unable to tolerate enteral feeding regardless of intestinal absorptive capacity. Specific foods that cause GI complaints should be avoided. However, it is important to evaluate objectively the validity of these complaints to prevent the unnecessary withdrawal of nutritious foods.

The goal of feeding is to provide the patient with all recommended nutritional requirements. The amount of ingested nutrients needed to reach this goal can be estimated based on the normal recommended dietary allowances modified by an estimate of absorptive function and intestinal losses. This usually requires ingestion of large amounts of fluid, calories, protein, vitamins, and minerals. Even in patients with severe short-bowel syndrome, TPN may not be needed when vitamin and mineral supplements and large amounts of calories and protein are provided enterally.[49,50] In general, most patients with severe malabsorption must ingest 40 to 60 kcal/kg/day and 1.2 to 1.5 g protein/kg/day.[51,52] Specific vitamin and mineral supplementation must be tailored to meet individual needs, but all patients should receive a general multivitamin and mineral supplement daily.

Energy Intake

The composition of the calorie source best suited for patients with short-bowel syndrome has been debated. One approach recommends a low-fat, high-carbohydrate diet because malabsorbed long-chain fatty acids (LCFAs) can cause steatorrhea, colonic water secretion, higher fecal output, greater loss of divalent ions, and hyperoxaluria.[53-56] However, carbohydrate malabsorption can also cause diarrhea,[57] and limiting fat intake usually translates into decreased caloric intake. In other studies total fluid, energy, nitrogen, sodium, potassium, and

TABLE 34–5   Commonly Prescribed Medications that May Cause Osmotic Diarrhea

Magnesium-Containing Products
Magnesium carbonate
  Maalox suspension
  Mylanta Gelcaps
Magnesium hydroxide
  Maalox Antacid Plus Antigas
  Extrastrength Maalox Antacid Plus Antigas suspension
  Maalox TC suspension
  Mylanta liquid
  Milk of Magnesia
  Ascriptin and Arthritis Pain Ascriptin
Magnesium sulfate
  Amoxicillin capsules
Magnesium stearate
  Dipentum (olsalazine)
Magnesium aluminum silicate
  Dilantin suspension (phenytoin)

Sorbitol-Containing Products
Zovirax suspension (acyclovir)
Symmetrel syrup (amantidine)
Bactrim suspension
Tegretol suspension (carbamazepine)
Theolair solutions or liquids (theophylline)
Reglan syrup (metoclopramide)
Septra suspension
Tagamet liquid (cimetidine)
Tylenol liquid (acetaminophen)

Mannitol-Containing Products
Prilosec (omeprazole)

divalent ion absorption were found to be the same with either a high-fat, low-carbohydrate or a low-fat, high-carbohydrate diet.[51, 58-61] The reason for these dichotomous results may be related to differences in patient populations. Most patients evaluated in the former studies had ileal resection and ileocolonic anastomoses. Most patients evaluated in the latter studies had more extensive small bowel resections with colectomies. Limiting fat intake in patients with an intact colon and severe steatorrhea will often reduce GI discomfort and diarrhea and may increase total energy absorption.[62] However, fat intake should not be restricted in patients who have had colectomy or who tolerate normal dietary fat ingestion.

Calorie intake can be enhanced by the use of medium-chain triglycerides (MCTs). Dietary supplementation with MCT oil may be beneficial in patients with severe steatorrhea, because MCTs do not require bile salts and micelle formation for hydrolysis and absorption.[63] However, many patients do not find MCT oil palatable. Furthermore, MCTs are ketogenic, and large doses can cause nausea, vomiting, abdominal discomfort, and osmotic diarrhea, which limits their usefulness. The maximum amount normally tolerated is limited to approximately 1 tablespoon (15 ml), four times daily, which provides 460 kcal. The oil can be ingested alone or with other foods, such as in salad.

Predigested Formulas

Predigested formulas (i.e., monomeric [elemental] and oligomeric formulas) have been recommended for patients with short-bowel syndrome. Theoretically, these formulas, which contain nitrogen in the form of free amino acids or small peptides, are absorbed more efficiently over a shorter length of intestine than polymeric formulas or whole food. However, the clinical efficacy of these formulas is not clear. Two prospective trials, using a randomized cross-over design, have evaluated the use of predigested formulas in patients with a jejunostomy and less than 150 cm of residual small bowel.[59,64] McIntyre and coworkers[59] found no difference in nitrogen or total calorie absorption between a polymeric or an oligomeric diet. In contrast, Cosnes and colleagues[64] found that nitrogen, but not total calorie, absorption was greater with a peptide-based diet than a diet containing whole proteins. However, it is not known whether the increase in nitrogen absorption led to an improvement in protein metabolism or nitrogen balance, because these parameters were not measured. Blood urea nitrogen and urinary urea excretion were greater during peptide-based diet feeding than during whole-protein diet ingestion, suggesting that the absorption of additional amino acids stimulated amino acid oxidation. Therefore, at present there is not sufficient clinical evidence to justify the routine use of expensive predigested formulas in patients with short-bowel syndrome.

Oral Rehydration Therapy

A subset of patients with severe short-bowel syndrome are able to absorb adequate protein and calories but cannot maintain fluid and electrolyte homeostasis. In particular, fluid, sodium, and magnesium balances are difficult to achieve. These patients may benefit from the principles used in oral rehydration therapy by frequently ingesting small-volume feedings of an isotonic glucose or starch-based electrolyte solution.[65] Oral rehydration therapy takes advantage of the sodium-glucose cotransporter present in the brush border of intestinal epithelium.[66] Thus, sodium is actively transported across the intestine, while water and additional sodium follow passively by solvent drag.[67]

The World Health Organization (WHO) developed a solution for oral rehydration therapy based on the results of studies in patients with cholera. This solution is made by mixing 3.5 g of sodium chloride, 2.9 g of sodium bicarbonate, 1.5 g of potassium chloride, and 20 g of glucose in 1 L of water. However, the composition of the ideal oral rehydration formula for patients with short-bowel syndrome is more controversial.

The appropriate concentration of sodium is perhaps the most important issue. The WHO formula has a sodium concentration of 90 mmol/L based on balance studies in patients with cholera. Because sodium loss in cholera is higher than in most other diarrheal illnesses, using the WHO formula could result in hypernatremia. Oral rehydration solutions that contain a wide variety of sodium concentrations have been used safely and effectively in many clinical studies. Data from studies in animals and patients with short-bowel syndrome suggest that sodium and water absorption is maximal from solutions containing 90 to 120 mmol/L of sodium.[68] Therefore, 90 to 120 mmol/L of sodium may be necessary to achieve sodium and fluid balance in patients with severe short-bowel syndrome and large volume intestinal output.

There are numerous oral rehydration formulas commercially available, and their electrolyte concentrations, including sodium, vary (Table 34–6). Sports drinks and commercially available defined liquid formulas have limited sodium concentrations and are inappropriate for electrolyte replacement. Patients already receiving an enteral formula may benefit from sodium added to the solution.

The potassium concentration in most oral rehydration formulas is 20 mmol/L, which is less than the potassium concentration of the stool of many patients with diarrhea. Therefore, it may be beneficial to increase the potassium content to 30 or 35 mmol/L.[69,70]

Most oral rehydration solutions are iso-osmolar. Replacement of glucose with polymeric forms of carbohydrate, such as rice syrup solids, provides a hypotonic solution that may be more effective than glucose-based solutions in decreasing stool volume. Infants with acute diarrhea given an oral rehydration formula containing rice syrup had greater retention of elec-

TABLE 34–6   Characteristics of Selected Oral Rehydration Solutions, Sport Drinks, and Defined Liquid Formula Diets

Solution	Sodium mmol/L	Potassium mmol/L	Chloride mmol/L	Base Equivalents mmol/L	Carbohydrate mmol/L (g/L)	Osmolality mOsm/L
Oral Rehydration Solutions						
WHO glucose based	90	20	80	30	111 (20)	330
Rice-based	50	25	45	10	167 (30)	200
Gastrolyte	50	20	52	18	100 (18)	240
Pedialyte	45	20	35	30	139 (25)	270
Rehydralyte	75	20	65	30	139 (25)	330
Sport Drinks						
Gatorade	20	3	27	3	278 (50)	330
Gatorade light	15	3	20	3	139 (25)	200
Exceed (FRED)	9	5	10	3	390 (70)	250
10-K	10	3	4	2	333 (60)	300
Liquid Formula Diets						
Ensure	37	40	41	—	805 (145)	470
Isocal	23	34	30	—	738 (133)	300
Osmolite	28	26	24	—	805 (145)	300
Sustacal	41	54	44	—	778 (140)	620
Vivonex TEN	20	20	23	—	1145 (206)	630

trolytes and less fecal output than infants given a similar formula containing glucose.[65]

In summary, the available data suggest that the most effective oral rehydration solution for patients with short-bowel syndrome should contain glucose, 100 to 150 mmol/L or rice syrup solids, 30 g/L; sodium, 60 to 120 mmol/L; potassium, 20 to 35 mmol/L; chloride, 45 to 80 mmol/L; and base (citrate or bicarbonate), 10 to 30 mmol/L. Daily oral administration of 1 to 2 L of rehydration solutions has been used successfully to correct fluid and electrolyte abnormalities and allow intravenous supplementation to be discontinued in patients who have had extensive intestinal resection.[68,71-73] In some patients oral rehydration therapy has decreased ostomy output by 4 L/day.[73]

Nutrient Delivery

Ingestion of large amounts of nutrients can often overcome impaired absorption and permit maintenance of a normal nutritional status. Furthermore, increasing the time food is in contact with the intestine can enhance nutrient absorption. Therefore, total dietary intake should be divided into at least six meals/day. In addition, defined liquid formulas can be used as supplements between meals and continuous tube feedings can be given at night. Some data show that aggressive oral or enteral feeding obviates the need for parenteral nutrition in patients with short-bowel syndrome receiving home-based TPN.[49,50,74] These recommendation have been challenged.[59]

Macrominerals

Several macrominerals are poorly absorbed and should be supplemented as indicated by plasma concentration or urinary excretion. Replacing magnesium is problematic because magnesium salts are cathartic and increase diarrhea. Do not use enteric-coated magnesium supplements because their delayed release reduces contact time with the intestine for absorption.[75] Soluble magnesium salts, such as magnesium gluconate (Magonate), are better tolerated and absorbed than other magnesium complexes. In some patients, magnesium is best given in liquid form added to one of the more hypotonic oral rehydration solutions in doses of 15 to 30 mmol (365 to 730 mg elemental magnesium)/day. Liquid magnesium sulfate is not as useful because of its cathartic effects. Magnesium is primarily an intracellular cation, and therefore normal serum magnesium levels do not exclude the presence of magnesium deficiency. The percentage of infused magnesium excreted in urine, normally more than 80 percent of the intravenous dose, may be a better index of body stores, but this has not been confirmed.[76]

Supplemental calcium is given routinely because of both impaired intestinal absorption and the limited calcium intake in patients who are consuming low-lactose diets. Plasma levels of calcium are usually maintained by mobilizing bone stores unless there is concurrent magnesium or vitamin D deficiency. Therefore, urinary calcium excretion, which should be more than 2 mg/kg/24 hours, is a more reliable index of calcium absorption. Bone densitometry is helpful to assess body calcium stores. Abnormalities in calcium status indicate that more aggressive treatment must be initiated, such as increasing vitamin D and calcium intake or starting estrogen therapy in postmenopausal women. Most patients require 1.5 to 2 g of elemental calcium daily. Although calcium citrate may be absorbed more easily than calcium carbonate,[77] most studies do not demonstrate any differences in bioavailability from calcium ingested as a carbonate, citrate, gluconate, lactate, or sulfate salt.[78,79] However, the amount of elemental calcium present in each calcium salt differs, influencing the number of tablets needed each day (Table 34–7).

When diarrhea is severe, potassium and bicarbonate are lost, resulting in hypokalemia and metabolic acidosis. An alkalinizing salt of potassium, given in liquid form to enhance absorption, helps restore both potassium and bicarbonate homeostasis. Further supplementation with either liquid potassium, as a chloride or gluconate salt, or base, as Shohl's (sodium citrate) solution, may be necessary to maintain normal plasma electrolyte concentrations.

Trace Minerals

Data regarding trace mineral requirements in patients with short-bowel syndrome are limited. Absorption of trace minerals from the diet and a multimineral supplement is often adequate to prevent overt deficiency syndromes. However, patients with short-bowel syndrome may develop zinc deficiency because zinc absorption is poor,[80] and zinc losses can be high.[51] Therefore, oral zinc replacement should include at least 100 mg of elemental zinc/L of intestinal output in addition to basal requirements of approximately 25 mg/day. Zinc gluconate is better tolerated than zinc sulfate, which may cause gastric distress. If possible, do not give zinc supplementation with meals, because food may decrease its absorption.[81]

Vitamins

Patients with malabsorption can usually absorb adequate amounts of most water-soluble vitamins, but patients with steatorrhea and bile acid depletion have difficulty absorbing fat-soluble vitamins. All patients with fat malabsorption should receive calcium and vitamin D supplementation to decrease the risk of osteopenia and osteomalacia. Adequate calcium replacement must be documented with a 24-hour urine collection. Large doses of vitamins A, D, and E may also be required to maintain normal body concentrations.

The need for specific therapy is guided by an assessment of body vitamin stores or functional evidence of deficiency (Tables 34–3 and 34–4). Large doses of vitamins A, E, and K should only be given if deficiencies are documented. Because intestinal bacteria synthesize vitamin K, deficiency is rarely a clinical problem, unless patients are receiving antibiotics. It is important to know the retinol-binding protein level when evaluating vitamin A status, be-

TABLE 34–7   Calcium Content of Selected Calcium Salts

Calcium Salt	Elemental Calcium (mg/g)	Representative Products	Calcium Content (mg/tablet)
Acetate	250	Phos-Lo	169
Carbonate	400	Alka-Mints	340
		Caltrate 600	600
		Nephro-Calci	600
		Oscal 250 + D	250
		Oscal 500	500
		Rolaids	220
		TUMS	250
Citrate	211	Citracal	200
Glubionate	64	Neo-Calglucon	115*
Gluconate	96	Generic 500 mg	48
		Generic 1000 mg	96
Lactate	130	Generic 325 mg	42
		Generic 650 mg	84
Phosphate (dibasic)	234	Dical D	117
Phosphate (tribasic)	400	Posture	600

*mg/5 ml.

cause retinol-binding protein is necessary to mobilize vitamin A. Patients with subnormal levels of retinol binding protein may have low serum levels of vitamin A, despite normal or high liver stores. Liquid vitamins present in water-miscible and water-soluble forms are preferable because they are better absorbed than pills. Water-miscible forms of vitamins still require bile acids and micelle formation for absorption, whereas the water-soluble forms do not.

In patients with severe fat malabsorption, daily supplementation with vitamin A (10,000 to 50,000 units [3000 to 15,000 retinol equivalents] of Aquasol A), vitamin D (50,000 units two to three times a week), and vitamin E (30 units [34 mg] Liqui-E) is often necessary. The amount of vitamin D needed depends in part on the patient's exposure to sunlight. The ultraviolet radiation from sunlight converts 7 dehydro-cholesterol present in skin to vitamin D_3. Patients who have renal dysfunction may be unable to metabolize 25 hydroxy vitamin D to its active form and require daily therapy with 1,25 dihydroxy vitamin D (0.25 to 0.50 µg of Rocaltrol). If hypoprothrombinemia is present, a large dose of vitamin K (10 to 25 mg of Mephyton) is given initially, followed by maintenance therapy as needed.

Patients who have had ileal resections may need vitamin B_{12} supplementation. The decision to give vitamin B_{12} is based on the history of ileal resection, serum vitamin B_{12} levels, or a Schilling's test. Note that peripheral neuropathy may be seen before the serum level of B_{12} falls below the lower limit of normal.[82,83] Treatment can be provided orally or parenterally. If there is enough remaining small bowel, large daily oral doses (1 mg/day) can overcome the absorptive defect and maintain normal vitamin B_{12} status. Appropriate supplementation can be guaranteed with intramuscular vitamin B_{12} injections, given as 100 to 500 µg every 1 to 2 months. Providing larger doses of parenteral B_{12} is not necessarily more effective, because once tissue stores are saturated, excess vitamin B_{12} is excreted in urine. Furthermore, providing parenteral B_{12} at intervals longer than every 2 months may not prevent deficiency, even when large doses are given, because there is continual loss of B_{12} through biliary secretions.[84]

Recommendations for vitamin and mineral supplementation are outlined in Table 34–8. A daily large-dose vitamin and mineral complex, such as a prenatal multivitamin with minerals, as well as vitamin D and calcium should probably be given to all patients with short-bowel syndrome. Specific vitamin and mineral needs can only be determined by careful assessment of nutrient status.

TABLE 34–8 Recommendations for Vitamin and Mineral Supplementation

Supplement (Representative Product)	Dose	Route
Multivitamin with minerals*	1 prenatal vitamin/day q d	PO
Vitamin D*	50,000 U 2–3 times/week	PO
Calcium*	500 mg of elemental calcium tid or qid	PO
Vitamin B_{12}[†]	1 mg q d	PO
	100–500 µg/1–2 months	IM
Vitamin A[†] (Aquasol A)	10,000 to 50,000 U/day	PO
Vitamin K[†] (Mephyton;	5 mg/day	PO
AquaMEPHYTON)	5–10 mg/week	SC/IM/IV
Vitamin E[†] (Liqui E)	30 U/day	PO
Magnesium gluconate[†] (Magonate)	54 mg of elemental magnesium tid or qid	PO
Magnesium sulfate[†]	290 mg of elemental magnesium 1–3 times/week	IM/IV
Zinc gluconate or zinc sulfate[†]	25 mg of elemental zinc/day plus 100 mg/L intestinal output	PO
Ferrous sulfate[†]	60 mg of elemental iron tid	PO
Iron dextran[†]	≤ 100 mg of elemental iron/day based on formula or table	IV

PO = oral; SC = subcutaneous; IM = intramuscular; IV = intravenous; tid = three times daily; qid = four times daily.
*Recommended routinely for all patients.
†Recommended for patients with documented nutrient deficiency or malabsorption.

Parenteral Support

Parenteral nutrition may be necessary to provide fluids, specific nutrients, or complete nutritional requirements in patients who cannot maintain normal hydration, electrolyte balance, or nutritional status with oral feeding. Some general guidelines are useful in deciding which patients require parenteral therapy. Patients in whom urine output is less than 1 L/day are at increased risk for developing renal dysfunction and should receive intravenous fluids. Adequate levels of certain minerals, such as magnesium, potassium, and zinc, and fat-soluble vitamins, are difficult to maintain with oral feedings in patients with severe steatorrhea or large intestinal fluid output and may require parenteral supplementation. Magnesium sulfate can be injected intramuscularly at a dosage of 12 mmol (290 mg of elemental magnesium) one to three times per week if attempts at oral therapy are unsuccessful. Intravenous infusion of magnesium is preferred, however, because intramuscular injections are painful and can cause sterile abscesses. Regular intramuscular injections of vitamin B_{12} are required in patients who malabsorb vitamin B_{12}. Five to 10 mg of vitamin K should be given subcutaneously or intravenously each week to patients who have evidence of, or are at high risk for, vitamin K-associated hypoprothrombinemia. In some patients, total parenteral nutrition may be needed to limit diarrhea and achieve an acceptable quality of life. As the intestine continues to adapt over months to years, the need for parenteral nutrition may decrease, and some patients have been weaned off TPN 5 years after intestinal resection.

COMPLICATIONS OF THE SHORT-BOWEL SYNDROME

Patients with short-bowel syndrome are at high risk for certain medical complications. Patients who have fat malabsorption and an intact colon are predisposed to developing hyperoxaluria and renal oxalate stones.[85] Hyperoxaluria is caused by increased absorption of oxalate by the colon. Unabsorbed fatty acids bind calcium in the small intestine, thereby preventing the formation of calcium oxalate, which is insoluble and poorly absorbed. A 24-hour urine collection for oxalate can identify high-risk patients. If urinary oxalate excretion is greater than 50 mg/day, consider a low-oxalate diet (Table 34–9), increased dietary calcium intake, and citrate supplementation to prevent renal stone formation. Dehydration with low urine output can lead to renal dysfunction and when present must be corrected by increasing oral or intravenous fluids. Cholelithiasis is common in patients who have had ileal resection, presumably because of alterations in bilirubin metabolism, bile salt depletion, and gallbladder stasis.[86,87] As in other patients who have gallstones, treatment is not indicated unless symptoms are present. The clinician must have a high index of suspicion for gallbladder and biliary disease in patients with right upper quadrant abdominal pain or abnormal liver biochemistries. D-lactic acidosis caused by anaerobic bacterial fermentation of malabsorbed carbohydrate can cause severe alterations in mental status, including slurred speech, ataxia, stupor, and coma. The diagnosis can be confirmed by measuring D-lactic acid in the blood using a specific enzymatic assay (D-lactate dehydrogenase). Most standard tests for lactic acidosis measure L-lactic acid only.[88,89] Treatment involves administration of antibiotics with anaerobic coverage and initiation of a low-carbohydrate diet.

SUMMARY

The clinical manifestations of short-bowel syndrome are protean and sometimes difficult to predict. Understanding the pathophysiologic alterations caused by massive intestinal resection is essential for developing an appropriate treatment plan. Meticulous attention must be paid to details to prevent nutrient deficiencies and medical complications. The therapeutic approach must also be flexible to maintain patient compliance and to adapt to alterations in clinical status.

TABLE 34–9   Oxalate Content in Selected Foods

Very High	*Moderate*
Spinach	Parsley
Rhubarb	Green beans
Cocoa	Collards
Chocolate	Kale
Tea	Turnip greens
	Beets
High	Brussel sprouts
Potatoes	Bread
Raw nuts	
Strawberries	
Figs	
Oranges	
Instant coffee	
Cola beverages	

REFERENCES

1. Greenberger NJ: The management of patients with short bowel syndrome. Am J Gastroenterol 1978;70: 528–540.
2. Weser E: The management of patients after small bowel resection. Gastroenterology 1976;71:146–150.
3. Ziegler MM: Short bowel syndrome in infancy: etiology and management. Clin Perinatol 1986;13:163–173.
4. Schwartz MZ, Maeda K: Short bowel syndrome in infants and children. Pediatr Clin North Am 1985;32: 1265–1279.
5. Goulet OJ, Revillon Y, Jan D et al: Neonatal short bowel syndrome. J Pediatr 1991;119:18–23.
6. Dowling RH: Update on intestinal adaptation. Triangle 1988;27:149–164.
7. Williamson RCN, Chir M: Intestinal adaptation: structural, functional and cytokinetic changes. N Engl J Med 1978;298:1393–1402.
8. Porus RL: Epithelial hyperplasia following massive small bowel resection in man. Gastroenterology 1965; 48:753–757.
9. Williamson RCN, Chir M: Intestinal adaptation: mechanisms of control. N Engl J Med 1978;298:1444–1450.
10. Buts J-P, Morin CL, Ling V: Influence of dietary components on intestinal adaptation after small bowel resection in rats. Clin Invest Med 1979;2:59–66.
11. Weser E, Fletcher JT, Urban E: Short bowel syndrome. Gastroenterology 1979;77:572–579.
12. Shanbhogue LKR, Molenaar JC: Short bowel syndrome: metabolic and surgical management. Br J Surg 1994;81:486–499.
13. Lentze MJ: Intestinal adaptation in short-bowel syndrome. Eur J Pediatr 1989;148:294–299.
14. Dworkin LD, Levine GM, Farber NJ et al: Small intestinal mass of the rat is partially determined by indirect effects of intraluminal nutrition. Gastroenterology 1976;71:626–630.
15. Richter GC, Levine GM, Shiau TF: Effects of luminal glucose versus nonnutritive infusates on jejunal mass and absorption in the rat. Gastroenterology 1983;85: 1105–1112.
16. Spector MH, Levine GM, Deren JJ: Direct and indirect effects of dextrose and amino acids on gut mass. Gastroenterology 1977;72:706–710.
17. Byrne TA, Morrissey TB, Ziegler TR et al: Growth hormone, glutamine, and fiber enhance adaptation of remnant bowel following massive intestinal resection. Surg Forum 1992;43:151–153.
18. Borgstrom B, Dahlquist A, Lundh G et al: Studies of intestinal digestion and absorption in the human. J Clin Invest 1957;36:1521.
19. Read NW, McFarlane A, Kinsman RI et al: Effect of infusion of nutrient solutions into the ileum and gastrointestinal transit and plasma levels of neurotensin and enteroglucagon. Gastroenterology 1983;86:274–280.
20. Nightingale JM, Kamm MA, van der Sijp JR et al: Disturbed gastric emptying in the short bowel syndrome. Evidence for a "colonic brake." Gut 1993;34: 1171–1176.
21. Debongnie JC, Phillips SF: Capacity of the colon to absorb fluid. Gastroenterology 1978;84:698–703.
22. Royall D, Wolever TM, Jeejeebhoy RN: Evidence for colonic conservation of malabsorbed carbohydrate in short bowel syndrome. Am J Gastroenterol 1992;87: 751–756.
23. Hammer HF, Fine KD, Santa Ana CA et al: Carbohydrate malabsorption. Its measurement and its contribution to diarrhea. J Clin Invest 1990;86:1936–1944.
24. Bond JH, Currier BE, Buchwald M et al: Colonic conservation of malabsorbed carbohydrates. Gastroenterology 1980;78:444–447.
25. Roediger WE: Role of anaerobic bacteria in the metabolic welfare of the colonic mucosa in man. Gut 1980;21:793–798.
26. Bowling TE, Raimundo AH, Grimble GK et al: Reversal by short-chain fatty acids of colonic fluid secretion induced by enteral feeding. Lancet 1993;342:1266–1268.
27. Dowling RH, Booth CC: Structural and functional changes following small intestinal resection in the rat. Clin Sci 1967;32:139–149.
28. Weser E, Hernandez MH: Studies of small bowel adaptation after intestinal resection in the rat. Gastroenterology 1971;60:69–75.
29. Mekhjian HS, Phillips SF, Hoffmann AF: Colonic secretion of water and electrolytes induced by bile acids: perfusion studies in man. J Clin Invest 1971;50:1569.
30. Nightingale JM, Lennard-Jones JE, Walker ER et al: Jejunal efflux in short bowel syndrome. Lancet 1990;336:765.
31. Gouttebel MC, Saint-Aubert B, Astre C et al: Total parenteral nutrition needs in different types of short bowel syndrome. Dig Dis Sci 1986;31:718.
32. Dudrick SJ, Latifi R, Fosnocht DE: Management of the short-bowel syndrome. Surg Clin North Am 1991;71: 625–643.
33. Green JH, Heatley RV: Nutritional management of patients with short-bowel syndrome. Nutrition 1992;8: 186–190.
34. Straus E, Gerson CD, Yalow RS: Hypersecretion of gastrin associated with the short bowel syndrome. Gastroenterology 1974;66:175–180.
35. Meyers WC, Jones RS: Hyperacidity and hypergastrinemia following extensive intestinal resection. World J Surg 1979;3:539–544.
36. Williams NS, Evans P, King RFGJ: Gastric acid secretion and gastrin production in the short bowel syndrome. Gut 1985;26:914–919.
37. Cortot A, Fleming CR, Malagelada J-R: Improved nutrient absorption after cimetidine in short-bowel syndrome with gastric hypersecretion. N Engl J Med 1979;300:79–80.
38. Nightingale JM, Walker ER, Farthing MJ et al: Effect of omeprazole on intestinal output in the short bowel syndrome. Aliment Pharmacol Ther 1991;5:405–412.
39. Saunders DR, Saunder MD, Sillery JK: Beneficial effects of glucose polymer and an H2-receptor blocker in a patient with a proximal ileostomy. Am J Gastroenterol 1989;84:192–194.
40. Ladefoged K, Christensen KC, Hegnhoj J et al: Effect of a long acting somatostatin analogue SMS 201-995 on jejunostomy effluents in patient with severe short bowel syndrome. Gut 1989;30:943–949.
41. Cooper JC, Williams NS, King RFGJ et al: Effects of a long-acting somatostatin analogue in patients with severe ileostomy diarrhea. Br J Surg 1986;73: 128–131.
42. O'Keefe SJ, Peterson ME, Fleming CR: Octreotide as an adjunct to home parenteral nutrition in the management of permanent end-jejunostomy syndrome. J Parenter Enter Nutr 1994;18:26–34.
43. Witt K, Pedersen NT: The long-acting somatostatin analogue SMS 201-995 causes malabsorption. Scand J Gastroenterol 1989;24:1248–1252.
44. Fisher RS, Rock E, Levin G et al: Effect of somatostatin on gallbladder emptying. Gastroenterology 1987;92: 885–890.
45. O'Keefe SJ, Haymond MW, Bennet WM et al: Long-acting somatostatin analogue therapy and protein metab-

olism in patients with jejunostomies. Gastroenterology 1994;107:379–388.

46. Thompson JS, Nguyen BLT, Harty RF: Somatostatin analogue inhibits intestinal regeneration. Arch Surg 1993;128:385–389.

47. Arrigoni E, Marteau P, Briet F et al: Tolerance and absorption of lactose from milk and yogurt during short-bowel syndrome in humans. Am J Clin Nutr 1994; 60:926–929.

48. Edes TE, Walk BE, Austin JL: Diarrhea in tube-fed patients: feeding formula not necessarily the cause. Am J Med 1990;88:91.

49. Levy E, Frileux P, Sandrucci S et al: Continuous enteral nutrition during the early adaptive stage of the short bowel syndrome. Br J Surg 1988;75:549–553.

50. Cosnes J, Gendre J-P, Evard D et al: Compensatory enteral hyperalimentation for management of patients with severe short bowel syndrome. Am J Clin Nutr 1985;41:1002.

51. Woolf GM, Miller C, Kurian R et al: Nutritional absorption in short bowel syndrome. Evaluation fluid, caloric, and divalent cation requirements. Dig Dis Sci 1987; 32:8.

52. Messing B, Pigot F, Rongier M et al: Intestinal absorption of free oral hyperalimentation in the very short bowel syndrome. Gastroenterology 1991;100:1502–1508.

53. Andersson H, Isaksson B, Sjogren B: Fat-reduced diet in the symptomatic treatment of small bowel disease. Gut 1974;15:351.

54. Andersson H, Jagenberg R: Fat-reduced diet in the treatment of hyperoxaluria in patients with ileopathy. Gut 1974;15:360.

55. Zurier RB, Campbell RG, Hashim SA et al: Use of medium-chain triglyceride in management of patients with massive resection of the small intestine. N Engl J Med 1966;274:490–493.

56. Ovesen L, Chu R, Howard L: The influence of dietary fat on jejunostomy output in patients with severe short bowel syndrome. Am J Clin Nutr 1983;38:270–277.

57. Ameen VZ, Powell GK, Jones LA: Quantitation of fecal carbohydrate excretion in patients with short bowel syndrome. Gastroenterology 1987;92:493.

58. Woolf GM, Miller C, Kurian R et al: Diet for patients with a short bowel: high fat or high carbohydrate? Gastroenterology 1983;84:823.

59. McIntyre PB, Fitchew M, Lennard-Jones JE: Patients with a high jejunostomy do not need a special diet. Gastroenterology 1986;91:25–33.

60. Simko V: Short bowel syndrome. Gastroenterology 1986;78:190.

61. Simko V, Linscheer WG: Absorption of different elemental diets in a short-bowel syndrome lasting 15 years. Dig Dis 1976;21:419–425.

62. Nordgaard J, Hansen BS, Mortensen PB: Colon as a digestive organ in patients with short bowel. Lancet 1994;343:373–376.

63. Bochenek W, Rodgers JB, Balint JA: Effects of changes in dietary lipids on intestinal fluid loss in the short bowel syndrome. Ann Intern Med 1970;72:205–213.

64. Cosnes J, Evard D, Beaugerie L et al: Improvement in protein absorption with a small-peptide-based diet in patients with high jejunostomy. Nutrition 1992;8: 406–411.

65. Pizarro D, Posada G, Sandi L et al: Rice-based oral electrolyte solutions for the management of infantile diarrhea. N Engl J Med 1991;324:517–521.

66. Schultz SG: Sodium-coupled solute transport of small intestine: a status report. Am J Physiol 1977;233: E249.

67. Fordtran JS: Stimulation of active and passive sodium absorption by sugars in the human jejunum. J Clin Invest 1975;55:728.

68. Lennard-Jones JE: Oral rehydration solutions in short bowel syndrome. Clin Ther 1990;12:129.

69. da Cunha Ferreira RMC, Walker-Smith JA: Controversies in oral rehydration therapy: a way forward. Gastroenterol J Club 1989;1:2.

70. Nalin DR, Harland E, Ramlal A et al: Comparison of low and high sodium and potassium content in oral rehydration solutions. J Pediatr 1980;97:848.

71. Griffin GE, Hodgson EF, Chadwick VS: Enteral therapy in the management of massive gut resection complicated by chronic fluid and electrolyte depletion. Dig Dis Sci 1991;27:902.

72. Laustsen J, Fallingborg J: Enteral glucose-polymer-electrolyte solution in the treatment of chronic fluid and electrolyte depletion in short-bowel syndrome. Acta Chir Scand 1983;149:787–788.

73. MacMahon RA: The use of the World Health Organization's oral rehydration solution in patients on home parenteral nutrition. J Parenter Enter Nutr 1984;8: 720–721.

74. Heymsfield SB, Smith-Andrews JL, Hersh T: Home nasoenteric feeding for malabsorption and weight loss refractory to conventional therapy. Ann Intern Med 1983;98:168–170.

75. Fine KD, Santa Ana CA, Porter JL et al: Intestinal absorption of magnesium from food and supplements. J Clin Invest 1991;88:396.

76. Rude RK, Singer FR: Magnesium deficiency and excess. Ann Rev Med 1981;32:245.

77. Nicar MJ, Pak CY: Calcium bioavailability from calcium carbonate and calcium citrate. J Clin Endocrinol Metab 1985;61:391.

78. Patton MB, Sutton TS: Utilization of calcium from lactate, gluconate, sulfate and carbonate salts by young college women. J Nutr 1952;48:443.

79. Recker RR: Calcium absorption and achlorhydria. N Engl J Med 1985;313:70.

80. Engels LGJ, van den Hamer CJA, van Tongeren JHM: Iron zinc, and copper balance in short bowel patients on oral nutrition. Am J Clin Nutr 1984;40:1038–1041.

81. Brewer GJ, Ellis F, Bjork L: Parenteral depot method for zinc administration. Pharmacology 1981;23:254.

82. Lindenbaum J, Rosenberg IH, Wilson PW et al: Prevalence of cobalamin deficiency in the Framingham elderly population. Am J Clin Nutr 1994;60:2–11.

83. Healton EB, Savage DG, Brust JC et al: Neurologic aspects of cobalamin deficiency. Medicine 1991;70: 229–245.

84. Green R, Jacobsen DW, Van Tonder SV et al: Enterohepatic circulation of cobalamin in the non human primate. Gastroenterology 1981;81:773–776.

85. Dobbins JW, Binder HJ: Importance of the colon in enteric hyperoxaluria. N Engl J Med 1977;296:298.

86. Roslyn JJ, Pitt HA, Mann LL et al: Gallbladder disease in patients on long term parenteral nutrition. Gastroenterology 1983;84:148–154.

87. Sitzman JV, Pitt HA, Steinborn PA et al: Cholecystokinin prevents parenteral nutrition induced biliary sludge in humans. Surg Gynecol Obstet 1990;170:25–31.

88. Stolberg L, Rolfe R, Gitlin N et al: D-Lactic acidosis due to abnormal gut flora: diagnosis and treatment of two cases. N Engl J Med 1982;306:1344–1348.

89. Traube M, Bock JL, Boyer JL: D-Lactic acidosis after jejunoileal bypass: identification of organic anions by nuclear magnetic resonance spectroscopy. Ann Intern Med 1983;98:171–173.

35

Enteral Nutrition and Dying: Ethical Issues in the Termination of Enteral Nutrition in Adults

TIMOTHY O. LIPMAN*

"An act has no ethical quality whatever unless it be chosen out of several all equally possible."

William James (1842–1910)
The Principles of Psychology

"Man is an animal with primary instincts of survival. Consequently, his ingenuity has developed first and his soul afterwards. Thus, the progress of science is far ahead of man's ethical behavior."

Sir Charles Spencer Chaplin (1899–1977)
My Autobiography

A classic scene in the movies, novels, drama, and opera is the death of a loved one. The dying individual is held in the succoring arms of his or her companion and given a sip of water as he or she takes a last breath or

*I am not an ethicist but rather a clinician asked to ponder and present the ethical issues involved with terminating enteral nutrition at the end of life. I have tried to approach the subject with an open mind, hold my own biases in check, and present a balanced survey of the conflicting ethical viewpoints. To this end, I certainly do not claim to present an exhaustive bibliography of the extensive literature on the topic, but I think I have provided a representative sample of the opinions involved, so that the clinician and health care worker can understand with sensitivity the conflicting and strongly felt issues involved.

sings a final aria. Of course, this no longer happens. Now, if the problem is acute, after a call to 911, the patient is rushed to the local emergency room for extensive resuscitation. If the problem is chronic, one gets the latest in appropriate antibiotics or chemotherapy. With further progression of disease comes dialysis, respiratory intubation, or organ transplantation. Finally, to maintain life throughout all, the patient is maintained with artificial nutrition and hydration through a feeding tube, gastrostomy, or intravenously. With high likelihood, this individual will die in a hospital or nursing home.

Because we are keeping patients alive with technology and pharmacology that did not exist decades ago, a host of ethical issues have surfaced over the same period,[1] involving truly fully informed consent, limits of patient refusal, brain death, coma, persistent vegetative states, "do not resuscitate" orders, suicide (with or without medical assistance or complicity), assisted death, and withholding or withdrawing artificial nutrition and hydration. All these ethical issues have received major discussion as a result of advancing medical technology.

ETHICS OVERVIEW

The ethical quandary involving enteral nutrition concerns the withholding or withdrawing of enteral nutrition when a patient cannot sustain himself or herself with oral intake. Much of literature on this subject focuses on court cases and legal issues. The law cannot be ignored, but in this chapter I wish to separate legal discussions from ethical discussions; with one exception, I will not discuss court cases or legal issues. I will focus instead on ethical analysis.

Withholding/withdrawing enteral nutrition involves three competency situations associated with two clinical scenarios. In the first competency situation, the patient can make his or her own decisions and can make these decisions known. In the second, the patient currently is incapable of making a decision but has made his or her wishes known in some prior format. In the third, the patient is incapable of decision making, and prior wishes are unknown. These above-mentioned decision elements are formulated in one of the two following clinical scenarios: (1) the patient has a terminal illness of which he or she will die despite ongoing enteral nutrition (e.g., terminal cancer, end-stage acquired immunodeficiency syndrome [AIDS]) or (2) the patient has a condition that does not permit eating but will not lead to death as long as nutrition and hydration are continued (e.g., coma, persistent vegetative state).

Ethics can be defined as the "branch of philosophy that deals with morality. Ethics is concerned with distinguishing between good and evil in the world, between right and wrong human actions, and between virtuous and nonvirtuous characteristics of people."[2] Medical ethics can be defined further as the study of human values as applied to the practice of medicine.[3] If all humans had the same value systems, there would be no need for study of ethical issues in medicine. However, different religious, cultural, and philosophical beliefs often lead to disagreement and dissent over how to approach patients. The study of ethics as applied to medicine allows analysis of competing values in a rational fashion.

As I understand current status of ethical thinking, a basic precept of medical ethics is the concept of self-determination or patient autonomy—that a competent patient capable of making decisions has the right to determine his or her own destiny by refusing or accepting any and all medical care—that medical care or intervention cannot be forced without consent.[3] In general, although not without controversy, enteral nutrition through tube or gastrostomy is considered a subset of artificial nutrition and hydration and a part of medical care, no different than antibiotics, chemotherapy, endoscopy, dialysis, or mechanical ventilation; as such, it may be accepted or refused by any competent individual.

The ethical issues arise when the patient is noncompetent (i.e., incapable of making a decision regarding care) and, usually, the patient has a disease for which enteral nutrition could significantly prolong survival (e.g., permanent coma or persistent vegetative state). If the patient's prior wishes are known explicitly, and it is known explicitly that these wishes included refusal of enteral nutrition with permanent coma or persistent vegetative state, then the patient's surrogates should ethically refuse enteral nutrition. When a patient's prior wishes are not known, or when there is severe disability without coma or vegetative state (e.g., multiple strokes with paresis and aphasia), the decision process is much more difficult, and the ethical issues become paramount. Here, societal norms (most people not wanting life-sustaining treatment if permanently incompetent) conflict with religious norms (honoring the sanctity of life) as well as with state norms (protecting life at all costs by preventing suicide, euthanasia, and murder).[4]

Before we can delve into the specific ethical conflicts, certain relevant concepts need discussion. These include the process of death without food and water as well as definitions of terminal conditions, medical futility, and medical benefits and burdens.

DEATH WITHOUT FOOD AND WATER

Of prime importance in the ethical discussion is the nature of death when food and water are withheld. Is this a cruel and painful demise, full of suffering, for which anyone supporting compassionate care for the dying, comatose, or vegetative patient could, in good conscience, not advocate? There is scant literature addressing this issue. However, the existing documentation suggests that death accompanied by dehydration and starvation is, in fact, painless and humane.

Case reports and case series document peaceful, comfortable, pain-free, and compassionate deaths when food and water are provided only for comfort. Sullivan[5] describes a 78-year-old fully competent woman with recurrent intestinal obstruction after extensive surgery and radiotherapy for uterine cancer. She refused further surgical intervention and intravenous therapy but allowed nasogastric suction for persistent vomiting. She was given ice chips and swabs for thirst plus morphine for sedation and sleep. She survived 29 days in this condition, remaining comfortable, participating in her own care, writing, and visiting with friends. Finally, she drifted into semiconsciousness, then coma, and death, all within a 1-day period. She never complained of pain or discomfort.

A prospective study of 32 terminal cancer patients over 12 months in an in-patient hospice setting in which food and water were given as requested, but without "force," revealed that 20 patients never experienced any hunger while the rest experienced hunger only initially.[6] Similarly, 20 patients never, or only initially, experienced thirst during their stay. In all patients hunger, thirst, or dry mouth could be alleviated by small amounts of food or fluids, ice chips, and lip lubrication. Narcotics were used in almost all 32 patients for comfort.

Other cases are described[7-9] in which death is without discomfort or pain in the absence of artificial nutrition and hydration. Hospice workers frequently observe that terminal dehydration leads to reduced secretions and excretions, therefore decreasing respiratory problems, vomiting, and urinary and fecal incontinence.[10]

With absolute starvation and dehydration, the metabolism of body fat produces both water, which may maintain circulation for weeks, as well as ketone bodies, which appear to have an analgesic effect, blocking hunger.[5] With initial good renal function and adipose stores, patients with terminal dehydration may live for weeks, experiencing no pain and often mild euphoria. In fact, providing some carbohydrates, electrolytes, and fluids can lead to pain and hunger from both the IV itself (the needle and infiltration) and blockage of ketone body production. Preterminally, patients may have azotemia, hypernatremia, or hypercalcemia, all of which have sedative and analgesic effects.

The most common patient care problems are dry mouth, sore and cracked gums, and thirst. These symptoms can be treated by sips of water and other fluids, ice chips, petroleum jelly to lips and gums, and good mouth care. The clinical manifestations of terminal dehydration and appropriate clinical responses are outlined in Table 35–1.

The important point in the discussion is that the death that occurs without forcing food and fluids can be part of total humane care for a patient. Usually, death is not immediate. Life may continue for weeks or months. Moreover, this clinical stance does not mean that food is being withheld; it means that food is not being forced. Intake will be insufficient to maintain life over a prolonged period, but food intake can continue as part of comfort care.

SOME DEFINITIONS

Definitions and descriptions of other terms pertinent to the ethical discussions are necessary. For the rest of the chapter I will refer to enteral nutrition, which can mean tube, gastrostomy, or jejunostomy feeding. Much of the literature refers to artificial nutrition and hydration, usually referring to some form of enteral nutrition, but often encompassing intravenous fluids and occasionally intravenous parenteral nutrition. In the ethical analysis here, enteral nutrition means all forms of nutritional food and fluid delivered in any manner other than oral intake.

Determining whether a patient is terminal may be easy or difficult. Dictionary definitions state "appearing at or contributing to the end of life" or "of or in the final stages of a fatal disease." In a medical sense, *terminal* encompasses or equates with the dying process—a "time in the course of an irreversible illness when treatment will no longer influence it."[3]

TABLE 35–1 Clinical Manifestations of Dehydration at the End of Life

Symptoms	Suggested Response
Analgesia	None
Lethargy	None
Weakness	None
Dry mouth	Ice chips, fluids, mouth care
Thirst	Ice chips, fluids, mouth care

Adapted from Printz LA: Terminal dehydration, a compassionate treatment. Arch Intern Med 1992;152:697–700. Copyright 1992, American Medical Association.

Terminal has also been defined as an incurable or irreversible condition with high probability of death within a relatively short time (less than a year) with or without treatment.[4] Many would be uncomfortable defining as terminal a condition that allows another year of life yet would readily accept a definition encompassing 1 week. Another definition sets a time frame of 3 to 6 months.[11] Certainly, clinicians would be more comfortable if they thought they could truly predict the natural history of terminal disease and time the onset of death within a week. Last, by definition of the terminal state, enteral nutrition should not significantly affect a terminal patient's survival.

Persistent vegetative state, the source of much ethical controversy, has been defined by a multisociety task force as

A clinical condition of complete unawareness of the self and the environment, accompanied by sleep-wake cycles, with either complete or partial preservation of hypothalamic and brain-stem autonomic functions. In addition, patients in a vegetative state show no evidence of sustained, reproducible, purposeful, or voluntary behavioral responses to visual, auditory, tactile, or noxious stimuli; show no evidence of language comprehension or expression; have bowel and bladder incontinence; and have variably preserved cranial-nerve and spinal reflexes.[12]

The clinical course and outcome of the persistent vegetative state depends on the cause. Functional recovery from acute traumatic brain injuries is unlikely after 12 months and from nontrauma is unlikely after 3 months. Life expectancy is shortened, usually to 2 to 5 years and rarely more than 10 years. Death occurs in weeks with withdrawal of food and hydration but may be prolonged significantly with enteral nutrition.

Coma is a condition in which the patient appears to be asleep and "is at the same time incapable of being aroused by external stimuli and inner needs....There are variations in the degree of coma.... Coma is always a potentially dangerous condition, often with a fatal outcome, whereas lesser degrees of impaired consciousness have a better prognosis."[13] Some patients in coma may be maintained alive with enteral nutrition for prolonged periods.

Medical futility is a concept frequently used in ethical discussions and is acquiring its own literature. In the dictionary, futility means "useless, ineffectual, vain...lacking in purpose...serving no useful purpose." Medically, one is concerned whether an intervention is "futile." Definitions of futility in the medical literature encompass the notion that an intervention does not have a desired effect, or it may be defined as an intervention without benefit, even though there is an effect.

Levels of futility exist,[14] and one winds up with definition by example. A truly futile treatment may be one in which it is impossible to achieve a desired effect—such as mechanical ventilation to restore life in the dead or antibiotics to eradicate a viral infection. Medical futility may involve achieving a physiologic effect but not reversing a functional disorder—thus oxygenating a brain-dead individual will not reverse the brain death. Finally, medical futility may involve some accrual of benefit to the patient but not a sufficient quantity to reverse the impression of futility—dialysis in an intensive care unit (ICU) patient may temporarily reverse hyperkalemia but will not alter the steady deterioration of multiple organ function in a critically ill individual.

One proposal suggests that futility can be defined quantitatively and qualitatively and offers as a definition of futile—when physicians conclude based on shared experience, their own experience, or published data that an intervention has been useless—has not worked—in the past 100 attempts, then that treatment is futile.[15] The definition relates to an objective quality of an action and differs from expressions such as "uncommon, rare, or hopeless." Furthermore, it is suggested, reports of rare miracles do not counteract objective notions of futility if they occur against a background of multiple failures.

The sources of dissension concerning notions of futility involve (1) truly trying to decide that an intervention is futile, (2) addressing the level of possible futility, and (3) deciding whose opinion counts most when there is disagreement. More specifically, enteral nutrition may maintain or prolong life, but under many clinical conditions it will not improve functional status or quality of life. Is the intervention of enteral nutrition then futile for not affecting performance, or is it not futile because it maintains life?

The last terms in the lexicon of medical ethics involving enteral nutrition relate to the concept of benefits and burdens. Does the intervention provide a benefit to or for the patient, or is it associated with inordinate burden or harm? Operation to remove an inoperable cancer is an obvious example of treatment without benefit but potential burdens. The issues in enteral nutrition are less clear-cut; it has proved quite difficult to agree on what constitutes a benefit and what a burden.

LETTING DIE OF DISEASE PROGRESS VS KILLING BY WITHHOLDING NUTRITION AND FLUIDS

The ultimate conflict of values, which drives the ethical debate, is the controversy over whether withholding or withdrawing enteral nutrition constitutes the end stage of a natural disease progression in which oral intake is no longer possible or whether withholding or withdrawal is a murderous act that terminates the life of an individual who would otherwise live with the enteral nutrition.[16] The context of the debate must be understood. Few, if any, are talking about forcibly withholding food and water from a healthy individual in circumstances of an individual conflict, coercion, war, concentration camps, and so on. Nor does the debate center around an otherwise healthy, clinically depressed individual who wishes to commit suicide by refusing intake. Rather, the issue concerns the necessity of providing enteral nutrition to a patient with a terminal condition (e.g., cancer or AIDS) or an incapacitated patient who cannot eat because of an underlying condition (e.g., prolonged coma or severe neurologic injury).

One of the difficulties arising from the ethical arguments surrounding decisions concerning enteral nutrition at the end of life is the frequent failure to distinguish two fairly distinct patient types in the ethical arguments. One is the patient who is truly terminal with or without enteral nutrition and will die no matter what is done. The other is the patient whose life course has been altered so much that existence depends on enteral nutrition; this patient can be expected to survive for a considerable time with enteral nutrition but will die shortly after its cessation. I will try to address the arguments as if both patients were the same, but I recognize that they are not.

THE ARGUMENT AGAINST WITHHOLDING OR WITHDRAWING ENTERAL NUTRITION

The overriding argument for providing enteral nutrition focuses on the primacy of human life—that life is inherently good and that it is never morally right to kill another person under any circumstances.[17,18] Because food and fluids universally are needed to sustain life, it is immoral to withdraw sustenance from any person. To do so is an act of killing—at best euthanasia by omission. Nutrition and hydration are such fundamentally different forms of treatment from all other possible medical ther-

apies that to deny enteral nutrition is a de facto death sentence. Judeo-Christian tradition teaches the sanctity of life, with the physician given a "divine license" to heal, not to hasten death.[19]

With respect to benefits and burdens, enteral nutrition provides the benefit of life and of itself does not decrease the quality of life. Burdens of continued care may fall more on the family, health care team, or society, but not excessively on the patient.[20] Because life is inherently good and because maintaining life is the healer's ultimate goal, maintaining life should not and cannot be viewed as a burden.[17] It is dangerous, the argument goes, to judge that a person's quality of life is so low that it must be ended. No Western society should ever impose, encourage, or tolerate this type of analysis.[21] Enteral nutrition may involve irritants but does not result in great burdens of pain, suffering, or damage to body self-image. Furthermore, if pain is not or cannot be perceived in comatose or persistent vegetative states, then enteral nutrition cannot be thought of as causing the burden of pain and suffering.

Maintenance of life vs quality of the maintained life lies at the heart of the ethical debate. Those arguing against withholding/withdrawing enteral nutrition focus on the importance and integrity of life itself. They note that one cannot judge and act on the quality of another person's life. The so-called burdens of a "low-quality" existence are insufficient justification for denial or cessation of enteral nutrition. Enteral nutrition is not futile because it maintains life.

Another major thrust against withholding or withdrawing enteral nutrition concerns discrimination against the disabled and the aged.[22] Of concern is that enteral nutrition is being terminated because someone else believes that a disability is so great or someone is so old that life is not worth living. This is a value judgment being imposed on the affected individual because of his or her infirmities or age. We do not deny crutches, wheelchairs, or other necessary appliances to those with disabilities. Why should we deny food and water?

Another concern is the "slippery slope."[23] If we can let some die who are "ready to die," the argument goes, why not assist these people to die and hasten their death with lethal injection? Furthermore, if the individual has a "right to die," will it be long before we regard the same patient as having a "duty to die" to provide resources for other societal needs? If it becomes acceptable to kill some by omission, this will be extended further to others with severe incapacities, or the senile, or the retarded, or the bedridden. Society then becomes like that which existed under Nazism, which wanted to eliminate those it considered "socially unacceptable." Furthermore, the physician becomes the physician of Nazism, a universally regarded perpetrator of unethical behavior. Finally, if the patient or family feels that the physician no longer has the patient's best interest at heart, because the patient now has a duty to die, the physician-patient relàtionship has been destroyed. This creates an environment of distrust and suspicion that could destroy the medical profession's integrity.

A final argument looks at the technology and symbolism of food. The distinction between eating and enteral nutrition as artificial nutrition is itself artificial. With modern technology and food processing, virtually all we eat is technically "artificial," and its delivery mode should not be made an important distinction. Providing food and fluid is fundamentally distinct from all other forms of medical therapy, and the differences in delivery methodology should not cloud the distinction. Food and water are basic foundations of caring support for an individual, no different than turning, talking, reading, or just listening. Finally, food and water have basic symbolic connotations fundamental to our humanity, culture, religion, and values—witness biblical injunctions, the Catholic communion, the Passover seder, a variety of holiday and festival meals, and ethnic eating patterns, while withholding and withdrawing nutrition are associated with famine, forced starvation, and concentration camps. The symbolism and connotations of providing and depriving food are too great to allow us to accept enteral nutrition as simply a medical intervention like all other medical interventions.

THE CASE FOR WITHHOLDING OR WITHDRAWING ENTERAL NUTRITION

The argument for terminating enteral nutrition looks at the same patient under the same conditions with a different value emphasis. No longer is preserving life paramount, but more important is the quality or viability of that life. Mere existence is not the goal, but rather the mode of that existence.

The argument for termination suggests that we all will die, and that if a pathologic process results in the inability to eat (be it end-stage cancer, AIDS, debilitating strokes, or severe head trauma), it is the disease process and not the withholding or withdrawing of enteral nutrition that is the cause of death. If the pathologic process that caused inability to eat is irreversible, than enteral nutrition prolongs the dying process initiated by the initial insult or disease.[24] Enteral nutrition is a medical technology that should be viewed no more or less a cause of death in a patient than denial of mechanical ventilation or dialysis is a cause of death in a patient with respiratory or renal failure.

The concept of benefit to the patient and what constitutes a benefit becomes important. Even though enteral nutrition may maintain life, it will not restore the quality of life existing before the pathologic process. Therefore, because viability and quality cannot be restored, enteral nutrition may be considered medically futile, providing no benefit to the patient.[25]

Additionally, there are burdens to enteral nutrition. A full discussion of complications of both tube and enterostomy feeding is handled elsewhere (Chapters 11, 12, and 14), but enteral nutrition is associated with significant morbidity and mortality. Moreover, the common complication of aspiration in the neurologically impaired may be higher with enteral nutrition than with careful spoon feeding.[26] Suggested reasons for high complication rates with enteral nutrition in the neurologically impaired include recumbency, reduced esophageal peristalsis and sphincter incompetence with reflux, and delayed gastric emptying. Aspiration and pneumonia are common terminal events from enteral nutrition in these patients. Spoon feeds with nutrient dense products can be successfully accomplished with proper training of the support staff. Nonavailability of staff or training to accomplish this level of patient care is a separate issue.

Additionally, there is high potential for misuse of enteral nutrition.[27] Often patients are provided enteral nutrition when they do not need it, perhaps because of staffing inadequacies. Often an impression is given that there is no viable alternative when oral feeding may be a perfectly acceptable alternative. Patients need full evaluation for rehabilitation. Responsible use of enteral nutrition includes knowledge of when patients can live without it.

The other major burden accruing to a patient receiving enteral nutrition is the frequent need to tie him or her down. If forceful restriction from pulling out a tube is the only means by which nutrition can be delivered, then many would consider this a burdensome affront to human dignity.

If enteral nutrition is burdensome and futile because it is without the benefit of improving life quality or viability, and the patient can be made comfortable, then the "slippery slope" concerns are problematic, because actions with respect to enteral nutrition reflect an increased sensitivity to, rather than disregard of, dying patients. The degrading nature of permanent unconsciousness in a previously viable individual may be sufficient to justify withholding or withdrawing enteral nutrition and does not a priori endanger other conscious disabled or unconscious persons, whose prior wishes to maintain life with enteral nutrition are known.[24]

With respect to the symbolic issues of food, enteral nutrition is factually different from feeding. It is a medical intervention that has been engendered as a result of body dysfunction and requires bodily invasion, medical expertise, and monitoring. Withholding or withdrawing of enteral nutrition connotes the denial of food to someone who is requesting food. Actually, it is honoring a request not to be fed artificially. Food can be given orally in many circumstances.

Caregivers and family must focus on the goals of intervention, which may be cure of disease, control of disease progression, or providing comfort at the end of life. Withholding or withdrawing enteral nutrition is compatible with the goals of comfort care. I have discussed previously the euphoric and analgesic effects of total starvation. Withholding or withdrawing enteral nutrition does not preclude giving oral food and fluid as well as other comfort care of family contact, verbal communication, turning, and skin care.[7]

Several suggestions have been put forward to try to resolve some of the ethical dilemmas, especially with coma and persistent vegetative states. The prime concern with these two conditions revolves around the fact that the patient is neither dead nor dying, and withholding or withdrawing enteral nutrition seems like intentional killing, no matter how hard the rationalization. However, duty to provide enteral nutrition may be overridden when we are morally certain that the condition is irreversible—usually, one arrives at this clinical decision by a combination of time course and etiology.[20] The treatment then becomes truly futile and the clinician has discharged his or her moral obligations to the patient; further care can ethically be directed toward comfort measures. If the family wishes continued feeding, this may be done at home. Another approach is to change the burden of proof.[28] Rather than assume a patient would want all efforts to be kept alive, assume he or she would *not* want to be main-tained in coma or a persistent vegetative state—the prevalent view reflected in national opinion poles. The new standard of care would be to stop after determination of irreversibility, with the family having to prove that the patient would want ongoing care.

ECONOMIC ISSUES AND ETHICS

Mixing economic analysis or fiscal realities with a discussion of ethical issues in medicine makes many uncomfortable, but the issues should be addressed. "Ethics consultations" in hospitals involving enteral nutrition may be generated by financial concerns or economic conflicts in patient care.[29] Problems may arise when medical indications conflict with third party sources of financing, if physicians or hospitals are financially affected by a decision regarding enteral nutrition, or if there is a wish to save "society" or family money by withholding enteral nutrition. Concern has been expressed that the combination of "death with dignity" and the "right to die" and cost containment will merge, such that withholding or withdrawing enteral nutrition becomes the treatment of choice for financial reasons.[1]

It is argued that it is perfectly ethical to weigh economic costs against the risk of loss of life and to make tradeoffs between lives and economic costs.[30] It is argued further that refraining from actions that can save lives is immoral. If an economic analysis of scarce resource utilization might point to ways to save more lives, then it may be immoral and unethical not to address explicitly the crucial tradeoffs involved with these areas of difficult choices.

One final area in which ethics and economics intermix is the significant financial advantages that accrue to nursing homes to encourage enteral nutrition. They are reimbursed for enteral nutrition but not for feeding patients, which actually is more labor intensive and thus more costly. The extent to which providing enteral nutrition is driven by increased reimbursement is unknown, but it has been suggested that the occurrence is real, with adverse impact on patients and their families.[27] Certainly, in my own institution I often hear that a percutaneous gastrostomy is necessary in a patient because nursing homes will not take a patient without one.

A FEW LEGAL ISSUES

I promised at the outset to avoid a discussion of law, but a review of "legal myths" specifically addressing termination of life support, applicable to withholding or withdrawing enteral nutrition, is germane.[31]

Legal Myth No. 1. *Anything that is not specifically permitted by law is prohibited.* In fact, it is impossible to legislate all behavior; this approach leads to conservative advice by lawyers. Litigation challenging termination of life support is rare, with only some 60 cases existent by the early 1990s. Most cases are undertaken to establish necessity of continuing feeding or permissibility of terminating feeding, not to find professional negligence or liability. The lack of specific legislation regarding termination does not render it illegal.

Legal Myth No. 2. *Termination of life support is murder or suicide.* Obviously, this question goes to the crux of the major ethical issue under concern. In general, courts have recognized a distinction between killing and letting die, with three judicial justifications: (1) the patient's condition rather than termination of life support is the cause of death, (2) the intent of termination is relief of suffering, and (3) ultimately, the courts recognize the individual's right to refuse any treatment.

Legal Myth No. 3. *Stopping enteral nutrition is legally different from stopping other treatments.* Again, this is related to no. 2 above and is a highly controversial, emotionally charged subject directly relating to the ethical issues. With few exceptions, all appellate courts have regarded enteral nutrition as a medical treatment that may be discontinued in the same manner as any other treatment.

Legal Myth No. 4. *A patient must be terminally ill for life support to be stopped.* Again, courts have tended to focus on quality of life rather than mere existence of life. However, to varying degrees, courts have insisted on knowing the patient's prior wishes.

Legal Myth No. 5. *It is permissible to withhold treatment, but once started, it must be continued.* There is no such law. It is often psychologically harder to stop once started, but there is no legal distinction between withholding and withdrawing. In fact, withholding initiating a treatment because of a fear of being unable to withdraw may be detrimental to the patient's best interests.

Legal Myth No. 6. *Stopping life support or withholding or withdrawing enteral nutrition requires going to court.* Three steps involved in the decision-making process include (1) assessing the patient's decision-making capacity, (2) designating an appropriate surrogate decision maker, and (3) deciding to terminate treatment. This is an informal clinical process that does not need a judicial imprimatur nor a court-approved surrogate. Courts are not the place to resolve clinical issues involving individual families; going to court is the action everyone involved in patient care should want to avoid.

Be aware of two caveats associated with this brief overview of some legal issues. First, I am not a lawyer and have no legal training. Second, there are probably lawyers who would disagree with this assessment.

CLINICAL GUIDELINES IN ETHICAL CARE

The decision-making process surrounding withholding or withdrawing enteral nutrition in the terminally ill or neurologically impaired is fraught with emotional difficulties. However, if the underlying clinical goals and ethical issues are understood, then one hopes the dilemmas can be approached meaningfully.[32,33] Several concepts intertwine and are of equal importance.

Realistic goals of therapy must be established. Is the goal elimination of disease, control of disease, or comfort care? How will enteral nutrition contribute to each of these goals?

Understand that the patient can refuse any medical therapy. On the other hand, a patient may express wishes to start or continue with enteral nutrition. Although still controversial, in general, enteral nutrition is regarded as any other therapy, be it coronary artery angioplasty, surgery, dialysis, mechanical ventilation, or antibiotics. The patient's wishes are paramount, and the patient's conception of medical futility should be paramount.

Encourage patients to make their preferences known while they can do so. If the patient cannot make preferences known, then seek evidence for the patient's prior expressed wishes from the patient's surrogates—family or a close friend if there is no family; consider any reliable evidence for prior wishes. When prior wishes are not known or surrogates are not available, then act in "the best interests of the patient."[34] Here conflicting value systems may collide, and the physician, other members of the health care team, and the institutional provider must be careful not to impose arbitrarily their own value system. If there are apparent conflicts between the physician and family's value system, discuss and resolve them before a crisis occurs. Often a patient may need transfer to another facility where the value systems do not conflict. If transfer is not possible, let the patient's preferences take precedence over the health system.[32]

TABLE 35–2   Lay Organizatons Involved with Ethical Issues of Withholding and Withdrawing Enteral Nutrition

The Hemlock Society USA
PO Box 101810
Denver, CO 80250
Telephone: 303-639-1202 or 800-247-7421
FAX: 303-639-1224
Mission Statement: "The Hemlock Society USA believes terminally ill people should have the right to self-determination for all end-of-life decisions. Because Hemlock reveres life, dying people must be able to retain their dignity, integrity and self-respect. We encourage, through a program of education and research, public acceptance of voluntary physician aid-in-dying for people with terminal illnesses."

Choice in Dying, Inc.
200 Varick Street
New York, NY 10014
Telephone: 212-366-5540 or 800-989-WILL
FAX: 212-366-5337
Statement: "Choice in Dying, Inc is [an]...organization dedicated to protecting the rights and serving the needs of dying patients and their families. We advocate patients' rights to make decisions about medical treatment, and to receive compassionate and dignified care at the end of life."
"Eight out of ten of us can expect to die in a hospital or nursing home. In these settings, the dying process is likely to involve a decision about whether to withhold or withdraw some form of life support. Such uniquely personal decisions should be based upon the wishes and values of the patient, not of doctors, judges or hospital administrators."
"Choice in Dying uses many means to promote advance planning and patients' rights, including distributing state-specific advance directives."

National Right to Life Committee, Inc.
Suite 500
419 7th Street, NW
Washington, DC 20004-2293
Telephone: 202-626-8800
FAX: 202-737-9189 or 202-347-5907
Statement: "For those who wish to help ensure that they receive assisted feeding and hydration, or lifesaving medical treatment, when no longer able to speak for themselves, the National Right to Life Committee makes available "Wills to Live," advance directive (durable power of attorney) forms tailored to the laws of each of the 50 states and D.C., expressing such an intent.
"The National Right to Life Committee also works to enact legislation protecting against involuntary denial of nutrition, hydration, or lifesaving medical treatment pending transfer to a provider willing to abide by patient or surrogate wishes to obtain them. Its state affiliates or General Counsel can also work to find legal representation to assist those threatened with such involuntary denial."

National Legal Center for the Medically Dependent & Disabled, Inc.
50 South Meridian
Suite 200
Indianapolis, IN 46204
Telephone: 317-632-6245
FAX: 317-632-6542
Statement: "The National Legal Center is a not-for-profit public interest law office and national support center funded through the Legal Services Corporation. The National Legal Center has... [a goal to]...protect the rights of indigent persons who have disabilities or serious medical needs to secure essential medical treatment, regardless of age, health, function, or condition of dependency or disability;
"Some persons with disabilities are cognitively impaired, unconscious, or otherwise legally incompetent when critical, lifesaving medical decisions must be made. These individuals may reside in nursing homes and hospitals.
"With these concerns in mind, the National Legal Center recently adopted the following revised priorities:
   Provision of essential nutrition and hydration;
   Provision of essential medical treatment;
"The National Legal Center offers the following services:
   Technical Assistance
   Direct Assistance
   Informational Assistance"

TABLE 35–3 Professional Organizations with Statements Addressing the Ethical Issues of Withholding or Withdrawing Enteral Nutrition

President's Commission for the Study of Ethical Problems in Medicine and Biomedical and Behavioral Research: Deciding to forego life-sustaining treatment: a report on the ethical, medical, and legal issues in treatment decisions. Washington, DC, Government Printing Office, 1983:171–192.

American Medical Association: Council on Scientific Affairs and Council on Ethical and Judicial Affairs. Persistent vegetative state and the decision to withdraw or withhold life support. JAMA 1990;263:426–430.

American Society for Parenteral and Enteral Nutrition: Guidelines for the use of parenteral and enteral nutrition in adult and pediatric patients. Section IX: Ethical and legal issues in specialized nutrition support. J Parenter Enter Nutr 1993;17/4(suppl):50SA–52SA.

Position paper. American College of Physicians Ethics Manual, Part 2: The Physician and Society; Research; Life-sustaining treatment; Other Issues. Ann Intern Med 1989;111:327–335.

Position of the American Academy of Neurology on certain aspects of the care and management of the persistent vegetative state patient: adopted by the Executive Board, American Academy of Neurology, April 21, 1988, Cincinnati, OH. Neurology 1989;39:125–126.

ANA Committee on Ethical Affairs: Persistent vegetative state: report of the American Neurological Association Committee on Ethical Affairs. Ann Neurol 1993;33:386–390.

Position of the American Dietetic Association: Issues in feeding the terminally ill adult. J Am Diet Assoc 1992;92:996–1005.

American Nurses Association: Position statement on foregoing artificial nutrition and hydration. Washington, DC: ANA, 1992.

Determine within reasonable medical certainty that the patient is terminal or has an underlying irreversible condition that would render enteral nutrition futile with respect to altering the underlying condition. Because it is permissible to withdraw enteral nutrition after starting, it is often better to err on the side of starting if the prognosis is uncertain, knowing that the treatment can be stopped in the future.

If a terminal or severely incapacitated individual decides against tube or gastrostomy feeding, be sure that treatable physiologic problems such as nausea or pain or psychological problems such as depression do not exist. Absent these and with competency, a rational individual has the recognized right to refuse feeding. Quality of life issues are important. Ultimately it is the patient or the surrogates, or the clinician acting in the patient's best interests, who must weigh the benefit of living vs the quality of living vs the quality of dying.

There should be a full discussion of the pros and cons of enteral nutrition, outlining the true benefits and burdens. Other supportive care including pain control, personal hygiene, skin care, and treatment of thirst and hunger with mouth care, ice chips, oral fluids, and spoon feeding must be presented, and it must be emphasized that cessation of enteral nutrition does not represent abandonment of the patient. The diagnosis should be as certain as it can be, without holding hope for miracles. It should be known that a terminal condition truly exists or that reversibility of a persistent vegetative state or coma has become highly unlikely.

Table 35–2 lists four lay organizations that span the ethical ideological spectrum and that provide information and support to patients or families. Table 35–3 provides a partial list of professional organizations that have formulated statements of ethics concerned with withholding or withdrawing enteral nutrition.

SUMMARY

Ethical conflicts in medicine arise because of competing value systems. Withholding or withdrawing enteral nutrition at the end of life is one of the many dilemmas that can cause great family and professional anguish. Resolution requires understanding the conflicts as well as understanding the goals of therapy, alternative therapies, concepts of medical futility, benefits and burdens, and the patient's right of refusal.

REFERENCES

1. Siegler M, Shiedermayer DL: Should fluid and nutritional support be withheld from terminally ill patients? Tube feeding in hospice settings. Am J Hospice Care 1987;4:32–35.
2. Hirsch Jr ED, Kett JF, Trefil J: The Dictionary of Cultural Literacy. Boston: Houghton Mifflin Company, 1988;90.
3. Boisaubin EV: Ethical issues in the nutritional support of the terminal patient. J Am Diet Assoc 1984;84: 52–54.
4. Snyder L: Artificial feeding and the right to die: the legal issues. J Leg Med 1988;9:349–375.

5. Sullivan Jr RJ: Accepting death without artificial nutrition or hydration. J Gen Intern Med 1993;8:220–224.

6. McCann RM, Hall WJ, Groth-Juncker A: Comfort care for terminally ill patients: the appropriate use of nutrition and hydration. JAMA 1994;272:1263–1266.

7. Printz LA: Terminal dehydration; a compassionate treatment. Arch Intern Med 1992;152:697–700.

8. Zerwekh JV: The dehydration question. Nursing 1983;13:47–51.

9. Oliver D: Terminal dehydration. Lancet 1984;2:631.

10. Andrews MR, Levine AM: Dehydration in the terminal patient: perception of hospice nurses. Am J Hospice Care 1989;Jan-Feb:31–34.

11. Position paper. American College of Physicians Ethics Manual, Part 2: The Physician and Society; Research; Life-sustaining treatment; Other issues. Ann Intern Med 1989;111:327–335.

12. The Multi-Society Task Force on PVS: Medical aspects of the persistent vegetative state. N Engl J Med 1994;330:1499–1508, 1572–1579.

13. Adams RD, Victor M: Principles of Neurology. 5th edition. New York: McGraw-Hill, 1993:302.

14. Gillon R: Persistent vegetative state and withdrawal of nutrition and hydration. J Med Ethics 1993;19:67–68.

15. Schneiderman LJ, Jecker NS, Jonsen AR: Medical futility: its meaning and ethical implications. Ann Intern Med 1990;112:949–954.

16. Schaffner KF: Philosophical, ethical, and legal aspects of resuscitation medicine. II. Recognizing the tragic choice: food, water, and the right to assisted suicide. Crit Care Med 1988;16:1063–1068.

17. May WE, Barry R, Griese O et al: Feeding and hydrating the permanently unconscious and other vulnerable persons. Issues Law Med 1987;3:203–217.

18. Studebaker ME: The ethics of artificial feeding. N Engl J Med 1988;319:306.

19. Rosner F: Withdrawing fluids and nutrition: an alternate view. NY State J Med 1987;87:591–593.

20. Mitchell KR, Kerridge IH, Lovat TJ: Medical futility, treatment withdrawal and the persistent vegetative state. J Med Ethics 1993;19:71–76.

21. Derr PG: Nutrition and hydration as elective therapy: Brophy and Jobes from an ethical and historical perspective. Issues Law Med 1986;2:25–38.

22. Uddo BJ: The withdrawal or refusal of food and hydration as age discrimination: some possibilities. Issues Law Med 1986;2:39–59.

23. Schiedermayer DL: The withdrawal of fluids and nutrition: a case presentation and ethical analysis. Wis Med J 1987;86:7–10.

24. Cantor NL: The permanently unconscious patient, non-feeding and euthanasia. Am J Law Med 1989;15:381–487.

25. Lynn J, Childress JF: Must patients always be given food and water? Hastings Cent Rep 1983;13:17–21.

26. Campbell-Taylor I, Fisher RH: The clinical case against tube feeding in palliative care of the elderly. J Am Geriatr Soc 1987;35:1100–1104.

27. Scofield GR: Artificial feeding: the least restrictive alternative? J Am Geriatr Soc 1991;39:1217–1220.

28. Angel M: After Quinlan: the dilemma of the persistent vegetative state. N Engl J Med 1994;330:1524–1525.

29. Schiedermayer DL, La Puma J, Miles SH: Ethics consultations masking economic dilemmas in patient care. Arch Intern Med 1989;149:1303–1305.

30. Keeney RL: Decisions about life-threatening risks. N Engl J Med 1994;331:193–196.

31. Meisel A: Legal myths about terminating life support. Arch Intern Med 1991;151:1497–1502.

32. Steinbrook R, Lo B: Artificial feeding—solid ground, not a slippery slope. N Engl J Med 1988;318:286–290.

33. Dresser RS, Boisaubin EV Jr: Ethics, law, and nutritional support. Arch Intern Med 1985;145:122–124.

34. Annas GJ: At law: precatory prediction and mindless mimicry: the case of Mary O'Connor. Hastings Cent Rep December 1988;31–33.

BIBLIOGRAPHY

Ahronheim JC, Mulvihill M: Refusal of tube feeding as seen from a patient advocacy organization: a comparison with landmark court cases. J Am Geriatr Soc 1991;39:1124–1127.

Annas GJ: Do feeding tubes have more rights than patients? Hastings Cent Rep 1986;16:26–28.

Annas GJ: Elizabeth Bouvia: whose space is this anyway? Hastings Cent Rep 1986;16:24–25.

Bleich JD: Providing nutrition and hydration for terminally ill patients. Issues Law Med 1986;2:117–131.

Bopp Jr J: Choosing death for Nancy Cruzan. Hastings Cent Rep Jan-Feb 1990;20:42–44.

Burt RA: Withholding nutrition and mistrusting nurturance: the vocabulary of In re Conroy. Issues Law Med 1987;2:317–340.

Colburn D: Is it ethical to withhold food and water from a terminally ill patient? Washington Post Health January 26, 1988:15.

Curran WJ: Defining appropriate medical care: providing nutrients and hydration for the dying. N Engl J Med 1985;313:940–942.

Grisez G: Should nutrition and hydration be provided to permanently unconscious and other mentally disabled persons. Issues Law Med 1989;5:165–179.

Hansen-Flaschen J: Choosing death or 'mamba' in the ICU: where there's life, there's hope is not necessarily true. Washington Post/Health Section May 8, 1990.

Horan DJ: Failure to feed: an ethical and legal discussion. Issues Law Med 1986;2:149–155.

Lynn J (ed): By No Extraordinary Means: The Choice to Forgo Life-Sustaining Food and Water. Bloomington & Indianapolis: Indiana University Press, 1986.

Lo B, Dornbrand L: The case of Claire Conroy: will administrative review safeguard incompetent patients? Ann Intern Med 1986;104:869–873.

Meilaender G: The confused, the voiceless, the perverse: shall we give them food and drink? Issues Law Med 1986;2:133–148.

Meyers DW: Legal aspects of withdrawing nourishment from an incurably ill patient. Arch Intern Med 1985;145:125–128.

Miles SH: Futile feeding at the end of life: family virtues and treatment decisions. Theor Med 1987;8:293–302.

National Legal Center Staff: Medical treatment for older people and people with disabilities: 1988 developments. Issues Law Med 1989;4:427–454.

Paris JJ: When burdens of feeding outweigh benefits. Hastings Cent Rep 1986;16:30–32.

Paris JJ, Crone RK, Reardon F: Physicians' refusal of requested treatment: the case of baby L. N Engl J Med 1990;322:1012–1014.

Paris JJ, Reardon FE: Court responses to withholding or withdrawing artificial nutrition and fluids. JAMA 1985;253:2243–2245.

Printz LA: Is withholding hydration a valid comfort measure in the terminally ill? Geriatrics 1988;43:84–88.

Siegler M, Weisbard AJ: Against the emerging stream: should fluids and nutritional support be discontinued? Arch Intern Med 1985;145:129–131.

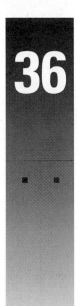

36

Managed Care

BARBARA T. MCKINNON
MARY KATHRYN WOLFSON
PHILLIP GEORGE

Today managed care has become firmly entrenched in the U.S. health care industry as an attempt to reduce costs and improve quality of health care delivery. However, it is really not a very recent phenomenon. It began in 1929 when Baylor University Hospital offered a group of teachers a prepaid health care plan, followed in 1938 by Kaiser-Permanente's development of a prepaid plan for construction workers building the Grand Coulee Dam. Kaiser went on to develop a comprehensive health maintenance organization (HMO) for the public at the end of World War II. The first Independent Practice Organization (IPA) for physicians began in 1954. Preferred provider organizations (PPOs) were next to enter the emerging market for managed health care.[1] In 1965 the federal government attempted price controls in the Medicare program through utilization review and in 1985 focused further on price controls vis-a-vis diagnosis-related groups (DRGs). In 1973 Congress passed the Federal HMO Act to create a less costly alternative to the unlimited demand in fee-for-service indemnity plans, and the HMOs attempted to better control provider usage through the dual combination of utilization review and case management. However, all these efforts have been limited in their effectiveness in controlling overall health care costs, and it is hoped that more recent

evolutions in managed care, including practice guidelines based on outcomes research, will be more effective.

The escalating costs of medical care and the increasing numbers of uninsured Americans have contributed to a push to reform the current U.S. health care system. Although Congress failed to pass a substantial health care reform package in its most recent legislative session, health care reform is already ongoing. It is happening at a local and state level as payors, providers, and the public search for ways to manage costs, access, and quality of health care.[2] As payors focus on controlling the rising costs of health care, providers seek to retain their market share, and patients worry about access to health care, the security of the health care system that we know seems threatened. Dr. David Zilz explains society's reaction to the health care crisis in this way: "When we need security, we are willing to trade in some freedom."[3] Thus it is that most of the new systems for health care delivery under a managed care system offer a lower cost—at the price of reduced freedom of choice.

Managed health care involves administrative firms that manage the allocation of health care benefits. This means that managed care organizations (MCOs) exert some level of control over the allocation of health care services for their patient populations. The degree of control is predicted by many experts to increase as managed care grows with the help of health care reform. MCOs exist to administer financial resources in such a way to maximize the quality of patient outcomes while ensuring that only the appropriate levels of service are used. To facilitate positive clinical and financial outcomes, most MCOs employ case managers.

MCOs differ from conventional indemnity insurers that did not manage the delivery of medical services—they simply paid for them. MCOs today have a meaningful role in determining what services will be covered and, most important, how much providers will be compensated for their services. One way MCOs control cost and delivery of health care services is by contracting with selected providers to furnish a comprehensive set of health care services to members. Explicit standards are used to choose these providers, and formal quality assurance and utilization review programs are established to monitor their clinical and financial performance. Significant financial incentives are implemented to encourage members to use the plan's providers and procedures. Currently, even traditional indemnity plans are following the MCOs' lead and becoming more active in governing the delivery of care.

TYPES OF MANAGED CARE ORGANIZATIONS

HMOs

HMOs are unique in that they are both payors and providers of services. HMOs have management responsibility for providing comprehensive health care services with an emphasis on preventive care on a prepayment or capitated basis to voluntarily enrolled persons within a designated population.[4] Enrollment in HMOs means enrollees will pay reduced fees and minimal out-of-pocket or copay expenses but will have limited access to and choice of hospitals, doctors, and other providers and incur dramatic financial penalties if they use out-of-plan providers.[5]

The HMO is a form of health insurance in which members prepay a premium for a comprehensive range of health services. Many employers have turned to HMOs charging a set premium, or fee per enrollee, to reduce their overall health care costs. Patients voluntarily enroll in HMO programs and generally receive care at a reduced out-of-pocket cost. Patients

usually only pay a small copay per visit and do not fill out insurance forms.

The prepayment for services represents the sole source of revenue for the HMO. The larger the HMO's enrollment, the greater the availability of financial resources. The HMO, like other MCOs, must find ways to hold onto as much of its premium revenues as possible. One way is to reduce the use of unnecessary procedures or tests, because profits are greater if fewer services are needed. Therefore, the HMO assumes the risk of its patient population. Healthier populations will likely require less utilization of services, whereas unhealthy populations may create a significant drain on the HMO's financial resources.

Traditional HMOs will not reimburse patients who receive services from providers outside the patient's HMO network. This effectively limits employees' choice of provider while strengthening employees' incentive to work within the network.

Not every organization managing the delivery of health care services can call itself an HMO. Under the federal HMO act, an entity must have three characteristics to call itself an HMO:

1. An organized system for providing health care or otherwise ensuring health care delivery in a geographic region
2. An agreed-on set of basic and supplemental health maintenance and treatment services
3. A voluntarily enrolled group of people

The basic components of an HMO include hospital and medical care benefits, providers (i.e., hospitals, physicians), members, and a plan manager (the HMO itself). There are five basic types of HMOs.

Staff Model

The staff model HMO is the purest form of managed care. This type of HMO was popularized by Kaiser-Permanente, one of the pioneers of the HMO movement. In the staff model, all physicians are employees of the organization and typically do not practice independently on a fee-for-service basis. Doctors, pharmacists, and other clinicians practice at a centralized site owned by the HMO.

The staff model is a popular model for many practitioners because it allows the doctors to concentrate on practicing medicine while someone else worries about business details. However, the physician is responsible for managing enrollees' total care needs and is financially at risk for the cost of their care. Thus, the physician must avoid overutilization of services such as laboratory tests, outside referrals, and hospitalization.

Traditional HMOs, such as staff model HMOs, will not reimburse patients who receive services from providers outside the patient's HMO network. This effectively limits the employees' choice of providers, while strengthening their incentive to work within the network.

IPA Model

The IPA contracts with independent physicians who work in their own private practices and see fee-for-service patients along with HMO enrollees. Physicians belonging to the IPA guarantee that they will not charge more than a prenegotiated fee to care for each patient under the plan.

Group Model

This model currently has the largest enrollment of all the HMO models. In the group model, the HMO contracts with a physician group, which is paid a fixed amount per patient to provide specific services. The administration of the group practice then decides how the HMO payments are distributed to each member physician. This type of HMO is usually located in a hospital or clinic setting and may include a pharmacy. These physicians usually do not have any fee-for-service patients.

Network Model

The network model is composed of a network of physician-group practices under the administration of one HMO. The HMO selects the group(s) it wants to participate and handles the necessary administration of the patient population. This allows the HMO to cover a larger geographic service area.

Point-of-Service Plan

The point-of-service (POS) plan is sometimes referred to as an "open-ended" HMO. The POS model is one in which the patient can receive care either from physicians contracting with the HMO or from those not contracting with the HMO. The deductible or copay agreements are more expensive if enrollees go outside the HMO agreements. A nonparticipating physician who sees an HMO patient is paid according to services performed.

PPOs

PPOs involved direct contractual relationships among hospitals, physicians, insurers, employers, or third-party administrators (also known as intermediaries) that form a network in which providers negotiate with group purchasers to provide health services for a defined population at a negotiated price.[4] These arrangements can be self-insured or self-funded. Patients can use a physician or other provider outside the PPO, but they must bear some portion of the fee. Financial penalties for PPO patients receiving "out-of-plan" care are not as severe as those imposed on HMO patients.

The beneficiaries of a PPO are given a financial incentive to use the services of certain providers. Providers negotiate lower fees in exchange for increased patient volume. The providers are paid on a fee-for-service schedule that is typically discounted 10 to 20 percent below normal fees. Providers in a PPO are not required to share risk. The preferred providers may be subject to monitoring of service utilization and the appropriateness of care. This monitoring and fee structure introduces an element of control that does not exist for an independent practitioner, but it leads to greater patient volume and the opportunity for higher income. These agreements usually state that the provider must follow guidelines for hospital admissions and other services and resources. This arrangement helps to ensure a more cost-effective delivery of care.

A growing trend is the use of daily fee payments, known as per diem payments, to hospitals or home care providers. These DRG-like payments put the providers more at risk for the cost of services provided.[6]

Physician-Hospital Organization

Another entrant into the prepaid health plan forum is the physician-hospital organization (PHO). These organizations are formed by groups of hospitals and their doctors with both parties assuming the financial risk for the care of patients. Currently, these groups compete with other MCOs for employers and their enrollees. PHOs may offer low, all-inclusive fees in the form of bundled bills. In this scenario, the financial risk for obtaining reimbursement for services is placed on the physicians and the hospital.

Networks

Networking or strategic partnering is a business strategy to reach more customers. Small independent health care providers can band together into a network as a strategy for growth. This is important not only to offer greater geographic coverage when contracting with large managed care entities, but also to provide the convenience of "one stop shopping" in which only one phone call is required to arrange a number of services. Single product networks are horizontal alliances containing a single health care product (e.g., intravenous [IV] infusion services). The main purpose of this alliance is to achieve greater geographic coverage. Multiproduct networks contain a combination of different product lines such as home nursing, IV infusion services, and durable medical equipment. The purpose of this multiproduct line alliance is to meet payors' requirements for a continuum of care and for the convenience of "one stop shopping."[7] Newer networking strategies include manufacturers or suppliers in risk-sharing agreements so that the network entity can compete for capitated business. Manufacturers' purchases of pharmacy benefits' management companies illustrate today's fully integrated networks.[8]

IMPACT OF MANAGED COMPETITION

Although the health care of today is mainly delivered through a fragmented group of providers, managed competition is emerging rapidly. The progression into managed competition has been described as a four-step process by Schaffer.[6] In the first stage, independent practitioners and hospitals exist without any organized payors. In the second stage, loose frameworks of managed care networks and provider networks begin to form. The third stage, known as consolidation, involves the emergence of a few large purchasers of health care. Health systems predominate, and private practices begin to disappear. Finally, in the fourth, or managed competition, stage, physicians, hospitals, and insurers join to form fully integrated networks.

Managed care's impact is felt in a multitude of ways. Manufacturers seek to design products and services tailored to MCOs' needs.[9] From computer software programs to risk-sharing product purchasing agreements, managed care is driving the innovations in health care products and services. Patients learn to live with the reduced freedom of choice, as long as it is matched with reduced health care out-of-pocket costs. Finally, as many areas of the country are experiencing health care consolidation, providers scramble to join the managed care networks rather than be left out of the business potential of these large patient groups.

MANAGED CARE STRATEGIES

MCOs use a variety of strategies to hold down the costs of patient care and to ensure that payment is made only for covered services. For HMOs to be financially successful, they must emphasize early detection and preventive services, emphasize outpatient care and minimize hospitalization, use medical rather than surgical treatment whenever possible, and promote use of home care or alternate site services. Finally, both cost per unit of service and use of services must be controlled to achieve an overall cost savings.

Case Management

MCOs accommodate large numbers of people; case management applies to a relatively small population—the high-cost users. Case management is a systematic approach for identifying high-risk/high-cost patients and allocating resources to the most appropriate and effective forms of care. It involves assessing and choosing treatment options and developing treatment plans to improve quality and efficacy while controlling costs. Additionally, case management ensures the smooth flow of care through the health care system and avoids fragmentation or duplication of care. Case management involves managing a patient's total care to achieve an optimal outcome.[10]

An important goal in case management is to evaluate high-acuity patients' individual health care needs and compare these needs with the individual's insurance coverage. The objective is to conserve the total benefit dollars (known as the lifetime maximum) for chronic cases. To meet this objective, case managers often have the flexibility to use different portions of a patient's insurance coverage to cover expenses and to select lower cost providers. For example, if a particular patient can be managed more cost effectively by using home care services, but the patient does not have home care benefits, the case manager can use the major medical (or hospital) portion of the patient's benefits to pay for the home care. However, case managers are not permitted to exceed the lifetime maximum for the patient.[11]

The individual who performs the case management function can be a physician or nurse or some other individual with a specific clinical background. Case managers are trained and can become certified. Internal case managers are employees of an insurance provider, self-insured company, or governmental agency. Because they follow the patient long term, they may be more concerned about quality and long-term benefits of therapies, such as nutritional support. External case managers are individuals or case management firms hired by an insurance company to manage identified high-cost patients. Sometimes external case managers are used to manage only one spell of illness; thus their focus is mainly on coordinating care and immediate cost savings. Reimbursement for external case management may be by the hour, by the case, or as a percentage of cost savings. With health care reform and the constant pressures to reduce costs, case managers will take on an even more important role in the future delivery of health care (Table 36–1).

Utilization Review

Utilization review encompasses a variety of techniques used to review prospectively, concurrently, and retrospectively the appropriateness of care to avoid the cost of unnecessary or inappropriate care. Preadmission screening is used to determine whether hospital stays or other intended health care procedures are appropriate and whether they are within the plan's stated benefits. For example, surgery for cosmetic purposes is rarely covered by managed care benefits plans.

Preacceptance screening is used by providers to verify that a planned service will be covered. Home care providers typically will check patients for active status in the payment plan and

TABLE 36–1 Role of the Case Manager

Identifies high-risk/high-cost patients
Develops the plan for patient care interventions and outcomes
Is accountable for seeing that interventions and outcomes are met by collaborating with the health care team and the patient/family
Identifies, documents, and analyzes variances if interventions and outcomes are not met and takes appropriate action
Follows the patient throughout the entire episode of illness, crossing all levels of care
Enhances collaboration, communication, and coordination among members of the health care team
Enhances the quality of life and satisfaction of patients and their families

for plan benefits before accepting a patient and providing costly services that might not be reimbursed. For example, some benefits plans do not include home enteral nutrition because they consider it to be food, not a medical therapy.

Concurrent utilization review is used by payors to ensure that care is still needed and to move the patient forward into the most appropriate level of care. The patient's progress is compared with the expected plan of care, and necessary interventions are planned to achieve the desired clinical and cost outcome. For example, case managers may recommend moving patients into a skilled nursing facility or may arrange for home health assistance to allow the care plan to be continued at home.

Formularies

A primary focus of cost containment in managed care is to attain the best therapeutic outcome for the least amount of money. One proven way to accomplish this goal is through the use of a formulary, which is a list of the therapeutic agents available that meet the needs of the MCO and its patients. Traditionally, formularies were based on the principle that health care providers should use the safest and most cost-effective prescription drugs. This logic has been extended to selecting the most appropriate enteral formula through use of a formulary. Hospitals have for some time used formularies to consolidate purchasing of enteral formulas and obtain volume purchasing discounts. MCOs can mandate the use of a particular product line to monitor more closely the appropriateness and cost of enteral formula selection as well as to obtain purchasing discounts. Some formularies are "open," providing for relative ease of access to nonformulary items, sometimes through a review and approval process involving case management. Other formularies are quite restrictive, with severe prohibitions against the use of costly formulas.

One of the main drivers of development of formularies are financial incentives in the form of rebates. Managed care entities demand rebates from manufacturers who have products on the formulary. The rebate system encourages participation in the program from manufacturers whose products are not on the formulary. Manufacturers are then motivated to direct their marketing efforts toward gaining a greater market share. The rebates help MCOs to lower their per member per month drug costs.

Formularies should be based on a sound scientific review of the effectiveness and cost of the available therapeutic classes of formulas. The issue of therapeutic substitution should be addressed—can a generically equivalent formulation be substituted for the prescribed formula? Follow-up review is important to ensure that the selected agents are being used and are meeting the desired therapeutic objectives and to allow for inclusion of significant therapeutic advances. Education of prescribers is necessary to achieve compliance with the formulary. Additionally, quality assurance activities should focus on appropriate use of the formulas included on the formulary.

Outcomes Monitoring

Outcomes management is a technology for measuring patient experiences designed to help patients, payors, and providers make rational medical care–related choices based on better insight into the effect of these choices on the patient's life.[12] Outcomes management interrelates the systemic collection and analysis of patient data with techniques for cost analysis and with current practice standards and guidelines.[13] It draws from a number of techniques associated with performance improvement, including continuous quality improvement, benchmarking, and critical paths. The human side of medical care is emphasized, with measures of patient satisfaction and quality of life.

Outcomes monitoring can be helpful in establishing what resources are required to reach a desired outcome; assess the success rates of providers with particular procedures, therapies, or patient groups; and enhance patient satisfaction through more effective use of limited resources. Outcome measures are being used to compare performance among providers of health care service as a basis of awarding business. For example, managed care publications compare HMOs by their patient satisfaction rates, and home care providers are compared by standardized indicators such as rates of catheter infection and rehospitalization.

Pharmacoeconomic Analyses

The marketplace must move away from a reliance on price alone, because health care costs will continue to rise unless use is also limited. To put it more simply—a 20 percent discount on an unnecessary or ineffective product or service is not much of a bargain. The tools for this paradigm shift come from the field of pharmacoeconomics.[14,15]

The pharmaceutical drug manufacturing industry has led the shift from promoting acquisition costs, which are not true economic analyses, to promoting outcome-based or cost-effectiveness analyses. The pharmaceutical industry is not focusing on outcome-based indicators for its drug products, such as length of hospital stay, length of stay in the critical care unit, mean time to return to work, etc. These provide a more accurate analysis of the overall cost impact of new products, because the cheapest product in terms of acquisition costs may not be the most effective.

Cost-Minimization Analysis

Cost-minimization analysis compares the costs of two or more alternatives that have equivalent outcomes. In this model, the alternatives are assumed to be identical, and the objective is to identify the least expensive alternative, thereby minimizing cost. This is the basis for the common practice of "shopping" for the best price through competitive price bidding. A limitation of this method is that the alternatives may in fact not be identical in terms of quality and outcomes.

Cost-Benefit Analysis

Cost-benefit analysis compares the cost and consequences of two or more alternatives with different outcomes. This type of analysis assumes that limited dollars are available, and it compares alternatives to determine which has the most favorable cost:benefit ratio. In this model costs and consequences are measured in dollars. For example, this could be used to compare price quotes from two home care providers if rates of rehospitalization and average cost per rehospitalization are known.

Cost-Effectiveness Analysis

Cost-effectiveness analysis compares the costs and consequences of alternative approaches to obtaining a common objective. In this model, alternatives have similar but not identical outcomes, which are measured in natural units (e.g., mm Hg, pounds of weight gained or lost, laboratory values, nitrogen balance). This method is often used to compare the cost effectiveness of different products in the same therapeutic category.

Cost-Utility Analysis

Cost-utility analysis is similar to cost-effectiveness analysis except that outcomes are adjusted for patient preferences. Results are expressed as cost per quality adjusted unit of outcome. The limitation of this type of analysis is the difficulty in objectively assessing patient preference.

Outcome: The Future

In the future, with contracted network agreements and capitated reimbursement systems, price is becoming a level playing field. In this scenario, outcomes will be the differentiating factor between providers.

Critical Pathways

Critical pathways are documentation tools that are an abbreviated version of the interventions that must occur in proper sequence and in a timely fashion to achieve anticipated goals for length of stay or resource utilization for a given diagnosis or treatment. The interventions outlined in a critical pathway include those employed by physicians, nurses, and other members of the health care team. Critical pathways are usually revised to meet individual patients' needs within the first 24 hours. Thereafter, any variances from the critical pathway are documented and analyzed. Multiple diagnoses may necessitate merging the appropriate critical pathways involved in the patient's care.

Critical pathways are used to describe the usual or typical patient, generally only about 75 to 80 percent of patients in a specified case type. Critical pathways function as a quality guide to identify undesirable outcomes in individual patients or trends and patterns in aggregate patients that represent poor quality. The health care team meets to identify and discuss trends and patterns and plans methods to improve care for the individual patient or for all patients with a specific case type. The effects of implemented interventions can continue to be monitored in subsequently admitted patients through use of the critical pathway.

Critical paths were initially used in health care delivery as tools to assist in managed care and case management in the acute care setting. More recently, critical pathways have been used in the chronic care setting not only as cost containment and outcomes management tools but also as cost and pricing tools. Cost can be calculated when all the resources (services, drugs, products, supplies, equipment) necessary to implement the interventions are identified from the pathway, and the unit cost and the number of units of each resource utilized are identified. Once cost is known, a pricing

strategy can be developed to support contract negotiations with third-party payors in the increasingly competitive managed care environment.

Clinical Guidelines

Clinical guidelines are the distillation of the best collective thinking from literature, practicing physicians, and academic experts on how to treat a particular medical situation. The terms *clinical guidelines*, *practice parameters*, or *practice protocols* are used interchangeably to describe "strategies for patient management designed to assist clinicians in clinical decision making."[16]

The development of clinical guidelines by private organizations has been spurred by the creation of the Agency for Health Care Policy and Research (AHCPR) in Rockville, MD.[17] Currently, the AHCPR has issued 12 guidelines that recommend provider interventions for diagnosing, preventing, treating, and managing a variety of diseases and disorders. AHCPR's guidelines are peer reviewed and are based on extensive literature reviews and actual clinical evaluations. They incorporate analyses of the use and cost of health care resources. Development of these guidelines has been viewed by some as a potential protection against physician malpractice suits, and legislation in Maine, Vermont, Minnesota, and Florida includes use of practice guidelines as an affirmative defense in malpractice suits. However, guidelines may in fact be used against providers because plaintiff's attorneys use the guidelines to demonstrate that care delivered did not meet the standard of care.[17]

As MCOs, government regulations, and health care reform prompt health care payors to cut deeper and deeper, a definition of the standard of care is necessary to avoid deterioration of quality of care in the interest of cost savings. Professionals should educate MCOs about guidelines such as the ASPEN Guidelines for Nutrition Support,[18] which evaluate the current literature on nutrition support and provide expert opinion in those areas where clinical data are not available or clear-cut. Private insurers are examining the guidelines to serve as the basis for their parenteral and enteral nutrition coverage guidelines. However, these guidelines are a good example of the limitations of the guideline development process. References cited in the guidelines were coded according to a method used by the AHCPR. The system rated evidence from meta-analysis of randomized clinical trials as most valid and from expert committee reports, opinions, and clinical experiences as least valid. However, prospective clinical trials evaluating nutrition therapy were often made difficult because investigators could not ethically randomize nutrition support for the most severely malnourished patients. For this reason, many of the guidelines rely on expert opinion and concensus.

Although the use of clinical practice guidelines is being widely promoted to assist practitioners in making appropriate patient care decisions, whether this actually produces improved clinical outcomes remains to be seen.[19] Critical pathways and clinical guidelines have been criticized by some as "cookbook medicine" because they ignore the tremendous variation inherent in patient care.[17,20,21] However, MCOs viewed them as a means to standardize care, reduce omissions and duplications of care, and give well-planned support to clinical decision-making processes.

Report Card

As consumers and MCOs demand information to help them select and evaluate providers of health care services, the concept of a "report card" for the health care systems has arisen.[22] The report card is based on the concept of outcomes monitoring, with the important difference that results of monitoring are made available to the public. Basically, information on performance measures of health care is collected by various providers. Standardized performance measures are designed to be valid but easily understandable. Compilation of results from several providers allows purchasers of health care to evaluate and compare health care systems or providers. This should promote accountability of health care delivery systems in terms of delivering quality care, consumer satisfaction, and cost-effective services.

The Joint Commission on Accreditation of Healthcare Organizations (JCAHO) has embraced the report card concept with its national performance data base, which is currently undergoing beta testing. Information on standardized indicators will be required to be reported by all accredited providers, probably by telephone modem. Indicators of nutrition performance will include achievement of a goal weight and rates of catheter-related infections. When the system is fully implemented (anticipated for 1997), case managers or consumers will likely have access to the results of the performance measures.

Capitation

Capitation means that product or service providers receive a fixed fee per enrollee or beneficiary in a managed care plan. All the services required are delivered to patients for the base rate. The rationale for such a system is that it naturally reduces use. This is the result of paying a limited fee such that the provider is actually harmed by providing more services than are required. Capitation payments are typically made at the beginning of the month and are divided into a per member per month basis. If the capitation rates are set above actual expenses, the provider earns a profit. If they are set below the actual expenses, the provider loses money. The issue of quality is treated totally separately.[6]

The main problem with capitation from a provider's perspective is that it is very difficult to set appropriate capitation payments, because it is difficult to predict the future use of a product or service. Ways to minimize risk in contracting for capitated payments would include monitoring use for a given time before signing the contract, establishing a set margin of use above which the capitated rate would be renegotiated, or setting up capitation rates for short periods and renegotiating them frequently.

MANAGED CARE IMPLICATIONS FOR NUTRITION SUPPORT PRACTICE

The proliferation of managed care in the health care system of today and tomorrow offers nutrition support professionals both challenges and opportunities. Although the traditional multidisciplinary nutrition support team may be endangered, it is not extinct. The current environment may allow nutrition practitioners to broaden their horizons, practicing in new ways and in new settings. Nutrition practitioners must accept the challenge and focus their energies on providing preventive services, documenting both the quality and cost effectiveness of care, and on obtaining reimbursement for services to be successful in the new era.[23] No matter what one's practice site may be, managed care is sure to have an influence. The following may be viewed as strategies for success, or at least for survival, in a managed care environment.

Hospital

Network

Teamwork will be essential, not only among nutrition support team members but among nutrition practitioners and physicians, hospital administrators, and other members of the health care system. The independent nutrition team, much like the solo physician practitioner, will not have the negotiating clout to participate independently in the new managed care system. Successful practitioners will affiliate with other providers in a variety of ways to gain strength in numbers. One method is to create large provider groups that can negotiate with MCOs. Another strategy is to become part of a managed care organization, such as a PHO, in which the new entity can negotiate directly with large employer groups for access to their populations. A different method of networking is to get involved with other practice sites and new services, such as providing outpatient nutrition counseling and wellness services such as weight control programs or sports nutrition programs, or to provide services by contracting with physicians' offices, dialysis centers, or home care organizations. Additionally, some dietitians have established relationships with PPOs so that they can obtain reimbursement for nutrition services as a preferred provider.[24]

Nutrition Screening Programs

These programs may be marketed as a value-added service to help hospitals negotiate provider contracts with MCOs. Malnutrition commonly occurs in hospitalized patients[25,26] and adds significantly to costs[27-30] and complications.[30,31] It is important to train hospital staff to identify the presence of malnutrition and to implement early nutritional interventions in patients identified as at risk of malnutrition. Additionally, nutritional screening is now required by new JCAHO standards.[32] A variety of methods have been developed for nutritional screening.[31-34] It is often best to develop a screening tool and protocol based on the literature but adapted to your own institution's needs.

One efficient way to accomplish screening is to train all nurses who perform admission history and physical examinations to screen for malnutrition.[35] Monitoring of poor nutritional intake should be an ongoing screening activity. If malnutrition or factors causing a high risk of nutritional compromise are detected, nutrition support professionals should be contacted to assess the patient. Documenting how many patients are identified through the screening program, and the interventions used to improve nutritional outcomes, can help demonstrate to MCOs the importance of nutrition support.

Document the Outcomes of Care

Managed care entities have taken note of reports that recent increases in health care costs have occurred without a commensurate improvement in health care outcomes.[36] MCOs are demanding to see the value of what they pay for. They are interested specifically in improvements in health status and patient satisfaction and in evaluating cost per utilization.[37] Outcomes, such as length of stay, achievement of a positive nitrogen balance, or achievement of a goal enteral formula intake, may be effective in demonstrating the quality and value of nutrition support services to MCOs.

Publicize Your Efforts

Hospital administrators, financial officers, case managers, or others responsible for managed care contracting and reimbursement will not know the value of your services unless you tell them. Consider a newsletter of your own, or contribute to an existing hospital newsletter. Make sure the managed care entities you deal with are on the mailing list. Try putting together a seminar and invite key physicians and hospital administrators. Publish a nutrition support manual or get involved in publishing outcomes of your work in professional journals. Do not forget to let others know about your activities in everyday settings as well, such as patient rounds, medical staff conferences, and committee meetings. Be organized and prepared to report on the numbers of patients you managed and the outcomes achieved.

Practice Cost Effectively

Ellwood notes that "expensive therapies with little medical benefit will not stand the test of case managers and medical review bureaucracies. Successful providers will be able to improve patient outcomes cost-effectively."[12] Table 36–2 lists strategies for cost-effective provision of enteral nutrition in hospitals.[38-43]

HMOs

Nutrition practitioners in MCOs, such as HMOs, have an advantage in understanding the managed care mind set from an insider's perspective. The focus of care is on prevention—encouraging lifestyle changes to prevent the development of diseases or to manage chronic disease conditions. Jenifer Buechner notes:

One reason preventive care works well in the HMO model is because HMO staff dietitians have an ex-

TABLE 36–2 Ideas for Cost Effective Provision of Enteral Nutrition

Utilize enteral, rather than parenteral, nutrition whenever the gut works.

Train nurses to include nutrition screening as a part of routine admission procedures and to alert nutrition professionals whenever nutritional deficits are identified.

Consider computerizing the nutritional assessment.

Purchase formulas through a buying group to obtain the best possible volume discounts.

Establish an enteral nutritional formulary. Using the nutrition committee or pharmacy and therapeutics committee, define generically equivalent formulas and substitute them whenever appropriate. Develop a mechanism for review and approval of nonformulary requests for products.

Evaluate costs for enteral containers, supplies, and preparation time based on buying contracts.

Cross-train nutrition support professionals to become multifunctional.

Standardize enteral nutrition order forms and order protocols to achieve calorie intake goals more rapidly.

Standardize nutrition support laboratory test panels and days of ordering laboratory values for stable patients.

Avoid wasting formula whenever appropriate; start orders for changes in enteral formulas with the next container to be fed for asymptomatic patients.

Move stable patients to alternate sites of care (e.g., home care, hospice care) when a suitable environment and a trainable, willing caregiver are available.

Work with local enteral formula manufacturer's representatives, public nutrition programs, home care providers, and hospital administration to develop a program to provide home enteral nutrition formula for uninsured patients who are hospitalized solely because they depend on nutritional support.

---

tended period of time to get to know patients and develop relationships. The focus is less on simply giving information and more on developing trust and rapport to help the patient supply the information. Because some patients may have no restrictions on the number of visits to the dietitian, there is a real opportunity to provide continuing monitoring, support and follow-up.[33]

Disease management is accomplished in the HMO by getting patients involved in taking control of their own care and becoming more responsible for the outcome of health care. This in turn saves money for the HMO as the patient is managed with cost-effective preventive services rather than more costly acute care services.

Home Care

Develop Relationships with Case Managers

In home care, business may be awarded on a case-by-case basis by case managers or by national or local contracts. In either case, it is important to work with the case manager to provide information, not only at the start of care, but also whenever significant changes occur and when care is completed. Case managers may award business on the basis of price bidding (cost-minimization analysis). However, because outcomes of care are not identical, it is necessary to educate case managers about the value of services a particular home care company may provide that may improve the effectiveness of care. For example, initial and ongoing nutritional assessments, training patients to monitor and detect complications before they become severe, selecting the most cost-effective enteral formula, and giving patients the less expensive bolus route of administration when possible are ways of providing value-added services.

Document the Plan of Care

A written plan of care is required for home care providers who wish to become accredited by the JCAHO.[32] Sharing this plan of care with the case manager is helpful to demonstrate that home enteral nutrition includes not only a product, but also services such as training, monitoring, and home delivery. The plan of care should include specific nutritional problems, planned interventions, measurable goals, and time expected to meet goals. For example, "lose 5 pounds within 3 months" or "maintain serum glucose between 80 and 120 mg/dl" are examples of measurable goals. Stating the plan objectively helps the case manager to understand clearly when goals are achieved and to recognize the effectiveness of services provided.

Document the Outcomes of Care

Monitoring of performance indicators is necessary not only to satisfy JCAHO requirements but also to meet the requirements for contracting with many MCOs. Although present contracts often require JCAHO accreditation for inclusion as a contracted provider, the trend is toward reviewing specific indicators of actual performance and selecting providers who can provide the best performance at an affordable price (cost effectiveness). In this type of analysis, the cheapest price may not always win out because poor quality costs more in the long run. Outcomes are of particular importance to home care practitioners to document that home care can produce patient outcomes equivalent to or better than those achieved in inpatient settings at a lower cost and with improved quality of life for the patient.

Consider the Appropriateness of Care

Home nutrition practitioners must face difficult ethical issues in providing nutrition support to patients with terminal illnesses. Starting aggressive nutrition support, such as parenteral nutrition, very late in the disease process for a patient with a terminal illness may not be effective or cost effective, while early intervention, such as early enteral feeding in trauma,[34] may not only be effective nutritionally but may prevent other complications. Use of practice guidelines may help determine when nutrition support is most appropriate.[35]

Analyze the Cost of Services

Costs associated with training and assessment, dispensing of formulas, home delivery, and billing and collections can be substantial. As profit margins shrink in home care, it becomes imperative to know the costs of providing services before deciding to sign on to managed care contracts with fixed, discounted pricing. Knowledge of both costs of services and of actuarial use of services is necessary to consider capitated or other risk-sharing contracts.

Provide an Appropriate Level of Services

The days of providing "extras" to patients, such as nursing visits to obtain specimens for laboratory tests for ambulatory patients, are disappearing rapidly. The telephone, the facsimile machine, and the computer modem are replacing duplicate visits by the physician, home pharmacy, and home health nurse. Communication among the home care team is essential to avoid omission or duplication of services and to provide optimal continuity of care.

Assess Patient Satisfaction

One of the most significant benefits of home care is the improvement in patient quality of life. Patient satisfaction surveys can assess both quality of life as well as quality of services provided. It is important to consider the patient's perspective because even clinically effective care will not be viewed positively by the patient if it is provided in an inconvenient or inconsiderate manner. Patient satisfaction results are extremely important to managed care entities, because they do not want to lose patients from their program because contracted providers have offered poor quality services.

Get Involved with Legislative and Regulatory Issues

The recent revision of the Medicare Durable Medical Equipment Regional Carriers (DMERC) guidelines for Durable Medical Equipment, Prosthetics, Orthotics, and Supplies (DMEPOS) illustrates the impact of regulatory changes on home care practice. Medicare governs care and reimbursement for services for a large segment of the home care market. The recent DMERC revision eliminated coverage for enteral nutrition patients with Alzheimers' disease who have a cognitive rather than a functional impairment of swallowing.[44] Perhaps a more organized lobbying effort by the home nutrition community would have been effective in changing this regulation. Although this is speculative, it is certain that knowledge of regulatory changes is an essential business practice to avoid accepting patients for services without acceptable reimbursement.

Develop Expertise in Reimbursement Issues

Many hospital-based nutrition practitioners have been recruited actively by the home care industry because home nutrition support is important to this marketplace. However, in the home care arena, clinical management skills must be matched with business management skills. Knowledge of reimbursement practices is necessary to avoid financial disasters. For example, many insurance payors do not cover home enteral formula because it is considered "food," and the payor would not normally purchase food for patients in outpatient settings.

Network

Networking has become a critical survival skill for home care organizations ranging from small independent providers to large, multisite, national chains. Figure 36–1 illustrates networking options for home infusion companies. These including risk-sharing purchase agreements with manufacturers or suppliers, horizontal networking with providers of other types of home care services, networking with providers of similar home care services to achieve greater geographic coverage, and networking with referral sources, either through joining a PHO, managed care contracting, or

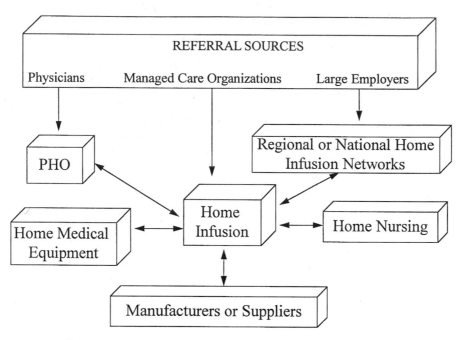

FIGURE 36–1 Networking options for a home infusion company.

through direct agreements with physician groups or large employers.

THE FUTURE

To succeed in a managed care environment, practitioners must understand the managed care organization's motivation. MCOs seek to reduce per member per month costs through preventive health care services, use of less costly outpatient services, preadmission screening, use of formularies, and other techniques. In the future, nutrition practitioners may benefit from calculating their costs per patient per day (for hospitals) or per month (home care or HMO). Trending this over several months may be a useful starting point to further investigate the cost effectiveness of services. Further questions should be asked to assess whether the cost was truly effective, such as achievement of a positive nitrogen balance (hospitals) or achievement of a goal weight (home care or HMO). Costs of complications such as aspiration pneumonia or tube site infections should also be considered. Finally, costs for increased length of stay (hospitals) or readmissions (home care or HMO) could be included. Although assessing the costs of these variables may be difficult, many quality assurance programs in nutrition support already include achievement of nutritional goals, read-

missions, or complications as a part of their routine monitoring. Assessment of costs of care for different patient groups, different processes of care, and different outcomes of care will be an important focus of future research for nutrition professionals.

CONCLUSION

Through the many means of managing America's health care ills, none has demonstrated itself to be a panacea for controlling the rising cost of health care, although certain forms of HMOs have proved most successful in reducing costs. Traditional attempts at managed care have been only marginally effective in the past, but many believe that a new paradigm is developing and consequently will be the model of health care delivery in the future. Under this new structure, managed care providers are offering their clients more of a coordinated clinical approach through an integration of multiple managed care components, while using more of an outcomes-based approach to high-cost, high-volume medical procedures. This type of delivery system can minimize health care expense through reduced administrative costs and better control of use while improving the quality of care by basing treatment on clinical guidelines designed to obtain the optimum medical outcome possible.

REFERENCES

1. Vogenberg FR: Managed care organizations: an introduction. Hosp Pharm 1995;30:40–44.
2. Spiller K: Shifting with the paradigm: a primer for embracing managed care. Remington Rep 1995;(Feb./Mar.):18–20.
3. Zilz D: Health care reform: future trends in industrial pharmacy. ASHP Midyear Clinical Meeting, Miami Beach, FL: December 6, 1994.
4. Kelly M, Bacon GT, Mitchell J: Glossary of managed care terms. J Ambulatory Care Manage 1994;17:70–76.
5. Morselander K: Selling to HMOs varies by model. Homecare 1994;March:42:161–162.
6. Schaffer C: Case management's role in networks. Continuing Care 1995;Jan-Feb:21–22.
7. Coleman JF, Algie BA: Health care reform: redefining care delivery systems produces opportunities for providers. Remington Rep 1994;(Feb-Mar):5–9.
8. Solovy A: New power strategies: the battle for control. Hosp Health Networks 1994;(Dec):24–34.
9. Saladow JM: Managed care and technology: a critical partnership under scrutiny. Remington Rep 1995;Feb-Mar:36–40.
10. Desimone BS: The case for case management. Cont Care 1988;(Jul):23.
11. Cherney A: Marketing products and services to managed care. Rancho Palos Verdes, CA: Cherney and Associates;1993.
12. Ellwood PM: Outcomes management: a technology of patient experience. N Engl J Med 1988;318:1549–1556.
13. Johnson N, Nash DB: The key players in an outcomes management program. P and T 1993;Sept.:883–887.
14. McDonald RC: An introduction to health economics. Indianapolis IN: Eli Lilly, 1993.
15. Sanchez LA: Evaluating the quality of published pharmacoeconomic evaluations. Hosp Pharm 1995;30:146–152.
16. Hirshfield EB: Practice parameters versus outcome measurements. How will prospective and retrospective approaches to quality management fit together? Nutr Clin Pract 1994;9:201–216.
17. Bergman R: Getting the goods on guidelines. Hosp Health Networks 1994;Oct:70–74.
18. ASPEN Board of Directors. Guidelines for the use of parenteral and enteral nutrition in adult and pediatric patients. J Parenter Enter Nutr 1993;17:1SA–52SA.
19. Bergman R: Getting the goods on guidelines. Hosp Health Networks 1994;Oct.:70–74.
20. Bothe A: Guidelines for nutrition support: guideline, cookbook, or coupon book? Nutr Clin Pract 1994;9:205–206.
21. Dans PE: Credibility, cookbook medicine, and common sense: guidelines and the College. Ann Intern Med 1994;120:966–968.
22. O'Leary DS: The measurement mandate: report card day is coming. Am J Hosp Pharm 1994;51:757–761.
23. Gillespie S: Finding your niche in the managed care market. Columbus, OH: American Dietetic Association/Ross Products Division, 1993.
24. Tootell M: Opportunities in managed care. Finding your niche in the managed care market. Columbus, OH: American Dietetic Association/Ross Products Division, 1993.
25. Bistrian BR, Blackburn GL, Vitale J et al: Prevalence of malnutrition in general medical patients. JAMA 1976;235:1567–1570.
26. Detsky AS, Baker JP, O'Rourke K et al: Perioperative parenteral nutrition: a meta-analysis. Ann Intern Med 1987;107:195–203.
27. Christensen KS, Gstundtner KM: Hospital-wide screening improves basis for nutrition intervention. J Am Diet Assoc. 1985;85:704–706.
28. Christensen KS: Hospitalwide screening increases revenue under prospective payment system. J Am Diet Assoc 1986;86:1234–1235.
29. Robinson G, Goldstein M, Levine GM: Impact of nutritional status on DRG length of stay. J Parenter Enter Nutr 1987;11:49–51.
30. Reilly JJ, Hull SF, Albert N et al: Economic impact of malnutrition: a model system for hospitalized patients. J Parenter Enter Nutr 1988;12:3721–3776.
31. Buzby GP, Mullen JL, Matthews DC et al: Prognostic nutritional index in gastrointestinal surgery. Am J Surg 1980;139:160–167.
32. Joint Commission on Accreditation of Healthcare Organizations: Accreditation Manual for Home Care. Oakbrook Terrace, IL: The Joint Commission of Accreditation of Healthcare Organizations, 1994.
33. Buechner J: Perspective: RDs on the HMO Staff. Finding your niche in the managed-care market. Columbus, OH: American Dietetic Association/Ross Products Division, 1993.
34. Detsky AS, McLaughlin JR, Baker JP et al: What is subjective global assessment of nutritional status? J Parenter Enter Nutr 1987;11:8–13.
35. Messner RL, Stephens N, Sheeler WE et al: Effect of admission nutritional status on length of hospital stay. Gastroenterol Nurs 1991;13:202–205.
36. Schroeder SA: Strategies for reducing medical costs by changing physicians behavior. Intl J Technology Assessment Health Care 1987;3:39–50. In Schaffer C: Case management's role in networks. Cont Care 1995;(Jan-Feb):21–22.
37. Handley MR: An evidence-based approach to evaluating and improving clinical practice: guideline development. HMO Pract 1994;10:19.
38. Mirtallo JM, Powell CR, Campbell SM et al: Cost-effective nutrition support. Nutr Clin Pract 1987;2:142–151.
39. Kudsk KA, Croce MA, Fabian TC et al: Enteral versus parenteral feeding: effects on septic morbidity after blunt and penetrating abdominal trauma. Ann Surg 1992;215:503–513.
40. Roberts MF, Levine GM: Nutrition support team recommendations can reduce hospital cost. Nutr Clin Pract 1992;7:227–230.
41. Twomey PL, Patching SC: Cost-effectiveness of nutrition support. J Parenter Enter Nutr 1985;9:3–10.
42. Viall CD, Crocker KS, Hennessy KA et al: High tech home care: surviving and prospering in a changing environment. Nutr Clin Pract 1995;10:32–36.
43. Chapman G, Curtas S, Meguid MM: Standardized enteral orders attain caloric goals sooner: a prospective study. J Parenter Enter Nutr 1992;18:96–98.
44. Medicare Region C Durable Medical Equipment Regional Carriers Manual: Columbia, SC: Palmetto Government Benefits Administrators, 1995.

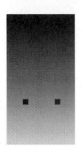

Index

Page numbers in *italics* refer to illustrations; page numbers followed by t refer to tables.

ISBN 0-7216-2155-4